HANDBOOK OF PHYSIOLOGY

SECTION 10: Skeletal Muscle

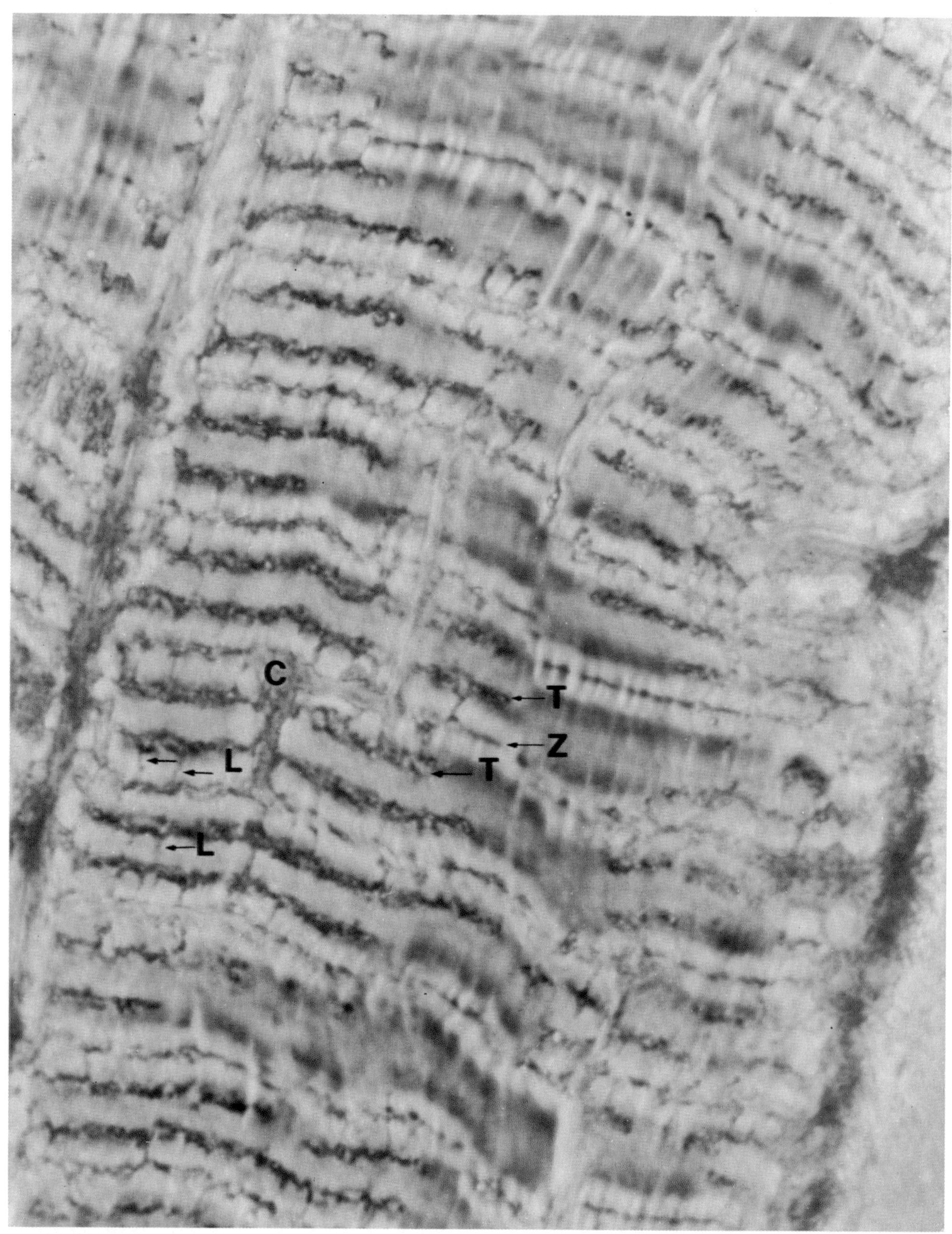

Longitudinal view of long-sarcomere, tonic-type muscle fiber from walking leg of crayfish (*Astacus fluviatilis*). For a complete description, see Fig. 5 legend, p. 28.

HANDBOOK OF PHYSIOLOGY

A critical, comprehensive presentation of physiological knowledge and concepts

---

SECTION 10: Skeletal Muscle

Section Editor: LEE D. PEACHEY

Associate Editor: RICHARD H. ADRIAN

Executive Editor: STEPHEN R. GEIGER

American Physiological Society, BETHESDA, MARYLAND, 1983

Library of Congress Catalog Card No. 78-315956

International Standard Book Number 0-683-06805-9

Printed in the United States of America by Waverly Press, Inc., Baltimore, Maryland 21202

Distributed by The Williams & Wilkins Company, Baltimore, Maryland 21202

Laurie S. Chambers, Elizabeth M. Cowley,
Susie P. Mann, Barbara E. Patterson,
Katherine S. Rogers, *Editorial Staff*

Brenda B. Rauner, *Production Manager*

Constantine J. Gillespie, *Indexer*

Preface

Scanning the history of science, we see how keen has been the animus to investigate the structure of contractile elements in the hope of discovering the secret mechanism of the most important phenomenon of animal life—movement!

Studies on muscle tissue by anatomists and physiologists throughout the years number in the hundreds. These studies have been conducted with diverse methods—each more perfect than the last, as technology became enriched with instruments, more precise methods of observation and measurement, and new contrivances capable of revealing the most minute structural details—and conducted with diverse objectives, as general notions on animal organization were modified. These studies represent many generations' steadfast pursuit of the solution to a great problem in biology.

And still we are far from reaching the goal.

Emilio Veratti, 1902
(transl. 1959; see chapt. 2 for refs.)

The *Handbook of Physiology: Skeletal Muscle* appears eight decades after Veratti wrote the above, yet the enthusiasm for contractile systems that he felt seems undiminished in the authors of this volume. Furthermore the goal of a full understanding of the workings of a muscle cell does not seem any closer to us than it did to Veratti. This is the nature of scientific investigation; each time we piece together some answers, we uncover new questions, and all the while we advance. In the last 25 years we have seen unprecedented growth in our knowledge of biological structure and function at the cellular and subcellular level. Clearly these advances have depended on high levels of scientific interest and adequate funding for research. At least equally important has been the availability of powerful new microscopic, mechanical, electronic, and chemical techniques. I think Veratti, were he alive today, would have enjoyed immensely seeing the networks he so elegantly described in muscle cells as we now see them in the high-voltage electron microscope. During his lifetime Veratti's ideas were not as widely accepted as they are now. To be fair, however, in 1902 it would have been difficult to know how real his observations were, without the information we now have. Each era has its mysteries, its limited tools for investigating them, its failures, and its successes. Often only in retrospect can we tell the successes from the failures. Thus we must continually review the state of our knowledge, look back at past results, and plan future experiments. These are the goals of this book.

During the last 25 years, muscle tissue has been probed as deeply and studied as thoroughly with many modern techniques as any other tissue. Two reasons for this are the large size of muscle cells and their high degree of functional and structural specialization, which make them particularly well suited for study with the newer biophysical and biochemical instruments and techniques. The organization of a striated muscle cell in repeating structural units (fibrils and sarcomeres) allows microscopists to concentrate on these small units in detail, looking at the whole fiber as an assembly of many such parts. The repeating structural pattern allows diffractionists to join in as well, and both X-ray–diffraction and light-diffraction techniques are contributing to our present knowledge of muscle structure and function.

When muscle cells are activated, they produce mechanical signals of considerable amplitude, thus permitting studies of the contractile system itself. Muscle cells also produce electrical signals with large amplitudes, often more than 0.1 V in total excursion, and with time scales easily recorded by modern electronic instruments. These signals are expressions of the activities of membranes that control the contractile state of the cell, and detailed understanding of them is needed before we can fully understand how a muscle cell works. Finally, because of the high degree of specialization of muscle cells, the common contractile proteins are present in such abundance in the cell that simple extraction gives an already rather well-purified product for biochemical studies.

Thus it is not surprising that biophysicists, physiologists, biochemists, and anatomists have been attracted in such large numbers to the study of skeletal muscle and that they have had such remarkable success. Many questions that excited Veratti and his colleagues at the turn of the century have been answered and replaced with new questions, which a new generation with new techniques is trying to answer. There is much to keep the animus, and the anima, keen.

The central purpose of *Skeletal Muscle*, like that of

earlier books in this series, is to present an integrated view of the history, recent research, present state, and possible future of several aspects of its central topic. The chapters have been prepared by eminent authorities in the field and are directed at an audience of professional physiologists, including graduate or research students, who desire a working knowlege of the field, perhaps as a preface to planning and executing a research project in muscle or a related area. It is hoped that the material will provide a precise statement of the present state of the field and help to bring into focus the experiments waiting to be done. The book also should prove useful as an authoritative and up-to-date review for teachers and students in advanced courses. The articles are intended to be more comprehensive and integrative than a typical annual review but no less authoritative and critical. Authors were not discouraged from emphasizing their own areas of greatest interest or the work from their own laboratories. The chapters are not intended as substitutes for journal articles or for presentations at scientific meetings. They differ from most textbook chapters by being more analytical, more current, more authoritative, and less simplified, especially in the treatment of difficult and controversial issues. The first group of chapters starts with structural studies and leads to the mechanics of force generation and biochemistry of the contractile proteins. Chapters on the basic electrical properties of muscle fibers then introduce discussion of excitation-contraction coupling and the biochemistry of the sarcoplasmic reticulum. Finally, discussions of specialized insect muscles, development, adaptation, and muscle diseases round out this *Handbook*.

STRUCTURE

Advances in microscopy, especially the development of the various forms of electron microscopes and their introduction into biological research in the last 30 years, have provided structural information that could hardly have been imagined at the turn of the century. The history of biological science abounds with instances of new insight into the structure of a biological system revolutionizing thinking about the physiology of that system and leading to new and highly rewarding research. In muscle research, this has happened both for the contractile mechanism and for the membrane systems that control the contraction state in the muscle cell. The 1954 light-microscopic observations of striation-pattern changes in shortening myofibrils by Hanson and H. E. Huxley and in actively shortening intact muscle fibers by A. F. Huxley and Niedergerke, along with electron-microscopic observations of interdigitating thick and thin filaments, led rather directly to the sliding-filament hypothesis for contraction. According to this hypothesis, length changes in striated muscle take place by a relative sliding of separate sets of thick and thin filaments, and both the force generated and the work done by the muscle result from action of cross bridges extending from the set of thick filaments attaching to and pulling on the set of thin filaments. The electron-microscopic discovery of the sarcoplasmic reticulum only a few years later provided the basis for our present ideas of the intracellular control of the contractile state of the cell through electrochemical activity of internal membrane systems. These were landmarks, or turning points, in the mainstream of muscle research.

The first three chapters of this book focus on results from electron-microscopic studies. Scanning electron microscopy provides three-dimensional views of natural or artificially produced surfaces in muscle cells at a resolution 100 times better than light microscopy. In chapter 1, Drs. Ishikawa, Sawada, and Yamada present images of capillary networks, muscle fiber surfaces, and internal structures in muscle fibers taken by scanning electron microscopy. The views of the fiber ends and of the neuromuscular junctions should be particularly intriguing to people interested in these parts of the fiber, because such views have never been obtained by any other technique. Transmission electron microscopy of thin sections, the conventional method of electron microscopy, provides the highest available image resolution of internal structures in muscle cells. This work is covered in chapter 2 by Drs. Peachey and Franzini-Armstrong, especially as related to the membrane systems that control contraction. Extensions of this approach, freeze-fracture and high-voltage electron miscroscopy, are also included. In chapter 3, Dr. B. Eisenberg discusses the structure and function of all the major organelles in a muscle fiber, presents data on the quantity of these elements in muscle cells of a variety of types (derived from morphometric electron microscopy), and discusses the general question of muscle fiber diversity. These important studies contribute interesting comparative data and also provide quantitative base lines to which diseased or otherwise altered tissue can be compared.

Although the optical resolution of the light microscope has not been improved in more than a century, light-microscopic techniques in biological research have advanced tremendously in the last decades through the development of procedures for fine-scale localization of specific chemical components in cells. Immunological and immunohistochemical methods provide the highest degree of sensitivity and specificity for the microscopic localization of proteins in cells; results from these methods are summarized by Dr. Pepe in chapter 4. The extension of these methods to electron microscopy provides a still higher level of resolution.

Microscopic methods provide pictures of the objects studied. Their interpretation is an extension of our everyday visual processes. The preparation of specimens for microscopy, especially electron microscopy, requires killing the cells by means of chemical and physical treatments that may introduce structural changes (artifacts). These preparation methods also eliminate the possibility of observing dynamic events in the contraction of a living muscle cell. On the other hand, X-ray–diffraction studies can be done on living cells without structural alteration. The full and true interpretation of diffraction patterns, however, requires sophisticated methods and a thorough understanding of the mathematical transformations involved. Beyond this, diffraction methods are restricted to repeating or crystalline structures and thus cannot be applied to all types of cells. Fortunately, skeletal muscle cells are highly suitable for study by diffraction methods because of the regularity and repeating nature of their structure. In chapter 5, Dr. Haselgrove presents the basic structure of the contractile apparatus and the results from X-ray diffraction of muscles in various physiological states.

CONTRACTION

The raison d'être of a muscle cell is to produce force and shortening. Over the years many types of mechanisms have been suggested as the basis for the contractile action of muscle. For almost three decades the cross-bridge theory has dominated all others, and the evidence favoring this theory now seems so strong that it is very likely to be, at least in broad terms, the true mechanism. Virtually all papers recently published in this area, if not lending support to the theory, at least discuss their results in its terms. Four chapters of this *Handbook* are devoted to the contraction mechanism. Drs. Podolsky and Schoenberg review the history and present thinking on the mechanical and biochemical aspects of cross-bridge action in chapter 6. This includes discussion of probably the most sophisticated mechanical experiments done in biology. Time-resolved mechanical measurements on single, isolated skeletal muscle fibers with controlled force or with controlled length (mechanical equivalents of voltage-clamp and current-clamp experiments in electrophysiology) have uncovered at least four separate dynamic steps in the cycle of cross-bridge action. Ultimately these steps need to be understood in terms of molecular energy and the motion and bonding of the cross bridges and to be related to the various states envisioned by the biochemists.

Energetic considerations have been important not only in providing understanding of the energy sources of muscle cells but also in providing data that limit and guide thinking about underlying mechanisms. Forty years ago, A. V. Hill's pioneering measurement of heat production in muscles undergoing carefully controlled contractions set the standard for this field and firmly brought thermodynamics into muscle research. Much work has subsequently been done to relate quantitatively the underlying biochemical reactions to mechanical shortening, work, and heat production. Complexity arises in these analyses from the multitude of reactions going on simultaneously, from dependence of internal reactions on the external forces applied to the muscle and on its speed of shortening, and from a nontrivial contribution of entropy in the overall energy balance. Muscle energetics is reviewed in chapter 7 by Dr. Kushmerick in terms of its historical background and the most recent use of modern methods, such as nuclear magnetic resonance, for noninvasive analysis.

The energy from a muscle that appears externally as mechanical work and heat is provided by the free energy of ATP hydrolysis. It has long been known that the stoichiometry of the cross-bridge reaction is such that one ATP is hydrolyzed for each cycle of activity. What has been more elusive is the identification of the particular step or steps in the biochemical cycle of reactions whereby the energy is transferred from ATP into the contractile proteins and then is converted into mechanical work. More generally, one wishes to know with some certainty about each step in the cross-bridge cycle, its rate constants and controls, and what limits the overall rate of the reaction under different physiological conditions. In chapter 8, Drs. Webb and Trentham concentrate on the roles played by ATP and relate these to the contractile mechanism. In chapter 9, Drs. Gergely and Seidel address the conformational changes that myosin is capable of and how these can be related to the molecular motions involved in force generation.

EXCITATION-CONTRACTION COUPLING

The next group of chapters is devoted to various aspects of the elaborate control system that exists in the skeletal muscle cell. As a first step in excitation-contraction coupling, electrical activity on the cell surface, initiated at the motor end plate by a nerve impulse, spreads over and along the surface of the fiber and then transversely into the fiber interior along the tubules of the T system. Chapter 10, by Dr. Adrian, the associate editor of this volume, covers the electrical properties and the activity of the surface membrane and T system from the points of view of cable analysis and ionic permeability. In their basic form these studies are direct extensions of the analysis of nerve fibers initiated by Cole, Hodgkin, and A. F. Huxley. However, the more complex geometry of the muscle fiber compared with the nerve axon makes this extension far from trivial, either mathematically or experimentally. The complex muscle structure must be represented in a geometric form simple enough to be treated theoretically, and often several different options can be chosen at this step. In chapter 11, Dr. R. Eisenberg discusses the principles of electrical impedance analysis of muscle cells. When the impedance data have sufficient precision, careful fitting of theoretical predictions to experimental measurements allows selection of certain models in preference to others. These models in turn provide important links between quantitative electron-microscopic studies of the T system and functional studies of the inward spread of activation.

In the next step in excitation-contraction coupling, the depolarized T system induces the sarcoplasmic reticulum to release calcium into the myoplasm, where it initiates the contraction. Radial spread of depolarization in the T system occurs, in typical fibers, in a few milliseconds. Most recording methods, electrical and mechanical, average or sum the activity at all depths in the fiber, even though these are not synchronous on a millisecond time scale. Dr. Gonzalez-Serratos reviews this inward spread of activation and its underlying mechanism in chapter 12.

Until recently it seemed impossible to dissect the events in excitation-contraction coupling taking place thoughout the cell volume except in a rather crude way provided by the time resolution of the records obtained electrically from the fiber surface and mechanically from the fiber ends. These measurements show that surface depolarization precedes the onset of contraction by a rather considerable latent period. The various optical probes introduced over the last few years offer a solution to this dilemma and a possible understanding of the individual, sequential steps in excitation-contraction coupling. The idea behind this approach is that certain chemical probes can be introduced into the fiber and that these will report back, through optical signals, on individual localized events, either through a selective response of the dye to a specific underlying event or through a selective localization of the dyes to a specific fiber structure. Intrinsic birefringence changes also provide signals, without the need to introduce dyes; these too can be thought of as probing internal events during excitation-contraction coupling. For example, both membrane potential and calcium concentration have been considered likely sources for the signals from particular probes, although responses to changes in pH or other ion concentrations must be ruled out carefully or understood and corrected for before the signals can be interpreted fully and accurately. I think it would be fair to say that at present none of these signals is totally understood, though some are gaining a firmer base all the time. The understanding of some of these signals is more than a little uncertain with regard both to the nature of the cellular event producing the signal and to the localized source within the cell of the signal recorded. Dr. Baylor, in chapter 13, discusses this rapidly developing and important field concerning the use of optical methods for studying excitation-contraction coupling. Pharmacological intervention, defined broadly to include not only natural and synthetic drugs but also normal tissue constituents such as ions, has been a powerful tool in muscle research, especially for studies of excitation-contraction coupling; this area is covered by Dr. Caputo in chapter 14.

The transport of calcium from the myoplasm back into the sarcoplasmic reticulum returns the muscle to the relaxed state. Here muscle biochemists have drawn on the experience of their colleagues in the use of cell-fractionation techniques. They have been aided by the presence within muscle fibers of large quantities of some elements of the coupling system, notably the membranes of the sarcoplasmic reticulum, and by the presence of a calcium-ATPase as the overwhelmingly predominant protein in those membranes. They also have been plagued by the structural disruption necessary to perform the isolations from a cell whose function is so intimately tied to intricate structural relationships. Considerable versatility in protein chemistry, analytical techniques, and even electron microscopy has been needed to make progress in this field, which is reviewed by Drs. Martonosi and Beeler in chapter 15.

SPECIALIZATION, ADAPTATION, AND DISEASE

The final five chapters cover a variety of important and broader topics in skeletal muscle. Insect flight muscles represent a high degree of specialization, with properties differing in some useful and informative ways from vertebrate skeletal muscles. Powering flight in these small animals requires particular muscle performance characteristics of speed, timing, and power output. The adaptations observed include a higher degree of mechanical feedback on the activation of the contractile system itself than has been seen in any vertebrate muscle. Virtually every type of study done on other muscles has been repeated for insect flight muscles, and the results are very useful for understanding how muscle systems in general work. Dr. Tregear discusses these and related topics in chapter 16.

Although the properties of muscle fibers often are considered to be specific, well determined, and fixed in time, this is far from true. A complex and interesting set of property changes takes place as an animal develops, much of the change occurring after birth, when muscle use increases dramatically. Dr. Kelly, in chapter 17, discusses the development of muscle, with special consideration of how the various fiber types in skeletal muscles emerge. Even once formed, skeletal muscle is hardly static and fixed in its properties. Dr. Goldspink, in chapter 18, discusses the structural changes that occur when muscles are subjected to changes in activity and environmental conditions. This topic is carried to the level of the whole muscle and the adaptability of the organism in chapter 19 by Drs. Saltin and Gollnick. Finally, Drs. Edwards and Jones discuss muscle diseases in chapter 20. Ultimately we hope and expect that the vast amount of basic information on muscle structure and function reviewed in this *Handbook* will be brought to bear on the important problems of human muscle diseases. This will be a long and arduous task for a number of reasons, not the least of which are the wide variety of diseases that occur and the obvious difficulties that arise in this study of human subjects compared with experimental animals. Nevertheless much progress has been made. Some of the most sophisticated procedures and instruments, once thought to belong only in the basic research laboratory, now are being applied to the study of abnormal human muscle tissue. Results and new insights from these clinical studies are feeding back into basic research, so this is a two-way path. This overview of the large topic of muscle diseases should help to promote communication along these lines.

This *Handbook* is a compendium of a wide variety of topics on skeletal muscle. This tissue, which represents the single greatest mass in the body and lies in the direct line of all animal behavior, has been looked at by a distinguished group of authors. The coverage has been restricted largely to a few types of muscles—those most studied in recent years. Although similar coverage of a broader spectrum of muscles is needed, including study of unusual forms of muscle found in diverse and sometimes obscure animal species, this has not been attempted here. Instead this volume brings together results obtained on a few types of muscles with a wide variety of experimental methods, resulting in a highly readable and authoritative review and analysis of the current state of the field.

LEE D. PEACHEY

Contents

CHAPTER 1

Surface and internal morphology of skeletal muscle

HARUNORI ISHIKAWA
HAJIME SAWADA
EICHI YAMADA

Department of Anatomy, Faculty of Medicine, University of Tokyo, Tokyo, Japan

CHAPTER CONTENTS

THE ELECTRON MICROSCOPE is responsible for our present understanding of the structure and function of skeletal muscles. Much of what we know about the ultrastructure of muscle fibers has been learned from thin-section electron microscopy. Examination of thin sections of plastic-embedded materials, however, has provided principally two-dimensional structural profiles of cells and tissues. Over the last 10 years, several other techniques have been developed and widely applied to electron microscopy. Among them, scanning electron microscopy (SEM) is especially useful in direct visualization of three-dimensional morphology of various cells and tissues. This approach was not entirely new when it was first used in biology, but it held limited attraction for electron microscopists, who had been busy in extensive application of thin sections to ultrastructural studies. Recent improvements in specimen preparation as well as advances in instrumentation have greatly increased the usefulness of SEM.

Specimens for SEM should be prepared so that the surfaces to be examined are freely exposed. Thus surface morphology deals not only with the natural surfaces of organisms, tissues, and cells but also with artificially exposed surfaces. Similarly the freeze-replica technique also can be used for relatively three-dimensional observation of cells and cell organelles, because such replicas are prepared from surfaces exposed by freeze-fracturing with or without etching.

In this chapter the surface and internal morphology of skeletal muscle fibers as revealed mainly by SEM is described in correlation with findings obtained by other methods and discussed with special reference to muscle physiology.

METHODS FOR SURFACE MORPHOLOGY

Scanning Electron Microscopy

In SEM the images are obtained by scanning a finely condensed electron beam (electron microprobe) on a specimen surface and collecting the secondary electrons emitted. The secondary-electron current varies depending on geometrical features (topography) of a specimen surface and on constituent substances. Hence SEM is well suited for the study of surface morphology with relatively better resolution and greater depth of focus than the light microscope. The recent advent of field-emission types of SEM has made possible high-resolution SEM studies. For SEM observation of cells and tissues, specimens should be able to withstand the high vacuum in the microscope and have sufficient electric conductivity not to be charged during exposure to the electron beam. Certain frozen specimens may fulfill these two specimen requirements without chemical fixation and metal coating, but the application of this approach to SEM still is limited.

In the standard preparative procedure for SEM observation, muscle tissues are dissected out, fixed in buffered glutaraldehyde, and then dehydrated in graded concentrations of ethanol. After dehydration, the tissues are substituted with isoamyl acetate and dried in a critical-point dryer. The dried tissues are torn with a pair of forceps or cut longitudinally with a razor blade, coated with gold in an ion-sputtering

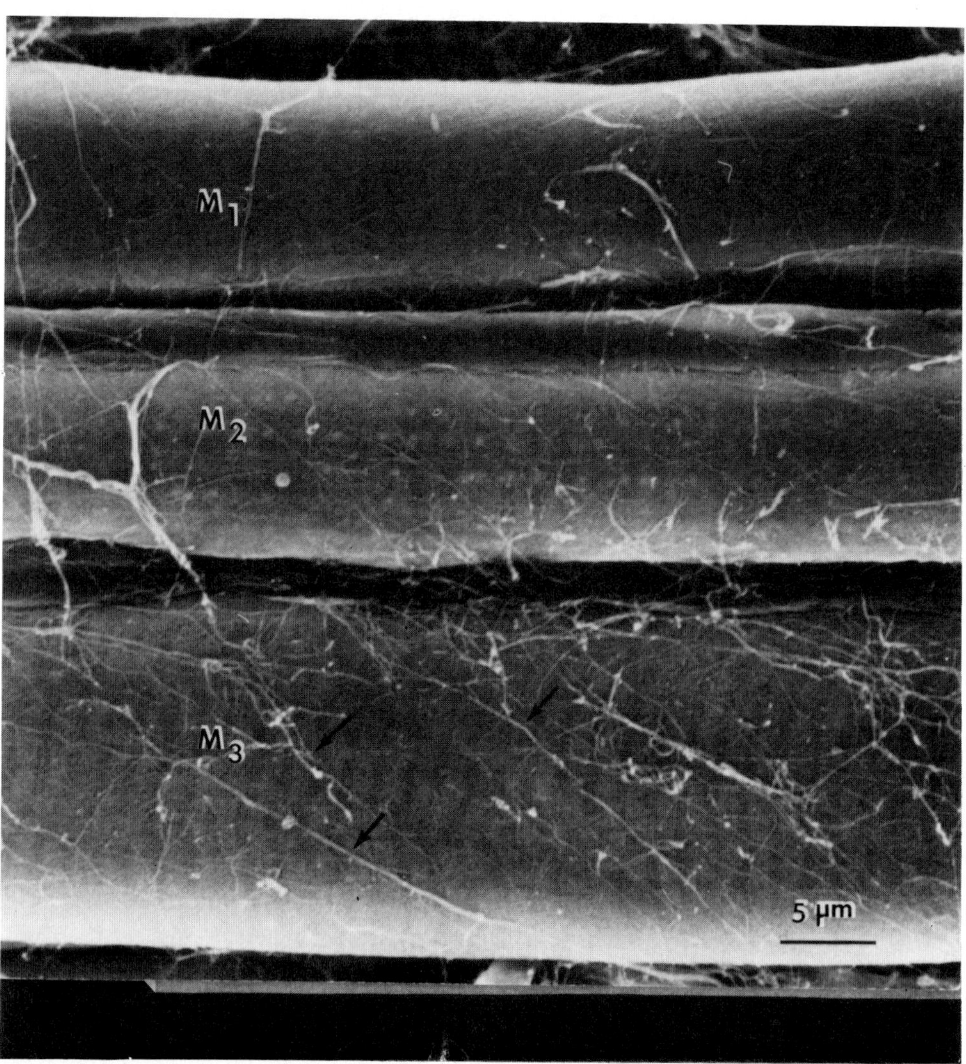

FIG. 1. Skeletal muscle fibers (M_1, M_2, M_3) appear as cylindrical units aligned in parallel bundles. Faint cross striations are visible along individual fibers. Coarse collagenous fibers of the endomysium run in various directions over and between muscle fibers (*arrows*). Teased preparation of frog sartorius muscle fixed with tannic acid–OsO_4.

device, and examined in an SEM at accelerating voltages of 5–25 kV. Although an SEM image is inherently three-dimensional, the specimen is often tilted at about $\pm 5°$ to take stereo-pair micrographs for better three-dimensional visualization.

Various preparative procedures have been used for specific or selective observations of the structure of muscle fibers. Depending on the information desired, one chooses an appropriate procedure. The fiber interior as well as the fiber surface can better be visualized when tissues are treated sequentially and often repeatedly with tannic acid and OsO_4 and torn after critical-point drying (52). The tannic acid–OsO_4 treatment, which is known as the conductive staining method, is especially useful for high-resolution SEM because metal coating can be much reduced (36, 37). Freeze-fracturing or freeze-cracking tissue blocks immersed in glycerol (39), epoxy resin (59), ethanol (17, 22), or stylene (60) can be used to examine the fiber interior. Prolonged treatment of tissues with OsO_4 after freeze-fracturing in dimethyl sulfoxide selectively preserves certain organelles inside cells (61). For SEM examination of the fiber interior, thick Epon sections are etched with an iodine-acetone solution (40). Likewise paraffin-embedded tissues are cut in thick sections from which the paraffin is removed for SEM specimens in correlative examination between light microscopy and SEM (33, 38, 43). Paraplast-embedded muscle tissues can also be used for comparative examination by SEM and scanning transmission electron microscopy (STEM) (13).

The true outer surface of the sarcolemma can be seen only in specimens from which connective tissue components are dissolved by chemical treatment with

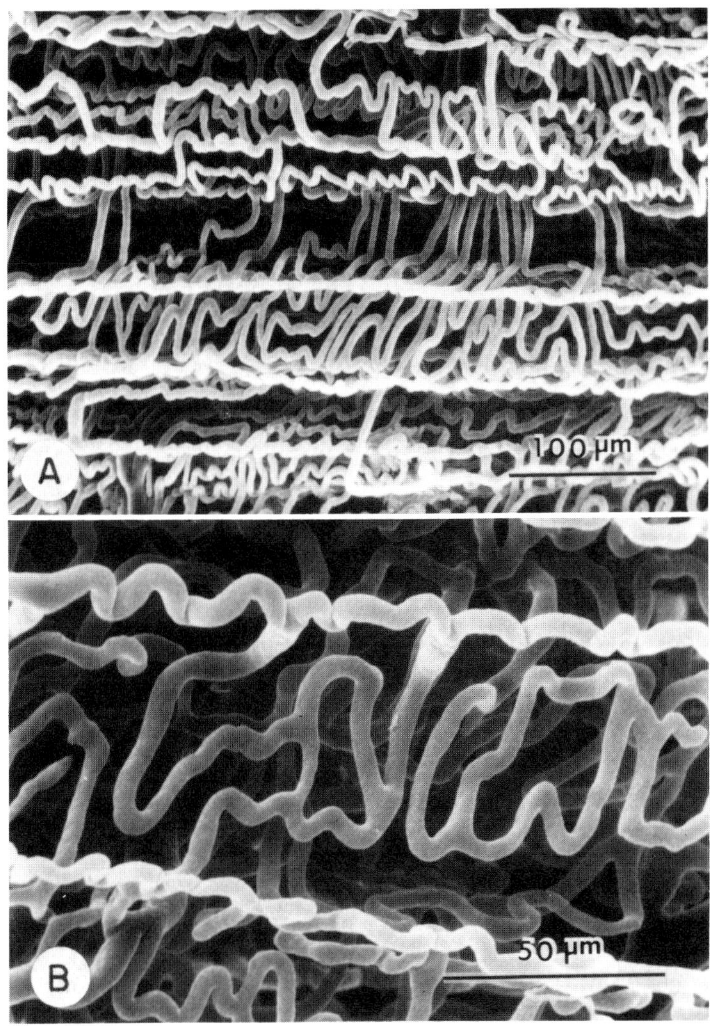

FIG. 2. Vascular corrosion cast of mouse soleus muscle. *A*: low-power SEM. *B*: high-power SEM. Capillary networks show a ladderlike pattern in this contracted state of muscle and are arranged in layers surrounding individual muscle fibers, which are dissolved away with all other tissue components. Note few occurrences of broken ends in the capillary casts. (From M. Kurotaki, unpublished observations.)

collagenase (4, 62), HCl and collagenase (11), or HCl (9). When any surfaces observed in the SEM are not identifiable, the same specimens are further processed for examination in thin-section electron microscopy (64).

Freeze-Replica Technique

Tissues are rapidly frozen with liquid nitrogen and then fractured in a high vacuum evaporator. The fractured surfaces are, with or without etching, shadow-cast by evaporating heavy metals such as platinum. The metal layer is backed with evaporated carbon, recovered as a replica film by dissolving the tissue, and examined in a transmission electron microscope (34). Tissues are usually fixed with glutaraldehyde and immersed in 20%–30% glycerol, a cryoprotectant. Fresh tissues may be frozen directly without pretreatment, although there is the danger of the introduction of artifacts due to ice-crystal formation.

In freeze-fractured specimens the fracture plane tends to follow along the membrane, often exposing a vast area of the cell surface. According to the present interpretation (5), the fracture plane passes through the middle of the membrane, thus splitting the membrane into two halves, the protoplasmic (P-face) and the external (E-face) leaflets. This indicates that any exposed membrane surface in this method is neither true outer surface nor true inner surface of the membrane. Nevertheless freeze-fracture replicas are often useful to examine the overall morphology of muscle fibers including intracellular membranous organelles. In freeze-fracture etching, water in frozen specimens is sublimated to expose the true membrane surface and many other structures that otherwise are covered with water.

A method has recently been developed in which fresh, unfixed tissues are rapidly frozen by contact with a metal block cooled by liquid nitrogen or helium to minimize ice-crystal formation (21). In this rapid-freezing method, the fracture surface is deeply etched and then coated by rotary shadowing with metal to form replica films. This method is particularly useful

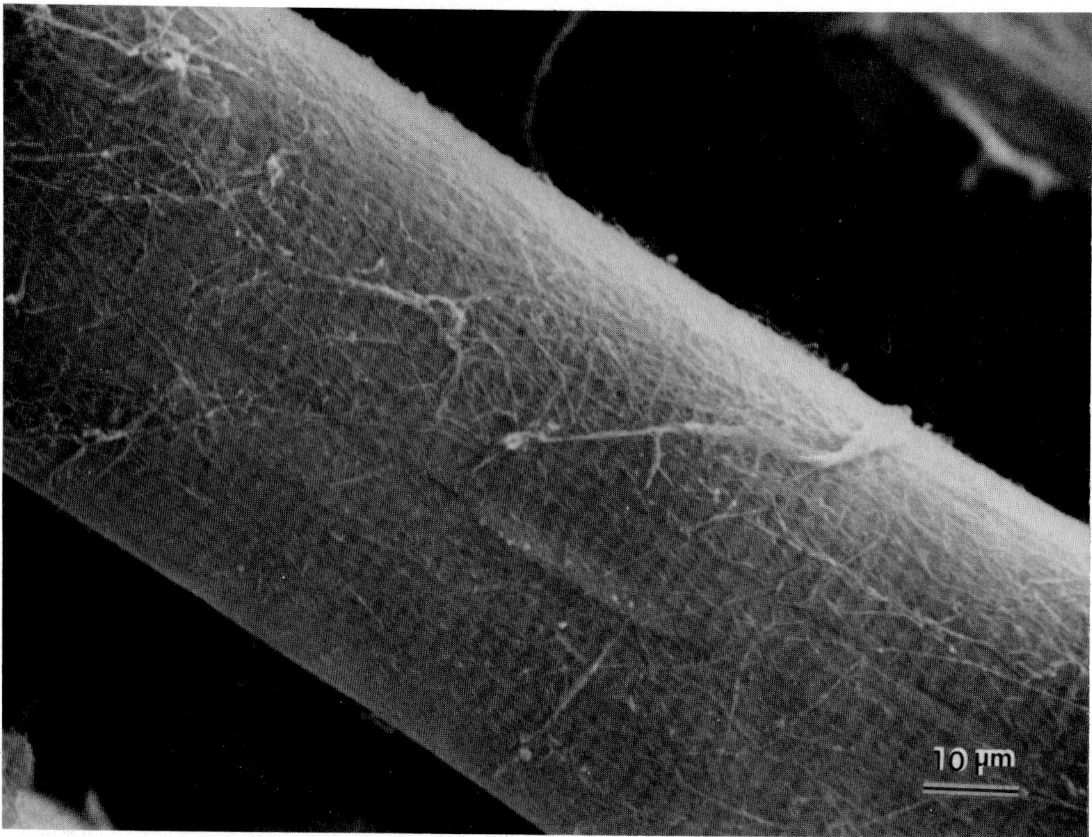

FIG. 3. Frog sartorius muscle fiber. Fiber surface is covered by a fibrous layer, through which cross striations are visible.

for the study of the three-dimensional distribution of fibrous structures (19).

ORGANIZATION OF MUSCLE TISSUE

Muscle fibers, usually 10–20, are grouped into bundles called fascicles. The endomysium, a delicate connective tissue, invests and separates individual muscle fibers within a fascicle, which is surrounded by the perimysium, a thicker connective tissue.

In SEM of teased or split preparations of muscle tissues, cylindrical units identified as muscle fibers are arranged in parallel bundles and are covered by varying amounts of collagenous connective tissues [Fig. 1; (31, 51, 52)]. In the contracted state of muscle, highly tortuous bundles of collagen fibrils run in various directions around the fibers, whereas in the stretched state, the collagenous bundles tend to take a straight and longitudinal course. The distribution pattern of collagenous bundles seems to permit a certain degree of length change of muscle fibers during contraction-relaxation cycles. In SEM of tissues treated with tannic acid–OsO_4, muscle fiber surfaces can be readily identified because they appear to be cross striated through the investing connective tissue layer. This transparency effect may be the result of a significant amount of secondary electrons also being emitted from subsurface structures such as myofibrils.

In teased muscle tissues, blood vessels and nerves can also be seen, although they are not always easy to identify. They can be tentatively identified under the SEM by their outline, dimension, and course. However, blood capillaries are clearly recognized when erythrocytes are seen through their thin walls or when the broken ends of rodlike structures appear as tubes. Skeletal muscle has a rich blood supply, although the degree of richness varies in different types of muscles.

The distribution pattern of blood capillaries in the endomysium can best be demonstrated in the SEM of vascular corrosion casts. Blood vessels in a muscle are first perfused with physiological saline to remove blood and then injected with a rapidly polymerizable methyl methacrylate mixture (35). After polymerization the tissues are completely dissolved by potassium hydroxide treatment. When the vascular cast thus obtained is coated with metal and examined under the SEM, an extensive network of capillaries can be seen in three dimensions, leaving a vacant space corresponding to muscle fibers. As demonstrated in mouse leg muscles (29), the capillaries show a ladderlike network extending longitudinally for a long distance

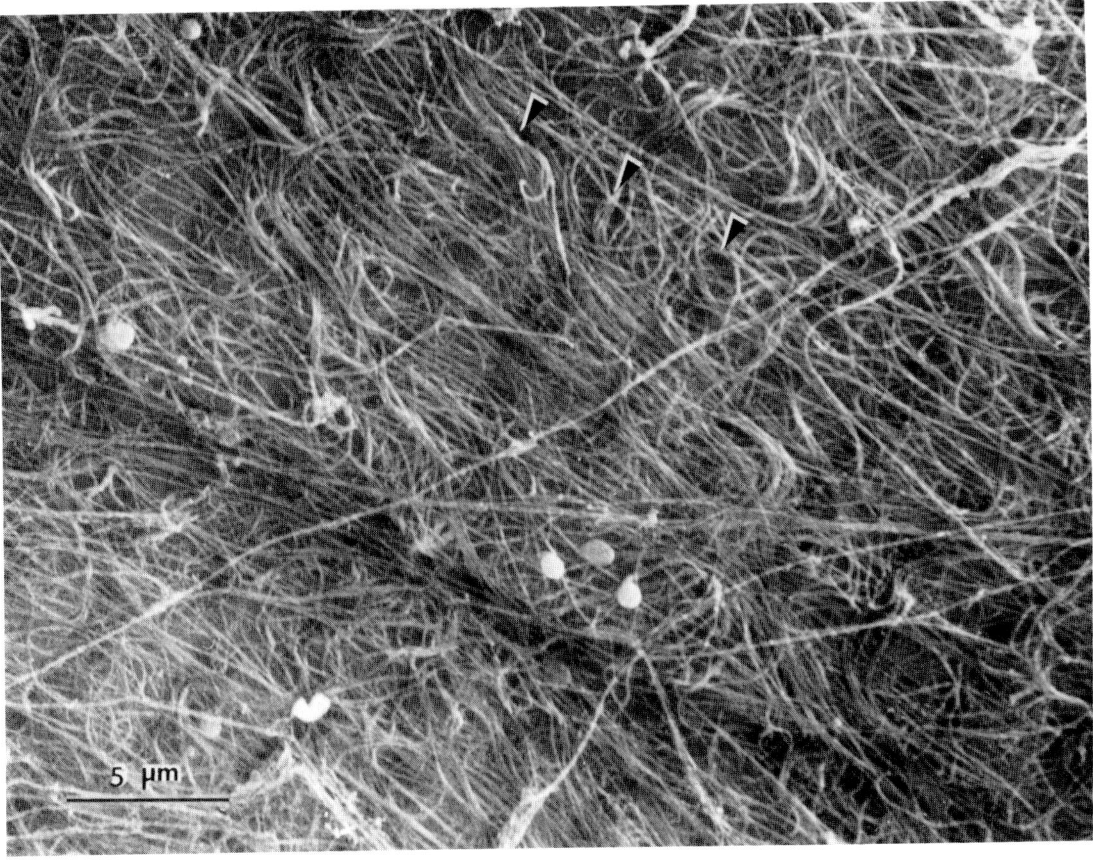

FIG. 4. Fibrous layer on surface of frog sartorius muscle fiber. Collagenous fibrils densely cover muscle fiber and take a predominantly longitudinal course. Cross striations can be seen through fibrous layer (*arrowheads*).

around or between individual muscle fibers. Such a ladderlike pattern is prominent in the contracted state (Fig. 2*A*, *B*). The network is composed of longitudinal and transverse segments, each of which takes a tortuous course. In the stretched state the network is pulled longitudinally, resulting in the disappearance of the ladderlike pattern. Interestingly the capillaries basically are arranged in layers in muscle tissues so that one layer of the network may be separated from the neighboring layers. This implies that anastomoses of capillaries in skeletal muscle do not function very efficiently.

FIBER SURFACE

Endomysium

Thin-section electron microscopy shows that the surface of a muscle fiber is composed of three components: the endomysial fibrous network, the basal lamina, and the plasmalemma (sarcolemma) (30, 50). These components form a complex that is not easily separated mechanically.

A muscle fiber in SEM is seen to be completely covered with a layer of fibrous networks [Fig. 3; (31, 52)]. This network forms part of the endomysial connective tissue and is composed mainly of two types of filaments, thicker filaments ~50 nm in diameter and thinner ones ~20 nm. The thicker filaments are identified as typical collagen fibrils, based on their distribution, size, and characteristic periodicity along the filaments. The collagen fibrils tend to form bundles taking a somewhat tortuous course (Fig. 4). Although the collagen fibrils may run in various directions, they predominantly are longitudinally arranged. The arrangement pattern of the collagen fibrils around the muscle fiber seems to reflect their roles as mechanical support for the fiber surface and as an elastic device for contraction-relaxation cycles. The amount of collagen fibrils in the endomysium varies in different types of muscles. For example, fibers in frog sartorius muscle are separated by a small amount of collagenous tissue, whereas fibers in mouse gastrocnemius muscle are tightly bound to each other by a thick network of collagenous bundles.

The thinner filaments appear to intermingle with

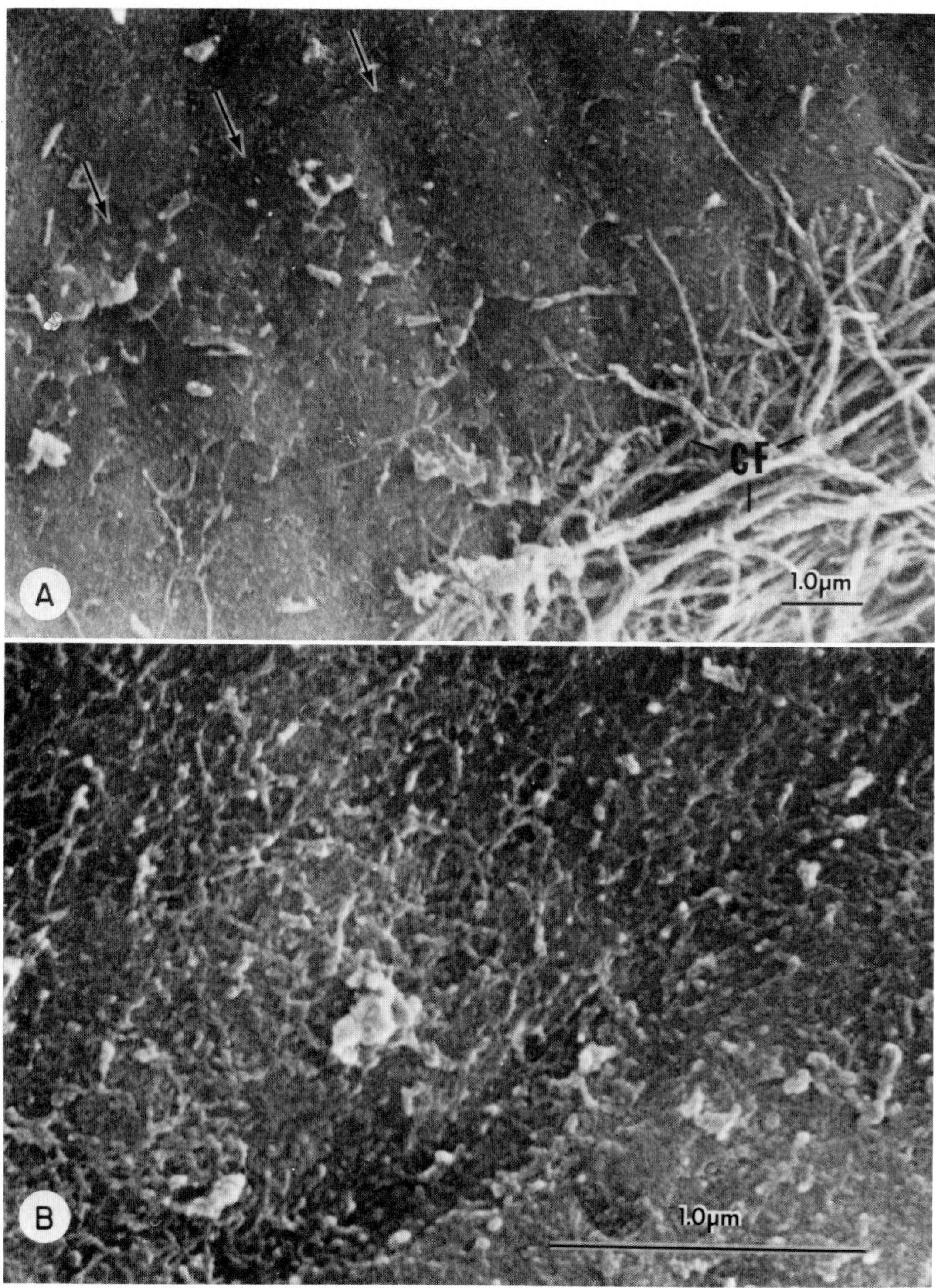

FIG. 5. Outer aspect of basal lamina of a frog sartorius muscle fiber. *A*: low-power SEM. Basal lamina is exposed where fibrous layer (*CF*) is stripped off. Cross striations (*arrows*) can be seen more clearly through the lamina than through the fibrous layer. *B*: high-power SEM. Outer aspect of basal lamina shows a feltlike structure, in which fine filamentous networks appear to be embedded in granular and amorphous materials.

the collagen fibrils. Although there is no periodicity found along these filaments, they probably represent immature forms of collagen fibrils, as demonstrated in thin-section electron microscopy (18).

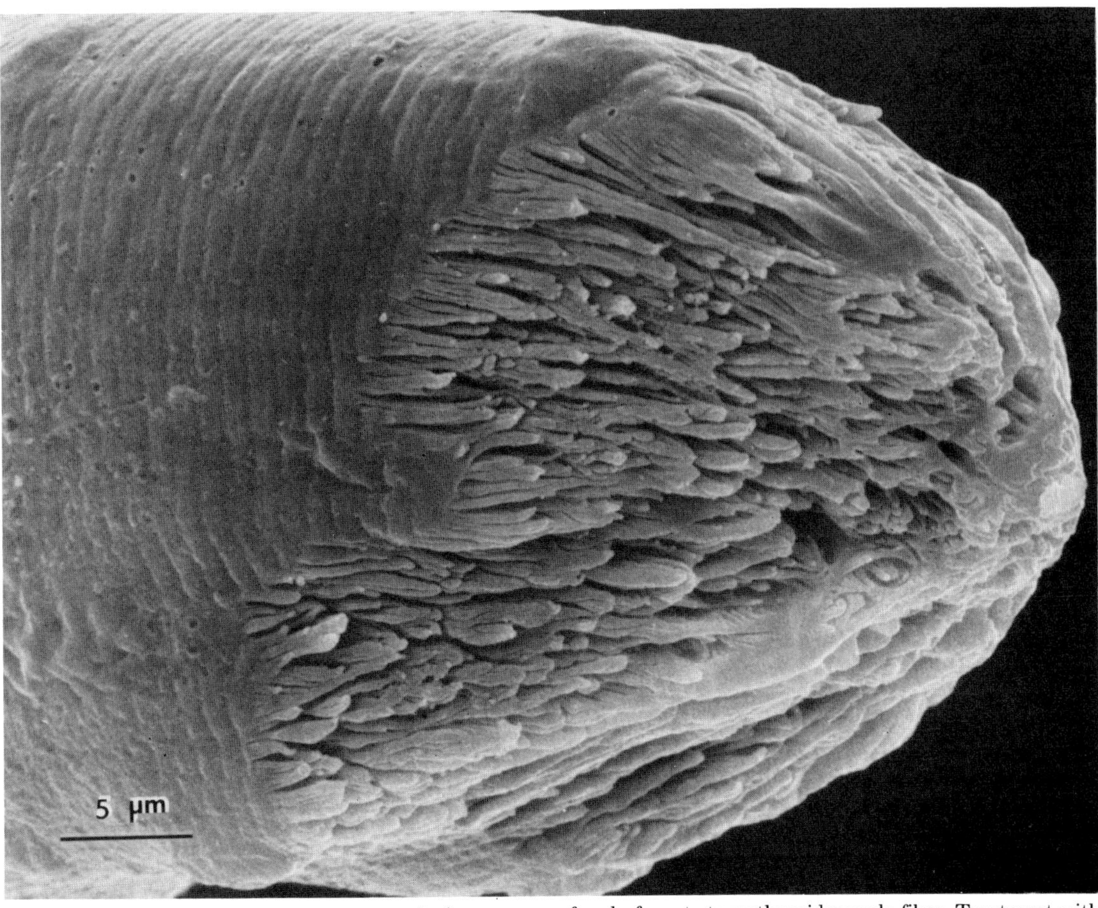

FIG. 6. Appearance of end of a rat sternothyroid muscle fiber. Treatment with HCl after fixation completely removes connective tissue components from surface of muscle fiber. At the myotendon junction the conical end of a muscle fiber is characterized by formation of many longitudinal processes, clefts, and invaginations. Fingerlike processes are predominant at the peripheral portion. (From J. Desaki and Y. Uehara, unpublished observations.)

Basal Lamina

In SEM a continuous feltlike surface appears to cover the muscle fiber in regions where the collagenous fibrous layer happens to be stripped off (52). As seen in frog sartorius muscle, this type of surface forms a substratum for collagen fibrils (Fig. 5*A*), and thus is interpreted to represent the outer aspect of the basal lamina (or basement membrane). Typical collagen fibrils never penetrate this layer. At higher magnification, fine filamentous materials are adhered and embedded, forming a feltlike layer (Fig. 5*B*). Characteristic cross striations can be seen more clearly through this layer than through the collagenous network.

A similar feltlike surface can also be observed, though rarely, in freeze-fracture replicas of frog sartorius muscle (26). This surface is cross striated, being different in appearance from any cleaved faces of the sarcolemma. Furthermore this surface appears to be composed of extremely fine filamentous and granular materials. This surface shows an association with irregularly running collagen fibrils, which are directly visualized beyond the lateral edges of the surface. This surface is thought to be exposed by cleavage along the basal lamina, probably through the lamina or between the lamina and the sarcolemma.

Sarcolemma

In SEM specimens the basal lamina can never be stripped from the sarcolemma by mechanical procedures in any preparative steps. This may reflect the tight connection between these two structures. The only way to expose the true outer surface of the sarcolemma is chemical treatment before or after fixation (52). The connective tissue and basal lamina have been successfully removed from the muscle fibers by treatment with bacterial collagenase (4). Desaki and Uehara (9) recently found that after glutaraldehyde-OsO_4 fixation the treatment with 8 N HCl alone for 20–40 min at 60°C removes the intramuscular connective tissue components, including collagen fi-

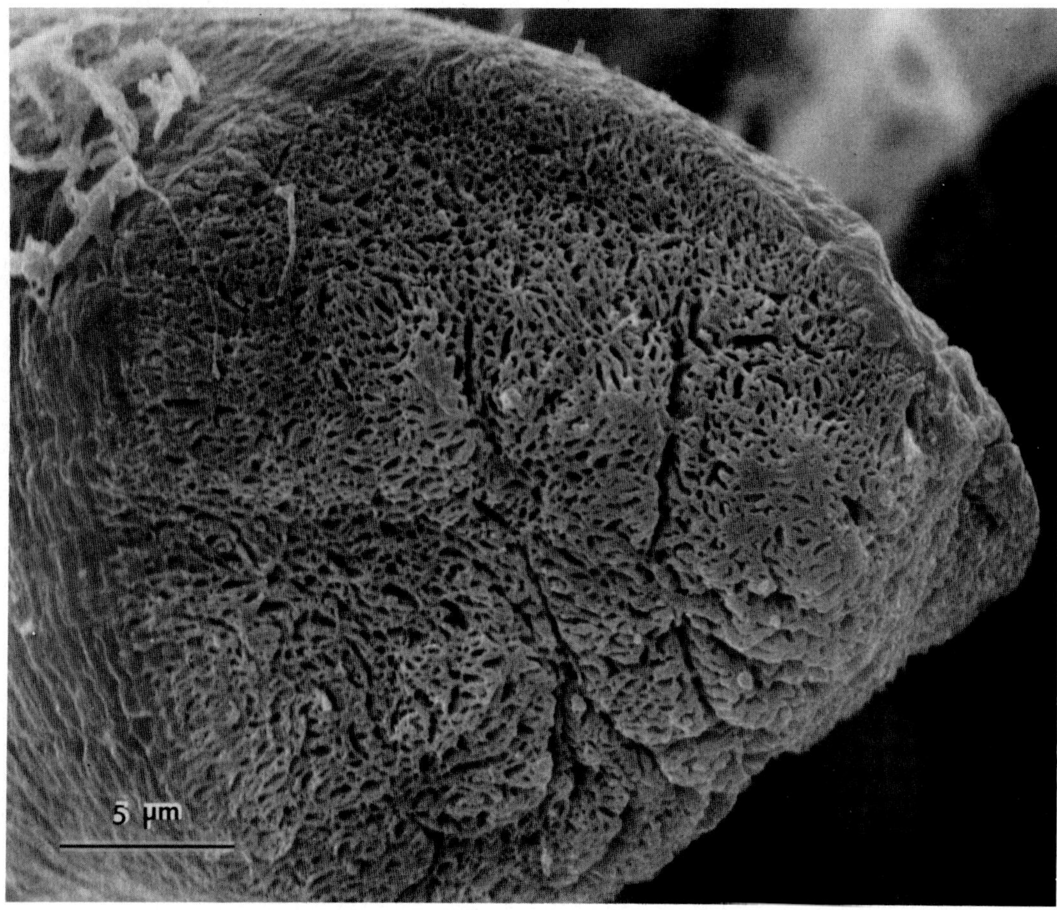

FIG. 7. Appearance of end of a frog extensor digitorum longus muscle fiber. End of this muscle fiber is characterized predominantly by invaginations and clefts. (From J. Desaki and Y. Uehara, unpublished observations.)

brils and basal lamina. This treatment exposes the true surface of the muscle fiber, showing a smooth membrane with a cross-striation pattern that conforms to the underlying myofibrils. Typical bandings of the A, I, and Z bands are clearly discernible on the fiber surface. The A and Z bands are slightly protruded compared with the I bands. Such surface striations are laterally aligned in register. The surface contour of the sarcolemma, such as cross striations and folds, varies in different degrees of fiber stretching before and during fixation.

Blood vessels, nerves with neuromuscular junctions, connective tissue cells, and myosatellite cells can also be observed with SEM in the same preparations. After prolonged exposure to OsO_4, the connective tissue can also be removed, revealing the fiber surface together with myosatellite cells (55). Chemical treatment separates the end of the muscle fiber from its tendon (4). The method of Desaki and Uehara (9) is particularly superior in demonstrating the end of the muscle fiber free of collagen fibrils (Figs. 6 and 7). At the myotendinous junction the end of the muscle fiber abruptly tapers, forming many longitudinal processes, clefts, and invaginations, as observed in thin-section electron microscopy (15, 24). Thus peripheral myofibrils terminate onto the sarcolemma before central myofibrils do. Which kind of the fiber-end specializations—processes or invaginations—is predominantly formed seems to depend on animal species and muscle types (Figs. 6 and 7).

Freeze-fracture replicas clearly reveal the openings of the T tubules on the fiber surfaces in mammalian cardiac muscles (47, 48), fish skeletal muscles (3), and insect striated muscles (56). In skeletal muscles of higher animals such as frog and mouse, however, T-tubule openings cannot be identified on freeze-fracture replicas (10, 26, 49) because the T-tubule openings are similar in size to those of caveolae. To examine the T-tubule openings with SEM, specimens are similarly prepared by freeze-fracturing glycerol-immersed tissues. Such specimens reveal extensive areas of the cleaved sarcolemma, either P or E face as seen in freeze-fracture replicas [Fig. 8; (52)]. Numerous round pits are seen on the P face of exposed surfaces, being distributed preferentially at the I-band level and in the interfibrillar region (Fig. 9*A*). From their distri-

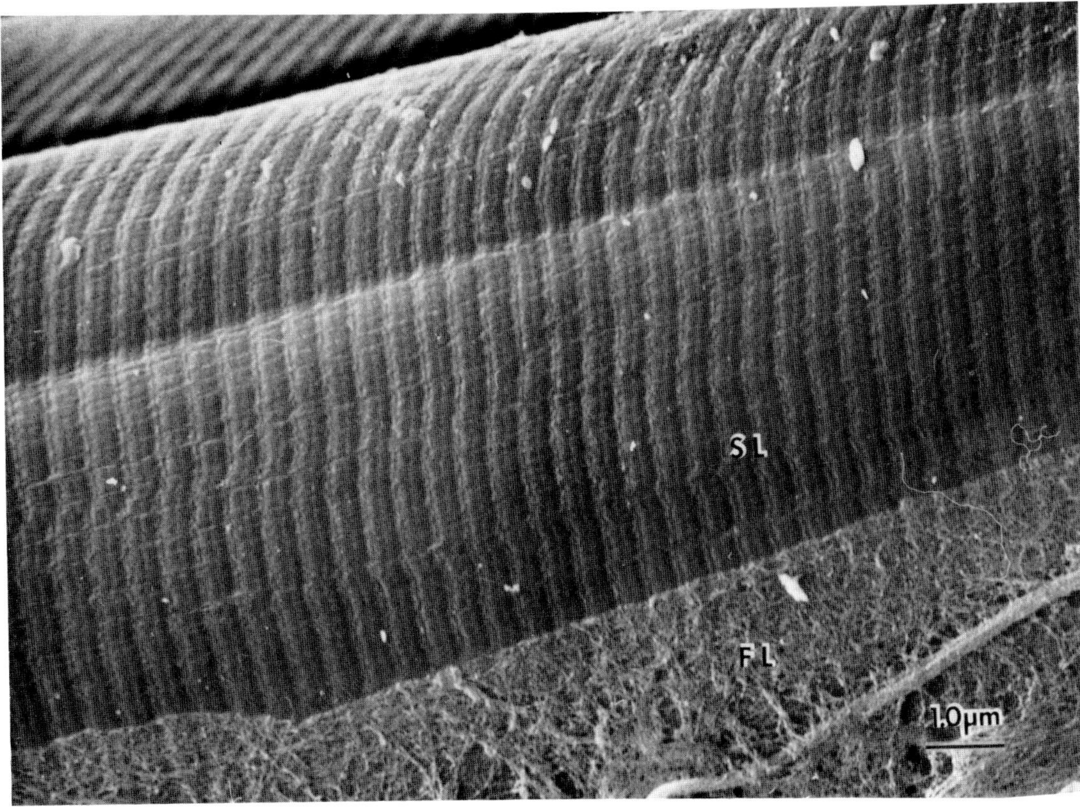

FIG. 8. Appearance of frog sartorius muscle sarcolemma exposed by freeze-fracture. Freeze-fracture of glycerol-immersed muscle can cleave the sarcolemma in a wide expanse. Exposed surface represents P face of sarcolemma and clearly shows characteristic cross striation of underlying myofibrils. Fibrous layer (*FL*) is seen where the fracture plane leaves the sarcolemma (*SL*). [From Sawada, Ishikawa, and Yamada (52).]

bution and comparison with the findings on freeze-fracture replicas (Fig. 9*B*), these pits are considered to represent the openings of both caveolae and T tubules. The size of these openings is not uniform, varying from 80 nm to unmeasurable pointlike depressions, but there is no clue to distinguish between the two types. The number of openings seen with SEM is much less than that of freeze-fracture replicas. Large openings in SEM specimens may be derived from coalescence and enlargement of individual openings during preparation. Nevertheless it is interesting that such pits are distributed predominantly at the level of the Z band. Surface openings of caveolae and T tubules have not been observed in chemically exposed fiber surfaces.

On rare occasions the true inner surfaces are seen where patches of the sarcolemma are peeled and reflected during tissue teasing [Fig. 10*A*, *B*; (52)]. Such surfaces are characterized by clusters of small spherical vesicles and tubules, which are somewhat regularly distributed in banding patterns corresponding to the cross striation. This particular feature can be observed only with SEM. The vesicles have a uniform diameter of ~60 nm and are regarded as the caveolae of the sarcolemma. Many of the caveolae are linked together to form tubular and rosettelike configurations. Some tubular structures apparently extend from the caveolae, suggesting that these are T tubules. This finding is consistent with results of thin-section electron microscopy (41). In fact the T tubules often open to the sarcolemma via caveolae (25, 41). Saccular structures, which are seen closely associated with the tubules, may represent the sarcoplasmic reticulum (SR). On this true inner surface of the sarcolemma, filamentous components of varying thickness are also seen running in various directions (Fig. 10*B*).

FIBER INTERIOR

Exposure of Fiber Interior

When the muscle tissue is longitudinally torn or fractured at various preparative steps, breaks occasionally occur along regions of least resistance, resulting in exposure of the fiber interior. Such specimens permit us to examine myofibrils and membranous organelles such as the SR, T tubules, and mitochondria. The features of the fiber interior vary among different preparations. To expose the intact myofibrils and membranous organelles, simple teasing of dried

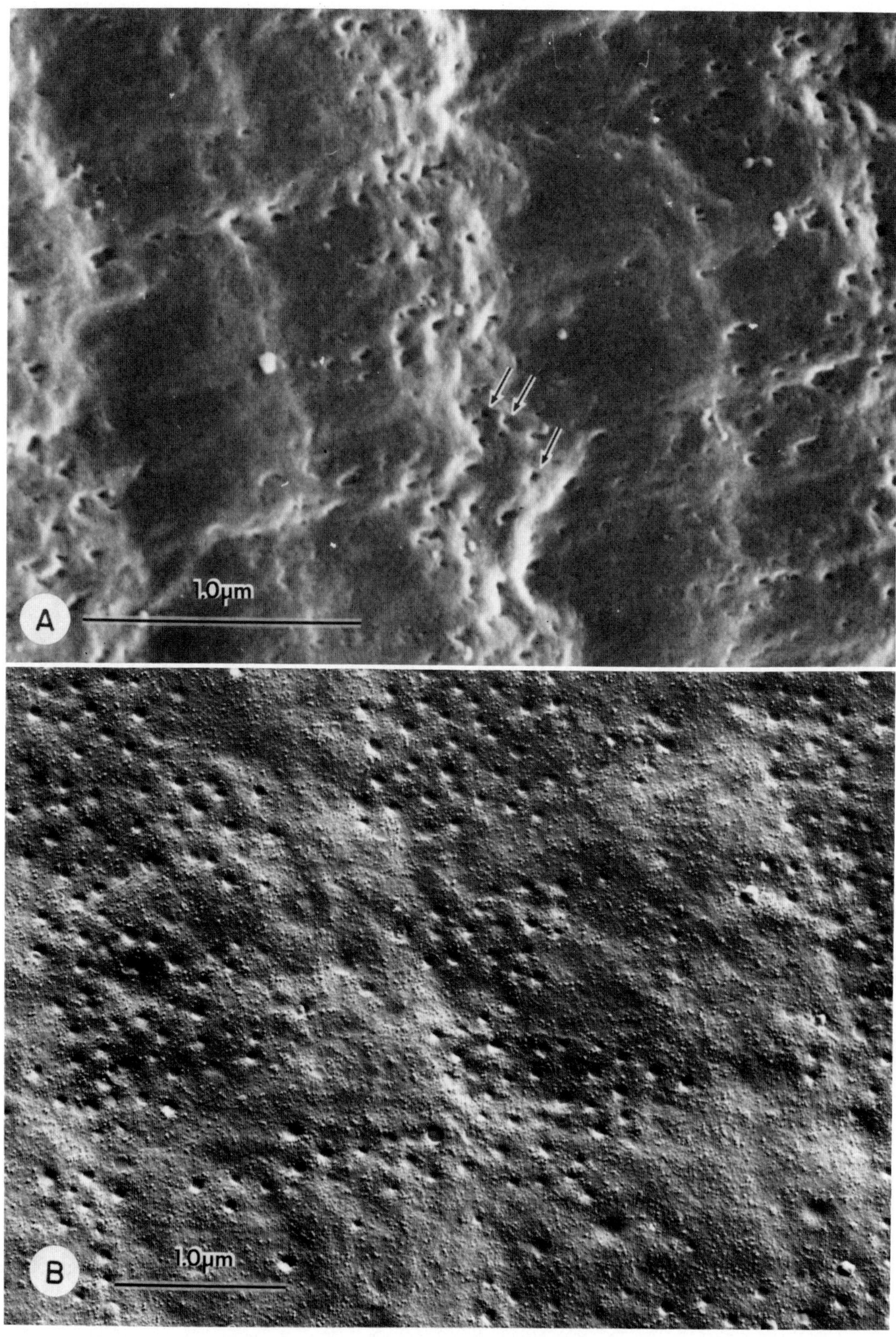

FIG. 9. Frog sartorius muscle sarcolemma exposed by freeze-fracture. *A*: numerous pits are seen on the P face, distributed predominantly at the level of the I band and in interfibrillar regions. *B*: freeze-fracture replica. A similar distribution of pits is observed in replica preparations. These pits represent surface openings of T tubules and caveolae. *Arrows* indicate level of Z band.

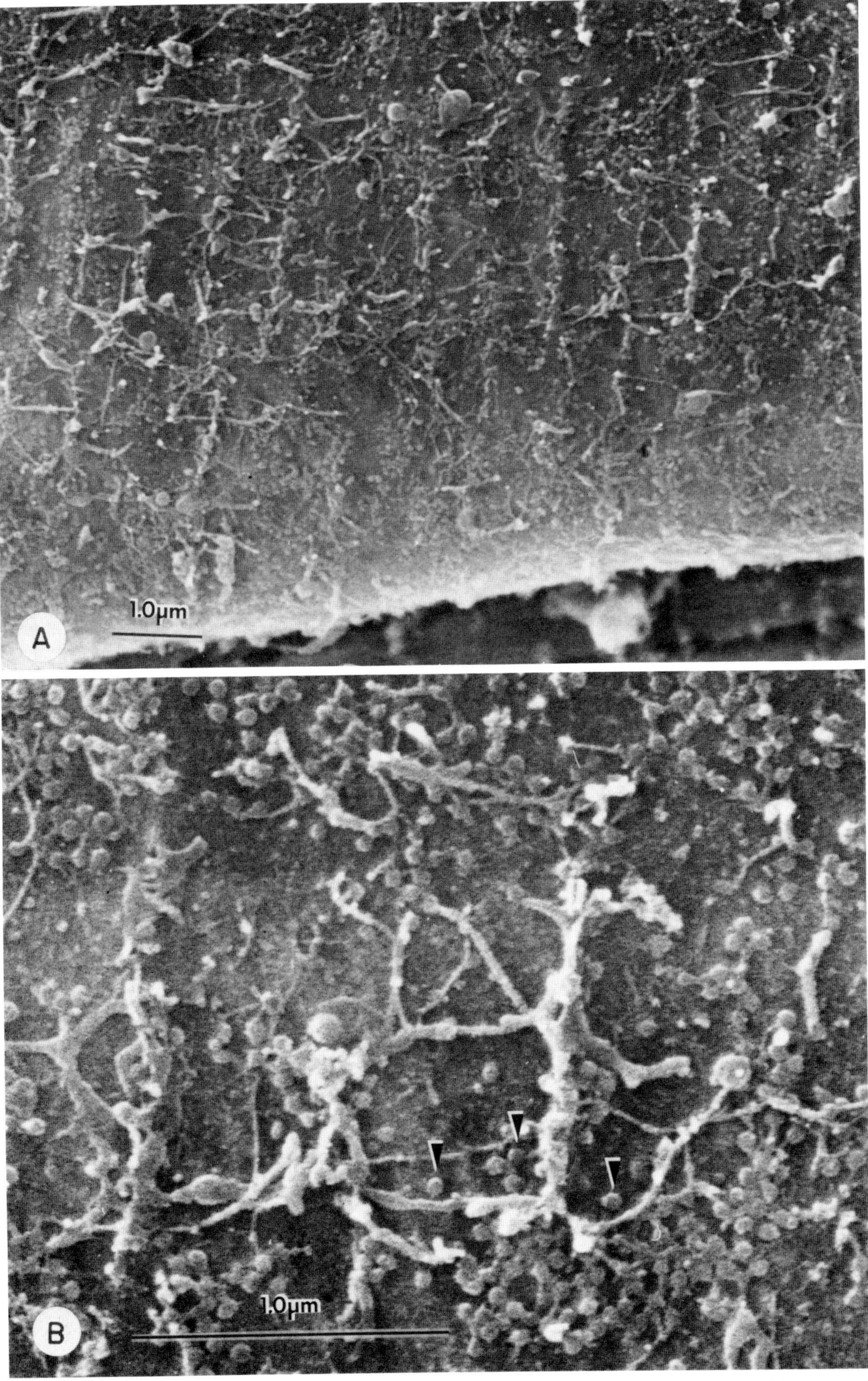

FIG. 10. Inner surface of frog sartorius muscle sarcolemma. *A*: low-power SEM. True inner surface is characterized by clusters of small spherical vesicles, which represent caveolae, and by tubular and saccular structures attached on the surface. These structures tend to be distributed in a cross-striated pattern. *B*: high-power SEM of part of *A*. Caveolae show a uniform diameter of 60 nm (*arrowheads*) and often are linked to form rosettelike clusters. Tubular structures are closely associated with caveolae. Filaments appear to adhere to the surface.

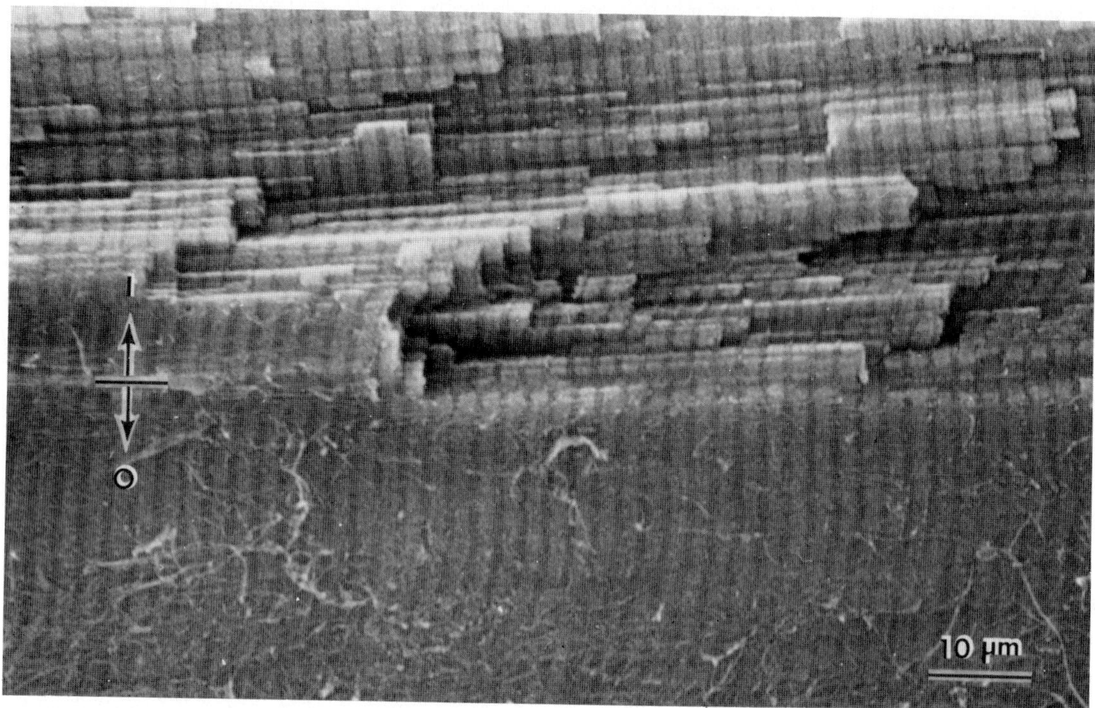

FIG. 11. Appearance of muscle fiber interior. Interior is partly exposed (*I*), showing closely packed, cross-striated myofibrils. Outer surface is covered by a filamentous layer (*O*). [From Sawada, Ishikawa, and Yamada (52).]

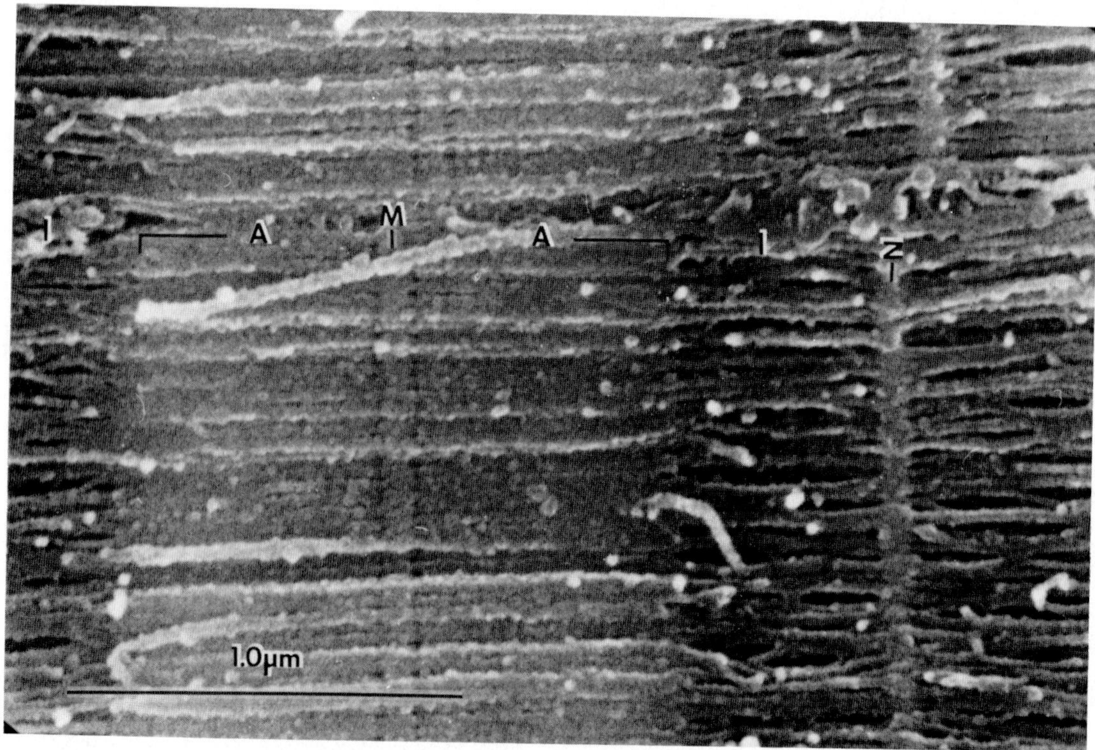

FIG. 12. Appearance of myofibril. Where myofibrils are longitudinally split, characteristic sarcomere pattern (*A*, *I*, *Z*, *M*) and filament organization clearly are seen.

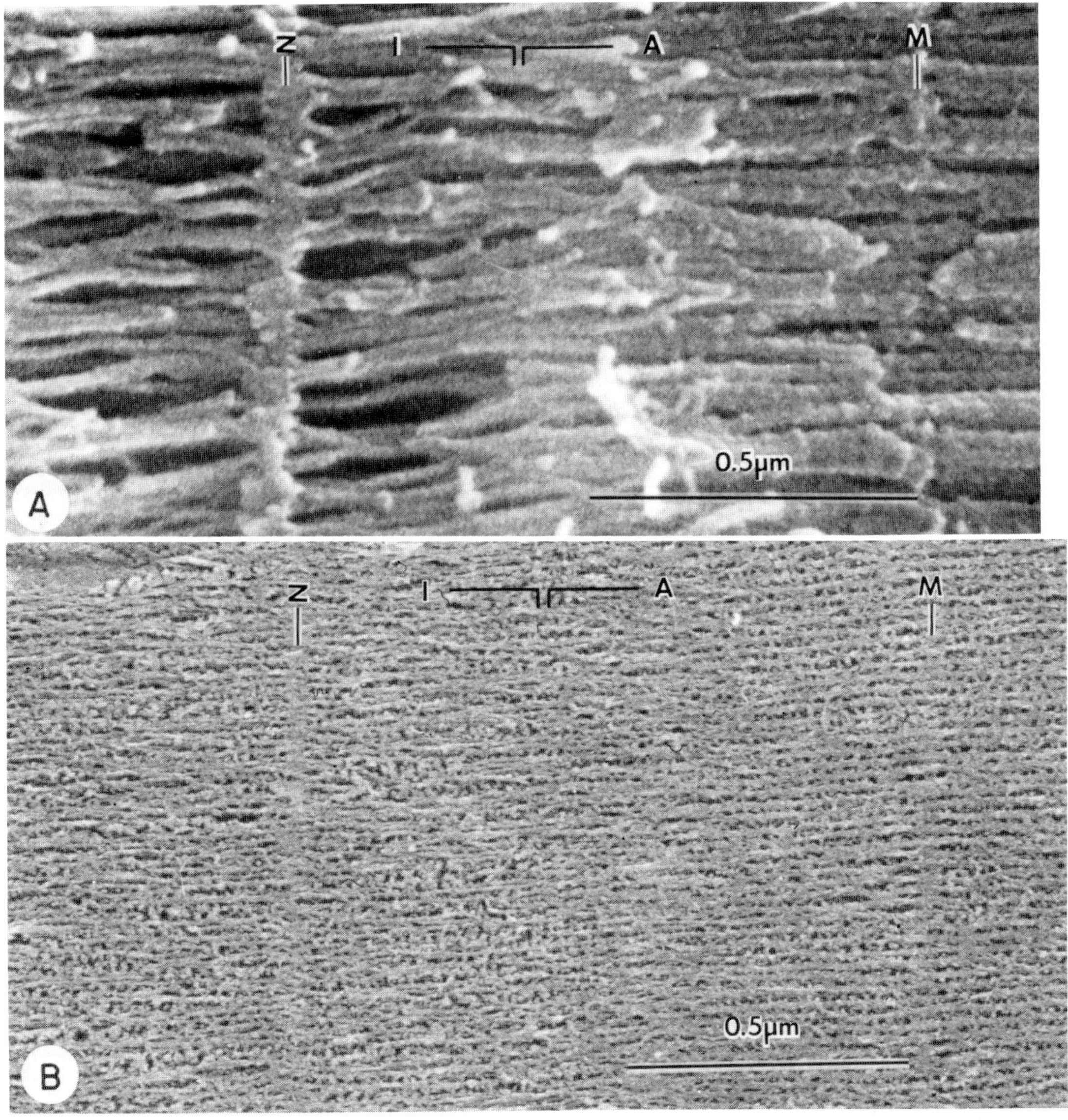

FIG. 13. Myofibrils of frog sartorius muscle. *A*: SEM. *B*: freeze-etch replica. Replica prepared by rapid freezing of an unfixed, fresh tissue and by rotary shadowing after freeze-fracture etching. Note banding pattern of myofibrils (*A, I, Z, M*) in different preparations.

tissues is more useful than other methods, such as freeze-fracturing and resin-cracking. In our experience the best result is obtained when the tissue is treated with tannic acid–OsO_4, probably because of the resulting increased firmness of intercellular connections [Fig. 11; (52)]. In freeze-fracturing (53) or resin-cracking (52, 65), fracture planes often pass through individual myofibrils as in thin sections, and therefore the surface is too flat to obtain three-dimensional images with SEM.

Myofibrils

When dried tissues are torn to expose the fiber interior and then examined with SEM, myofibrils are seen closely packed against each other (Fig. 11). Individual myofibrils show a typical banding pattern of A, I, Z, and M bands (Fig. 12). The surface of the myofibril is slightly depressed in the I bands, with the elevated Z bands in the middle. The myofibril tends to break off in the I band near the Z band. With high-resolution SEM, one can clearly recognize the individual thick and thin myofilaments that constitute the myofibril (52). The thick filaments are ~20 nm in diameter and take a straight course, which suggests their stiff nature. They are characterized by a regularly beaded contour. The beading is ~40 nm in periodicity, which roughly corresponds to that of the cross bridges on one plane in X-ray diffraction (23). Measurements with SEM are not as accurate as those in other anal-

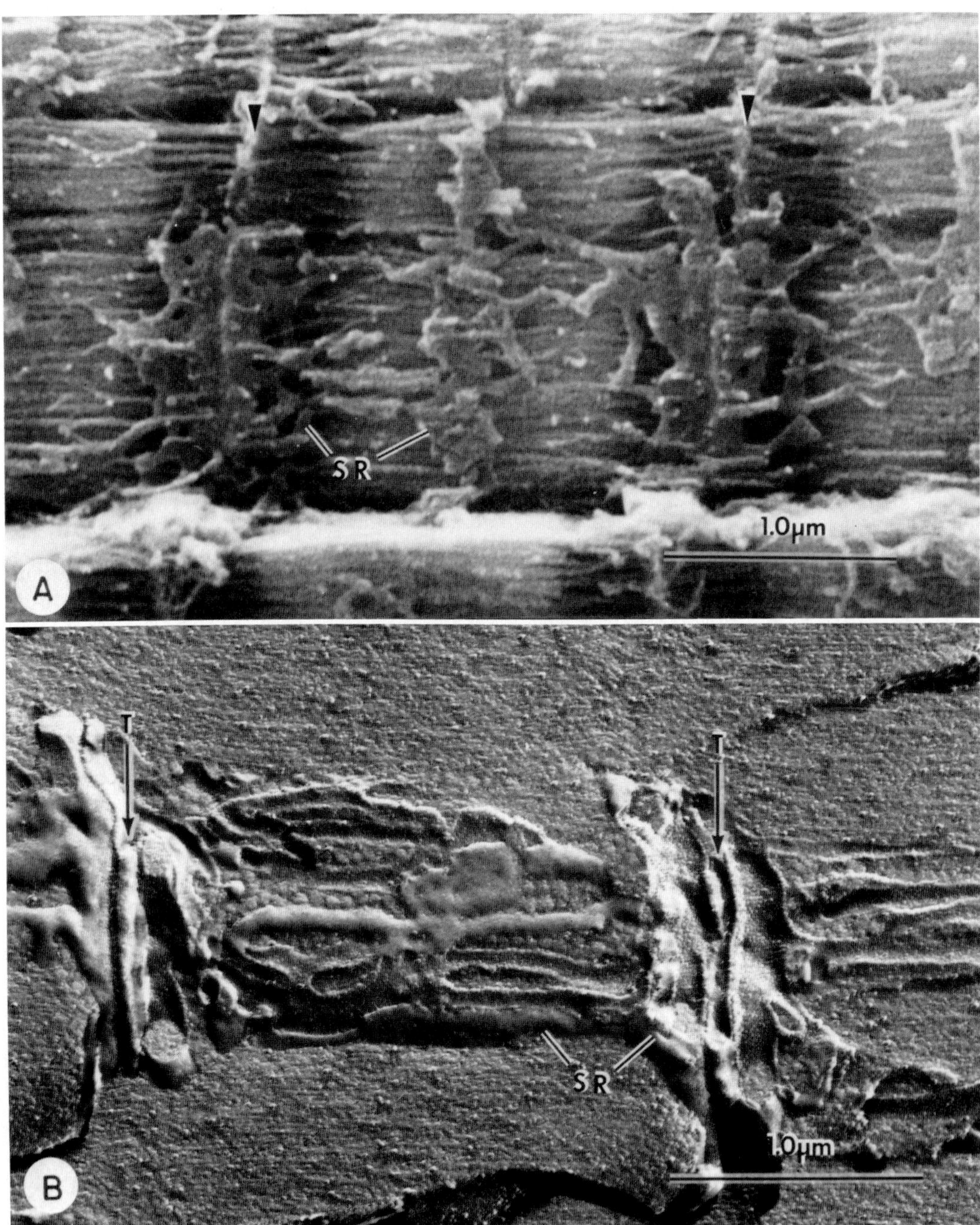

FIG. 14. Frog sartorius muscle sarcoplasmic reticulum and T tubule. *A*: SEM. *B*: freeze-fracture replica. Regional differentiation of sarcoplasmic reticulum (*SR*) is clearly discernible in both preparations [see Peachey (41)]. *T*, T tubule.

yses mainly because of the great shrinkage of specimens as a whole. The heads of myosin molecules project from the filament in a helical array (23, 42). With high-resolution SEM, it may be possible to directly visualize the three-dimensional arrangement of the myosin heads along the individual filaments. In the middle of the A band the M line is clearly seen connecting the thick filaments (Fig. 12). Each thick filament possesses narrow and smooth segments just lateral to the M line as seen in thin sections. Isolated myofibrils can be examined by SEM (7).

Under SEM the thin myofilaments are ~10 nm in diameter and appear as rather smooth filaments taking a slightly wavy course. They often form small bundles in the I band and split into individual filaments to connect with the Z band. In high-resolution

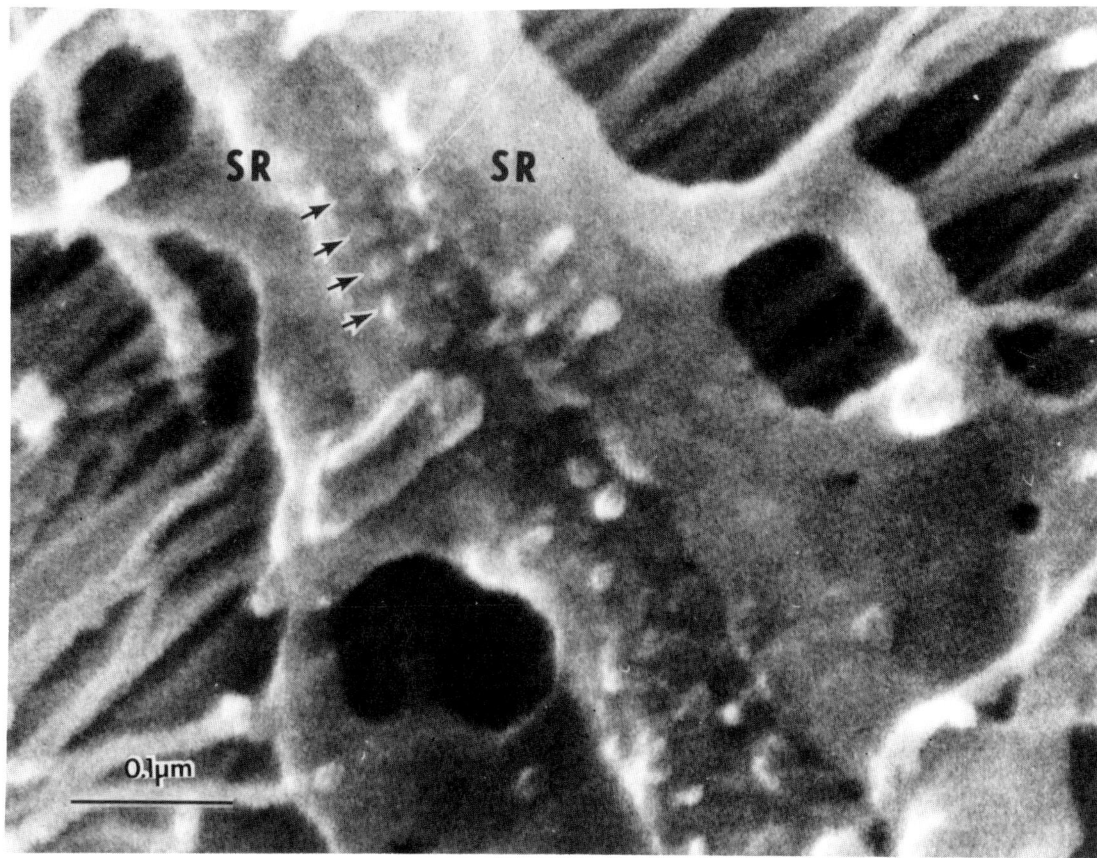

FIG. 15. Frog sartorius muscle triad. Note granular projections (*arrows*) on terminal cisternae of sarcoplasmic reticulum (*SR*) facing the T tubule. Behind these structures are thin myofilaments in the I band. [From Sawada, Ishikawa, and Yamada (52).]

SEM the thin filaments in the I band often have a somewhat beaded appearance (Fig. 13*A*). The Z band shows a zigzag pattern with the thin filaments extending from both sides of the sarcomere, but the mode in which the thin filaments attach to the Z band is not clearly visualized.

Freeze-fracture–etching replicas can be used for the study of the myofibrils (44, 45). More promising is the recently developed rapid-freezing method (21), in which fresh, unfixed tissues are rapidly frozen, fractured, and then deeply etched followed by rotary shadowing to obtain replicas [Fig. 13*B*; (63)].

Sarcoplasmic Reticulum and T System

In some SEM preparations the network of the SR and T tubules can be observed overlying the myofibrils [Fig. 14*A*; (14, 16, 52)]. Although complete images of the SR networks are rarely obtained in SEM observations, the regional differentiation of the SR into terminal cisternae, longitudinal tubules, and fenestrated collars (41) is clearly recognized (52). The SR networks are best demonstrated in tannic acid–OsO_4 specimens, although fragments of myofilaments are often left on the SR surface.

The SEM can be used to examine the distribution of the T tubules in skeletal muscles (53) and in cardiac muscles (1, 14, 32, 38, 58). The T tubules often are seen bridging adjacent myofibrils at a particular level of the sarcomere, for example the level of the Z band in frog and fish skeletal muscles and in mammalian cardiac muscles. In most of the studies, T tubules have been identified as continuous elements running transversely over several myofibrils at the level expected. Like mammalian cardiac muscles, fish skeletal muscles contain large T tubules; these are more easily recognized than those in amphibian, reptilian, avian, and mammalian skeletal muscles, which are of small caliber. Seen in high-resolution SEM, a slender T tubule is interposed between the dilated terminal cisternae of the SR forming a triad [Fig. 15; (52)]. A characteristic feature of the triad is the granular structures 5–12 nm in diameter on the terminal cisterna of the SR. Such granular structures are found only on the surface facing the T tubule and often arranged in a linear fashion. These structures are not fragments of myofilaments or the Z band and hence may correspond to the dimples or feet, the structures bridging the SR and T tubule (12, 27, 28). Three-dimensional images of the SR, T tubules, and triads can also be obtained with

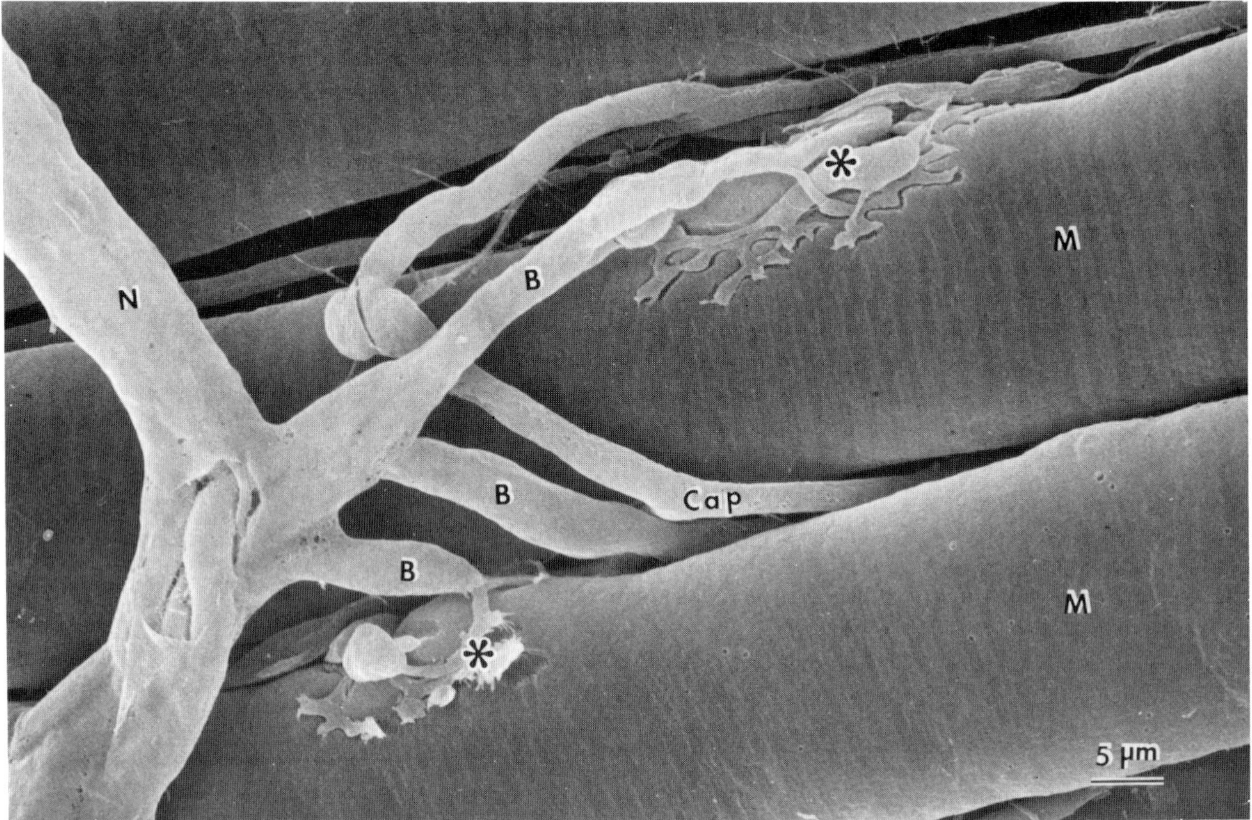

FIG. 16. Innervating nerve and neuromuscular junction of Chinese hamster sternothyroid muscle. Nerve (*N*) forms side branches (*B*) that terminate on muscle fibers (*M*) to form neuromuscular junctions (*asterisks*). *Cap*, capillary. [From Desaki and Uehara (9).]

freeze-fracture replicas [Fig. 14*B*; (2, 3, 6, 28, 46, 54)]. Although the exposed surface is not true outer or inner surface, these replicas also provide the overall morphology of fiber surface with additional information (at higher resolution than SEM), including the distribution of intramembranous particles.

Mitochondria

Mitochondria in muscle fibers are easily recognizable in SEM by their shape, size, and distribution. They are round, oval, or cylindrical and show smooth outer surfaces. Confirming findings from thin-section electron microscopy, SEM also reveals that mitochondria vary in quantity among different muscles and in different types of muscle fibers. Red muscle fibers are rich in mitochondria, often arranged in rows between myofibrils and in aggregates beneath the sarcolemma, in addition to their common distribution at the level of the I bands. Mitochondria in white fibers are considerably reduced in quantity and localized at the level of the I bands in mouse muscles and only scattered and much fewer in number in frog sartorius muscle. In some mouse muscles, elongated mitochondria are arranged perpendicular to the fiber axis in pairs on both sides of the Z band. Distribution of mitochondria in cardiac muscles has been examined in some detail by SEM (38, 57, 58). Cardiac muscle cells possess some morphological features of mitochondria common to red skeletal muscle fibers in quantity and distribution. Mitochondria seem to be distributed in close relation to the sarcomere pattern of myofibrils and change their form during the contraction-relaxation cycles.

NEUROMUSCULAR JUNCTION

The overall structure of neuromuscular junctions has been beautifully demonstrated by SEM after removal of connective tissue components by treatment with HCl after glutaraldehyde-OsO_4 fixation (9). The surface topography of intramuscular nerve fibers with their branchings and of terminal arborization of axons can be visualized in three dimensions while their structural integrity is well preserved (Fig. 16). In the vicinity of the neuromuscular junctions, nerves ramify repeatedly into terminal branches that abruptly taper by losing the myelin sheaths to give rise to nerve endings, as confirmed by thin-section electron microscopy (Fig. 17*A*). Where the nerve endings are pulled away from the muscle fiber, subneural apparatuses

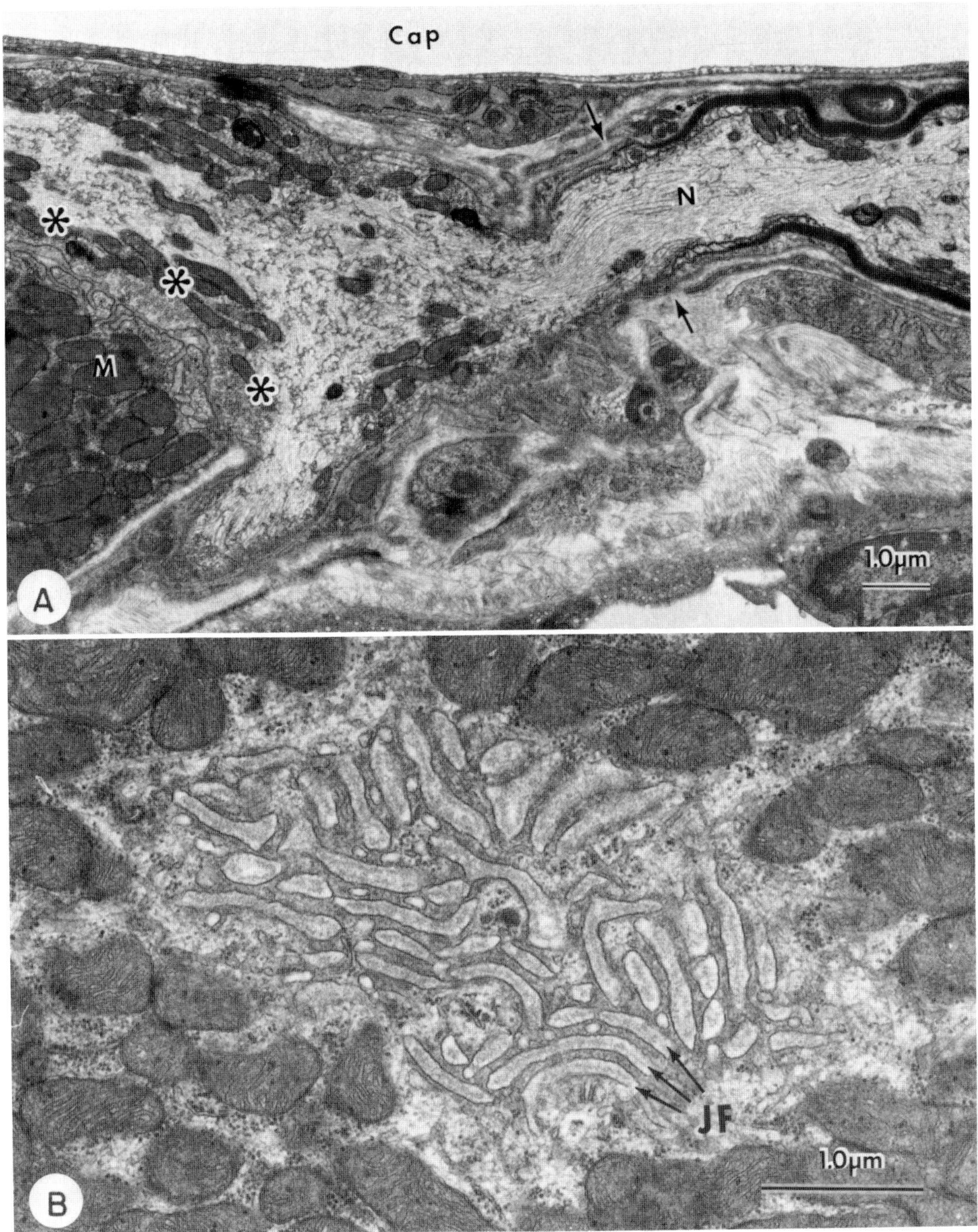

FIG. 17. Thin-section electron micrographs of neuromuscular junction of mouse diaphragm. *A*: branch (*N*) of a motor axon approaches a muscle fiber (*M*) to form neuromuscular junction (*asterisks*). Myelin sheath is lost just before terminal arborization (*arrows*). *Cap*, capillary. Compare with Fig. 16. *B*: *en face* view of subneural apparatus showing characteristic pattern of junctional folds (*JF*). Compare with Fig. 18*A*.

composed of synaptic troughs with junctional folds are seen *en face* (Figs. 18 and 19).

The shape and arrangement of the nerve endings and the complexity of the subneural apparatuses vary considerably in different animal species and muscle types, as determined by light microscopy (8) and electron microscopy (66). The SEM observation is especially useful in understanding the developmental and comparative aspects of neuromuscular junctions (Figs. 18 and 19). Arrangement of synaptic troughs corresponds to that of nerve endings. In mammalian muscles, terminal branches overlap and join to form a

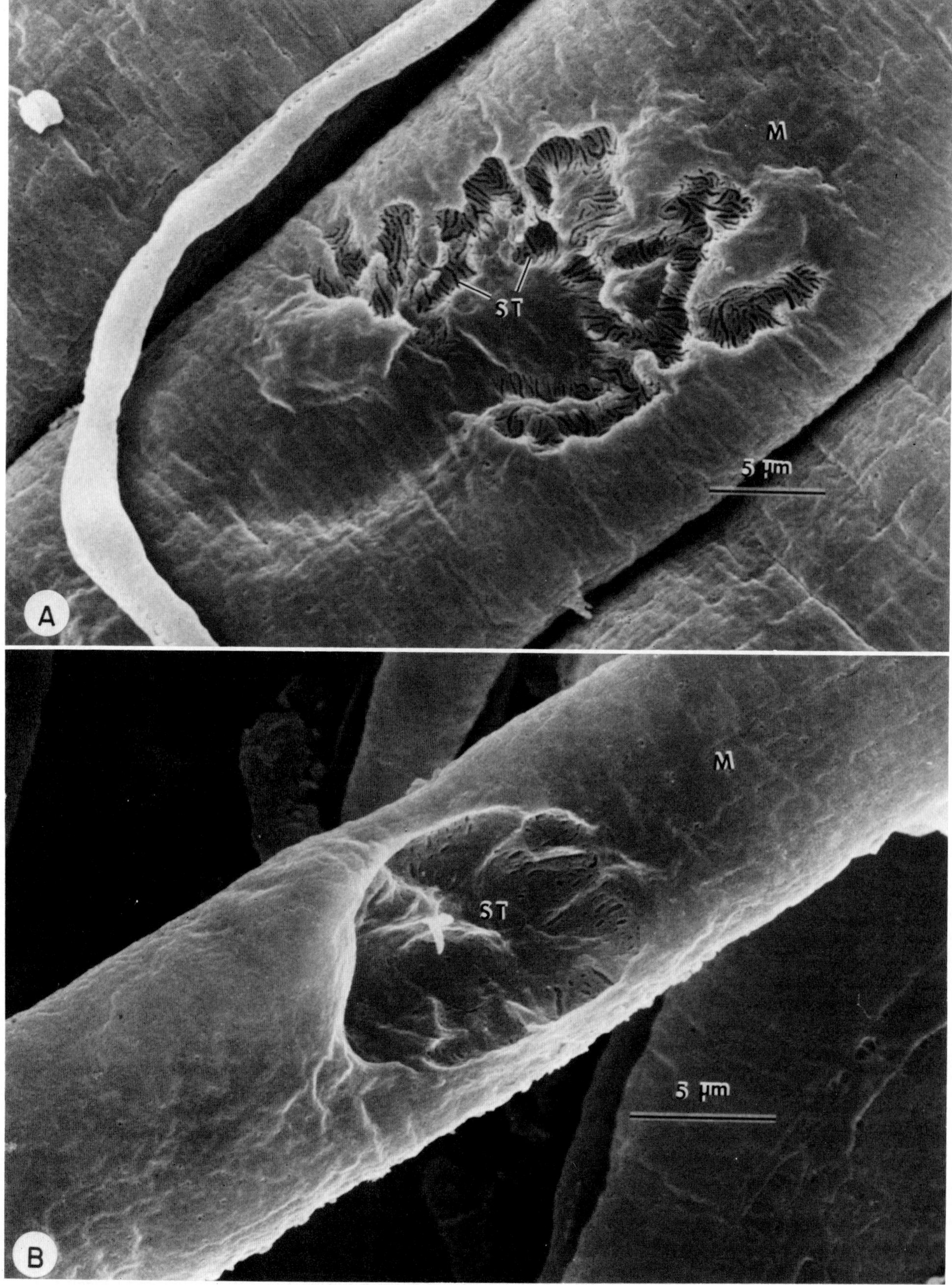

FIG. 18. Neuromuscular junction. *En face* views of subneural apparatuses from adult (*A*) and 10-day-old (*B*) rats. Note extent of elaboration of synaptic troughs (*ST*) with junctional folds in adult and developing muscles. *M*, muscle fiber. (From J. Desaki and Y. Uehara, unpublished observations.)

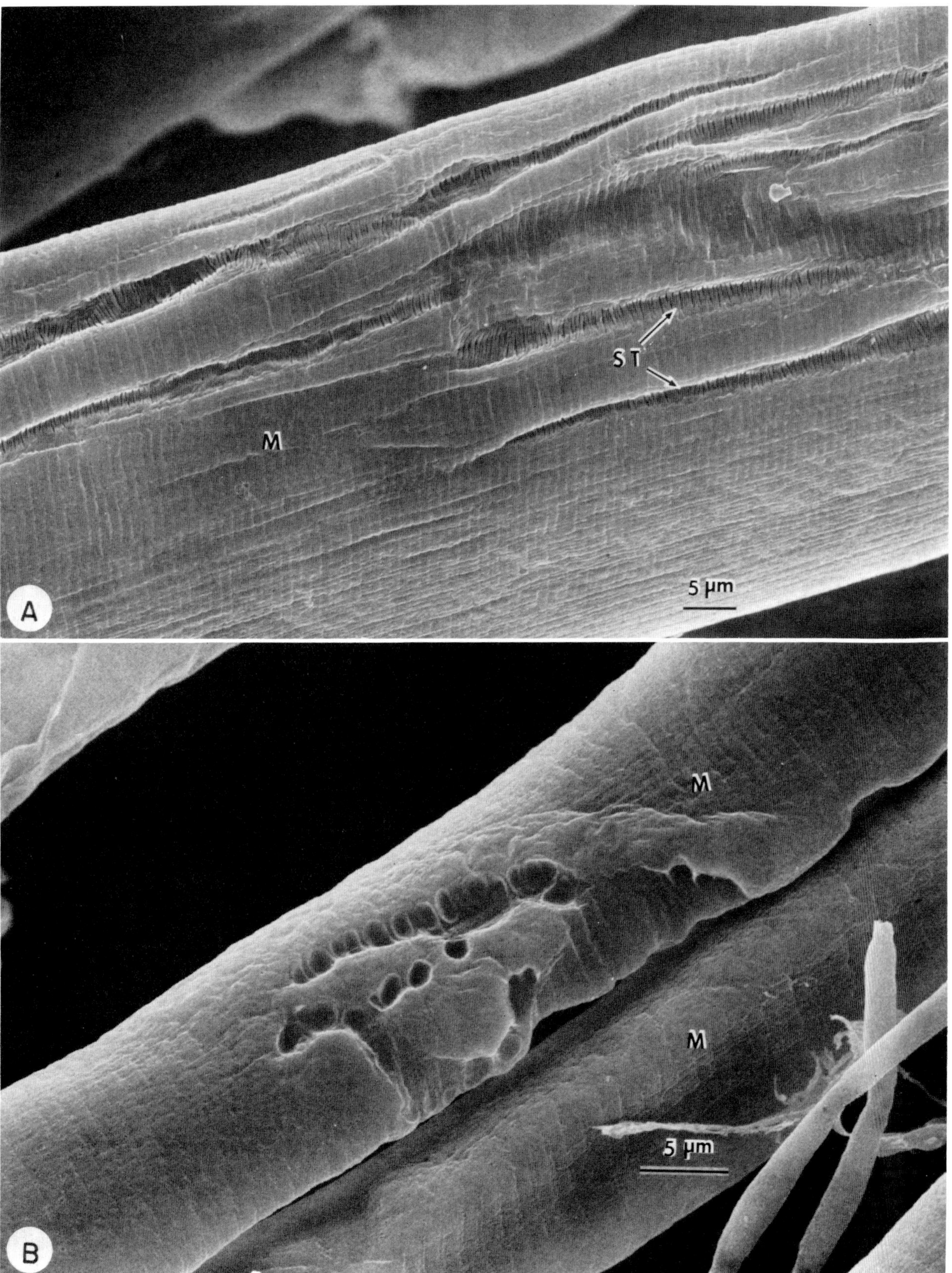

FIG. 19. Neuromuscular junction. *A*: frog sartorius muscle. Subneural apparatus reflects *en plaque* type of nerve ending. Synaptic troughs (*ST*) are elongated along the muscle fiber (*M*). *B*: finch latissimus dorsi anterior muscle. *En grappe* type of nerve ending. (From J. Desaki and Y. Uehara, unpublished observations.)

complicated pattern over an oval area of about 15 μm by 30 μm [Fig. 18A; (9)]. In frog sartorius muscle, each nerve ending is arranged in a ribbonlike strand with a fairly constant width and running parallel to the long axis of the muscle fiber [Fig. 19A; (9, 55)], whereas in finch posterior latissimus dorsi muscle the nerve ending ramifies into several branches with varicose swellings (Fig. 19B). In frog sartorius muscle, the nerve endings possess small lateral projections of the covering Schwann cells (9). It would be interesting to know if the projections may be related to the beltlike extensions of the Schwann cell in the synaptic trough seen in thin sections (20).

In adult rat muscles, junctional clefts or folds in the postsynaptic sarcolemma have a highly elaborate pattern (Fig. 18A), in agreement with images in thin-section electron micrographs (Fig. 17B). Within each synaptic trough the junctional clefts that differ in pattern among different animal species, muscle types, and stages of development are clearly seen. In frog sartorius muscles a series of junctional clefts traverse the trough at regular intervals of ~0.5 μm (9, 55). However, the clefts are not always straight across the trough: some clefts are branched or shorter.

SUMMARY

The surface structure of skeletal muscle fibers has been described. Morphological details vary in different muscle fibers, and the SEM observations presented are limited to several kinds of muscles. However, one expects these observations to illustrate basic features common to many other muscles.

As described above, SEM has great potential for the study of the surface morphology of striated muscles. It not only shows the three-dimensional aspects of structure, supplementing observations with the light microscope and transmission electron microscope, but also adds new information. The usefulness of the SEM depends largely on proper and suitable specimen preparation. One should choose or even develop methods of specimen preparation suitable for the particular purposes of the study.

We thank Drs. Yasuo Uehara and Junzo Desaki of Ehime University, Japan, and Dr. Mitsuaki Kurotaki of Hirosaki University, Japan, for kindly providing plates for inclusion in this chapter.

REFERENCES

1. Ashraf, M., and H. D. Sybers. Scanning electron microscopy of ischemic heart. In: *Scanning Electron Microscopy/1974*, edited by O. Johari and I. Corvin. Chicago: Illinois Inst. Technol. Res. Inst., 1974, p. 722–728.
2. Beringer, T. A freeze-fracture study of sarcoplasmic reticulum from fast and slow muscle of the mouse. *Anat. Rec.* 184: 647–664, 1975.
3. Bertaud, W. S., D. G. Rayns, and F. O. Simpson. Freeze-etch studies on fish skeletal muscle. *J. Cell Sci.* 6: 537–557, 1970.
4. Boyde, A., and J. C. P. Williams. Surface morphology of frog striated muscle as prepared for and examined in the scanning electron microscope. *J. Physiol. London* 197: 10–11, 1968.
5. Branton, D. Fracture faces of frozen membranes. *Proc. Natl. Acad. Sci. USA* 55: 1048–1056, 1966.
6. Bray, D. F., and D. G. Rayns. A comparative freeze-etch study of the sarcoplasmic reticulum of avian fast and slow muscle fibers. *J. Ultrastruct. Res.* 57: 251–259, 1976.
7. Cohen, S. H. Dry Ice fixation of myofibrils for scanning electron microscopy. *Stain Technol.* 51: 43–45, 1976.
8. Couteaux, R. Motor end-plate structure. In: *The Structure and Function of Muscle*, edited by G. H. Bourne. New York: Academic, 1960, vol. 1, p. 337–380.
9. Desaki, J., and Y. Uehara. The overall morphology of neuromuscular junctions as revealed by scanning electron microscopy. *J. Neurocytol.* 10: 101–110, 1981.
10. Dulhunty, A. F., and C. Franzini-Armstrong. The relative contributions of the folds and caveolae to the surface membrane of frog skeletal muscle fibres at different sarcomere lengths. *J. Physiol. London* 250: 513–539, 1975.
11. Evan, A. P., W. G. Dail, D. Dammrose, and C. Palmer. Scanning electron microscopy of cell surface following removal of extracellular material. *Anat. Rec.* 185: 433–446, 1976.
12. Franzini-Armstrong, C. Studies of the triad. IV. Structure of the junction in frog slow fibers. *J. Cell Biol.* 56: 120–128, 1973.
13. Geissinger, H. D., and I. Gringer. Correlated scanning electron microscopy in transmission (STEM) and reflection (SEM) on sections of skeletal muscle. *Mikroskopie* 32: 329–333, 1976.
14. Geissinger, H. D., S. Yamashiro, and C. A. Ackerly. Preparation of skeletal muscle for intermicroscopic (LM, SEM, TEM) correlation. In: *Scanning Electron Microscopy/1978*, edited by R. P. Becker and O. Johari. O'Hare, IL: SEM Inc., 1978, vol. II, p. 267–274.
15. Gelber, D., D. H. Moore, and H. Ruska. Observations of the myo-tendon junction in mammalian skeletal muscle. *Z. Zellforsch. Mikrosk. Anat.* 52: 396–400, 1960.
16. Gunji, T., M. Wakita, and S. Kobayashi. Conductive staining in SEM with especial reference to tissue transparency. *Scanning* 3: 227–232, 1980.
17. Hamano, M., T. Otaka, T. Nagatani, and T. Tanaka. A frozen liquid cracking method for high resolution scanning electron microscopy. *J. Electron Microsc.* 22: 298, 1973.
18. Hayes, R. L., and E. R. Allen. Electron-microscopic studies on a double-stranded beaded filament of embryonic collagen. *J. Cell Sci.* 2: 419–434, 1967.
19. Heuser, J. E., and M. W. Kirschner. Filament organization revealed in platinum replicas of freeze-dried cytoskeletons. *J. Cell Biol.* 86: 212–234, 1980.
20. Heuser, J. E., and T. S. Reese. Evidence for recycling of synaptic vesicle membrane during transmitter release at the frog neuromuscular junction. *J. Cell Biol.* 57: 315–344, 1973.
21. Heuser, J. E., T. S. Reese, M. J. Dennis, Y. Jan, L. Jan, and L. Evans. Synaptic vesicle exocytosis captured by quick freezing and correlated with quantal transmitter release. *J. Cell Biol.* 81: 275–300, 1979.
22. Humphreys, W. J., B. O. Spurlock, and J. S. Johnson. Critical point drying of ethanol-infiltrated, cryofractured biological specimens for scanning electron microscopy. In: *Scanning Electron Microscopy/1974*, edited by O. Johari and I. Corvin. Chicago: Illinois Inst. Technol. Res. Inst., 1974, p. 276–282.
23. Huxley, H. E., and W. Brown. The low angle X-ray diagram

of vertebrate striated muscle and its behavior during contraction and rigor. *J. Mol. Biol.* 30: 383–434, 1967.
24. ISHIKAWA, H. The fine structure of myo-tendon junction in some mammalian skeletal muscles. *Arch. Histol. Jpn.* 25: 275–296, 1965.
25. ISHIKAWA, H. Formation of elaborate networks of T-system tubules in cultured skeletal muscle with special reference to the T-system formation. *J. Cell Biol.* 38: 51–66, 1968.
26. ISHIKAWA, H., Y. FUKUDA, AND E. YAMADA. Freeze-replica observations on frog sartorius muscle. I. Sarcolemmal specialization. *J. Electron Microsc.* 24: 97–107, 1975.
27. KELLY, D. E. The fine structure of skeletal muscle triad junctions. *J. Ultrastruct. Res.* 29: 37–49, 1969.
28. KELLY, D. E., AND A. M. KUDA. Subunits of the triadic junction in fast skeletal muscle as revealed by freeze fracture. *J. Ultrastruct. Res.* 68: 220–233, 1979.
29. KUROTAKI, M. Observations on blood capillary arrangements in the striated muscle by plastic injection method. *Acta Anat. Nippon* 55: 336, 1980.
30. MAURO, A., AND W. R. ADAMS. The structure of the sarcolemma of the frog skeletal muscle fiber. *J. Biophys. Biochem. Cytol. Suppl.* 10: 177–185, 1961.
31. MCCALLISTER, L. P., AND R. HADEK. Transmission electron microscopy and stereo ultrastructure of the T-system in frog skeletal muscle. *J. Ultrastruct. Res.* 33: 360–368, 1970.
32. MCCALLISTER, L. P., V. R. MUMAW, AND B. L. MUNGER. Stereo ultrastructure of cardiac membrane system in the rat heart. In: *Scanning Electron Microscopy/1974,* edited by O. Johari and I. Corvin. Chicago: Illinois Inst. Technol. Res. Inst., 1974, p. 714–719.
33. MCDONALD, L. W., R. F. W. PEASE, AND T. L. HAYES. Scanning electron microscopy of sectioned tissue. *Lab. Invest.* 16: 532–538, 1967.
34. MOOR, H., AND K. MÜHLETHALER. Fine structure in frozen-etched yeast cells. *J. Cell Biol.* 17: 609–628, 1963.
35. MURAKAMI, T. Application of the scanning electron microscope to the study of the fine distribution of the blood vessels. *Arch. Histol. Jpn.* 32: 445–454, 1971.
36. MURAKAMI, T. A metal impregnation method of biological specimens for SEM. *Arch. Histol. Jpn.* 35: 323–326, 1973.
37. MURAKAMI, T. A revised tannin-osmium method for noncoated SEM specimens. *Arch. Histol. Jpn.* 36: 189–193, 1974.
38. MYKLEBUST, R., H. DALEN, AND T. S. SAETERSDAL. A comparative study in the transmission electron microscope and scanning electron microscope of intracellular structures in sheep heart muscle cells. *J. Microsc. Oxford* 105: 57–65, 1975.
39. NEMNIC, M. K. Critical point drying, cryofracture, and serial sectioning. In: *Scanning Electron Microscopy/1972,* edited by O. Johari. Chicago: Illinois Inst. Technol. Res. Inst., 1972, p. 297–304.
40. PACHTER, B. R., J. DAVIDOWITZ, B. ZIMMER, AND G. M. BREININ. Scanning electron microscopy of etched Epon extraocular muscle sections. *J. Microsc. Oxford* 99: 85–90, 1973.
41. PEACHEY, L. D. The sarcoplasmic reticulum and transverse tubules of the frog's sartorius. *J. Cell Biol.* 25: 209–231, 1965.
42. PEPE, F. A. Stucture of the myosin filament of striated muscle. *Prog. Biophys. Mol. Biol.* 22: 75–96, 1971.
43. POH, T., R. L. J. ALTENHOFF, S. ABRAHAM, AND T. HAYES. Scanning electron microscopy of myocardial sections originally prepared for the light microscopy. *Exp. Mol. Pathol.* 14: 404–407, 1971.
44. RAYNS, D. G. Myofilaments and cross-bridges as demonstrated by freeze-fracturing and etching. *J. Ultrastruct. Res.* 40: 103–121, 1972.
45. RAYNS, D. G. Freeze-fracturing and freeze-etching of cardiac myosin filaments. *J. Microsc. Oxford* 103: 215–226, 1975.
46. RAYNS, D. G., C. E. DEVINE, AND C. L. SUTHERLAND. Freeze fracture studies of membrane systems in vertebrate muscle. I. Striated muscle. *J. Ultrastruct. Res.* 50: 306–321, 1975.
47. RAYNS, D. G., F. O. SIMPSON, AND W. S. BERTAUD. Transverse tubule apertures in mammalian myocardial cells: surface array. *Science* 156: 656–657, 1967.
48. RAYNS, D. G., F. O. SIMPSON, AND W. S. BERTAUD. Surface features of striated muscle cells. I. Guinea-pig cardiac muscle. *J. Cell Sci.* 3: 467–474, 1968.
49. RAYNS, D. G., F. O. SIMPSON, AND W. S. BERTAUD. Surface features of striated muscle cells. II. Guinea-pig skeletal muscle. *J. Cell Sci.* 3: 475–482, 1968.
50. ROBERTSON, J. D. Some features of the ultrastructure of reptilian skeletal muscle. *J. Biophys. Biochem. Cytol.* 2: 369–394, 1956.
51. SAKURAGAWA, N., T. SATO, AND T. TSUBAKI. Scanning electron microscopic study of skeletal muscle. Normal, dystrophic, and neurogenic atrophic muscle in mice and humans. *Arch. Neurol. Chicago* 28: 247–251, 1973.
52. SAWADA, H., H. ISHIKAWA, AND E. YAMADA. High resolution scanning electron microscopy of frog sartorius muscle. *Tissue Cell* 10: 179–190, 1978.
53. SCHALLER, D. R., AND W. P. POWRIE. Scanning electron microscopic study of skeletal muscle from rainbow trout, turkey and beef. *J. Food Sci.* 36: 552–559, 1971.
54. SCHMALBRUCH, H. The membrane systems in different fibre types of the triceps surae muscle of cat. *Cell Tissue Res.* 204: 187–200, 1979.
55. SHOTTON, D. M., J. E. HEUSER, B. F. REESE, AND T. S. REESE. Postsynaptic membrane folds of the frog neuromuscular junction visualized by scanning electron microscopy. *Neuroscience* 4: 427–435, 1979.
56. SMITH, D. S., AND H. C. ALDRICH. Membrane systems of freeze-etched striated muscle. *Tissue Cell* 3: 261–281, 1971.
57. SYBERS, H. D., AND M. ASHRAF. Scanning electron microscopy of cardiac muscle. *Lab. Invest.* 30: 441–450, 1974.
58. SYBERS, H. D., AND C. A. SHELDON. SEM techniques for cardiac cells in fetal, adult and pathologic heart. In: *Scanning Electron Microscopy/1975,* edited by O. Johari and I. Corvin. Chicago: Illinois Inst. Technol. Res. Inst., 1975, p. 276–280.
59. TANAKA, K. Freezed resin cracking method for scanning electron microscopy of biological materials. *Naturwissenschaften* 59: 77, 1972.
60. TANAKA, K. Application of secondary electron and backscattered electron images for biological research. *J. Electron Microsc.* 29: 76, 1980.
61. TANAKA, K., A. IINO, AND T. NAGURO. Stylene resin cracking method for observing biological materials by scanning electron microscopy. *J. Electron Microsc.* 23: 313–315, 1974.
62. UEHARA, Y., AND K. SUYAMA. Visualization of the adventitial aspect of the vascular smooth muscle cells under the scanning electron microscope. *J. Electron Microsc.* 27: 157–159, 1978.
63. USUKURA, J., H. ISHIKAWA, AND E. YAMADA. Fine structure of unfixed frog sartorius muscle as revealed by deep-etch-replica and freeze-substitution methods. *J. Electron Microsc.* 30: 237, 1981.
64. WICKHAM, M. G., AND D. M. WORTHEN. Correlation of scanning and transmission electron microscopy on the same tissue sample. *Stain Technol.* 48: 63–68, 1973.
65. WOODS, P. S., AND M. C. LEDBETTER. Cell organelles and uncoated cryofractured surfaces as viewed with the scanning electron microscope. *J. Cell Sci.* 21: 47–58, 1976.
66. ZACKS, S. I. *The Motor Endplate.* Philadelphia, PA: Saunders, 1964.

CHAPTER 2

Structure and function of membrane systems of skeletal muscle cells

LEE D. PEACHEY
CLARA FRANZINI-ARMSTRONG

Departments of Biology and Anatomy, University of Pennsylvania, Philadelphia, Pennsylvania

CHAPTER CONTENTS

THIS CHAPTER BEGINS with a discussion of the surface and internal structure of skeletal muscle fibers, partly covered in the chapter by Ishikawa, Sawada, and Yamada in this *Handbook*. Attention then focuses on the structure and function of the internal membranes of striated muscle fibers, the sarcoplasmic reticulum (SR), and the transverse tubules or T-system (T-tubule or T) networks. General principles are described with examples and a few especially interesting variations found in different types of muscles in different species. This chapter is not a comprehensive review of muscle cell membrane structure or function but does discuss most of the important principles and some of the historical development of this knowledge. Other chapters in this volume and recent books and reviews contain additional information (1, 26, 37, 43, 44, 60–64, 74, 81, 103, 109, 124, 147, 190, 196, 201, 211, 219, 251, 262, 269, 282, 306, 309, 314).

STRUCTURAL COMPONENTS OF SKELETAL MUSCLE FIBERS

A coarse division can be made between those structures in a muscle fiber that are directly involved in the contractile activity (force production) of the muscle cell and those structures that perform supportive functions, e.g., controlling the state of contraction or providing metabolic energy. The contractile components of the muscle cell are the assembly of myofibrils and the myofilaments of which the myofibrils are built.

The surface membrane of the fiber, the T-system membranes, and the SR control contraction. Mitochondria, glycolytic enzymes, and high-energy phosphate intermediates, including adenosine 5′-triphosphate (ATP) and creatine or arginine phosphate, provide metabolic energy. Metabolic substrates are found in the form of glycogen deposits and fat droplets.

Sarcomeres, Striations, and Fibrils

The sarcomere is the basic repeating unit of structure along the longitudinal axis of the striated muscle fiber. The myofibril is the basic unit in the transverse plane. Van Leeuwenhoek (184) first detected sarcomeres in 1712 when he described "circular rings" around the surfaces of air-dried muscle fibers from a whale (see quote in the chapter by B. R. Eisenberg in this *Handbook*, p. 79). William Bowman (32) first described fibrils (or myofibrils) in skeletal and cardiac muscles from a variety of species in 1840 (Fig. 1). Bowman correctly pointed out that the fibrils fill the interiors of the fibers and are striated (show a sarcomere pattern). Thus the striations are not just on the fiber surface where van Leeuwenhoek had observed them. Bowman suggested that van Leeuwenhoek had seen circular impressions on the surface of a dried muscle fiber made by the bands of the underlying myofibrils. Such surface details are observed now in the scanning electron microscope (Fig. 2; see also the chapter by Ishikawa, Sawada, and Yamada in this *Handbook*).

The approximate shape of a single sarcomere unit

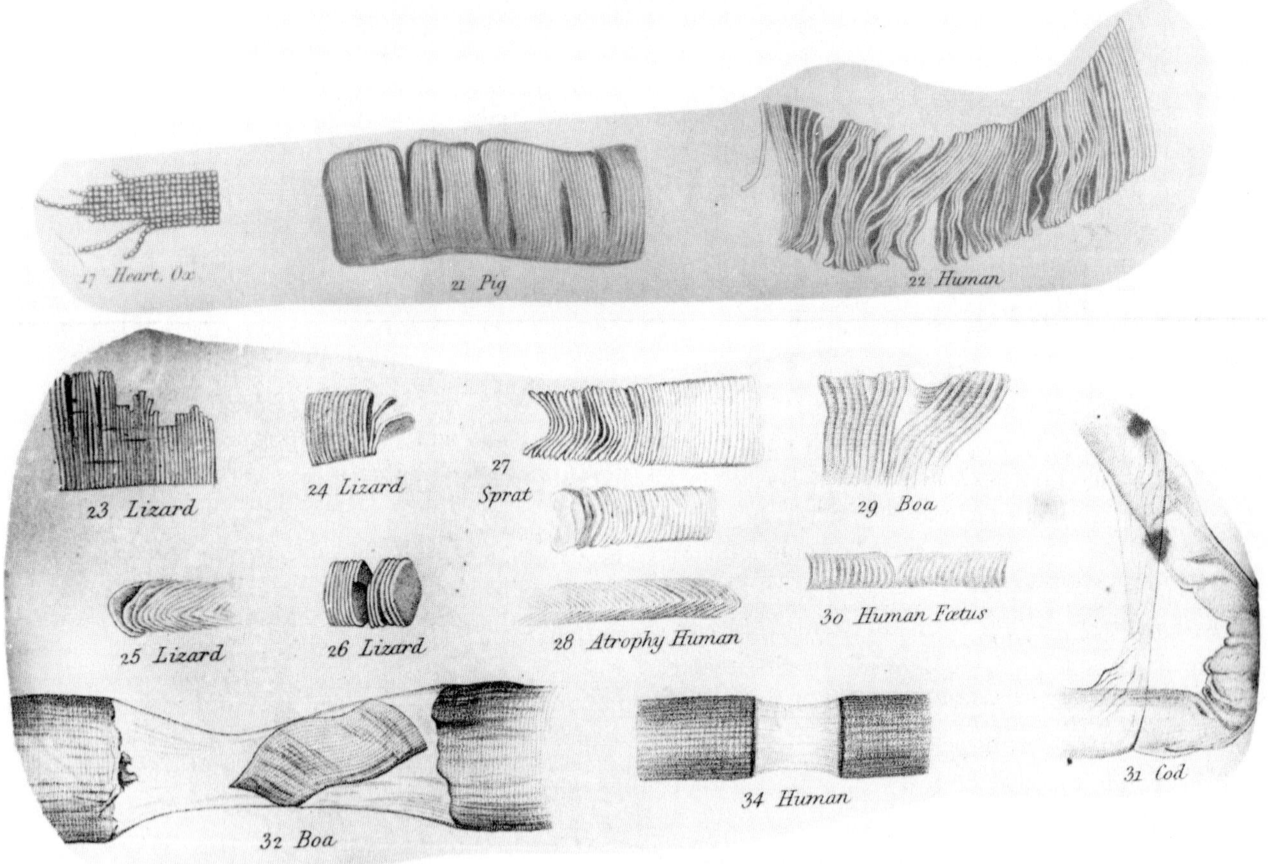

FIG. 1. Bowman (32) was hesitant to accept the fibrillar nature of muscle fibers because the "fibrillae" were so small and thus difficult to separate from one another without "suffering an unnatural mutilation" and because of the difficulties of interpreting optical images of such small objects. He believed, however, that the internal structure of muscle fibers basically is fibrillar. Bowman depicted the fibrils from a macerated ox heart (*17*) as periodically beaded; this was the basis for his belief that muscle fiber striations are not just on the surface, as van Leeuwenhoek (183) observed earlier, but come from the banded nature of the fibrils inside the fiber. Bowman also depicted a tendency for muscle fibers from a variety of species to disintegrate under certain conditions into transverse disks (*21–30*), which led him to challenge van Leeuwenhoek's interpretation of muscle striations as helical. *31, 32, 34*: Bowman's view of the sarcolemma in regions where the fiber had broken internally and the fibrillar mass retracted, leaving an empty sarcolemmal tube covering the surface of a muscle fiber. [From Bowman (32).]

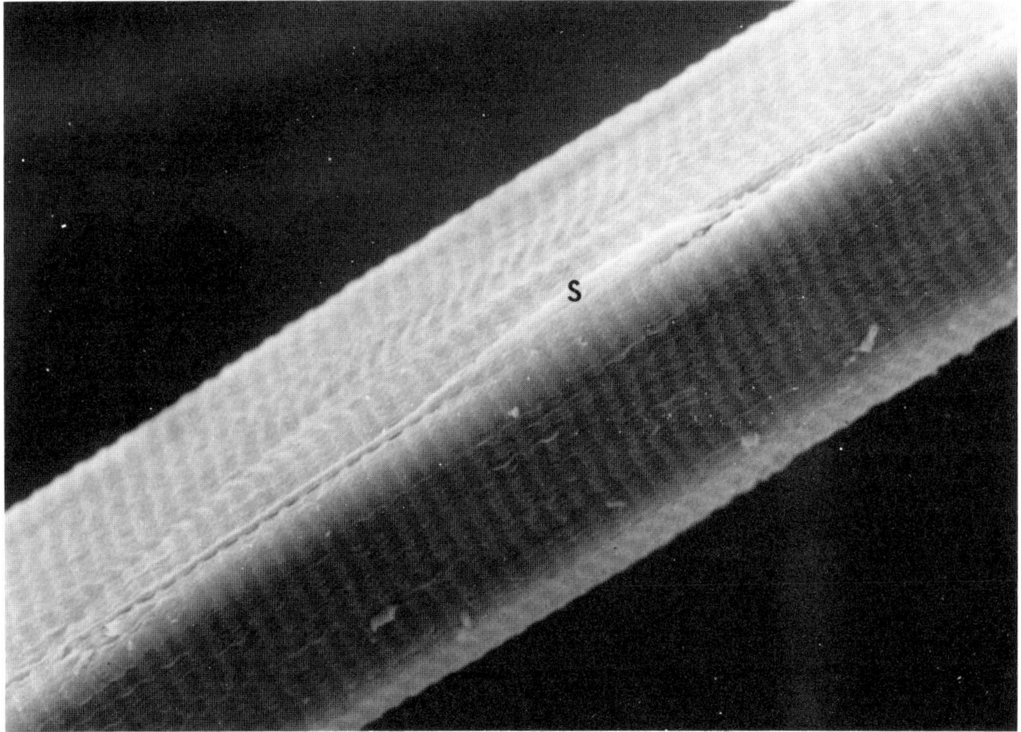

FIG. 2. Scanning electron micrograph of portion of a single muscle fiber from frog sartorius muscle. Sarcolemma shows a series of ridges around circumference of fiber. Ridges must be similar to what van Leeuwenhoek observed in his light microscope more than 250 years ago. Satellite cell (*S*) lies in longitudinal groove in surface of muscle fiber. (Courtesy of R. Mazanet.)

in a vertebrate skeletal muscle is that of a cylinder ~1 μm in diameter and ~3 μm long. However, these dimensions are different in different types of fibers and in different species and change as the muscle fiber is shortened or stretched. Also the cross section of a myofibril rarely is circular or close to circular. More often the myofibrils are pressed together and take on various polygonal shapes in cross section. This varies in different types of fibers; in some types where fibrils are loosely packed an approximately circular cross section is seen. However, in some other types of fibers, e.g., in amphioxus fibers (93, 94, 203, 231), in some fibers in extraocular muscles of mammals (7, 198, 207, 248), in some fish fibers (111), in arachnid fibers (13, 104, 113, 287), and in the cross-striated adductor muscle of the scallop (208, 277), the fibrils are ribbon shaped and present an elongated profile in cross sections.

The structural organization of the contractile apparatus of the muscle fiber is important in this discussion because a variety of other organelles occupy the spaces between the myofibrils. The shape and disposition of these organelles, which carry out a variety of important functions in the muscle cell other than contraction, are considerably influenced by their confinement to the interfibrillar spaces and their need for close functional and structural association with the myofibrils. Mitochondria, SR, T tubules, and glycogen granules are thus confined. Most of the other organelles, including some of the mitochondria, are in perinuclear and subsarcolemmal positions or in a central core of sarcoplasm without fibrils when such a core is present. Modern microscopic methods, e.g., transmission, high-voltage, and scanning electron microscopy, have allowed the visualization and description of these cell structures and have contributed greatly to our understanding of important structure-function correlations in muscle biology.

Membranes

The primary subjects of this chapter are the membranes in the muscle cell. One of these (the plasmalemma) covers the fiber's outer surface; two others (the SR and T tubules) are within the fiber, surrounding and lying between the myofibrils. In several important ways the membranes are structurally and functionally related to the myofibrils. Often this can be seen as a repeating structural pattern in the internal membranes with the same period and in registration with the sarcomere repeat of the adjacent myofibrils. In the transverse plane within the fiber, the membranes are located between the myofibrils, resulting in a complex and three-dimensional branching network pattern. Functionally these membranes play key roles in the control of activation and relaxation of the

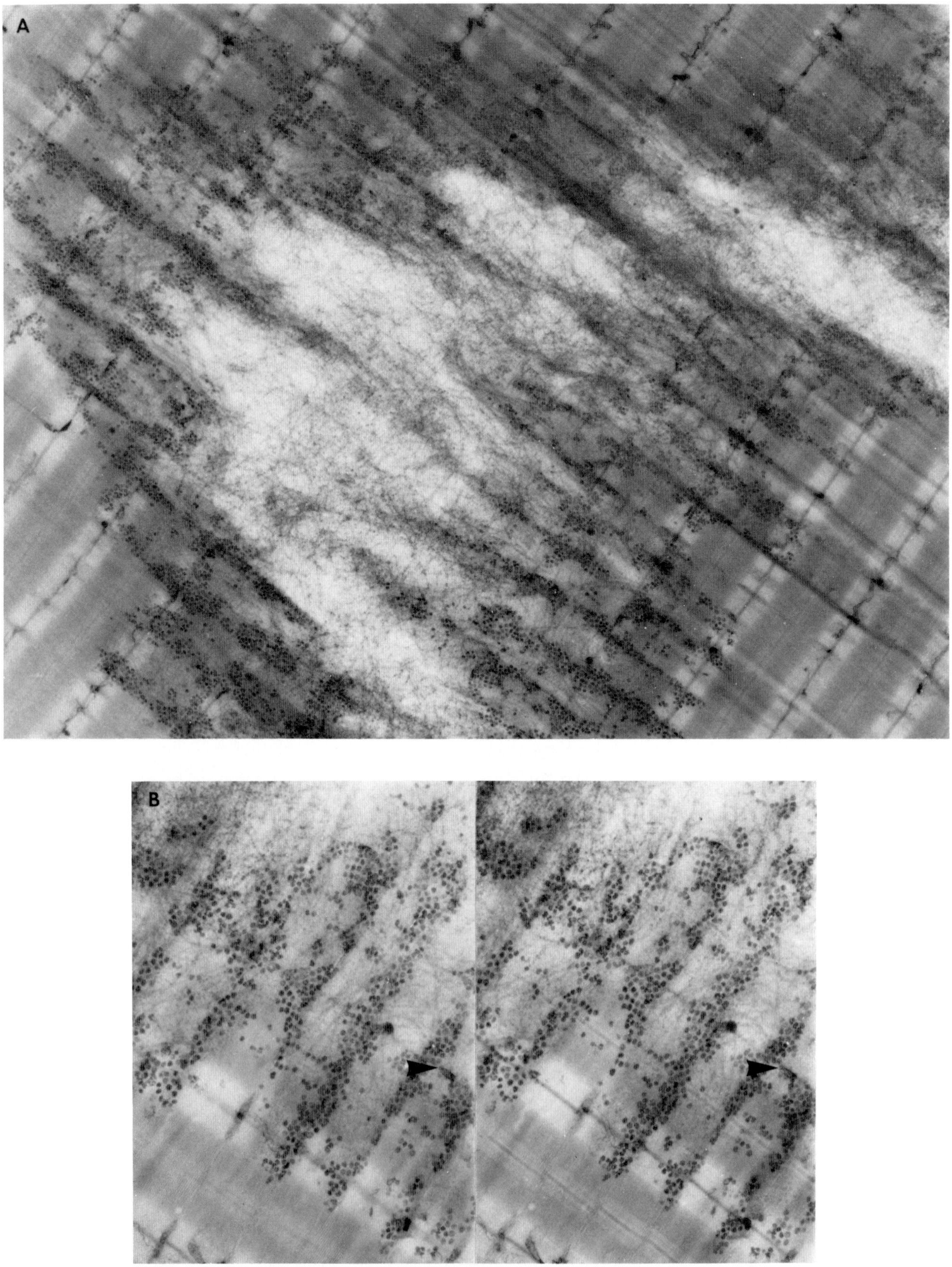

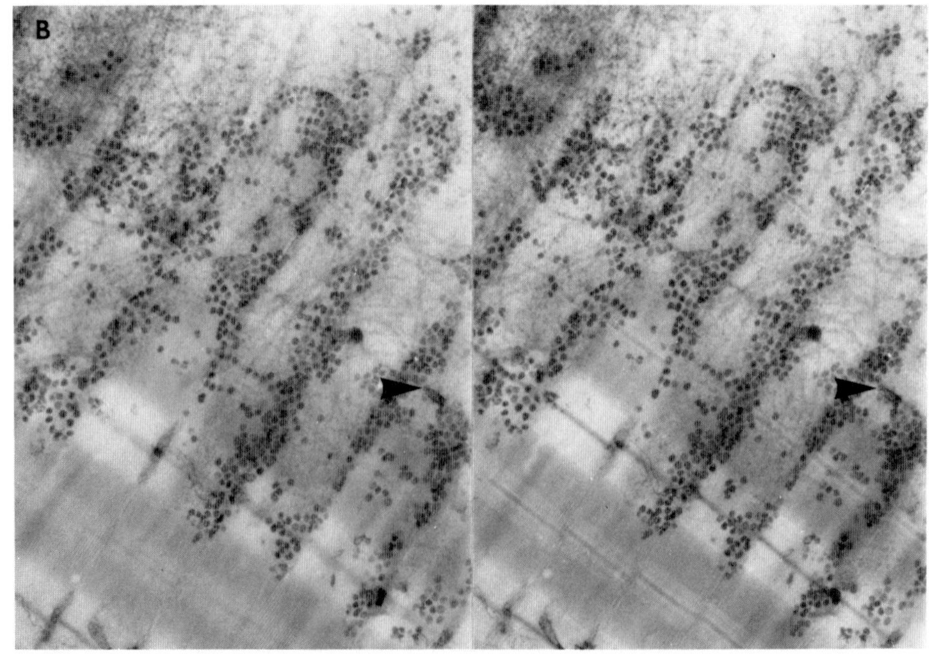

FIG. 3. High-voltage electron micrographs of longitudinal sections ~ 1 μm thick of frog sartorius muscle, lanthanum colloid method. *A*: low magnification. Surfaces of 2 adjacent muscle fibers pass

contractile fibrils (see the chapters by Gonzalez-Serratos, Adrian, R. S. Eisenberg, Baylor, Caputo, and Martonosi and Beeler in this *Handbook*).

A close relationship between the structure of the membrane networks in muscle cells and their function is widely accepted. Researchers have expended considerable effort in the last 25 years, after the first application of the electron microscope to these studies, in the search for clues in the structure to help explain the function. Correlation with physiology and with biochemical studies is still an important component of this work.

SARCOLEMMA. The sarcolemma of a muscle fiber is a multicomponent structure covering the entire surface of the fiber. At the ends of the fiber, where the sarcolemma attaches to tendon, it has a different structure than at the free, lateral surfaces of the fiber.

The sarcolemma first was observed as a separate structural entity in early light-microscopic studies of muscle (32, 183). Anthony van Leeuwenhoek was probably first to refer to a "membrane" covering individual muscle fibers, which he refers to as "Flesh Particles" (184, p. 443):

> In these Discoveries it was very remarkable, that each of the before-mention'd Flesh Particles appear'd to me as if they were wrapt about with a little thin Membrane, which I observ'd in a thousand several Places; and the more easily, because as the Flesh Particles grew dryer, these fine Skins or Membranes were separated from them.

The "Membrane" van Leeuwenhoek refers to probably did not include the plasma membrane but only the fibrous outer layers of the fibers.

The sarcolemma of a muscle fiber is especially apparent in the light microscope when the fibers are damaged so that a retraction of the contractile and other internal structures in the fiber occurs, leaving an empty sarcolemmal tube (197), which was observed by Bowman (32) in 1840 (see Fig. 1; panels 31, 32, 34). The sarcolemma has considerable strength, as seen in these damaged fibers, where it is the only continuous structure holding the fiber intact and transmitting tension in the longitudinal direction (311).

The sarcolemma stains with the periodic acid–Schiff method, with thorium dioxide, and with ruthenium red (96, 118, 119, 186, 187), and therefore contains a component of mucopolysaccharide. The sarcolemma can be divided into its innermost component, the plasma membrane (the true external boundary of the muscle cell), and an overlying basement membrane consisting of an inner basal lamina and an external reticular lamina. The feltlike basal lamina contains laminin, fibronectin, and collagen IV. The more fibrous reticular lamina contains fibronectin, collagen V, and another collagenous protein, high-salt-soluble protein (HSP) (276).

A population of mononucleated satellite cells can be found lying between the basal lamina and the plasma membrane of the muscle cell (49, 196, 197, 199). These satellite cells are thought to be dormant myoblasts that are able to activate and participate in fusion and differentiation of a new muscle fiber when the original has been damaged. Invasive cells, thought to originate from the circulatory system, also penetrate across the basal lamina and into the bulk of the muscle fiber but do not fuse with it (38).

PLASMA MEMBRANE AND CAVEOLAE. Knowledge of the form of the plasma membrane in muscle cells and especially quantitative knowledge of its surface area is important in relation to impedance measurements (see *Relation of Total Surface Area to Fiber Capacitance*, p. 32, and the chapter by R. S. Eisenberg in this *Handbook*). Early measurements of the low-frequency capacitance of muscle fibers (89) suggested that the area of the true membrane covering a muscle fiber must be considerably greater than the area of a smooth cylinder that would cover the same muscle fiber. The latter area has been called the "apparent area" by Dulhunty and Franzini-Armstrong (57). The presence of folds, invaginating caveolae, and T tubules makes the area of the true membrane several times larger than the apparent area in most types of vertebrate muscle fibers. In large invertebrate fibers an even greater augmentation of surface area is achieved by gross folding of the fiber surface and extensive T-tubular networks, though caveolae are not present.

Caveolae are ellipsoidal inpocketings of the plasma membrane connected to the exterior of vertebrate muscle fibers through a narrow neck (24, 57, 156, 210, 278, 328). Caveolae can be found singly but are often clustered in groups of two or three, connecting to the extracellular space through a common neck. In at least some types of fibers, caveolae are not found uniformly distributed over the surface of the fiber but in circumferential and longitudinal bands often associated with the I-band regions of the underlying myofibrils (57). This clustering of caveolae is illustrated in Figure 3, which shows a high-voltage electron micrograph of a section of frog muscle stained with the lanthanum

obliquely through section in this region. Light space between 2 fibers in center of figure shows collagen fibrils. Caveolae in each fiber are filled with dense lanthanum material, making them especially apparent. T tubules also appear dark because of their lanthanum content. 1,000 kV; × 8,400. *B*: higher magnification and stereo. (Stereoscopic images should be viewed with a simple stereoscope, by diverging the eyes until both images are fused, or by crossing the eyes, in which case front and rear of image will be reversed from description in legends.) Caveolae appear as small, approximately circular structures underlying fibrous connective tissue layer on surface of fiber and plasmalemma and overlying myofibrils. Caveolae groups follow undulations of fiber surface and concentrate in I-band regions. *Arrow,* probable connection of T tubule to fiber surface. Total tilt 24°; 1,000 kV; × 12,000.

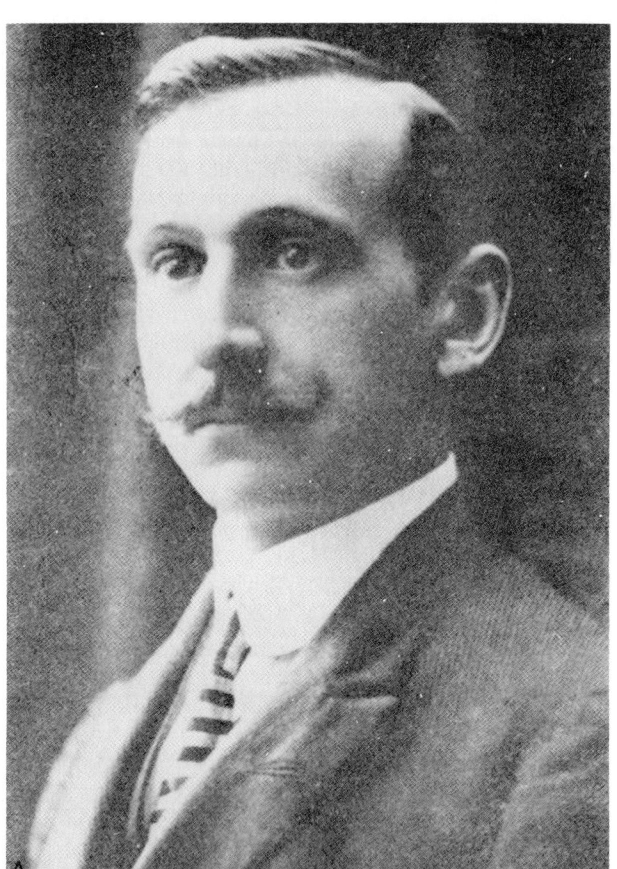

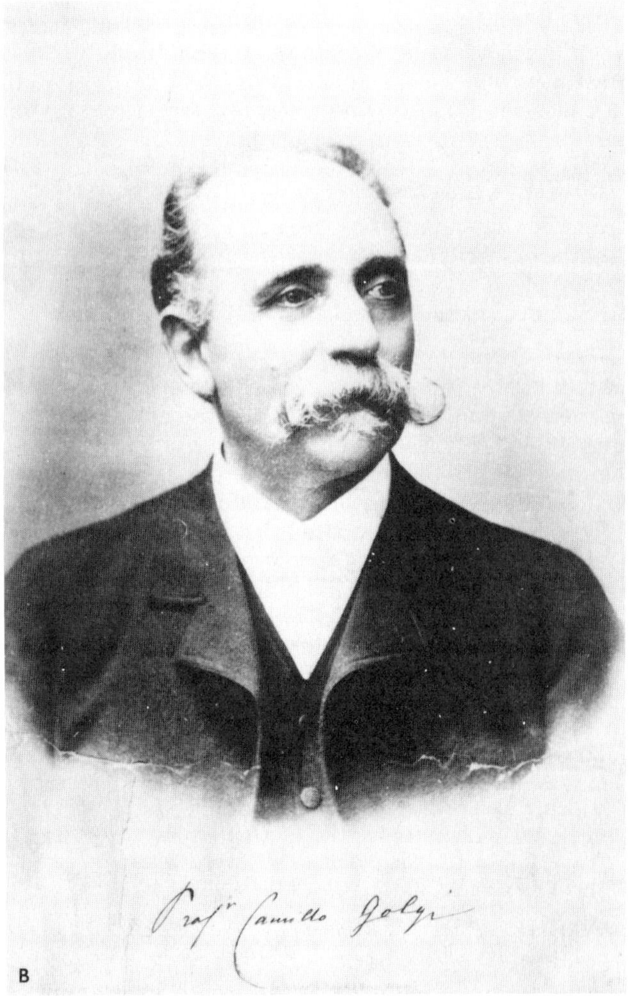

FIG. 4. *A*: Emilio Veratti (born in Varese, Italy, Nov. 24, 1872) was a student of medicine at the University of Pavia, where he worked with Camillo Golgi for 5 yr and then spent 1 yr at the University of Bologna, where he obtained his degree (Laurea in Medicina e Chirurgia) in 1896. He was appointed Aiuto of Histology in 1896 and of General Pathology in 1906, both at the University of Pavia. He died in Varese, February 28, 1967, in the same house in which he was born. *B*: Camillo Golgi, Veratti's professor. Golgi's black-reaction staining technique, used by Veratti, was recently adapted for use in high-voltage electron-microscopic studies of muscle cells (110).

FIG. 5 (frontispiece). Phase-light micrograph of section 1–2 μm thick prepared using a modification of the Golgi black reaction as used by Veratti. Longitudinal view of long-sarcomere, tonic-type muscle fiber from walking leg of crayfish (*Astacus fluviatilis*). Large regions of extracellular space appear orange. Orange region at *lower right*, surface of muscle fiber: orange region at *upper left*, deep infolding or cleft in fiber surface. Smaller clefts enter fiber from surface at *right* and from large cleft at *left*. Finer terminations of these smaller clefts tend to lie in a longitudinal position corresponding to Z line of nearby sarcomeres. *C*, cleft with zigzag profile near micrograph center. Two classes of tubules extend from all fiber surfaces, including those of the clefts. One class is called Z tubules (*Z*) because of its sarcomeric location (229). Second class of tubular invaginations from various fiber surfaces is found in 2 sets per sarcomere near ends of A bands (*T*). Because latter tubules form dyadic associations with sarcoplasmic reticulum (*SR*), they represent true T tubules of these muscle fibers. Longitudinally oriented tubules (*L*) connect from individual Z tubules to adjacent T tubules in these muscle fibers, though not as frequently as in some other types of crustacean muscle fibers. × 2,752. (Micrograph by Franzini-Armstrong, Eastwood, and Peachey.)

method and thick enough to include many caveolae in a single field of view.

The contribution of folds and caveolae to the surface area of a frog skeletal muscle fiber was analyzed quantitatively by Dulhunty and Franzini-Armstrong (57) using freeze-fracture preparations and by Mobley and Eisenberg (210) using stereological methods. Together the folds and caveolae can almost double the surface area of a frog fiber at short sarcomere lengths. There can be many caveolae per square micrometer of fiber surface; the number observed decreases as the fiber is stretched beyond the length where the folds disappear. This suggests that the folds and the caveolae represent reservoirs of membrane that are recruited as the fiber stretches, though most of the effects observed experimentally occur at muscle lengths that could never be achieved with the muscle still attached to the skeleton; the in vivo physiological importance of this effect is not clear.

LIGHT-MICROSCOPIC OBSERVATIONS OF INTERNAL RETICULA. Several observers in the nineteenth century reported reticular networks inside muscle cells, but it seems unlikely that these early observers were seeing evidence of the same reticular networks, T tubules, and/or SR that we know today (291). The sarcoplasmic space between the closely packed myofibrils in most muscles has a honeycomb pattern, similar to what often was described as reticula. In 1888 Rollet (266) stained the sarcoplasm of muscle fibers from the sea horse (*Hippocampus*) with gold chloride, the stain used for many of the earlier observations of supposed reticula. The sea horse muscle fibers have a very restricted distribution of fibrils and a very abundant cytoplasm. In Rollet's preparations the sparse myofibrils appeared in negative contrast against the dark background of the highly stained sarcoplasm, supporting the conclusion that the earlier observations were of sarcoplasm and not of an internal reticulum. The German anatomist Gustav Retzius (261) made probably the first observation of reticular networks within muscle fibers in muscles from beetles and hagfish stained with a chrome-osmium method. Cajal (35) applied the Golgi silver-impregnation method to insect muscles and observed similar networks, though he incorrectly interpreted them as fine extensions of the tracheal system (291). The best of the several light-microscopic descriptions of true reticula in muscle cells of this period is that of the Italian histologist Emilio Veratti [Fig. 4*A*; (316)]. Veratti used the *reazione nera* (black-reaction) staining method of Camillo Golgi (Fig. 4*B*) to examine a wide selection of muscle fiber types by light microscopy. Veratti described a variety of patterns of delicate, transversely oriented reticula often linked longitudinally by fine strands of stained material, which he called *un reticolo transversale* (316).

The beauty of these preparations can be appreciated only by examining Veratti's lovely engravings or by looking at specimens prepared similarly (110). The color plate in Figure 5 (frontispiece; see legend on p. 28) shows one such preparation. The muscle fiber shown, which will be described in more detail later, is from a leg muscle of a crayfish and is a fiber of the long-sarcomere, tonic type. These fibers are large, often 0.5 mm or more in diameter, and the sarcolemma is folded to form a number of large, longitudinally oriented clefts (50, 235, 286), which appear orange in these micrographs. Tubular invaginations, which appear darker and smaller than the clefts, extend into the muscle fiber from all of its surfaces. The tubular invaginations appear to be in groups of three in these muscles, when viewed in longitudinal sections, as in Figure 5. Veratti accurately drew the complex network each set of tubules forms in the transverse plane. Veratti drew double and single sets of transverse reticula in other muscle fiber types, though apparently he believed that all muscles had three networks and only failure of the staining procedure prevented him from seeing all three in every case. Today we can say with certainty that some muscles do contain three networks of invaginating tubules in each sarcomere, but that there are muscles with two or only one network per sarcomere.

Little functional significance was attributed to these networks before electron-microscopic observations; often they were dismissed as preparation artifacts induced by the special staining procedures used to demonstrate them (see discussions in refs. 148 and 291). Interestingly, the staining procedure used by Veratti has been resurrected in modified form in the most recent high-voltage electron-microscopic observations. There now seems to be no basis for believing that the networks are artifactual. Rather, they are widely believed to be real cell structures with important functional significance in the control of the contractile activity of the cell.

EARLY ELECTRON-MICROSCOPIC OBSERVATIONS OF RETICULA. Elaborate internal reticular networks of membranes appeared in electron micrographs of thin sections of striated muscles of a variety of types in the 1950s, drawing attention again to their complex, elegant structure and possible functional significance (25, 254). Veratti's paper of 1902 was "rediscovered" and reprinted in English in 1961 (317), launching a new period of extensive morphological study of membranes in muscle cells.

The early electron-microscopic observations of membrane-bound cisternae and tubules inside muscle cells were made soon after Porter and Palade (254) described the endoplasmic reticulum in nonmuscle cells and the term *sarcoplasmic reticulum* was applied to the equivalent system in muscle cells. Even though specimen preparations at that time were somewhat crude, the major points made in the early electron-microscopic descriptions of the SR are still valid.

Early electron-microscopic observations did not distinguish between the SR and the membrane networks that correspond to Veratti's transverse reticulum, now called the T system or transverse-tubular network. The T tubules, called the intermediary vesicles, were included in the description of the SR and were not thought to be continuous across the fiber in the transverse plane (254). Andersson-Cedergren (9) used reconstructions from serial thin sections of mouse skeletal muscle fibers fixed with osmium tetroxide to show that these vesicles formed continuous tubules across the fiber in the transverse direction, at least for distances of several micrometers. After the use of glutaraldehyde for fixation for electron microscopy, this continuity was more readily apparent. Fixation with osmium tetroxide results in convoluted and vesicular T tubules. Osmium tetroxide used after glutaraldehyde primary fixation leads to images of tubules as continuous profiles. Tormey (315) observed similar fixation effects in sheetlike plasma membrane invaginations in the ciliary epithelial cells of the eye; presumably fixation with osmium tetroxide leads to an artifactual disruption and vesiculation of these membrane structures. Problems remained in obtaining good, three-dimensional views of the T-system networks, even with glutaraldehyde fixation, because only short lengths of tubules appeared in the thin sections. However, it was generally and correctly believed that T tubules form continuous networks across the width of the fiber (111, 221, 232, 292).

A second problem in T-system structure also was not easily resolved. Although physiological evidence (local activation experiments and impedance measurements) strongly suggested that T tubules were connected to the surface of the muscle fiber, this was not easily demonstrated in electron micrographs, at least in muscle fibers of vertebrates. Openings of T tubules to the extracellular space at the surfaces of the fibers were clearly visualized electron microscopically in one insect muscle (292) and in cardiac muscle fibers (213, 289). In vertebrate muscle fibers the geometry of the T tubules near their connections to the fiber surface is complex and difficult to visualize in thin sections. The tubules often are narrow and take a tortuous course just before joining the fiber surface and may open into caveolae (42, 100, 145, 153, 200, 319, 328). This may be a consequence of the way T tubules form during cellular differentiation (79, 168, 280). However, Franzini-Armstrong and Porter (111) visualized T-tubule openings in a fish muscle with relative ease in thin sections, because the tubules follow a relatively straight course as they approach the fiber surface.

Indirect evidence for T-tubule connection to the fiber surface became available at the same time with the visualization of an extracellular tracer (ferritin) within T tubules in electron micrographs (152, 220, 247) and of fluorescent dyes in the region of T tubules with light microscopy (73).

PHYSIOLOGICAL CORRELATES

During this same period, physiologists were interested in discovering how excitation at the surface of a large muscle fiber can lead to activation of myofibrillar contraction deep in the fiber in the short latent periods observed. In the 1940s Hill (135, 136) measured the time between a stimulus and the response of the deepest myofibrils in two types of muscle fibers and calculated the amount of a diffusible substance that might be expected to reach the center of the fiber from its surface in that time. Hill concluded that diffusion was much too slow to account for the inward communication of the stimulus to the myofibrils. The problem of how such communication takes place has become known as the excitation-contraction (EC) coupling problem [(274, 275); see also the chapter by Gonzalez-Serratos in this *Handbook*].

Local Activation Experiments

A. F. Huxley and R. E. Taylor (150, 151) designed and performed a series of clever and important physiological experiments on living skeletal muscle fibers that provided the first clue to a likely function for the T tubules. These local activation experiments depolarized a small patch (~1 μm diam) of the surface of an isolated muscle fiber while recording cinematographically any resulting contractions through a polarizing or interference light microscope. The researchers believed that if a special structure or a localized activity accounted for the inward spread of activation, then only when the depolarized area lay over certain sensitive spots where this structure or activity was located would a contraction be observed.

FROG TWITCH FIBERS. Huxley and Taylor (151) initially studied twitch muscle fibers from the frog in this way and found that contractions could be elicited only when the depolarized spot included a portion of the Z disk of the striation pattern. Only the I band embracing the Z disk under the depolarized patch of membrane shortened (Fig. 6*A*). Furthermore the shortening always was equal in the two half I bands flanking the Z disk, even when the depolarized patch was displaced more over one half I band than over the other half I band. The activation could spread radially into the fiber as far as 10 μm but never spread to longitudinally adjacent I bands, although these were considerably closer to the depolarized patch of surface than 10 μm. These results suggested that some process occurring in the plane of the Z disk at the center of each I band resulted in the spread of contraction activation specifically in the radial direction and never longitudinally.

By themselves the local activation results on frog twitch muscle fibers were not very useful in helping formulate a specific hypothesis to explain the inward spread of contraction activation. The early suggestion was that Krause's membrane, the light-microscopic designation of the Z line, was the likely structural substrate for contraction activation (150). However, the electron-microscopic information that soon became available suggested a more likely interpretation of the physiological experiments (see discussion in ref. 147). With the electron microscope it could be seen that Krause's membrane is a discontinuous structure, the optical image of the Z disks of the individual myofibrils, which are separated by sarcoplasmic space. The SR and the membranes we now call the T tubules, however, provide a continuous link transversely across the fiber and therefore seemed structurally more suitable to play a role in conducting activation into the fiber.

LIZARD FIBERS. The real confirmation of this role came when the local activation experiments were extended to another muscle fiber type, the skeletal muscle fibers of a lizard. When these fibers were subjected to the same sort of surface local depolarization, the results were different from those obtained with frog fibers. Activation of contraction was not observed when the depolarized area was over the Z disk but only when the depolarization was over a region near the edge of an A band where it adjoins an I band. Furthermore the contractions observed were not symmetrical with respect to the Z line but could occur more strongly in the half I band nearer the pipette than in the half I band on the other side of the same Z line. These results strongly suggested that, in contrast to frog fibers, structures found in the regions of the Z lines were not responsible for the inward spread of contraction activation in lizard fibers.

The correlation between the physiological results and the structure of the lizard fibers came when A. F. Huxley (see discussion in ref. 147) presented the results of the local activation experiments to the Physiological Society in England. A morphologist in the audience, J. David Robertson, pointed out that some membranous structures, which we now call triads, could be seen in pairs near the junctions between the A bands and I bands in lizard fibers, just where the local activation experiments gave positive results. This suggested that some component of the triad was involved in EC coupling. This location for triads in lizard muscles was confirmed in later studies by Forbes and Sperelakis (97), among others.

Thus triads were found in both frog and lizard muscle to be localized where local depolarization of the surface membrane led to contraction, even though this happened at two different locations in the sarcomere pattern in the two fiber types. This correlation was subsequently corroborated in two other fiber types, though full understanding of the results in these two cases requires knowledge not available in the late 1950s.

CRAB FIBERS. Huxley and Taylor (151) subjected muscle fibers from the walking legs of marine crabs to the

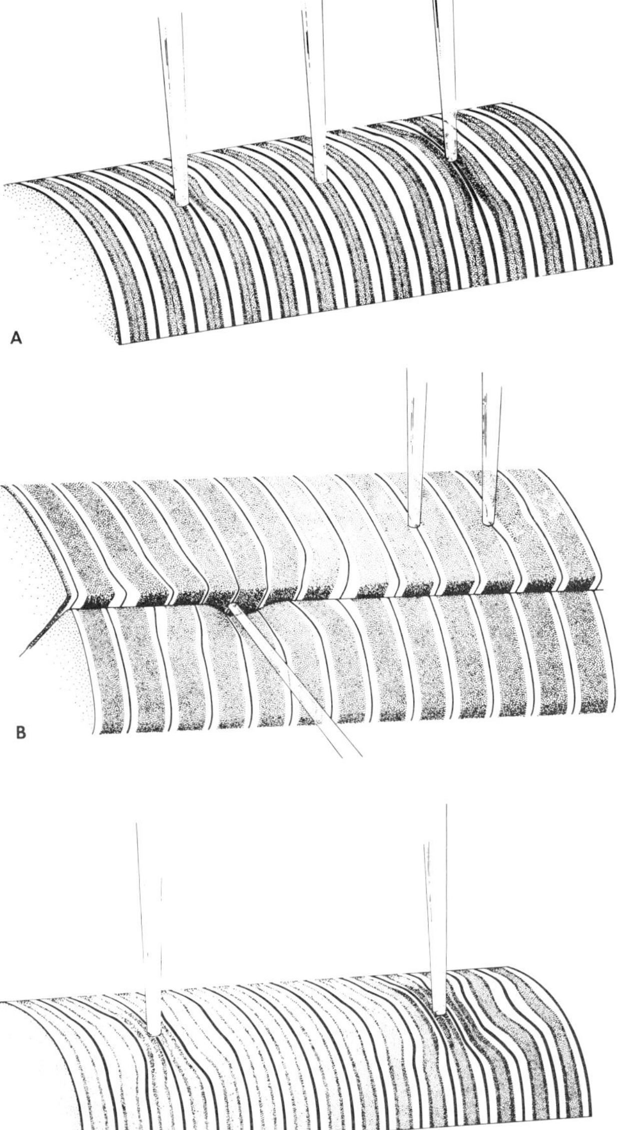

FIG. 6. Results of local activation experiments on 3 kinds of muscle fibers by A. F. Huxley and co-workers (147, 149–151, 243). In actual experiments a single pipette depolarized small patches of surface of an isolated muscle fiber; resulting contractions observed with light microscope. *A*: frog twitch muscle fibers. *Right*, contractions obtained only when depolarized patch of membrane is adjacent to Z line of underlying striation pattern. *Left*, contraction seen is always symmetric on 2 sides of Z line, even when pipette is displaced to 1 side of Z line. *Center*, contractions never seen when pipette is over an A band. *B*: results from local activation experiments on crab muscle fibers (149, 151). In these fibers and in lizard fibers, contractions observed only when an area over a region near junction of A bands and I bands was depolarized; resulting contraction always asymmetric and stronger in half I band closer to pipette. Extensive attempts (149) to obtain contractions when a region over Z line and within I band was depolarized gave negative results (center pipette). Extensive longitudinal clefts in sarcolemma of crab fibers; when pipette passes current into these clefts, contractions involving several sarcomeres are seen, regardless of pipette placement with respect to striations. Pipette cannot be considered sealed well enough against fiber surface to restrict depolarization to a small area of membrane. This result shows only that activation can be obtained by depolarization of the membrane within clefts. *C*: results from local activation experiments on frog slow fibers (243). Fibers behaved quite differently from twitch fibers of same species. Although not all areas of fiber surface led to contraction when depolarized, as was also true with twitch fibers, sensitive spots were found at all levels of the striation pattern in slow fibers. Furthermore, contraction often spread as far longitudinally as radially and thus could involve several sarcomeres. Lack of precise localization of sensitivity and lack of specific spread of activation in the radial direction can be correlated with a similarly imprecise arrangement of T tubules and peripheral couplings in these muscle fibers (221, 244).

same type of local activation experiments. These muscle fibers were chosen because they have sarcomere lengths more than three times greater than frog and lizard fibers, allowing more precise exploration of the sarcomere pattern. The results on the crab fibers were similar to those obtained with lizard muscles; two regions of sensitivity were found in each sarcomere near the ends of the A bands, and the I bands could be made to contract asymmetrically by stimulating over only one sensitive region (Fig. 6*B*). The early electron-microscopic observations on these same muscles (229), however, were difficult to reconcile with the physiological results and the hypothesis that triad or triadlike structures were responsible for the radial spread of activation into the fiber. Structures thought to be equivalent to triads were found in crab fibers in the correct position, i.e., near the ends of the A bands. The difficulty was that a set of tubules clearly patently open to the extracellular space at the surface of the fiber was found specifically near the Z lines, and these Z tubules, as they were called, seemed ideally suited for the inward spread of activation.

Because of this uncertainty Huxley and Peachey (149, 245) repeated the local activation experiments and extended the morphological studies using better fixation methods. These results confirmed the earlier results, and extensive attempts to activate crab fibers by depolarization of the fiber surface near the Z line failed. The newer structural studies, however, suggested that the Z line tubules, although real and present, lack one feature that is essential for a role in activation. The Z tubules do not form close and specific associations with the SR, as are formed by the tubular system entering in the A bands. More recent results, using high-voltage electron microscopy and freeze fracture, further clarify the structural relationships between these membrane systems, as discussed later in T-SYSTEM–SARCOPLASMIC RETICULUM COUPLINGS, p. 51. Tubular invaginations and association of the invaginating tubules with the SR are necessary for the inward spread of activation from surface depolarization to contraction.

FROG SLOW FIBERS. The second case where both local activation and electron-microscopic studies on the same fiber type helped to explain the inward spread of activation was in slow (tonic) muscle fibers of the frog. These special muscle fibers have been known for some time to be involved in the maintenance of tension for long periods of time, as in posture maintenance and amplexus (230). Regions of muscles that contain these fibers, termed *tonus bundles*, respond to dilute acetylcholine solutions with slow, long-lasting contractions in addition to twitches (307). Krüger (174) found fibers with a special structural appearance in the same regions in the light microscope and termed this histological appearance *Felderstruktur*. In the electron microscope, individual fibers specifically identified physiologically as of the slow or tonic contractile type show broad myofibrils incompletely separated by SR (244). Slow fibers have a transverse network of T tubules that is not as precisely limited to the Z-disk plane as in twitch fibers but extends longitudinally over the middle of the I band. Triads are oriented longitudinally and transversely (16, 92, 103, 221). These fibers also have surface couplings, structures in which the SR couples directly to the plasma membrane at the fiber surface.

Local activation experiments on frog slow fibers showed that activation could occur with depolarization at all levels of the sarcomere and that the spread of contraction activation was in the longitudinal and transverse direction (Fig. 6*C*), in contrast to the more localized and specifically radial responses observed in twitch fibers of the same species (243). The lack of precision in the structural arrangement in slow fibers, the presence of surface couplings at various levels of the sarcomere, and the corresponding irregularity in the physiological results again suggested a relationship between the structural arrangement and location of SR and/or T tubules and the inward spread of contraction activation.

Comparison of Slow-Acting and Fast-Acting Muscle Fibers

During the early period of interest in the internal membranes of skeletal muscle cells, a series of comparative electron-microscopic studies of muscles with different speeds of contraction indicated a general correlation between rapidity of the contractile cycle and the content level of the SR and T system (84, 91, 221–223, 229, 246, 259, 263, 292). These observations supported the idea that membrane networks are involved in the control of the contractile cycle.

Relation of Total Surface Area to Fiber Capacitance

It had been known for some time before the first electron-microscopic studies on the T system that muscle fibers have an unusually high specific capacitance. Most cells, including nerve cells from a variety of species, have specific membrane capacitances of ~1 $\mu F/cm^2$. When the capacitance of muscle cells was determined at low frequency and expressed as capacitance per unit of fiber surface area, values of 4–8 $\mu F/cm^2$ were obtained for frog muscle fibers (85, 88, 166) and up to more than 50 $\mu F/cm^2$ for crab and crayfish fibers (12, 85, 87). To explain these data, muscle cells had to have either membranes differing in thickness (thinner) or composition (higher dielectric constant) from those of nerve cells or more surface membrane than was estimated by considering only their cross-sectional profile and length. Researchers soon realized that the latter was true; the extra membrane and therefore the extra capacitance were due to extensive augmentation of the surface area of the muscle fiber by invaginating clefts and tubules. When the measured low-frequency capacitance was divided by the total surface and surface-connected membrane, values of specific capacitance comparable to those of nerve cells were obtained (71, 85, 233). Subsequently the extent of T tubules in frog slow fibers (92, 221) and the capacitance of the same fibers (4, 116) were determined. Slow fibers have about half the capacitance of frog twitch fibers per unit of outer surface area; this correlates with their lower content of T tubules.

The surface membranes of muscle cells thus seem to have specific properties much like those of other cells, with specific capacitances of ~1 $\mu F/cm^2$ but a more complex form and a total surface area that can be considerably greater than suggested by the cell size and shape. More detailed analysis of muscle fiber capacitance, its relationship to membrane structure, and its dispersion with frequency is covered in the chapter by R. S. Eisenberg in this *Handbook*.

Glycerol-Shock Experiments

Support for the hypothesis that T tubules are involved in the inward spread of excitation from the fiber surface to sites in the vicinity of the myofibrils has come from the so-called glycerol-shock experiments (66, 112, 142, 154, 173, 212, 227). After exposure to solutions made severalfold hypertonic by the addition of glycerol or some other slowly penetrating solute and sudden return to isotonic medium, the fibers become mechanically uncoupled. These fibers are electrically excitable, though their electrical capacitance is reduced and their action potentials differ from normal (72, 154), but they do not respond mechanically when stimulated. The osmotic treatment disrupts the functional continuity of the T system and its ability to convey activation into the fiber and disrupts the structural continuity of the T tubules to the extent that peroxidase and ferritin can no longer enter from the outside solution (66, 212).

MICROSCOPIC METHODS IN STUDY OF CELLULAR MEMBRANE STRUCTURE

Some of the cellular organelles that consist structurally of membranes could be seen and were studied extensively in the light microscope, including mitochondria, the Golgi apparatus, the surface of the cell itself, and, as discussed in LIGHT-MICROSCOPIC OBSERVATIONS OF INTERNAL RETICULA, p. 29, the T-system networks of skeletal muscle cells. However, the reality and true nature of cellular membranes was uncertain before they were studied in the electron microscope, beginning in the 1950s. The early electron-microscopic studies used transmission electron microscopes operating with accelerating voltages of 80 kV or less. This required ultrathin specimens, e.g., parts of cells or sections of embedded tissues with thicknesses not much more than 0.1 μm. The kinds of specimens that could be examined were limited, and although high-quality two-dimensional information was obtained, three-dimensional information required an indirect approach. Muscle biologists now have a wider variety of electron microscopes at their disposal and various specimen preparation methods for each microscope. A rich variety of views of membranes in muscle cells now is available, allowing us to go well beyond the early understanding of membrane structure in these cells.

Scanning Electron Microscopy

The main differences between scanning electron microscopy (SEM) and transmission electron microscopy (TEM) are that SEM provides views of the surfaces of objects and much less severely limits the size of objects that can be examined. Macroscopic objects as large as groups of whole muscle cells or whole tissue cultures can be examined effectively in ordinary scanning electron microscopes. The resolution achieved by SEM is intermediate between that achieved in TEM and that in light microscopy. The chapter by Ishikawa, Sawada, and Yamada in this *Handbook* reviews the achievements of SEM in the study of muscle cells.

High-Voltage Electron Microscopy of Thick Sections

The high-voltage electron microscope (HVEM) is a transmission electron microscope that operates at an accelerating voltage in the range of 1–3 million V, rather than the 100,000 V common in ordinary TEM. The major advantage of the higher accelerating voltage for our purposes is the ability of the higher energy beam to penetrate thicker specimens. Thus sections of embedded muscle tissue up to several micrometers thick can be examined effectively in the HVEM.

The images obtained from such thick preparations are very different from those from thin sections. Often these micrographs are difficult to interpret because the images of structures at various depths in the section are superimposed in the micrograph. Two techniques are useful in this regard. If the images are not too complex and cluttered, stereoscopic electron microscopy can be very helpful (237). A pair of micrographs of the same area of the specimen is made with the specimen tilted an appropriate angle between the two exposures. When these two images are presented to the viewer so that each eye views a different image, the parallax between the two images, caused by the relative tilt and the different depths of different structures, gives an impression of depth and three-dimensionality. The result can be a dramatic and highly informative view of a structure at electron-microscopic resolution but without the two-dimensional appearance characteristic of thin sections. The viewer is able to distinguish structures at different depths in the specimen and to sort out certain three-dimensional details of the structures and their relationships to each other.

When even stereoscopic methods leave the image too confusing to be useful, it becomes necessary selectively to enhance the visibility of certain structures over that of others. The use of dense tracer molecules that are confined to the extracellular space has been particularly useful for the T system in muscle cells. Two such extracellular tracers are colloidal lanthanum and peroxidase. The muscles are fixed briefly before exposure to the tracer because the lanthanum preparations are toxic. The lanthanum colloid is dense and requires no additional staining. When peroxidase is used a dense precipitate must be generated in those regions where the peroxidase is present, because the peroxidase itself does not have a high density. The procedure used involves incubation with hydrogen peroxide and 3,3′-diaminobenzidine tetrahydrochloride after brief fixation (66, 122). The resulting precipitate binds osmium from the fixative, resulting in density observable in the electron microscope. Sometimes this is intensified by adding potassium ferricyanide to the osmium fixative used after the incubation.

An alternative to molecular tracers is the use of true stains, i.e., substances that specifically bind to selected structures physically and/or chemically. Ruthenium red (96, 119, 186, 187) and tannic acid (31, 297) both have been used as stains for the T system. A difficulty with the use of such stains for identifying extracellular spaces, such as the T tubules, is that the small molecules may cross the surface membrane, enter the fiber, and be found in intracellular compartments not connected to the extracellular space. Stains thought to be specific for the extracellular space have been found in the SR. These results are discussed later in *Functional Mechanism of Coupling Between T Tubules and Sarcoplasmic Reticulum*, p. 57.

The Golgi black reaction used by Veratti, as specified by Smith (292) and modified slightly (108, 110, 241, 279), has been a reliable and useful marker for high-voltage electron microscopy on muscle cells for studies of the T-system network at relatively low magnification. Details of tubule shape and association with the SR in triads and dyads, which often are not visible in these preparations because of the punctate nature of the marker deposit, must be obtained with other methods, e.g., lanthanum. However, large areas of T-tubule networks and sometimes SR are visible with the Golgi method, even in slices of embedded muscles up to 10 μm thick.

Freeze-Fracture Electron Microscopy

Fracturing of frozen specimens splits membranes along the planes of their hydrophobic interiors and allows visualization of intrinsic membrane proteins, i.e., protein molecules that extend into or across the normally hydrophobic inner layer of the membrane. An extension of this method (deep-etch) reveals details of structures deeper in the specimen below the fracture planes, i.e., true membrane surfaces, the content of organelles, myofilaments, etc.

T SYSTEM

Definition, Development, and Function

The T system of a muscle cell is a network or a series of networks of tubular invaginations (T tubules) of the plasma membrane of the cell that forms specific, functional associations with the SR (Fig. 7). This definition is restrictive because only those invaginations of the muscle surface associating specifically with the SR are included. Folds and clefts in the sarcolemma, caveolae of the plasma membrane, and some tubular invaginations that do not form SR couplings in invertebrate muscles are excluded.

Images suggesting two different mechanisms for the formation of T tubules during cell differentiation have been obtained; it seems possible that developing muscle cells use both mechanisms. In one case early T tubules are seen as tubes with periodic swellings or grapelike clusters of interconnected vesicles, the size of the swellings and vesicles approximating the size of caveolae, as if the formation of multiple caveolae at a single site on the membrane had occurred (79, 155, 280). In extreme cases, elaborate three-dimensional networks of these structures are observed in developing or regenerating muscle cells (155, 192, 281). Similar structures have been observed in pathological muscles and muscles undergoing atrophy (76–78, 250, 284). Ishikawa and Ezerman (79, 155) used ferritin as an extracellular marker to confirm the extracellular continuity of both the simple, developing T tubules and the elaborate networks. The developing T tubules make contacts with the developing SR in a form reminiscent of that of mature T-SR couplings, though more irregularly arranged (155, 192, 281). According to this scheme, coupling with SR is a secondary event, occurring after the formation of the T tubules. Other images of developing T tubules suggest a primary event in which SR couples to the surface membrane of the cell and invaginations form subsequently (65, 168).

The T system has the function of carrying electrical depolarization into the cell to activate contraction by causing calcium release from the SR. This discussion of the T system presents information from both structural and functional points of view. Some historical information is provided, but the discussion is not always historically arranged.

T-Tubule Networks

The T tubules in frog twitch muscle fibers form transversely oriented networks extending completely across the width of the fiber and localized specifically in close relation to the Z lines of the striation pattern of the myofibrils (Figs. 7 and 8). This somewhat simplified view contains some geometric errors, and ex-

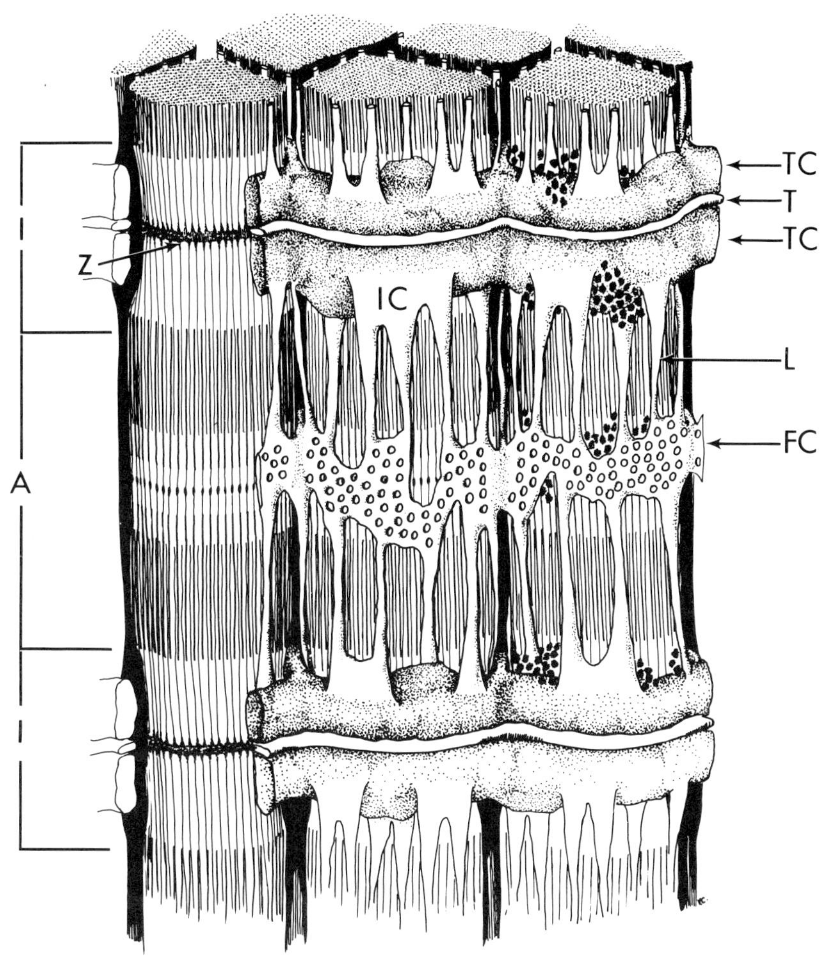

FIG. 7. T system and SR of frog twitch fiber. Longitudinal axis of fiber is vertical, as drawn. Slightly more than 1 sarcomere length of fiber shown. SR forms a 3-dimensional network of cisternae and tubules around myofibrils, with specific structural differentiation of membrane forms adjacent to specific bands of myofibrillar striations. Two levels of T-tubular networks shown, adjacent to Z lines within I bands of myofibrils and forming central elements of 3-part structures (triads), which also include 2 SR terminal cisternae (TC). TC of SR connect to SR longitudinal tubules (L) either directly or through SR intermediate cisternae (IC). Near center of A band, longitudinal tubules join fenestrated collar (FC) of SR. [From Peachey (232), by copyright permission of The Rockefeller University Press.]

ceptions will be discussed in detail in SPECIAL GEOMETRY OF T SYSTEM, p. 61.

Peachey and Eisenberg (239) used the extrinsic peroxidase method to stain T tubules selectively and examined serial transverse sections in the HVEM. They reconstructed an entire T-tubular network of a frog twitch muscle fiber as projected into the transverse plane (Fig. 9). The network is not entirely closed, in that free ends of tubules were found, but otherwise the network is much as had been expected from studies of thin sections. Eisenberg and Peachey (70) also determined the network parameters of the T systems of these fibers. The average length of a T tubule between nodes (branch points) is 0.9 μm with an average of 5.4 nodes around each myofibril. The most common nodes had three branches (68%), with four-branch nodes accounting for 22% of the total number of nodes. The remaining 10% of the nodes had five, six, or zero branches (free end).

A difficulty with the peroxidase method is the relatively low density of the resulting deposit in the embedded specimens, which limits the useful specimen thickness for the HVEM. The visibility of the T tubules in transverse sections is too low for reliable identification beyond a thickness of ~0.75 μm (239). The lanthanum infiltration method and the Golgi stain produce a much denser precipitate and thus can be used for greater thicknesses of slices (240, 241). Figures 10 and 11 demonstrate how well the Golgi stain depicts the form of the T-system network over extensive transverse areas of the muscle fiber, without the need for serial reconstruction. The degree to which the planes occupied by the T-system networks undulate and dislocate is clear in these low-magnification micrographs of Golgi-stained muscles when viewed stereoscopically.

Mammalian muscles present a similar appearance when stained with the Golgi method and examined by HVEM of thick sections [Fig. 12; (241)]. The major difference from the frog muscle fibers is the presence of two T-system networks per sarcomere (Fig. 13). Figure 12 shows the faster-contracting, primarily glycolytic, white type of mammalian skeletal muscle fiber; Figure 13 illustrates the slower, primarily oxidative, red fiber. Both fibers are twitch fibers, so neither resembles either structurally or functionally the true slow fibers of amphibians and reptiles discussed earlier in FROG SLOW FIBERS, p. 32. The differences between the fast-twitch and slow-twitch fibers of mammals are discussed in the chapter by B. R. Eisenberg in this *Handbook*.

Two muscle fiber types have been studied exten-

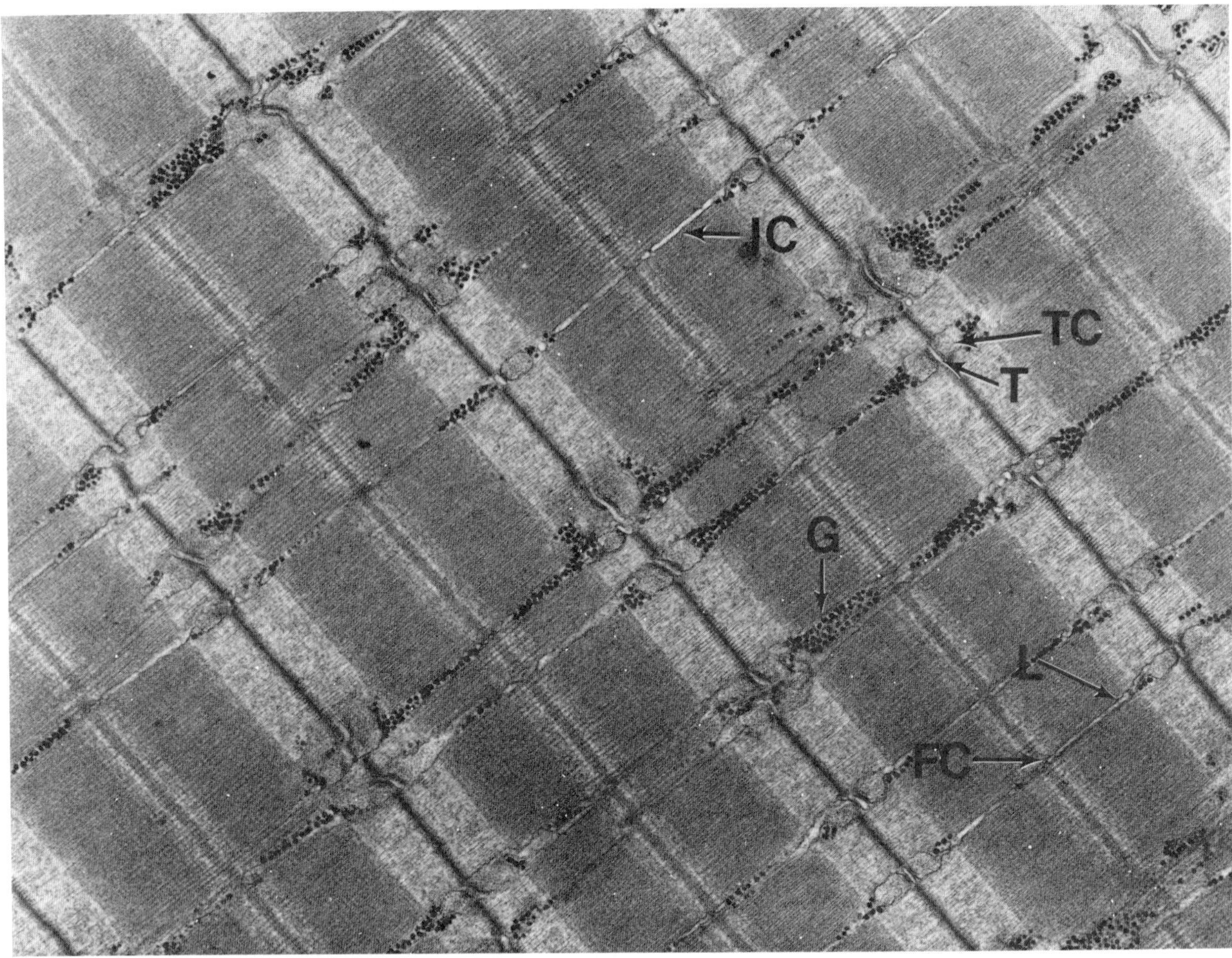

FIG. 8. Longitudinal section of frog sartorius muscle fiber, seen in thin section in electron microscope. *T*, T tubules; *TC*, terminal cisternae; *IC*, intermediate cisternae; *L*, longitudinal tubules; *FC*, fenestrated collar. Glycogen granules (*G*) intermingled with SR elements between myofibrils. × 23,000.

sively in crabs and crayfish and can be used to illustrate the structure of the T system in crustacea (108). The walking legs of crustacea contain one type of muscle fiber that has unusually long sarcomeres, up to 12–15 μm in length. These muscle fibers are tonic in function, i.e., they contract and relax rather slowly. One tonic fiber already has been illustrated in a Golgi preparation in the light microscope in the color micrograph of Figure 5. A tonic fiber is also illustrated in a high-voltage electron micrograph in Figure 14. The T system of these fibers is represented by the two transversely oriented networks in the A bands that flank the Z-tubular network located at the center of the I band. Some longitudinal connections among these networks is observed, particularly between the Z-tubular network and two longitudinally adjacent T tubules, with fewer connections between the two T-tubule networks across the center of the A band.

A faster, phasic-type fiber with shorter sarcomeres from a crayfish is illustrated in Figure 15. The prominent feature of the T system here is its approximately equal proportion of longitudinally and transversely oriented tubules, providing a ladderlike appearance.

T-Tubule Shapes

The T tubules have two different cross-sectional shapes (16, 56, 102, 104, 113, 221, 223, 228, 287, 294). The more common shape in amphibian twitch fibers is that of flattened or ribbon-shaped tubules. The less common cross section is circular with a diameter about equal to the smaller of the two dimensions of the flattened form. The circular form is found as short connectors between flattened elements, predominantly at or near junctions in the network, but also forming longitudinal elements connecting one sarcomere level to the next. The circular form does not form specific associations with the SR, although the flattened form does.

Figure 16 shows a field of a frog muscle fiber stained

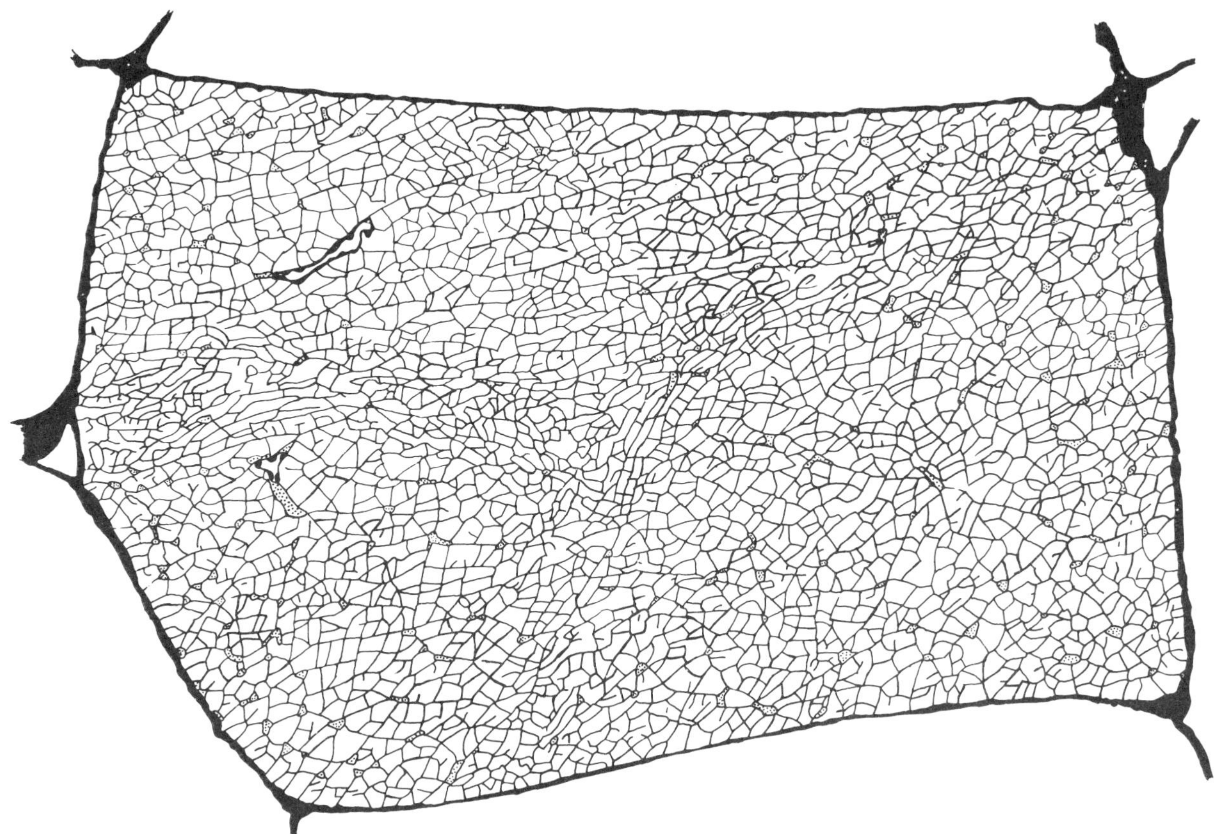

FIG. 9. Reconstruction of T system of frog twitch muscle fiber made by tracing T tubules stained with peroxidase method in series of high-voltage electron micrographs of serial transverse sections 0.7 μm thick. T tubules projected into transverse plane of fiber. 1,000 kV; × 1,800. [From Peachey and Eisenberg (239), by copyright permission of the Biophysical Society.]

with the Golgi method. The two forms of T tubule—the round tubular form and the flat ribbon form—are easily distinguished. This figure clearly shows that the flat form is predominant in these muscle fibers. In contrast, a greater length of tubular than flattened form of T tubule is found in frog slow fibers (16, 92).

SARCOPLASMIC RETICULUM

Definition, Development, and Function

Structurally the SR is a completely internal membrane system not in continuity with the plasma membrane of the muscle cell. The SR is the muscle cell's equivalent of the smooth-surfaced endoplasmic reticulum of cells of other types. It is related to and often continuous with the nuclear membrane (232), a property it shares with endoplasmic reticula in general. The SR is continuous transversely across the fiber, at least at some level of the striations, and longitudinally continuous within a single sarcomere, part of a sarcomere, or over long distances, depending on the muscle.

During cell differentiation the SR is formed from the rough-surfaced endoplasmic reticulum and develops simultaneously with the formation of the myofibrils and T tubules. In embryonic muscle cells the early SR is seen as tubular evaginations from the ER, which immediately form reticular networks and wrap around the developing myofibrils (79). Walker and coworkers (318, 321) observed an early association specifically with the Z lines of the myofibrils. At first these early SRs form irregular associations with the developing T tubules; later they take on the mature form of triads (157, 168, 169, 185, 280). The mature fully differentiated form of the SR appears only as the entire mature architecture and interrelationships among the SR, the T tubules, and the myofibrils form in a coordinated way (47, 65, 280).

The SR plays a major role in controlling the state of activation of the contractile machinery of the muscle cell by regulating the concentration of calcium in the sarcoplasmic space, which contains the contractile myofilaments and myofibrils. The SR engages in two separate activities while carrying out this important function. First, the SR pumps calcium into its interior and holds it there, thus lowering the free calcium concentration in the sarcoplasmic space below $\sim 10^{-7}$ M (see the chapter by Martonosi and Beeler in this *Handbook*). At this concentration little calcium will

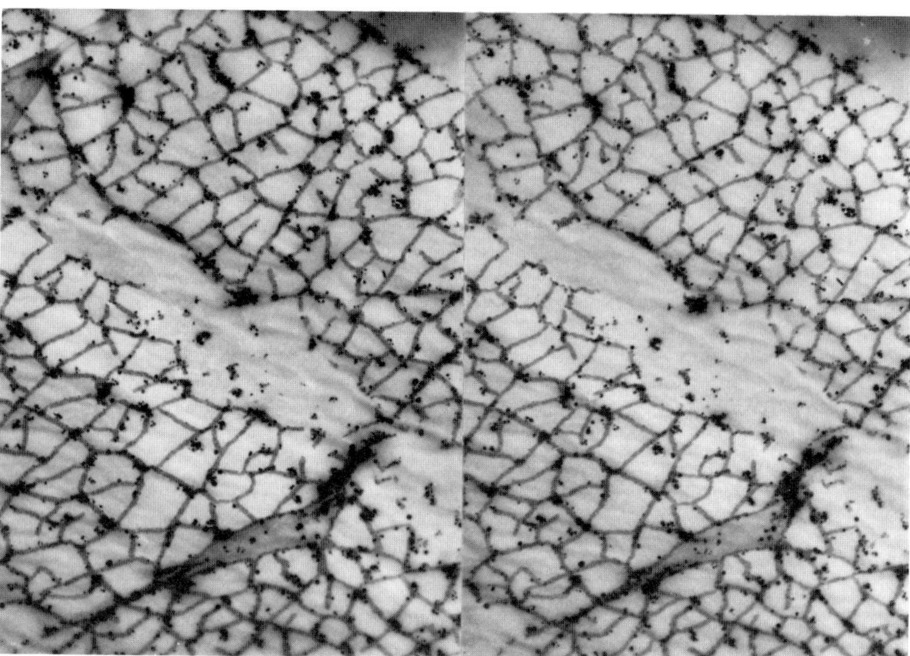

FIG. 10. Stereoscopic high-voltage electron micrograph of frog twitch skeletal muscle fiber, Golgi stain. Section 1.5 μm thick. Only T tubules stained in this region. Some artifactual precipitate from stain is found outside T tubules. Nucleus near figure *bottom*. T-system networks lie at an oblique angle within thickness of transverse section. Viewed stereoscopically, T tubules do not confine themselves to a flat plane but wander considerably in longitudinal direction of fiber. Total tilt 30°; 1,000 kV; × 6,000. [From Franzini-Armstrong and Peachey (110); micrograph incorrectly described when originally published.]

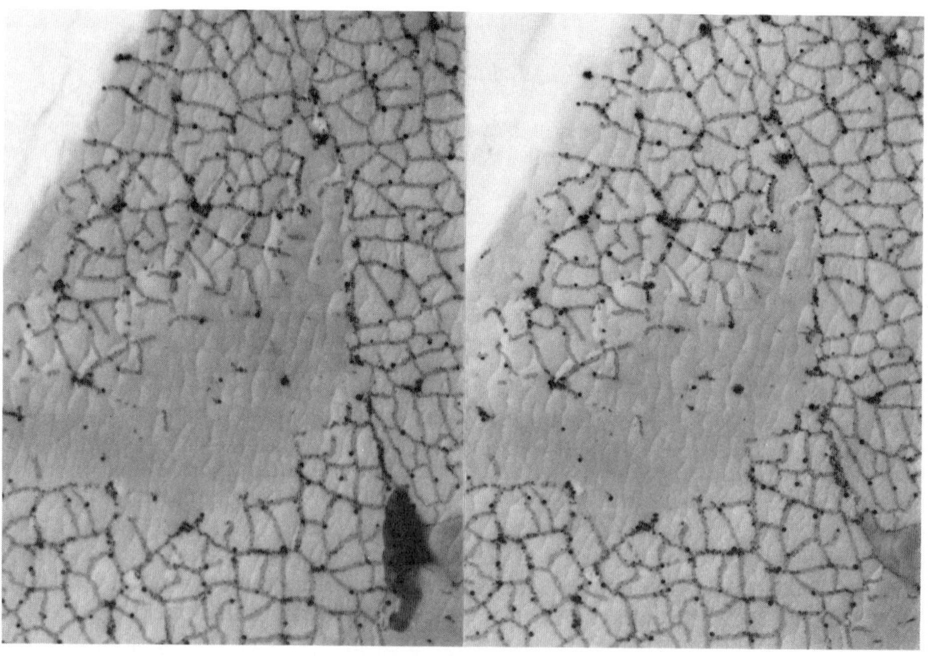

FIG. 11. Stereoscopic high-voltage electron micrograph of frog twitch muscle fiber, Golgi stain. Section 1.5 μm thick. T-system plane undulates through entire thickness of section within small area represented in micrograph. Total tilt 30°; 1,000 kV; × 5,000.

be complexed to troponin, and the contractile proteins will be inactivated. Second, SR releases sufficient calcium into the sarcoplasm to bind to troponin and thus release the contraction inhibition. The pumping activity of the SR takes place continuously. The release function is triggered only when the muscle cell is stimulated. Autoradiographic evidence suggests that the release takes place primarily from a specific part

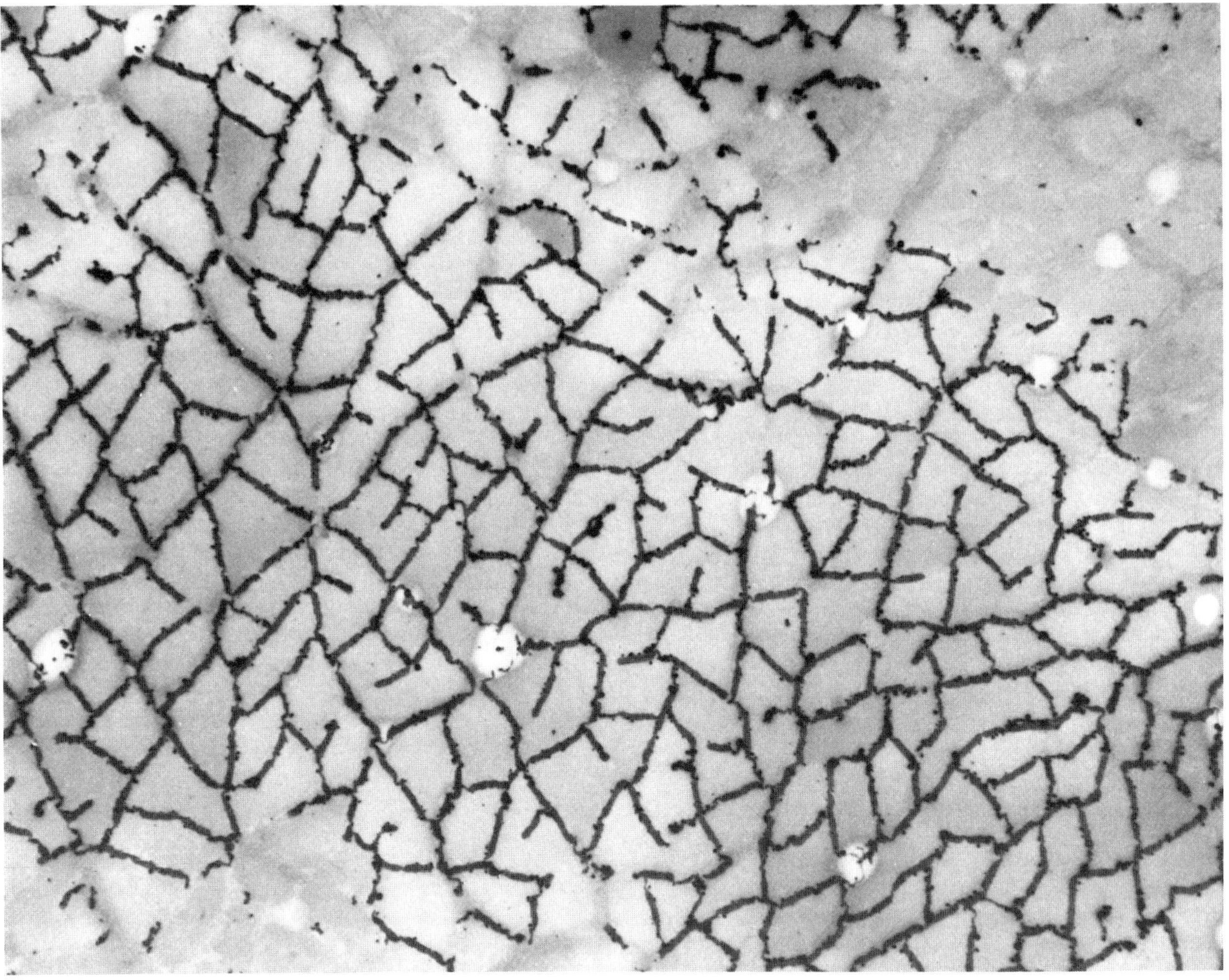

FIG. 12. Transverse section 0.25–0.5 μm thick of rat white muscle fiber from sternomastoid muscle, Golgi stain. At this thickness, only part of single layer of T system is seen. *Clear areas,* lipid droplets. 100 kV; × 11,000.

of the SR, the terminal cisternae (325, 326). Calcium is repumped into the SR during the relaxation phase of the contraction cycle.

Each cycle of calcium release and accumulation results in a brief period of tension production called a twitch. The calcium release and accumulation cycles can be repeated at frequencies that can be tens of times per second or faster in some fiber types. Above a certain frequency, called the fusion frequency and characteristic for different types of fibers, the calcium concentration in the sarcoplasmic space stays relatively high, the contractile apparatus is in a state of constant activation, and the contraction becomes a tetanus.

Structural Relationship to Myofibrils and Striations

The SR in most striated muscle cells lies in close proximity to the contractile myofibrils of the cell and shows a structural periodicity with the same spacing as that of the myofibrils. This periodicity is reasonably closely aligned with the myofibrillar striations. Filamentous connections between Z lines of adjacent myofibrils or between Z lines and adjacent SR have been observed with electron microscopy (23, 167, 223, 303, 322) and recently confirmed with freeze-etch techniques (217). This location coincides with the region where a protein characteristic of intermediate-sized filaments has been found with immunocytochemical techniques (23, 180–182). This evidence suggests the presence of structural elements that link myofibrils and SR into a mechanical unit.

Form of Sarcoplasmic Reticulum

The SR structure in any type of muscle fiber can be understood in terms of the extent of development and distribution of three or four typical structural regions: terminal cisternae, flattened intermediate cisternae, tubules, and fenestrated cisternae. These structural regions are connected and share a common interior

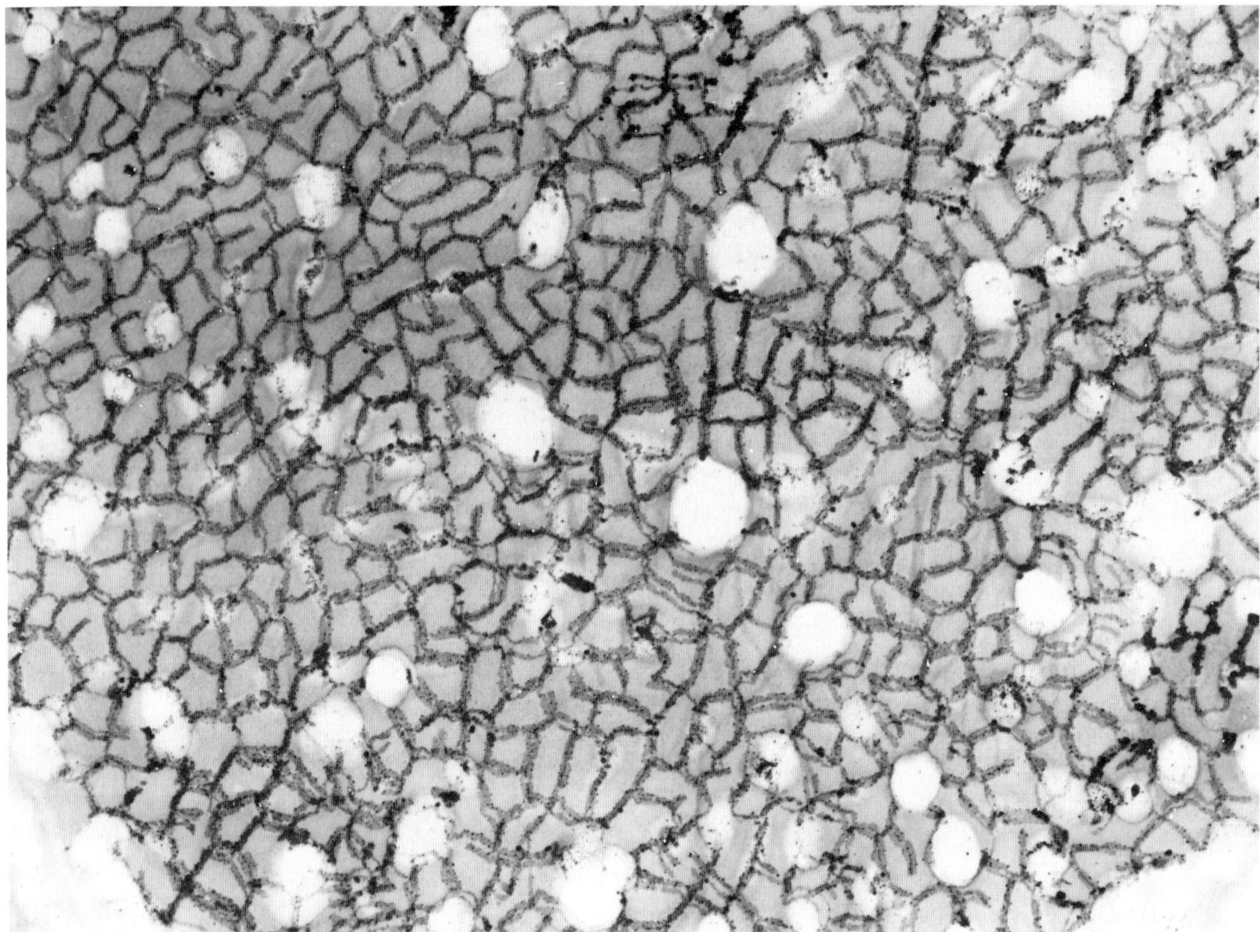

FIG. 13. Transverse section 2.5 μm thick of red muscle fiber from rat sternomastoid muscle, Golgi stain. Two layers of T-system networks lie within section thickness, resulting in a double image in some regions. *Clear areas*, lipid droplets, numerous in these red fibers. 1,000 kV; × 9,000.

phase, although it is clear that molecular species, e.g., calsequestrin (162), can be preferentially located in one region. Researchers also propose that constriction of the lumen or other barriers may restrict diffusion from one part of the SR to another (141, 232, 305, 325, 326).

In frog skeletal muscle fibers of the twitch type, the four regions are found in sequence in each half sarcomere, with terminal cisternae near each Z line at the center of the I band and fenestrated cisternae at the M line at the center of the A band (Fig. 17). The terminal cisternae, or terminal sacs, near the Z lines are the part of the SR in frog twitch muscle that forms specific junctions with the T tubules. The usual arrangement is two cisternae of SR on either side of a single T tubule, forming a structure called a triad because of its three parts. Other arrangements are also found, e.g., pentads, with three SR elements alternating with two T tubules, and occasionally dyads, with one SR element missing.

Attached to the terminal cisternae in some muscles, including frog twitch fibers, are flattened cisternae called intermediate cisternae (232) because of their location between the terminal cisternae and the longitudinal tubules (Fig. 17). The special function of these elements or why they are present in some muscles and not in others is not known. Several interesting features are known, however. They are the only part of the SR that contains cholesterol in its membranes (301), and they have a greater tendency to collapse under certain conditions of preparation for electron microscopy (Fig. 18). These conditions include exposure to ruthenium red (140, 141, 305) and rapid freezing [J. Heuser, personal communication; (303)]. In the collapsed state the membranes on either side of the lumen of the intermediate cisternae fuse, obliterating the normally narrow lumen of this component. This phenomenon is not very constant, and the degree of collapse can vary greatly from preparation to preparation and in different regions within one preparation. Whether or not the phenomenon occurs in vivo is unknown.

In some vertebrate muscles a marked restriction of the SR lumen where the terminal cisternae join the

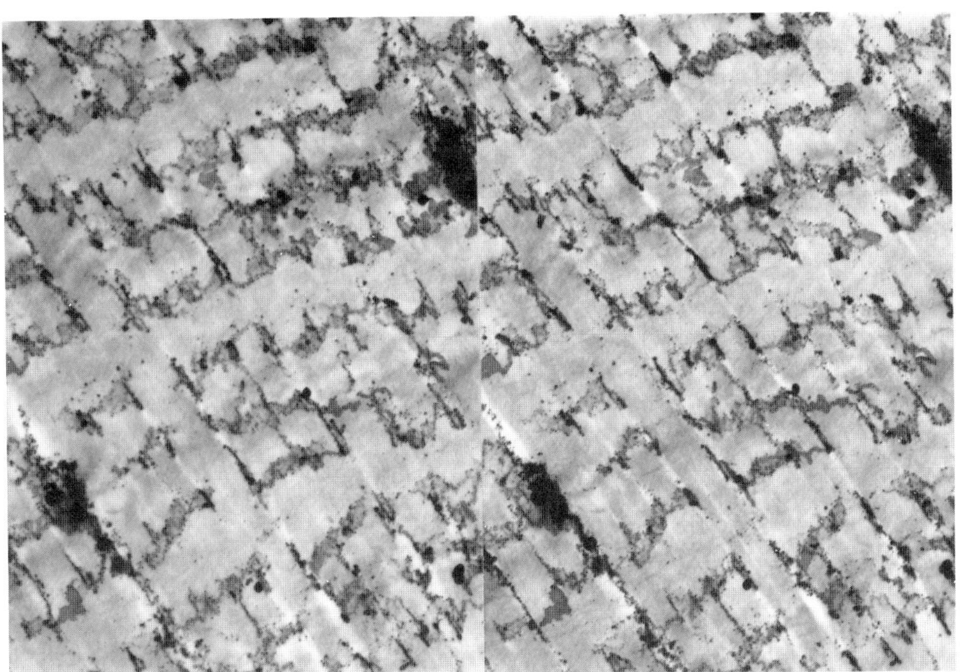

FIG. 14. Stereoscopic high-voltage electron micrograph of longitudinal section of tonic, long-sarcomere muscle fiber from flexor muscle of crayfish leg. Groups of 3 transverse reticula extend transversely across fiber, approximately horizontally. Central of the 3, found at level of Z lines of myofibrils, consists of Z tubules, which do not directly form contacts with SR. Remaining 2 reticula in each sarcomere are T tubules, located near ends of myofibrillar A bands. Occasional longitudinal connections from one network to the next. Section 2 μm thick. Total tilt 14°; 1,000 kV; × 6,000. (Micrograph by Franzini-Armstrong, Eastwood, and Peachey.)

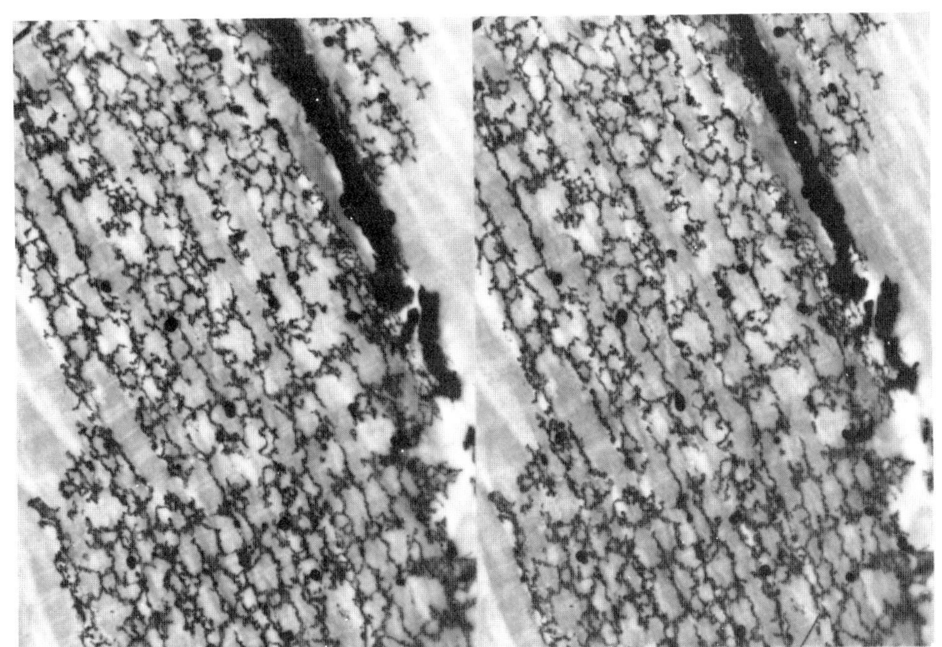

FIG. 15. Stereoscopic high-voltage electon micrograph of longitudinal section of phasic muscle fiber from abdominal flexor muscle of crayfish. Only T tubules are seen, forming a network with frequent longitudinal elements and tubules oriented transversely. Section 1 μm thick. Total tilt 30°; 1,000 kV; × 4,000. (Micrograph by Franzini-Armstrong, Eastwood, and Peachey.)

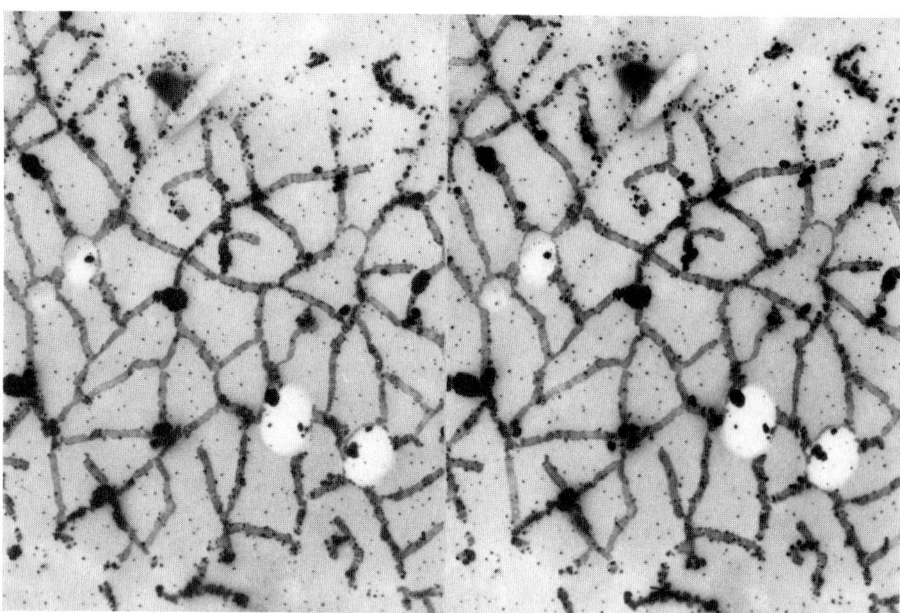

FIG. 16. Stereoscopic high-voltage micrograph of transverse section of frog twitch muscle fiber showing 2 forms of T tubules. Flattened ribbonlike tubules predominate, but short segments of round tubules also are seen, especially near nodes in network. Round tubules appear narrower in this transverse view. Section 0.5 μm thick. Total tilt 40°; 1,000 kV; × 10,000.

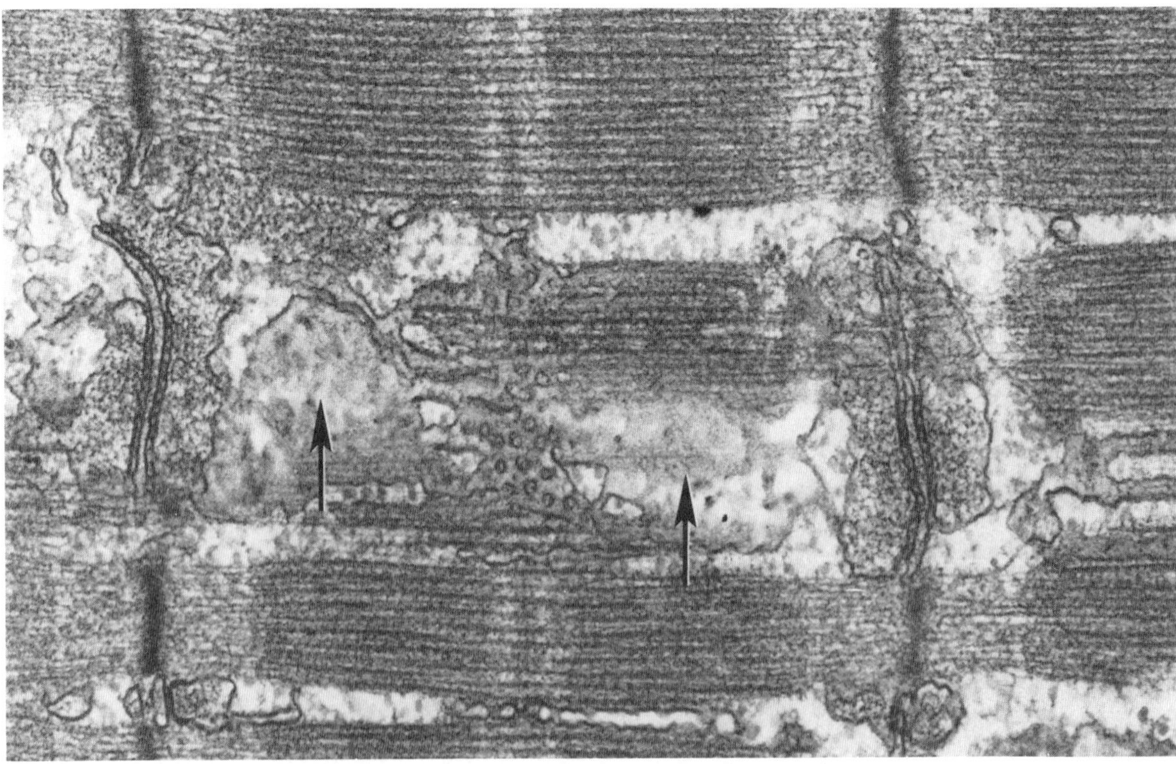

FIG. 17. Longitudinal section of frog sartorius fiber. Grazing view of SR and T tubules near image center. Terminal cisternae (lateral sacs of triad) face T tubules and contain a dense meshwork of calsequestrin. Intermediate cisternae (*arrows*) are flat and join lateral sacs to longitudinal tubules. Fenestrated collar opposite sarcomere center. × 45,000.

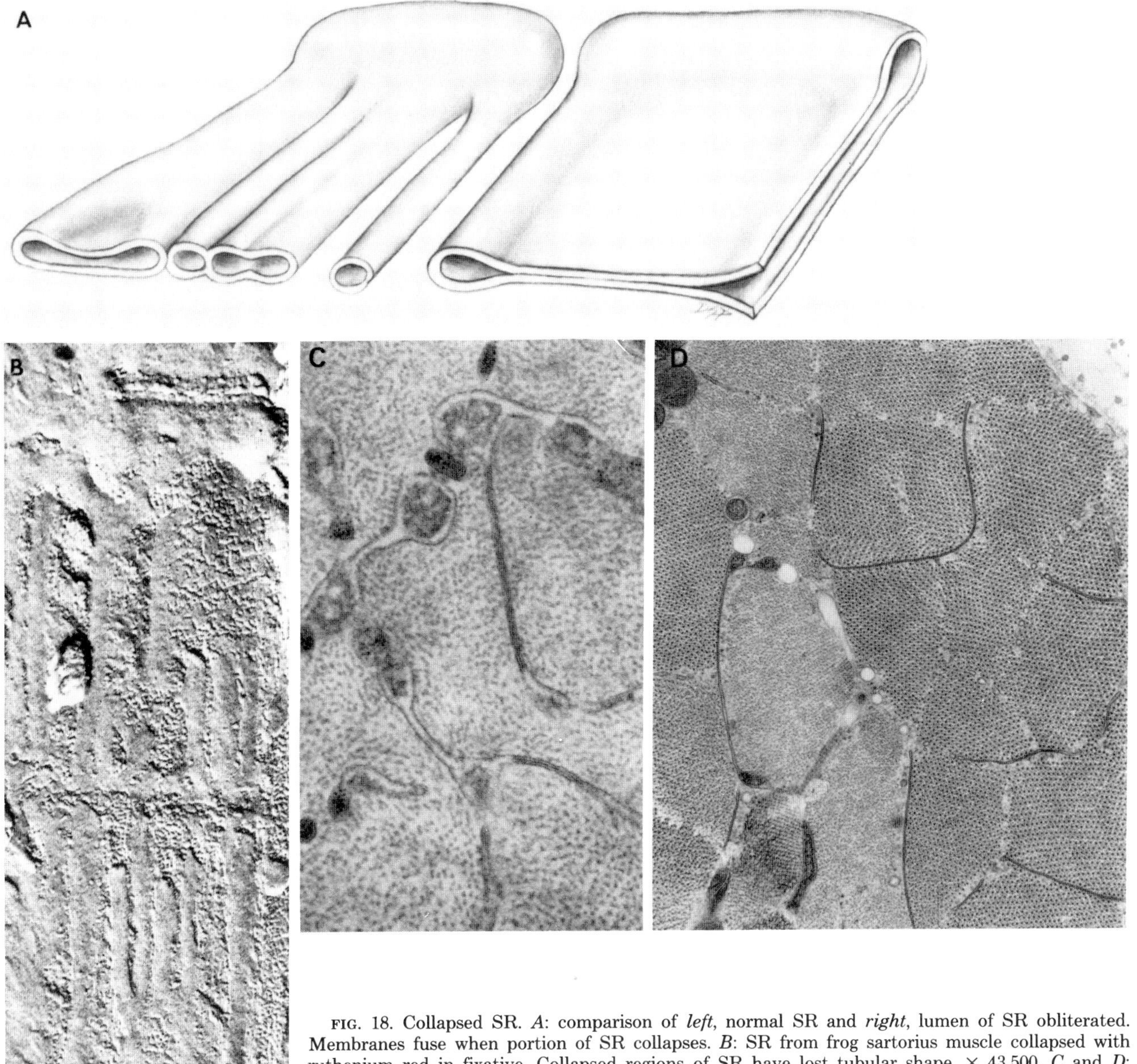

FIG. 18. Collapsed SR. *A*: comparison of *left*, normal SR and *right*, lumen of SR obliterated. Membranes fuse when portion of SR collapses. *B*: SR from frog sartorius muscle collapsed with ruthenium red in fixative. Collapsed regions of SR have lost tubular shape. × 43,500. *C* and *D*: transverse sections of fibers from frog cutaneous pectoris muscle, frozen rapidly and freeze substituted. Collapse of SR wherever SR membranes have flat shape and SR lumen is obliterated. *C*, × 42,600; *D*, × 21,300. [*A* courtesy of J. Sommer; *B* from Sommer et al. (305a); *C* and *D* courtesy of J. Heuser.]

intermediate cisternae or the longitudinal tubules is commonly observed (141, 232–234, 305). In other muscles no such constriction is apparent (111, 234).

The tubules in the next portion of the SR run somewhat irregularly in the longitudinal direction and fuse in a transitional zone near the center of the A band to form a fenestrated region of the SR (Fig. 17). The latter structure, often referred to as the fenestrated collar, is a flat cisternal element perforated by pores, usually of round cross section but sometimes elongated. The pores are formed by fusion of the membranes from either side of the SR, so the opening of the pore extends completely across the SR from cytoplasm to cytoplasm and not into the SR from the cytoplasm.

In transverse sections in the electron microscope, the SR is seen surrounding the myofibrils and occupying the space between them (Fig. 19). It is possible to identify each component of the SR and deduce the general appearance of the entire reticulum in three dimensions from the information from longitudinal and transverse views (Fig. 7).

In comparison, the striated muscle fibers of crustacea have SR with extensive fenestrated cisternae in

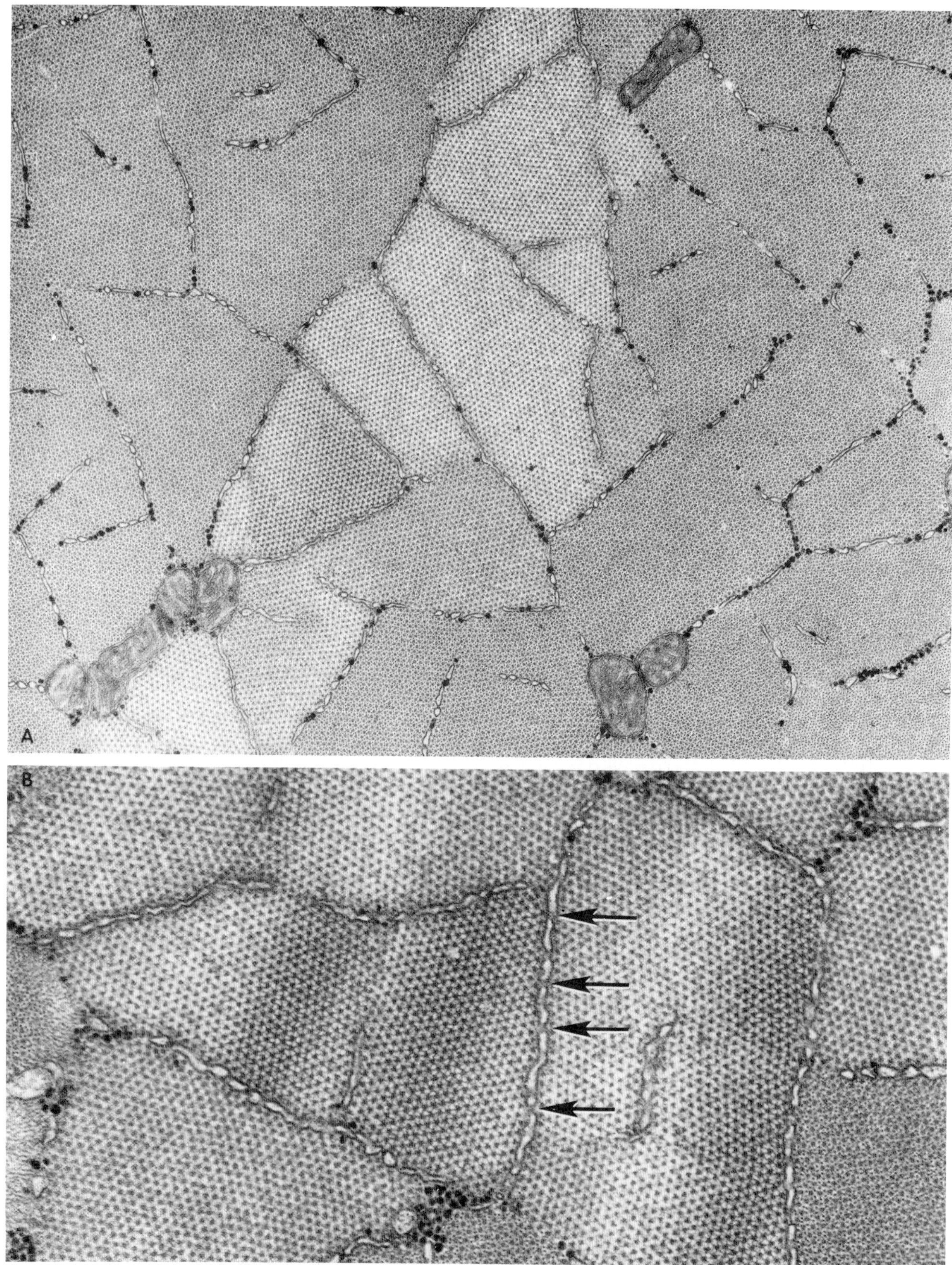

FIG. 19. Cross sections of frog sartorius fibers at sarcomere center. *A*: area within A band, except for small area at *lower right*, in I band. H zone extends vertically in middle of figure. Overlap regions of A band on either side. Transversely cut longitudinal tubules separate myofibrils in overlap region. Fenestrated collar surrounds fibrils opposite H zone. × 31,000. *B*: most of image occupied by H zone. Pores of fenestrated collar entire SR (*arrows*) as can be seen at this higher magnification. × 60,000.

both A bands and I bands and patchlike cisternae that form dyad contacts with the T tubules (34, 144, 179, 235, 260). The SR of the long-sarcomere, tonic type of fiber is illustrated with the Golgi stain in Figure 20. Figure 21 shows the phasic fiber type from these crustacea; compared to the tonic fiber type, these fibers have less of the fenestrated cisternae. The patches of cisternae are connected longitudinally by tubular SR regions and form generally larger patches of dyadic contact with the T tubules.

Content of Sarcoplasmic Reticulum

A property of the SR in all muscle cells that is critical for its function is its division of the muscle cell into two major compartments: the internal space of the SR and the sarcoplasm outside the SR. Electron-microprobe analysis (146, 183, 288) of muscle cells prepared by cryoultramicrotomy (125, 165, 300) has confirmed that these compartments differ in ionic composition (298). Thus the internal compartment of the SR is not in equilibrium with the extracellular fluid, a point debated until recently (130, 214, 265). Chloride concentrations in terminal cisternae of frog muscle resemble intracellular values and are significantly lower than extracellular values (299). Additionally, approximately two-thirds of the total calcium in the fiber is localized in the terminal cisternae in resting frog skeletal muscle fibers. Clearly the content of the SR differs in ionic content both from the cytoplasm and the extracellular space of the fiber.

Calcium Movements

The amount of calcium cycled by the SR must be large enough for near saturation of troponin with calcium when the fiber is maximally activated in a tetanus. In some fibers the presence of significant amounts of other calcium-binding proteins, e.g., parvalbumins (121, 129), with binding constants similar to those of troponin (114, 128, 255) increases the amount of calcium that must be released to approach saturation of contractile control proteins.

Electron-microprobe analysis of frozen frog semitendinosus muscles gave an average value of 117 mmol/kg dry wt for the calcium of terminal cisternae of the SR (298). After fibers were tetanized for 1.2 s at 4°C, frozen, and analyzed by this method, the terminal cisternae contained only 69 mmol/kg dry wt for a net release to the cytoplasm of 59% of the original calcium content. If the terminal cisternae have a volume of ~5% of the fiber volume (210, 232), this amount of released calcium would increase the cytoplasmic concentration by 3–4 mmol/kg dry wt, almost exactly equal to that found in the cytoplasm by microprobe analysis of the tetanized fibers. This cytoplasmic calcium is equivalent to ~1 mM concentration in the fiber water, which is roughly equivalent to the concentration of binding sites of troponin (324) and parvalbumin (121) in these muscles.

Somlyo et al. (298) also investigated the ions that move into or out of the terminal cisternae at the same time as calcium in the tetanized fibers. Sodium and chlorine levels in the terminal cisternae are not changed significantly, but both magnesium and potassium in the terminal cisternae are increased, suggesting that the latter two ions may move into the SR as calcium exits. The amount of charge carried into the SR by magnesium and potassium is significantly less than that carried out by calcium. The reason for this discrepancy is not known, although the charge unaccounted for could be carried by protons entering the SR or by some other charged species undetected by microprobe analysis.

Any consideration of calcium movements and binding in skeletal muscle must consider the calcium-binding protein calsequestrin, the major extrinsic protein associated with the SR (Fig. 22). Calsequestrin has been identified within terminal cisternae in intact fibers and in purified heavy SR fractions, which contain predominantly vesicles from terminal cisternae (36, 134, 162, 191, 202). Calsequestrin, as its name implies, is a calcium-binding protein and probably buffers the free calcium concentration within the SR and aids pumping and retention of calcium by the SR.

INTRINSIC MEMBRANE PROTEINS

Sarcoplasmic Reticulum

The freeze-fracture technique is useful in the description of the internal architecture of a membrane, since it reveals its hydrophobic interior by splitting the membrane along its middle (Fig. 23). Myofibrils can be identified, and in longitudinal views their various bands can be distinguished sufficiently well for orientation with respect to the equivalent thin-section image. All the longitudinally oriented components of the SR, including the intermediate cisternae, the longitudinal tubules, and the fenestrated region (Fig. 24), contain a uniform distribution of intrinsic protein particles ~8 nm in diameter on the cytoplasmic leaflet (48, 106, 258, 294, 295, 304). The particles are not in a regular pattern, though they are essentially packed closely throughout the SR in most twitch fibers. Similar particles are seen in freeze-fracture preparations of isolated SR fractions (53) and vesicles reconstituted from isolated adenosine triphosphatase (ATPase) [(189); see also the chapter by Martonosi and Beeler in this *Handbook*]. Probably this is the calcium-pump protein, or Ca^{2+}-Mg^{2+}-ATPase, because it is the predominant protein found in isolated SR preparations (190). Indirect immunofluorescence studies show Ca^{2+}-Mg^{2+}-ATPase distributed throughout the sarcomere (162, 163). These results suggest that the pumping ability of the SR for calcium is relatively evenly distributed.

In the freeze-fracture studies, particles in the SR membranes are found exclusively on the membrane half-leaflet that faces the cytoplasm in the muscle cell and not on the half-leaflet that faces the SR lumen.

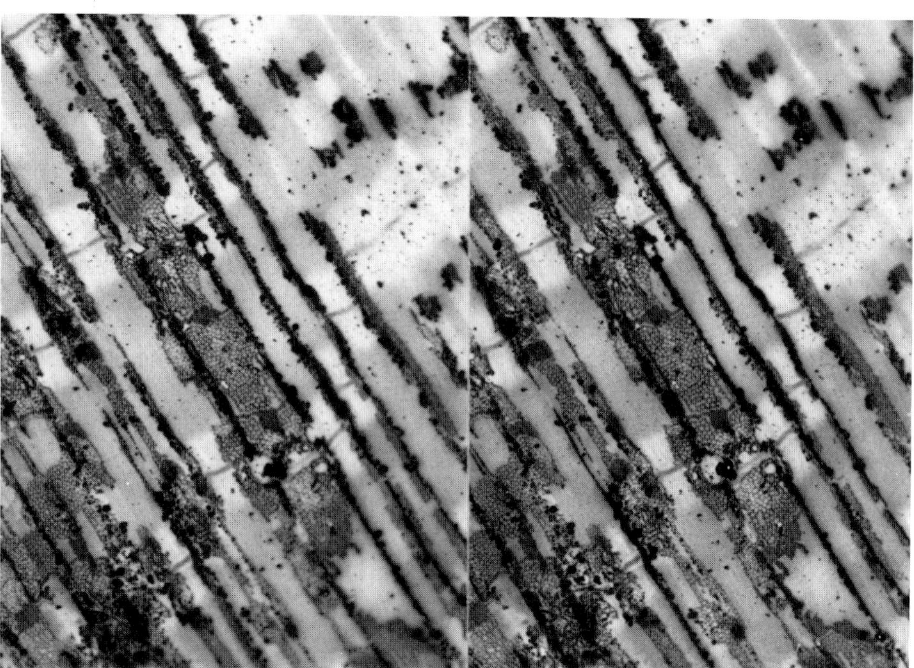

FIG. 20. Stereoscopic high-voltage electron micrograph of Golgi-stained crab tonic muscle fiber with SR stained. T tubules, stained more densely than SR, show both transversely oriented tubules and flattened disklike regions that form dyad contacts with SR. SR in form of fenestrated cisternae in both A bands and I bands. Section 0.5 μm thick. Total tilt 12°; 1,000 kV; × 6,000. (Micrograph by Franzini-Armstrong, Eastwood, and Peachey.)

This suggests an asymmetric positioning of the protein molecules within the membrane and agrees both with the observation by X-ray diffraction of a strong asymmetry in electron density of SR membranes (58, 131) and with the greater sensitivity of the SR ATPase to tryptic digestion when the enzyme is presented from the cytoplasmic side than when presented from the luminal side. This result also supports the identification of the particles seen in the SR by freeze fracture with the SR ATPase, because the two show the same sort of asymmetric positioning in the membrane (see the chapter by Martonosi and Beeler in this *Handbook*).

A small proportion of SR membranes faces directly toward T-tubule membranes in the junctional complex, and these junctional SR membrane areas have a different appearance in freeze-fracture preparations compared to the free SR that is not in junctional contact with T tubules. The luminal leaflet of junctional SR has very prominent, deep pits and, in invertebrate muscles, a fairly large number of particles. The cytoplasmic leaflet of junctional SR shows particles that are both larger and less densely packed than the particles on the corresponding leaflet of free SR. Thus junctional SR is decidedly different in its intrinsic protein content than SR membranes not participating in junctions with the T tubules.

T Tubules

Two types of surfaces must be distinguished when discussing membrane particles in T-tubule membranes. A portion of the T-tubule membrane faces into the junctional area with the SR and is called the junctional T membrane. The rest of the T-tubule membrane either is in portions of the network not participating in junction formation or, although within a junctional portion of the tubule, faces away from the junction itself. All these membrane areas are called free T membranes. Junctional T membranes contain a population of large particles that remain preferentially with the cytoplasmic leaflet when the membrane splits, though they appear on the luminal leaflet to a varying degree. These particles have a distribution regularity that can be related to the distribution of feet in the junction, as discussed in *Structural Details*, p. 54. The free T membrane appears in freeze-fracture replicas with either no particles or a few shallow, wide particles on the luminal leaflet and a smooth cytoplasmic leaflet, which is very different from the appearance of the junctional T membranes. The T membranes have fewer particles overall than either surface or SR membranes.

COMPARATIVE STRUCTURE OF SARCOPLASMIC RETICULUM AND T SYSTEM

Comparative structural studies suggest which structural features of a cellular component are essential for its function and how much structural variability can be tolerated without loss of function. This approach has had considerable success in studies of the complex

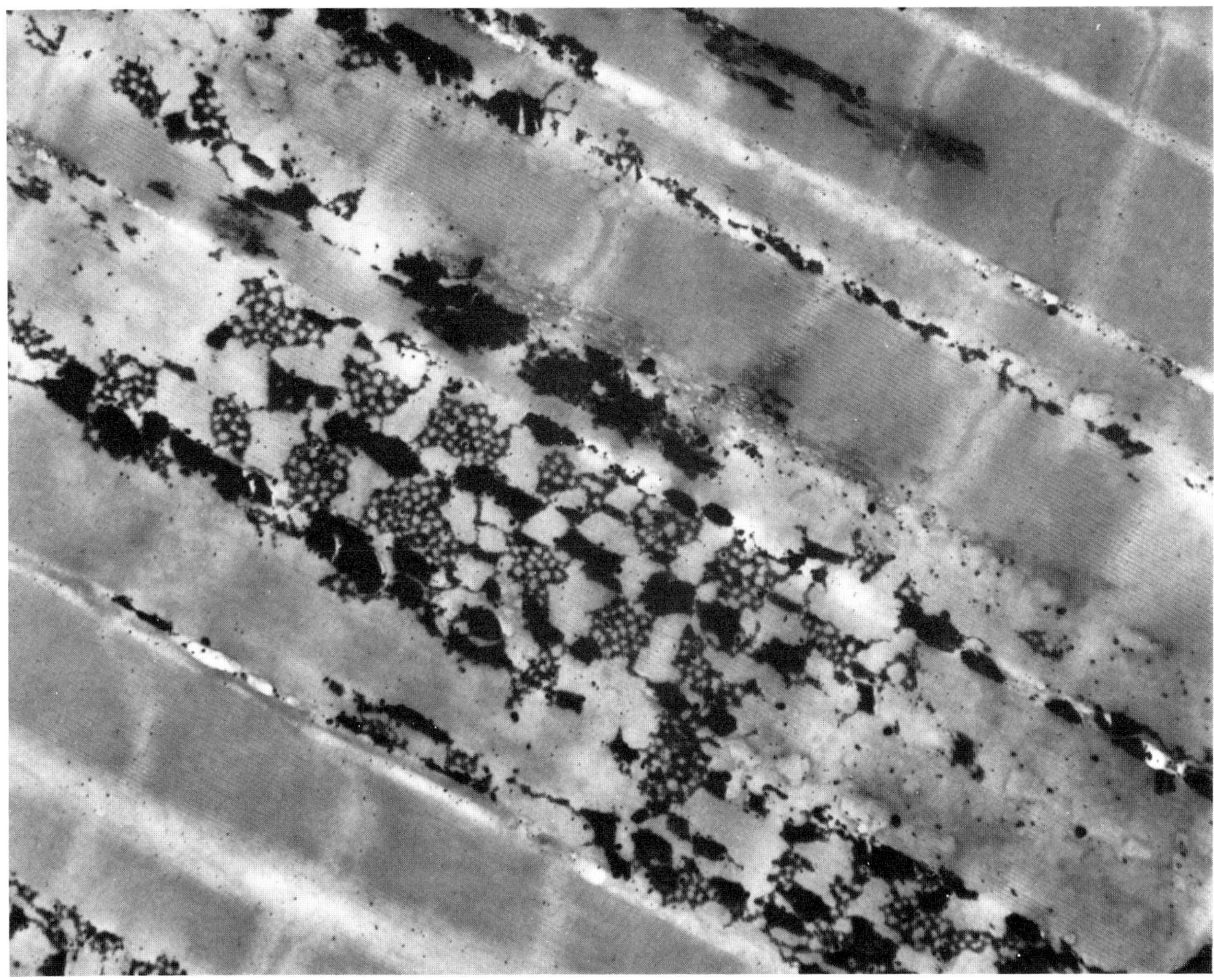

FIG. 21. Golgi-stained preparation from phasic fiber from crayfish abdominal flexor muscle. Only SR is stained. Numerous flat cisternae of SR match similar regions of T-tubule network (Fig. 15) with which they form triads and dyads. Fenestrated cisternae of SR less prominent than in tonic fibers. Section 0.5 μm thick. 100 kV; × 15,000. (Micrograph by Franzini-Armstrong, Eastwood, and Peachey.)

networks of membranes in skeletal muscle cells. Comparisons are usually made across species lines, though sometimes they are made between normal and experimentally altered muscles or between muscles altered in different ways. The method is most successful when good physiological information is available on the same muscles.

A normal muscle fiber is assumed in these studies to be structurally uniform along its length so that a microscopic sample taken anywhere is representative of the fiber as a whole. This assumption seems reasonable because the segments of the fiber mechanically are in series and should act similarly to avoid instabilities that would result if one part of the fiber stretched another segment of the same fiber. An exception is found in the intrafusal muscle fibers in sensory spindles, where stretch of a fiber segment during activity and movement is understood to be part of the sensory mechanism. A clearly documented example of variation in fiber diameter and organelle content along the length of a fiber thought to be extrafusal, i.e., not sensory, is found in a small population of muscle fibers in rabbit extraocular muscles (41, 51, 52). These results indicate that caution is called for in structural studies where the fibers are not sampled at various points along their lengths, though variability of structure as extreme as this does seem unusual.

As discussed in *Comparison of Slow-Acting and Fast-Acting Muscle Fibers*, p. 32, one early clue to the role of the T system and SR in EC coupling was the observation that relatively fast muscles tended to contain larger quantities of SR and T-tubule membrane systems than slower muscles. Comparative morphological and physiological studies continue to support that relationship and allow discussion of the relationship among size of fibers and fibrils, speed of contraction activation and relaxation, and extent of development of T tubules and SR.

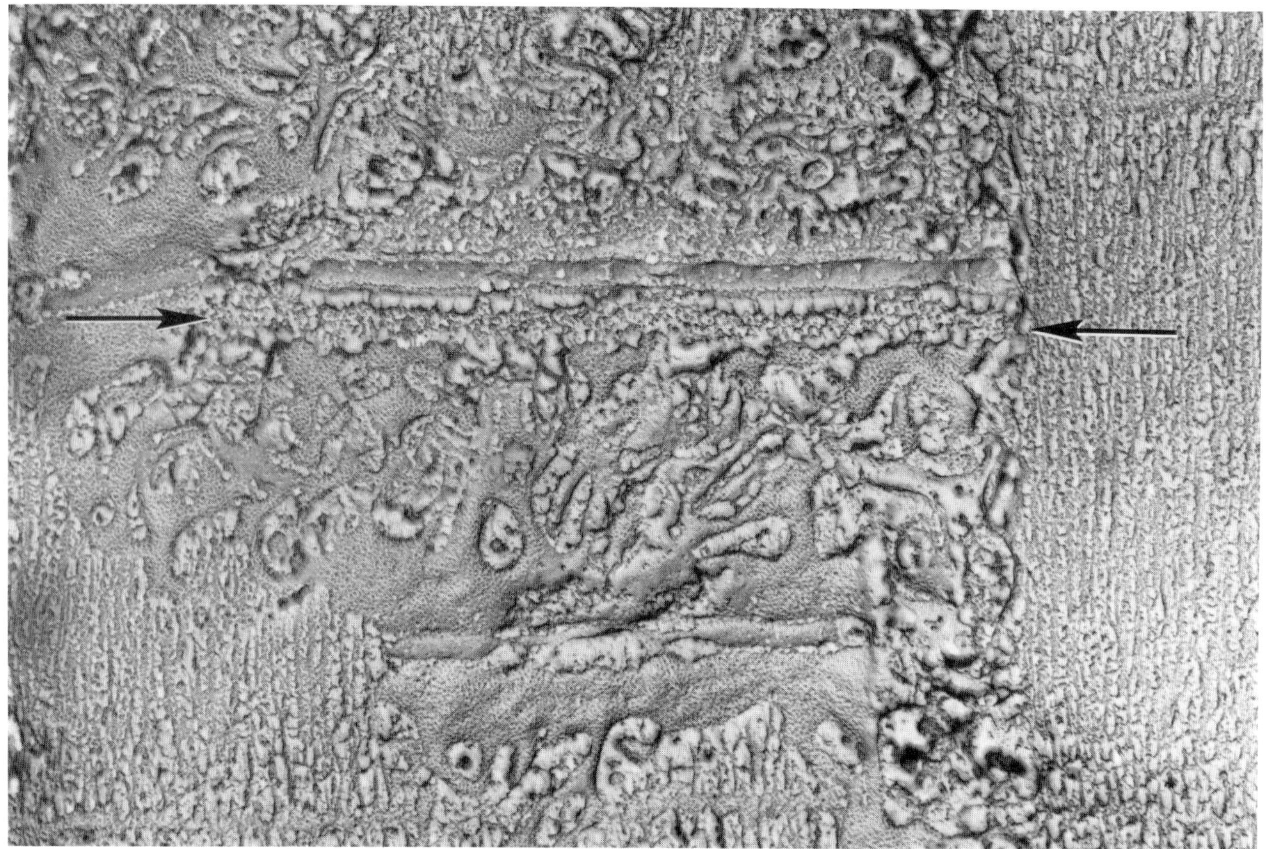

FIG. 22. Freeze-fractured deep-etched image of SR in toadfish swimbladder muscle. Between *arrows* fracture splits interior of lateral sac of triad. Calsequestrin content of cisternae and its connections to SR membrane revealed. × 39,000. (From M. G. Nunzi and C. Franzini-Armstrong, unpublished observations.)

Fibers With One Small Dimension and No T System

The muscle fibers of lower invertebrates and of the lowest vertebrate apparently achieve their speed of EC coupling by maintaining a small distance between the fiber surface and the contractile element most distant. These fibers have only one myofibril per muscle fiber, which is flattened so that the maximum distance from surface to interior is small. These fibers are a simple form of contractile-activation system: calcium entering through the fiber surface or released from SR sites very close to the surface diffuses to the contractile proteins and activates them directly.

The muscle fibers forming the body musculature of the primitive chordate, amphioxus *Branchiostoma lanceolatum*, fall into this group. Early light- and electron-microscopic examination of these muscle fibers (93, 94, 123, 229, 231) showed that each fiber or cell is in the form of a broad flat sheet ~1 μm thick and contains only one myofibril (Fig. 25). Although it was first thought that there is no SR in amphioxus body muscles, this error was corrected when improved fixation methods were used and a small amount of SR forming surface couplings was found (94, 126). Even so, the amount of SR present is relatively small, and there is no T system in these simply constructed fibers. No part of the contractile myofibril is more than ~0.5 μm away from the surface of the cell because of the flat planar shape of these muscle cells. Thus the diffusion distance for calcium entering the cell through its surface or released from surface couplings is small enough for diffusion to be essentially complete in a very short time, probably less than a millisecond (246). This is well within the delay time between excitation and contraction observed in vertebrate muscle fibers. Therefore these specialized fibers would require no special conducting system, such as a T system, which agrees with the electron-microscopic observations that found no T system.

Also included in this group are, among others, the smooth and striated portions of the adductor muscles of scallops (208, 218, 268, 277) and fibers from annelids (268). These muscles have peripheral couplings of SR to the interior surface of the plasma membrane and fibrils of flattened form similar to those of the amphioxus.

Vertebrate smooth muscle cells can also be included in this group, though they differ in shape. Their contractile material is not clearly subdivided into fibrils,

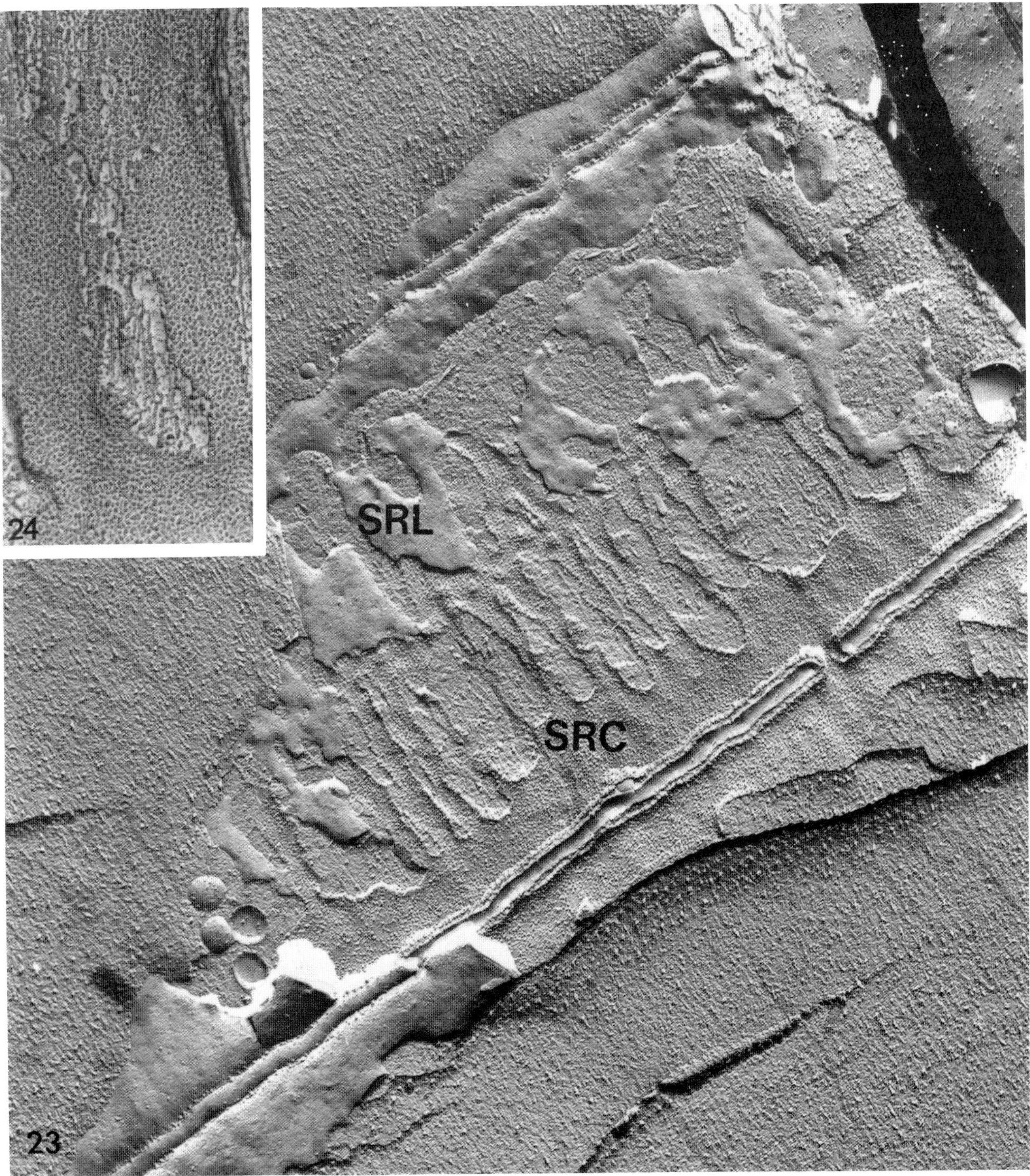

FIG. 23. Longitudinal fracture along SR of fish muscle (guppy). Myofilaments barely identifiable in this standard freeze-fracture image. Membranes very visible (see also Fig. 28). Fracture plane preferentially follows membranes, splitting them into 2 leaflets. Cytoplasmic leaflet (*SRC*) in SR decorated by uniformly distributed population of small particles of variable size thought to represent aggregates of calcium-pump proteins. Luminal leaflet (*SRL*) is smooth. Nonjunctional regions only of T tubules shown; very few particles on either leaflet. × 50,000. [From Franzini-Armstrong (105).]

FIG. 24 (*top left*). Detail of cytoplasmic leaflet of SR in frog sartorius fiber. Rotary shadowing allows better visibility of numerous intramembranous particles. × 88,000.

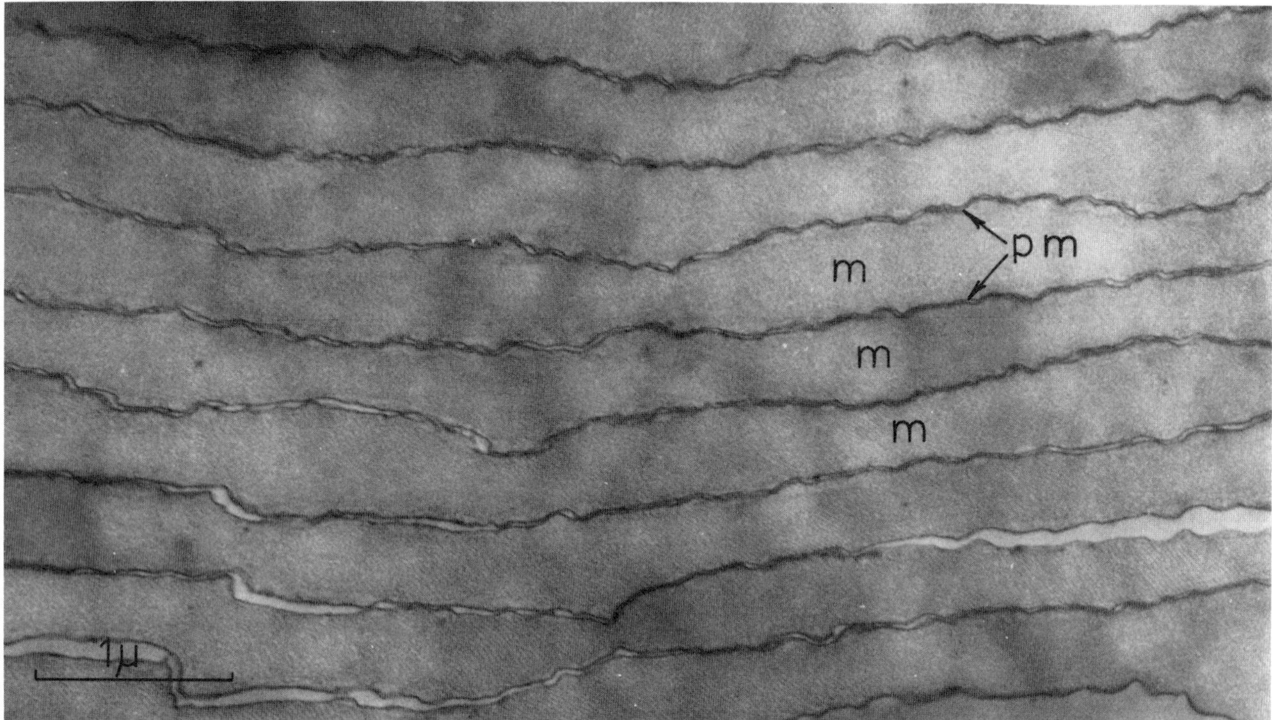

FIG. 25. Transverse section of body musculature of amphioxus. Each flat myofibril (*m*) forms a muscle fiber, completely covered by plasma membrane (*pm*). × 26,600. [From Peachey (231), by copyright permission of The Rockefeller University Press.]

the cells are relatively small, and contraction is slow enough that an elaborate conduction system involving T tubules inside the cell is not needed (54, 296). The scanty SR forms junctions with the plasmalemma that are similar to those of skeletal muscle cells (297), and these SR elements accumulate calcium (253). Ventricular cardiac muscle cells in frogs also essentially fit this structural pattern (224) and are thought to have calcium entry from the external medium as a major source of activator calcium (215, 216, 224). Some mammalian atrial cells also lack T tubules (99), as do Purkinje fibers in a variety of mammalian species (302).

Fibers With Low Speed and Small Quantity of Membranes

Compared to twitch fibers of the same species, the slow fibers of amphibians (16, 92, 176, 221, 223), birds (223), and reptiles (145) contract more slowly and have quantitatively less T and SR membrane. The total T-system membrane area present in fibers of comparable size differs only by a factor of ~2 between frog twitch and slow fibers, but there is a larger difference in the quantity of T-SR junctional area because a larger proportion of the T-tubule length is nonjunctional in the slow fibers. In twitch fibers most of the T-tubule length is in the form of a flattened tubule embedded in triad junctions with SR. In the slow fibers the junctional T areas are approximately circular patches of flattened tubule separated by considerable lengths of nonjunctional T tubules. Fawcett and McNutt (90) compared mammalian ventricular papillary muscle cells to amphibian slow fibers and found them similar structurally. Fewer membranes overall, less junctional area, a less precise organization of membranes, and larger fibrils are associated with slower speeds of contraction and relaxation.

Fibers With High Speed and Large Quantity of Membranes

Electron-microscopic examinations of several muscle types notable for the high speed of their contractile cycle have found a remarkably large amount of precisely arranged internal membranes, both SR and T tubules, and small fibrils, which is the opposite of the slow fibers discussed above. The muscle fibers in the wall of the gas bladder of a teleost fish, the toadfish *Opsanus tau* or *O. beta* (91, 107, 217), have narrow flat fibrils that are radially arranged. This arrangement is advantageous for several types of structural studies. The membrane systems are confined between the myofibrils to flat planes oriented perpendicular to the fiber surface. Extensive views of them are relatively common. The longitudinal SR tubules form multiple layers, resulting in a large total quantity of membranes. The maximum diffusion distance into the deepest point in the myofibrils also is very small because of the narrow myofibrils. The ability of these muscle fibers to contract very rapidly when producing the sounds characteristic of this group of fish is related to this small diffusion distance (290).

Not only is the quantity of SR increased in these fast-acting fish fibers but the protein composition of the SR also is different. Sodium dodecyl sulfate–polyacrylamide gel electrophoresis studies of the *Opsanus tau* swimbladder muscle and of the slower body muscles of the same fish show differences in proteins between the two muscle types, suggesting molecular adaptation of SR in extremely fast muscles (129). These studies also show a greatly increased parvalbumin content in the very fast muscle compared to the slower one. This calcium-binding protein may be closely associated with the SR.

A second very fast-acting muscle is the cricothyroid muscle of the bat, which modulates the frequency of its ultrasonic echolocation cry. The rapid relaxation of this muscle during the cry relaxes tension on the vocal chords, reducing the cry frequency. The larger-than-usual content of SR in these fibers supports the contention that the SR is involved in causing relaxation of an activated fiber (263).

A variety of physiological types of striated muscle fibers is in the extrinsic eye muscles (extraocular muscles) of mammals, fish, birds, and perhaps other groups (11, 15, 133, 252, 259). Included in these is a group of particularly fast-acting fibers, probably the fastest fibers in mammals. Although the correlation has not been done on a fiber-for-fiber basis, as was done for the slow and twitch fibers of the frog (244), the extraocular muscles also contain a population of muscle fibers that have unusually narrow flattened fibrils and unusually abundant T- and SR-membrane systems (7, 33, 132, 198, 207, 236, 248). The tentative conclusion, based on their structure, is that these are the rapidly contracting fibers (Fig. 26). The opposite situation also seems true in these unusual muscles. Fibers that contract slowly and are multiply innervated are present (15, 133, 195, 252). Fibers structurally resembling the slow fibers of amphibians are also found (7, 8, 132, 198, 207, 236, 248). The direct correlation between structure and function has not been made, though a technique for doing this has been developed (14, 242).

Fast-acting fibers with highly developed membrane systems are also found in invertebrates, including crustacea, several examples of which Fahrenbach (82–84) and Rosenbluth (267) studied.

Variation in Speed and Quantity of Membranes in Mammalian Fibers

In other mammalian muscles not associated with eye movements, the differences in contraction speed and simultaneously in content of SR and T tubules are less dramatic, but speed still tends to correlate with membrane content. In these cases precise measurement of contraction speeds and quantitative electron-microscopic assessments of membrane content are necessary. This subject is discussed in the chapter by B. R. Eisenberg in this *Handbook*.

Invertebrate Fibers

Invertebrate muscles show considerably more variety in the structural arrangement of the internal membrane systems than do vertebrate muscles (103, 127, 143, 158, 256, 267, 291, 292). In insects, for example, a major division is found between synchronous and asynchronous fibers. Asynchronous fibers do not have a separate excitatory event for each contraction (see the chapter by Tregear in this *Handbook*) and generally have less SR than do the synchronous fibers. Although the frequency of contractions of an asynchronous fiber can be high (up to 1,000/s), the speed of its activation-inactivation cycle is low because the muscle is part of a resonant mechanical system with a high resonant frequency and stays activated through many mechanical cycles of shortening and lengthening (257). Correspondingly, the content of SR in the asynchronous fibers is low. In synchronous fibers each contraction is activated by its own excitatory event, as in vertebrate twitch fibers, and more internal membranes are present than in the asynchronous fibers.

T-SYSTEM–SARCOPLASMIC RETICULUM COUPLINGS

Basic Form

The common form of association between T tubules and SR in muscle fibers of vertebrates is a triadic structure with a single T tubule in the center flanked by two cisternal elements of SR (Figs. 7, 8, 17, 22, and 23). In invertebrate muscles the equivalent structure commonly is the dyad, consisting of one T tubule and one cisternal element of SR. Less common in invertebrate muscles are triads or, in some very unusual muscles, higher order complexes with multiple SR elements associated with one T tubule (83).

In the junctional region between the T tubule and the SR the membranes are usually rather flat, and often the plane of the junctional region has a preferred orientation with respect to the fiber axis. In most vertebrate fibers the junctional plane is transversely oriented, although the common orientation in invertebrate fibers is longitudinal. Variations from these general rules and irregularity in junction orientation are sometimes found, e.g, in amphibian slow fibers.

An interesting structural variation among muscle fibers of different species and even among different muscles in the same species is the location of T-SR junctional structures with respect to the striation pattern of the adjacent myofibrils. In the frog twitch fibers already described, triads are found at the level of the Z lines of each sarcomere. In mammalian skeletal muscle fibers, triads are located about midway

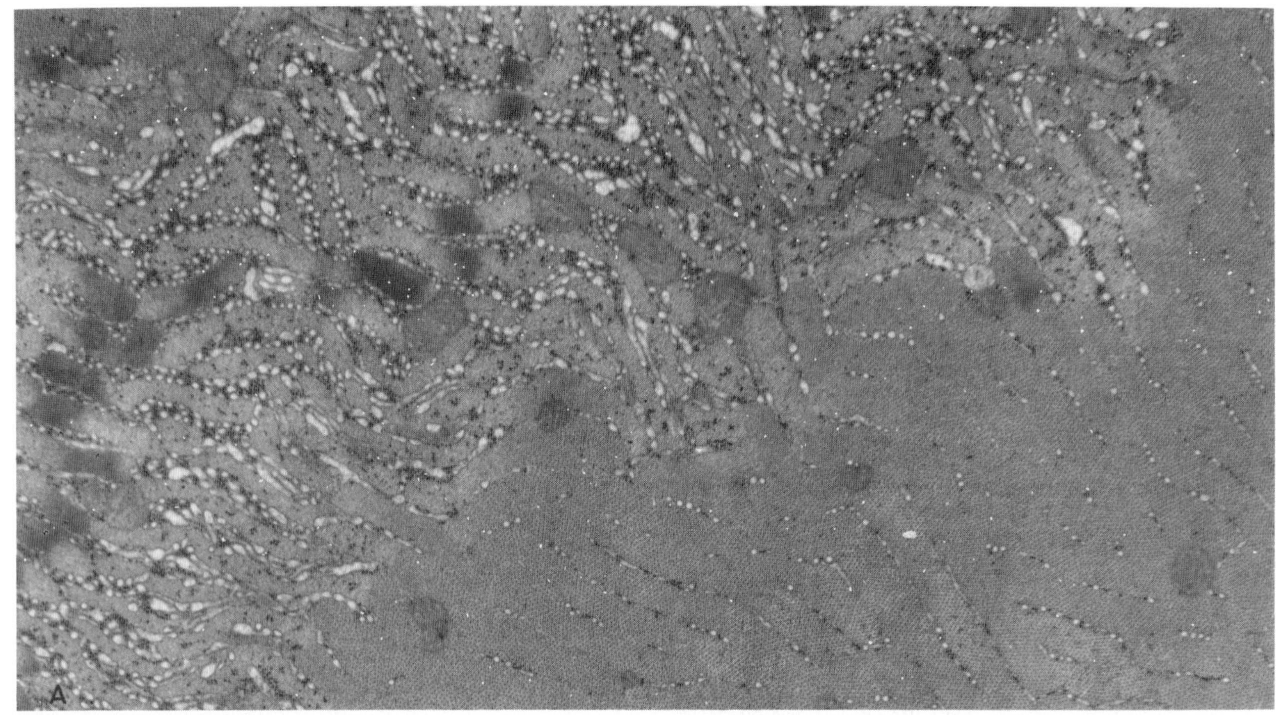

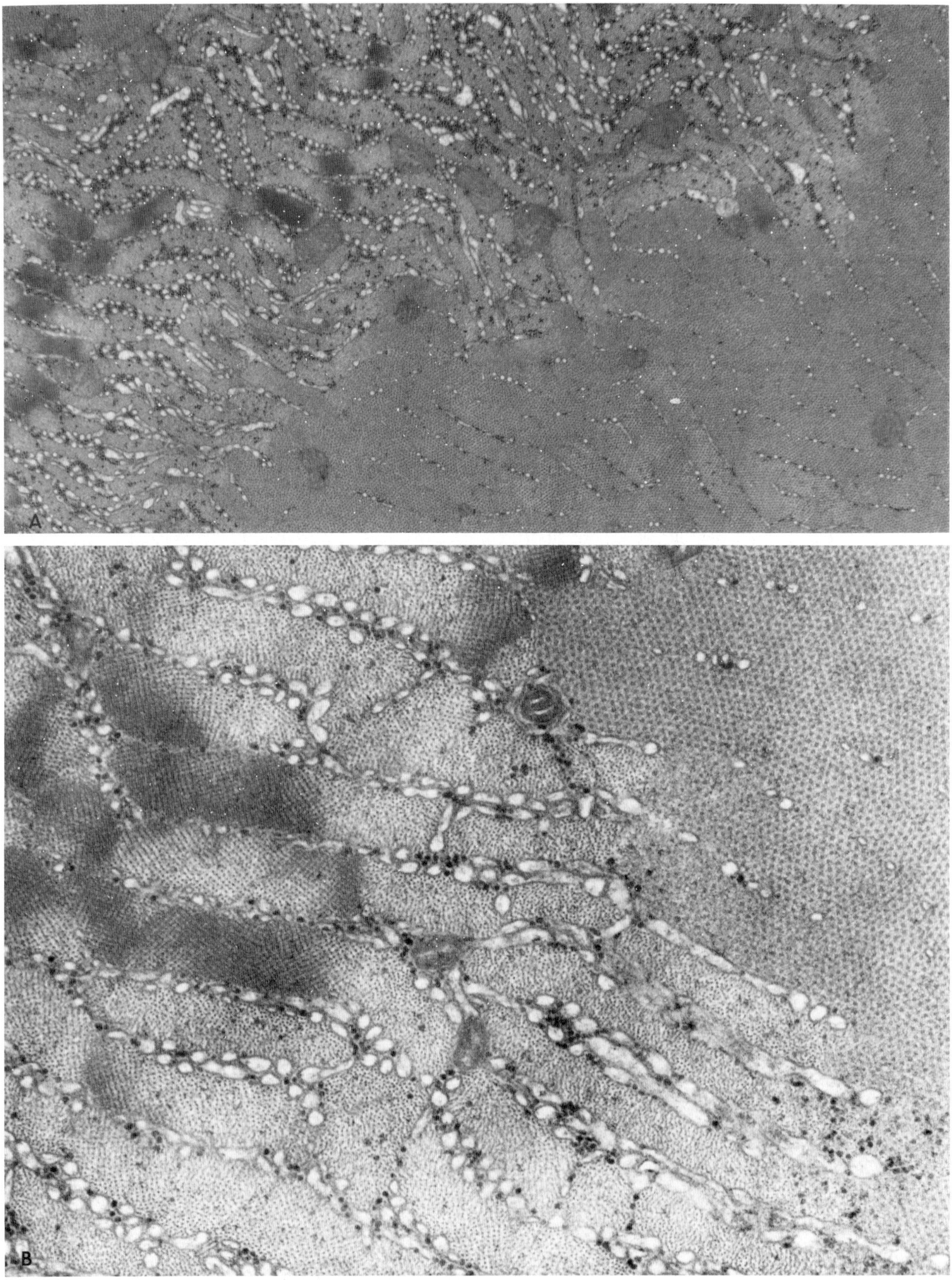

B

FIG. 26. Transverse sections of muscle fiber from superior rectus (extraocular) muscle of domestic cat. Ribbon-shaped myofibrils and abundant SR arranged in multiple layers between myofibrils, especially in I bands. *A*, × 20,000; *B*, × 52,000.

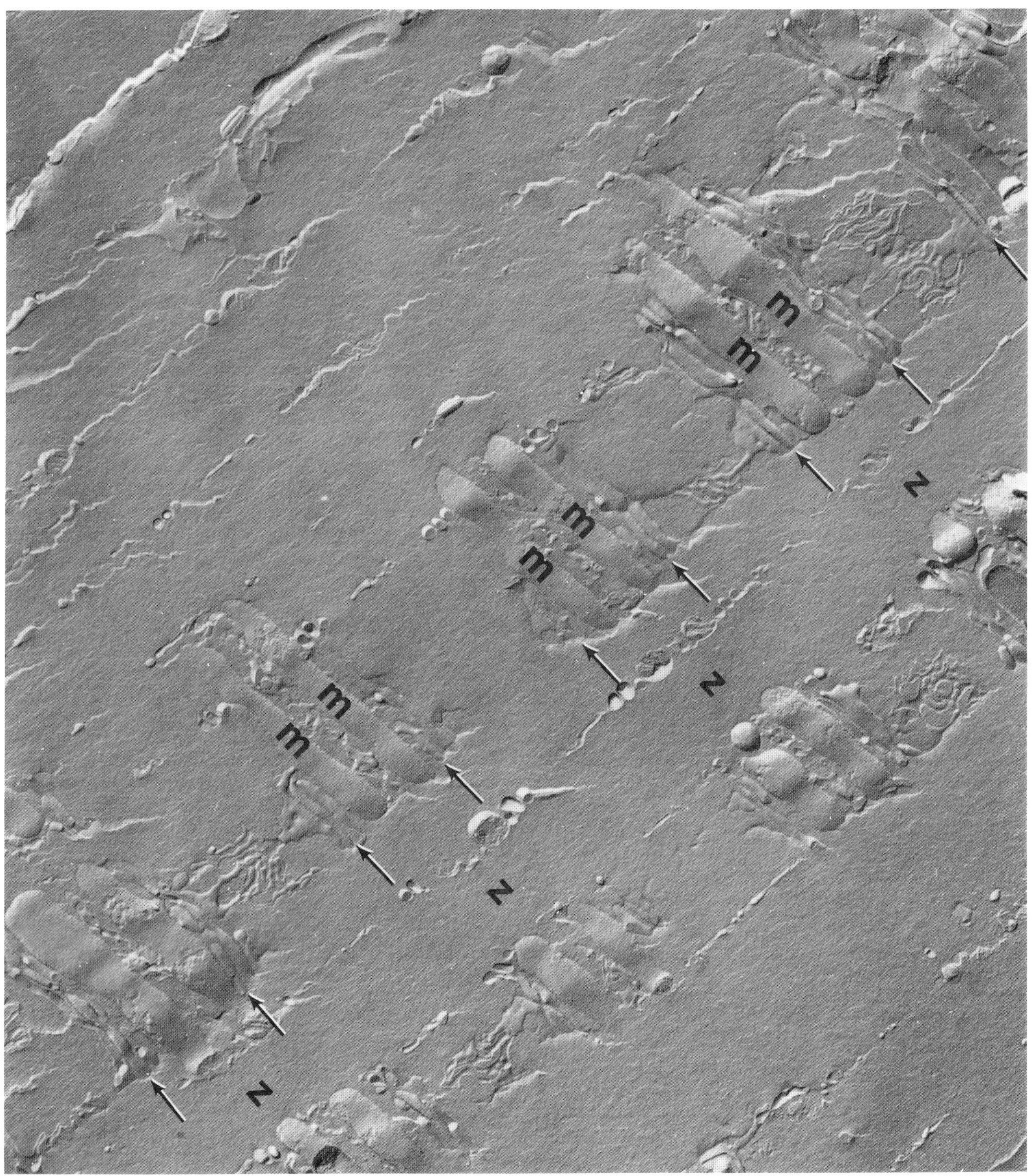

FIG. 27. Longitudinal fracture along fiber from red portion of rat sternomastoid muscle. Location of Z lines (*Z*) detectable on myofibrils. As in most mammalian fibers, triads (*arrows*) located at A-I junction. Extensions of mitochondria (*m*) encircle myofibrils at I-band level, immediately adjacent to triads. (See also Fig. 28.) × 25,000. (From R. Mazanet and C. Franzini-Armstrong, unpublished observations.)

between the Z line and the middle of the A band (Figs. 27 and 28). Thus mammalian fibers have two triads in each sarcomere. This arrangement also results in an additional longitudinal linkage in the I-band area of the SR, consisting of a second fenestrated collar around each myofibril.

The distribution of triads with the mammalian position among different biological groups is interesting

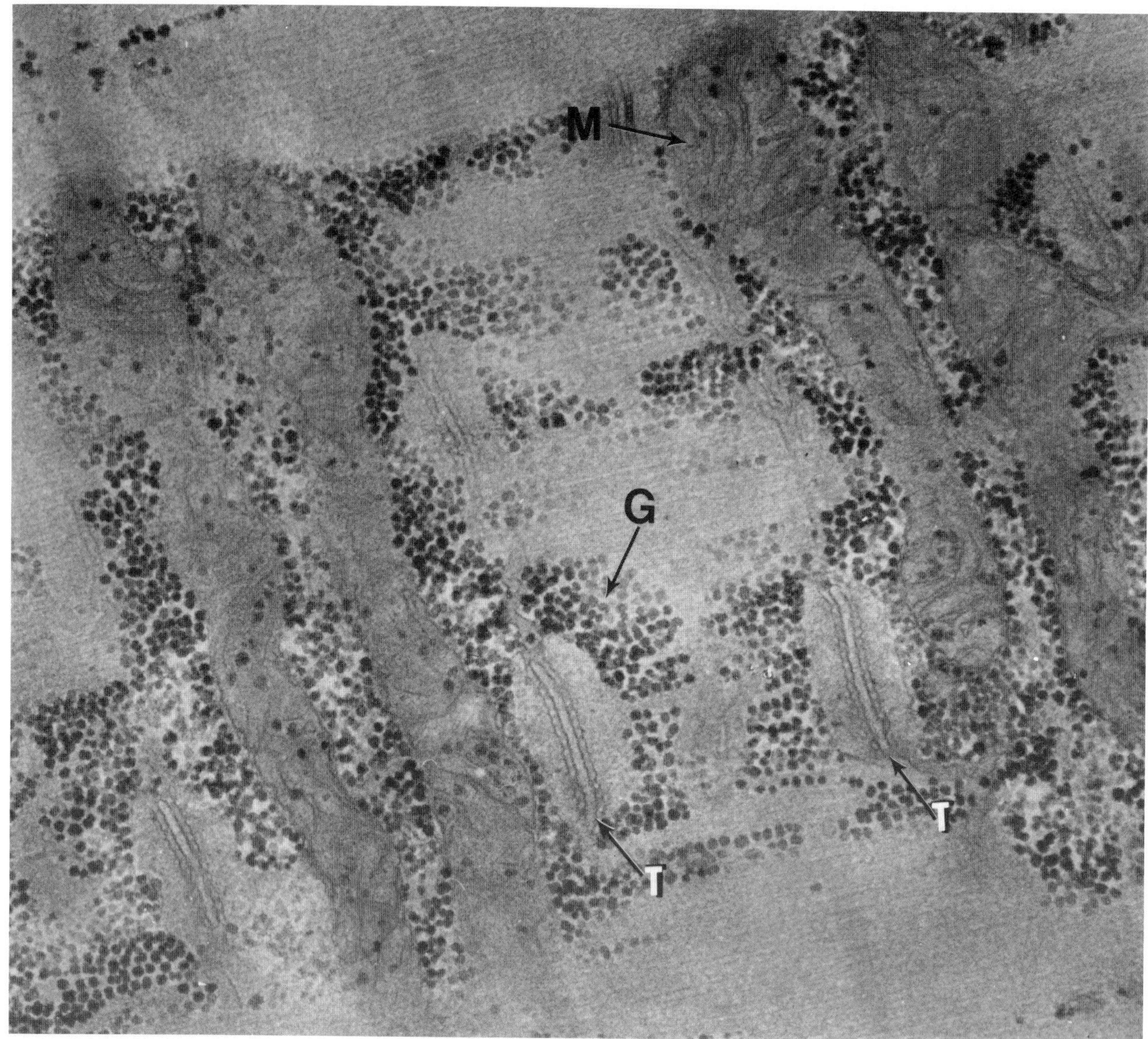

FIG. 28. Longitudinal thin section of human skeletal muscle showing 2 triads (*T*) in each sarcomere, large mitochondria (*M*) in I bands, and large accumulations of glycogen granules (*G*). × 60,000. (From biopsy material supplied by D. Schotland.)

but not understood in regard to function. Among the vertebrates, two triads per sarcomere are found in reptile muscles, in some but not all fish and bird muscles, and in all mammalian skeletal muscles. The location of triads, dyads, and peripheral couplings is more variable in invertebrate fibers, where a complete range from a fixed to a random positioning can be found.

Structural Details

Regularly disposed feet link the membranes of the T tubule with those of the SR in the region where the flattened membranes face each other within the triad [Fig. 29; (67, 105, 161, 170, 297, 320)]. These feet seem to function in mechanical adhesion because the junctions remain intact even when fibers are swollen and distorted osmotically. The feet may also be involved in EC coupling as possible sites for the molecular movements or ionic currents required in the various coupling mechanisms proposed.

The T-SR junctions are not morphologically identical to nexuses (55) or gap junctions (264), which provide electrical coupling between two cells, e.g., smooth muscle and epithelial cells, sharing in junction formation. The spacing of the T-SR junction is larger than that of a typical gap junction (99). Two different types of membranes participate in forming the T-SR junction, and the T-SR junction appears asymmetric in electron micrographs.

The arrangement of junctional feet and the size of the junctional gap between T and SR membranes are remarkably similar in all muscles studied (59, 95, 102,

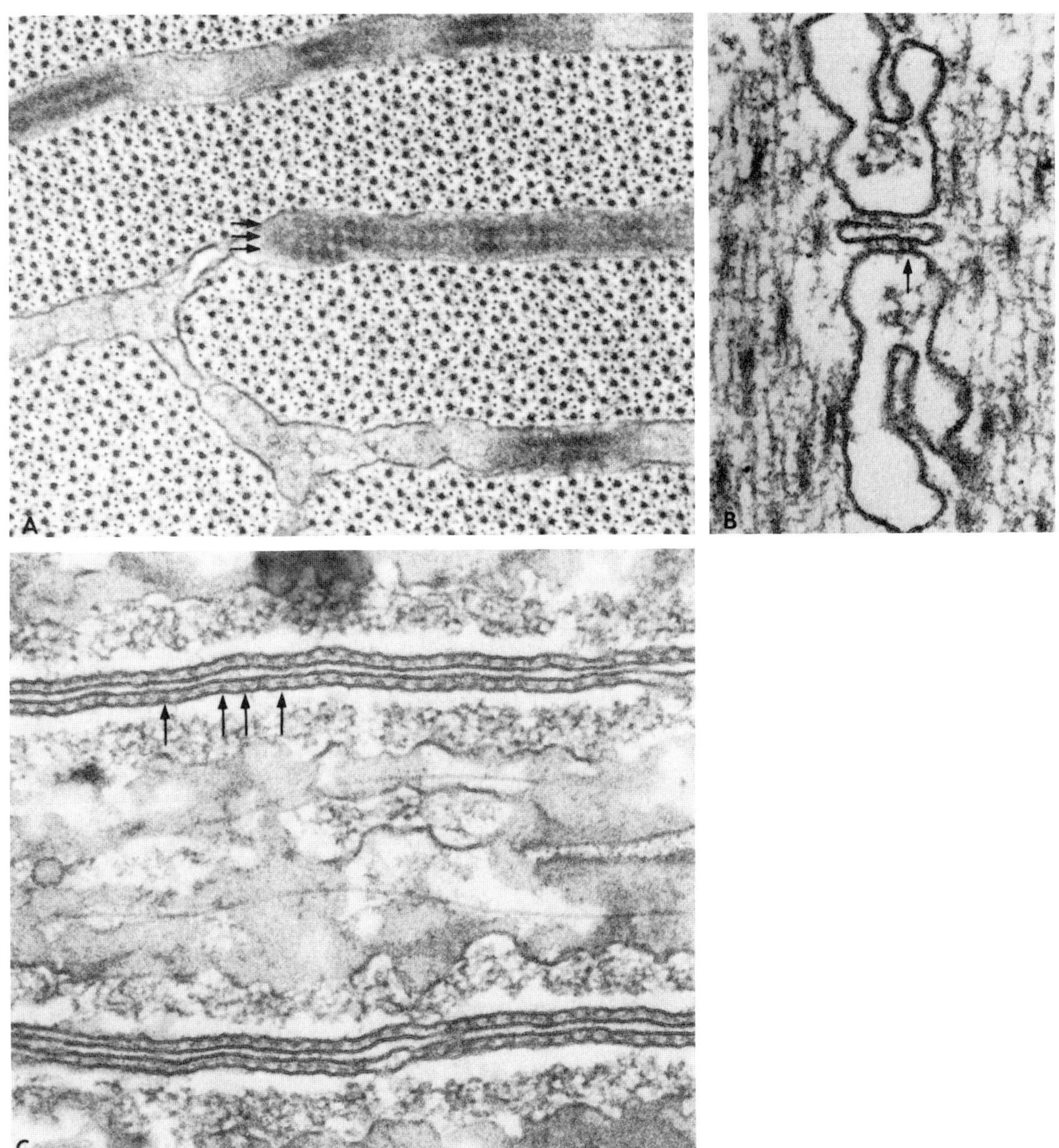

FIG. 29. Three views at right angles of junctional feet in triads from toadfish swimbladder. *A*: grazing view of junction; 2 or 3 parallel rows of feet in tetragonal arrangement. × 36,000. *B*: section at right angle to long axis of T tubule. Double set of feet covers both flat junctional surfaces of T tubules. × 114,000. *C*: section approximately parallel to row of feet, showing their periodic arrangement. × 90,000. Feet have different appearances, 2 most frequently illustrated in the literature being a hollow-cored appearance (*arrow, B*) and a line parallel to 2 junctional membranes (*arrows, C*). [*C* from Franzini-Armstrong (107).]

105, 160, 285, 287, 293). Junctional feet are arranged tetragonally in two or more rows of varying length, depending on the size and shape of the junctional membrane. Structurally the feet are more closely associated with the SR membrane than with the T-tubule membrane, as seen most clearly in some muscles where feet exist extrajunctionally on the SR (160, 287). Experiments in which T tubules detached from SR are made to reattach in vitro provide evidence for specific attachment sites on T tubules for feet. Thus the feet clearly have a structural association with the T tubules (177, 178).

The appearance of T-SR feet in thin sections varies and is quite sensitive to orientation and plane of section. Some appear elongated in a direction parallel to the adjacent T-tubule and SR membranes and may appear to contact one or both membranes, usually in their central region. Others appear as a narrow column connecting the two membranes. This column may or may not have an apparently less-dense core extending perpendicular to the membranes. Eisenberg and Gilai (68) called this open-core appearance a pillar and present evidence supporting the idea that pillars are a morphological correlate of open ionic channels between T tubules and SR during EC coupling (see *Functional Mechanism of Coupling Between T Tubules and Sarcoplasmic Reticulum*, p. 57).

Freeze-fracture replicas of the junctional T-tubule membrane show large prominent particles with a somewhat variable degree of regularity in their pattern (Fig. 30*A*). A similar pattern is seen in the plasma membrane where it forms peripheral couplings with the SR (Fig. 30*B*). The pattern commonly seen on the cytoplasmic leaflet of the surface T-tubule membrane in these junctional regions is groups of four particles in two rows extending along the long axis of the tubule. Individual particles or whole groups may be missing, which contributes to making the pattern less obvious than it would be if all elements were present. Interestingly, the spacing along the tubule between groups corresponds closely to twice the spacing between feet, suggesting a possible function of the particle groups as attachment sites for pairs of feet. The pattern of feet also is represented in freeze-fracture images of the SR. The slight scalloping of the junctional surface of the SR associated with the pattern of the feet can sometimes be seen in freeze-fracture replicas, and a faint pit is seen at each attachment site (171).

Figure 31 is a three-dimensional representation of the structure of the triad and T-SR junction in frog skeletal muscle fibers, as derived from study of thin sections and freeze-fracture preparations.

Role of T-Tubular Calcium Current in Excitation-Contraction Coupling

In his 1952 review of EC coupling, Sandow (274) proposed a direct relationship between depolarization of the surface membrane of a muscle fiber and the liberation into the myoplasm of an activating substance, presumably calcium. Flux measurements (28) and electrophysiological methods (21, 22) have been used to measure calcium influx related to activity. However, frog twitch muscle fibers produce normal twitches in external media with low calcium concentrations buffered with ethylene glycol-bis(β-aminoethylether)-*N,N′*-tetraacetic acid (EGTA) (10), support-

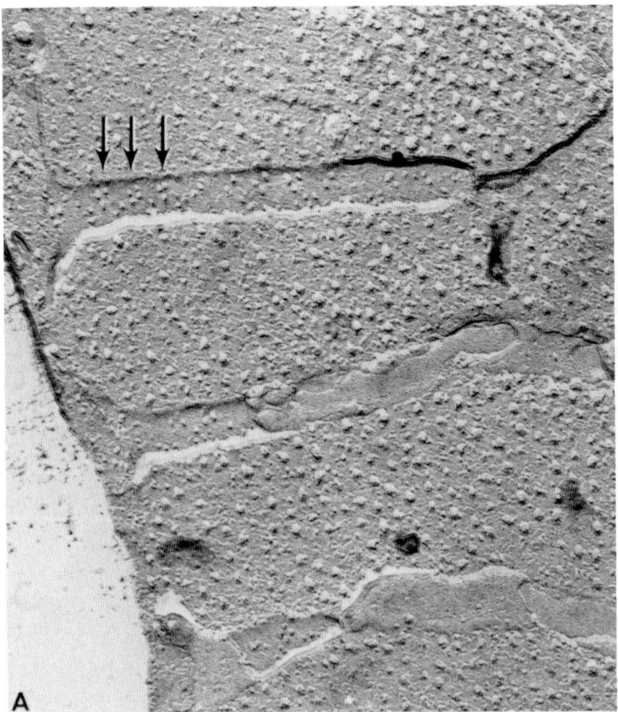

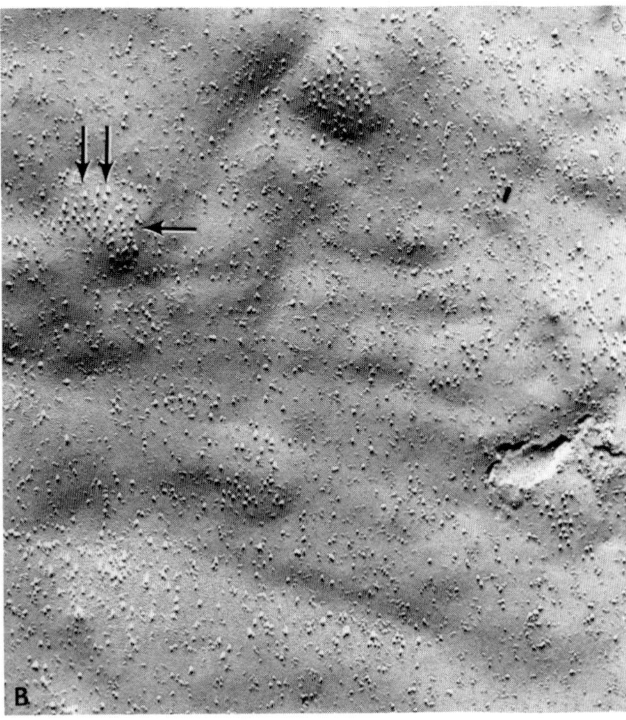

FIG. 30. Cytoplasmic leaflets of junctional T-tubule membrane (*A*) and plasmalemma at sites of peripheral couplings (*B*) occupied by similar-looking large and tall particles. Where most regularly arranged (*arrows*), particles form groups of 4 separated by twice the distance that separates junctional feet. *A*: × 74,500; *B*: × 44,600. [*A* from Franzini-Armstrong and Nunzi (108a). *B* from Eastwood, Franzini-Armstrong, and Peracchia (59).]

ing the idea that entry of calcium per se is not necessary for the initiation of EC coupling processes and that intracellular storage sites in the SR are the source of the calcium that activates contraction. This result was questioned when it was observed that potassium contractures were smaller and briefer in low-calcium solutions (308) and that higher concentrations of EGTA, although causing depolarization of the fibers, led to action potentials without twitches when the fibers were repolarized with injected current and then stimulated (17). Later experiments, however, found that substitution of magnesium for calcium in the low-calcium solutions resulted in normal twitches even in the presence of very low external calcium concentrations (188). This rules out calcium moving from the lumen of the T tubule into the fiber as a link in EC coupling, but does not rule out calcium released from binding sites on the cytoplasmic side of the T-tubule membrane or some other transmitter substance that enters the fiber from the T tubules from playing this role.

In addition, the inward calcium current that occurs during activity is too small and too late to account for the early phases of activation (225, 273). This calcium may aid in the maintenance of contraction in a tetanus or in a potassium contracture. This agrees with the observation that the aequorin signal, thought to measure myoplasmic calcium concentration, is decreased in a tetanus in a low-calcium solution but not in a twitch (30).

Essentially parallel experiments on frog slow fibers produced similar results. Direct application of calcium to the interiors of frog slow fibers resulted in characteristically slow contractions (46). Miledi et al. (204, 206) observed calcium transients in slow fibers during membrane depolarization and determined that the general voltage dependence of these transients is similar to that in twitch fibers, though their time course is slower. External calcium does not appear to be necessary for mechanical activation of slow fibers (115), as in twitch fibers.

Thus the calcium that enters a vertebrate skeletal muscle fiber as a measurable current during a twitch probably does not directly account for setting off the events leading to contraction activation. This does not rule out a role for a calcium release that would not appear as a current, i.e., calcium released in exchange for other ions from sites within the membrane or on the cytoplasmic side of the T-tubule membrane. This is discussed next.

Functional Mechanism of Coupling Between T Tubules and Sarcoplasmic Reticulum

The junctions between the T tubules and the SR are the sites of an important step in EC coupling, the transmission of a signal from the T tubules to the SR (see the chapters by Adrian, Baylor, and Caputo in this *Handbook*). The nature of this transmission step is presently unknown; in every other step in the coupling process at least the general nature of the process is known.

Three mechanisms have been or are being considered for this coupling step. *1)* In a chemical mechanism, a small amount of a trigger substance is released from the T tubules during the action potential and diffuses the short distance across the T-SR gap, leading to calcium release from the SR. This is a calcium-induced calcium-release mechanism when calcium itself is considered the trigger substance (28, 74, 98). *2)* In an electrical mechanism, conductance channels in the T-SR junction open and a small amount of ionic current passes into the SR, where a process induced by depolarization of the SR membrane leads to calcium release from the SR (75); this is an ionic current coupling mechanism (194). *3)* In a mechanical mechanism, an electrostatically driven conformation change or movement in one or more molecules extending across the T-SR gap in turn opens calcium channels in the SR; this is a charge-movement mechanism (1, 283).

For the chemical (calcium-induced calcium-release) mechanism to work, the small amount of calcium that can reasonably be expected to be released from the T tubules during activity must diffuse to and sufficiently influence the SR to trigger the next step in the sequence. There is no structural evidence either for a barrier to such diffusion or for a restricted diffusion space between T tubules and SR that might aid in the effectiveness of this mechanism. The region between the two membranes, excluding that occupied by the feet, is accessible to large molecules placed in the sarcoplasm (69, 101), supporting the idea that a trigger substance could diffuse across this space. However, the openness of this space could lead to loss of trigger substance released from the T tubules before it reached and acted on the SR membranes, unless the diffusion pathway is within the feet.

There also is physiological evidence relating to the possible role played by calcium-induced calcium release in EC coupling in skeletal muscle fibers. Blocking agents, e.g., procaine, that inhibit calcium-induced calcium release do not prevent a contraction when the fiber is depolarized by increasing the external potassium concentration (74). This mode of stimulation is thought to work via the normal route of activation involving depolarization of the surface and T-tubule membranes (137), which is evidence against a role for calcium-induced calcium release in the normal route of EC coupling.

Other experiments suggest that calcium-induced calcium release may play a role in the nonphysiological activation of muscle fibers by agents such as caffeine that can cause calcium release from the SR in the absence of depolarization of the surface or T-tubule membranes (M. Endo, personal communication). Calcium-induced calcium release also may be important

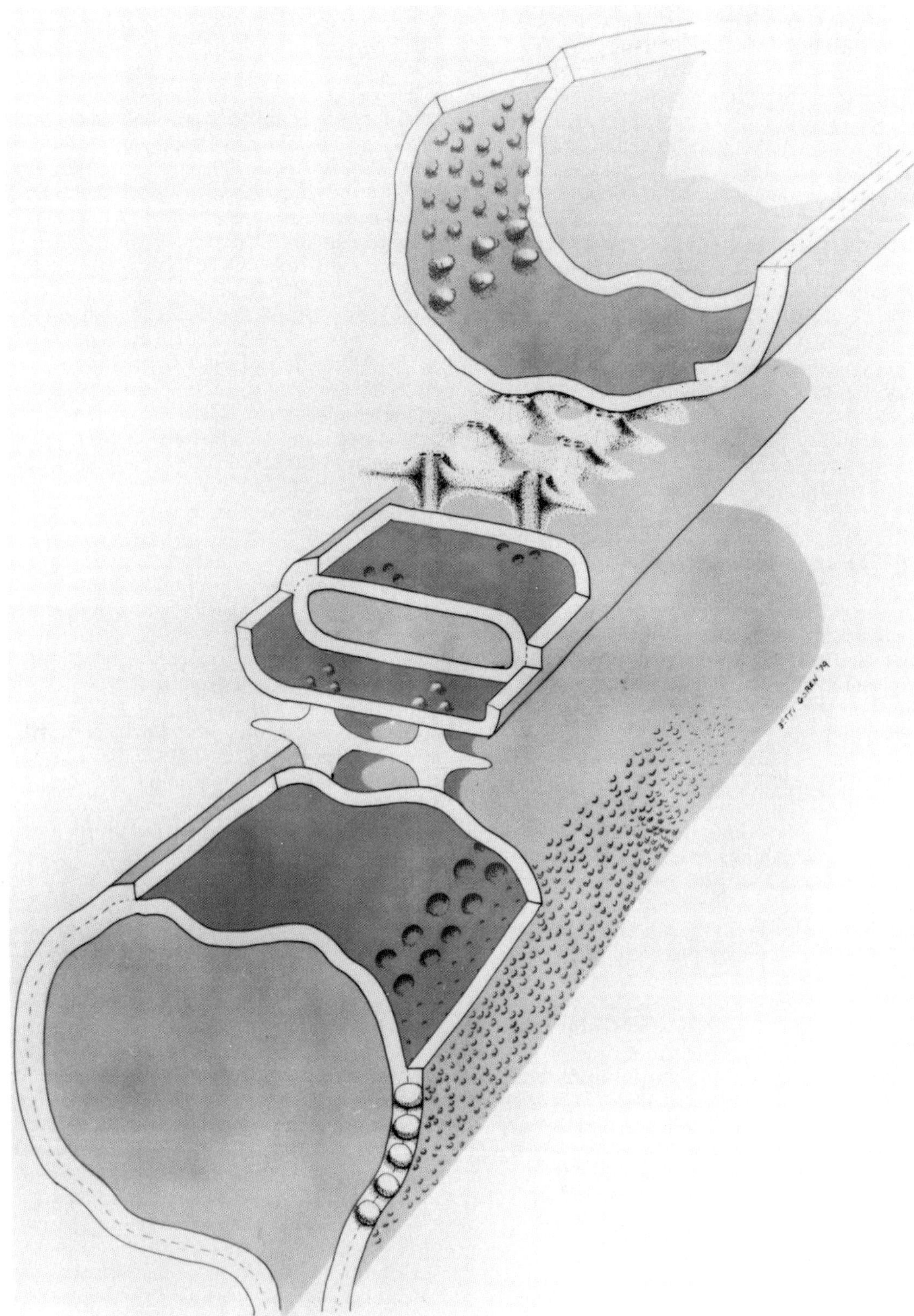

FIG. 31. Triad in frog skeletal muscle. Results from both thin sections and freeze-fracture preparations. [From Franzini-Armstrong and Nunzi (108a).]

in the normal activation of cardiac cells (80, 81) and other muscle and nonmuscle cells. However, a faster or more effective mechanism apparently has evolved in skeletal muscles.

The second T-SR coupling mechanism involves the conductance pathway for ionic current, presumably not carried by calcium, from the T tubule into the SR. This current is thought to trigger a release of calcium from the SR. Early solute distribution studies suggested the presence within muscle fibers of a special space with a volume of about 15% of the volume of the fiber that equilibrates with extracellular fluid (130) and suggested that this space might be the SR (29, 153). The existence of such a space within the fiber in continuity with the extracellular space would support the concept of a conductance pathway between T tubules and SR, as required by the electrical coupling mechanism. However, kinetic flux data on solutes with widely varying size do not support the conclusion that there is equilibration between extracellular space and the SR interior. A space comparable to the one observed by Harris (130) was seen in whole muscles but not in single fibers. Thus the special space observed earlier probably is the extracellular space between the fibers, at least in a large part (214).

Electrical evidence on the impedance of muscle fibers determined with intracellular electrodes, discussed earlier in *Relation of Total Surface Area to Fiber Capacitance*, p. 32, has been used to argue against continuity from the lumen of T tubules into the SR. The fiber surface areas and areas of T tubules and SR membranes in several types of muscles agree rather well with capacitance measurements if it is assumed that only the surface membrane and the T tubules contribute to the low-frequency capacitance and fit very poorly if the SR membrane is included. However, capacitance measurements usually are done in resting fibers; if the junction opened only transiently, the SR capacitance could be missed. Furthermore, if a relatively high resistance existed in series with the SR, given the large expected capacitance of the SR membrane the time constant characteristic of this element would be very long and perhaps missed in the impedance analysis.

Early measurements with extracellular electrodes of the transverse electrical impedance of whole muscles (86) suggested the presence of a transverse electrical pathway with a capacitance of $\sim$50 $\mu F/cm^2$ of sarcolemmal surface area, a number consistent with the SR surface area (210, 232). However, similar experiments measuring the transverse impedance of single fibers (209) showed a capacitance of only $\sim$5 $\mu F/cm^2$, consistent with the area of the T system. Again, no evidence for a conductance pathway from T tubules to SR in resting fibers was found.

As discussed in MICROSCOPIC METHODS IN STUDY OF CELLULAR MEMBRANE STRUCTURE, p. 33, sometimes stains or tracers thought specific for extracellular space and compartments continuous with the extracellular space are observed in the SR, usually in the terminal cisternae of the triad or dyad. Initially these observations seemed to warrant concluding that free communication exists from the lumen of the T tubules into the interior of the SR through the triad junction. However, in every case where SR staining was observed with presumed extracellular stains or tracers, the density in the SR could be explained as an artifact.

With ruthenium red, staining is observed in T tubules, as expected, and also in SR and perinuclear cisternae (187). However, staining of lipid droplets is also observed, suggesting that ruthenium red must slowly infiltrate the sarcoplasm and then accumulate in SR and lipid droplets. Application of ruthenium red to skinned fibers, with the surface membrane removed so that the stain has direct access to the sarcoplasm, results in staining of the SR within a few minutes, which confirms this interpretation (Fig. 32).

Staining of the SR has also been observed after exposure of intact fibers to horseradish peroxidase, another presumed extracellular marker, followed by an incubation to localize the enzyme. Rubio and Sperelakis (270) and Kulczycky and Mainwood (175) found reaction products used to localize the enzyme in SR and T tubules. Histochemical incubation alone, without preincubation of the muscle in exogenous peroxidase, was subsequently found sufficient for staining of the SR. Thus it cannot be concluded that peroxidase molecules had penetrated through the T-SR junction (249, 322). Finally, Waugh et al. (323) report fortuitous contrasting of SR of cardiac muscle by lanthanum colloid but do not conclude that their results support the idea that the SR is open to the extracellular space. Electron-microprobe analysis of the ionic content of the SR is discussed in *Content of Sarcoplasmic Reticulum*, p. 45.

Despite the lack of evidence for direct communication between the lumen of the T tubule and the SR interior in resting fibers, a conductance channel that opens transiently during activity and participates in EC coupling has not been ruled out. The experiments of Eisenberg, Eisenberg, and Gilai (67, 68) suggest a structural reorganization of the feet in the T-SR junction during activity. Mathias et al. (194) have argued for the electrophysiological plausibility of a mechanism involving a transient ionic current flow from T tubules to SR depolarizing the SR and triggering calcium release through the SR membrane to the sarcoplasm (see also the chapter by B. R. Eisenberg in this *Handbook*).

Both calcium-induced calcium-release mechanisms and electrical coupling mechanisms assume a regenerative release of calcium from the SR. This is inherent in the calcium-induced calcium-release mechanism because appearance of a small amount of trigger calcium

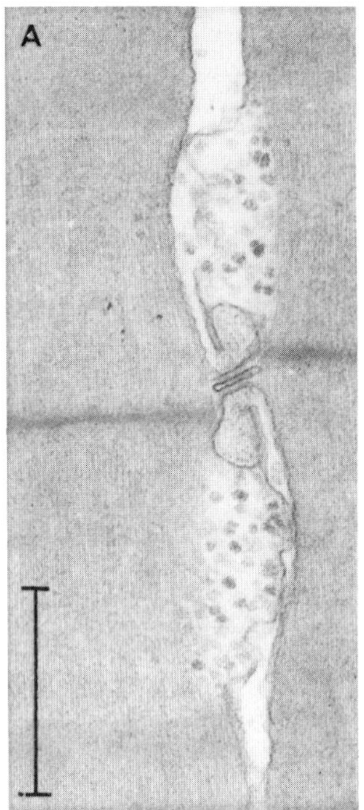

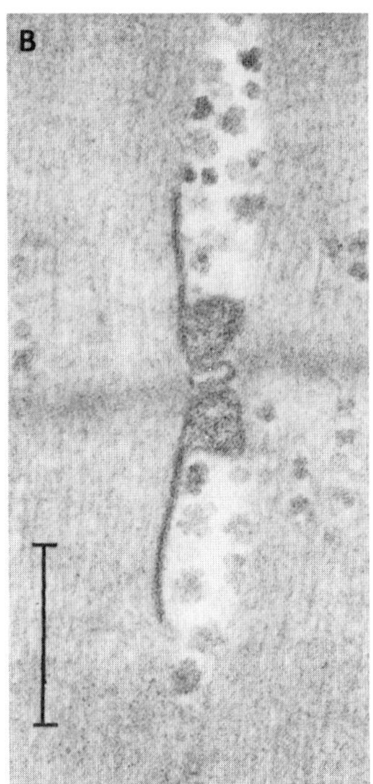

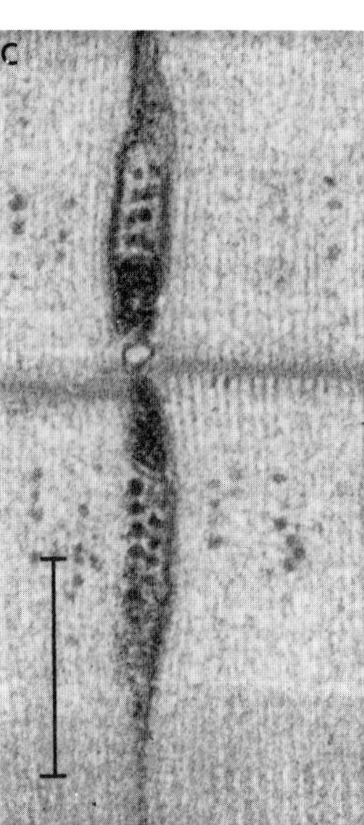

FIG. 32. Triads in muscle fibers from frog semitendinosus muscles. *A*: control untreated with ruthenium red. *B* and *C*: muscles treated with ruthenium red after and before glutaraldehyde fixation, respectively. Uptake of ruthenium red by SR and fusion of SR membranes at intermediate cisternae level. *A*, × 48,000; *B*, × 94,000; *C*, × 48,000. [From Howell (141), by copyright permission of the Rockefeller University Press.]

at the surface of the SR starts the process, and calcium leads to its own release. The electrical model proposed by Mathias et al. (194) employs a regenerative, voltage-dependent calcium-release process initiated by a depolarization of the SR membrane by the current flowing into the SR from the T tubules. Miledi et al. (205) found that calcium release detected with the dye arsenazo III is a smooth function of membrane potential over a rather wide potential range, an unexpected result if calcium release from the SR is regenerative. Baylor et al. (20), however, found a steeper relationship between calcium release and potential in the T tubules, a result more consistent with regenerative release.

Costantin and Podolsky (45) and Stephenson and Podolsky (310) obtained evidence for calcium release from SR induced by depolarization with increased chloride concentrations in skinned fibers. Electric currents applied to skinned fibers also induce contraction (45), possibly by depolarizing part of the SR. Best et al. (27) found an optical signal tentatively thought to reflect an SR membrane voltage change associated with calcium release, although whether this signal is the cause of calcium release and not a result of it is not yet established. These results are consistent with the basic idea of electrically induced calcium release, though they do not prove that it is an important mechanism in the intact muscle cell. Thus we can presently neither reject nor accept a mechanism in which the T tubules and SR are coupled by a process involving direct electrical communication between T tubules and SR during activity. Additional discussion of this mechanism is in the chapters by Baylor and by Martonosi and Beeler in this *Handbook* and in several articles from a recent symposium (124).

The third mechanism, the charge-movement hypothesis, supposes that molecules or assemblies of molecules lie partly within the T-tubule membrane and extend across the junction to the SR membrane. When the T membrane is depolarized to the contraction threshold, these molecules sense the voltage change across the T membrane and move or change shape in such a way as to induce the SR to release calcium (2, 3, 6, 39, 40, 117, 138, 139, 283). The movement of these charged molecules within the T membrane is detected as a nonlinear capacitance or charge movement that is seen when the muscle fiber is depolarized through the range of membrane potentials around the mechanical threshold. The timing and voltage dependence of this signal is such that it could be causally related to the release of calcium into the myoplasm, as detected by calcium-sensitive indicator dyes [(172); see also the chapter by Baylor in this *Handbook*].

The feet are visible structures that extend across the junction from one membrane to the other; the molecules required by the charge-movement mechanism could exist within the feet. The membrane particles in the junctional T tubule, or rather the intrinsic proteins they represent, could be the SR terminal ends of the voltage-sensing molecules proposed by the charge-movement hypothesis. Schneider and Chandler (283) estimated the number of charged groups detected per square micrometer of surface and T membrane. Their estimate agrees within a factor of ~2 with the number of feet in the same area (100). However, this correspondence should not be taken too seriously, because some of the charge moved could be unrelated to EC coupling activity. Similarly, the particles seen in the T membrane could be no more than attachment sites for feet, and feet could serve only the mechanical function of holding the junction together. The structural evidence available now does not allow acceptance or rejection of the mechanical charge-movement model for EC coupling.

Even if the mechanical (molecular) movements proposed in this mechanism do not occur or do not activate the SR to release calcium, whatever the mechanism triggering calcium release is, it does depend on voltage changes across the external membrane of the muscle fiber, including the membranes of the T tubules. A voltage-sensing mechanism must exist, and a gating-current or a charge-movement type of phenomenon must be involved in this voltage-sensing mechanism. Probably this phenomenon is part of what has been seen in the electrical records, though this is not entirely certain now. The next step in the process, the mechanism that passes the effect of the voltage sensor on to the SR, remains most open to interpretations.

SPECIAL GEOMETRY OF T SYSTEM

Longitudinal T Tubules

Longitudinal connections from one T-tubular network to the next one along the muscle fiber in the longitudinal direction are fairly common in invertebrate muscles, e.g., crab muscle fibers (Figs. 14 and 15). They have been described in mammalian cardiac muscle cells (e.g., ref. 99); they are less common in skeletal muscle fibers of vertebrates, where Veratti clearly showed them (316), and rarely seen in electron micrographs of thin sections (159). Such longitudinal T tubules are more easily demonstrated and studied in thick sections (238, 240). They are very apparent in stereoscopic high-voltage electron micrographs of thick sections of muscles infiltrated with the colloidal lanthanum method (264). Figure 33 is a stereoscopic high-voltage electron micrograph showing numerous longitudinal T tubules in a frog muscle. Such longitudinal T tubules are not evenly distributed throughout the volume of the muscle fiber. More common in regions where there are dislocations in the sarcomere banding pattern, they are found only rarely where the bands are well aligned.

Helicoids

Peachey and Eisenberg (239) observed helicoids in the planes of the T-tubule networks in HVEM studies using peroxidase. These three-dimensional, sloped spirals in the T system connect from one sarcomere to the next. Previously it was thought that there were one or two independent T-tubular networks in each sarcomere along the length of a muscle fiber, though there was no direct evidence for or against this. It was thought that the striations were independent planes, and because the striations and the T networks were so precisely aligned, the T networks should also be independent planes. Although researchers observed T tubules connecting longitudinally from one triad to another, it was generally accepted that aside from

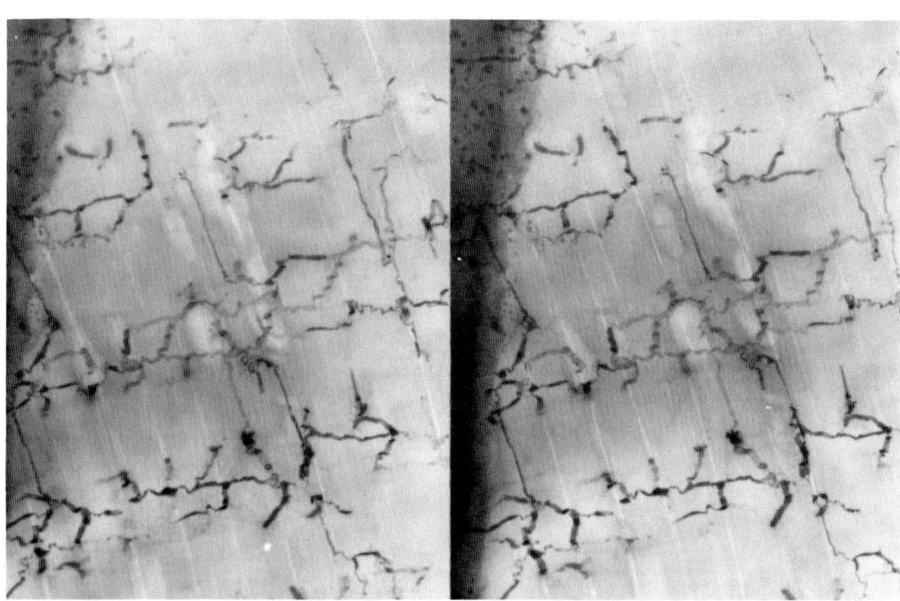

FIG. 33. Stereoscopic high-voltage electron micrograph of an approximately longitudinal section 3 μm thick of frog sartorius muscle fiber. Lanthanum colloid method used to show T tubules. Several longitudinal connections of T tubules from one network to the next. *Left*, fiber surface. Total tilt 10°; 1,000 kV; × 10,000.

such direct longitudinal connections each T-tubule network was independent of its two longitudinally adjacent neighbors and separated from them by the length of a sarcomere. The helicoids, however, suggest that the entire T-tubule population of a muscle fiber may be joined into one continuous unit.

Helicoids can be seen directly in transverse sections of sufficient thickness to include at least one full turn of the helicoid when the muscle is stained with the Golgi method and examined in the HVEM. Figure 34 shows an example of this for a frog twitch fiber. Figure 35 shows the double, interlocking helicoids observed in mammalian muscles with two T systems per sarcomere.

Structural and Functional Implications

ELECTRICAL. Looked at in simple terms, the effects of longitudinal T tubules and helicoids on the measurable electrical properties of muscle fibers must be negligible. The extra membrane and luminal volume introduced by these geometric variations from ideal are only a very small fraction of the total membrane and volume present, so their presence is not detected in measurements of, for example, fiber capacitance. The maximum voltage gradient present from one sarcomere to the next, i.e., in the longitudinal direction along the fiber, is small compared to the maximum voltage gradient in the radial direction during an action potential (5); thus the currents carried by longitudinal T tubules or carried down the ramps of helicoids are always small compared to the larger currents in the radial direction that account for radial spread of the action potentials.

Mathias (193), who made a more complete and rigorous analysis of the electrical effects of helicoids in the T system, concludes that only very minor changes in the function of the T system electrically or in electrical signals recorded with microelectrodes would be expected as a result of the presence of the helicoids.

A possible physiological importance of longitudinally oriented T tubules and helicoids is the electrical continuity they provide across dislocations in the plane of the T-system networks. Propagation around a dislocation at the center of a helicoid might be slower in the absence of longitudinal T tubules than in their presence. In some forms of dislocation a portion of the T-system network could be completely isolated from the rest of the T system were it not for longitudinal T tubules in the dislocation plane. The myofibrils surrounded by the dislocation would be poorly activated at best.

HELICAL BANDING. The helicoidal arrangement of the T-system networks implies that the band patterns of the myofibrils are also arranged helicoidally because of the close relationship between the positions occu-

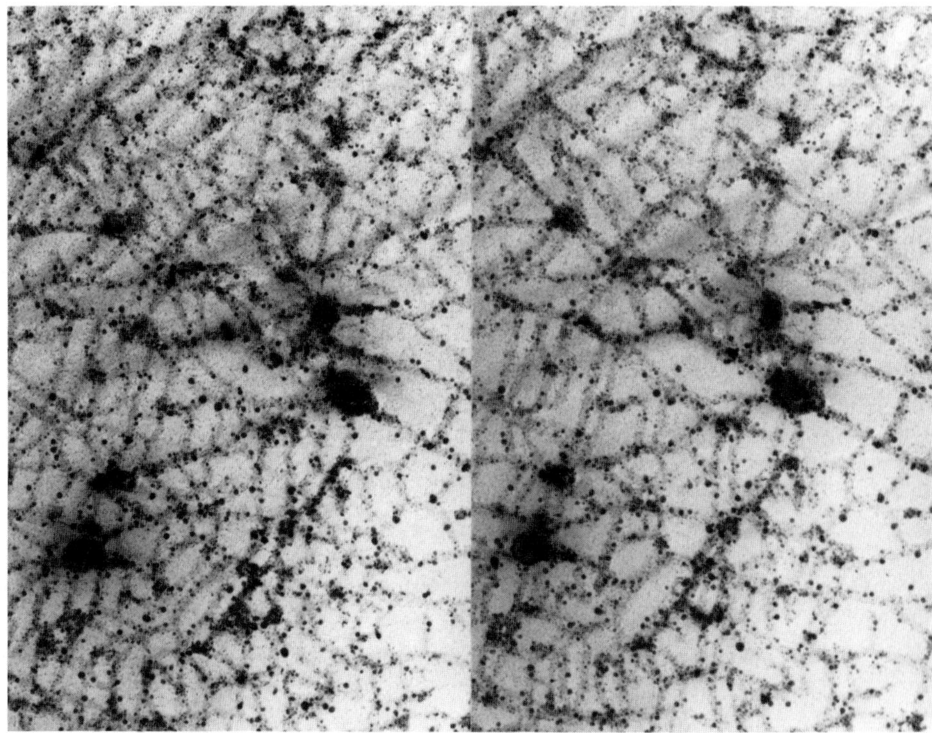

FIG. 34. Stereoscopic high-voltage electron micrograph of transverse section of frog muscle fiber, Golgi stain. Region of fiber with helicoid. Almost 2 turns of helicoid within section 5 μm thick. Total tilt 10°; 1,000 kV; × 8,000.

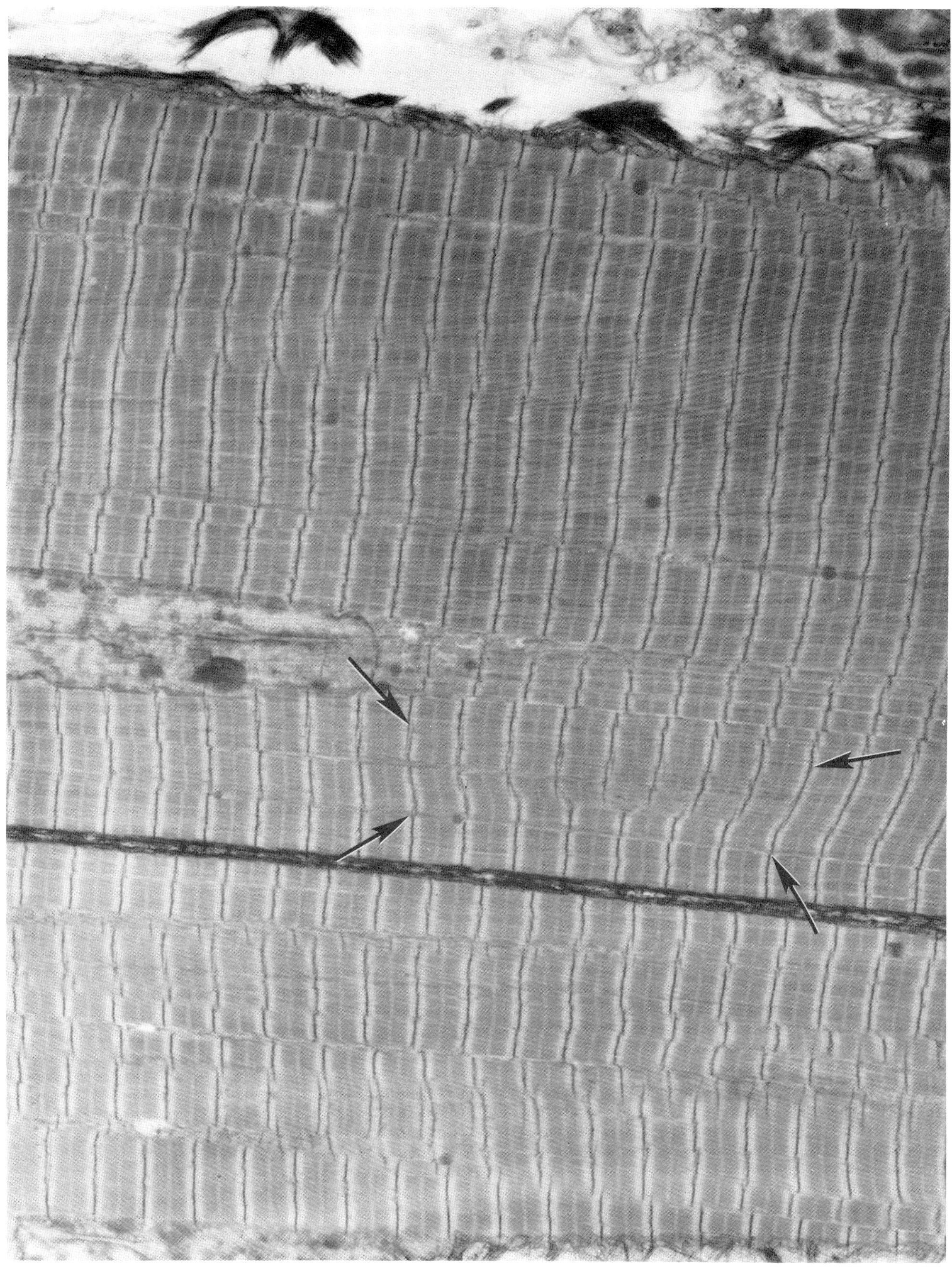

FIG. 36. High-voltage electron micrograph of longitudinal section of frog twitch muscle fiber. Muscle stained with method for SR staining (322), though staining does not show. Displacement of myofibrillar striations occurs, including a vernier displacement between *arrows*. One more sarcomere between 2 *upper arrows* than between *lower arrows*. Section 1 μm thick. 1,000 kV; × 4,000.

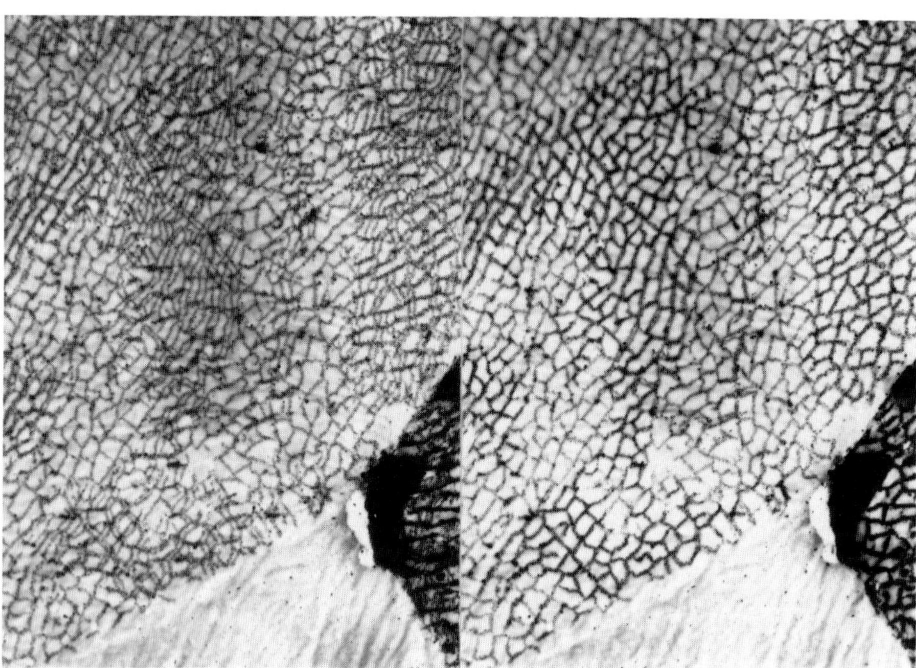

FIG. 35. Stereoscopic high-voltage electron micrograph of transverse section 3 μm thick from rat white muscle fiber, Golgi stain. Double helicoid with 2 T-system networks in sarcomere, each completing slightly more than a single turn of the helicoid. Total tilt 16°; 1,000 kV; × 4,000.

pied by the major elements of the T system and the bands of the immediately adjacent myofibrils. Although T tubules are not easily and commonly observed in light microscopy, the bands are; therefore it would be surprising if the helicoidal arrangement had not at some time been observed, especially by the careful light-microscopic observations of the late nineteenth and early twentieth centuries. A search of the literature that appeared just after the discovery of helicoids in high-voltage electron micrographs (239) revealed no such surprise. In 1955 the well-known Australian entomologist, O. W. Tiegs (313), reviewed a series of his studies in the 1920s in which he observed helicoids in fibers from a variety of species by focusing up and down through thick preparations, following the bands visually and in a series of photographs. Tiegs quotes van Leeuwenhoek, who in 1718 apologized for having said in 1712 that the rings he observed around muscle fibers were circular and corrected his interpretation to a helical model. Bowman (32) called this interpretation "fanciful."

MECHANICAL. At first glance, there seem to be no mechanical implications for the helicoidal arrangement of bands in a muscle fiber. A simple helicoid results in relative longitudinal displacement of the bands of adjacent sarcomeres, but to the extent that adjacent fibrils act as independent force generators in parallel, this displacement should not have an effect on the force produced at the ends of the fibers. However, some helicoids are clearly associated with vernier displacements of the myofibrillar bands; this could introduce some mechanical anomalies. A vernier has two different spacings on the two sides of the dislocation (Fig. 36), implying two populations of sarcomere lengths in the region of the vernier displacement. Because the force generated by a myofibril depends on its sarcomere length (120), two populations of myofibrils at two different sarcomere lengths will produce two different tensions. Whether the magnitude of this effect and the frequency of occurrence of verniers is sufficient to produce measurable effect is not now known, but the effect is worthy of attention.

DIFFRACTION ANOMALIES. Inclined striations, helicoids, and vernier formations in the striations of skeletal muscle fibers can be expected to have considerable influence on the diffraction of light by the fiber. The muscle fiber, instead of acting as a coherent volume grating with fixed spacing and angle, acts as a group of such gratings of different volumes and with different spacings and angles. Diffraction from this ensemble of gratings causes the observed diffraction pattern. Variation of diffraction intensities in contracting fibers and asymmetries between left and right halves of the diffraction pattern are expected in this case and have been observed (18, 19, 164, 226, 271, 272, 312, 327).

The authors' research is supported by National Institutes of Health Grant HL-15835 (to the Pennsylvania Muscle Institute) and by the Muscular Dystrophy Association of America (to the Henry M. Watts Neuromuscular Disease Research Center).

REFERENCES

1. Adrian, R. H. Charge movements in the membrane of striated muscle. *Annu. Rev. Biophys. Bioeng.* 7: 85–112, 1978.
2. Adrian, R. H., and W. Almers. Charge movement in the membrane of striated muscle. *J. Physiol. London* 254: 339–360, 1976.
3. Adrian, R. H., W. K. Chandler, and R. F. Rakowski. Charge movement and mechanical repriming in striated muscle. *J. Physiol. London* 254: 361–388, 1976.
4. Adrian, R. H., and L. D. Peachey. The membrane capacity of frog twitch and slow muscle fibres. *J. Physiol. London* 181: 324–336, 1965.
5. Adrian, R. H., and L. D. Peachey. Reconstruction of the action potential of frog sartorius muscle. *J. Physiol. London* 235: 103–131, 1973.
6. Adrian, R. H., and A. R. Peres. Charge movement and membrane capacity in frog muscle. *J. Physiol. London* 289: 83–97, 1979.
7. Alvarado, J. A., and C. van Horn. Muscle cell types of the cat inferior oblique. In: *Basic Mechanisms of Ocular Motility and Their Clinical Applications,* edited by G. Lennerstrand and P. Bach-y-Rita. Oxford, UK: Pergamon, 1975, p. 15–43.
8. Alvarado-Mallart, R.-M. Ultrastructure of muscle fibers of an extraocular muscle of the pigeon. *Tissue Cell* 4: 327–339, 1972.
9. Andersson-Cedergren, E. Ultrastructure of motor end-plate and sarcoplasmic components of mouse skeletal muscle fiber. *J. Ultrastruct. Res. Suppl.* 1: 1–191, 1959.
10. Armstrong, C. M., F. M. Bezanilla, and P. Horowicz. Twitches in the presence of ethylene glycol bis (β-aminoethyl ether)-*N,N'*-tetraacetic acid. *Biochim. Biophys. Acta* 267: 605–608, 1972.
11. Asmussen, G. The properties of the extraocular muscles of the frog. I. Mechanical properties of the isolated superior oblique and superior rectus muscles. *Acta Biol. Med. Ger.* 37: 301–312, 1978.
12. Atwood, H. L. Differences in muscle fibre properties as a factor in "fast" and "slow" contraction in *Carcinus. Comp. Biochem. Physiol.* 10: 17–32, 1963.
13. Auber, M. Remarques sur l'ultrastructure des myofibrilles chez des scorpions. *J. Microsc. Paris* 2: 233–236, 1963.
14. Bach-y-Rita, P. Structural-functional correlations in eye muscle fibers. Eye muscle proprioception. In: *Basic Mechanisms of Ocular Motility and Their Clinical Implications,* edited by G. Lennerstrand and P. Bach-y-Rita. Oxford, UK: Pergamon, 1975, p. 91–109.
15. Bach-y-Rita, P., and F. Ito. *In vivo* studies on fast and slow muscle fibers in cat extraocular muscles. *J. Gen. Physiol.* 49: 1177–1198, 1966.
16. Bailey, C. H., and L. D. Peachey. High voltage electron microscopy of the T-system in slow fibers of the frog cruralis muscle. *Annu. Proc. Electron Microsc. Soc. Am., 33rd, Las Vegas, Nevada, 1975,* p. 554–555.
17. Barrett, J. N., and E. F. Barrett. Excitation-contraction coupling in skeletal muscle: blockade by high extracellular concentration of calcium buffers. *Science* 200: 1270–1272, 1978.
18. Baskin, R. J., R. L. Lieber, T. Oba, and Y. Yeh. Intensity of light diffracted from striated muscle as a function of incident angle. *Biophys. J.* 36: 759–773, 1981.
19. Baskin, R. J., K. P. Roos, and Y. Yeh. Light diffraction study of single skeletal muscle fibers. *Biophys. J.* 28: 45–64, 1979.
20. Baylor, S. M., W. K. Chandler, and M. W. Marshall. Arsenazo III signals in singly dissected frog muscle fibres. (Abstract). *J. Physiol. London* 287: 23P–24P, 1979.
21. Beaty, G. N., and E. Stefani. Inward calcium current in twitch muscle fibres of the frog (Abstract). *J. Physiol. London* 260: 27P–28P, 1976.
22. Beaty, G. N., and E. Stefani. Calcium dependent electrical activity in twitch muscle fibres of the frog. *Proc. R. Soc. London Ser. B* 194: 141–150, 1976.
23. Bennett, G. S., S. A. Fellini, Y. Toyama, and H. Holtzer. Redistribution of intermediate filament subunits during skeletal myogenesis and maturation in vitro. *J. Cell Biol.* 82: 577–584, 1979.
24. Bennett, H. S. The structure of striated muscle as seen by the electron microscope. In: *The Structure and Function of Muscle* (1st ed.), edited by G. H. Bourne. New York: Academic, 1960, vol. 1, p. 137–150.
25. Bennett, H. S., and K. R. Porter. An electron microscope study of sectioned breast muscle of the domestic fowl. *Am. J. Anat.* 932: 61–105, 1953.
26. Berne, R. M., and N. Sperelakis (editors). *Handbook of Physiology. Cardiovascular System.* Bethesda, MD: Am. Physiol. Soc., 1979, sect. 2, vol. I.
27. Best, P. M., J. Asayama, and L. E. Ford. Membrane voltage changes associated with calcium movement in skinned muscle fibers. In: *Regulation of Muscle Contraction: Excitation-Contraction Coupling,* edited by A. D. Grinnell and M. A. B. Brazier. New York: Academic, 1981, p. 161–170.
28. Bianchi, C. P., and A. M. Shanes. Calcium influx in skeletal muscle at rest, during activity, and during potassium contracture. *J. Gen. Physiol.* 42: 803–815, 1959.
29. Birsk, R. I., and D. F. Davey. Osmotic responses demonstrating the extracellular character of the sarcoplasmic reticulum. *J. Physiol. London* 202: 171–188, 1969.
30. Blinks, J. R., R. Rüdel, and S. R. Taylor. Calcium transients in isolated amphibian skeletal muscle fibres: detection with aequorin. *J. Physiol. London* 277: 291–323, 1978.
31. Bonilla, E. Staining of transverse tubular system of skeletal muscle by tannic acid-glutaraldehyde fixation. *J. Ultrastruct. Res.* 58: 162–165, 1977.
32. Bowman, W. On the minute structure and movements of voluntary muscle. *Philos. Trans. R. Soc. London* 130: 457–501, 1840.
33. Brandt, D. E., and C. R. Leeson. Structural differences of fast and slow fibers in human extraocular muscle. *Am. J. Ophthalmol.* 62: 478–487, 1966.
34. Brandt, P. N., J. P. Reuben, L. Girardier, and H. Grundfest. Correlated morphological and physiological studies on isolated single muscle fibers. I. Fine structure of the crayfish muscle fiber. *J. Cell Biol.* 25: 233–260, 1965.
35. Cajal, S. R. Coloration par la méthode de Golgi des terminaisons des trachées et des nerfs dans les muscles des ailes des insectes. *Z. Wiss. Mikrosk.* 7: 332–342, 1890.
36. Campbell, K. P., C. Franzini-Armstrong, and A. E. Shamoo. Further characterization of light and heavy sarcoplasmic reticulum vesicles. *Biochim. Biophys. Acta* 602: 97–116, 1980.
37. Caputo, C. Excitation and contraction processes in muscle. *Annu. Rev. Biophys. Bioeng.* 7: 63–83, 1978.
38. Castillo de Maruenda, E., and C. Franzini-Armstrong. Satellite and invasive cells in frog sartorius muscle. *Tissue Cell* 10: 749–772, 1978.
39. Chandler, W. K., R. F. Rakowski, and M. F. Schneider. A non-linear voltage dependent charge movement in frog skeletal muscle. *J. Physiol. London* 254: 245–283, 1976.
40. Chandler, W. K., R. F. Rakowski, and M. F. Schneider. Effects of glycerol treatment and maintained depolarization on charge movement in skeletal muscle. *J. Physiol. London* 254: 285–316, 1976.
41. Chiarandini, D. J., and J. Davidowitz. Structure and function of extraocular muscle fibers. In: *Current Topics in Eye Research,* edited by J. A. Zadunaisky and H. Davson. New York: Academic, 1979, vol. 1, p. 91–142.
42. Clark, A. W., and E. Schultz. Rattlesnake shaker muscle. II. Fine structure. *Tissue Cell* 12: 335–351, 1980.
43. Costantin, L. L. Contractile activation in skeletal muscle. *Prog. Biophys. Mol. Biol.* 29: 197–224, 1975.
44. Costantin, L. L. Activation in striated muscle. In: *Handbook of Physiology. The Nervous System,* edited by J. M. Brookhart and V. B. Mountcastle. Bethesda, MD: Am. Physiol. Soc., 1977, sect. 1, vol. I, pt. 1, chapt. 7, p. 215–259.

45. Costantin, L. L., and R. J. Podolsky. Depolarization of the internal membrane system in the activation of frog skeletal muscle. *J. Gen. Physiol.* 50: 1101–1124, 1967.
46. Costantin, L. L., R. J. Podolsky, and L. W. Tice. Calcium activation of frog slow muscle fibres. *J. Physiol. London* 188: 261–271, 1967.
47. Crowe, L. M., and R. J. Baskin. Stereological analysis of developing sarcotubular membranes. *J. Ultrastruct. Res.* 58: 10–21, 1977.
48. Crowe, L. M., and R. J. Baskin. Freeze-fracture of intact sarcotubular membranes. *J. Ultrastruct. Res.* 62: 147–154, 1978.
49. Cull-Candy, S. G., R. Miledi, Y. Nakajima, and O. D. Uchitel. Visualization of satellite cells in living muscle fibres of the frog. *Proc. R. Soc. London Ser. B* 209: 563–568, 1980.
50. D'Ancona, U. Per la miglior conoscenza delle terminazione nervose nei muscole somatici dei crostacei decapodi. *Trav. Biol. Univ. Madrid* 23: 393–423, 1925.
51. Davidowitz, J., G. Philips, and G. M. Breinin. Organization of the orbital surface layer in rabbit superior rectus. *Invest. Ophthalmol.* 16: 711–729, 1977.
52. Davidowitz, J., G. Philips, and G. M. Breinin. Variation of mitochondrial volume fraction along multiply innervated fibers in rabbit extraocular muscle. *Tissue Cell* 12: 449–457, 1980.
53. Deamer, D. W., and R. J. Baskin. Ultrastructure of sarcoplasmic reticulum preparations. *J. Cell Biol.* 42: 269–307, 1969.
54. Devine, C. E., A. V. Somlyo, and A. P. Somlyo. Sarcoplasmic reticulum and excitation-contraction coupling in mammalian smooth muscle. *J. Cell Biol.* 52: 690–718, 1972.
55. Dewey, M. M., and L. Barr. A study of the structure and distribution of the nexus. *J. Cell Biol.* 23: 553–585, 1964.
56. Dulhunty, A. F. The effect of chloride withdrawal on the geometry of the T-tubules in amphibian and mammalian muscle. *J. Membr. Biol.* 67: 81–90, 1982.
57. Dulhunty, A. F., and C. Franzini-Armstrong. The relative contributions of the folds and caveolae to the surface membrane of frog skeletal muscle fibres at different sarcomere lengths. *J. Physiol. London* 250: 513–538, 1975.
58. Dupont, Y., S. C. Harrison, and W. Hasselbach. Molecular organization in the sarcoplasmic reticulum studied by X-ray diffraction. *Nature London* 244: 555–558, 1973.
59. Eastwood, A. B., C. Franzini-Armstrong, and C. Peracchia. Freeze-fracture of crustacean muscle. *J. Muscle Res. Cell Motil.* 3: 273–294, 1982.
60. Ebashi, S. Excitation contraction coupling. *Annu. Rev. Physiol.* 38: 293–313, 1976.
61. Ebashi, S. The Croonian Lecture, 1979. Regulation of muscle contraction. *Proc. R. Soc. London Ser. B* 207: 259–286, 1980.
62. Ebashi, S., and M. Endo. Calcium and muscle contraction. *Prog. Biophys. Mol. Biol.* 18: 123–183, 1968.
63. Ebashi, S., M. Endo, and I. Ohtsuki. Control of muscle contraction. *Q. Rev. Biophys.* 2: 351–384, 1969.
64. Ebashi, S., K. Maruyama, and M. Endo (editors). *Muscle Contraction: Its Regulatory Mechanisms.* Berlin: Springer-Verlag, 1980.
65. Edge, M. B. Development of apposed sarcoplasmic reticulum at the T system and sarcolemma and the change in orientation of triads in rat skeletal muscle. *Dev. Biol.* 23: 634–659, 1970.
66. Eisenberg, B. R., and R. S. Eisenberg. Selective disruption of the sarcotubular system in frog sartorius muscle: a quantitative study with exogenous peroxidase as a marker. *J. Cell Biol.* 39: 451–467, 1968.
67. Eisenberg, B. R., and R. S. Eisenberg. The T-SR junction in contracting single skeletal muscle fibers. *J. Gen. Physiol.* 79: 1–19, 1982.
68. Eisenberg, B. R., and A. Gilai. Structural changes in single muscle fibers after stimulation at a low frequency. *J. Gen. Physiol.* 74: 1–16, 1979.
69. Eisenberg, B. R., R. T. Mathias, and A. Gilai. Intracellular localization of markers within injected or cut frog muscle fibers. *Am. J. Physiol.* 237 (*Cell Physiol.* 6): C50–C55, 1979.
70. Eisenberg, B. R., and L. D. Peachey. The network parameters of the T-system in frog muscle measured with the high voltage electron microscope. *Annu. Proc. Electron Microsc. Soc. Am., 33rd, Las Vegas, Nevada, 1975,* p. 550–551.
71. Eisenberg, R. S. The equivalent circuit of single crab muscle fibers as determined by impedance measurements with intracellular electrodes. *J. Gen. Physiol.* 50: 1785–1806, 1967.
72. Eisenberg, R. S., and P. W. Gage. Frog skeletal muscle fibers: changes in electrical properties after disruption of transverse tubular system. *Science* 158: 1700–1701, 1967.
73. Endo, M. Entry of fluorescent dyes into the sarcotubular system of frog muscle. *J. Physiol. London* 185: 224–238, 1964.
74. Endo, M. Calcium release from the sarcoplasmic reticulum. *Physiol. Rev.* 57: 71–108, 1977.
75. Endo, M., and Y. Nakajima. Release of calcium induced by "depolarization" of the sarcoplasmic reticulum membrane. *Nature London New Biol.* 246: 216–218, 1973.
76. Engel, A. G. Morphologic and immunopathologic findings in myasthenia gravis and in congenital myasthenic syndrome. *J. Neurol. Neurosurg. Psychiatry* 43: 577–589, 1980.
77. Engel, A. G., and R. D. McDonald. Ultrastructural reactions in muscle disease and their light microscopic correlates. In: *Proc. Int. Congr. Muscle Dis., Milan, 1969.* Amsterdam: Excerpta Med., 1969, p. 71–89. (Int. Congr. Ser. No. 199.)
78. Engel, A. G., T. Santa, and H. H. Stonnington. Morphometric studies of skeletal muscle ultrastructure. *Muscle Nerve* 2: 229–237, 1979.
79. Ezerman, E. B., and H. Ishikawa. Differentiation of the sarcoplasmic reticulum and T system in developing chick skeletal muscle in vitro. *J. Cell Biol.* 35: 405–420, 1967.
80. Fabiato, A. Myoplasmic free calcium concentration reached during the twitch of an intact isolated cardiac cell and during calcium-induced release of calcium from the sarcoplasmic reticulum of a skinned cardiac cell from the adult rat or rabbit ventricle. *J. Gen. Physiol.* 78: 457–497, 1981.
81. Fabiato, A., and F. Fabiato. Calcium and cardiac excitation-contraction coupling. *Annu. Rev. Physiol.* 41: 473–484, 1979.
82. Fahrenbach, W. H. The sarcoplasmic reticulum of striated muscle of a cyclopoid copepod. *J. Cell Biol.* 17: 629–640, 1963.
83. Fahrenbach, W. H. A new configuration of the sarcoplasmic reticulum. *J. Cell Biol.* 22: 477–481, 1964.
84. Fahrenbach, W. H. The fine structure of fast and slow crustacean muscle. *J. Cell Biol.* 35: 69–79, 1967.
85. Falk, G., and P. Fatt. Linear electrical properties of striated muscle fibres observed with intracellular electrodes. *Proc. R. Soc. London Ser. B* 160: 69–123, 1964.
86. Fatt, P. An analysis of the transverse electrical impedance of striated muscle. *Proc. R. Soc. London Ser. B* 159: 606–651, 1964.
87. Fatt, P., and B. L. Ginsborg. The ionic requirements for the production of action potentials in crustacean muscle fibres. *J. Physiol. London* 142: 516–543, 1958.
88. Fatt, P., and B. Katz. An analysis of the end-plate potential recorded with an intra-cellular electrode. *J. Physiol. London* 115: 320–370, 1951.
89. Fatt, P., and B. Katz. The electrical properties of crustacean muscle fibres. *J. Physiol. London* 120: 171–204, 1953.
90. Fawcett, D. W., and N. S. McNutt. The ultrastructure of the cat myocardium. *J. Cell Biol.* 42: 1–45, 1969.
91. Fawcett, D. W., and J. P. Revel. The sarcoplasmic reticulum of a fast-acting fish muscle. *J. Biophys. Biochem. Cytol.* 1(4), Suppl.: 89–109, 1961.
92. Flitney, F. W. The volume of the T-system and its association with the sarcoplasmic reticulum in slow muscle fibres of the frog. *J. Physiol. London* 217: 243–257, 1971.
93. Flood, P. R. Structure of the segmental trunk muscle in amphioxus. With notes on the course and "endings" of the so-called ventral root fibres. *Z. Zellforsch. Mikrosk. Anat.* 84: 389–416, 1968.
94. Flood, P. R. The sarcoplasmic reticulum and associated plasma membrane of trunk muscle lamellae in *Branchiostoma lanceolatum* (Pallas). A transmission and scanning electron microscopic study including freeze-fractures, direct replicas

and X-ray microanalysis of calcium oxylate deposits. *Cell Tissue Res.* 181: 169–196, 1977.

95. FORBES, M. S., AND N. SPERELAKIS. Myocardial couplings: their structural variations in the mouse. *J. Ultrastruct. Res.* 58: 50–65, 1977.
96. FORBES, M. S., AND N. SPERELAKIS. Ruthenium red staining of skeletal and cardiac muscles. *Cell Tissue Res.* 200: 367–382, 1979.
97. FORBES, M. S., AND N. SPERELAKIS. Membrane systems in skeletal muscle of the lizard, *Anolis carolinensis. J. Ultrastruct. Res.* 73: 245–261, 1980.
98. FORD, L. E., AND R. J. PODOLSKY. Intracellular calcium movements in skinned muscle fibres. *J. Physiol. London* 223: 21–33, 1972.
99. FORSSMANN, W. G., AND L. GIRARDIER. A study of the T system in rat heart. *J. Cell Biol.* 44: 1–19, 1970.
100. FRANZINI-ARMSTRONG, C. Studies of the triad. I. Structure of the junction in frog twitch fibers. *J. Cell Biol.* 47: 488–499, 1970.
101. FRANZINI-ARMSTRONG, C. Studies of the triad. II. Penetration of tracer into the junctional gap. *J. Cell Biol.* 49: 196–203, 1971.
102. FRANZINI-ARMSTRONG, C. Studies of the triad. IV. Structure of the junction in frog slow fibers. *J. Cell Biol.* 56: 120–128, 1973.
103. FRANZINI-ARMSTRONG, C. Membranous systems in muscle fibers. In: *The Structure and Function of Muscle* (2nd ed.) edited by G. H. Bourne. New York: Academic, 1973, vol. 2, p. 531–619.
104. FRANZINI-ARMSTRONG, C. Freeze-fracture of striated muscle from a spider. Structural differentiations of sarcoplasmic reticulum and transverse tubular membranes. *J. Cell Biol.* 61: 501–520, 1974.
105. FRANZINI-ARMSTRONG, C. Membrane particles and transmission at the triad. *Federation Proc.* 34: 1382–1389, 1975.
106. FRANZINI-ARMSTRONG, C. The comparative structure of intracellular junctions in striated muscle fibers. In: *Pathogenesis of Muscular Dystrophies, Proc. Int. Conf. Muscular Dystrophy Assoc., 5th, Durango, Colorado, June 21–25, 1976,* p. 612–625.
107. FRANZINI-ARMSTRONG, C. Structure of the sarcoplasmic reticulum. *Federation Proc.* 39: 2403–2409, 1980.
108. FRANZINI-ARMSTRONG, C., A. B. EASTWOOD, AND L. D. PEACHEY. A new view of Veratti's "reticulum" in crustacean muscle fibers (Abstract). *J. Cell Biol.* 79: 330a, 1978.
108a. FRANZINI-ARMSTRONG, C., AND G. NUNZI. Junctional feet and particles in the triads of a fast twitch muscle fiber. *J. Muscle Res. Cell Motil.* In press.
109. FRANZINI-ARMSTRONG, C., AND L. D. PEACHEY. Striated muscle—contractile and control mechanisms. *J. Cell Biol.* 91: 166s–186s, 1981.
110. FRANZINI-ARMSTRONG, C., AND L. D. PEACHEY. A modified Golgi black reaction method for light and electron microscopy. *J. Histochem. Cytochem.* 30: 99–105, 1982.
111. FRANZINI-ARMSTRONG, C., AND K. R. PORTER. Sarcolemmal invaginations constituting the T-system in fish muscle fibers. *J. Cell Biol.* 22: 675–696, 1964.
112. FUJINO, M., T. YAMAGUCHI, AND K. SUZUKI. Glycerol effect and the mechanism linking excitation of the plasma membrane with contraction. *Nature London* 192: 1159–1161, 1961.
113. GILAI, A., AND I. PARNAS. Electromechanical coupling in tubular muscle fibers. I. The organization of tubular muscle fibers in the scorpion *Leiurus quinquestriatus. J. Cell Biol.* 52: 626–638, 1972.
114. GILLIS, J. M., A. PIRONT, AND C. GOSSELIN-REY. Parvalbumins. Distribution and physical state inside the muscle cell. *Biochim. Biophys. Acta* 585: 444–450, 1979.
115. GILLY, W. F., AND C. S. HUI. Mechanical activation in slow and twitch skeletal muscle fibres of the frog. *J. Physiol. London* 301: 137–156, 1980.
116. GILLY, W. F., AND C. S. HUI. Membrane electrical properties of frog slow muscle fibres. *J. Physiol. London* 301: 157–173, 1980.
117. GILLY, W. F., AND C. S. HUI. Voltage-dependent charge movement in frog slow muscle fibres. *J. Physiol. London* 301: 175–190, 1980.
118. GOLDSTEIN, M. A. A morphological and cytochemical study of sarcoplasmic reticulum and T system of fish extraocular muscle. *Z. Zellforsch. Mikrosk. Anat.* 102: 31–39, 1969.
119. GOLDSTEIN, M. A. Anionic binding of ruthenium red in fish extraocular muscle. *Z. Zellforsch. Mikrosk. Anat.* 102: 459–465, 1969.
120. GORDON, A. M., A. F. HUXLEY, AND F. J. JULIAN. The variation of isometric tension with sarcomere length in vertebrate muscle fibres. *J. Physiol. London* 184: 170–192, 1966.
121. GOSSELIN-REY, C., AND C. GERDAY. Parvalbumins from frog skeletal muscle (*Rana temporaria* L.); isolation and characterization; structural modifications associated with calcium binding. *Biochem. Biophys. Acta* 492: 53–63, 1977.
122. GRAHAM, R. C., AND M. J. KARNOVSKY. The early stages of absorption of injected horseradish peroxidase in the proximal tubules of mouse kidney: ultrastructural cytochemistry by a new technique. *J. Histochem. Cytochem.* 14: 291–302, 1966.
123. GRENACHER, H. Beiträge zur nähern Kenntniss der Muskulatur der Cyclostoma und Leptocardier. *Z. Wiss. Zool.* 17: 577–597, 1867.
124. GRINNELL, A. D., AND M. A. BRAZIER (editors). *The Regulation of Muscle Contraction: Excitation-Contraction Coupling.* New York: Academic, 1981.
125. GUPTA, B. L., AND T. A. HALL. The X-ray microanalysis of frozen-hydrated sections in scanning electron microscopy. *Tissue Cell* 13: 623–643, 1981.
126. HAGIWARA, S., M. P. HENKART, AND Y. KIDOKORO. Excitation contraction coupling in amphioxus muscle cells. *J. Physiol. London* 219: 233–251, 1971.
127. HAGOPIAN, M., AND D. SPIRO. The sarcoplasmic reticulum and its association with the T system in an insect. *J. Cell Biol.* 32: 535–545, 1967.
128. HAIECH, J., J. DERANCOURT, AND J. G. DEMAILLE. Magnesium and calcium binding to parvalbumins: evidence for differences between parvalbumins and an explanation of their relaxing function. *Biochemistry* 13: 2752–2758, 1979.
129. HAMOIR, G., AND B. FOCANT. Proteinic differences between the sarcoplasmic reticulums of the superfast swimbladder and the fast skeletal muscles of the toadfish *Opsanus tau. Mol. Physiol.* 1: 353–359, 1981.
130. HARRIS, E. J. Distribution and movement of muscle chloride. *J. Physiol. London* 166: 87–109, 1963.
131. HERBETTE, L., J. MORQUART, A. SCARPA, AND J. K. BLASIE. A direct analysis of lamellar X-ray diffraction from hydrated oriented multilayers of fully-functional sarcoplasmic reticulum. *Biophys. J.* 20: 245–272, 1977.
132. HESS, A. The structure of slow and fast extrafusal muscle fibers in the extraocular muscles and their nerve endings in guinea pigs. *J. Cell. Comp. Physiol.* 58: 63–79, 1961.
133. HESS, A., AND G. PILAR. Slow fibres in the extraocular muscles of the cat. *J. Physiol. London* 169: 780–798, 1963.
134. HIDALGO, C., AND N. IKEMOTO. Disposition of proteins and amino phospholipids in the sarcoplasmic reticulum membrane. *J. Biol. Chem.* 252: 8446–8454, 1977.
135. HILL, A. V. On the time required for diffusion and its relation to processes in muscle. *Proc. R. Soc. London Ser. B* 135: 446–453, 1948.
136. HILL, A. V. The abrupt transition from rest to activity in muscle. *Proc. R. Soc. London Ser. B* 136: 399–420, 1949.
137. HODGKIN, A. L., AND P. HOROWICZ. The effect of sudden changes in ionic concentrations on the membrane potential of single muscle fibres. *J. Physiol. London* 153: 370–385, 1960.
138. HOROWICZ, P., AND M. F. SCHNEIDER. Membrane charge movement in contracting and non-contracting skeletal muscle fibres. *J. Physiol. London* 314: 565–593, 1981.
139. HOROWICZ, P., AND M. F. SCHNEIDER. Membrane charge moved at contraction thresholds in skeletal muscle fibres. *J. Physiol. London* 314: 595–633, 1981.
140. HOWELL, J. N. A lesion of the transverse tubules of skeletal muscle. *J. Physiol. London* 201: 515–533, 1969.

141. HOWELL, J. N. Intracellular binding of ruthenium red in frog skeletal muscle. *J. Cell Biol.* 62: 242–247, 1974.
142. HOWELL, J. N., AND D. J. JENDEN. T-tubules of skeletal muscle: morphological alterations which interrupt excitation-contraction coupling (Abstract). *Federation Proc.* 26: 553a, 1967.
143. HOYLE, G. Comparative aspects of muscle. *Annu. Rev. Physiol.* 31: 43–84, 1969.
144. HOYLE, G., P. A. MCNEILL, AND A. I. SELVERSTON. Ultrastructure of barnacle giant muscle fibers. *J. Cell Biol.* 56: 74–91, 1973.
145. HOYLE, G., P. A. MCNEILL, AND B. WALCOTT. Nature of invaginating tubules in *Felderstruktur* muscle fibers of the garter snake. *J. Cell Biol.* 30: 197–201, 1966.
146. HUTCHINSON, T. E. Determination of subcellular elemental composition through ultrahigh resolution electron microprobe analysis. *Int. Rev. Cytol.* 58: 115–158, 1979.
147. HUXLEY, A. F. The Croonian Lecture, 1967. The activation of striated muscle and its mechanical response. *Proc. R. Soc. London Ser. B* 178: 1–27, 1971.
148. HUXLEY, A. F. Looking back on muscle. In: *The Pursuit of Nature,* edited by A. L. Hodgkin, et al. Cambridge, UK: Cambridge Univ. Press, 1977, p. 23–64.
149. HUXLEY, A. F., AND L. D. PEACHEY. Local activation of crab muscle (Abstract). *J. Cell Biol.* 23: 107A, 1964.
150. HUXLEY, A. F., AND R. E. TAYLOR. Function of Krause's membrane (Abstract). *Nature London* 176: 1068, 1955.
151. HUXLEY, A. F., AND R. E. TAYLOR. Local activation of striated muscle fibres. *J. Physiol. London* 144: 426–441, 1958.
152. HUXLEY, H. E. Evidence for continuity between the central elements of the triads and extracellular space in frog sartorius muscle. *Nature London* 202: 1067–1071, 1964.
153. HUXLEY, H. E., S. PAGE, AND D. R. WILKIE. An electron microscopic study of muscle in hypertonic solutions (Appendix to M. Dydynska and D. R. Wilkie). *J. Physiol. London* 169: 312–329, 1963.
154. ILDEFONSE, M., J. PAGER, AND O. ROUGIER. Analyse des propriétés de rectification de la fibre musculaire squelettique rapides aprés traitement au Glycérol. *C. R. Acad. Sci. Paris* 268: 2783–2786, 1969.
155. ISHIKAWA, H. Formation of elaborate networks of T-system tubules in cultured skeletal muscle with special reference to the T-system formation. *J. Cell Biol.* 38: 51–66, 1968.
156. ISHIKAWA, H., Y. FUKUDA, AND E. YAMADA. Freeze-replica observations on frog sartorius muscle. I. Sarcolemmal specializations. *J. Electron Microsc.* 24: 97–107, 1975.
157. ISHIKAWA, H., AND E. YAMADA. Differentiation of the sarcoplasmic reticulum and T-system in developing mouse cardiac muscle. In: *Developmental and Physiological Correlates of Cardiac Muscle,* edited by M. Lieberman and T. Sano. New York: Raven, 1971, p. 21–35.
158. JAHROMI, S. S., AND H. L. ATWOOD. Correlation of structure, speed of contraction and total tension in fast and slow abdominal muscles of the lobster (*Homarus americanus*). *J. Exp. Zool.* 171: 25–38, 1969.
159. JASPER, D. Body muscles of the lamprey: some structural features of the T system and sarcolemma. *J. Cell Biol.* 32: 219–227, 1967.
160. JEWETT, P. H., J. R. SOMMER, AND E. A. JOHNSON. Cardiac muscle. Its ultrastructure in the finch and hummingbird with special reference to the sarcoplasmic reticulum. *J. Cell Biol.* 49: 50–65, 1971.
161. JOHNSON, E. A., AND J. R. SOMMER. A strand of cardiac muscle. Its ultrastructure and the electrophysiological implications of its geometry. *J. Cell Biol.* 33: 103–129, 1967.
162. JORGENSEN, A. O., V. KALNINS, AND D. H. MACLENNAN. Localization of sarcoplasmic reticulum proteins in rat skeletal muscle by immunofluorescence. *J. Cell Biol.* 80: 372–384, 1979.
163. JORGENSEN, A. O., A. C. Y. SHEN, D. H. MACLENNAN, AND K. T. TOKUYASHI. Ultrastructural localization of the $Ca^{2+} + Mg^{2+}$-dependent ATPase of sarcoplasmic reticulum in rat skeletal muscle by immunoferritin labeling of ultrathin frozen sections. *J. Cell Biol.* 92: 409–416, 1982.
164. JUDY, M. M., V. SUMMEROUR, T. LECONEY, R. L. ROA, AND G. H. TEMPLETON. Muscle diffraction theory. Relationship between diffraction subpeaks and discrete sarcomere length distributions. *Biophys. J.* 37: 475–487, 1982.
165. KARP, R., J. C. SILCOX, AND A. V. SOMLYO. Cryoultramicrotomy: evidence against melting and the use of a low temperature cement for specimen preparation. *J. Microsc.* 125: 157–165, 1982.
166. KATZ, B. The electrical properties of the muscle fibre membrane. *Proc. R. Soc. London Ser. B* 135: 506–534, 1948.
167. KELLY, A. M. Myofibrillogenesis and Z-band differentiation. *Anat. Rec.* 163: 403–426, 1968.
168. KELLY, A. M. Sarcoplasmic reticulum and T-tubules in differentiating rat skeletal muscle. *J. Cell Biol.* 49: 335–344, 1971.
169. KELLY, A. M. T tubules in neonatal rat soleus and extensor digitorum longus muscles. *Dev. Biol.* 80: 501–505, 1980.
170. KELLY, D. E. The fine structure of skeletal muscle triad junctions. *J. Ultrastruct. Res.* 29: 37–49, 1969.
171. KELLY, D. E., AND A. M. KUDA. Subunits of triadic junctions in fast skeletal muscle as revealed by freeze-fracture. *J. Ultrastruct. Res.* 68: 220–233, 1979.
172. KOVACS, L., E. RIOS, AND M. F. SCHNEIDER. Calcium transients and intramembrane charge movements in skeletal muscle fibers. *Nature London* 279: 391–396, 1979.
173. KROLENKO, S. A. Changes in the T system of muscle fibers under the influence of influx and efflux of glycerol. *Nature London* 221: 966–968, 1969.
174. KRÜGER, P. *Tetanus und Tonus der guergestreiften Skeletmuskeln der Wirbeltiere und des Menschen.* Leipzig, East Germany: Akad. Verlagsgesellschaft, 1952.
175. KULCZYCKY, S., AND G. W. MAINWOOD. Evidence for a functional connection between the sarcoplasmic reticulum and the extracellular space in frog sartorius muscle. *Can. J. Physiol. Pharmacol.* 50: 87–89, 1972.
176. LÄNNERGREN, J. Structure and function of twitch and slow fibers in amphibian skeletal muscle. In: *Basic Mechanisms of Ocular Motility and Their Clinical Implications,* edited by G. Lennerstrand and P. Bach-y-Rita. New York: Pergammon, 1975, p. 63–84.
177. LAU, Y. H., A. H. CASWELL, AND J. P. BRUNSCHWIG. Isolation of transverse tubules by fractionation of triad junctions of skeletal muscle. *J. Biol. Chem.* 252: 5565–5574, 1977.
178. LAU, Y. H., A. H. CASWELL, J. P. BRUNSCHWIG, R. J. BAERWALD, AND M. GARCIA. Lipid analysis and freeze-fracture studies on isolated transverse tubules and sarcoplasmic reticulum fractions of skeletal muscle. *J. Biol. Chem.* 254: 540–546, 1979.
179. LAVALLARD, R. *Estudo com o microscópio eletrônico do retículo endoplasmático em fibras musculares de carangueijos.* São Paulo, Brazil: Univ. of São Paulo, 1960, Bull. 260, Zool. 23, p. 141–169.
180. LAZARIDES, E. The distribution of desmin (100 Å) filaments in primary cultures of embryonic chick cardiac cells. *Exp. Cell Res.* 112: 265–273, 1978.
181. LAZARIDES, E. Intermediate filaments as mechanical integrators of cellular space. *Nature London* 283: 249–256, 1980.
182. LAZARIDES, E., AND B. H. HUBBARD. Immunological characterization of the subunit of 100 Å filaments from muscle cells. *Proc. Natl. Acad. Sci. USA* 73: 4344–4348, 1976.
183. LECHENE, C. Electron probe microanalysis of biological soft tissues: principles and technique. *Federation Proc.* 39: 2871–2880, 1980.
184. LEEUWENHOEK, A. VAN. A letter from Mr. Anthony van Leeuwenhoek, F.R.S. Containing his observations upon the seminal vesicles, muscular fibres, and blood of whales. *Philos. Trans. R. Soc. London Ser. B* 27: 438–446, 1712.
185. LUFF, A. R., AND H. L. ATWOOD. Changes in the sarcoplasmic reticulum and transverse tubular system of fast and slow skeletal muscles of the mouse during postnatal development. *J. Cell Biol.* 51: 369–383, 1971.

186. LUFT, J. H. Fine structure of nerve and muscle cell membrane: permeability to ruthenium red. *Anat. Rec.* 154: 379–380, 1966.
187. LUFT, J. H. Ruthenium red and violet. II. Fine structural localization in animal tissues. *Anat. Rec.* 171: 369–415, 1971.
188. LÜTTGAU, H. C., AND W. SPIECKER. The effects of calcium deprivation upon mechanical and electrophysiological parameters in skeletal muscle fibres of the frog. *J. Physiol. London* 296: 411–429, 1979.
189. MACLENNAN, D. H. Purification and properties of an adenosinetriphosphatase from the sarcoplasmic reticulum. *J. Biol. Chem.* 245: 4508–4518, 1970.
190. MACLENNAN, D. H., AND P. C. HOLLAND. Calcium transport in sarcoplasmic reticulum. *Annu. Rev. Biophys. Bioeng.* 4: 377–404, 1975.
191. MACLENNAN, D. H., AND P. T. S. WONG. Isolation of a calcium-sequestering protein from sarcoplasmic reticulum. *Proc. Natl. Acad. Sci. USA* 68: 1231–1235, 1971.
192. MARTONOSI, A., D. ROUFA, E. REYES, AND T. W. TILLACK. Development of sarcoplasmic reticulum in cultured chicken muscle. *J. Biol. Chem.* 252: 318–332, 1977.
193. MATHIAS, R. T. An analysis of the electrical properties of a skeletal muscle fiber containing a helicoidal T system. *Biophys. J.* 23: 277–284, 1978.
194. MATHIAS, R. T., R. A. LEVIS, AND R. S. EISENBERG. Electrical models of excitation-contraction coupling and charge movement in skeletal muscle. *J. Gen. Physiol.* 76: 1–31, 1980.
195. MATYUSHKIN, D. P., AND T. M. DRABKINA. Electrophysiological characteristics of tonic fibers of the extrinsic ocular muscles. *Fiziol. Zh. SSSR* im. I.M. Sechenova 56: 563–569, 1970.
196. MAURO, A. (editor). *Muscle Regeneration.* New York: Raven, 1979.
197. MAURO, A., AND W. R. ADAMS. The structure of the sarcolemma of the frog skeletal muscle fiber. *J. Biophys. Biochem. Cytol.* 10(4), Suppl.: 177–185, 1961.
198. MAYR, R. Structure and distribution of fibre types in the external eye muscles of the rat. *Tissue Cell* 3: 433–462, 1971.
199. MAZANET, R., B. F. REESE, C. FRANZINI-ARMSTRONG, AND T. S. REESE. Variability in the shapes of satellite cells in normal and injured frog sartorius muscle. *Dev. Biol.* 93: 22–27, 1982.
200. MCCALLISTER, L. P., AND R. HADEK. Transmission electron microscopy and stereo ultrastructure of the T system in frog skeletal muscle. *J. Ultrastruct. Res.* 33: 360–368, 1970.
201. MEIS, L. DE. *The Sarcoplasmic Reticulum. Transport and Energy Transduction.* New York: Wiley, 1981.
202. MEISSNER, G. Isolation and characterization of two types of sarcoplasmic reticulum vesicles. *Biochim. Biophys. Acta* 389: 51–68, 1975.
203. MELZER, W. Die Activierung der Myotome von Branchiostoma lanceolatum. Bochum, West Germany: Ruhr-Universität Bochum, 1980. Dissertation.
204. MILEDI, R., E. PARKER, AND G. SCHALOW. Calcium transients in frog slow muscle fibres. *Nature London* 268: 750–752, 1977.
205. MILEDI, R., E. PARKER, AND G. SCHALOW. Measurement of calcium transients in frog muscle by the use of arsenazo III. *Proc. R. Soc. London Ser. B* 198: 201–210, 1977.
206. MILEDI, R., E. PARKER, AND G. SCHALOW. Calcium transients in normal and denervated slow muscle fibres of the frog. *J. Physiol. London* 318: 191–206, 1981.
207. MILLER, J. E. Cellular organization of *Rhesus* extraocular muscle. *Invest. Ophthalmol.* 6: 18–39, 1967.
208. MILLMAN, B. M., AND P. M. BENNETT. Structure of the cross-striated adductor muscle of the scallop. *J. Mol. Biol.* 102: 439–467, 1976.
209. MOBLEY, B. A., AND G. EIDT. Transverse impedance of single frog skeletal muscle fibers. *Biophys. J.* 40: 51–59, 1982.
210. MOBLEY, B. A., AND B. R. EISENBERG, Sizes of components in frog skeletal muscle measured by methods of stereology. *J. Gen. Physiol.* 66: 31–45, 1975.
211. MORAD, M. (editor). *Biophysical Aspects of Cardiac Muscle.* New York: Academic, 1978.
212. NAKAJIMA, S., Y. NAKAJIMA, AND L. D. PEACHEY. Speed of repolarization and morphology of glycerol-treated frog muscle fibres. *J. Physiol. London* 234: 465–480, 1973.
213. NELSON, D. A., AND E. S. BENSON. On the structural continuities of the transverse tubular system of rabbit and human myocardial cells. *J. Cell Biol.* 16: 217–313, 1963.
214. NEVILLE, M. C. The extracellular compartments of frog skeletal muscle. *J. Physiol. London* 288: 45–70, 1979.
215. NIEDERGERKE, R. Movements of Ca in frog heart ventricles at rest and during contractures. *J. Physiol. London* 167: 515–550, 1963.
216. NIEDERGERKE, R., AND R. K. ORKAND. The dual effect of calcium on the action potential of the frog's heart. *J. Physiol. London* 184: 291–311, 1966.
217. NUNZI, M. G., AND C. FRANZINI-ARMSTRONG. Trabecular network in adult skeletal muscle. *J. Ultrastruct. Res.* 73: 21–26, 1980.
218. NUNZI, M. G., AND C. FRANZINI-ARMSTRONG. The structure of smooth and striated portions of the adductor muscle of the valves in a scallop. *J. Ultrastruct. Res.* 76: 134–148, 1981.
219. OETLIKER, H. An appraisal of the evidence for a sarcoplasmic reticulum membrane potential and its relation to calcium release in skeletal muscle. *J. Muscle Res. Cell Motil.* 3: 247–272, 1982.
220. PAGE, S. G. The organization of the sarcoplasmic reticulum in frog muscle (Abstract). *J. Physiol. London* 175: 10P–11P, 1964.
221. PAGE, S. G. A comparison of the fine structures of frog slow and twitch muscle fibres. *J. Cell Biol.* 26: 477–497, 1965.
222. PAGE, S. G. Fine structure of tortoise skeletal muscle. *J. Physiol. London* 197: 709–715, 1968.
223. PAGE, S. G. Structure and some contractile properties of fast and slow muscles of the chicken. *J. Physiol. London* 205: 131–145, 1969.
224. PAGE, S. G., AND R. NIEDERGERKE. Structures of physiological interest in the frog heart ventricle. *J. Cell Sci.* 11: 179–203, 1972.
225. PALADE, P. T., AND W. ALMERS. Slow Na and Ca currents across the membrane of frog striated muscle fibres (Abstract). *Biophys. J.* 21: 168a, 1978.
226. PAOLINI, P. J., K. P. ROOS, AND R. J. BASKIN. Light diffraction studies of sarcomere dynamics in single skeletal muscle fibers. *Biophys. J.* 20: 221–232, 1977.
227. PAPIR, D. The effect of glycerol treatment on crab muscle fibres. *J. Physiol. London* 230: 313–330, 1973.
228. PASQUALI-RONCHETTI, I. The ultrastructural organization of femoral muscles in *Musca domestica* (Diptera). *Tissue Cell* 2: 339–354, 1970.
229. PEACHEY, L. D. Morphological Pathways for Impulse Conduction in Muscle Cells. New York: Rockefeller Inst., 1959. PhD Thesis.
230. PEACHEY, L. D. Structure and function of slow striated muscle. In: *Biophysics of Physiological and Pharmacological Actions,* edited by A. M. Shanes. Washington, DC: Am. Assoc. Adv. Sci., 1961, p. 391–411.
231. PEACHEY, L. D. Structure of the longitudinal body muscles of amphioxus. *J. Biophys. Biochem. Cytol.* 10 (4), Suppl.: 159–176, 1961.
232. PEACHEY, L. D. The sarcoplasmic reticulum and transverse tubules of the frog's sartorius. *J. Cell Biol.* 25 (3, pt. 2): 209–231, 1965.
233. PEACHEY, L. D. Transverse tubules in excitation-contraction coupling. *Federation Proc.* 24: 1124–1134, 1965.
234. PEACHEY, L. D. Structure of the sarcoplasmic reticulum and T-system of striated muscle. In: *Proc. Int. Congr. Physiol. Sci., 23rd, Tokyo, 1965,* vol. 4, p. 388–398.
235. PEACHEY, L. D. Membrane systems in crab fibers. *Am. Zool.* 7: 505–513, 1967.
236. PEACHEY, L. D. The structure of the extraocular muscle fibers of mammals. In: *The Control of Eye Movements,* edited by P. Bach-y-Rita, C. C. Collins, and J. E. Hyde. New York: Academic, 1971, p. 47–66.

237. PEACHEY, L. D. Stereoscopic electron microscopy: principles and methods. *Bull. Electron Microsc. Soc. Am.* 8: 15–21, 1978.
238. PEACHEY, L. D. Three-dimensional structure of the T-system of skeletal muscle cells. In: *Proc. Int. Congr. Physiol. Sci., 28th, Budapest, 1980,* vol. 14, p. 299–311.
239. PEACHEY, L. D., AND B. R. EISENBERG. Helicoids in the T system and striations of frog skeletal muscle fibers seen by high voltage electron microscopy. *Biophys. J.* 22: 145–154, 1978.
240. PEACHEY, L. D., AND C. FRANZINI-ARMSTRONG. Three-dimensional visualization of the T-system of frog muscle using high voltage electron microscopy and a lanthanum stain. *Annu. Proc. Electron Microsc. Soc. Am., 35th, Boston, 1977,* p. 570–571.
241. PEACHEY, L. D., AND C. FRANZINI-ARMSTRONG. Observation of the T-system of rat skeletal muscle fibers in three dimensions using high voltage electron microscopy and the Golgi stain (Abstract). *Biophys. J.* 21: 61a, 1978.
242. PEACHEY, L. D., C. HUDSON, AND P. BACH-Y-RITA. Marking extraocular muscle fibers for physiological-morphological correlation (Abstract). *Proc. Int. Congr. Physiol. Sci., 25th, Munich, 1971,* vol. 9, p. 443.
243. PEACHEY, L. D., AND A. F. HUXLEY. Local activation and structure of slow striated muscle fibers of the frog (Abstract). *Federation Proc.* 19: 257, 1960.
244. PEACHEY, L. D., AND A. F. HUXLEY. Structural identification of twitch and slow striated muscle fibers of the frog. *J. Cell Biol.* 13: 177–180, 1962.
245. PEACHEY, L. D., AND A. F. HUXLEY. Transverse tubules in crab muscle (Abstract). *J. Cell Biol.* 23: 70a–71a, 1964.
246. PEACHEY, L. D., AND K. R. PORTER. Intracellular impulse conduction in muscle cells. *Science* 129: 721–722, 1959.
247. PEACHEY, L. D., AND R. F. SCHILD. The distribution of the T-system along the sarcomeres of frog and toad sartorius muscles. *J. Physiol. London* 194: 249–258, 1968.
248. PEACHEY, L. D., M. TAKEICHI, AND A. C. NAG. Muscle fiber types and innervation in adult cat extraocular muscles. In: *Exploratory Concepts in Muscular Dystrophy II.* Amsterdam: Excerpta Med., 1974, p. 246–254.
249. PEACHEY, L. D., R. A. WAUGH, AND J. R. SOMMER. High voltage electron microscopy of sarcoplasmic reticulum (Abstract). *J. Cell Biol.* 63: 262a, 1974.
250. PELLEGRINO, C., AND C. FRANZINI. An electron microscope study of denervation atrophy in red and white skeletal muscle fibers. *J. Cell Biol.* 17: 327–349, 1963.
251. PETTE, D. (editor). *Plasticity of Muscle.* Berlin: Gruyter, 1980.
252. PILAR, G. Further study of the electrical and mechanical responses of slow fibers in cat extraocular muscles. *J. Gen. Physiol.* 50: 2289–2300, 1967.
253. POPESCU, L. M., AND I. DICULESCU. Calcium in smooth muscle sarcoplasmic reticulum *in situ.* Conventional and X-ray analytical electron microscopy. *J. Cell Biol.* 67: 911–918, 1975.
254. PORTER, K. R., AND G. E. PALADE. Studies on the endoplasmic reticulum. III. Its form and distribution in striated muscle cells. *J. Biophys. Biochem. Cytol.* 3: 269–300, 1957.
255. POTTER, J. D., J. D. JOHNSON, AND F. MANDEL. Fluorescence stopped flow measurements of Ca^{2+} and Mg^{2+} binding to parvalbumin (Abstract). *Federation Proc.* 37: 1608, 1978.
256. PRINGLE, J. Arthropod muscle. In: *The Structure and Function of Muscle* (2nd ed.), edited by G. H. Bourne. New York: Academic, 1972, vol. 1, p. 491–562.
257. PRINGLE, J. W. S. The muscles and sense organs involved in insect flight. In: *Insect Flight,* edited by R. C. Rainey. Oxford, UK: Blackwell, 1976, p. 3–15. (Symp. R. Entomol. Soc. London, 7th.)
258. RAYNS, D. G., C. E. DEVINE, AND C. L. SUTHERLAND. Freeze-fracture studies of membrane systems in vertebrate muscle. I. Striated muscle. *J. Ultrastruct. Res.* 50: 306–321, 1975.
259. REGER, J. F. The fine structure of neuromuscular junctions and the sarcoplasmic reticulum of extrinsic eye muscles of *Fundulus heteroclitus. J. Biophys. Biochem. Cytol.* 10(4), Suppl.: 111–121, 1961.
260. REGER, J. F. A comparative study on striated muscle fiber of the antenna and the claw muscle of the crab *Primixie sp. J. Ultrastruct. Res.* 20: 72–82, 1967.
261. RETZIUS, G. Muskelfibrille und Sarcoplasma. *Biol. Unters. Neue Folge* 1: 51–88, 1890.
262. REUBEN, J. P., D. P. PURPURA, M. V. L. BENNETT, AND E. R. KANDEL (editors). *Electrobiology of Nerve, Muscle and Synapse.* New York: Raven, 1976.
263. REVEL, J. P. The sarcoplasmic reticulum of the bat cricothyroid muscle. *J. Cell Biol.* 12: 571–588, 1962.
264. REVEL, J. P., AND M. KARNOVSKY. Hexagonal array of subunits in intercellular junctions of the mouse heart and liver. *J. Cell Biol.* 33: C7–C12, 1967.
265. ROGUS, E., AND K. L. ZIERLER. Sodium and water contents of sarcoplasm and sarcoplasmic reticulum in rat skeletal muscle: effects of anisotonic media, ouabain and external sodium. *J. Physiol. London* 233: 227–270, 1973.
266. ROLLET, A. Über die Flossenmuskeln des Seepferdchens (*Hippocampus antiquorum*) und über Muskel Struktur in Allgemeinen. *Arch. Mikrosk. Anat.* 32: 233–266, 1888.
267. ROSENBLUTH, J. Sarcoplasmic reticulum of an unusually fast-acting crustacean muscle. *J. Cell Biol.* 42: 534–547, 1969.
268. ROSENBLUTH, J. Oblique striated muscle. In: *The Structure and Function of Muscle* (2nd ed.), edited by G. H. Bourne. New York: Academic, 1972, vol. 1, p. 389–420.
269. ROWLAND, L. P. (editor). *Pathogenesis of Human Muscular Dystrophies.* Amsterdam: Excerpta Med., 1976. (Int. Congr. Ser. 404.)
270. RUBIO, R., AND N. SPERELAKIS. Penetration of horseradish peroxidase into the terminal cisternae of frog skeletal muscle fibers and blockade of caffeine contracture by Ca^{++} depletion. *Z. Zellforsch. Mikrosk. Anat.* 124: 57–71, 1972.
271. RÜDEL, R., AND F. ZITE-FERENCZY. Interpretation of light diffraction by cross-striated muscle as Bragg reflection of light by the lattice of contractile proteins. *J. Physiol. London* 290: 317–330, 1979.
272. RÜDEL, R., AND F. ZITE-FERENCZY. Efficiency of light diffraction by cross-striated muscle fibers under stretch and during isometric contraction. *Biophys. J.* 30: 507–516, 1980.
273. SANCHEZ, J. A., AND E. STEFANI. Inward calcium current in twitch muscle fibres of the frog. *J. Physiol. London* 283: 197–209, 1978.
274. SANDOW, A. Excitation-contraction coupling in muscular response. *Yale J. Biol. Med.* 25: 176–201, 1952.
275. SANDOW, A. Excitation-contraction coupling in skeletal muscle. *Pharmacol. Rev.* 17: 265–320, 1965.
276. SANES, J. R. Laminin, fibronectin, and collagen in synaptic and extrasynaptic portions of muscle fiber basement membrane. *J. Cell Biol.* 93: 442–451, 1982.
277. SANGER, J. W. Sarcoplasmic reticulum in the cross striated adductor muscle of the bay scallop *Aquipecten iridians. Z. Zellforsch. Mikrosk. Anat.* 118: 156–161, 1971.
278. SAWADA, H., H. ISHIKAWA, AND E. YAMADA. High resolution scanning electron microscopy of frog sartorius muscle. *Tissue Cell* 10: 179–190, 1978.
279. SCALES, D. J., AND T. YASUMURA. Stereoscopic views of a dystrophic sarcotubular system: selective enhancement by a modified Golgi stain. *J. Ultrastruct. Res.* 78: 193–205, 1982.
280. SCHIAFFINO, S., AND A. MARGRETH. Coordinated development of the sarcoplasmic reticulum and T system during postnatal differentiation of rat skeletal muscle. *J. Cell Biol.* 41: 855–875, 1969.
281. SCHMALBRUCH, H. Regeneration of soleus muscles of rat autografted *in toto* as studied by electron microscopy. *Cell Tissue Res.* 177: 159–180, 1977.
282. SCHNEIDER, M. F. Membrane charge movement and depolarization-contraction coupling. *Annu. Rev. Physiol.* 48: 507–517, 1981.
283. SCHNEIDER, M. F., AND W. K. CHANDLER. Voltage dependent charge movement in skeletal muscle: a possible step in excitation-contraction coupling. *Nature London* 242: 244–246, 1973.
284. SCHOTLAND, D. L. An electron microscopic investigation of myotonic dystrophy. *J. Neuropathol. Exp. Neurol.* 29: 241–253, 1970.

285. SCHULTZ, E., A. W. CLARK, A. SUZUKI, AND R. G. CASSENS. Rattlesnake shaker muscle. II. Fine structure. *Tissue Cell* 12: 335–351, 1980.
286. SELVERSTON, A. Structure and function of the transverse tubular system in crustacean muscle. *Am. Zool.* 7: 515–525, 1967.
287. SHERMAN, R. G., AND A. R. LUFF. Structural features of the tarsal claw muscles of the spider *Euripelma marxi* Simon. *Can. J. Zool.* 49: 1549–1556, 1971.
288. SHUMAN, H., A. V. SOMLYO, AND A. P. SOMLYO. Quantitative electron probe microanalysis of biological thin sections: methods and validity. *Ultramicroscopy* 1: 317–339, 1976.
289. SIMPSON, F. O., AND S. J. OERTELIS. Relationship of the sarcoplasmic reticulum to sarcolemma in sheep cardiac muscle. *Nature London* 189: 758–759, 1961.
290. SKOGLUND, C. R. Functional analysis of swim-bladder muscles engaged in sound production of the toadfish. *J. Biophys. Biochem. Cytol.* 10 (4), Suppl.: 187–200, 1961.
291. SMITH, D. S. Reticular organization within the striated muscle cell. An historical survey of light microscopic studies. *J. Biophys. Biochem. Cytol.* 10 (4), Suppl.: 61–87, 1961.
292. SMITH, D. S. The structure of insect fibrillar flight muscle. A study made with special reference to the membrane systems of the fiber. *J. Biophys. Biochem. Cytol.* 10: 123–158, 1961.
293. SMITH, D. S. The organization of flight muscle fibers in the odonata. *J. Cell Biol.* 28: 109–126, 1966.
294. SMITH, D. S., AND H. C. ALDRICH. Membrane systems of freeze-etched striated muscle. *Tissue Cell* 3: 261–281, 1971.
295. SMITH, D. S., R. J. BAERWALD, AND M. A. HART. The distribution of orthogonal assemblies and other intercalated particles in frog sartorius and rabbit sacrospinalis muscle. *Tissue Cell* 7: 369–382, 1975.
296. SOMLYO, A. P., A. V. SOMLYO, AND H. SHUMAN. Electron probe analysis of vascular smooth muscle: composition of mitochondria, nuclei, and cytoplasm. *J. Cell Biol.* 81: 316–335, 1979.
297. SOMLYO, A. V. Bridging structures spanning the junctional gap at the triad of skeletal muscle. *J. Cell Biol.* 80: 743–750, 1979.
298. SOMLYO, A. V., H. GONZALEZ-SERRATOS, H. SHUMAN, G. MCCLELLAN, AND A. P. SOMLYO. Calcium release and ionic changes in the sarcoplasmic reticulum of tetanized muscle: an electron-probe study. *J. Cell Biol.* 90: 577–594, 1981.
299. SOMLYO, A. V., H. SHUMAN, AND A. P. SOMLYO. Elemental distribution in striated muscle and the effects of hypertonicity. *J. Cell Biol.* 74: 828–857, 1977.
300. SOMLYO, A. V., AND J. SILCOX. Cryoultramicrotomy for electron probe analysis. In: *Microbeam Analysis in Biology,* edited by C. Lechene and R. Warner. New York: Academic, 1979, p. 535–555.
301. SOMMER, J. R., P. C. DOLBER, AND I. TAYLOR. Filipin-cholesterol complexes in the sarcoplasmic reticulum of frog skeletal muscle. *J. Ultrastruct. Res.* 72: 272–285, 1980.
302. SOMMER, J. R., AND E. A. JOHNSON. Cardiac muscle. A comparative study of Purkinje fibers and ventricular fibers. *J. Cell Biol.* 36: 497–526, 1968.
303. SOMMER, J. R., AND E. A. JOHNSON. Ultrastructure of cardiac muscle. In: *Handbook of Physiology. The Cardiovascular System,* edited by R. M. Berne and N. Sperelakis. Bethesda, MD: Am. Physiol. Soc., 1979, sect. 2, vol. I, chapt. 5, p. 113–186.
304. SOMMER, J. R., R. L. STEERE, E. A. JOHNSON, AND P. H. JEWETT. Ultrastructure of cardiac muscle. A comparative review with emphasis on the muscle fibers of the ventricles. In: *Hibernation and Hypothermia: Perspectives and Challenges,* edited by F. E. South, J. P. Hannon, J. R. Willis, E. T. Pengelley, and N. R. Alport. Amsterdam: Elsevier, 1972, p. 255–291.
305. SOMMER, J. R., N. R. WALLACE, AND W. HASSELBACH. The collapse of the sarcoplasmic reticulum in skeletal muscle. *Z. Naturforsch.* 33: 561–573, 1978.
305a. SOMMER, J. R., N. R. WALLACE, AND J. JUNKER. The intermediate cisterna of the sarcoplasmic reticulum of skeletal muscle. *J. Ultrastruct. Res.* 71: 126–142, 1980.
306. SOMMER, J. R., AND R. A. WAUGH. The ultrastructure of the mammalian cardiac muscle cell with special emphasis on the tubular membrane systems. A review. *Am. J. Pathol.* 82: 192–221, 1976.
307. SOMMERKAMP, H. Das Substrat der Dauerverkürzung am Froschmuskel. *Arch. Exp. Pathol. Pharmakol.* 128: 99–115, 1928.
308. STEFANI, E., AND D. J. CHIARANDINI. Skeletal muscle: dependence of potassium contractures on extracellular calcium. *Pfluegers Arch. Gesamte Physiol. Menschen Tiere* 343: 143–150, 1973.
309. STEPHENSON, E. W. Activation of fast skeletal muscle: contributions of studies on skinned fibers. *Am. J. Physiol.* 240 (*Cell Physiol.* 9): C1–C19, 1981.
310. STEPHENSON, E. W., AND R. J. PODOLSKY. Influence of magnesium on chloride-induced calcium release in skinned muscle fibers. *J. Gen. Physiol.* 69: 17–35, 1977.
311. STREET, S. F., AND R. W. RAMSAY. Sarcolemma: transmitter of active tension in frog skeletal muscle. *Science* 149: 1379–1380, 1965.
312. TAMEYASU, T., N. ISHIDE, AND G. H. POLLACK. Discrete sarcomere length distributions in skeletal muscle. *Biophys. J.* 37: 489–492, 1981.
313. TIEGS, O. W. The flight muscles of insects—their anatomy and histology; with some observations on the structure of striated muscle in general. *Philos. Trans. R. Soc. London Ser. B* 238: 221–348, 1955.
314. TODA, M., T. YAMAMOTO, AND Y. TONOMURA. Molecular mechanism of active calcium transport by sarcoplasmic reticulum. *Physiol. Rev.* 58: 1–79, 1978.
315. TORMEY, J. M. Differences in membrane configuration between osmium tetroxide-fixed and glutaraldehyde-fixed ciliary epithelium. *J. Cell Biol.* 23: 658–664, 1964.
316. VERATTI, E. Ricerche sulla fine struttura della fibra muscolare striata. *Mem. Ist. Lombardo Cl. Sci. Mat. Nat.* 19: 87–133, 1902.
317. VERATTI, E. Investigations on the fine structure of the striated muscle fiber. *J. Biophys. Biochem. Cytol.* 10(4), Suppl.: 3–59, 1961. (Paper from 1902, transl. by C. Bruni, H. S. Bennett, F. deKoven, and D. deKoven.)
318. WALKER, S. M., AND M. B. EDGE. The sarcoplasmic reticulum and development of Z lines in skeletal muscle fibers of fetal and postnatal rats. *Anat. Rec.* 169: 661–677, 1971.
319. WALKER, S. M., AND G. R. SCHRODT. Continuity of the T system with the sarcolemma in rat skeletal muscle fibers. *J. Cell Biol.* 27: 671–677, 1965.
320. WALKER, S. M., AND G. R. SCHRODT. Triads in skeletal muscle fibers of 19-day fetal rats. *J. Cell Biol.* 37: 564–569, 1968.
321. WALKER, S. M., G. R. SCHRODT, AND M. BINGHAM. Evidence for connections of the sarcoplasmic reticulum with the sarcolemma and with the Z line in skeletal muscle fibers of fetal and newborn rats. *Am. J. Phys. Med.* 48: 63–77, 1969.
322. WAUGH, R. A., J. R. SOMMER, AND L. D. PEACHEY. Cardiac sarcoplasmic reticulum: distribution and ultrastructure revealed by selective staining. *Circulation* 50: III-13, 1974.
323. WAUGH, R. A., T. L. SPRAY, AND J. R. SOMMER. Fenestrations of sarcoplasmic reticulum. Delineation by lanthanum acting as a fortuitous tracer and *in situ* negative stain. *J. Cell Biol.* 59: 254–260, 1973.
324. WEBER, A. M., R. HERZ, AND I. REISS. Study of the kinetics of calcium transport by isolated fragmented sarcoplasmic reticulum. *Biochem. J.* 345: 329–369, 1966.
325. WINEGRAD, S. Intracellular calcium movements of frog skeletal muscle during recovery from tetanus. *J. Gen Physiol.* 51: 65–83, 1968.
326. WINEGRAD, S. The intracellular site of calcium activation of contraction in frog skeletal muscle. *J. Gen. Physiol.* 55: 77–88, 1970.
327. YEH, Y., R. J. BASKIN, R. L. LIEBER, AND K. P. ROOS. Theory of light diffraction by single skeletal muscle fibers. *Biophys. J.* 29: 509–522, 1980.
328. ZAMPIGHI, E. G., J. VERGARA, AND F. RAMON. The connection between the T-tubules and the plasma membrane in frog skeletal muscle *J. Cell Biol.* 64: 734–740, 1975.

CHAPTER 3

Quantitative ultrastructure of mammalian skeletal muscle

BRENDA R. EISENBERG | *Department of Physiology, Rush Medical College, Chicago, Illinois*

CHAPTER CONTENTS

MUSCLE FIBERS EXIST IN SPECIES throughout the animal kingdom and allow directed movements to be performed at the command of the nervous system. Physiologically the muscle cell generates force and shortening at the tendons; both require energy. Anatomically a coordinated movement is produced by structural specializations of the nervous and muscular systems. This chapter deals with the anatomy within the muscle fiber. There is a great diversity in muscle ultrastructure, just as there is a great diversity in the mechanical outputs of muscles. The diversity presumably optimizes the directed movements the animal commands.

The history of research into muscle has been reviewed in a splendid book by Needham (207). She covers all the earliest papers and devotes special attention to breakthroughs made in this century. A historical perspective of the contractile system is given by A. F. Huxley (140) and of the structure of muscle by Andersson-Cedergren (3) and Bennett and Porter (13). Much of the interest in muscle this century can be traced to the influence of A. V. Hill, whose autobiography (126) is also most valuable. A recently published book by Squire (306) gives a complete review of the structural basis of muscular contraction.

Muscle fibers are grouped into functional units by their innervation. One neuron can control hundreds of muscle fibers, and this functional unit is called the motor unit, the properties of which have been reviewed by Buchthal and Schmalbruch (24). The muscle cells usually have a single motor end plate that elicits a single muscle action potential. Therefore the mechanical response of the fiber is much the same each time the motor nerve is stimulated. Furthermore fibers innervated by the same nerve contract together even though they are physically apart. Thus it is not surprising that all muscle fibers in a motor unit are biochemically alike (26–31, 209, 210).

Skeletal muscles with multiple innervation on a single fiber are found in invertebrates, frogs, birds, and in the extraocular muscles of mammals. Multiple motor end plates on single fibers allow graded potentials to spread over the whole length of a muscle fiber. Thus the propagating, all-or-none action potential is not needed, and graded end-plate potentials can be used to produce graded mechanical activity. These multiply innervated fibers are called tonic or slow-tonic muscles. All slow fibers discussed in this chapter are of the singly innervated slow-twitch type, not of the slow-tonic variety. This chapter concentrates on the subcellular arrangement of organelles within a mammalian muscle cell and on how these organelles meet physiological demands.

The nervous system of every animal apparently recruits motor units in a restricted, stereotyped fashion, and the resultant response of the muscle fibers is therefore specialized. Fibers do not show complete diversity but rather are grouped according to the particular functional demands they meet.

The classification of mammalian skeletal muscle fibers has challenged scientists from several disciplines because of the evident diversity of mammalian muscle. It is difficult to compare the classification scheme of one scientist measuring one property of muscle with that of another scientist measuring a different property. Additional information correlating the two properties is needed. The classification of fibers used to be considered simple: all slow fibers were thought to be red, and all fast fibers were thought to be white (207, 243); the real situation, however, is far more complicated. The population of muscle fibers can be divided into different numbers of types: for example, two (82), three (232), eight (256), and even a continuous spectrum (119). Table 1 presents some of the different terminologies. Numerous reviews summarize and attempt to correlate the classification scheme of one discipline with that of another, working from a single viewpoint. [For the perspective of physiology, see Close (36); for that of histochemistry, see Khan (167, Spurway 305), and Stein and Padykula (310); for that of biochemistry, see Peter et al. (232); and for that of electron microscopy, see Gauthier (101).] In some of these attempts, such as the work of Peter and his colleagues (10, 11, 59, 231, 232), the histochemical properties have been directly related to the biochemical and contractile properties by analyzing whole muscles containing fibers predominantly of a single histochemical type (see also the chapter by Gergely and Seidel in this *Handbook*). These muscles of the guinea pig were also used by Eisenberg and colleagues (60–62, 66–70) to compare the ultrastructure with contractile and biochemical properties.

Burke and colleagues (28, 29) related physiological properties and histochemical characteristics of a mixed muscle. He stimulated a motoneuron going to the mixed muscle and later identified the type of the corresponding motor unit histochemically by observing glycogen depletion. Analysis of fiber types has direct clinical application because the classification of the histochemical fiber type (52, 82) is a most useful tool in aiding the diagnosis of neuromuscular diseases. Perhaps a fuller understanding of the nature and extent of fiber types and of their changes in disease will better help us to understand the disease process itself.

In recent years attention has been paid to the changes that occur in fibers in local regions of normal muscle (133) during pathological stress (233, 323), in development (see the chapter by Kelly in this *Handbook*), during exercise (10, 119), during chronic stimulation (307), during cross innervation (255, 256), after denervation (104, 228), and during disease (41, 52). It is often difficult to fit these changes into a particular restricted scheme for fiber types. As A. F. Huxley presciently stated (138):

> Evidently mammals possess more than two types of fibre distinguishable on these microscopic and physiological criteria; it remains to be seen whether there is a finite number of types or a whole spectrum varying continuously as regards structure, innervation, speed of contraction, and type of electrical response.

If the mechanical properties of muscle cover a continuous range of function, then the anatomical composition of the muscle fibers might also cover a spectrum rather than be grouped into distinct types. Every organelle within a muscle fiber could vary in amount, and thus one might expect a myriad of slightly different muscle cells within one animal. To study the extent of the spectral diversity it is necessary to collect

TABLE 1. *Terminologies for Describing Fibers of Mammalian Muscle*

Method	Fiber Spectrum			Reference
Histology and physiology	Slow red	Fast white	Fast white	Ranvier (243)
Oxidative enzymes, phosphorylase	I	II	II	Dubowitz and Pearse (53), Engel (82)
Mitochondrial distribution, ATPase	B	C	A	Stein and Padykula (310)
Histochemical profile	III	II	I	Romanul (256)
Mitochondrial distribution	Intermediate	Red	White	Padykula and Gauthier (217)
Z-line width	Red	Intermediate	White	Gauthier (100)
Oxidative enzymes, ATPase	I	IIA	IIB	Brooke and Kaiser (22)
	β	αβ	α	Yellin and Guth (338)
	β-Red	α-Red	α-White	Ashmore and Doerr (8)
Motor unit physiology and histochemistry	S	FR	FF	Burke et al. (29)
Homogeneous muscle: physiology, histochemistry, biochemistry	Slow twitch, oxidative	Fast twitch, oxidative, glycolytic	Fast twitch, glycolytic	Peter et al. (232)

Table modified from Eisenberg (61).

data cell by cell for every system. The resulting histograms can be analyzed to see whether clustered fiber types or a continuous spectrum does occur. Cell-by-cell analysis is needed to test this "cluster" hypothesis; that is why quantitative single-cell studies have been done recently by physiologists (9, 28–30, 36, 51, 176), biochemists (15, 48, 150, 233, 240, 324, 327, 328), anatomists (44, 45, 56, 60, 61, 66–68, 70, 100–104, 168, 169, 317), and histochemists (10, 21, 22, 58, 59, 82, 105, 107, 167, 232, 272, 305, 320).

A major theme of this chapter is the quantitative distribution of organelles within a muscle fiber and their relationship to physiological function. I consider the major functional mechanisms in the same order they are used during a twitch. The first mechanism couples the muscle action potential to calcium release by the sarcoplasmic reticulum (SR). This mechanism is called excitation-contraction (EC) coupling and is accomplished by the membrane systems within the muscle, viz. the sarcolemma, transverse tubular (T) system, and SR (Fig. 1).

The second system to be used physiologically is the contractile machinery, viz the actin and myosin filaments, and the Z, M, and N lines. These work together to produce a mechanical twitch that has a given time course, output of force, and resistance to fatigue.

The third functionally important system is the metabolic system, which supplies the energy to maintain contraction and EC coupling. Contraction is energized directly by ATP (buffered by the creatine/creatine phosphate system); EC coupling is energized by concentration gradients across the surfaces of the T and SR membranes, which are in turn maintained by ATP-dependent pumps. The organelles involved directly in

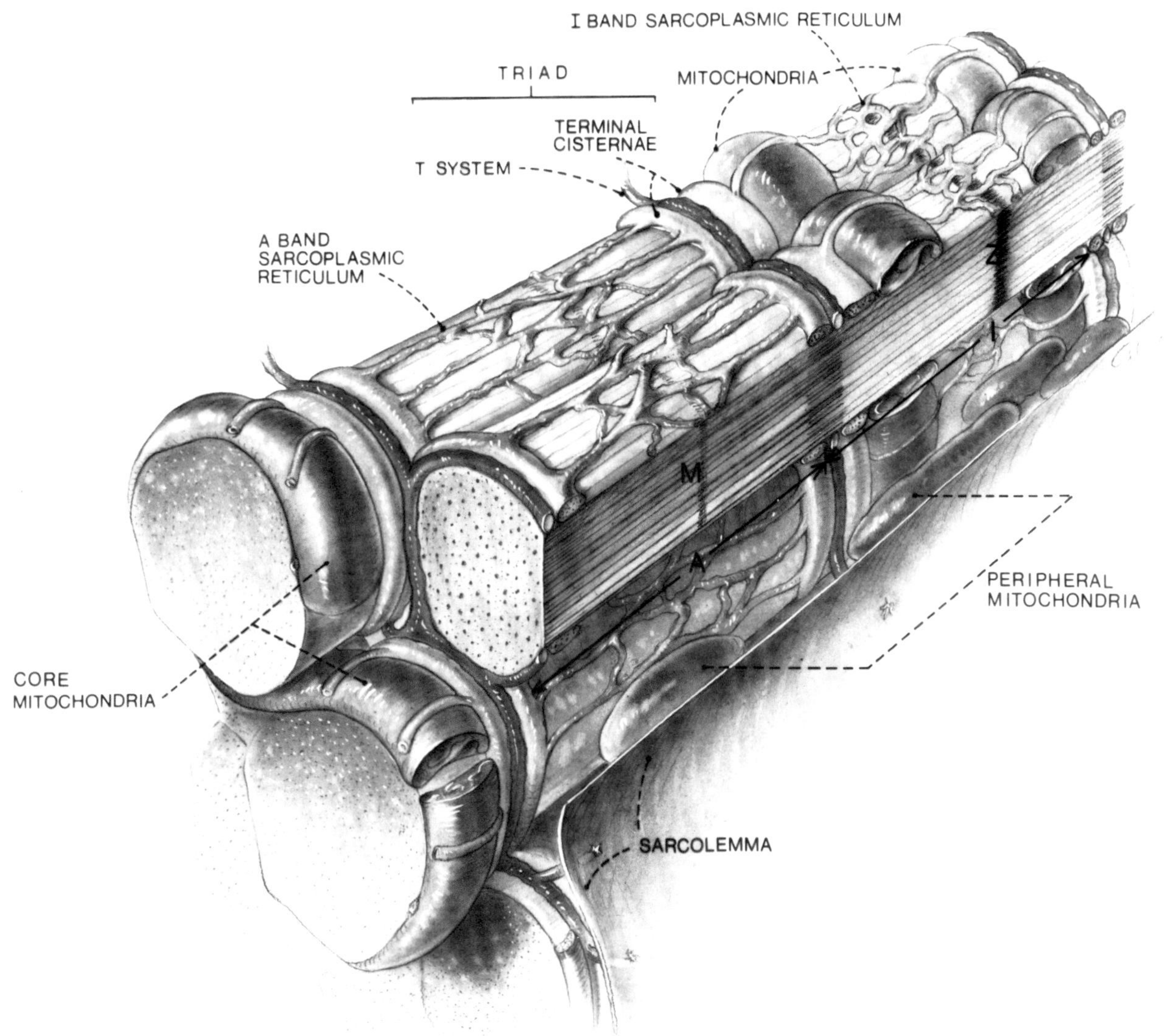

FIG. 1. Schematic drawing of part of a mammalian skeletal muscle fiber showing relationship of sarcoplasmic reticulum, terminal cisternae, T system, and mitochondria to a few myofibrils. [From Eisenberg et al. (70).]

oxidative and glycolytic metabolism are the mitochondria, glycogen granules, and lipid droplets. The blood system supplies the muscle cell with the necessary oxygen and other nutrients.

PHYSIOLOGICAL FUNCTIONS

Excitation-Contraction Coupling

SARCOLEMMA. During development many small myoblast cells fuse together to form long cylindrical multinucleate muscle fibers (Fig. 2). The fibers in young animals are loosely packed and have a nearly circular cross section. With time, however, the fibers pack more closely and take on an irregular polyhedral form (Fig. 3). Both fiber length and fiber diameter are highly variable. Adult mammalian fibers can be up to one-half meter (500 mm) in length and up to 0.1 mm in diameter. The largest fiber has a surface area of at least 160 mm^2. In fact, since the fibers are neither circular nor smooth, the actual surface area could be much more. The surface membrane of a muscle fiber was named the *sarcolemma* (Greek *sarc*, "flesh") by Bowman in 1840 (19).

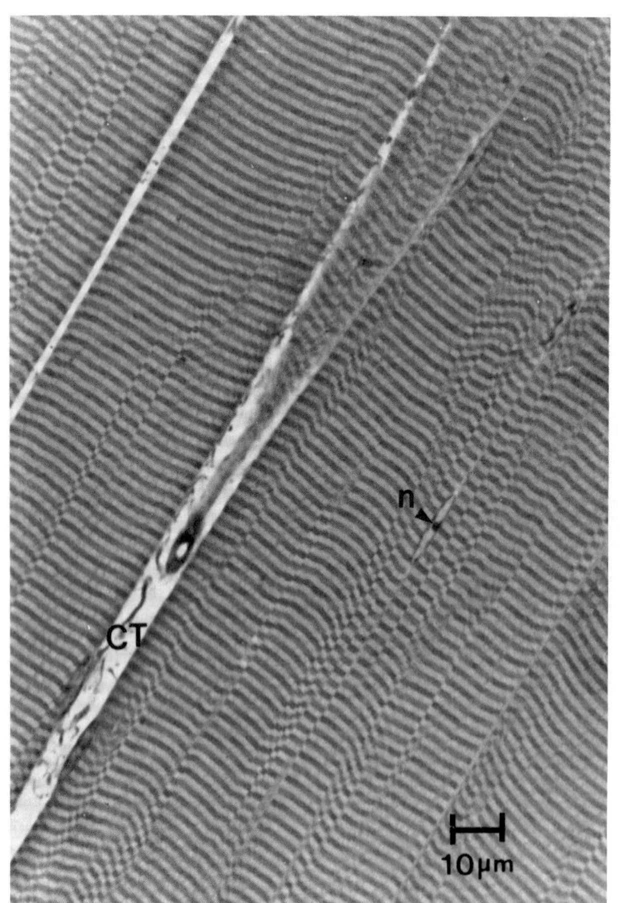

FIG. 2. White vastus muscle of the guinea pig. Light micrograph of plastic-embedded muscle cut in a 0.5-μm-thick longitudinal section. Fibers are striated with dark (A) and light (I) bands. Note peripherally located nuclei (*n*) and connective tissue (*CT*).

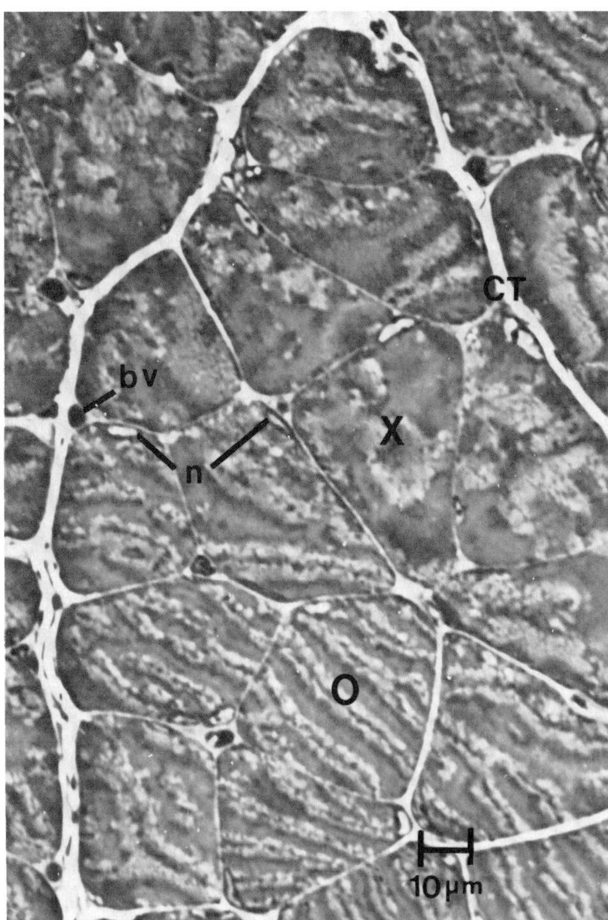

FIG. 3. Soleus muscle from guinea pig. Light micrograph of plastic-embedded muscle cut as a 0.5-μm-thick cross section. Fibers are irregularly shaped and contain peripheral nuclei (*n*). Note small blood vessels (*bv*) and connective tissue (*CT*). Dark A band, light I band, and Z disk vary in orientation from one fiber to another, giving fibers a marbled appearance. Pattern in fiber *X* is formed from only one A and one I band, indicating a nearly true cross section, whereas in fiber *O*, striation patterns indicate an oblique section. [From Eisenberg et al. (70).]

The first transmission electron micrographs of the sarcolemma were made by Bennett and Porter (13), who described the sarcolemma as "a thin membrane . . . applied to the outside of the fiber, and embraced on the outside by a closely adherent loose irregular collagenous network."

The ultrastructure of the sarcolemma is best viewed with the techniques of freeze fracture or scanning electron microscopy. Both techniques reveal large expanses of curved membrane, compared to the small amount of membrane seen in the flat thin sections used in transmission electron microscopy. Replication and scanning electron microscopy allow the outer surface (273) and T-system openings to be seen [(197); see also the chapter by Ishikawa, Sawada, and Yamada in this *Handbook*]. Freeze fracture (247) takes us between the lipid bilayers and allows observation of the particles embedded in the membrane (248, 249, 275, 276). Traditional transmission electron microscopy gives the best view of the structures just below the membrane within the cell. Numerous spherical pockets lie just under the membrane (339) and have been called caveolae by Dulhunty and Franzini-Armstrong (55). Their function is unknown. They are not pinocytotic in function because extracellular markers lodge in them but are not absorbed later.

The sarcolemma in a healthy muscle is homogeneous throughout its length except at the neuromuscular junction and the tendon insertions. Specializations at the tendon have not been thoroughly studied. More attention should be paid to the anatomy of this region, particularly in the frog, because voltage clamping is often done in the terminal segment of a single frog fiber [see Almers review (2)]. The neuromuscular junction has been very well explored. The sarcolemma is thrown into deep clefts with a different distribution of intramembraneous particles at the shoulders and in the valleys (245, 246). Mitochondria are more concentrated near the neuromuscular junction.

The plasmalemma covers the peripheral muscle surface, the T system, and the caveolae. Of these, the area of the peripheral surface, the sarcolemma, is often estimated by the apparent fiber diameter seen with a light microscope. Contracted fibers have larger diameters and more wrinkling, whereas stretched fibers are narrower and smoother (55). Fiber diameters are generally smaller in small animals than in large. Within the same species the diameter can vary with fiber type. For example, in rat the slow-twitch, oxidative (red) fibers are about 45 μm and the fast-twitch, glycolytic (white) fibers are about 65 μm (100). In larger animals, such as humans, however, the diameters of all fiber types are similar and sex dependent and are about 50–70 μm (21). The diameter of a fiber is readily altered by growth (214, 261) and by exercise or disuse [see review by Salmons and Henriksson (265)].

T SYSTEM. It has been clear for many years that skeletal muscle fibers must contain a specialized system for linking excitation of the surface membrane with contraction in the depths of the fiber (125). Indeed in frog skeletal muscle, Huxley and Taylor (142) postulated a specialized conduction system located at the Z line before the fine structure of muscle had been properly examined in the electron microscope. The structure of this conducting system is now known (3, 225). In frog sartorius muscle and in many heart cells, a system of tubules arises as invaginations of the sarcolemma and invades the fiber in the plane of the Z disk, branching to surround the myofibrils. The network of tubules is called the T system.

In mammalian skeletal muscle, inpockets of sarcolemma invade at each side of the A band, twice a sarcomere. Although the reason for the variation of location of the T system in muscles of different animals is not yet known, the fact of variation was established by Verrati in 1902 using light microscopy of silver-stained preparations (321). Morphological evidence shows that the tubular lumen is open and thus that the tubular membrane is continuous with the sarcolemma: various extracellular markers fill the lumen of the T tubules (80, 127, 144, 220, 221, 225). Detailed structural information obtained by high-voltage electron microscopy and other methods (73, 97–99, 226, 325) is reviewed by Peachey in his chapter in this *Handbook*. Electrophysiological studies have confirmed that the muscle's action potential is actively conducted radially through the T system (37, 205). The radial spread of current within the T system is reviewed by Gonzalez-Serratos in his chapter in this *Handbook*.

At an early stage of myotube development, a large number of caveolae fuse below the surface into a complex regular labyrinth (39, 161). This labyrinth is also seen in muscle grown in tissue culture (148). At this stage the contractile filaments are already organized into regular bands. A review of developing muscle is given in the chapter by Kelly in this *Handbook*.

COUPLINGS BETWEEN OUTER AND INNER MEMBRANE SYSTEMS: T-SR JUNCTION. The outer cell membrane of the T system makes intimate contact with the inner membrane system of the SR. The region of contact is usually named the T-SR junction, although it also has been called the triadic junction or T-TC junction (13, 227, 238–240). Recently the terms junctional SR (JSR) and peripheral JSR and interior JSR couplings have been used (302) because morphologically similar regions of contact also occur between the sarcolemma and the SR. Few if any peripheral JSR couplings occur in most normal adult mammalian fibers, although both are quite common in skeletal muscle of some species, in cardiac muscle, in slow-tonic muscle fibers, and in some neurons (122, 335).

The microscopic anatomy of the T-SR junction has been extensively studied by Franzini-Armstrong and others (64, 65, 71, 88–96, 163, 165, 225, 239, 301). Despite all this work, the relationship of structure to function is not yet known. The three anatomical components of the junction are *1*) the outer T membrane (which conducts the muscle action potential); *2*) the central gap containing pillars, bridges, and/or feet; and *3*) the inner SR membrane (Figs. 4 and 5).

Our laboratory is presently testing the hypothesis that the pillars undergo a molecular reorganization when the T membrane is depolarized. The reorganization is then supposed to produce a transient electrical coupling between T system and TC. Then, after the TC depolarizes, calcium is released from the SR. The hypothesis is based on interpreting a mass of electrophysiological data (193, 194). It is supported by structural experiments in frog muscle that suggest that the frequency of pillars connecting the T and TC

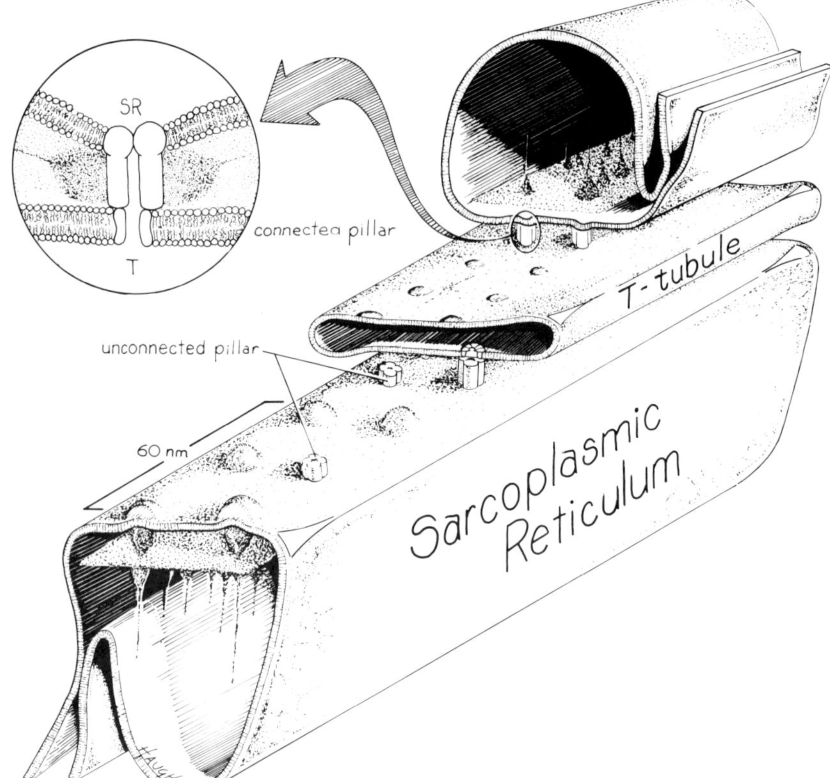

FIG. 4. Arrangement of structures in T-SR junction. This diagram is a fanciful melding of morphological data [Eisenberg (64, 65, 71), Franzini-Armstrong (96), Kelly and Kuda (165), and Somlyo (301)] with the electrical model of T-SR coupling [Mathias et al. (193, 194)]. Fine structure of pillar shown in *inset* is certainly beyond the practical resolution of the electron microscope. [Adapted from Eisenberg and Eisenberg (64).]

membranes is greater in activated muscle than in muscle at rest (64, 65).

Alternative mechanisms of T-SR coupling, such as a direct remote control of calcium release by a voltage sensor in the T membrane (33), are considered more plausible by many workers.

The T-SR junctional regions are remarkably similar throughout the animal kingdom (95, 96) and even occur in nonmuscle tissue where calcium ions are relevant to function (122, 335).

SARCOPLASMIC RETICULUM: TERMINAL CISTERNAE AND FREE SR. The sarcoplasmic reticulum (Latin *rete*, "mesh") is an internal endoplasmic reticulum that abuts the T system at the T-SR junction. The saccular region of SR abutment has had several names. In longitudinally sectioned muscle, one sees a triad, with a central T element and two adjacent sacs first named lateral cisternae (13, 227, 238–240). However, when it was found that these sacs were really the ends of the reticulum running between two T systems, the distal elements of the triad were renamed terminal cisternae (TC). In mammalian twitch fibers, most of the T system has an adjacent TC, whereas in slow-tonic frog fibers most of the T system is bare. In mammals the TC is also a network lying on both sides of the T system, occurring twice a sarcomere at the A-I junction (Figs. 6*A* and *B*), and there are four TC systems per sarcomere.

The lumen of the TC contains granular material that is almost certainly calsequestrin. This protein is present in large amounts and has a large capacity to bind calcium. The binding constant for calcium is relatively low, and so calcium can be readily released (see the chapter by Martonosi and Beeler in this *Handbook*). Inside the TC there seems to be a dense plate of calsequestrin about 200 Å away from the part of the TC membrane facing the T system (65). Strands spread away from this plate like bristles from a brush, and some strands spread toward the T-SR pillars (see ref. 301, Fig. 4). These anatomical arrangements have not yet been related to the molecular mechanisms involved in calcium storage and release.

The cisternal structure of the wide TC contrasts markedly with the tubular organization of the remainder of the SR. The remaining SR is free of granular material, has no junctions, and has sometimes been called free SR (96, 302). In frog muscle a narrow neck, called the intermediate cisternae (225), separates free SR from the TC. Analogous regions can be found in mammalian fibers. The remaining free SR meanders as longitudinally oriented meshes from one TC to the next. Some SR lies in the A band and some in the I band. The free SR can be thought of as an irregular fluid structure that probably distorts readily to accommodate the dynamic changes of contraction. Fusion of the SR membranes can be demonstrated in material "fixed" with ruthenium red and in rapidly frozen normal muscle (135, 303). Sommer et al. (303) have proposed the novel idea that the tubules can fuse to from

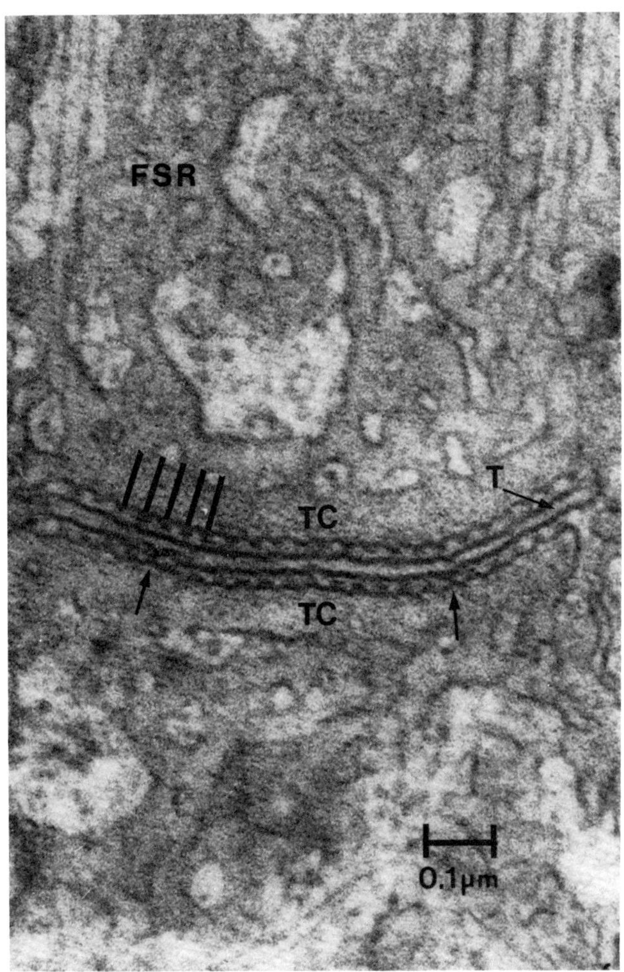

FIG. 5. Electron micrograph of T-SR junctional region from longitudinally sectioned mouse extensor digitorum longus muscle (fast twitch) fixed with oxygenated glutaraldehyde (155). T-system membrane (*T*) lies between 2 terminal cisternae (*TC*). Free SR (*FSR*) extends beyond the *TC*. Note projections from *TC* membranes (indicated by *lines*), some of which form connecting T-SR pillars (*arrows*). (Micrograph courtesy of J. E. Rash.)

flattened sheets; they speculate that this process is involved in squeezing calcium back into the TC from the free SR after a twitch.

The entire SR membrane is richly studded with calcium ATPase uptake sites (85) that can be localized by immunofluorescence (157) and are visible in freeze-fractured replicas. Counts of particles per unit area on the intact SR (14, 20, 40, 320) and in SR-vesicle preparations have been made (270). The technology of freeze fracture may be criticized if the estimates of particle and pit density are not equal; in that case, contamination, distortion, and other artifacts must be suspected (247). The published values of particle density are probably on the low side. A comprehensive review of the membrane systems within muscle is given in the chapter by Martonosi and Beeler in this *Handbook*.

Contractile System

Van Leeuwenhoek was the earliest anatomist to use a light microscope to view muscle, and an English translation appeared in 1712 [(183), p. 441]:

> Now, in order to demonstrate the fineness or slenderness of the Parts of the Flesh, length-ways, of so great a Creature as the Whale is (for this was above 50 Foot long) I placed one of the Hairs of my Beard by one of the Flesh Particles of the Whale, and I judg'd that the said Hair was at least Nine times thicker than one of those which I may call a little Flesh Muscle, it being again composed of other long Particles or Fibres

He also noted a banding pattern twisting around the muscle fibers [(183), p. 442]:

> When I cut the afore-mention'd long slender Flesh Particles, either across or obliquely with a sharp Knife, I could see therein a vast number of exceeding small Particles, of which one of those Flesh Particles did consist, and they were also cut across: And Through the Microscope it appear'd to me just as if one should see with the naked Eye small Grains of Sand lying upon them; and I also could discover the ends of them. In these my Observations there appear'd to me a great many Flesh Particles, surrounded with little Figures like Rings, and very close to one another, just as if you should take a common Iron Wire, and twist it about with another very fine one: And such circular Flesh Particles have I formerly observ'd in the Muscular part of the Paw or Foot of an Gnat; but the Rings were closer to one another in the Flesh Particles of a Whale, than in those of a Gnat; and if I remember right, the Flesh Particles (or Fibres) of a Gnat, were as thick as those of a Whale. How wonderful are such Conjextures!

The spiraling rings were later declared to be disks by Bowman in 1840 (19), although in fact van Leeuwenhoek (183) appears to have been correct (226, 315, 316). The striation pattern of the alternating dark and light bands form the structural basis of contractile activity. The names A and I band were coined by Brücke (23) for the dark anisotropic and light isotropic striations of muscle when viewed with polarizing optics. The striated appearance of a fiber in longitudinally sectioned muscle is shown in Figure 2. In cross section (Fig. 3) the fiber appears marbled because the striations are not in perfect register.

Force is developed when the actin filaments from the I band are slid between the myosin filaments of the A band by the cross bridges. Much research on muscle has been aimed at understanding how force is generated by mechanics and energetics (86, 141, 292) and has been reviewed elsewhere [A. F. Huxley (137–139), H.E. Huxley (145–147)].

SARCOMERE. The sarcomere is the physiologically defined contractile unit whose structure seen in longitudinal section stretches from one Z disk to the next. The Z disk is the thin, dense structure in the center of every I band.

Filaments. In electron micrographs of longitudinally sectioned muscle, we see that the A band is composed

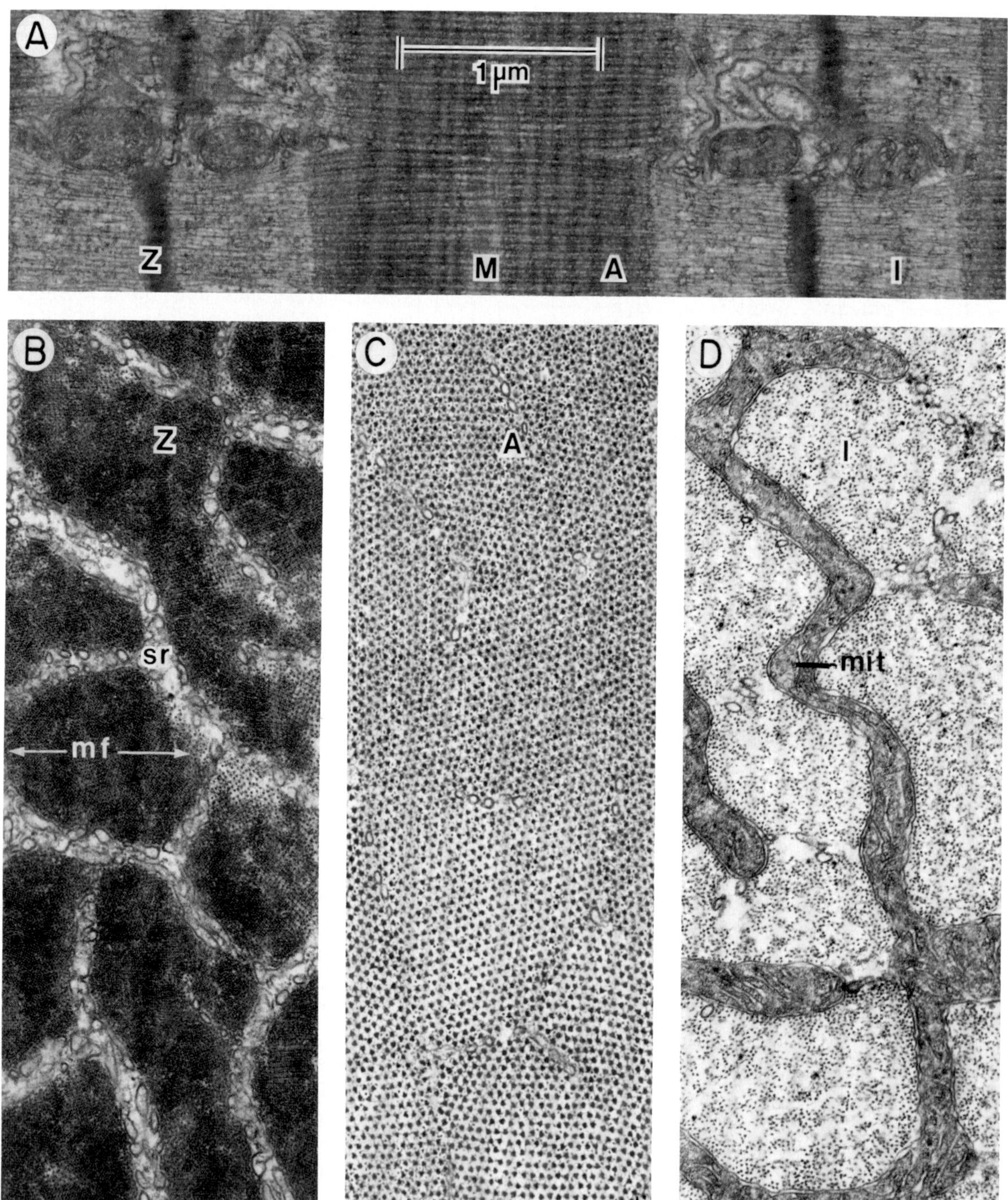

FIG. 6. Slow-twitch fibers from guinea pig soleus muscle. Micrographs are at the same magnification. *A*: longitudinal section showing paired mitochondria on either side of the Z line (*Z*), extensive SR in I band (*I*), lack of mitochondria and SR around the A band (*A*), and M line (*M*) in center. *B*: cross section entirely in plane of Z disk showing extensive SR (*sr*) that divides the *Z* disk into irregular myofibrils (*mf*). *C*: cross section in A band (*A*). Note thick myosin filaments, sparse mitochondria, and SR. Myofibrils are ill-defined. *D*: cross section in I band (*I*). Note thin actin filaments and elongated mitochondria (*mit*) almost encircling myofibrils. [From Eisenberg et al. (69).]

of thick, straight myosin filaments. The I band is composed of thin actin filaments (Fig. 6*A*). When a muscle fiber shortens, the actin filaments slide farther into the A band, decreasing the I-band length, increasing the filament overlap, and decreasing the myosin region without actin filaments, named the H band after Hensen (124) who first described it in 1868. In cross-sectioned slow-twitch muscle the filaments are seen as regular arrays of dots (Figs. 6*B*, *C*, and *D*). The electron microscope has not yet revealed any specialization in the thin and thick filaments in different mammalian fibers (297) corresponding to the many isozymes that have been demonstrated biochemically or immunologically (105, 198, 236, 271). Electron micrographs of longitudinal and cross-sectioned fast-twitch muscle (Fig. 7*A–C*) show a similar filament array to that of the slow-twitch muscle (Fig. 6*A–D*).

Z disk. The I band has a dense structure in its center, called the Z disk (from German *Zwischen*, "between"). In longitudinally oriented muscle the Z disk appears as a narrow dark Z line and was observed with the light microscope by Dobie in 1849 (49) and by Krause in 1868 (174). In the early 1950s the Z disk was thought to be a membrane responsible for the inward spread of excitation (142, 143). In electron micrographs of longitudinally sectioned muscle, the Z disk appears as a dense, interrupted Z line [Fig. 7*A*; (171)]. In cross sections, the Z disk is seen as a flat plate, apparently a basket weave of filaments (Figs. 6*B* and 7*B*). Reconstruction from longitudinal and transverse images shows that the Z disk is a complex three-dimensional lattice of filaments that join the actin filaments of one sarcomere to actins of opposite polarity in the adjacent sarcomere. Several papers describe the arrangement of the Z-filament lattice within the disk (92, 114–118, 164, 178, 179, 251, 260, 298, 319, 337).

The Z disks of fast-twitch fibers are narrower than those of slow-twitch fibers [Fig. 8; (67, 102)]. Alterations of thickness of the Z line are probably produced by the addition of subunits to the Z lattice [Fig. 9; (115, 118, 266)].

M disk. Groups of myosin filaments are joined to each other in a hexagonal array in the middle of the A band by the M line (German *Mittellinie*, "midline") (Fig. 8). The structure is also called the M band or M disk. In transverse sections prepared for electron microscopy, M-band bridges connect the hexagonally packed myosin filaments in the center of the myosin filaments (172, 230). In longitudinal sections, three to five layers of M bridges are found. The number of layers seems to be related to fiber type (296, 297). The M-band protein is readily extracted from stretched fibers (177) and has been studied biochemically (57, 312). Further information is given by Pepe in his chapter in this *Handbook*.

Function of Z disk and M disk. The function of Z and M disks is presumably to hold the filaments in the desired three-dimensional array so that efficient sliding may occur. It is usually claimed that the Z disks also hold the striations in register. In fact, since the Z disk is discontinuous, this function is probably accomplished by the intermediate desmin or skeletin filaments that connect the individual parts of the Z disk (180–182, 314).

The M and Z disks must also support radial forces, which develop as a fiber fattens on shortening, to maintain a constant fiber volume (78, 79). The thickness and structure of the Z and M disks are specialized in different fiber types. Perhaps these differences can be understood in terms of the different mechanical stresses developed. The Z-disk width changes during chronic stimulation of the fiber (74, 75, 264), although this takes 2–3 wk to occur and seems to be accomplished by fibrillar reorganization. The Z-band width also has been shown to increase after tenotomy (35, 252), when the fibers are shortening in an unloaded situation. However, there is no increase in Z width when a muscle is both denervated and tenotomized so that the shortened muscle remains unused (159). Experimentally induced hypoxia is claimed to increase the Z-band width in cardiac muscle (118), although this has been disputed (34). The work load of the heart is increased in hypoxia.

It is not yet known what mechanical stresses and strains are borne by the Z and M bands; perhaps when these are known it will be possible to understand how the structures adapt to them. During active tension development some changes in the Z lattice do occur (178). Normal sarcomere length changes do not produce changes in the width of the Z band (75, 264), but the effect of extreme sarcomere length changes on Z- and M-band structure has not been studied.

Etlinger and Fischman (84) suggested that the components of the M and Z bands may be necessary for the assembly of myofibrils. The recent work of Peng (229), however, shows that myofibrils develop from the long actin filaments of stress fibers. Nonetheless there is much more to be learned about myofibril assembly, and one can expect that some structures of the adult muscle will prove to be relics of the assembly process without any other functional role.

N lines. In addition to the well-known Z and M bands, there are less visible N lines (German *Nebenscheibe*: *neben*, "adjacent" + *Scheibe*, "slice") found at varying distances from the Z line within the I band (see Fig. 10). The actin filaments are straight and tetragonally arranged from the Z to the N_1 line. The actin filaments form an irregular array in the rest of the I band but are forced into a hexagonal lattice by the myosin filaments of the A band (87). To my knowledge, no function or molecular basis has been ascribed to N lines, but the N_2 protein has been identified (326).

MYOFIBRIL. The contractile filaments seem to be bundled into small threads in teased or squashed fresh preparations of single muscle fibers (19). Early light microscopy of formaldehyde-fixed, paraffin-embedded muscle also showed these threads. Kolliker (173) in 1888 called the threads myofibrils and the spaces between them sarcoplasm. The size and shape of the myofibrils are quite variable. In fast-twitch and slow-twitch mammalian muscles the myofibrils have small, roughly circular profiles and form *Fibrillenstruktur*. In cardiac and slow-tonic muscles the myofibrils form large irregular fields or *Felderstruktur* (175). In early electron micrographs the myofibrils were seen to con-

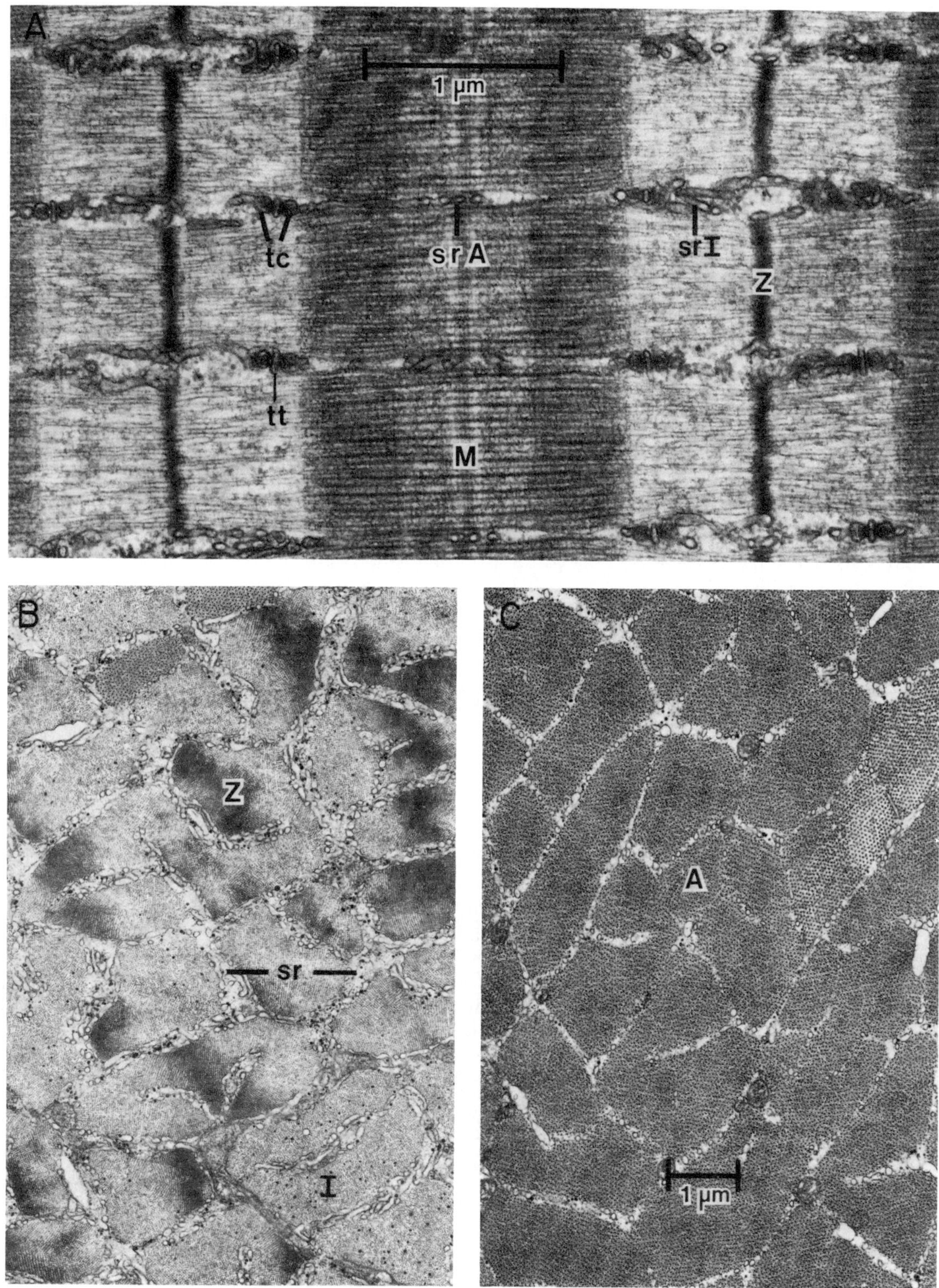

FIG. 7. Fast-twitch fiber from guinea pig white vastus lateralis muscle. *A*: longitudinal section showing SR in the A band (*srA*) and I band (*srI*). Terminal cisternae (*tc*) contain granular material and flank the elliptical T system (*tt*). Z line is thin, but note variation in width across several myofibrils. *M*, M line. [From Eisenberg and Kuda (66).] *B*, *C*: cross sections at a lower magnification showing extensive SR in Z-disk (*Z*) and I-band (*I*) regions and less SR in the A band (*A*). Myofibrils are irregular structures outlined by SR that are better defined in the I band than in the A band. (B. R. Eisenberg, unpublished micrographs.)

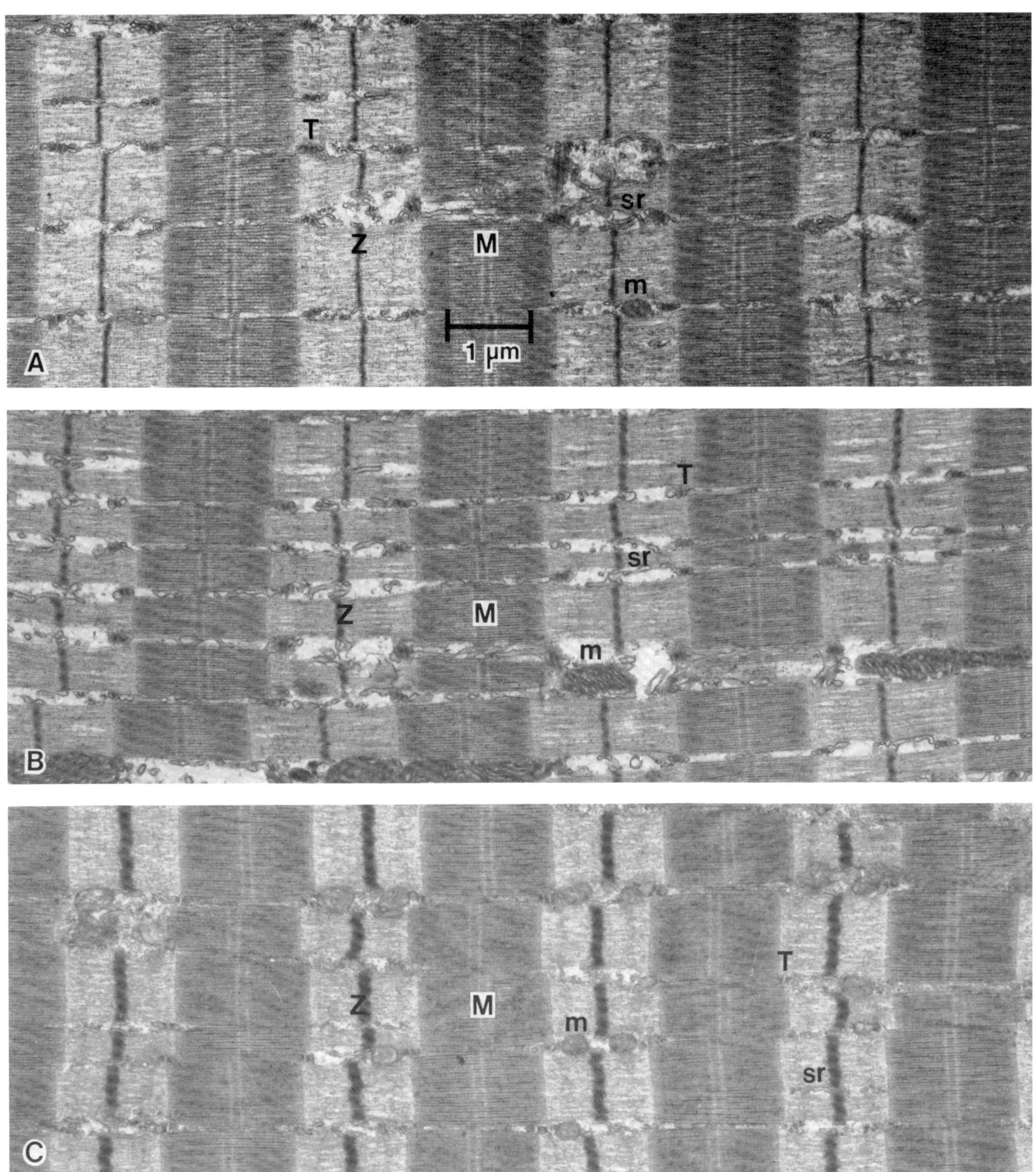

FIG. 8. Longitudinal section of parts of adult guinea pig muscle. *A*: white vastus (fast twitch, glycolytic). *B*: red vastus (fast twitch, oxidative, glycolytic). *C*: soleus (slow twitch, oxidative). Mitochondria (*m*) are sparse in the white vastus (*A*), intermediate to frequent in the red vastus (*B*), and intermediate in the soleus (*C*). Sarcoplasmic reticulum (*sr*) and T system (*T*) are more abundant in fast-twitch muscles of the white and red vastus (*A* and *B*) than in slow-twitch muscle of the soleus (*C*). Z-line (*Z*) widths are narrower in fast-twitch fibers (*A* and *B*) than in slow-twitch fiber (*C*). *M*, M lines. [From Eisenberg (60).]

sist of bundles of contractile filaments. The bundles were separated from each other by wide spaces containing cytoplasm and other subcellular organelles (13). The mesh of the T and TC systems also delineates fibrils. As fixation has improved, the spaces separating the myofibrils have narrowed! In many slow-twitch mammalian fibers no myofibrillar boundaries can be seen in the A band (Fig. 6*C*). Fibers that have

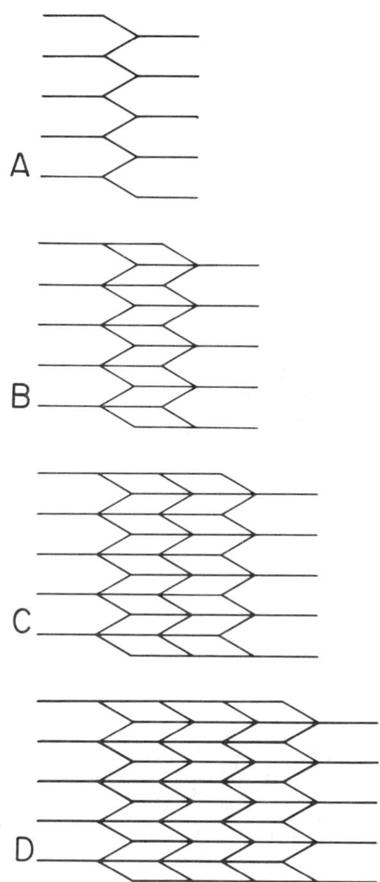

FIG. 9. Models of longitudinal sections through Z disks of different complexity. *A*: simplest Z disk has one layer of connecting filaments giving a zigzag appearance like that found in fish (92). *B*: another 38-nm segment added to each filament and a second layer of connecting filaments give an appearance more typical of mammalian skeletal Z lattice of fast-twitch, glycolytic muscle such as rat EDL or guinea pig white vastus. *C*: one more 38-nm layer is added to give 2 complete subunits. This Z lattice corresponds to Z widths found in fast-twitch, oxidative, glycolytic fibers and some slow-twitch, oxidative fibers. *D*: a final layer is added to give 3 complete subunits and a Z lattice typical for the soleus muscle (117) and canine cardiac muscle. Note that the number of subunits is not constant throughout an entire Z disk. Fast-twitch fibers usually have 1–2 or 2–3 subunits, whereas cardiac and slow-twitch have 2–4 subunits. [Figure was kindly provided by M. A. Goldstein, modified from Goldstein et al. (115).]

particularly large volumes of SR (253) or mitochondria (149) may have recognizable myofibrils in the A band as well (Fig. 12). Most studies that discuss myofibrillar size and shape are probably referring to spaces in the I-band or Z-disk regions where they impart the fibrillar appearance visible even with the light microscope.

Goldspink and colleagues (111–113, 284) suggest that the myofibrils are dynamic structures containing bundles of filaments that may split off or rejoin (see also the chapter by Goldspink in this *Handbook*).

Metabolic Systems

Cell metabolism is performed largely by soluble enzymes that cannot be resolved with structural techniques. However, subcellular organelles, visible in the electron microscope, are involved in metabolism and can be used as crude indices of the nature and extent of metabolism. For example, mitochondria support oxidative metabolism, and so the volume of mitochondria and surface area of their cristae are some measure of the oxidative metabolism of a fiber. Some cells store glycogen and lipid as reserve energy supplies. The amount of glycogen and lipid can be measured with morphometric techniques, and these measurements can also serve as an index of metabolism.

The color of muscle has long been used to classify fibers as red or white [e.g., in 1860 by Ranvier (243)]. The redness comes from the blood in capillaries and from myoglobin and mitochondria in the muscle fibers. All three red constituents are found in large amounts in muscles with a high oxidative capacity. Although historically it was thought that all red fibers were slow twitch, type I, this is false. There are also fast-twitch red fibers, and so any nomenclature based on color conveys limited information about speed. A recent exchange of letters on nomenclature can be consulted in this regard (208, 304).

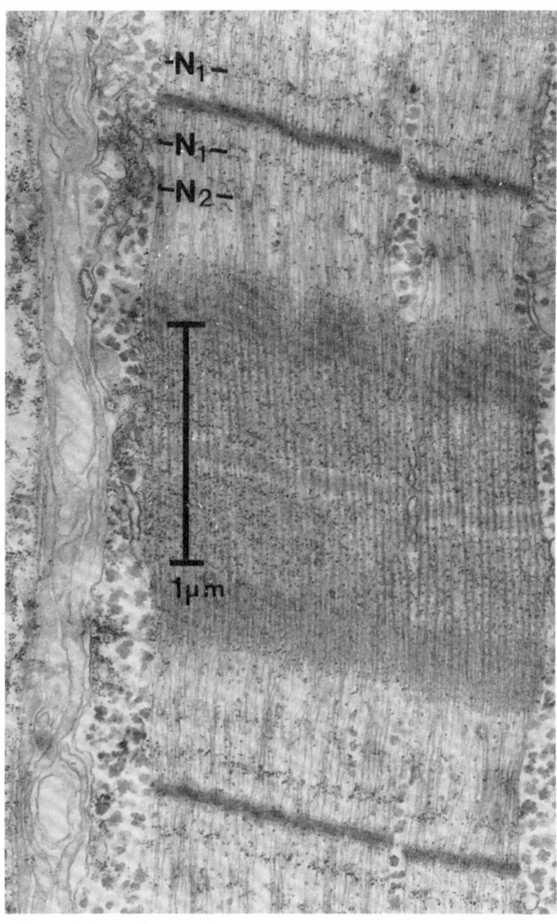

FIG. 10. Longitudinal section through a peripheral myofibril of a frog fiber that was skinned and exposed to a ferritin suspension. Positions of N_1 and N_2 lines are marked. Large granules between the fibrils are glycogen granules. Sarcomere length is 2.8 μm. [From Franzini-Armstrong (87).]

MITOCHONDRIA. The mitochondria in muscle cells are long cylindrical bodies. In mammalian muscle most of the mitochondrial population is found packed in between the myofibrils, and the remainder is found in peripheral locations. The distribution and amount of the mitochondria are remarkably constant throughout the length of the fibers, with a rare exception (46).

The mitochondria that accumulate at the periphery of the fiber are found in parallel clusters under the sarcolemma (Figs. 11 and 12). The largest subsarco-

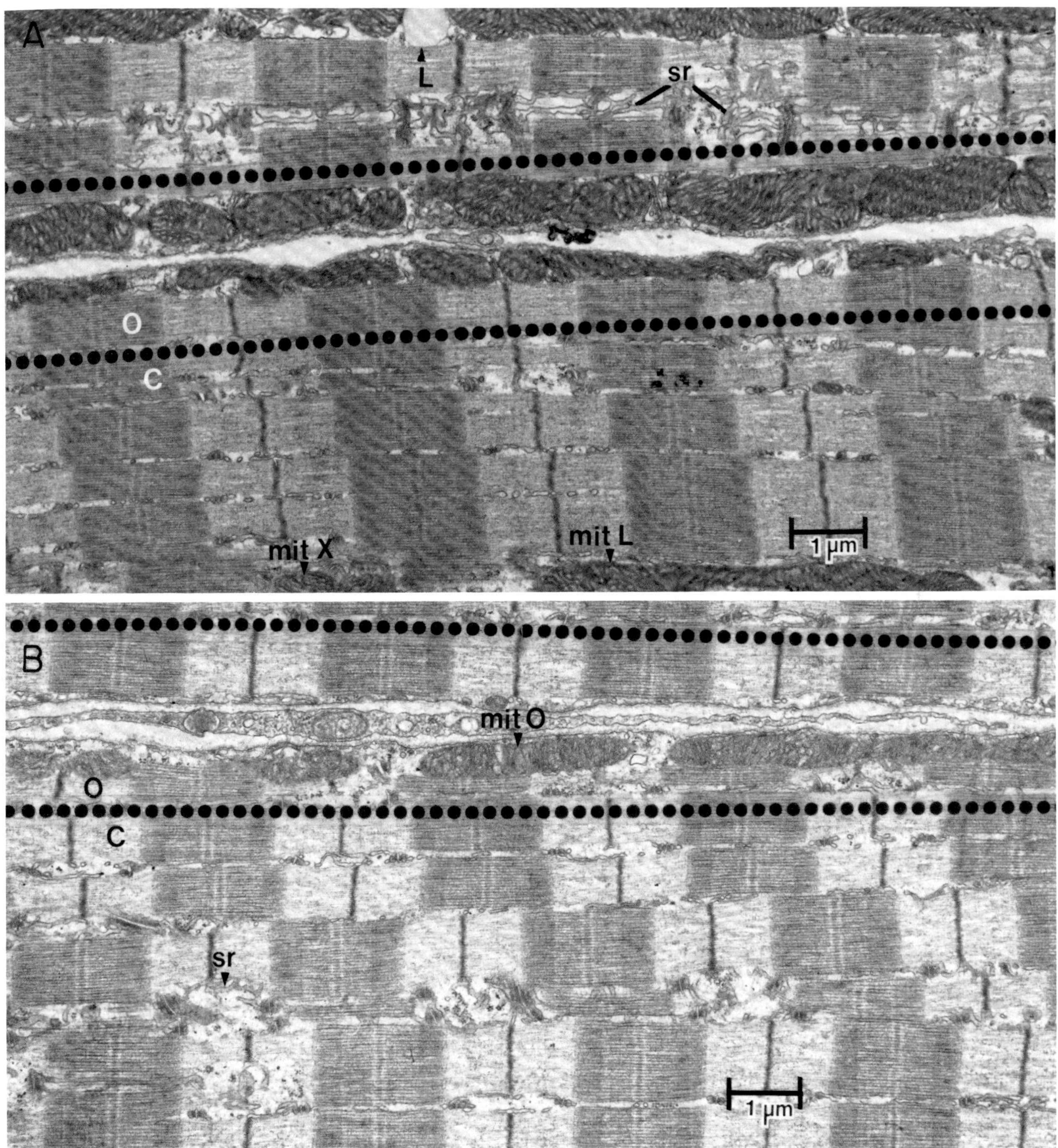

FIG. 11. Longitudinal sections through parts of vastus lateralis muscle of the adult guinea pig. *Dotted line* is drawn 1 µm from the sarcolemma to divide outer annulus (*O*) from fiber core (*C*). Mitochondria in outer annulus (*mitO*) are oriented longitudinally (*mitL*) and transversely (*mitX*) to fiber axis; *sr*, sarcoplasmic reticulum; *L*, lipid droplet. Both micrographs are at same magnification. *A*: red portion of vastus lateralis muscle is mainly composed of fast-twitch, oxidative, glycolytic fibers. *B*: white portion of vastus lateralis muscle is mainly composed of fast-twitch, glycolytic fibers. [*A* from Eisenberg and Kuda (67), *B* from Eisenberg and Kuda (66).]

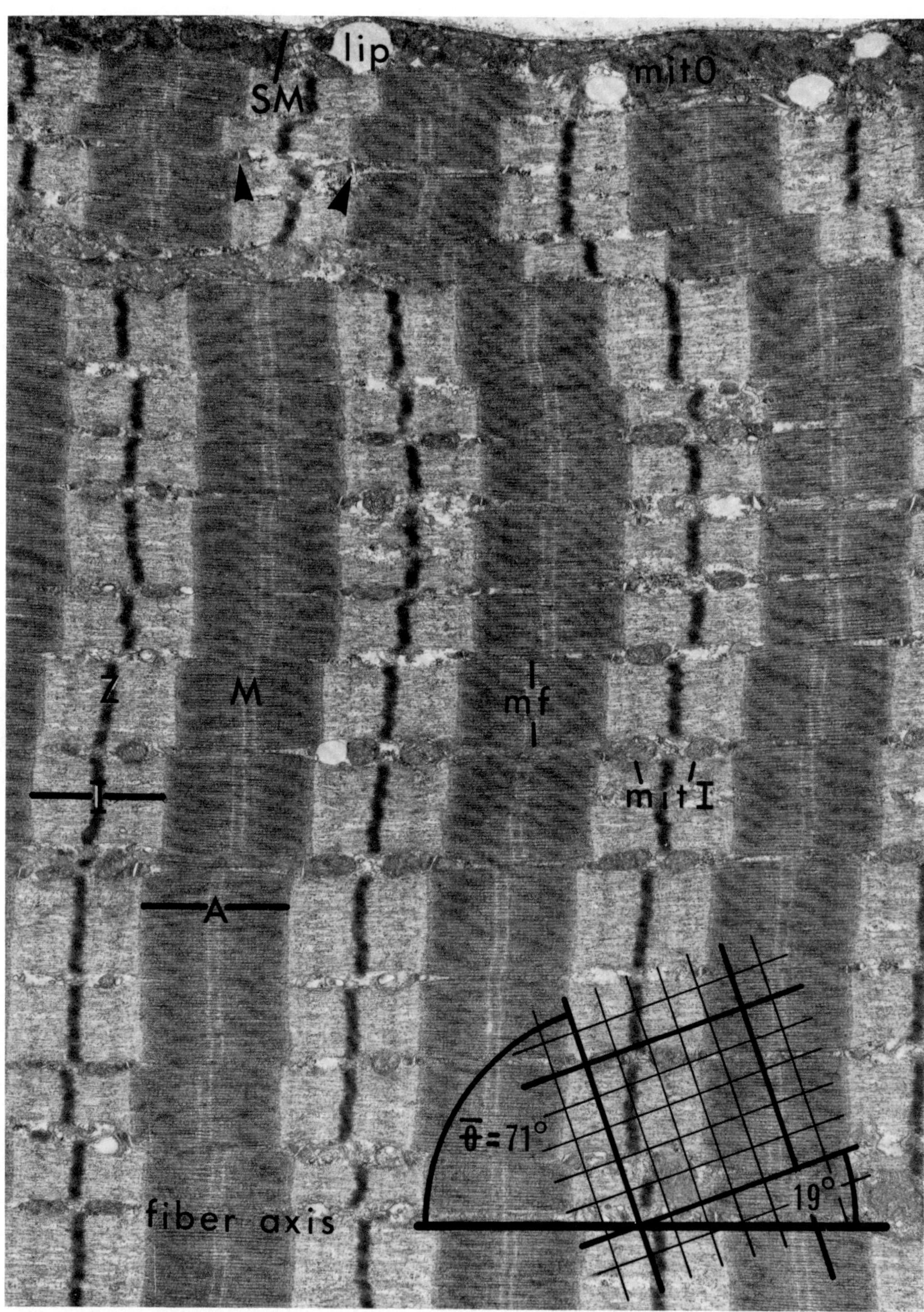

FIG. 12. Longitudinal section through part of a soleus muscle slow-twitch fiber of the guinea pig. Lipid droplets (*lip*) and mitochondria (*mitO*) lie close to sarcolemma (*SM*). Dense Z line (*Z*), moderate M line (*M*), dark A band (*A*), and light I band (*I*) give the fiber a regularly striated appearance. *Arrows* point to triads located at junction of A and I bands, between some, but not all, myofibrils (*mf*). Mitochondria in the I band (*mitI*) are often paired and A-band mitochondria are sparse. A portion of a stereological test grid is shown oriented at optimal angle $\theta = 19°$ and $71°$ (293). Light-line spacing ~0.4 μm and heavy-line spacing ~1.8 μm. [From Eisenberg et al. (70).]

lemmal clusters are said to be found near nerve terminals, near nuclei, and near capillaries (Fig. 13), where they presumably serve specialized local functions (133, 195). However, mitochondria also occur when no special adjacent structure is observed. The function of the subsarcolemmal mitochondria is not known, but they do seem to be associated with the general level of activity of the fiber (133, 195). In the

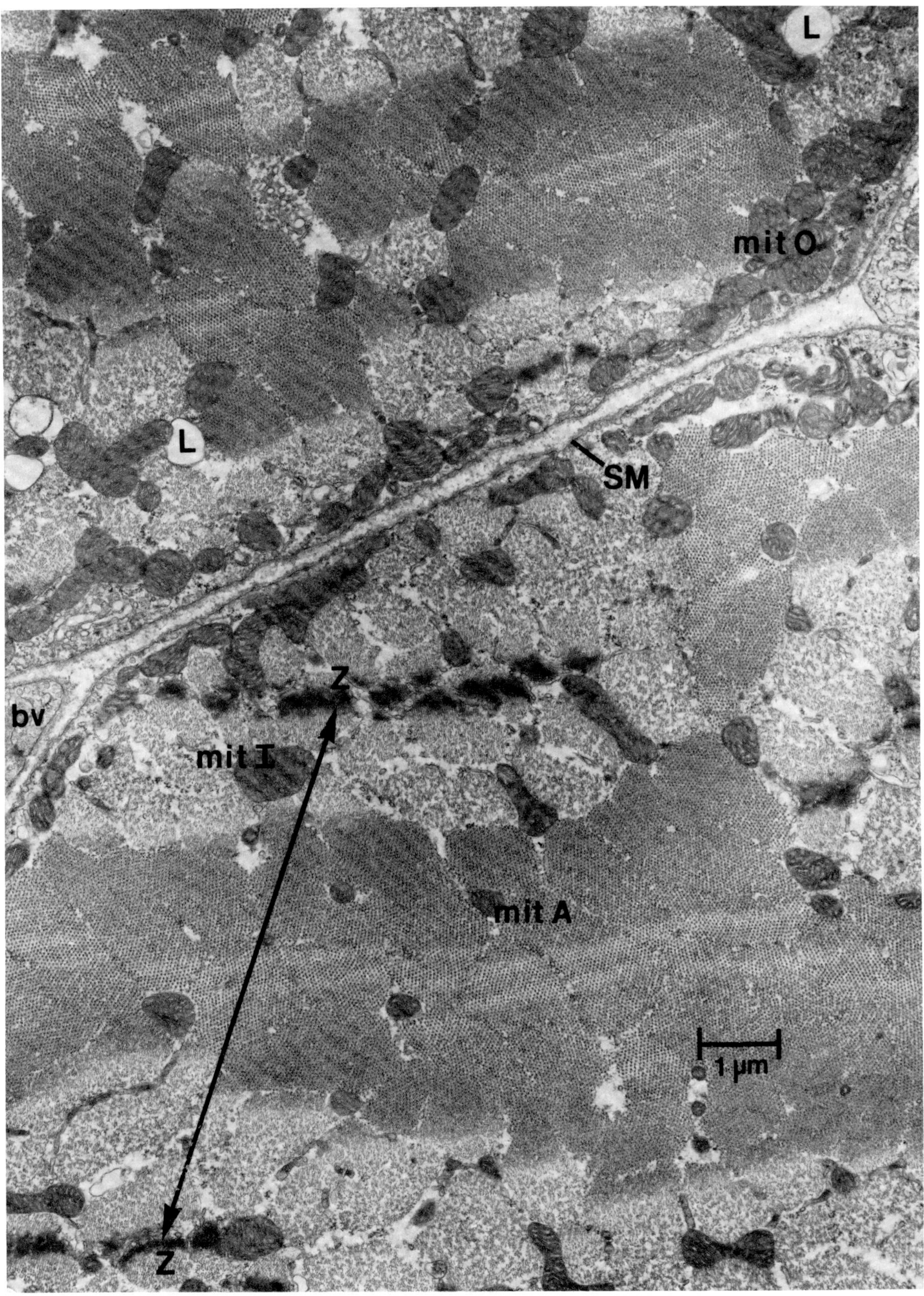

FIG. 13. Oblique section of soleus muscle from the guinea pig showing parts of 2 fibers and a capillary (*bv*). Note peripheral accumulation of mitochondria (*mitO*) near sarcolemma (*SM*), the numerous, large mitochondria in the I band (*mitI*), small mitochondria in the A band (*mitA*), and sarcomere repeats between Z disks (*Z*); note also spherical lipid droplets (*L*). [From Eisenberg et al. (70).]

diaphragm of different-sized mammals, high breathing rates and high metabolic activity are correlated with increased subsarcolemmal mitochondria (108).

Mitochondrial rearrangements are commonly seen in human muscle pathology (52, 158, 211). Increased subsarcolemmal accumulations of mitochondria are a feature of peripheral neuropathies where denervation and reinnervation are occurring. Subsarcolemmal masses also increase during fiber-type transformation (75).

The mitochondria packed in the contractile part of a fiber are forced to lie outside the contractile system. In slow-twitch mammalian muscle, the preferred location of mitochondria seems to be in a transverse plane between the triadic systems and the Z disk (Fig. 1). In cross section a mitochondrion can be seen to worm its way between several myofibrils (Fig. 6*D*). In longitudinal section, one sees pairs of circular profiles of mitochondria on either side of the Z line (Figs. 6*A*, 8, and 12). The mitochondria branch extensively in the transverse plane. Sometimes the branching is at right angles, and a mitochondrion runs for several sarcomeres in the longitudinal direction between the myofibrils. These longitudinally oriented mitochondria are most commonly found in muscles that have a high mitochondrial content and rely for the most part on oxidative metabolism, such as cardiac (5, 6, 219, 302) and pigeon flight muscles (149). It has been said that the type of a fiber can be recognized by the amount and distribution of the mitochondrial profiles (54, 102, 310). This is true in specific muscles. For example slow-twitch fibers in guinea pig have more transversely oriented mitochondria and fast-twitch fibers have more in the longitudinal orientation (67). In other muscles, however, such as in the human (223, 296), mitochondrial distribution is not as useful in determining fiber type.

GLYCOGEN GRANULES. Glycogen granules appear in electron micrographs as spherical particles about 200 Å in diameter, distributed in cytoplasmic spaces throughout the muscle. The most common location is in the I band in the region between the triad and the Z line (Figs. 6*A*, 7*A*, and 8). In some muscle the glycogen granules are found in rows between the I filaments (279). Schmalbruch has found that in human muscle only type I (slow-twitch) fibers have interfilament glycogen granules.

LIPID DROPLETS. Spherical lipid droplets about 0.25 μm in diameter are uniformly distributed throughout the muscle fibers in the intermyofibrillar spaces. Droplets are found more frequently in oxidative fibers (Figs. 11*A* and 12).

Other Systems

BLOOD SYSTEM. In general, muscles with a high oxidative capacity have a larger vascular bed (66, 67, 70, 133, 134, 257). In mixed muscles, the number of capillaries surrounding high-oxidative fibers is greater than the number surrounding low-oxidative fibers. Studies with the light microscope can be done with special stains (185, 200, 204, 237, 287–289) or thin plastic sections [Figs. 2, 3, and 14; (81)]. Electron microscopy has also been used [Fig. 13; (133, 134, 151, 153, 154, 203)]. Vascularization rapidly increases with exercise (265) and with chronic stimulation (50, 136).

CONNECTIVE TISSUE. Another level of anatomical complexity of muscle is evident in the connective tissue. The arrangement of groups of muscle cells and their attachment to the bones or exoskeleton of the animals via tendon determine the mechanical advantage of the movement. The subject is covered elsewhere (259). Epimysial connective tissue occurs in thick sheets or fascia around large bundles of muscle fibers (Fig. 14). The thinner endomysial connective tissue surrounds individual muscle fibers (Fig. 3). The amount of connective tissue varies greatly from one muscle to another. Connective tissue makes muscle strong and meat tough. One way to assess the connective tissue content is by the teeth, but other methods

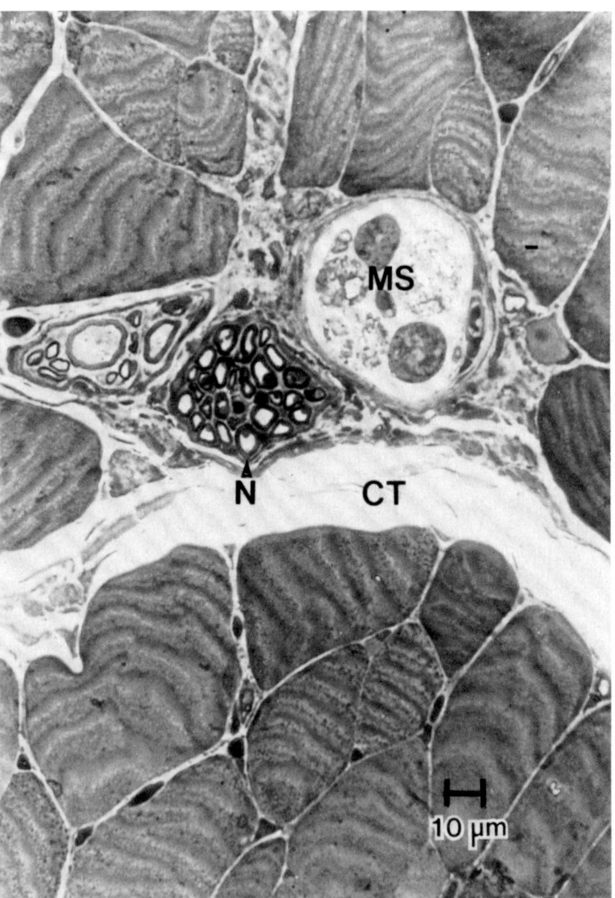

FIG. 14. Light micrograph of cross section through rabbit tibialis anterior muscle showing a nerve bundle (*N*) and a muscle spindle (*MS*) containing intrafusal muscle fibers. A thick layer of epimysial connective tissue (*CT*) wraps around a fascicle of muscle fibers.

are more scientific! Mechanical properties of the connective tissue are responsible for a large part of the passive length-tension behavior of muscle. Little seems to have been done to compare the distribution of connective tissue in fibers of different types.

More attention has been paid recently to the connective tissue that lies just outside the sarcolemma. Techniques such as transmission and scanning electron microscopy allow views of the collagen and basement membrane material (16, 206, 215, 322), and a great deal of complex architecture is present.

SATELLITE CELLS. The small satellite cells that nestle in the periphery of a muscle fiber under the protection of its basement membrane appear deceptively inert. Yet the satellite cells are responsible for muscle regeneration (1, 196) and development [(162, 214) and the chapter by Kelly in this *Handbook*]. There is little quantitative information about the numbers of satellite cells (32, 277, 278, 282). In young animals a third of the nuclei within the basal lamina are from satellite cells, and this fraction decreases with age (109) to only a few percent. Quantitative studies of satellite cells are scarce, probably because electron microscopy is needed for their recognition, yet large areas of tissue must be analyzed to find them.

SPINDLES. The anatomy of the spindle structure has been well studied (Fig. 14), but only a few morphometric references are available (192, 281).

NEUROMUSCULAR JUNCTION. Morphometric analysis of the membrane folds in the postjunctional region has been done in normal and denervated muscle and in mysasthenic patients (269). The sampling methods by which the sections are obtained have been criticized, however (245). The junction has a complex geometry (218, 246), and the estimates of membrane areas are quite sensitive to the plane and location of the section.

METHODS OF OBSERVATION

Having described the structures associated with EC coupling, contraction, and metabolism, I describe the methods by which these structures are observed and measured. It must be decided first which muscles are easiest to analyze when viewed with the electron microscope.

Selection of Muscle for Morphometric Analysis

The investigator's goal is to relate quantitative ultrastructural information with the physiological and biochemical properties of a single muscle fiber. This cannot readily be done for a fiber that comes from a muscle of mixed composition. Fortunately there are some muscles that are relatively pure or homogeneous in fiber type, the best known of which is surely the soleus muscle. This muscle is 100% slow-twitch, oxidative in the guinea pig and some 95% pure in the rat (7, 285, 286). The tibialis anterior and the extensor digitorum longus are widely used as the archetypes of pure fast-twitch muscle, although in rat only 84% of the fibers are in fact fast-twitch. The guinea pig provides three highly pure muscles, judged histochemically, biochemically, or physiologically (10, 11, 232), and these muscles were used in the ultrastructural studies of Eisenberg and colleagues (66, 67, 70). The sternomastoid muscle of the rat provides another histochemically well-defined muscle (54).

Instead of relying on supposedly pure muscles, methods have been developed that directly compare a fiber in the electron microscope and in an adjacent histochemically stained frozen section [see Fig. 15; (17, 68, 296)]. A stain for myoglobin (3,3′-diaminobenzidine) can be used on Epon sections, and identification of histochemical type by this method has been done (268). Mitochondrial distribution can be observed histochemically and with the electron microscope. In some species separate fiber types can be defined this way (102), whereas in other species this is not possible. The Z width and M-line structure have also been used as fiber-type indicators, although both have problems in some species (Z DISK, p. 97; M LINE, p. 98). A comparison of immunocytochemical results and morphometric parameters has also been made (103, 106, 230, 313).

Electron Microscopy

The electron microscope is the primary tool for observation of the ultrastructure of muscle because it is the only instrument with sufficient sensitivity and resolution. Electron beams do not penetrate thick preparations, and electrons are not well scattered by the atoms of low atomic number that comprise most biological tissue. Therefore muscle must be preserved, embedded in a hard plastic, sectioned into very thin slices, and heavily stained with metals before it can be seen with the electron microscope. There are many technical problems related to these preparative steps; these are discussed in numerous texts (47, 110, 121). Only the specific problems that arise from making measurements on micrographs are dealt with here.

Stereological Analysis

Collection of numerical data allows fiber classification to be based on statistical criteria rather than on subjective impressions of a single observer using a particular assay. Anatomy has been one of the last biological sciences to develop methods by which data could be readily accumulated in numerical form. Even today only a small fraction of the publications in major anatomical journals give results in numbers rather than in words or pictures. This is changing rapidly now that the basic measuring tools and analytical methods of stereology are available.

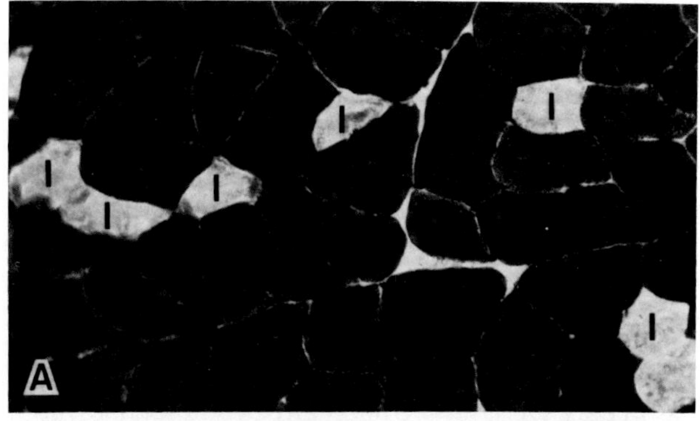

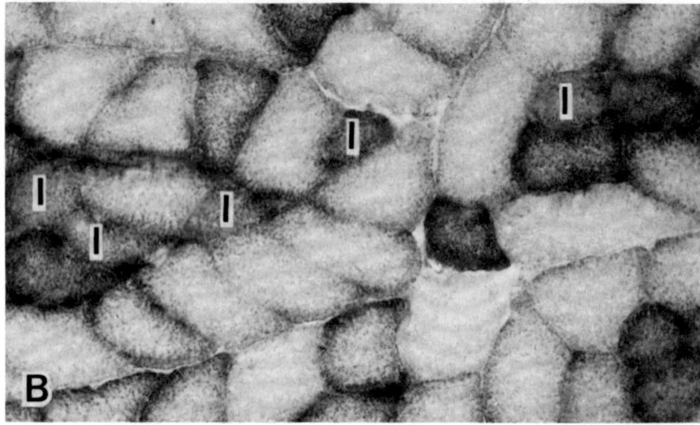

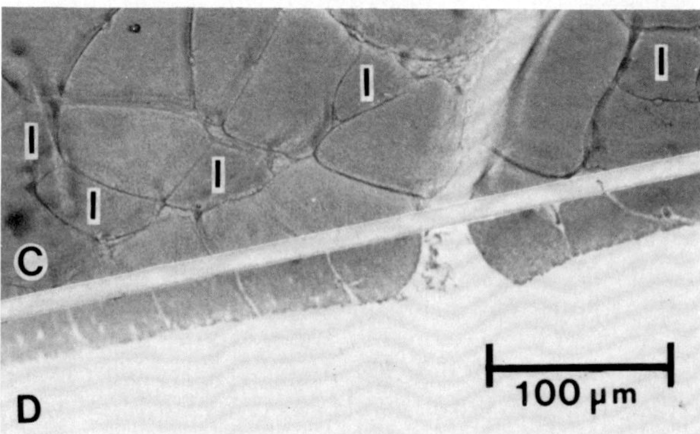

FIG. 15. Serial cross sections of guinea pig medial gastrocnemius muscle. *A*: section stained from myofibrillar ATPase at pH 9.4. Light fibers are type I or slow twitch; dark unlabeled fibers are type II or fast twitch. *B*: frozen section stained for succinic dehydrogenase. Note there is a continuous range in staining density of the fibers. Type I fibers from *A* all stain at darker end of the range. Type II fibers are distributed throughout whole density range. *C*: 30-μm frozen cross section thawed by immersion in glutaraldehyde fixative, postfixed in osmium tetroxide, embedded in Epon, and photographed through Epon block. *D*: narrow strip cut by rotating Epon block (*C*) through 90°. Fibers are longitudinally sectioned and about 30 μm in length. Alignment between fibers in *C* and *D* allows comparison between a cross and a longitudinal section of the same fibers. [From Eisenberg and Kuda (68), reprinted from *J. Histochem. Cytochem.* Copyright 1977 by The Histochemical Society, Inc.]

It must be stressed that tissue preparation and photomicrography are just as important as the actual method of measurement. The reader who wishes to make these measurements from good photomicrographs is referred to the didactic publications of Weibel (330–332) and other workers in the discipline known as morphometry or stereology. Morphometry is the measurement of form, shape, or size (Greek *morphe*, "form" + *metre*, "measurement"). Examples of morphometric parameters are the height of a person or the diameter of a cell. The term stereology deals with solids and dimensionality, has a rather diffuse etymology, and was coined by a group of scientists in 1961 [see Elias (76)]. Stereology is now defined as "the body of mathematical methods relating three-dimensional parameters defining a structure to two-dimensional measurements obtainable on sections of the structure" (330). The mathematical methods of geometric probability theory are used (300). The equations are usually derived with assumptions about the random distribution and orientation of structures viewed in infinitely thin sections. None of these conditions is valid for muscle and rederivation is necessary.

In classic stereological analysis, one considers a three-dimensional volume of tissue containing randomly oriented, homogeneously distributed organelles. The tissue is sectioned into flat slices for viewing in the electron microscope, and in a micrograph one observes numerous two-dimensional profiles of the organelles, which vary in shape, size, and orientation from picture to picture. The structure observed in the section is obviously related to that of the original tissue. For example, the probability of finding the profiles of mitochondria in the section is that of finding the total volume of the mitochondria in the cell volume. Furthermore the total boundary length (perimeter) of the mitochondrial profiles in the flat section bears a simple relationship to their surface area in the cell volume. Geometric probability theory can be used to calculate the average three-dimensional volumes and surface areas from the observed two-dimensional images of these isotropic structures. Note that the area ratio is an estimate of the volume ratio $A_1/A_2 = V_1/V_2$. This fraction is often written V_v (330). The derivation of the volume ratio (330) is not affected by orientation of structures except to the extent that section thickness and orientation interact (see SECTION THICKNESS, p. 92). Orientation affects the derivation of all equations involving surfaces. The equations for surface densities are given in Table 2. Inhomogeneous distribution of organelles can affect the sampling and must be taken into account when sample fields are selected, regardless of which equation is to be used (see SPATIAL INHOMOGENEITIES, p. 92). Inhomogeneous distributions are characteristic of organized structures like cells and must be considered in the design and implementation of morphometric experiments (283).

I now discuss the three main problems in stereology, which arise because muscle tissue does not fulfill the assumptions of standard stereological derivations: orientation, section thickness, and spatial inhomogeneities.

TABLE 2. *Surface-Density Equations*

	Surface-Density Equations for Planimetric Methods		Surface-Density Equations for Intersection-Counting Methods	
	Equation	Numerical constant	Equation	Numerical constant
Isotropic Random orientation	$\frac{S}{V}=\frac{4}{\pi}\cdot\frac{B}{A}$	1.27	$\frac{S}{V}=2\frac{I}{L}$	2
Anisotropic Fully oriented cylinders cut in longitudinal section	$\frac{S}{V}=\frac{\pi}{2}\cdot\frac{B}{A}$	1.57	$\frac{S}{V}=\frac{\pi^2}{4}\cdot\frac{I}{L}$	2.47
Fully oriented cylinders cut in cross section	$\frac{S}{V}=1\cdot\frac{B}{A}$	1	$\frac{S}{V}=\frac{\pi}{2}\cdot\frac{I}{L}$	1.57
Partially oriented cylinders cut in longitudinal section	$\frac{S}{V}=\frac{1}{\Lambda}\cdot\frac{B}{A}$	*	$\frac{S}{V}=\frac{\pi}{2\Lambda}\cdot\frac{I}{L}$	*
Fully oriented disks cut perpendicular to disks†	$\frac{S}{V}=1\frac{B}{A}$	1	$\frac{S}{V}=\frac{\pi}{2}\cdot\frac{I}{L}$	1.57

S, surface area of organelle; *V*, volume of muscle; *B*, boundary length of elements being measured; *A*, containing test area; *I*, number of intersection counts; *L*, total test-line length. See ref. 311. Λ, a constant defined in ref. 333. Note that $B/A = (\pi/2)\ (I/L)$, which is the Buffon (25) relationship. * Numerical constant depends on degree of orientation (62, 331, 333). † Disks cut parallel have a constant of 1/0 and cannot be evaluated (333).

ORIENTATION. The organelles of muscle are oriented with respect to one another; a single micrograph contains anisotropic profiles of the organelles that depend on the orientation of the section with respect to the organelle of interest. For example, when a volume contains cylinders, cross sections yield sets of circles, oblique sections yield ellipses, and longitudinal sections yield parallel lines. Nonetheless the profiles appearing in the section occur with the same frequency as the cylinders appear in the cell volume, and the volume of the cylinders is correctly estimated by the formula derived for the isotropic case. However, the relationship between the boundary length (perimeter) of the two-dimensional circles and the surface area of the three-dimensional cylinders is different from the isotropic case. Indeed the relationship must be quite different for sections in which the profiles are ellipses from sections in which the profiles are parallel lines. The exact relationship depends on the statistical distribution of the orientation and size of the cylinders; it also depends on the orientation of the sectioning plane.

Distributions of the size and shape of the cylinders make the problem of section thickness formidable and probably insoluble without additional experimental information. Anisotropy can be handled practically by using randomly oriented sections, circular test grids (18), and extensive sampling (201, 202). Anisotropy has also been handled theoretically in special cases by judicious assumption. A special shape, such as a cylinder, has been assumed, and the basic stereological equations were rederived for that geometry. This has been done for right circular, parallel cylinders (329) and later modified (77, 333). The equations for surface density are given in Table 2; results are presented for both the isotropic case and the case of cylinders oriented in either the parallel or perpendicular plane of section.

One must always remember that the surface density of a structure, which is the surface area of the organelle (*S*) per unit volume of muscle (*V*), is the same no matter which way the muscle is sliced because the property of surface density belongs to the solid three-dimensional body, not to the two-dimensional micrograph. The surface density is written as a fraction S/V or as S_v (330). However, in the two-dimensional micrograph the boundary length of the organelle profile (*B*) per unit area of muscle (*A*) depends on the geometry and section angle. The necessary integration constants are derived from geometric probability theory, and B/A must be multiplied by the correct constant to give the correct estimate of S/V. The equation for the isotropic case is $S/V = (4/\pi)(B/A)$. Other constants for nonisotropic cases are given in Table 2. One method of measuring B/A uses a modern planimeter, which electronically measures line length and enclosed area. This method requires tracing every profile, which is not practical for small contours like the SR. However, this tracing method is practical for larger structures such as nuclei or whole fibers.

A second, more efficient method was needed for assessment of small irregular profiles and was found to be useful for measurement of the larger profiles as well (128). Much stereology is now done by the statistical sampling approach with the intersection-counting method (330, 331). This method requires statistical equations relating the measured parameters I/L to B/A, where *L* is the length of the test line lying over the muscle and *I* is the number of intersections made between the test line and the boundary of the organelle (330). Intuitively one can see these ratios must be related since the number of intersection counts is clearly larger when an organelle has more membrane per unit area of micrograph. In fact, Buffon derived the relationship $B/A = (\pi/2)(I/L)$ in 1777 (25). He used this equation to measure π. We now know π and use the equation to estimate B/A. Buffon (25) derived the relationship from the consideration of randomly oriented test needles of small length thrown onto a parallel array of lines. It is important that the estimate of *I* be independent of orientation, which Buffon achieved by random averaging over all orientations of the needles. Modern treatments of the Buffon and orientations problems are given in reference 300 and in chapter 10 of reference 331.

Independence from orientation is easily achieved in biology because most organelles are randomly oriented (isotropic), so straight test lines can be used as test "needles." On the other hand, if the organelles are oriented (anisotropic), micrographs show that the membranes have straight parallel portions. Then a straight test system placed parallel with the membranes gives a low count (in fact, it gives $I = 0$); the same test system placed perpendicular to the membranes gives a high count. At angles in between, the value of I counted depends on the orientation. The angle that gives the correct or "optimal" count can be determined for a particular assumed structure (293). Measurements made at this angle were used in the measurement of muscle by Eisenberg [see portion of test grid drawn on Fig. 12; (67–69)]. Another way of introducing random orientation is to replace the test system of straight test needles with a test system of semicircles. Here the test grid is isotropic and, when placed over straight, oriented membranes, it introduces averaging over all orientations. The use of a semicircular test grid (199) averages over the orientation of the test lines instead of over the orientation of the membranes (18, 70).

As mentioned in the preceding paragraphs, B/A can be measured by tracing methods or intersection counting of I/L. In either case one must relate B/A to S/V by constants $4/\pi$ for isotropic surfaces, $\pi/2$ for cyclinders cut longitudinally, or 1 for cylinders cut transversely (Table 2).

Unfortunately one often encounters less simple geometries with only partial orientation. One cannot assume the degree and distribution of the orieintation of a particular organelle without empirical testing and theoretical analysis. Often one has to resort to experimentally determined constants. These can sometimes be obtained from comparison of data from more than one orientation (70, 201).

SECTION THICKNESS. The basic equations of stereology assume that the observed two-dimensional images lie on a true section plane, whereas in fact they are the projection of a thin slab onto a plane. The systematic error caused by the finite thickness of the section must be considered; these errors interact with the effects of orientation (331). A rule of thumb is that projection errors need correction when the section thickness is more than 10% of the size of the structure. Incidentally the section thickness is usually estimated by the interference color of the section floating on water as suggested by Peachey (224).

In muscle the section thickness problem is complex because the sarcolemma and SR tubules are longitudinally oriented and the TC and T tubules lie in an irregular transverse net. Therefore muscle sectioned longitudinally gives the best views of the T and TC membranes (and also of the Z band). Conversely muscle sectioned transversely gives the best view of the SR profiles and the worst view of the T and TC. Some correction factors (130, 330, 334) compensate for underestimation of membrane areas due to section thickness effects. However, these corrections always introduce a degree of uncertainty. Sectioning in both longitudinal and transverse planes can resolve the problem if structures can be recognized in both planes, but this doubles the work; nonetheless it has been done (70, 152, 311). Although sampling errors are minimal if oblique sections are taken (44, 329), such sections introduce systematic errors. Many membrane systems are difficult to resolve in such sections: a membrane at an angle of less than 30° to the plane of section will not be resolved (187). It is more efficient to restrict the sectioning to one orientation and to choose the one most appropriate to the particular study. For example, the Z band, M lines, and T system can only be observed well in longitudinal sections. The SR tubules are best resolved in transverse sections. Mitochondria and lipids are seen well in any orientation because they are large compared with the section thickness.

SPATIAL INHOMOGENEITIES. Classic stereology assumes that the organelles are randomly and homogeneously distributed through a cell. In muscle they are not. Organelles occur in different concentrations in the A band and the I band. Mitochondria are more concentrated in the cell periphery than in the core. One can average over the regional concentrations by pooling data from all regions and assuming that the pool is large enough so that all zones are uniformly represented (44, 45, 311). This is sensible when one only wishes to know the average organelle content and is not interested in regional concentrations. However, sometimes one wants to measure the concentrations in local regions because the functional behavior is related to the local concentration of the organelle. Averaging must be done with care!

One can collect the data in defined zones, such as the fraction of mitochondrial volume in the periphery V_{mitp}/V_p and the fraction of mitochondria in the core V_{mitc}/V_c. If one also collects the fractions of periphery and core to fiber, V_p/V_f and V_c/V_f, then one can calculate the total mitochondria (tot mit) per fiber from the equation

$$\frac{V_{\text{tot mit}}}{V_f} = \frac{V_{mitp}}{V_p}\cdot\frac{V_p}{V_f} + \frac{V_{mitc}}{V_c}\cdot\frac{V_c}{V_f}$$

Recent work on the distribution of mitochondria within a muscle fiber (133), however, leads to doubt that zones can be well defined.

CALIBRATION. The size of an object in an electron micrograph depends on distortion during fixation and sectioning and on calibration of the equipment used. One of the earliest and best discussions of absolute size in electron microscopy is given by Page and Huxley (222).

Glutaraldehyde is the most frequently used fixative and is a rapidly penetrating nonelectrolyte. Introduction of nonelectrolytes into saline solutions produces transient water flows across membranes, with the amount of water flow being determined by the reflection coefficient (43, 160, 309). Reflection coefficients are defined as the ratio of the osmotic flow produced by a concentration gradient of the test solute to the flow caused by the same concentration gradient of an impermeable solute. Thus the value of the reflection coefficient depends on the nature of both the membrane and the test solute. With time, fixatives change the permeability properties of membranes and also change the number of osmotically active particles within the cell. Thus further transient water flows can occur (201). For these reasons the observed size of organelles may not be the size of the living organelle. If possible, the structure should be compared with other preparative techniques, such as freeze fracture or scanning electron microscopy. Unbroken membranes are often used to indicate good fixation. In morphometry, I recommend that the living cell dimensions be compared with the sectioned cell dimensions. This gives an outer limit of cell shrinkage or swelling. However, one can never rule out the possibility that an organelle shrinks (or swells) while the muscle cell swells (or shrinks). This possibility exists because the nonelectrolyte permeabilities are probably different for the membranes of different organelles.

The real limit of morphometry is the uncertainty of preserving absolute size during processing. One must be compulsive about reproducing fixation, embedding, and sectioning procedures from day to day, in the hope that comparative data will be valid even if the absolute dimensions prove faulty.

The calibration of the electron microscope must be made frequently, and magnetic hysteresis in the lenses must be avoided. It has recently been brought to my attention that the calibration grid itself must be measured, since manufacturers' claims cannot all be believed. For instance, one waffle (square) calibration grid was actually rectangular with the length of one side 1.1 times the other, a 10% error! Many microscopists are only interested in relative sizes, and their calibration markers can be in error by ± 20%.

Several workers (45, 260, 274) have calibrated their instruments from the length of the myosin filament, 1.5–1.6 μm, and from the cross-bridge repeat of 14 nm. The myosin has been used as the calibration standard. Using this internal standard, kindly suggested to me by S. Page, I now conclude that the calibration grid that I used at UCLA was in error by 6%. Old tissue blocks were remeasured with new calibration grids and this error was confirmed. Note that volume fractions are dimensionless and therefore are not in error. However, all absolute areas are 12% too large and all lengths are 6% too large (60, 61, 66–70, 72). Ratios and relative values remain unchanged. These corrections have not been applied in the morphometric tables (Tables 3–10), although the calibration bars on the figure are now correct.

MORPHOMETRIC RESULTS

There is by now a sizable literature of morphometric studies of organelle composition in mammalian skeletal muscle (131). Tables 3–10 give average values for these data in a variety of different muscles from small laboratory animals: mouse (189, 290), rat (44, 45, 311), cat (274), rabbit (75), and guinea pig (66, 67, 70). Human muscle data are given in Table 5 and in references 4, 42, 132, 152, 169, 241, 294–296, 336. I have only included normal adult muscle and may have inadvertently omitted important work with normal

TABLE 3. *Volume of Cell Element as Percentage of Cell Volume in Mouse Cardiac Muscle and in Frog, Guinea Pig, and Rabbit Skeletal Muscle*

Cell Element	Mouse	Frog	Guinea Pig				Rabbit	
	Ventricle	Sartorius	Soleus	White vastus	Red vastus	SMA*	Anterior tibialis	Soleus
	Cardiac (302)	FG (201)	SO (70)	FG (66)	FOG (67)	SO†	FG, FOG (75)	SO (75)
Myofibrils	54.3	82.6	86.7	82.0	80.3			
Mitochondria								
Total	37.5	1.6	4.9	1.9	8.2	2.6		
Core‡			3.6	1.5	6.9		1.8	2.9
Periphery‡			18.6	10.6	25.0	12.0	11.9	11.1
T system	0.8	0.32	0.14	0.27	0.28	0.16		
Sarcoplasmic reticulum								
Total	0.6	9.1	3.15	4.59	3.26	1.40		
TC or JSR	0.2	4.1	0.92	1.62	1.24	0.46		
A band			0.51	0.95	0.81			
I band			1.72	2.02	1.21			
Free SR (A+I)	0.4	5.0	2.23	2.97	2.02	0.94		
Nucleus			0.86	0.15	0.96	0.86		
Lipid			0.18	0.012	0.12	0.25		
Blood vessels			2.05	0.8	2.4			

Reference numbers are in parentheses. F, fast twitch; G, glycolytic; S, slow twitch; O, oxidative; TC, terminal cisternae; JSR, junctional sarcoplasmic reticulum. * Semimembranosus accessorius (254). † B. R. Eisenberg, unpublished data. ‡ Mitochondria in the core as a percentage of the core volume; mitochondria in the periphery as a percentage of the peripheral volume.

TABLE 4. *Volume of Cell Element as Percentage of Cell Volume in Cat, Rat, and Mouse Muscle*

Cell Element	Cat (274)			Rat					Mouse			
	Gastrocnemius, medial		Soleus	EDL	Soleus			Gastrocnemius	Gastrocnemius (290)		EDL	Soleus
	F	S	SO	F (44, 45)	SO (44, 45)	SO[a]	SO[b] (311)	FG (311)	Crown FG	Medial FOG, SO	F (189)	SO (189)
Myofibrils							82	85			75	81
Mitochondria total	2.8	5.0	3.6	7.1[c]	10[c]	5.9	7.4	2.2	1–5	3–19	8	6
T system	d	d	d								0.4	0.22
Sarcoplasmic reticulum												
Total	1.28	0.72	0.63	9.3[c]	5.5[c]	3.3					5.5	2.9
A band	0.29[e]	0.28[e]	0.12[e]									
I band	0.95[e]	0.48[e]	0.50[e]									
Nucleus				1.1	2.6							
Lipid				0.1	0.4							

Reference numbers in parentheses. EDL, extensor digitorum longus; F, fast twitch; S, slow twitch; O, oxidative; G, glycolytic. [a] B. R. Eisenberg, unpublished data. [b] Data from longitudinal sections. [c] Means from two colonies of rats. [d] Included in SR. [e] Recalculated from (274) and expressed here as A-band or I-band SR per fiber volume.

TABLE 5. *Volumes of Cell Elements as Percentages of Fiber Volume in Human Muscle*

Cell Element	Vastus Lateralis, Mixed Fibers (131)		Vastus Lateralis, Mixed Fibers, Men (169, 170)	Mixed Muscle, Mixed Fibers, Men and Women (42)	Mixed Muscle, Mixed Fibers, Men and Women (151)	Quadriceps,* Men and Women		Anterior Tibialis, Men (4, 294, 296)		
	Men	Women				F	S	FOG	FG	SO
Myofibrils	85.9	87.4	79.8	83.3						
Mitochondria										
Total	5.19	4.08	4.6	5.14	3.4	1.14	3.03			
Core	4.96	3.97	2.14					3.6	3.1	4.7
Periphery	0.23	0.11								
T system	†	†		†	†	0.28	0.13			
Sarcoplasmic reticulum										
Total	3.78	3.78		1.59		1.94	1.22			
TC or JSR						1.20	0.67			
Free SR (A + I)						0.74	0.55			
Lipid	0.34	0.41	0.56	0.05–1.3	0.12	0.18	0.47			

Reference numbers in parentheses. F, fast twitch; S, slow twitch; O, oxidative; G, glycolytic; TC, terminal cisternae; JSR, junctional sarcoplasmic reticulum. * F fibers have Z width less than 100 nm; S fibers have Z width more than 100 nm. (B. R. Eisenberg, unpublished data.) † T system included in SR.

fibers, particularly if they were measured as controls. Many papers describe muscle during development, disease, and functionally or pharmacologically stressed situations, and it was impractical to search through all this literature for control data.

Each table gives the histochemical fiber type of the muscle being measured. The nomenclature used is slow-twitch, oxidative (SO); fast-twitch, oxidative, glycolytic (FOG); and fast-twitch, glycolytic (FG) as defined by Peter et al. (232). A useful reference for giving the proportions of these histochemical types in small mammals is that of Ariano et al. (7). Because there can be variability from one animal colony to another, it is wiser to correlate the ultrastructure with the histochemical properties in each study.

The reader should not assume that the values given in Tables 3–10 apply to each and every member of a species. There is considerable variation depending on housing conditions and many other factors (134, 156, 265). For example, Davey and Wong (45) compared the mitochondrial content of Wistar rats housed at Monash University, Australia with those housed in Sydney. In Monash the mitochondrial content was 80% higher in extensor digitorum longus (EDL) muscles and 40% higher in soleus! The SR, however, remained remarkably constant.

The volume fractions or volume density V/V are given in Tables 3, 4, and 5. The data are expressed as organelle volume per unit volume of muscle fiber, V_o/V_f. In some cases this required recalculation of published data. Volume fractions are not affected by errors in magnification or orientation (unless the structure is too small). Some ambiguity can occur in names of the membrane systems because SR includes T system in some cases, which are indicated by footnotes to the tables.

The surface density (S/V) is the surface of the organelle per unit volume of muscle fiber (S_o/V_f).

These values are large because large areas of membrane are needed to cover irregular objects. Surface densities are sensitive to errors in magnification and to orientation. Therefore Tables 6, 7, and 8 include information that can be used to assess whether those problems were correctly handled: the section orientation is given and the stereological equation is indicated. If longitudinal sections or A-band lengths are available, the length of the myosin filament is tabulated. Since this value should be 1.6 μm, errors in magnification can be detected.

The surface-to-volume ratios are available for some organelles, S_o/V_o (Table 9). These give the ratio of the surface membrane area of an organelle (S_o) to its own volume (V_o). They are subject to the same systematic errors as those for the calculations of surface density.

Finally, some absolute sizes are given in Table 10. The Z-band width is the most useful of these parameters.

The values in Tables 3–10 are averages. The sample size is usually tens to hundreds of electron micrographs taken randomly from many fibers in several animals. These values are useful when comparison from species to species or from muscle to muscle is being made. When one wants to study the distribution of parameters from fiber to fiber, however, the sample must

TABLE 6. *Ratio of Surface Area of Cell Element to Volume of Cell Comparing Technique for Measuring Surface Density in Mouse, Frog, and Guinea Pig*

	Mouse	Frog	Guinea Pig			
	Ventricle, Cardiac (88)	Sartorius, FG (90)	Soleus, SO (70)	White vastus lateralis, FG (66)	Red vastus lateralis, FOG (67)	SMA,[a] SO[b]
Technique						
Section angle	Random	LS	LS and XS	LS	LS	LS
A-band length, μm		1.7	1.8	1.7	1.7	1.7
Equation	c	d	d e	d	d	d
Cell element			*Surface density, μm²/μm³*			
Plasmalemma						
Total	0.50	0.314	0.177	0.243	0.245	0.133
Periphery	0.28	0.064	0.116	0.097	0.097	0.057
T system	0.22	0.22	0.064	0.146	0.148	0.076
Caveolae		0.03[f]				
Sarcoplasmic reticulum						
Total	0.84	2.03	0.97	1.32	0.98	0.57
TC	0.20	0.54	0.24	0.41	0.33	0.17
A band			0.162	0.30	0.27	
I band			0.566	0.61	0.38	
Free SR (A + I)	0.64	1.49	0.728	0.91	0.65	0.40

Reference numbers are in parentheses. F, fast twitch; S, slow twitch; O, oxidative; G, glycolytic; LS, longitudinal section; XS, cross section; TC, terminal cisternae. [a] Semimembranosus accessorius (242). [b] B. R. Eisenberg, unpublished data. [c] Isotropic equation. [d] Anisotropic equation for oriented cylinders cut in longitudinal section. [e] Anisotropic equation for cylinders cut in cross section. [f] Calculated from 47% S_F/V_F.

TABLE 7. *Ratio of Surface Area of Cell Element to Volume of Cell Comparing Technique for Measuring Surface Density in Cat, Rat, and Mouse*

	Cat (274)			Rat				Mouse		
	Gastrocnemius, medial, F	Gastrocnemius, medial, S	Soleus, S	EDL,[a] F (44, 45)	Soleus, S (44, 45)	Soleus, S (311)	Gastrocnemius, FG (311)	Gastrocnemius, crown, FG (291)	EDL,[a] F (189)	Soleus, S (189)
Technique										
Section angle	LS and XS[b]			XS		XS		LS	LS and XS	
A-band length, μm	1.5			1.4		1.6		1.5	1.6	
Equation	c			c		d		d	e	
Cell element					*Surface density, μm²/μm³*					
Mitochondria	0.40	0.69	0.55							
Plasmalemma										
Peripheral				0.21	0.21					
T system								0.26	0.41[f]	0.24[f]
Total SR	0.81	0.54	0.39	2.41	1.42	2.45	4.59			

Reference numbers in parentheses. F, fast twitch; S, slow twitch; G, glycolytic; LS, longitudinal section; XS, cross section. [a] Extensor digitorum longus. [b] Published data were given separately for I-band organelles from LS and for A-band organelles from XS. Values here are recalculated per fiber volume. The SR value includes T system. [c] Anisotropic equations for cylinders cut in cross section. [d] Isotropic equations. [e] Calculated from size times average number. [f] Calculated from their data for fiber diameter of 30 μm.

contain several micrographs from each fiber. Samples of these distributions can be presented as frequency histograms for individual parameters or as scattergrams for pairs of parameters. When larger numbers of parameters are involved, graphic representation is difficult and can be misleading, especially when some, but not all, parameters are highly correlated.

Membrane Systems

T SYSTEM. Fast-twitch fibers have a T system that is about twice as extensive as that of slow-twitch fibers of the same species. The T system can best be seen in longitudinally sectioned muscle and has not been estimated in oblique or cross-sectioned fibers. Unfortunately many papers lump the T system with the SR, despite their functional and structural separation. The total membrane system may be named the *sarcotubular system* or may even retain the name sarcoplasmic reticulum. The lumping of two different membrane systems is not sensible.

The amount of T system has been estimated by volume density and surface density (66, 67, 70, 189, 201, 291, 302) and length of T luminal axis per unit volume of muscle fiber (63, 75, 274). Of these measurements, the surface density probably has the most functional significance because the action potential travels over the surface. The surface density of the T system remains remarkably constant throughout the length of a fiber (with the exception of the neuromuscular junction and tendon and nuclear regions). However, the surface density of the T system varies quite considerably from one fiber to another. This can be seen in the histogram (Fig. 16) showing the similar distributions of the surface of the T system from the fibers of fast-twitch, glycolytic (white) and fast-twitch, oxidative (red) vastus lateralis of the guinea pig. The mean values from the fast fibers are about twice those of the slow-twitch, oxidative soleus fibers. The volume of the T system was highly correlated with the surface ($r = 0.81$) (67).

TABLE 8. *Ratio of Surface Area of Cell Element to Volume of Cell: Surface Density of Human Muscle and Method of Measuring*

	Vastus Lateralis, Mixed Fibers (131)		Mixed Muscle, Mixed Fibers, Men and Women (151)		Quadriceps[a], Men and Women	
	Men	Women			F	S
Technique						
Section angle	Oblique		LS	XS	LS	LS
A-band length, μm			1.6	1.6	1.7	1.7
Equation	b		c	c	c	c
Cell element	*Surface density, μm²/μm³*					
Mitochondria						
Outer	0.89	0.66				
Cristae	1.06	0.74				
T system					0.17	0.09
SR						
Total	1.69[d]	1.69[d]	1.24	1.92	0.66	0.42
Terminal cisternae					0.40	0.21
Free SR (A + I)					0.26	0.21

Reference numbers in parentheses. F, fast twitch; S, slow twitch; LS, longitudinal section; XS, cross section. [a] B. R. Eisenberg, unpublished data. [b] Equations not given, presumed isotropic. [c] Isotropic equations. [d] Presumed to include T system.

TABLE 10. *Other Morphometric Parameters for Guinea Pig*

Cell Element	Parameters	Soleus S*	White Vastus, FG†	Red Vastus, FOG‡
Myofibrils	Diameter, μm	1.06	1.12	1.19
Mitochondria§				
Transversely oriented	Area, μm²	0.16	0.14	0.20
Longitudinally oriented	Area, μm²	0.44	0.55	1.04
T system	Major diameter, nm	100	100	
	Minor diameter, nm	40	30	
Terminal cisternae	Diameter, nm	130	80	
Free SR	Minor diameter, nm	55	52	
Z line	Width, nm	142	61	88

* From Eisenberg et al. (70) † From Eisenberg and Kuda (66). ‡ From Eisenberg and Kuda (67). § Muscle cut in longitudinal section.

TABLE 9. *Ratio of Surface Area of Cell Element to Volume of Element*

Cell Element	Mouse Ventricle, Cardiac (302)	Frog Sartorius, F (201)	Guinea Pig Soleus, S (70)	Guinea Pig White vastus, FG (66)	Guinea Pig Red vastus, FOG (67)	Guinea Pig SMA,* S	Human Quadriceps, Mixed Type (131)
	Surface density, μm²/μm³						
Myofibrils		3.8	3.8†	3.6†	3.4†		
Mitochondria							17‡
T system	33.3	69	46	54	53	48	33
SR							
Total	140	22	30	29	30	41	17
Terminal cisternae	128	13	24	26	27	37	17
Free SR (A + I)	148	30	33	31	32	43	18

Reference numbers in parentheses. F, fast twitch; S, slow twitch; G, glycolytic; O, oxidative. * Semimembranosus accessorius. (B. R. Eisenberg, unpublished data.) † Calculated from myofibril-diameter data assuming that myofibrils have a circular cylindrical shape. ‡ Calculated from published data for volume and surface densities.

TERMINAL CISTERNAE. Fast-twitch fibers also have a more extensive TC system than do slow-twitch fibers. The T and TC systems cooperate functionally and the amounts of both systems within a given fiber are highly correlated ($r = 0.85$) (67). The extent of the T membrane facing the TC membrane has not been measured in mammals but is known in frog (201). The number of pillars per unit area of T system has also been measured in frog [(64); see review (94)]. Although this number might well be higher in fast-twitch than in slow-twitch fibers, it has not been measured in them. The volume and surface densities have been used to estimate the extent of the TC (66, 67, 70, 132, 201, 302). Figure 17 shows that the surface area of TC

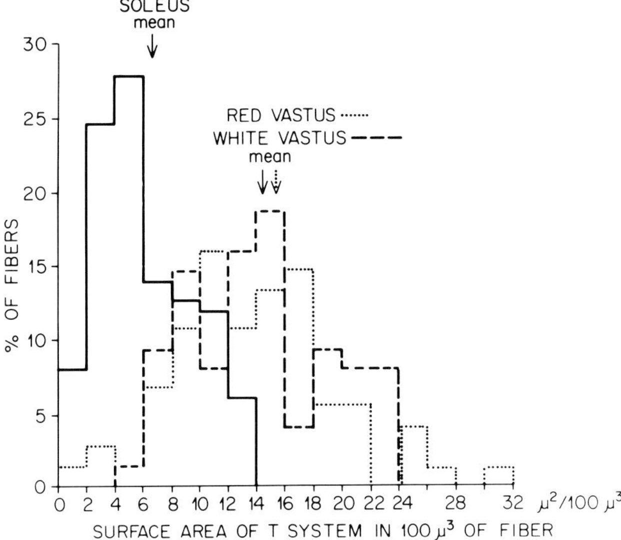

FIG. 16. Histograms of surface area of T system from 300 fibers in 3 muscles of the guinea pig. Note that fast-twitch red and white vastus fibers show identical distributions, but differ from slow-twitch soleus fibers. [From Eisenberg and Kuda (67).]

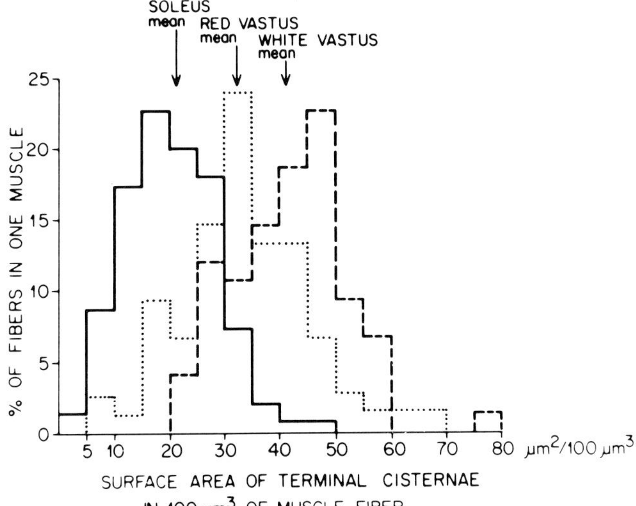

FIG. 17. Histograms of surface area of terminal cisternae from 3 muscles of the adult guinea pig. [From Eisenberg and Kuda (67).]

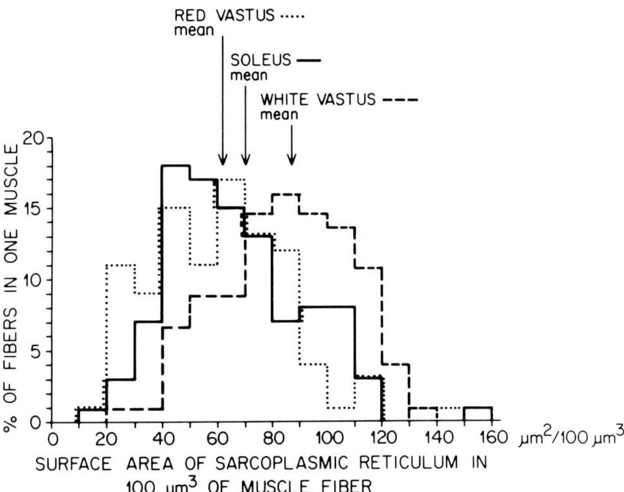

FIG. 18. Histograms of surface area of sarcoplasmic reticulum are similar for all 3 guinea pig muscles. [From Eisenberg and Kuda (67).]

per unit volume of fiber allows excellent separation of fast-twitch from slow-twitch fibers and even allows some separation between fast-twitch, oxidative (red) and fast-twitch, glycolytic (white) vastus fibers.

FREE SR. The portion of the SR that runs longitudinally between the TC and does not contain the granular material found in them is called the longtitudinal or free SR (96). Many papers lump the free SR with the TC. Morphometric values for free SR are given in Tables 3–10. The distributions for the surface area of the free SR (Fig. 18) are similar in guinea pig slow-twitch, oxidative; fast-twitch, oxidative; and fast-twitch, glycolytic muscles (67). Surprisingly the mean values are the same in the physiologically fast and slow muscles. However, note that the standard deviation is 30% of the mean, which implies the existence of a large biological variation or experimental error. Perhaps the error arose because the longitudinal, free-SR tubules are of comparable size to the section thickness and recognition errors were very high in longitudinally sectioned material. However, this does not appear to be the case because similar values were obtained from cross and longitudinal sections of soleus muscle (see the table on p. 750 in ref. 70).

Contractile Systems

MYOFIBRILS. The myofibrils occupy 75%–85% of the fiber volume (Tables 3–5) in most species and muscles. The size of myofibrils (111, 112), or perhaps more correctly the peripheral boundary around the thin filament bundle of the I band (67), has been estimated. Fast- and slow-twitch mammalian skeletal muscle have similar myofibril size.

Z DISK. The width of the Z disk in longitudinally sectioned muscles has long been used to classify fibers from electron micrographs (61, 67, 100, 101, 260, 264). Fast-twitch fibers have narrower Z disks than do slow-

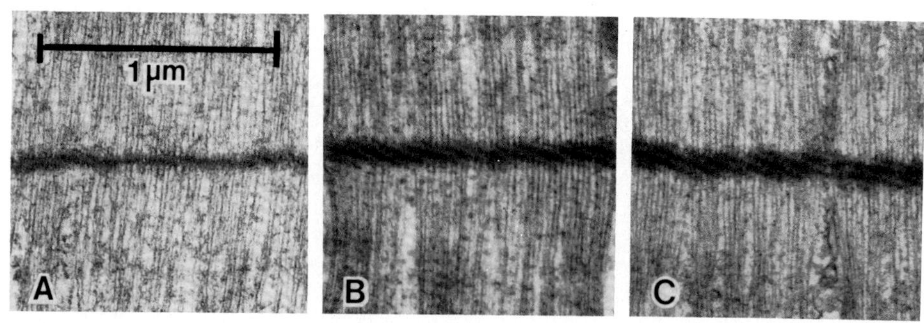

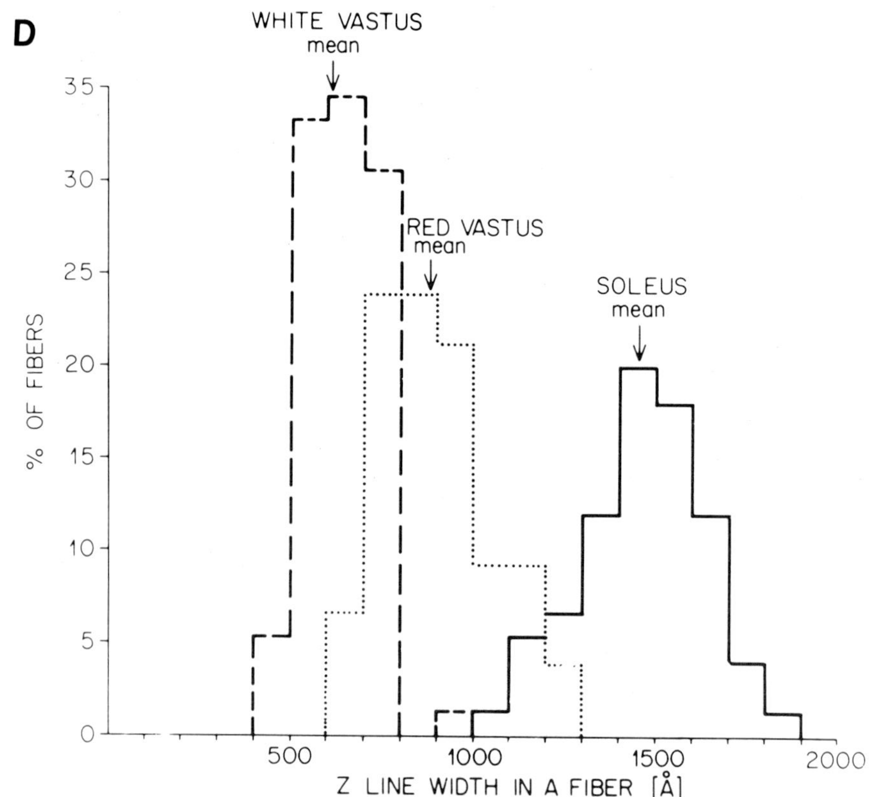

FIG. 19. Segments of Z-line structure from longitudinally sectioned muscle of the adult guinea pig. Range in width of Z line is seen: *A*, white vastus; *B*, red vastus; *C*, soleus muscle. *D*: histogram of widths of Z-line structure from segments of Z line similar to those in *A*, *B*, and *C*. The Z lines from 300 guinea pig fibers were measured. [From Eisenberg (60).]

twitch fibers (Fig. 19; Table 10). In most electron micrographs the orientation of the section is random with respect to the planes of the Z lattice. Furthermore dense material adheres to the Z lattice and obscures structural details. Therefore most estimates of Z-disk width are actually average measurements across some central dense zone (75, 279, 280). In certain orientations more revealing Z-overlap regions can be seen, which provide details of the Z-lattice spacings (114, 115, 117, 118, 264).

Nonetheless the Z disk can be reproducibly measured (100 ± 5 nm) (70) and has been found to be a most valuable structural parameter for discriminating fiber types [Table 10; (70, 296)]. The Z-line width is highly correlated to the surface and volume densities of the T and TC systems ($r \sim 0.6$) (67). The histogram of distributions for Z-line widths from three different guinea pig muscles (Fig. 19*D*) shows that slow-twitch and fast-twitch fibers are indeed from different populations. Within the fast-twitch population, however, there is considerable overlap between the two subtypes, the fast-twitch, glycolytic and fast-twitch, oxidative, glycolytic.

M LINE. The M lines vary in different fibers (173, 223, 296). In a recent study on human muscle, fibers were examined in the electron microscope and the same fiber was identified with histochemical techniques in the light microscope (296). Slow-twitch, oxidative (type I) fibers have five strong M lines. Fast-twitch, oxidative (type IIA) fibers have three strong central lines bordered by two weak lines. Fast-twitch, glycolytic (type IIB) fibers display only three strong central lines. These differences in M lines are not observed in all species. For example, different types of rabbit fibers are not readily distinguishable by their M-line structure, whereas rat fibers are (M. Sjöström, personal communication).

Metabolic Systems

MITOCHONDRIA. Mitochondria perform oxidative metabolism for their host muscle fiber. As expected, fibers with a high oxidative capacity have a high mitochondrial content, a rich capillary supply, and a red color. The low-oxidative (and high-glycolytic) fibers have a low oxidative capacity, a sparse blood supply, and a whiter color. Intermediate fibers have a pinkish color.

Much morphometry averages the mitochondrial content over many fibers in a whole muscle. Oxidative muscles have higher volumes of mitochondria per unit muscle volume, and glycolytic muscles have lower volume densities [Tables 3–10; (4, 44, 45, 66, 67, 70, 75, 132, 169, 170, 189, 201, 274, 294, 296, 302, 311)]. Individual fibers must be sampled in order to measure the intermediate mitochondrial content of pink fibers. Estimates of mitochondrial volume density should not be affected by the orientation of the section plane because the mitochondrial profiles are readily recognized in any orientation. Experimental comparisons confirm this expectation (70, 152). Care must be taken to sample the A and I bands in an unbiased way because more mitochondria are located in the I band than the A band. I believe that longitudinal sections provide the best sample of mitochondria, particularly if they are preferentially found in one band or the other. Systematic errors are readily corrected in longitudinal sections [see discussion in Eisenberg (62)].

Measurement of the concentration of mitochondria in nuclear and subsarcolemmal regions is also subject to sampling difficulties. Attention must also be paid to the denominator in the fraction estimated stereologically. Does it refer to the whole fiber, or has only the core of the fiber been included? Oblique or cross sections provide the least biased sampling over the core and periphery (44, 45, 329) and can retain information about the radial distribution of mitochondria (133). Longitudinal sections do not give a good estimate of the periphery for an individual fiber (70). However, longitudinal sections provide a millimeter or so of length of the fiber on the electron-microscopic grid, and thus a large enough area of a single fiber is available to provide an estimate of mitochondrial volume per unit volume (of the fiber core) for a single fiber.

Figure 20 shows histograms of mitochondrial content in the core of single guinea pig fibers. In human muscle a bimodal distribution allows easy separation into two populations of high-oxidative (red) and low-oxidative (white) fibers (Fig. 21). However, in guinea pig the distributions are far more complicated and

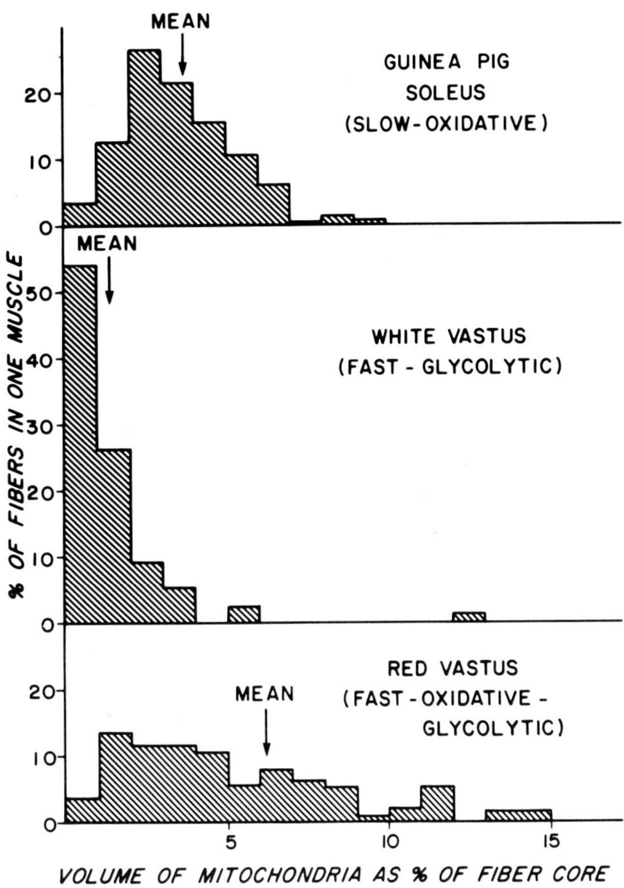

FIG. 20. Histograms of volume of mitochondria in fiber core from 300 fibers in 3 muscles of the guinea pig. Note large range and skewed distribution for fast-twitch fibers. [Redrawn from Eisenberg and Kuda (67).]

many of the fibers belong to an intermediate pink category (Fig. 20).

The mitochondrial content does not correlate in any way with the speed of an individual twitch, but it has been correlated with resistance to fatigue or with the frequency of action potentials within a burst of twitches. The mitochondrial content is readily altered by increased demands on the muscle (265).

The surface areas of the outer and inner mitochondrial membranes have been extensively estimated in cardiac muscle (5, 6, 213, 219, 302). However, in skeletal muscle there is little information published (132, 274). More attention seems to have been paid to the number of mitochondrial profiles per unit area (67, 152) and the average cross-sectional area of a mitochondrial profile (Table 10). Unfortunately these latter parameters do not yield stereological equations of numerical density, because the mitochondria have such a complex geometry in the third dimension. Branched structures cannot be reconstructed mathematically after cuts have been made experimentally!

LIPID DROPLETS. Lipid droplets are approximately spherical and their mean cross-sectional profile area has been measured (120, 222). The volume fraction of

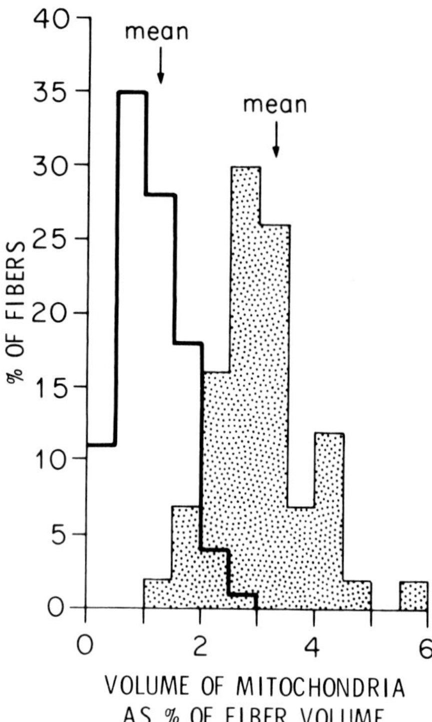

FIG. 21. Histogram of volume of mitochondria in fiber core of human muscle from quadriceps of adult males. Population was arbitrarily divided into 2 groups: stippled histogram is from fibers with a Z-line width >100 nm (presumed slow twitch), and empty histogram is of fibers with a Z-line width <100 nm (presumed fast twitch). (Unpublished data of B. R. Eisenberg.)

lipid has been estimated for different fiber types (Tables 3, 4, and 5) and fibers that have a high oxidative capacity also have higher lipid concentrations (67, 223, 241). Trained athletes also have higher lipid volumes, and it has been shown that there is an increased reliance on lipid as an energy source during prolonged exercise (38, 83, 123, 129, 184).

MUSCLE FIBER DIVERSITY

Historically most studies of mammalian muscle have assumed that restricted fiber types exist. This assumption arose in attempts to describe the diverse nature of muscle: it was simpler to classify into types than to deal with continuous distributions of muscle properties. However, when several properties were measured from the same muscles, the classifications scheme became anything but simple to apply. The problem was compounded when the time course of dynamic adaptation from one type to another was being studied, for example, adaptations caused by exercise, aging, or stimulation.

A contemporary hypothesis is that fibers are diverse in function and structure and that fibers respond to physiological demands by altering their diverse properties. Testing this hypothesis requires experimental data from populations of single fibers. The data ideally describe the physiological, biochemical, and structural properties of the same fiber. No one has yet achieved this goal. At present studies of whole muscle and the kinds of structure-function correlations that have been well established by other techniques must be relied on.

In the earlier part of this chapter three functional systems, the excitation-contraction coupling system, the contractile system, and the metabolic system, were related to three anatomical systems. These three systems and the anatomical structures that support them were discussed in the section PHYSIOLOGICAL FUNCTIONS, p. 76. These three systems do not function independently: all work together. Furthermore in an electron micrograph one does not see a single anatomical system: all are present. Thus electron micrographs of single muscle fibers provide useful data on the diverse systems within a muscle fiber. Few other techniques sample so many different biochemical and physiological systems of a muscle fiber.

An anatomist looking at a large group of electron micrographs taken from different muscles can sort them by eye into groups and guess their origin (67). The task might not be so easy if more muscles with less functional diversity were used. In sorting, the anatomist is unconsciously looking at many variables and evaluating them according to some previous scheme.

It is preferable to use an objective scheme based on the statistical theory of multivariate analysis. Useful statistical references (166, 244, 299) explain the difference between discrimination, classification, and dissection. In all cases many measurements from members of the population are made. In discrimination analysis the existence of two or more populations is given. The problem is to set up a rule that enables us to allocate some new individual to the correct population. In classification, the problem is to classify samples of individuals into groups that are as distinct as possible. In discrimination the existence of groups is given; in classification it is a matter to be determined. In dissection a sample or population is divided into groups, whether the border lines of subdivision are natural or not.

In our anatomical studies it would seem that classification is the statistical method of choice. In practice, however, there are problems in defining how tightly or loosely clustered a group should be. Therefore we used discriminant analysis in our studies (67): if the discriminator (i.e., the computer) could not place an unknown fiber or micrograph into the "fiber type" from which it was known to come, the concept of fiber type would be falsified. Discriminant analysis has an additional useful feature. It selects the structural parameters that best discriminate an unknown fiber and classify a fiber into a distinct group.

The analysis took data from many fibers of a known histochemical fiber type and then used discriminant analysis to reclassify them. The best discriminator was the Z-line width, followed by the mitochondrial volume, and then the surface area of the TC (67). Other parameters were weighted very lightly and were not of much use in determining the fiber type.

Gratifyingly the somewhat abstract discriminant analysis selected one anatomical discriminator for each of the three major systems of muscle: Z-line width for the contractile system, mitochondrial volume for the metabolic system, and TC area for the EC system. The majority of electron microscopists have also chosen the Z-line width and mitochondrial volume. The EC coupling system is the most difficult system to assess in practice. Most microscopists use a measure of the T system, although the discriminant analysis selected the surface area of the TC.

Once the best structural discriminators of fiber type are objectively known, the number of measurements needed on an unknown muscle is greatly reduced. If one had absolute confidence in the statistical analysis and its applicability to the unknown muscle being examined, one would only need to measure the discriminant variables.

It is not enough to study the variables of a multivariate system one by one, since correlations between variables often are the essence of a problem. Individual histograms of diameter and weight of a population of spheres do not permit conclusions about the distribution of density, a correlated variable. A population of spheres with a distribution of densities cannot be distinguished from a population of uniform density, with distributed diameter and weight, unless the correlation of volume and diameter is studied. For this reason, one must study the relation of Z-line width, mitochondrial volume, and (for example) TC area from fiber to fiber, thereby examining the interdependence of the various systems. Scattergrams, plots of one variable against another, illustrate such interdependence. The correlation coefficient of one variable with another is a numerical estimate of interdependence.

I now discuss some of the analyses of paired anatomical data and relate these to their physiological functions: *1*) the contractile and metabolic systems, *2*) the metabolic system and the EC coupling system, *3*) the contractile and EC coupling systems. In principle, one should look for higher-order correlations (among more than two variables); these are awkward to visualize and fortunately not necessary in our analysis.

Contractile and Metabolic Systems

To determine the correlation of Z-line width and the mitochondrial content paired data are taken from many fibers, thus testing whether these variables are dependent on each other. The speed of the fiber might be expected to correlate with the width of the Z line, and the fatigue resistance of the fiber might be expected to correlate with mitochondrial content.

When data from many fibers are considered, a low correlation coefficient is found between Z-line width and mitochondrial content ($r = 0.34$) (152). However, when only the fast-twitch population is considered, the correlation coefficient is increased ($r = 0.57$) (67). Perhaps this implies that within the group called fast fibers the Z disk and the mitochondria are both related to the underlying pattern of activity. The slow-twitch fibers, however, belong to a distinct group and for them the correlation fails.

In every case the scattergram has a large cloud of points (Fig. 22), each point representing the value of the Z-line width and mitochondrial volume for a single fiber (60, 67, 70, 152, 290). When additional information about the fibers is available, however, some clustering can be recognized. For example, fibers typed by histochemical means show distinct clusters (Fig. 23), as do fibers (Fig. 22) that come from muscles of relatively pure fiber type, judged biochemically, histochemically, and physiologically (232).

The physiological function of a fiber with a low mitochondrial content is to give a short, fast contraction. Presumably, fibers with the shortest duration of activity have the lowest mitochondrial content and narrowest Z band. In guinea pig these fibers are located in the lower left portion of the scattergram (Figs. 22 and 23). Some fibers have the same fast contraction time but a longer duration of activity (30). Perhaps these are higher in mitochondrial content, wider in Z-band width, and in the upper part of the fast-twitch fiber group. Scattergrams provide no evidence that two subtypes of fast-twitch fibers exist, namely fast-twitch, oxidative (red) and fast-twitch, oxidative, glycolytic (white) fibers. Rather, there seems to be a continuous rather broad distribution of properties with the fast-twitch type.

The clear separation between the slow-twitch and fast-twitch population is interesting (Figs. 22 and 23). The slow-twitch group in guinea pig is separated by both the expected increase in Z-disk width and an unexpected decrease in mitochondrial volume. The width of the Z disk may correlate linearly with speed, but the mitochondrial content clearly does not. Instead of continuing to grow more mitochondria to keep up with the increased energy being demanded, the fiber seems to change the contractile proteins from the fast-twitch to the slow-twitch kind. Perhaps there is a gain in efficiency and economy to the cell by changing this way.

In human muscle biopsies, diverse, mixed populations of fibers are examined, rather than the highly specialized muscles of the common laboratory animals. In humans one might expect more widely scattered plots. However, the scattergram of Z width and mitochondrial volume of some human muscle (241) is similar to that of the guinea pig. Muscle from sedentary humans [(152), B. R. Eisenberg, unpublished observations] contain very few high-oxidative, narrow Z fibers (FOG type). The proportion of FOG fibers increases in human long-distance runners but not in

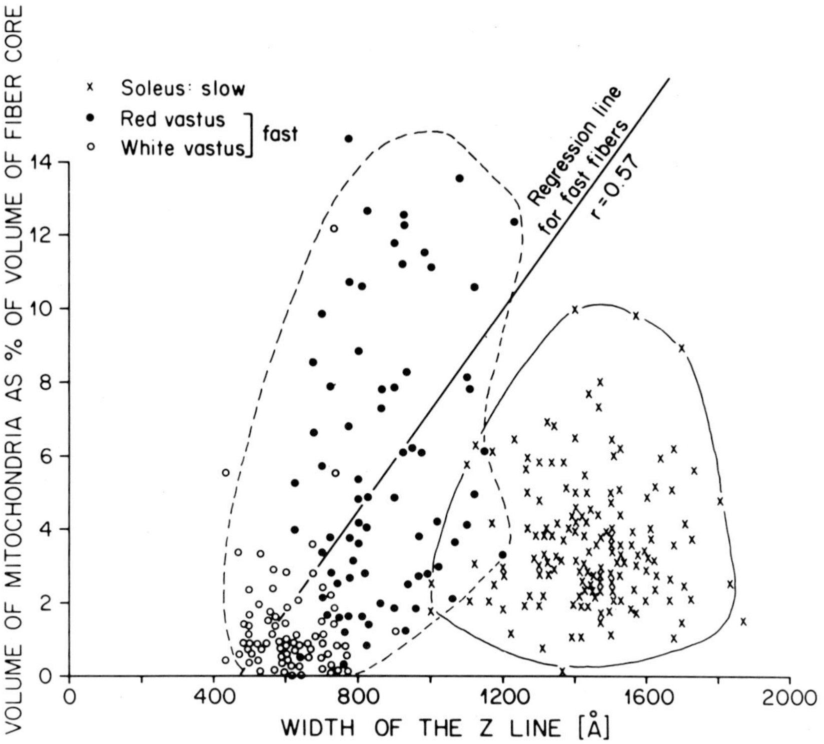

FIG. 22. Scattergram of Z-line width vs. mitochondrial volume in core of fibers. Slow-twitch soleus fibers form a separate cluster from fast-twitch red and white vastus fibers. Within fast-twitch fiber population there is some correlation (r = 0.57) between Z-line width and mitochondrial volume. [From Eisenberg (60).]

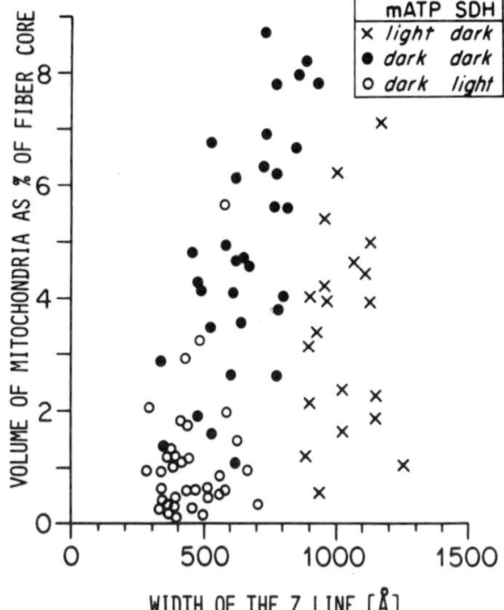

FIG. 23. Scattergram of Z-line width vs. mitochondrial volume measured from electron micrographs of medial gastrocnemius muscle fibers of the guinea pig that had been frozen, thawed, and then fixed. Serial cryostat sections were used to determine histochemical stains of myofibrillar ATP and succinic dehydrogenase (SDH) of each fiber to give the conventional fiber types: x, slow-twitch, oxidative; ●, fast-twitch, oxidative, glycolytic; and ○, fast-twitch, glycolytic (see Fig. 15). The 3 types form 1 large cluster that can be separated into 3 subclusters only by reference to histochemical profile of the fiber. [From Eisenberg and Kuda (68), reprinted from *J. Histochem. Cytochem.* Copyright 1977 by The Histochemical Society, Inc.]

power lifters (241), so there is clearly a large dynamic range. Scattergrams provide a good method for following dynamic or plastic events.

Metabolic and EC Coupling Systems

The volumes of mitochondria (of the metabolic system) have been frequently estimated, but the surface areas of membranes (of the EC coupling system) have been measured only occasionally (45, 67). It is not surprising that relationships between these two systems have not been well explored. Eisenberg and Kuda (67) studied guinea pig muscle and plotted the mitochondrial volume against the surface area of the TC (Fig. 24). They found that only 73% of the fibers could be correctly classified in a discriminant analysis. A much better reallocation (89%) is achieved with scattergrams of Z-band width and mitochondrial volume (67). Davey and Wong (45) plotted the mitochondrial content of rat muscle against the reciprocal of the fractional volume of the SR. They found a regression coefficient of some 0.6 for these parameters but no physiological implications were made. The pair of variables used by Davey and Wong (45) may prove particularly useful in future work because these variables can be measured in transverse sections.

Contractile and EC Coupling Systems

As discussed, the Z-line width seems to be related to the speed of contraction, as do measures of the EC

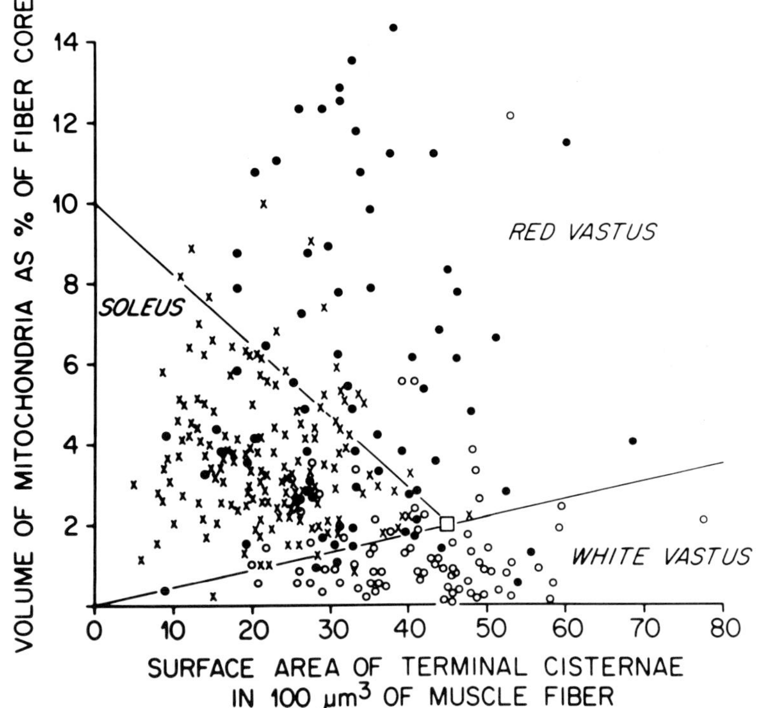

FIG. 24. Scattergram of surface area of terminal cisternae plotted against volume of the mitochondria for 300 fibers from guinea pig muscle. Ad hoc lines are drawn by eye to separate the 3 muscles into 3 areas. Tallies of correct fiber allocations are given in ref. 67. Note that soleus fiber symbols are tightly clustered. However, red vastus fiber symbols form a large cloud not readily separated from the white vastus fiber symbols. X, Soleus; ●, red vastus; ○, white vastus. [From Eisenberg and Kuda (67).]

coupling system. Both have been estimated several ways as discussed. Fibers with wide Z disks (slow contracting) have a lower amount of SR and T system, but correlation coefficients have not been given (75, 280).

The choice of variables in a scattergram depends on practical as well as theoretical considerations. Because T profiles can be counted much faster than areas of membrane can be determined (75), scattergrams have often used this variable as a measure of the EC system [see Fig. 25; (75, 279)].

MUSCLE FIBER PLASTICITY

A muscle fiber can adapt readily when different work output is demanded from it. The muscle fiber changes the specialized contractile proteins from which the filaments are built and also changes the amount and extent of the membrane and metabolic systems. Several reviews can introduce the reader to this extensive and rapidly growing area of research (156, 233, 265, 323). It is now well accepted that the activity of the muscle determines the type of the fiber. The nerve normally drives this activity. The fast-twitch fibers are under voluntary control and respond more rapidly to change in usage than do the slow-twitch fibers, which are mainly under reflex control. Because conversion of type can occur in denervated preparations (186), the very existence of neurotrophic (chemical) factors for a switch in muscle type is in question. However, the chemicals traveling up and down the neuron by axoplasmic transport are obviously essential for the maintenance of a healthy, functional neuromuscular junction.

The state of muscle has been manipulated in many ways, including cross innervation (255, 256), immobilization (113, 318), exercise (216, 265), and electrical stimulation (234, 235, 242, 258, 262–267, 307, 308). Development and aging also affect the state of a muscle (see the chapter by Kelly in this *Handbook*). For the most part, the new demands on the muscle have been drastic and the experiments have shown that the muscle fibers are capable of transforming from one fiber type to another.

The concept of a rigid, immutable fiber type has been discarded, and it is now time to study the mechanisms by which fiber plasticity is accomplished. Surely plasticity will prove a complex process involving every cellular function. An obvious first step in studying plasticity is to follow the time course of fiber transformation. Because it surveys so many systems of muscle, electron microscopy has been a useful technique (75).

Ultrastructural studies have been done on rabbit muscle in which the nerve to the normally fast-twitch tibialis anterior muscle receives chronic stimulation for many weeks (264, 267). The ultrastructure of the muscle transforms in every system. Eisenberg and Salmons (75) studied the time course of these changes and found that the transformation of the EC coupling system (as estimated by profiles of the T system) begins in a few days and is complete by 2 wk. The Z-band width increases between 1.5 and 3 wk. The

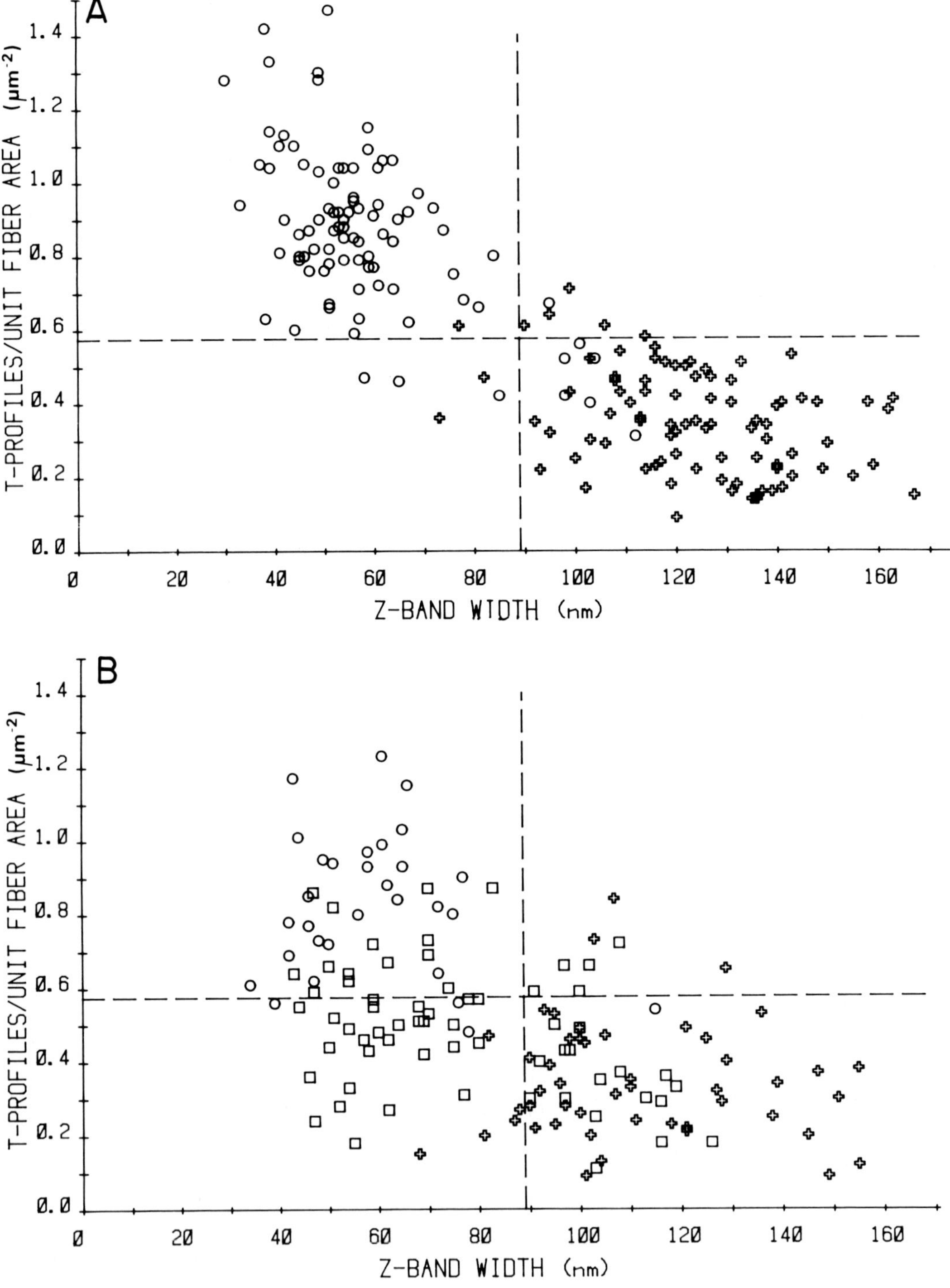

FIG. 25. Scattergram of Z-band width vs. number of T profiles per unit fiber area Q_T/A_F for rabbit muscle. *A: open circles* represent 80 control tibialis anterior (TA) fibers and *open crosses*, 89 control soleus fibers. Note that most TA control fibers are in *upper left quadrant*; most soleus fibers are in *lower right quadrant*. Quadrants are created by lines at Z = 90 nm and $Q_T/A_f = 0.58\ \mu m^{-2}$ computed at Gaussian crossover points. *B*: scattergram of Z-band width vs. number of T profiles for stimulated TA fibers from rabbit muscle. Symbols indicate duration of stimulation. *Open circles*, at an early stage (0–2 days) stimulated fibers occupy *upper left quadrant* (fast-twitch type); *squares*, at times for periods of stimulation from 5 to 12 days, most fibers occupy *lower left quadrant* (transitional type); *open crosses*, after 2 wk of stimulation most fibers occupy *lower right quadrant* (slow-twitch type). [From Eisenberg and Salmons (75).]

volume of mitochondria peaked during transformation (at 1–7 wk) and eventually reached a steady level, still above normal levels. The scattergram of the Z-band width plotted against the T-profile density (Fig. 25) shows clearly that the T system changes before the Z band (lower left quadrant) and that unusual fiber composition can occur during fiber transformation.

During fiber transformation, many cellular processes are affected. The membrane systems and metabolic systems are altered in quantity but not in kind, at least as judged in the electron microscope (which can not discriminate isoenzymes). The contractile machinery is being altered in kind. This transformation must involve suppression of genes for old proteins, perhaps it also involves an increase in the rate of degradation of the old proteins. Transformation also requires switching on genes to make new proteins. All of these processes must be triggered and controlled by the mechanical function of the fiber.

The mechanism of fiber transformation is as yet unknown, and there may be more than one way the fiber can transform. The task is now to apply biologically relevant challenges to a muscle and to monitor biochemical and structural changes relevant to the eventual physiological adaptation. The major relevant physiological properties are *1)* speed, either as the isometric time to peak tension or as the isotonic velocity of shortening; *2)* strength of the isometric tension, which is related to fiber size; *3)* distance of shortening, depending on both the resting sarcomere length and number of sarcomeres as well as on the duration of the active state; and finally, *4)* fatigue, which involves the balance of oxidative and glycolytic metabolism, the cross-bridge proteins, and perhaps the EC coupling system. At present, it is not clear which of these physiological properties of the twitch are functionally important in a given muscle. Most likely, different motor units have different physiological roles, and thus depend on different fundamental properties for their natural function. Some motor units are likely to have tension as their natural output; others, velocity of shortening; still others, an amount of shortening.

One current hypothesis concerning the mechanism of transformation is naive but testable. It assumes that *the twitch is the switch* controlling the long-term structural and functional character of a fiber. The problem is to understand how the mechanical twitch controls the molecular switch, which in turn governs the contractile abilities of the fiber, its natural output.

This research would not have been possible without the technical support of Aileen M. Kuda, Ruth Knopf, Mary Meus, and others and of the secretarial assistance of Alease Negron and Glenda A. Keaton. I am indebted to Drs. M. Ann Goldstein, John E. Rash, and Clara Franzini-Armstrong for supplying figures. I especially thank Dr. Robert S. Eisenberg for editing this review from the perspective of a related outsider.

I appreciate the grant support from the Muscular Dystrophy Association for the past 10 years.

REFERENCES

1. ALLBROOK, D. Skeletal muscle regeneration. *Muscle Nerve* 4: 234–245, 1981.
2. ALMERS, W. Gating currents and charge movements in excitable membranes. *Rev. Physiol. Biochem. Pharmacol.* 82: 97–190, 1978.
3. ANDERSSON-CEDERGREN, E. Ultrastructure of motor end-plate and sarcoplasmic components of mouse skeletal muscle fibre as revealed by three-dimensional reconstruction from serial sections. *J. Ultrastruct. Res. 1 Suppl.* 5: 1–191, 1959.
4. ÄNGQUIST, K. A., AND M. SJÖSTRÖM. Intermittent claudication and muscle fiber fine structure: morphometric data on mitochondrial volumes. *Ultrastruct. Pathol.* 1: 461–470, 1980.
5. ANVERSA, P., A. V. LOUD, F. GIACOMELLI, AND J. WIENER. Absolute morphometric study of myocardial hypertrophy in experimental hypertension. II. Ultrastructure of myocytes and interstitium. *Lab. Invest.* 38: 597–609, 1978.
6. ANVERSA, P., G. OLIVETTI, M. MELISSARI, AND A. V. LOUD. Morphometric study of myocardial hypertrophy induced by abdominal aortic stenosis. *Lab. Invest.* 40: 341–349, 1979.
7. ARIANO, M. A., R. B. ARMSTRONG, AND V. R. EDGERTON. Hindlimb muscle fiber population of five mammals. *J. Histochem. Cytochem.* 21: 51–55, 1973.
8. ASHMORE, C. R., AND L. DOERR. Comparative aspects of muscle fiber types in different species. *Exp. Neurol.* 31: 408–418, 1971.
9. BÁRÁNY, M. ATPase activity of myosin correlated with speed of muscle shortening. *J. Gen. Physiol.* 50: 197–216, 1967.
10. BARNARD, R. J., V. R. EDGERTON, T. FURUKAWA, AND J. B. PETER. Histochemical, biochemical, and contractile properties of red, white, and intermediate fibers. *Am. J. Physiol.* 220: 410–414, 1971.
11. BARNARD, R. J., V. R. EDGERTON, AND J. B. PETER. Effect of exercise on skeletal muscle. I. Biochemical and histochemical properties. *J. Appl. Physiol.* 28: 762–766, 1970.
12. BASKIN, R. J. Ultrastructure and calcium transport in microsomes from developing muscle. *J. Ultrastruct. Res.* 49: 348–371, 1974.
13. BENNETT, H. S., AND K. R. PORTER. An electron microscopic study of sectioned breast muscle of domestic fowl. *Am. J. Anat.* 93: 61–105, 1953.
14. BERINGER, T. A freeze-fracture study of sarcoplasmic reticulum from fast and slow muscle of the mouse. *Anat. Rec.* 184: 647–664, 1975.
15. BILLETER, R., H. WEBER, H. LUTZ, H. HOWALD, M. EPPENBERGER, AND E. JENNY. Myosin types in human skeletal muscle fibres. *Histochemistry* 65: 249–259, 1980.
16. BORG, T. K., AND J. B. CAULFIELD. Morphology of connective tissue in skeletal muscle. *Tissue Cell* 12: 197–207, 1980.
17. BORMIOLI, S. P., AND S. SCHIAFFINO. A procedure for correlated histological, histochemical and ultrastructural study of skeletal muscle tissue. *J. Submicrosc. Cytol.* 7: 361–371, 1975.
18. BOSSEN, E. H., J. R. SOMMER, AND R. A. WAUGH. Comparative stereology of the mouse and finch left ventricle. *Tissue Cell* 10: 773–784, 1978.
19. BOWMAN, W. On the minute structure and movement of voluntary muscle. *Philos. Trans. R. Soc. London Ser. B* 130: 457–501, 1840.
20. BRAY, D. F., D. G. RAYNS, AND E. B. WAGENAAR. Intramembrane particle densities in freeze-fractured sarcoplasmic reticulum. *Can. J. Zool.* 56: 140–145, 1978.
21. BROOKE, M. H., AND W. K. ENGEL. The histographic analysis of human muscle biopsies with regard to fiber types. 1. Adult male and female. *Neurology* 19: 221–233, 1969.
22. BROOKE, M. H., AND K. K. KAISER. Muscle fiber types: how

many and what kind? *Arch. Neurol. Chicago* 23: 369–379, 1970.

23. BRÜCKE, E. Untersuchungen über den Bau der Muskelfasern mit Hülfe des polarisierten Lichtes. *Denkschr. Acad. Wiss. Math-Naturw. Wien* 15: 69–84, 1858.
24. BUCHTHAL, F., AND H. SCHMALBRUCH. Motor unit of mammalian muscle. *Physiol. Rev.* 60: 90–142, 1980.
25. BUFFON, G. Essai d'arithmétique morale. *Suppl. Histoire Naturelle Paris* 4: 1777.
26. BURKE, R. E., AND V. R. EDGERTON. Motor unit properties and selective involvement in movement. *Exercise Sport Sci. Rev.* 3: 31–81, 1975.
27. BURKE, R. E., D. N. LEVINE, M. SALCMAN, AND P. TSAIRIS. Motor units in cat soleus muscle: physiological, histochemical and morphological characteristics. *J. Physiol. London* 238: 503–514, 1974.
28. BURKE, R. E., D. N. LEVINE, P. TSAIRIS, AND F. E. ZAJAC. Physiological types and histochemical profiles in motor units of the cat gastrocnemius. *J. Physiol. London* 234: 723–748, 1973.
29. BURKE, R. E., D. N. LEVINE, F. E. ZAJAC, P. TSAIRIS, AND W. K. ENGEL. Mammalian motor units: physiological-histochemical correlation in three types in cat gastrocnemius. *Science* 174: 709–712, 1971.
30. BURKE, R. E., AND P. TSAIRIS. Anatomy and innervation ratios in motor units of cat gastrocnemius. *J. Physiol. London* 234: 749–765, 1973.
31. BURKE, R. E., AND P. TSAIRIS. Trophic functions of the neuron. II. Denervation and regulation of muscle. The correlation of physiological properties with histochemical characteristics in single muscle unit. *Ann. NY Acad. Sci.* 228: 145–159, 1974.
32. CASTILLO DE MARUENDA, E., AND C. FRANZINI-ARMSTRONG. Satellite and invasive cells in frog sartorius muscle. *Tissue Cell* 10: 749–772, 1978.
33. CHANDLER, W. K., R. F. RAKOWSKI, AND M. F. SCHNEIDER. Effects of glycerol treatment and maintained depolarization on charge movement in skeletal muscle. *J. Physiol. London* 254: 285–316, 1976.
34. CHASE, D., K. DASSE, A. H. GOLDBERG, AND W. C. ULLRICK. Influence of acute hypoxia on Z-line width of cardiac muscle. *J. Mol. Cell. Cardiol.* 10: 1077–1080, 1978.
35. CHASE, D., AND W. C. ULLRICK. Changes in Z-disc width of vertebrate skeletal muscle following tenotomy. *Experientia* 33: 1177–1178, 1977.
36. CLOSE, R. I. Dynamic properties of mammalian skeletal muscles. *Physiol. Rev.* 52: 129–197, 1972.
37. COSTANTIN, L. L. Contractile activation in skeletal muscle. *Prog. Biophys. Mol. Biol.* 29: 197–224, 1975.
38. COSTILL, D., W. FINK, L. GETCHELL, J. IVY, AND F. WITZMANN. Lipid metabolism in skeletal muscle of endurance-trained males and females. *J. Appl. Physiol.* 47: 787–791, 1979.
39. CROWE, L. M., AND R. J. BASKIN. Stereological analysis of developing sarcotubular membranes. *J. Ultrastruct. Res.* 58: 10–21, 1977.
40. CROWE, L. M., AND R. J. BASKIN. Freeze fracture of intact sarcotubular membranes. *J. Ultrastruct. Res.* 62: 147–154, 1978.
41. CULLEN, M. J., AND J. J. FULTHORPE. Stages in fibre breakdown in Duchenne muscular dystrophy. An electron-microscopic study. *J. Neurol. Sci.* 24: 179–200, 1975.
42. CULLEN, M. J., AND D. WEIGHTMAN. The ultrastructure of normal human muscle in relation to fibre type. *J. Neurol. Sci.* 25: 43–56, 1975.
43. DAINTY, J. Water relations of plant cells. *Adv. Bot. Res.* 1: 279–326, 1963.
44. DAVEY, D. F., AND G. M. O'BRIEN. The sarcoplasmic reticulum and T-system of rat extensor digitorum longus muscles exposed to hypertonic solutions. *Aust. J. Exp. Biol. Med. Sci.* 56: 409–419, 1978.
45. DAVEY, D. F., AND S. Y. P. WONG. Morphometric analysis of rat extensor digitorium longus and soleus muscles. *Aust. J. Exp. Biol. Med. Sci.* 58: 213–230, 1980.
46. DAVIDOWITZ, J., G. PHILIPS, AND G. M. BREININ. Variation of mitochondrial volume fraction along multiply innervated fibers in rabbit extraocular muscle. *Tissue Cell* 12: 449–457, 1980.
47. DAWES, C. J. *Biological Techniques for Transmission and Scanning Electron Microscopy.* Burlington, VT: Ladd Research Industries, 1979.
48. DHOOT, G. K., AND S. V. PERRY. Distribution of polymorphic forms of troponin components and tropomyosin in skeletal muscle. *Nature London* 278: 714–718, 1979.
49. DOBIE, W. M. Observations on the minute structure and mode of contraction of voluntary muscular fibre. *Ann. Mag. Nat. Hist.* 3: 109–119, 1849.
50. DODD, L., S. D. GRAY, O. HUDLICKÁ, AND E. M. RENKIN. Evaluation of capillary density in relation to fibre types in electrically stimulated muscles. *J. Physiol. London* 301: 11P–12P, 1980.
51. DONALDSON, S. K. Single skinned skeletal fiber Ca^{2+} and H^+ sensitivities: comparison of the various histochemical types (Abstract). *Biophys. J.* 33: 57a, 1981.
52. DUBOWITZ, V., AND M. H. BROOKE. *Muscle Biopsy; a Modern Approach.* London: Saunders, 1973.
53. DUBOWITZ, V., AND A. G. E. PEARSE. Reciprocal relationship of phosphorylase and oxidative enzymes in skeletal muscle. *Nature London* 185: 701–702, 1960.
54. DULHUNTY, A. F., AND M. DLUTOWSKI. Fiber types in red and white segments of rat sternomastoid muscle. *Am. J. Anat.* 156: 51–61, 1979.
55. DULHUNTY, A. F., AND C. FRANZINI-ARMSTRONG. The relative contribution of the folds and caveolae to the surface membrane of frog skeletal muscle fibres at different sarcomere lengths. *J. Physiol. London* 250: 513–539, 1975.
56. EASTWOOD, A. B., M. SORENSON, J. A. LEAVENS, AND K. BOCK. Distinctive ultrastructural and biochemical characteristics of skinned fibers on mammalian fast- and slow-twitch muscles (Abstract). *Biophys. J.* 25: 107a, 1979.
57. EATON, B. L., AND F. A. PEPE. M band protein. Two components isolated from chicken breast muscle. *J. Cell Biol.* 55: 681–695, 1972.
58. EDGERTON, V. R., R. J. BARNARD, J. B. PETER, A. MAIER, AND D. R. SIMPSON. Properties of immobilized hind-limb muscles of the *Galago senegalensis. Exp. Neurol.* 46: 115–131, 1975.
59. EDGERTON, V. R., AND D. R. SIMPSON. The intermediate muscle fiber of rats and guinea pigs. *J. Histochem. Cytochem.* 17: 828–839, 1969.
60. EISENBERG, B. R. Can electron microscopy distinguish fiber types? In: *Recent Advances in Myology*, edited by W. G. Bradley, D. Gardner-Medwin, and J. N. Walton. Amsterdam: Excerpta Med. 1975, p. 316–321. (Int. Cong. Ser. 360.)
61. EISENBERG, B.R. Quantitative ultrastructural analysis of adult mammalian skeletal muscle fibers. In: *Exploratory Concepts in Muscular Dystrophy II*, edited by A. T. Milhorat. Amsterdam: Excerpta Med. 1974, p. 258–270. (Int. Cong. Ser. 333.)
62. EISENBERG, B. R. Skeletal muscle fibers: stereology applied to anisotropic and periodic structures. In: *Stereological Methods For Biological Morphometry. Practical Methods*, edited by E. R. Weibel. London: Academic, 1979, vol. 1, p. 274–284.
63. EISENBERG, B. R., AND R. S. EISENBERG. Selective disruption of the sarcotubular system in frog sartorius muscle. A quantitative study with exogenous peroxidase as a marker. *J. Cell Biol.* 39: 451–467, 1968.
64. EISENBERG, B. R., AND R. S. EISENBERG. The T-SR junction in contracting single skeletal muscle fibers. *J. Gen. Physiol.* 79: 1–19, 1982.
65. EISENBERG, B. R., AND A. GILAI. Structural changes in single muscle fibers after stimulation. *J. Gen. Physiol.* 74: 1–16, 1979.
66. EISENBERG, B. R., AND A. M. KUDA. Stereological analysis of mammalian skeletal muscle. II. White vastus muscle of the adult guinea pig. *J. Ultrastruct. Res.* 51: 176–187, 1975.
67. EISENBERG, B. R., AND A. M. KUDA. Discrimination between fiber populations in mammalian skeletal muscle by using ultrastructural parameters. *J. Ultrastruct. Res.* 54: 76–88, 1976.
68. EISENBERG, B. R., AND A. M. KUDA. Retrieval of cryostat sections for comparison of histochemistry and quantitative

electron microscopy in a muscle fiber. *J. Histochem. Cytochem.* 25: 1169–1177, 1977.

69. EISENBERG, B. R., A. KUDA, AND J. B. PETER. Morphometric analysis of the slow-twitch fibers of the guinea pig. *Proc. Annu. Meet. Electron Microsc. Soc. Am., 30th*, edited by C. J. Arcencaux. Baton Rouge, LA: Claitor's, 1972, p. 36–37.
70. EISENBERG, B. R., A. M. KUDA, AND J. B. PETER. Stereological analysis of mammalian skeletal muscle. I. Soleus muscle of the adult guinea pig. *J. Cell Biol.* 60: 732–754, 1974.
71. EISENBERG, B. R., R. T. MATHIAS, AND A. GILAI. Intracellular localization of markers within injected or cut frog muscle fibers. *Am. J. Physiol.* 237 (*Cell Physiol.* 6): C50–C55, 1979.
72. EISENBERG, B. R., AND B. A. MOBLEY. Size changes in single muscle fibers during fixation and embedding. *Tissue Cell* 7: 383–387, 1975.
73. EISENBERG, B. R., AND L. D. PEACHEY. The network parameters of the t-system in frog muscle measured with the high voltage electron microscope. *Proc. Annu. Meeting Electron Microscopy Soc. Am., 33rd*, edited by G. W. Bailey. Baton Rouge, LA: Claitor's, 1975, p. 550–551.
74. EISENBERG, B. R., AND S. SALMONS. Stereological analysis of sequential ultrastructural changes in the adaptive response of fast muscle to chronic stimulation. *Muscle Nerve* 3: 277, 1980.
75. EISENBERG, B. R., AND S. SALMONS. The reorganization of subcellular structure in muscle undergoing fast-to-slow type transformation: a stereological study. *Cell Tissue Res.* 220: 449–471, 1981.
76. ELIAS, H. Address of the President. In: *Proceedings First International Congress for Stereology*, edited by H. Haug. Vienna: Congressprint, 1963, p. 2.
77. ELIAS, H. Stereology of parallel, straight, circular cylinders. *J. Microsc. Oxford* 107: 199–202, 1976.
78. ELLIOTT, G. F. Donnan and osmotic effects in muscle fibres without membranes. *J. Mechanochem. Cell Motil.* 2: 83–89, 1973.
79. ELLIOTT, G. F. The muscle fiber: liquid-crystalline and hydraulic aspects. *Ann. NY Acad. Sci.* 204: 564–574, 1973.
80. ENDO, M. Entry of fluorescent dyes into the sarcotubular system of the frog muscle. *J. Physiol. London* 185: 224–238, 1966.
81. ENGEL, A. G., T. SANTA, H. H. STONNINGTON, F. JERUSALEM, M. TSUJIHATA, A. K. W. BROWNELL, H. SAKAKIBARA, B. Q. BANKER, K. SAHASHI, AND E. H. LAMBERT. Morphometric study of skeletal muscle ultrastructure. *Muscle Nerve* 2: 229–237, 1979.
82. ENGEL, W. K. The essentiality of histo- and cytochemical studies of skeletal muscle in the investigation of neuromuscular disease. *Neurology* 12: 778–794, 1962.
83. ESSEN, B. Intramuscular substrate utilization during prolonged excercise. *Ann. NY Acad. Sci.* 301: 30–43, 1977.
84. ETLINGER, J. D., AND D. A. FISCHMAN. M and Z band components and the assembly of myofibrils. *Cold Spring Harbor Symp. Quant. Biol.* 37: 511–522, 1972.
85. FIEHN, W., AND J. B. PETER. Properties of fragmented sarcoplasmic reticulum from fast twitch and slow twitch muscles. *J. Clin. Invest.* 50: 570–573, 1971.
86. FORD, L. E., A. F. HUXLEY, AND R. M. SIMMONS. The relation between stiffness and filament overlap in stimulated frog muscle fibres. *J. Physiol. London* 311: 219–249, 1981.
87. FRANZINI-ARMSTRONG, C. Details of the I band structure as revealed by the localization of ferritin. *Tissue Cell* 2: 327–338, 1970.
88. FRANZINI-ARMSTRONG, C. Studies of the triad. I. Structure of the junction in frog twitch fibers. *J. Cell Biol.* 47: 488–499, 1970.
89. FRANZINI-ARMSTRONG, C. Studies of the triad. II. Penetration of tracers into the junctional gap. *J. Cell Biol.* 49: 196–203, 1971.
90. FRANZINI-ARMSTRONG, C. Studies of the triad. III. Structure of the junction in fast twitch fibers. *Tissue Cell* 4: 469–478, 1972.
91. FRANZINI-ARMSTRONG, C. Studies of the triad. IV. Structure of the junction in frog slow fibers. *J. Cell Biol.* 56: 120–128, 1973.
92. FRANZINI-ARMSTRONG, C. The structure of a simple Z line. *J. Cell Biol.* 58: 630–642, 1973.
93. FRANZINI-ARMSTRONG, C. Freeze fracture of skeletal muscle from the tarantula spider. Structural differentiations of sarcoplasmic reticulum and transverse tubular system membranes. *J. Cell Biol.* 61: 501–513, 1974.
94. FRANZINI-ARMSTRONG, C. Membrane particles and transmission at the triad. *Federation Proc.* 34: 1382–1389, 1975.
95. FRANZINI-ARMSTRONG, C. The comparative structure of intracellular junctions in striated muscle fibers. In: *Pathogenesis of Human Muscular Dystrophies*, edited by L. P. Rowland. Amsterdam: Excerpta Med. 1977, p. 612–625. (Int. Cong. Ser. 404.)
96. FRANZINI-ARMSTRONG, C. Structure of sarcoplasmic reticulum. *Federation Proc.* 39: 2403–2409, 1980.
97. FRANZINI-ARMSTRONG, C., L. LANDMESSER, AND G. PILAR. Size and shape of transverse tubule openings in frog twitch muscle fibers. *J. Cell Biol.* 64: 493–496, 1975.
98. FRANZINI-ARMSTRONG, C., AND K. R. PORTER. Sarcolemmal invaginations constituting the T-system of fish muscle fibers. *J. Cell Biol.* 22: 675–696, 1964.
99. FRANZINI-ARMSTRONG, C., AND K. R. PORTER. Sarcolemmal invaginations and the T-system in fish skeletal muscle. *Nature London* 202: 355–357, 1964.
100. GAUTHIER, G. F. On the relationship of ultrastructural and cytochemical features to color in mammalian skeletal muscle. *Z. Zellforsch. Mikrosk. Anat.* 95: 462–482, 1969.
101. GAUTHIER, G. F. The structural and cytochemical heterogeneity of mammalian skeletal muscle fibers. In: *The Contractility of Muscle Cells and Related Processes*, edited by R. J. Podolsky. Englewood Cliffs, NJ: Prentice-Hall, 1971.
102. GAUTHIER, G. F. Some ultrastructural and cytochemical features of fiber populations in the soleus muscle. *Anat. Rec.* 180: 551–564, 1974.
103. GAUTHIER, G. F. Ultrastructural identification of muscle fiber types by immunocytochemistry. *J. Cell Biol.* 82: 391–400, 1979.
104. GAUTHIER, G. F., AND R. A. DUNN. Ultrastructural and cytochemical features of mammalian skeletal muscle fibers following denervation. *J. Cell Biol.* 12: 525–547, 1973.
105. GAUTHIER, G. F., AND S. LOWEY. Polymorphism of myosin among skeletal muscle fiber types. *J. Cell Biol.* 74: 760–779, 1977.
106. GAUTHIER, G. F., AND S. LOWEY. Distribution of myosin isoenzymes among skeletal muscle fiber types. *J. Cell Biol.* 81: 10–25, 1979.
107. GAUTHIER, G. F., S. LOWEY, AND A. W. HOBBS. Fast and slow myosin in developing muscle fibres. *Nature London* 274: 25–29, 1978.
108. GAUTHIER, G. F., AND H. A. PADYKULA. Cytological studies of fiber types in skeletal muscle. A comparative study of the mammalian diaphragm. *J. Cell Biol.* 28: 333–354, 1966.
109. GIBSON, M. C., AND E. SCHULZ. Skeletal muscle satellite cell populations decrease with age (Abstract). *J. Cell Biol.* 87: 264a, 1980.
110. GLAUERT, A. M. *Practical Methods in Electron Microscopy.* New York: Elsevier, 1974, vol. 3.
111. GOLDSPINK, G. The proliferation of myofibrils during postembryonic muscle fibre growth. *J. Cell Sci.* 6: 593–604, 1970.
112. GOLDSPINK, G. Changes in striated muscle fibres during contraction and growth with particular reference to myofibril splitting. *J. Cell Sci.* 9: 123–137, 1971.
113. GOLDSPINK, G., AND P. E. WILLIAMS. The nature of the increased passive resistance in muscle following immobilization of the mouse soleus muscle (Abstract). *J. Physiol. London* 289: 55P, 1979.
114. GOLDSTEIN, M. A., J. P. SCHROETER, AND R. L. SASS. Optical diffraction of the Z lattice in canine cardiac muscle. *J. Cell Biol.* 75: 818–836, 1977.
115. GOLDSTEIN, M. A., J. P. SCHROETER, AND R. L. SASS. The Z lattice in canine cardiac muscle. *J. Cell Biol.* 83: 187–204, 1979.
116. GOLDSTEIN, M. A., M. H. STROMER, J. P. SCHROETER, AND R.

L. Sass. Optical diffraction and reconstruction of Z bands in skeletal muscle (Abstract). *J. Cell Biol.* 87: 261a, 1980.
117. Goldstein, M. A., M. H. Stromer, J. P. Schroeter, and R. L. Sass. Optical reconstruction of nemaline rods. *Exp. Neurol.* 70: 83–97, 1980.
118. Goldstein, M. A., P. T. Thyrum, D. L. Murphy, J. H. Martin, and A. Schwartz. Ultrastructural and contractile characteristics of isolated papillary muscle exposed to acute hypoxia. *J. Mol. Cell. Cardiol.* 9: 285–295, 1977.
119. Guth, L., and H. Yellin. The dynamic nature of the so-called "fiber types" of mammalian skeletal muscle. *Exp. Neurol.* 31: 277–300, 1971.
120. Hayashida, Y., and H. Schmalbruch. Zur Grösse der Fettpartikel in mitochondrienreichen Skelettmuskelfasern der Ratte in Abhängigkeit von der Nahrungsaufnahme. *Z. Zellforsch. Mikrosk. Anat.* 127: 374–381, 1972.
121. Hayat, M. A. *Principles and Techniques of Electron Microscopy: Biological Applications.* New York: Van Nostrand Reinhold, 1970, vol. 1.
122. Henkart, M., D. M. D. Landis, and T. S. Reese. Similarity of junctions between plasma membranes and endoplasmic reticulum in muscle and neurons. *J. Cell Biol.* 70: 338–347, 1976.
123. Henriksson, J. Training induced adaptation of skeletal muscle and metabolism during submaximal exercise. *J. Physiol. London* 270: 661–675, 1977.
124. Hensen, V. Ueber ein neues Strukturverhältniss der quergestreiften Muskelfaser. *Arb. Kieler Physiol. Inst.* 1: 26, 1868.
125. Hill, A. V. On the time required for diffusion and its relation to processes in muscle. *Proc. R. Soc. London Ser. B* 135: 446–453, 1948.
126. Hill, A. V. *Trails and Trials in Physiology.* London: Arnold, 1965.
127. Hill, D. K. The space accessible to albumin within the striated muscle fibre of the toad. *J. Physiol. London* 175: 275–294, 1964.
128. Hillard, J. E. Assessment of sampling errors in stereological analyses. *Proc. Fourth Int. Congr. Stereology*, edited by E. E. Underwood, R. de Wit, and G. A. Moore. Washington, DC: U.S. Government Printing Office, Washington 1976, p. 59–67. (Natl. Bureau of Standards Spec. Publ. 431.)
129. Holloszy, J., M. Rennie, R. Hickson, R. Conlee, and J. Hägberg. Physiological consequences of the biochemical adaptations to endurance excercise. *Ann. NY Acad. Sci.* 301: 440–450, 1977.
130. Holmes, A. H. *Petrographic Methods and Calculations.* London: Murby, 1927.
131. Hoppeler, H. Structural quantification of muscle-tissue by stereological methods. *Ultramicroscopy* 5: 367–368, 1980.
132. Hoppeler, H., P. Lüthi, H. Claassen, E. R. Weibel, and H. Howald. The ultrastructure of the normal human skeletal muscle. A morphometric analysis on untrained men, women and well-trained orienteers. *Pfluegers Arch.* 344: 217–232, 1973.
133. Hoppeler, H., O. Mathieu, R. Kauer, H. Claassen, R. B. Armstrong, and E. R. Weibel. Design of the mammalian respiratory system. VI. Distribution of mitochondria and capillaries in various muscles. *Respir. Physiol.* 44: 87–112, 1981.
134. Hoppeler, H., O. Mathieu, E. R. Weibel, R. Krauer, S. L. Lindstedt, and C. R. Taylor. Design of the mammalian respiratory system. VIII. Capillaries in skeletal muscles. *Respir. Physiol.* 44: 129–150, 1981.
135. Howell, J. N. Intracellular binding of ruthenium red in frog skeletal muscle. *J. Cell Biol.* 62: 242–247, 1974.
136. Hudlická, O., and K. R. Tyler. Importance of different patterns of frequency in the development of contractile properties and histochemical characteristics of fast skeletal muscle. *J. Physiol. London* 301: 10P–11P, 1980.
137. Huxley, A. F. Muscle structure and theories of contraction. *Prog. Biophys. Biophys. Chem.* 7: 255–318, 1957.
138. Huxley, A. F. Muscle. *Annu. Rev. Physiol.* 26: 131–152, 1964.
139. Huxley, A. F. The Croonian lecture, 1967. The activation of striated muscle and its mechanical response. *Proc. R. Soc. London Ser. B* 178: 1–27, 1971.
140. Huxley, A. F. Looking back on muscle. In: *The Pursuit of Nature, Informal Essays on the History of Physiology.* Cambridge, UK: Cambridge Univ. Press, 1977, p. 23–64.
141. Huxley, A. F., and R. Niedergerke. Interference microscopy of living muscle fibres. *Nature London* 173: 971–973, 1954.
142. Huxley, A. F., and R. E. Taylor. Function of Krause's membrane. *Nature London* 176: 1068, 1955.
143. Huxley, A. F., and R. E. Taylor. Local activation of striated muscle fibres. *J. Physiol. London* 144: 426–441, 1958.
144. Huxley, H. E. Evidence for continuity between the central elements of the triads and extracellular space in frog sartorius muscle. *Nature London* 202: 1067–1071, 1964.
145. Huxley, H. E. The mechanism of muscular contraction. *Science* 164: 1356–1366, 1969.
146. Huxley, H. E. The Croonian lecture, 1970. The structural basis of muscular contraction. *Proc. R. Soc. London Ser. B* 178: 131–140, 1971.
147. Huxley, H. E., and J. Hanson. Changes in the cross-striations of muscle during contraction and stretch and their structural interpretation. *Nature London* 173: 973–976, 1954.
148. Ishikawa, H. Formation of elaborate networks of t-system tubules in cultured skeletal muscle with special reference to the t-system formation. *J. Cell Biol.* 38: 51–66, 1968.
149. James, N. T., and G. A. Meek. Stereological analyses of the structure of mitochondria in pigeon skeletal muscle. *Cell Tissue Res.* 202: 493–503, 1979.
150. Jenny, E., H. Weber, H. Lutz, and R. Billeter. Fibre populations in rabbit skeletal muscles from birth to old age. In: *Plasticity of Muscle*, edited by D. Pette. New York: de Gruyter, 1980, p. 97–109.
151. Jerusalem, F., A. G. Engel, and M. R. Gomez. Duchenne dystrophy. I. Morphometric study of the muscle microvasculature. *Brain* 97: 115–122, 1974.
152. Jerusalem, F., A. G. Engel, and H. A. Peterson. Human muscle fiber fine structure: morphometric data on controls. *Neurology* 25: 127–134, 1975.
153. Jerusalem, F., M. Rakusa, A. G. Engel, and R. D. MacDonald. Morphometric analysis of skeletal muscle capillary ultrastructure in inflammatory myopathies. *J. Neurol. Sci.* 23: 391–402, 1974.
154. Johansson, B. R. Quantitative ultrastructural morphometry of blood capilary endothelium in skeletal muscle. Effect of venous pressure. *Microvasc. Res.* 17: 118–130, 1979.
155. Johnson, T. J. A., and J. E. Rash. Glutaraldehyde chemistry: fixation reactions consume O_2 and are inhibited by tissue anoxia (Abstract). *J. Cell Biol.* 87: 231a, 1980.
156. Jolesz, F., and F. A. Sréter. Development, innervation, and activity-pattern induced changes in skeletal muscle. *Annu. Rev. Physiol.* 43: 531–552, 1981.
157. Jorgensen, A. O., V. Kalnins, and D. H. MacLennan. Localization of sarcoplasmic reticulum proteins in rat skeletal muscle by immunofluorescence. *J. Cell Biol.* 80: 372–384, 1979.
158. Kamieniecka, Z., and H. Schmalbruch. Neuro-muscular disorders with abnormal muscle mitochondria. *Int. Rev. Cytol.* 65: 321–357, 1980.
159. Karpati, G., S. Carpenter, and A. A. Eisen. Experimental core-like lesions and nemaline rods. A correlative morphological and physiological study. *Arch. Neurol. Chicago* 27: 237–251, 1972.
160. Katchalsky, A., and O. Kedem. Thermodynamics of flow processes in biological systems. *Biophys. J.* 2: 53, 1962.
161. Kelly, A. M. Sarcoplasmic reticulum and T tubules in differentiating rat skeletal muscle. *J. Cell Biol.* 49: 335–344, 1971.
162. Kelly, A. M. Perisynaptic satellite cells in the developing and mature rat soleus muscle. *Anat. Rec.* 190: 891–904, 1978.
163. Kelly, D. E. The fine structure of skeletal muscle triad junctions. *J. Ultrastruct. Res.* 29: 37–49, 1969.
164. Kelly, D. E., and M. A. Cahill. Filamentous and matrix components of skeletal muscle Z-disks. *Anat. Rec.* 172: 623–642, 1972.
165. Kelly, D. E., and A. M. Kuda. Subunits of the triadic junction

in fast skeletal muscle as revealed by freeze-fracture. *J. Ultrastruct Res.* 68: 220–233, 1979.

166. KENDALL, M. G., AND A. STUART. The advanced theory of statistics. In: *Design and Analysis and Time-Series.* New York: Hafner, 1968, p. 314–341.
167. KHAN, M. A. Histochemical characteristics of vertebrate striated muscle: a review. *Prog. Histochem. Cytochem.* 8: 1–48, 1976.
168. KIESSLING, K. H. Comparison between muscle morphology and metabolism. *Acta Agr. Scand.* S21: 39–46, 1979.
169. KIESSLING, K. H., L. PILSTRÖM, A.-C. BYLUND, B. SALTIN, AND K. PIEHL. Enzyme activities and morphometry in skeletal muscle of middle-aged men after training. *Scand. J. Clin. Lab. Invest.* 33: 63–69, 1974.
170. KIESSLING, K. H., L. PILSTRÖM, J. KARLSSON, AND K. PIEHL. Mitochondrial volume in skeletal muscle from young and old physically untrained and trained healthy men and from alcoholics. *Clin Sci.* 44: 547–554, 1973.
171. KNAPPEIS, G. G., AND F. CARLSEN. The ultrastructure of the Z disc in skeletal muscle. *J. Cell Biol.* 13: 323–335, 1962.
172. KNAPPEIS, G. G., AND F. CARLSEN. The ultrastructure of the M line in skeletal muscle. *J. Cell Biol.* 38: 202–211, 1968.
173. KÖLLIKER, A. V. Zur kenntnis der quergestreiften Muskelfasern. *Z. Wiss. Zool.* 47: 689–710, 1888.
174. KRAUSE, W. Mikroskopische Untersuchungen über die quergestreifte Muskelsubstanz. *Nachrichten Gesellsch. Univ. Goettingen Mitt Path Inst.* 17: 357, 1868.
175. KRÜGER, P. *Tetanus and Tonus der quergestreiften Skelettmuskeln der Wirbeltiere und des Menschen.* Leipzig: Akad. Verlags Geest & Portig, 1952.
176. KUGELBERG, E. Adaptive transformation of rat soleus motor units during growth. *J. Neurol. Sci.* 27: 269–289, 1976.
177. KUNDRAT, E., AND F. A. PEPE. The M band. Studies with fluorescent antibody staining. *J. Cell Biol.* 48: 340–347, 1971.
178. LANDON, D. N. Change in Z-disk structure with muscular contraction. *J. Physiol. London* 211: 44P–45P, 1970.
179. LANDON, D. N. The influence of fixation upon the fine structure of the Z-disk of rat striated muscle. *J. Cell Sci.* 6: 257–276, 1970.
180. LAZARIDES, E. Intermediate filaments as mechanical integrators of cellular space. *Nature London* 283: 249–256, 1980.
181. LAZARIDES, E., AND D. R. BALZER, JR. Specificity of desmin to avian and mammalian muscle cell. *Cell* 14: 429–438, 1978.
182. LAZARIDES, E., AND B. L. GRANGER. Fluorescent localization of membrane sites in glycerinated chicken skeletal muscle fibres and the relationship of these sites to the protein composition of the Z-disk. *Proc. Natl. Acad. Sci. USA* 75: 3683–3687, 1978.
183. LEEUWENHOEK, A. VAN. A letter from Mr. Anthony van Leeuwenhoek, F.R.S. Containing his observations upon the seminal vesicles, muscular fibres, and blood of whales. *Philos. Trans. R. Soc. Lond. Ser. B* 27: 438–446, 1712.
184. LITHELL, H., J. ÖRLANDER, R. SCHÉLE, T. SJÖDIN, AND J. KARLSSON. Changes in lipoprotein-lipase activity and lipid stores in human skeletal muscle with prolonged heavy exercise. *Acta Physiol. Scand.* 107: 257–261, 1979.
185. LOATS, J. T., A. H. SILLAU, AND N. BANCHERO. How to quantify skeletal muscle capillarity. In: *Oxygen Transport to Tissue III*, edited by I. A. Silver, M. Erecinska, and H. I. Bicher. New York: Plenum, 1978, p. 41–48.
186. LØMO, T., R. H. WESTGAARD, AND L. ENGEBRETSEN. Different stimulation patterns affect contractile properties of denervated rat soleus muscles. In: *Plasticity of Muscle*, edited by D. Pette. New York: de Gruyter, 1980, p. 297–309.
187. LOUD, A. V. Quantitative estimation of the loss of membrane images resulting from oblique sectioning. *Proc. Annu. Meet. Electron Microsc. Soc. Am., 25th*, edited by C. J. Arceneaux. Baton Rouge, LA: Claitor's, 1967, p. 144–145.
188. LUFF, A. R. Dynamic properties of the inferior rectus, extensor digitorum longus, diaphragm and soleus muscles of the mouse. *J. Physiol. London* 313: 161–171, 1981.
189. LUFF, A. R., AND H. L. ATWOOD. Changes in the sarcoplasmic reticulum and transverse tubular system of fast and slow skeletal muscles of the mouse during postnatal development. *J. Cell Biol.* 51: 369–383, 1971.
190. LUFF, A. R., AND H. L. ATWOOD. Membrane properties and contraction of single muscle fibers in the mouse. *Am. J. Physiol.* 222: 1435–1440, 1972.
191. LUTZ, H., H. WEBER, R. BILLETER, AND E. JENNY. Fast and slow myosin within single skeletal muscle fibers of adult rabbits. *Nature London* 281: 142–144, 1979.
192. MAIER, A., AND E. ELDRED. Postnatal growth of the extra- and intrafusal fibers in the soleus and medial gastrocnemius muscles of the cat. *Am. J. Anat.* 141: 161–178, 1974.
193. MATHIAS, R. T., R. A. LEVIS, AND R. S. EISENBERG. Electrical models of excitation-contraction coupling and charge movement in skeletal muscle. *J. Gen. Physiol.* 76: 1–31, 1980.
194. MATHIAS, R. T., R. A. LEVIS, AND R. S. EISENBERG. An alternative interpretation of charge movement in skeletal muscle. In: *UCLA Forum in Medical Sciences 22: The Regulation of Muscle Contraction: Excitation-Contraction Coupling*, edited by A. D. Grinnell and M. A. B. Brazier. New York: Academic, 1981, p. 39–52.
195. MATHIEU, O., R. KRAUER, H. HOPPELER, P. GEHR, S. L. LINDSTEDT, R. MCN. ALEXANDER, C. R. TAYLOR, AND E. R. WEIBEL. Design of the mammalian respiratory system. VII. Scaling mitochondrial volume in skeletal muscle to body mass. *Respir. Physiol.* 44: 113–128, 1981.
196. MAURO, A. *Muscle Regeneration.* New York: Raven, 1979.
197. MCCALLISTER, L. P., AND R. HADEK. Transmission electron microscopy and stereo ultrastructure of the T-system in frog skeletal muscle. *J. Ultrastruct. Res.* 33: 360–368, 1970.
198. MCDONALD, O. B., AND F. H. SCHACHAT. Multiple forms of structural proteins in rabbit skeletal muscles (Abstract). *J. Cell Biol.* 87: 264a, 1980.
199. MERZ, W. A. Streckenmessung an gerichteten Strukturen im Mikroskop und ihre Anwendung zur Bestimmung von Oberflächen-Volumen-Relationen im Knochengewebe. *Mikroskopie* 22: 132–142, 1967.
200. MINGUETTI, G., AND W. G. P. MAIR. Ultrastructure of human intramuscular blood vessels in development. *Arq. Neuro-Psiquiatr.* 37: 127–137, 1979.
201. MOBLEY, B. A., AND B. R. EISENBERG. Sizes of components in frog skeletal muscle measured by methods of stereology. *J. Gen. Physiol.* 66: 31–45, 1975.
202. MOBLEY, B. A., AND E. PAGE. The surface area of sheep cardiac Purkinje fibres. *J. Physiol. London* 220: 547–563, 1972.
203. MUSCH, B. C., T. A. PAPAPETROPOULOS, D. A. MCQUEEN, P. HUDGSON, AND D. WEIGHTMAN. A comparison of the structure of small blood vessels in normal, denervated and dystrophic human muscle. *J. Neurol. Sci.* 26: 221–234, 1975.
204. MYRHAGE, R. Microvascular supply of skeletal muscle fibres. A micro angiographic, histochemical and intravital study of hindlimb muscles in the rat, rabbit and cat. *Acta Orthop. Scand.* 48: 2–46, 1977.
205. NAKAJIMA, S., AND J. BASTIAN. Membrane properties of the transverse tubular system in amphibian skeletal muscle. In: *Electrobiology of Nerve, Synapse and Muscle*, edited by J. P. Reuben, D. P. Purpura, M. V. L. Bennett, and E. R. Kandel. New York: Raven, 1976, p. 243–268.
206. NAKAO, T. Fine structure of the myotendinous junction and terminal coupling in the skeletal muscle of the lamprey, *Lampetra japonica. Anat. Rec.* 182: 321–338, 1975.
207. NEEDHAM, D. M. *Machina Carnis. The Biochemistry of Muscular Contraction in its Historical Development.* Cambridge, UK: Cambridge Univ. Press, 1971.
208. NEMETH, P. M., AND D. PETTE. The limited correlation of myosin-based and metabolism-based classifications of skeletal muscle fibers. *J. Histochem. Cytochem.* 29, 89–90, 1981.
209. NEMETH, P. M. D. PETTE, AND G. VRBOVÁ. Malate dehydrogenase homogeneity of single fibres of the motor unit. In: *Plasticity of Muscle*, edited by D. Pette. New York: de Gruyter, 1980, p. 45–54.
210. NEMETH, P. M., D. PETTE, AND G. VRBOVÁ. Comparison of

enzyme activities among single muscle fibres within defined motor units. *J. Physiol. London* 311: 489–495, 1981.

211. NEVILLE, H. Ultrastructural changes in disease of human skeletal muscle. In: *Handbook of Clinical Neurology. Disease of Muscle*, edited by P. J. Vinken and G. W. Bruyn. Amsterdam: North-Holland, 1979, vol. 40, p. 63–123.
212. ODUSOTE, K., G. KARPATI, AND S. CARPENTER. An experimental morphometric study of neutral lipid accumulation in skeletal muscles. *Muscle Nerve* 4: 3–9, 1981.
213. OLIVETTI, G., P. ANVERSA, M. MELISSARI, AND A. V. LOUD. Morphometric study of the atrioventricular node in normal and hypertrophic rat heart. *Lab. Invest.* 40: 331–340, 1979.
214. ONTELL, M., AND R. F. DUNN. Neonatal muscle growth: a quantitative study. *Am. J. Anat.* 152: 539–556, 1978.
215. ORENSTEIN, J., D. HOGAN, AND S. BLOOM. Surface cables of cardiac myocytes. *J. Mol. Cell. Cardiol.* 12: 771–780, 1980.
216. ÖRLANDER, J., K. H. KIESSLING, J. KARLSSON, AND B. EKBLOM. Low intensity training in sedentary men. *Acta Physiol. Scand.* 101: 351–362, 1977.
217. PADYKULA, H. A., AND G. F. GAUTHIER. Morphological and cytochemical characteristics of fiber types in normal mammalian skeletal muscle. In: *Exploratory Concepts in Muscular Dystrophy and Related Disorders*, edited by A. T. Milhorat. New York: Excerpta Med., 1967, p. 117–131. (Int. Cong. Ser. 147.)
218. PADYKULA, H. A., AND G. F. GAUTHIER. The ultrastructure of the neuromuscular junctions of mammalian red, white, and intermediate skeletal muscle fibers. *J. Cell Biol.* 46: 27–41, 1979.
219. PAGE, E. Quantitative ultrastructural analysis in cardiac membrane physiology. *Am. J. Physiol.* 235 (*Cell Physiol.* 4): C147–C158, 1978.
220. PAGE, S. G. The organization of the sarcoplasmic reticulum in frog muscle (Abstract). *J. Physiol. London* 175: 10P, 1964.
221. PAGE, S. G. A comparison of the fine structure of frog slow and twitch muscle fibres. *J. Cell Biol.* 26: 477–497, 1965.
222. PAGE, S. G., AND H. E. HUXLEY. Filament lengths in striated muscle. *J. Cell Biol.* 19: 369–390, 1963.
223. PAYNE, C., I. STERN, R. CURLESS, AND L. HANNAPEL. Ultrastructural fiber typing in normal and diseased human muscle. *J. Neurol. Sci.* 25: 99–108, 1975.
224. PEACHEY, L. D. Thin sections 1. A study of section thickness and physical distortion produced during microtomy. *J. Biophys. Biochem. Cytol.* 4: 233–242, 1958.
225. PEACHEY, L. D. The sarcoplasmic reticulum and transverse tubules of the frog's sartorius. *J. Cell Biol.* 25: 209–231, 1965.
226. PEACHEY, L. D., AND B. R. EISENBERG. Helicoids in the T system and striations of frog skeletal muscle seen by high voltage electron microscopy. *Biophys. J.* 22: 145–154, 1978.
227. PEACHEY, L. D., AND K. R. PORTER. Intracellular impulse conduction in muscle cells. *Science* 129: 721–722, 1959.
228. PELLEGRINO, C., AND C. FRANZINI. An electron microscope study of denervation atrophy in red and white skeletal muscle fibers. *J. Cell Biol.* 17: 327–349, 1963.
229. PENG, B. H., J. J. WOLOSEWICK, AND P. C. CHENG. The development of myofibrils in cultured muscle cells. A wholemount and thin-section electron microscopic study. *Dev. Biol.* 88: 121–136, 1981.
230. PEPE, F. A. Structure of muscle filaments from immunohistochemical and ultrastructural studies. *J. Histochem. Cytochem.* 23: 543–562, 1975.
231. PETER, J. B. Histochemical, biochemical and physiological studies of skeletal muscle and its adaptation to exercise. In: *Contractility Of Muscle Cells And Related Processes*, edited by R. J. Podolsky. Englewood Cliffs, NJ: Prentice Hall, 1971.
232. PETER, J. B., R. J. BARNARD, V. R. EDGERTON, C. A. GILLESPIE, AND K. E. STEMPEL. Metabolic profiles of three fiber types of skeletal muscle in guinea pigs and rabbits. *Biochem.* 11: 2627–2633, 1972.
233. PETTE, D. (editor). *Plasticity of Muscle*. New York: de Gruyter, 1980.
234. PETTE, D., W. MULLER, E. LEISNER, AND G. VRBOVÁ. Time dependent effects on contractile properties, fibre population, myosin light chains and enzymes of energy metabolism in intermittently and continuously stimulated fast twitch muscle of the rabbit. *Pfluegers Arch.* 364: 103–112, 1976.
235. PETTE, D., B. U. RAMIREZ, W. MULLER, R. SIMON, G. U. EXNER, AND R. HILDEBRAND. Influence of intermittent longterm stimulation on contractile, histochemical and metabolic properties of fibre populations in fast and slow rabbit muscles. *Pfluegers Arch.* 361: 1–7, 1975.
236. PETTE, D., AND U. SCHNEZ. Myosin light change patterns of individual fast- and slow-twitch fibres of rabbit muscles. *Histochem.* 54: 97–107, 1977.
237. PLYLEY, M. J., AND A. C. GROOM. Geometrical distribution of capillaries in mammalian striated muscle. *Am. J. Physiol.* 228: 1376–1383, 1975.
238. PORTER, K. R. The sarcoplasmic reticulum in muscle cells of *Amblystoma* larvae. *J. Biophys. Biochem Cytol.* 2: 163–169, 1956.
239. PORTER, K. R. The sarcoplasmic reticulum: its recent history and present status. *J. Biophys. Biochem. Cytol.* 10: 219–226, 1961.
240. PORTER, K. R., AND G. E. PALADE. Studies on the endoplasmic reticulum. III. Its form and distribution in striated muscle cells. *J. Biophys. Biochem. Cytol.* 3: 269–300, 1957.
241. PRINCE, F. P., R. S. HIKIDA, F. C. HAGERMAN, R. S. STARON, AND W. H. ALLEN. A morphometric analysis of human muscle fibers with relation to fiber types and adaptations to exercise. *J. Neurol. Sci.* 49: 165–179, 1981.
242. RAMIREZ, B. U., AND D. PETTE. Effects of long-term electrical stimulation on sarcoplasmic reticulum of fast rabbit muscle. *FEBS Lett.* 49: 188–190, 1974.
243. RANVIER, M. L. Des muscles rouges et des muscles blancs chez les rongeurs. *C. R. Acad. Sci.* 77: 1030, 1873.
244. RAO, C. R. *Linear Statistical Inference and Its Applications*, edited by R. A. Bradley, J. S. Hunter, D. G. Kendall, and G. S. Watson. New York: Wiley, 1973.
245. RASH, J. E. Ultrastructure of normal and myasthenic endplates. In: *Myasthenia Gravis*, edited by E. Albuquerque and M. E. Eldifrawi. London: Chapman & Hall, 1982.
246. RASH, J. E., AND M. H. ELLISMAN. Studies of excitable membranes. I. Macromolecular specialization of the neuromuscular junction and the nonjunctional sarcolemma. *J. Cell Biol.* 63: 567–586, 1974.
247. RASH, J. E., AND C. S. HUDSON. *Freeze-Fracture: Methods, Artifiacts and Interpretations.* New York: Raven, 1979.
248. RAYNS, D. G., C. E. DEVINE, AND C. L. SUTHERLAND. Freeze fracture studies of membrane systems in vertebrate muscle. I. Striated muscle. *J. Ultrastruct. Res.* 50: 306–321, 1975.
249. RAYNS, D. G., F. O. SIMPSON, AND W. S. BERTAUD. Surface features of striated muscle. I. Guinea pig cardiac muscle. *J. Cell Sci.* 3: 467–474, 1968.
250. RAYNS, D. G., F. O. SIMPSON, AND W. S. BERTAUD. Surface features of striated muscle. II. Guinea pig skeletal muscle. *J. Cell Sci.* 3: 475–488, 1968.
251. REEDY, M. K. In discussion on "The physical and chemical basis of muscular contraction," by J. Hanson and J. Lowy. *Proc. R. Soc. London Ser. B* 160: 458–460, 1964.
252. RESNICK, J. S., W. K. ENGEL, AND P. G. NELSON. Changes in the Z disk of skeletal muscle induced by tenotomy. *Neurology* 18: 737–740, 1968.
253. REVEL, J.-P. The sarcoplasmic reticulum of the bat cricothyroid muscle. *J. Cell Biol.* 12: 571–588, 1962.
254. RICH, T. L., AND G. A. LANGER. A comparison of excitation-contraction coupling heart and skeletal muscle: an examination of "calcium-induced calcium release." *J. Mol. Cell. Cardiol.* 7: 747–765, 1975.
255. ROBBINS, N., G. KARPATI, AND W. K. ENGEL. Histochemical and contractile properties in the cross innervated guinea pig soleus muscle. *Arch. Neurol. Chicago* 20: 318–329, 1969.
256. ROMANUL, F. C. A. Enzymes in muscle. 1. Histochemical studies of enzymes in individual muscle fibers. *Arch. Neurol. Chicago* 11: 355–368, 1964.
257. ROMANUL, F. C. A. Capillary supply and metabolism of muscle fibers. *Arch. Neurol. Chicago* 12: 497–509, 1965.

258. ROMANUL, F. C. A., F. A. SRÉTER, S. SALMONS, AND J. GERGELY. The effects of a changed pattern of activity on histochemical characteristics of muscle fibres. In: *Exploratory Concepts in Muscular Dystrophy II*, edited by A. T. Milhorat. New York: Excerpta Med. 1974, p. 344-348. (Int. Cong. Ser. 333.)
259. ROSSE, C., AND D. K. CLAWSON. *The Musculoskeletal System in Health and Disease*. Hagerstown, MD: Harper & Row, 1980.
260. ROWE, R. W. D. The ultrastructure of Z disks from white, intermediate, and red fibers of mammalian striated muscles. *J. Cell Biol.* 57: 261-277, 1973.
261. ROWE, R. W. D., AND G. GOLDSPINK. Muscle fibre growth in five different muscles in both sexes of mice. I. Normal mice. *J. Anat.* 104: 519-530, 1969.
262. ROY, R. K., K. MABUCHI, S. SARKAR, C. MIS, AND F. A. SRÉTER. Changes in tropomyosin subunit pattern in chronic electrically stimulated rat fast muscles. *Biochem. Biophys. Res. Commun.* 89: 181-187, 1979.
263. RUBINSTEIN, N., K. MABUCHI, F. PEPE, S. SALMONS, J. GERGELY, AND F. A. SRÉTER. Use of type-specific antimyosins to demonstrate the transformation of individual fibers in chronically stimulated rabbit fast muscles. *J. Cell Biol.* 79: 252-261, 1978.
264. SALMONS, S., D. R. GALE, AND F. A. SRÉTER. Ultrastructural aspects of the transformation of muscle fibre type by long term stimulation: changes in Z discs and mitochondria. *J. Anat.* 127: 17-31, 1978.
265. SALMONS, S., AND J. HENRIKSSON. The adaptive response of skeletal muscle to increased use. *Muscle Nerve* 4: 94-105, 1981.
266. SALMONS, S., AND F. A. SRÉTER. Significance of impulse activity in the transformation of skeletal muscle type. *Nature London* 263: 30-34, 1976.
267. SALMONS, S., AND G. VRBOVA. The influence of activity on some contractile characteristics of mammalian fast and slow muscles. *J. Physiol. London* 201: 535-549, 1969.
268. SALTIS, L. M., AND J. R. MENDELL. The fine structural differences in human muscle fiber types based on peroxidase activity. *J. Neuropathol. Exp. Neurol.* 33: 632-640, 1974.
269. SANTA, T., AND A. G. ENGEL. Histometric analysis of neuromuscular junction ultrastructure in rat red, white and intermediate muscle fibers. In: *Developments in Electromyography and Clinical Neurophysiology*, edited by J. E. Desmedt. Basel: Karger, 1973, vol. 1, p. 41-54.
270. SCALES, D. J., AND R. SABBADINI. Microsomal T-system: a stereological analysis of purified microsomes derived from normal and dystrophic skeletal muscle. *J. Cell Biol.* 83: 33-46, 1979.
271. SCHACHAT, F. H., A. D. MAGID, D. D. BRONSON, O. B. MCDONALD, AND W. GARRETT. Gene expression in single muscle fibers from rabbit skeletal muscles (Abstract). *J. Cell Biol.* 87: 263a, 1980.
272. SCHIAFFINO, S., V. HANZLIKOVA, AND S. PIEROBON. Relations between structure and function in rat skeletal muscle fibers. *J. Cell Biol.* 47: 107-119, 1970.
273. SCHMALBRUCH, H. The sarcolemma of skeletal muscle fibres as demonstrated by a replica technique. *Cell Tissue Res.* 150: 377-387, 1974.
274. SCHMALBRUCH, H. The membrane systems in different fibre types of the triceps surae muscle of cat. *Cell Tissue Res.* 204: 187-200, 1979.
275. SCHMALBRUCH, H. Square arrays in the sarcolemma of human skeletal muscle fibers. *Nature London* 281: 145-146, 1979.
276. SCHMALBRUCH, H. Delayed fixation alters the pattern of intramembrane particles in mammalian muscle fibers. *J. Ultrastruct. Res.* 70: 15-20, 1980.
277. SCHMALBRUCH, H., AND U. HELLHAMMER. The number of nuclei in adult rat muscles with special reference to satellite cells. *Anat. Rec.* 189: 169-176, 1977.
278. SCHMALBRUCH, H., AND U. HELLHAMMER. The number of satellite cells in normal human muscle. *Anat. Rec.* 185: 279-288, 1976.
279. SCHMALBRUCH, H., AND Z. KAMIENIECKA. Fiber types in the human brachial biceps muscle. *Exp. Neurol.* 44: 313-328, 1974.
280. SCHMALBRUCH, H., AND Z. KAMIENIECKA. Histochemical fiber typing and staining intensity in cat and rat muscles. *J. Histochem. Cytochem.* 23: 395-401, 1975.
281. SCHRÖDER, J. M., P. T. KEMME, AND L. SCHOLZ. The fine structure of denervated and reinnervated muscle spindles: morphometric study of intrafusal muscle fibers. *Acta Neuropathol.* 46: 95-106, 1979.
282. SCHULTZ, E. A quantitative study of the satellite cell population in postnatal mouse lumbrical muscle. *Anat. Rec.* 180: 589-596, 1974.
283. SHAY, J. The economy of effort in electron microscopy morphometry. *Am. J. Pathol.* 81: 503-511, 1975.
284. SHEAR, C. R., AND G. GOLDSPINK. Structural and physiological changes associated with the growth of avian fast and slow muscle. *J. Morphol.* 135: 351-372, 1971.
285. SICKLES, D. W., AND C. A. PINKSTAFF. Comparative histochemical study of prosimian primate hindlimb muscles. I. Muscle fiber types. *Am. J. Anat.* 160: 175-186, 1981.
286. SICKLES, D. W., AND C. A. PINKSTAFF. Comparative histochemical study of prosimian primate hindlimb muscles. II. Populations of fiber types. *Am. J. Anat.* 160: 187-194, 1981.
287. SILLAU, A. H., AND N. BANCHERO. Effect of maturation on capillary density, fiber size and composition in rat skeletal muscle. *Proc. Soc. Exp. Biol. Med.* 154: 461-466, 1977.
288. SILLAU, A. H., AND N. BANCHERO. Visualization of capillaries in skeletal muscle by the ATPase reaction. *Pfluegers Arch.* 369: 269-271, 1977.
289. SILLAU, A. H., AND N. BANCHERO. Skeletal muscle fiber size and capillarity. *Proc. Soc. Exp. Biol. Med.* 158: 288-291, 1978.
290. SILVERMAN, H., AND H. L. ATWOOD. Increase in oxidative capacity of muscle fibers in dystrophic mice and correlation with overactivity in these fibers. *Exp. Neurol.* 68: 97-113, 1980.
291. SILVERMAN, H., AND H. L. ATWOOD. Surface density of T tubules in normal and dystrophic mouse muscle. *Exp. Neurol.* 70: 40-46, 1980.
292. SIMMONS, R. M., AND B. R. JEWELL. Mechanics and models of muscular contraction. In: *Recent Advances in Physiology*, edited by R. J. Linden. Edinburgh: Churchill Livingstone, 1974, p. 87-147.
293. SITTE, H. Morphometrische Untersuchungen an Zellen. In: *Quantitative Methods in Morphology*, edited by E. R. Weibel and H. Elias. New York: Springer-Verlag, 1967, p. 167-198.
294. SJÖSTRÖM, M., K. A. ÄNGQUIST, AND O. RAIS. Intermittent claudication and muscle fiber fine structure: correlation between clinical and morphological data. *Ultrastruct. Pathol.* 1: 309-326, 1980.
295. SJÖSTRÖM, M., AND J. HENRIKSSON. Abstracts of the international symposium on the functional specificity of human muscle fibers. *Muscle Nerve* 3: 263-279, 1980.
296. SJÖSTRÖM, M., S. I. W. KIDMAN, K. LARSÉN, AND K. A. ÄNGQUIST. Z and M band appearance in different histochemically defined types of human skeletal muscle fibers. *J. Histochem. Cytochem.* 30: 1-11, 1982.
297. SJÖSTRÖM, M., AND J. M. SQUIRE. Fine structure of the A-band in cryo-sections. The structure of the A-band of human skeletal muscle fibres from ultra-thin cryo-sections negatively stained. *J. Mol. Biol.* 109: 49-68, 1977.
298. SLINDE, E., AND H. KRYVI. Studies on the nature of the Z-discs in skeletal muscle fibres of sharks, *Etmopterus spinax* L. and *Galeus melastomus Rafinesque-Schmaltz*. *J. Fish Biol.* 16: 299-308, 1980.
299. SNEATH, P. H. A., AND R. SOKAL. *Numerical Taxonomy*, edited by D. Kennedy and R. B. Park. San Francisco: Freeman, 1973.
300. SOLOMON, H. Geometric probability. In: *Society for Industrial and Applied Mathematics*. Bristol, UK: Arrowsmith, 1978.
301. SOMLYO, A. V. Bridging structures spanning the junctional gap at the triad of skeletal muscle. *J. Cell Biol.* 80: 743-750, 1979.
302. SOMMER, J. R., AND E. A. JOHNSON. Ultrastructure of cardiac muscle. In: *Handbook of Physiology. The Cardiovascular System*, edited by R. Burns. Bethesda, MD: Am. Physiol. Soc., 1979, sec. 2, vol. I, chapt. 5, p. 113-186.

303. SOMMER, J. R., N. R. WALLACE, AND W. HASSELBACH. The collapse of the sarcoplasmic reticulum in skeletal muscle. *Z. Naturforsch.* 33: 561–573, 1978.
304. SPURWAY, N. Interrelationship between myosin-based and metabolism-based classifications of skeletal muscle fibers. *J. Histochem. Cytochem.* 29: 87–90, 1981.
305. SPURWAY, N. C. Objective characterization of cells in terms of microscopical parameters: an example from muscle histochemistry. *Histochem. J.* 13: 269–317, 1981.
306. SQUIRE, J. *The Structural Basis of Muscular Contraction.* New York: Plenum, 1981.
307. SRÉTER, F. A., J. GERGELY, S. SALMONS, AND F. ROMANUL. Synthesis of fast muscle of myosin light chains characteristic of slow muscle in response to long term stimulation. *Nature London New Biol.* 241: 17–19, 1973.
308. SRÉTER, F. A., F. C. A. ROMANUL, S. SALMONS, AND J. GERGELY. The effect of a changed pattern of activity on some biochemical characteristics of muscle. In: *Exploratory Concepts of Muscular Dystrophy II,* edited by A. T. Milhorat. 1974, p. 338–343. (Int. Cong. Ser. 333.)
309. STAVERMAN, A. J. The theory of measurement of osmotic pressure. *Recl. Trav. Chim. Pays-Bas* 70: 344–352, 1951.
310. STEIN, J. M., AND H. A. PADYKULA. Histochemical classification of individual skeletal muscle fibers of the rat. *Am. J. Anat.* 110: 103–104, 1962.
311. STONNINGTON, H. H., AND A. G. ENGEL. Normal and denervated muscle. A morphometric study of fine structure. *Neurology* 23: 714–724, 1973.
312. STREHLER, E. E., G. PELLONI, C. W. HEIZMANN, AND H. M. EPPENBERGER. Biochemical and ultrastructural aspects of M_r 165,000 M-protein in cross-striated chicken muscle. *J. Cell Biol.* 86: 775–783, 1980.
313. TE KRONNIE, G., C. W. POOL, G. SCHOLTEN, AND W. VAN RAAMSDONK. Myofibrillar differences among mammalian skeletal-muscle fibers at the ultrastructural level. A comparison of immunocytochemical and morphometrical parameters. *Eur. J. Cell Biol.* 22: 772–779, 1980.
314. THORNELL, L. E., L. EDSTRÖM, A. ERIKSSON, K. G. HENRIKSSON, AND K. A. ÄNGQUIST. The distribution of intermediate filament protein (skeletin) in normal and diseased human skeletal muscle. An immunohistochemical and electron-microscopic study. *J. Neurol. Sci.* 47: 153–170, 1980.
315. TIEGS, O. W. On the arrangement of the striations of voluntary muscle fibres in double spirals. *Trans. Proc. R. Soc. South Aust.* 46: 222–224, 1922.
316. TIEGS, O. W. The flight muscle of insects—their anatomy and histology: with some observations on the structure of striated muscle in general. *Philos. Trans. R. Soc. London Ser. B* 238: 221–348, 1955.
317. TOMANEK, R. J., C. R. ASMUNDSON, R. R. COOPER, AND R. J. BARNARD. Fine structure of fast-twitch and slow-twitch guinea pig muscle fibers. *J. Morphol.* 139: 47–65, 1973.
318. TOMANEK, R. J., AND D. D. LUND. Degeneration of different types of skeletal muscle fibers. II. Immobilization. *J. Anat.* 118: 531–541, 1974.
319. ULLRICK, W. C., P. A. TOSELLI, J. D. SAIDE, AND W. P. C. PHEAR. Fine structure of the vertebrate Z-disc. *J. Mol. Biol.* 115: 61–74, 1977.
320. VAN WINKLE, W. B., AND A. SCHWARTZ. Morphological and biochemical correlates of skeletal muscle contractility in the cat. I. Histochemical and electron microscopic studies. *J. Cell. Physiol.* 97: 99–120, 1978.
321. VERATTI, E. Investigations on the fine structure of striated muscle fiber [transl. from Italian]. *J. Biophys. Biochem. Cytol.* 10: 1–60, 1961.
322. VRACKO, R., AND E. P. BENDIT. Basal lamina: the scaffold for orderly cell replacement. *J. Cell Biol.* 55: 406–419, 1972.
323. VRBOVA, G., T. GORDON, AND R. JONES. *Nerve-Muscle Interaction.* New York: Wiley, 1978.
324. WAGNER, P. D., AND A. G. WEEDS. Studies on the role of myosin alkali light chains. *J. Mol. Biol.* 109: 455–473, 1977.
325. WALLACE, N., AND J. R. SOMMER. Fusion of sarcoplasmic reticulum with ruthenium red. *Proc. Annu. Meet. Electron Microsc. Soc. Am., 33rd,* edited by G. W. Bailey. Baton Rouge, LA: Claitor's, 1975, p. 500–501.
326. WANG, K., AND C. L. WILLIAMSON. Identification of an N_2 line protein of striated muscle. *Proc. Natl. Acad. Sci. USA* 77: 3254–3258, 1980.
327. WEEDS, A. Myosin light chains, polymorphism and fibre types in skeletal muscles. In: *Plasticity of Muscle,* edited by D. Pette. New York: de Gruyter, 1980, p. 55–68.
328. WEEDS, A. G., R. HALL, AND N. C. S. SPURWAY. Characterization of myosin light chains from histochemically identified fibres of rabbit psoas muscle. *FEBS Lett.* 49: 320–324, 1975.
329. WEIBEL, E. R. A stereological method for estimating volume and surface of sarcoplasmic reticulum. *J. Microsc. Oxford* 95: 229–242, 1972.
330. WEIBEL, E. R. *Stereological Methods. I. Practical Methods for Biological Morphometry.* New York: Academic, 1979.
331. WEIBEL, E. R. *Stereological Methods. II. Theoretical Foundations.* New York: Academic, 1980.
332. WEIBEL, E. R., AND R. P. BOLENDER. Stereological techniques for electron microscopic morphometry. In: *Principles and Techniques of Electron Microscopy,* edited by M. A. Hayat. New York: Van Nostrand Reinhold, 1973, p. 237–296.
333. WHITEHOUSE, W. J. A stereological method for calculating internal surface areas in structures which have become anisotropic as the result of linear expansions or contractions. *J. Microsc. Oxford* 101: 169–176, 1974.
334. WHITEHOUSE, W. J. Errors in area measurement in thick sections, with special reference to trabecular bone. *J. Microsc. Oxford* 107: 183–187, 1976.
335. WILEY, C. A., AND M. H. ELLISMAN. Rows of dimeric-particles within the axolemma and juxtaposed particles within glia, incorporated into a new model for the paranodal glial-axonal junction at the node of Ranvier. *J. Cell Biol.* 84: 261–280, 1980.
336. WROBLEWSKI, R., AND E. JANSSON. Fine structure of single fibres of human skeletal muscle. *Cell Tissue Res.* 161: 471–476, 1975.
337. YAMAGUCHI, M., M. H. STROMER, R. M. ROBSON, B. ANDERSON, AND W. D. ANDERSON. Studies on the basic structural unit of muscle Z lines (Abstract). *J. Cell Biol.* 87: 259a, 1980.
338. YELLIN, H., AND L. GUTH. The histochemical classification of muscle fibers. *Exp. Neurol.* 26: 424–432, 1970.
339. ZAMPIGHI, G., J. VERGARA, AND F. RAMÓN. On the connection between the transverse tubules and the plasma membrane in frog semitendinosus skeletal muscle. Are caveolae the mouth of the transverse tubule system? *J. Cell Biol.* 64: 734–740, 1975.

CHAPTER 4

Immunological techniques in fluorescence and electron microscopy applied to skeletal muscle fibers

FRANK A. PEPE | *Department of Anatomy, School of Medicine, University of Pennsylvania, Philadelphia, Pennsylvania*

CHAPTER CONTENTS

THIS CHAPTER REVIEWS how immunological techniques are being applied in fluorescence and electron microscopy to study the protein composition, structure, and molecular organization of skeletal muscle fiber components. The use of these techniques to study the development and regeneration of muscle fibers or the transformation of muscle fiber types is not considered because the subject is covered in other chapters of this *Handbook*. An earlier review (123) on the analysis of antibody-staining patterns of striated myofibrils covered some of the very early work on this subject. This chapter takes over where that review left off and emphasizes the refinements in interpretation that have occurred as a result of more recent findings. It is not the purpose here to present an exhaustive review of the literature, but rather to survey the important developments in the use of immunological techniques in fluorescence and electron microscopy.

Immunohistochemical studies of muscle fibers have not been limited to identifying the presence of muscle proteins but have also provided structural information on the molecular organization of muscle components. A major difficulty in the interpretation of immunological data has been establishing the specificity of the antibody. More sensitive methods of detecting the presence of contaminating antibodies and the use of properly screened monoclonal antibodies have made this less of a problem. Therefore it is becoming possible to take better advantage of the tremendous capabilities of immunological and immunohistochemical approaches for identifying proteins with their structural counterparts.

Comprehensive coverages of the most recent advances in immunochemical techniques (17, 182), the hybridoma technology of producing monoclonal antibodies (69), and techniques of immunocytochemistry (163) have been published. Some of the detailed information on the basic principles involved are compiled in these books. The specific application of some of these techniques to the study of skeletal muscle fibers is considered here.

Most of the studies of skeletal muscle fibers have involved the myofibrillar proteins. Although this highly organized system has considerable advantages, it also has disadvantages. The highly ordered system makes it possible to take advantage of the presence of regularly repeating structures to analyze the structural organization of the system; however, the small separation between the myofilaments in the zone of overlap of the thick and thin filaments precludes the use of antibodies labeled with an electron-dense tag because the labeled antibody becomes too large to penetrate between the filaments. It is possible to use unlabeled antibody to visualize periodically repeating antigenic determinants in electron microscopy by the change in structure produced with introduction of antibody protein. The disadvantage of this approach is that unlabeled antibody introduced in a nonperiodic fashion is more difficult to detect in electron microscopy and may therefore lead to erroneous conclusions. It is possible, however, to verify whether or not antibody has been introduced elsewhere in a nonperiodic fashion by comparing the staining pattern in electron microscopy with that in fluorescence microscopy (127). The visualization of antibody in fluorescence microscopy is dependent only on the amount of antibody introduced, and the immunofluorescence method is very sensitive. Thus maximum advantage is taken of the highly ordered structure of the system and the disadvantage of having to use unlabeled antibody is minimized by the use of the fluorescence approach in conjunction with electron microscopy. The detection of regularly repeating antigenic determinants and more randomly distributed determinants is separated in this way.

The use of immunological techniques to identify proteins with their structural counterparts is, of course, dependent on the availability of the antigenic determinants on the proteins for binding the antibody. It is possible that one or more of the antigenic determinants may be unavailable for binding of specific antibody, depending on the following: *1*) the structural organization in which the protein is involved, i.e., whether it is buried inside or is on the surface; *2*) the sites involved in protein-protein interactions, or *3*) the conformational state of part or all of the protein molecule. Therefore a negative result cannot be consid-

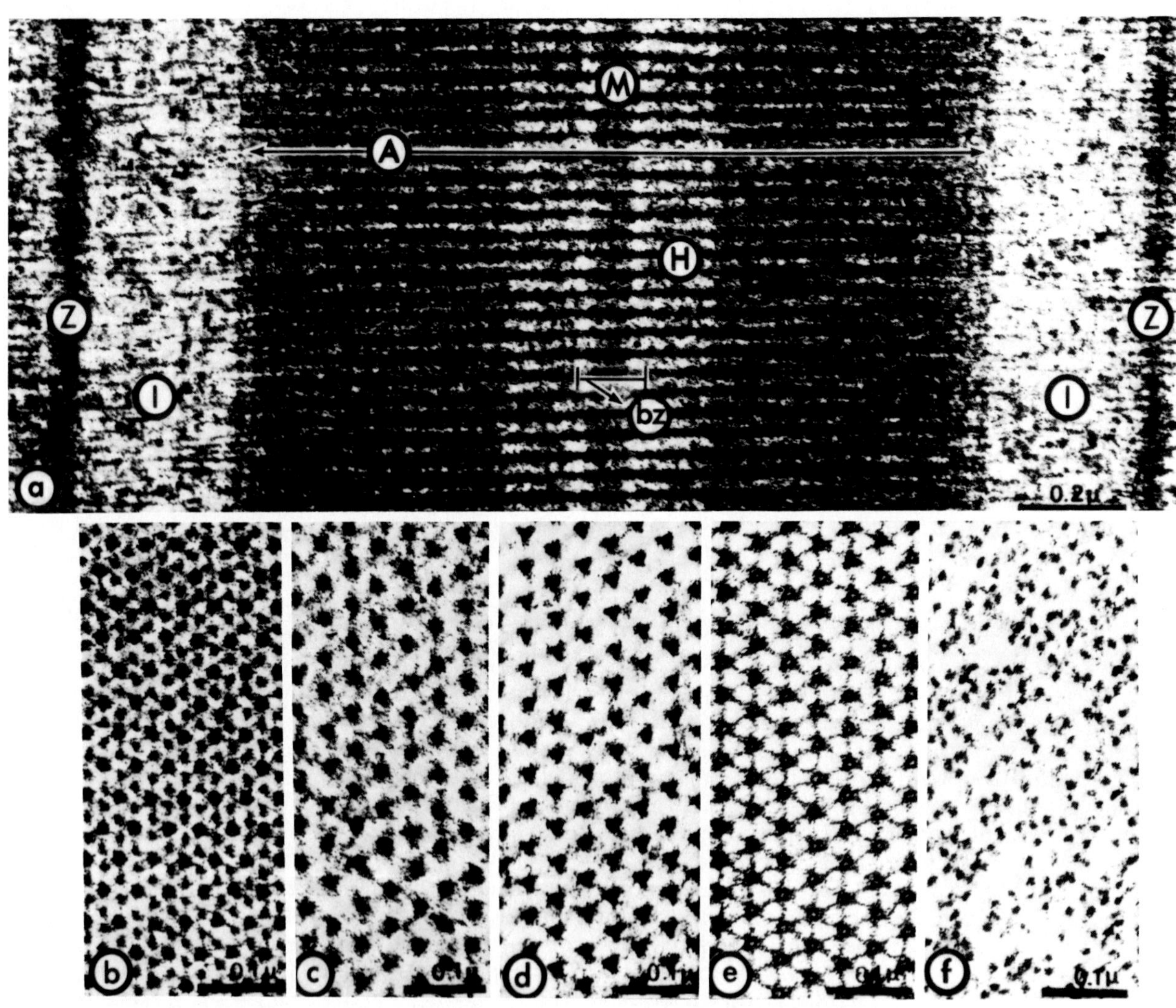

FIG. 1. Sarcomere (repeat unit of striated myofibril) from muscle of the freshwater killifish (*Fundulus diaphanus*). *a*: Longitudinal section. *Z*, Z band; *I*, I band; *A*, A band; *H*, H band; *bz*, bare zone; *M*, M band. *b*: Cross section through A band in region of overlap of thin and thick filaments. Thick filaments have solid circular profiles. Some appear to have triangular profiles. *c*: Cross section through A band in region of H band (nonoverlap region). Only thick filaments are present. Thick filaments have solid circular profiles. *d*: Cross section through A band in region of bare zone immediately adjacent to M band. Thick filaments have solid triangular profiles. *e*: Cross section through A band in region of M band. Each thick filament is connected to each of its 6 neighboring thick filaments by M bridges. Some filaments are clearly hollow and have circular profiles. *f*: Cross section through I band. Only thin filaments are present. [From Pepe (123a).]

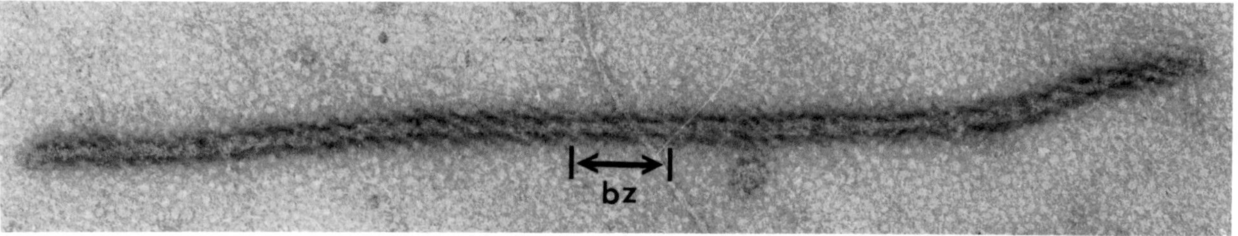

FIG. 2. Negative-stained natural myosin filaments. Note rough surface of filament where myosin cross bridges are present and smooth bare-zone region (*bz*) in middle of filament where there are no myosin cross bridges.

ered proof of the absence of a protein. The protein may be present but for one or more reasons the antigenic determinants on the protein may not be available for antibody binding. Although this at first appears to be a disadvantage, it can be used to advantage. For instance, antibody binding observed under one set of conditions and not under a different set of conditions can give information about changes in the structure being studied under a variety of different conditions. Changes in the interaction between structural components under different conditions may also be detectable in this way. This then becomes a very powerful tool for studying systems that can exist in a variety of different states.

MYOFIBRILLAR PROTEINS

The myofibrillar proteins make up the major portion of the proteins in muscle cells. The repeat unit of the striation pattern of cross-striated skeletal muscle myofibrils is the sarcomere shown in Figure 1. The sarcomere extends from Z band to Z band. The Z band is a narrow dense band that is in the middle of a less dense band, the I band. The I band therefore is half in one sarcomere and half in an adjacent sarcomere. The A band is a dense band in the middle of the sarcomere. The thick filaments (made up of myosin with other proteins associated with them) extend the length of the A band and are about 1.6 μm long (60). The thin filaments (made up of actin and the regulatory proteins tropomyosin and troponin) extend from the Z band into the sarcomere where they overlap with one-half of the thick filaments of the A band. They are about 1 μm long. The thin filaments attach to the Z band in a square lattice arrangement. The H band is the region in the middle of the A band where there is no overlap of the thick and thin filaments. Along the length of the thick filaments there are myosin cross bridges except for a bare-zone region in the middle of the filament that is about 149 nm long measured from longitudinal sections of the A band (18). A separated natural filament is shown in Figure 2 by negative staining with uranyl acetate. There is a rough surface on the filament where the myosin cross bridges are located, and the smooth bare zone in the middle of the filament can be seen. M-band proteins attach to the middle of the bare-zone region of the myosin filaments in the myofibril (Fig. 1) to form the M band, which is made up of five M lines (126, 158, 159). These lines are formed by proteins that bridge the myosin filaments at these five positions along the bare-zone region of the filament. The length of the M band is 86 nm (121, 158, 159). In traverse sections through the I band, the thin filaments are disorganized; in the region of overlap of the thin and thick filaments, there is a hexagonal packing arrangement with each thin filament equidistant from three thick filaments and with six thin filaments surrounding each thick filament. In the region of the A band where only the thick filaments are present, there is a simple hexagonal arrangement. In the bare-zone region immediately adjacent to the M band, the thick filaments appear to have triangular transverse profiles. In the M-band region, the thick filaments have circular profiles and a less-dense core and there are M bridges extending to each of the six neighboring thick filaments. It is only in the M-band region of the filament (86 nm long) that the filaments have a less-dense core. Everywhere else along the length of the filaments there is no evidence for a less-dense core. These are the general characteristics of the striated myofibril. The application of immunohistochemical techniques to study the protein composition and structural detail of the A band, M band, I band, and Z band is discussed separately.

A Band

Before discussing the application of immunological techniques in fluorescence and electron microscopy to studies of the A band of skeletal muscle, a little more detail about the structural organization and protein composition of the A band helps. The proteins of the A band are those of the thick filament, which is made up of myosin and other associated proteins. Starr and Offer (162) showed that myosin preparations that were purified by repeated reprecipitation at low ionic strength were contaminated with other proteins that coprecipitated with the myosin. It was later shown that at least one of these proteins, C protein, is associated with the myosin filament with evidence that at least two others may also be (19, 133). Morimoto and

Harrington (103) isolated native myosin filaments, which on analysis were shown to be free of other proteins except for C protein, and there is considerable evidence that the C protein is bound to the surface of the myosin filament (19, 133). Therefore the evidence is strong that the thick filament is made up of myosin and that other proteins are associated with the surface of the thick filament.

The structure of vertebrate skeletal myosin filaments has been studied by X-ray diffraction (61) as well as by electron microscopy (59, 61, 121, 129, 130, 131, 132, 164). From these studies, models have been proposed for myosin packing and for the helical arrangement of myosin cross bridges on the surface of the filament (61, 121, 161).

The X-ray–diffraction data clearly show that there are myosin cross bridges at intervals of 14 nm along the length of the filament and that there is a helical repeat of 43 nm (61). It is not possible to determine from the X-ray data whether the helix is two-, three-, or four-stranded.

A considerable amount of biochemical work has been done to pin down the myosin content of the vertebrate skeletal myosin filament. The myosin content would help decide strandedness of the helical arrangement. Values for myosin content have centered around three or four myosin molecules per 14-nm interval along the length of the filament. The value of three myosin molecules per 14-nm interval has been obtained by quantitative sodium dodecyl sulfate (SDS)–gel electrophoresis (139, 170), nucleotide-binding studies (89), hydrodynamic studies (32), and mass measurements with a scanning transmission electron microscope (STEM) (75, 140). The value of four myosin molecules per 14-nm interval has been obtained by quantitative SDS-gel electrophoresis (104, 134), nucleotide-binding studies (92, 181), hydrodynamic studies (68), and a particle-counting technique (104). Pepe and Drucker (134) have shown that the source of this discrepancy, for data obtained from quantitative SDS–polyacrylamide gel electrophoresis, appears to be related to whether or not actin (to which the myosin content was standardized) was properly resolved from two closely neighboring protein bands. When actin was properly resolved a value of four myosin molecules per 14-nm interval was obtained for the myosin content of vertebrate skeletal myosin filaments. Quantitative data must be good enough to clearly distinguish between this difference of only 25% between a value of three and four. Because of the relatively large uncertainties in all of the quantitative procedures used, it is not likely that a definitive value will come from these approaches. It is more likely that the correct quantitative results will eventually be accepted because of the force of structural information rather than the results of quantitative analytical techniques.

Electron-microscopic studies of the structure of vertebrate skeletal myosin filaments have been concentrated more heavily on the structure of the backbone than on the arrangement of the myosin cross bridges on the surface of the filaments because the cross-bridge arrangement is not easily preserved through preparations for electron microscopy. A comprehensive review of electron-microscopic studies of the backbone of the vertebrate skeletal myosin filament has been published recently (129). From studies of transverse sections of the myosin filament with optical diffraction of the images and from the effect of tilt on the optical-diffraction pattern, there is good evidence that the backbone of the filament is made up of parallel subfilaments spaced 4 nm apart and packed in an approximately hexagonal array (129, 131). A subfilament spacing of about 4 nm has also been observed from X-ray–diffraction studies of both vertebrate (98) and invertebrate muscle (188, 189). Computer-image analysis of electron micrographs of transverse sections of vertebrate skeletal myosin filaments has additionally shown that there are 12 subfilaments (129, 164), hexagonally packed with three located centrally and nine located peripherally as predicted by the model for the myosin filament proposed by Pepe (119, 121). Such an image is shown in Figure 3.

MYOSIN: HISTORICAL BACKGROUND. Antibodies to myosin have been used to study the A-band–staining patterns and their relation to the structure of the myosin filament and to identify myosin isozymes. The studies of the distribution of myosin isozymes among fiber types are treated in detail in other chapters of this *Handbook*. Note, however, that the first demon-

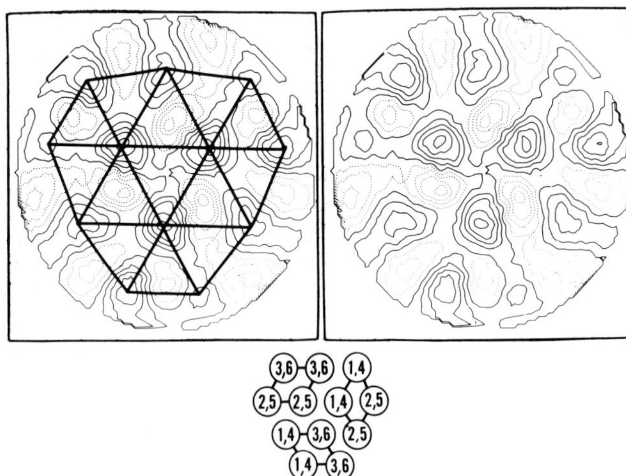

FIG. 3. Computer processing of images of transverse sections of individual myosin filaments by rational averaging. Contour density maps of rotational averaging of 6 combined images are shown. *Left*, bold straight lines join centers of subfilaments. *Right*, same map without these lines. There are 12 subfilaments hexagonally packed with 3 located centrally and 9 located peripherally, forming a triangular profile with a subfilament missing at each apex. Diagram at *bottom* is model proposed by Pepe (119, 121), in which the predicted arrangement and number of subfilaments are similar to those observed in the rotationally averaged images. [From Pepe (129).]

stration that there are immunochemically distinctive myosins in different muscle fibers came from studies in which the antibodies to one fiber type were obtained. These antibodies therefore stained some of the fibers but left other fibers unstained (45, 47). Antibodies to both fast-twitch and slow-twitch muscle myosins were first obtained by Arndt and Pepe (2) and were shown by immunodiffusion to be antigenically distinct (Fig. 4*A*, *B*). In addition fluorescent antibody staining exhibited complimentary staining patterns in frozen sections of muscles containing both fast- and slow-twitch fiber types (Fig. 4*C*, *D*). Similar studies were made by Gauthier and Lowey (38). Antibody prepared against fast-twitch muscle myosin has generally been used for structural studies. In this chapter only the structural studies are discussed.

In the early studies of antimyosin staining of vertebrate skeletal muscle myofibrils reviewed by Pepe (123), the staining observed in fluorescence microscopy was restricted to the A band. The myosin used as immunogen in this early work was purified by several reprecipitations at low ionic strength. Starr and Offer (162) showed by SDS–polyacrylamide gel electrophoresis that myosin purified in this way still contained appreciable amounts of other proteins. It was later shown that the antimyosins did indeed contain antibodies to other protein contaminants (125) and one of these, C protein, was studied further in considerable detail (19, 108, 125, 133).

The evolution of our understanding of the antimyosin-staining pattern of the A band and its relation to the structure of the sarcomere illustrates how structural information and immunological techniques applied in microscopy can be related. Marshall, et al. (88), in addition to using myosin, also used the myosin fragments heavy meromyosin (HMM) and light meromyosin (LMM) as immunogens. They found that whereas antimyosin stained the entire A band, anti-HMM stained more brightly in the middle of the A band, anti-LMM stained more brightly at the edges of the A band, and anti-LMM stained more brightly at the edges of the A band near each A-I junction. These authors suggested that the myosin molecule might be greatly extended in the A band to account for the distance between the antibody localization for the HMM and LMM portions of the molecule. Tunik and Holtzer (174) did a detailed study of how the pattern of A-band staining observed with these antibodies changed with change in sarcomere length. They found that with shortening sarcomere length, antimyosin staining became limited to the edges of the A band near each A-I junction as the unstained region in the middle of the A band became wider. The anti-LMM behaved similarly except that the unstained region in the middle of the A band at the longer sarcomere lengths was wider than with antimyosin and comparable to that observed with antimyosin at the shortest sarcomere length studied. With anti-HMM the brightest fluorescence was in a narrow band in the middle of the A band and this persisted at all sarcomere lengths with lighter staining elsewhere in the A band. They suggested that the discontinuous staining of antimyosin could be due either to movement of myosin in the A band with change in sarcomere length or to alteration in the availability of antigenic sites on the myosin molecule. They also obtained evidence that the narrow bright band observed with anti-HMM in the middle of the A band was due to the presence of antibody to a nonmyosin contaminant in the HMM preparation. Therefore at this point the most likely possibilities for the discontinuous staining pattern for antimyosin were that it could represent either a discontinuity in the distribution of myosin in the A band or an alteration in the availability of antigenic determinants in the A band. It was reasonably clear that at least some of the staining obtained with anti-HMM could be explained as staining of a nonmyosin component. How these observations and possibilities might be related to the structure of the A band as had been described by Huxley (59) was not clear.

A variation on the use of antibodies to study myofibrillar structure was introduced by Szent-Gyorgyi and Holtzer (168). From observations in phase microscopy, they showed that reaction of myofibrils with antibodies could insolubilize portions of the sarcomere preventing extraction of the portion of the myofibril to which the antibody bound. Antimyosin prevented extraction of the A bands of myofibrils with 0.6 M KI. Anti-LMM protected the edges of the A band along each A-I junction and anti-HMM protected the middle of the A band from extraction. With this method Pepe et al. (135) made similar observations in electron microscopy for antimyosin and anti-HMM stained fibers.

With antimyosin similar to that used in previous work (88, 174), Pepe (120) took a slightly different approach to the analysis of the antimyosin-staining pattern of the A band. He reasoned that if the myosin fragments, HMM and LMM, had some antigenic determinants in common, then using them directly as immunogens could produce antibodies that were shared by both the HMM and LMM. Therefore he obtained antibody specific for LMM by absorbing antimyosin with an excess of HMM and antibody specific for HMM by absorbing antimyosin with an excess of LMM. In this way the antibodies to common antigenic determinants would be absorbed out in each case leaving only antibodies specific for the other fragment. In addition, Pepe (120) reanalyzed the antimyosin-staining pattern. He found that when the amount of antimyosin used for staining was reduced, the A-band–staining pattern could be resolved into four bands, two in the middle of the A band and one at each edge of the A band near the A-I junction for sarcomeres about 2.5 μm in length (Fig. 5*A*). This pattern contrasted with that described for sarcomeres of about the same length by Tunik and Holtzer (174), who observed either uniform staining of the A band or a fluorescent A band with a more brightly stained

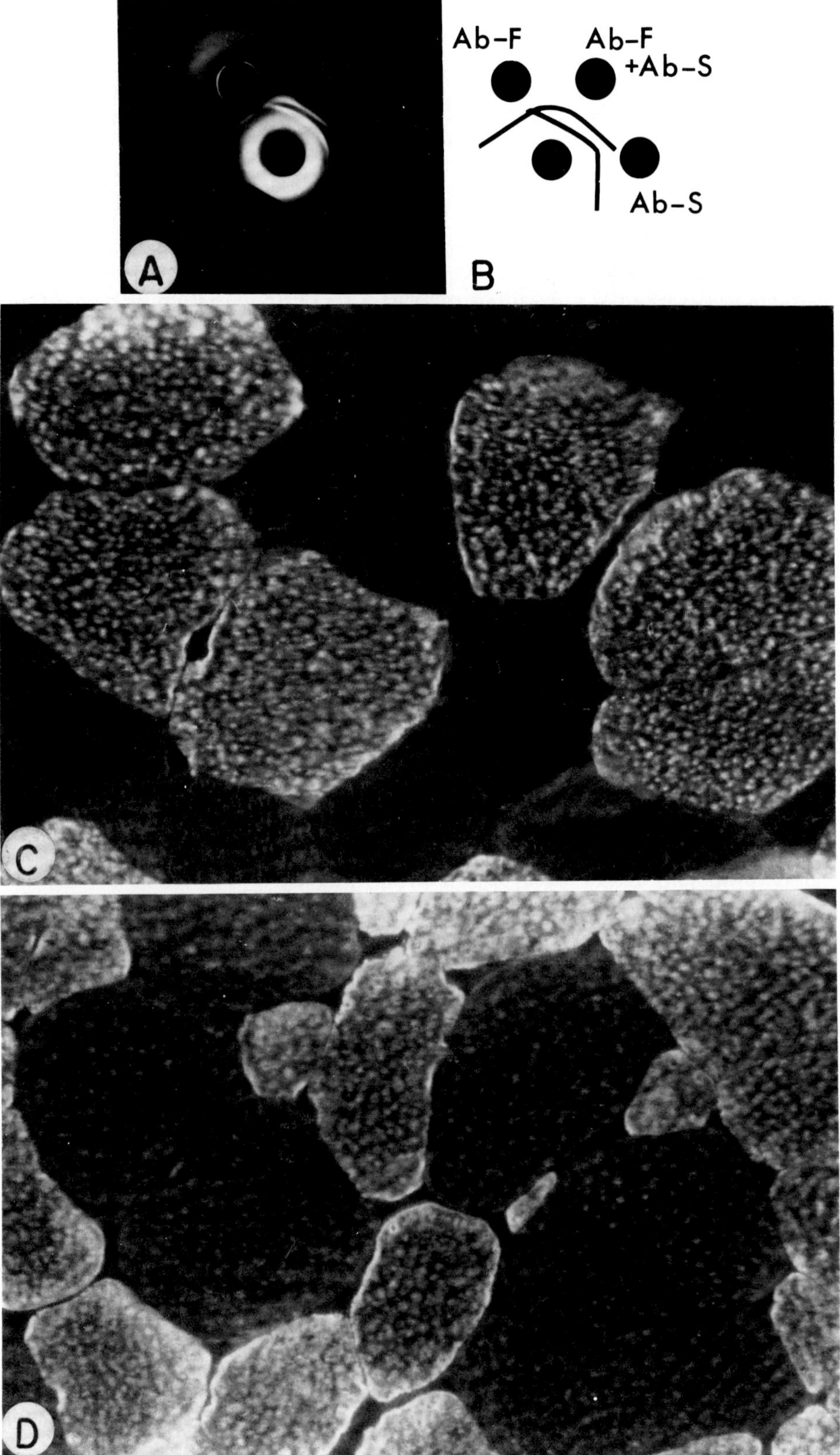

FIG. 4. Antibody specific for fast-twitch and slow-twitch myosins. *A* and *B*: specific antibody to fast-twitch myosin (*Ab-F*) gives a single precipitin line when immunodiffused against a mixture of fast-twitch and slow-twitch myosins (*central well*). This line fuses with 1 of the 2 lines obtained when a mixture of antibody to fast-twitch myosin (*Ab-F*) and slow-twitch myosin (*Ab-S*) is diffused against

band in the middle of the A band. The four bands in the A band observed by Pepe (120) seemed to represent the staining of different antigenic determinants because with reduction of the amount of antimyosin used for staining, the bands at the edges of the A band along each A-I junction were found to drop out while the medial bands remained bright. This difference in antigenicity was verified by the absorption studies. On absorbing the antimyosin with an excess of HMM, the medial bands were no longer observed and only the lateral-band staining was obtained (Fig. 5*B*). On absorbing with LMM the opposite was observed, i.e., the lateral-band staining was not obtained and only the medial bands were observed (Fig. 5*C*). Therefore, it was concluded that the two bands in the middle of the A band represented specific staining of antigenic determinants on HMM (Fig. 5*C*), whereas the other two bands represented specific staining of antigenic determinants on LMM (Fig. 5*B*). The LMM staining was therefore similar to that described previously (88, 174).

Pepe (120, 122) further studied the change in the pattern of A-band staining with change in sarcomere length. He found that the two bands in the middle of the A band that represent specific staining of HMM

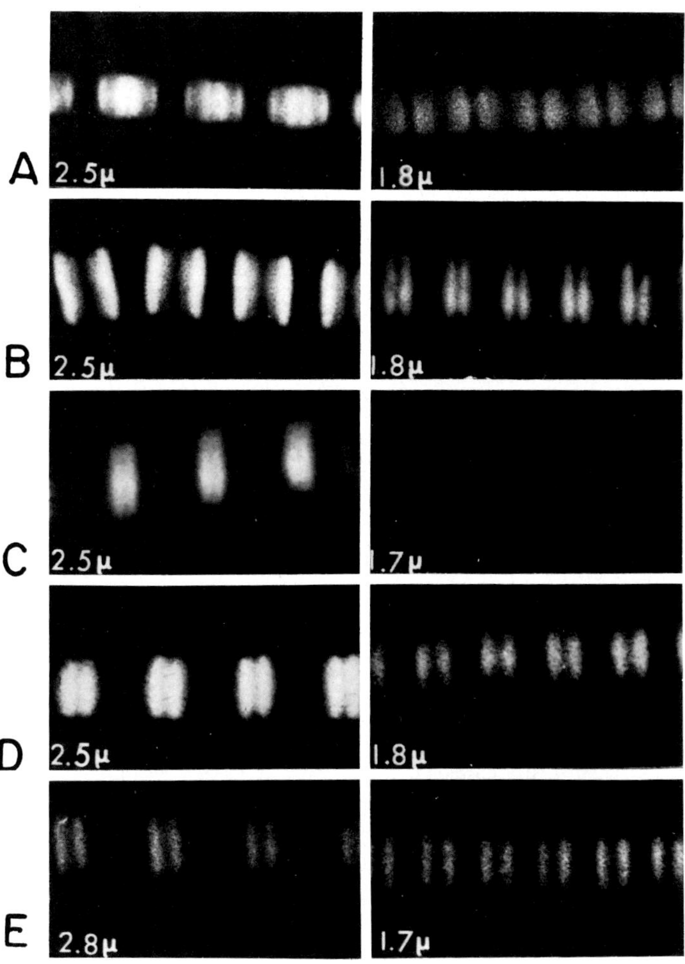

FIG. 5. Fluorescent antimyosin staining of chicken fibrils. All staining was done in 25% glycerol containing 7.5×10^{-2} M KCl, 7.5×10^{-4} M $MgCl_2$, 7.5×10^{-3} M phosphate buffer at pH 7.0. *A*: antimyosin contaminated with anti-C protein. Staining of fibrils at 2.5 μm and 1.8 μm sarcomere lengths. *B*: antilight meromyosin staining of fibrils obtained by absorption of antimyosin with heavy meromyosin contaminated with C protein. *C*: anti-heavy meromyosin staining of fibrils obtained by absorption of antimyosin with light meromyosin contaminated with C protein. *D*: anti-heavy meromyosin and anti-C-protein staining of fibrils obtained by absorption of antimyosin with light meromyosin that was not contaminated with C protein. *E*: specific anti-C protein isolated from antimyosin contaminated with anti-C protein. Same pattern is observed with specific anti-C protein isolated from IgG fraction of antiserum to C protein.

---

the mixture of the 2 myosins. The other line fuses with the single line obtained with specific antibody to slow-twitch myosin (*Ab-S*). Immunodiffusion patterns are shown in *A* and diagramed in *B*. *C*: frozen sections of chicken sartorius muscle stained with fluorescein-labeled Ab-S show that some cells contain slow-twitch myosin (bright fluorescent cells), whereas other cells do not (unstained cells). *D*: serial section of same muscle fibers now stained with Ab-F; the cells in *C* that contained slow myosin are unstained, whereas the cells in *C* that were unstained now stain brightly, indicating presence of fast myosin. Therefore in the sartorius muscle 2 types of muscle fibers are present: those containing fast-twitch myosin and those containing slow-twitch myosin. [*A* and *B* from Arndt and Pepe (2). Micrographs *C* and *D* courtesy of N. Rubinstein.]

antigenic determinants disappeared with decrease in sarcomere length; but the other two bands that represent specific staining of LMM antigenic sites did not. This was concluded from the change in the staining pattern with sarcomere length obtained with antimyosin (120, 122) as well as with antimyosin absorbed with either HMM or LMM (122). These findings (Fig. 5*A*, *B*, and *C*) made it possible to relate the antimyosin-staining pattern to the sliding-filament model for sarcomere shortening (62, 63). In the region of the A band where there is no overlap between myosin and actin filaments, the antigenic determinants on the myosin cross bridges (HMM portion of the myosin molecule) are available for antibody binding. The unstained bare-zone region in the middle of the filament where there are no myosin cross bridges makes the staining of the nonoverlap region appear as two bands in the middle of the A band. Everywhere else in the A band where the myosin cross bridges are bound to the overlapping actin filaments the antigenic determinants on the HMM are blocked by the interaction with actin and are not available for antibody binding. The LMM staining in the other two bands in the A band was not affected by the change in sarcomere length except that it appeared to increase in brightness with decrease in sarcomere length. The LMM antigenic sites were considered to be involved in the intermolecular interactions leading to aggregation of the myosin molecules to form the myosin filament and are therefore not available for antibody binding except for the region near the tapered end of the filament where some LMM sites become available due to loosening of the structure resulting from the attachment of the myosin cross bridges to the actin filaments. This explanation for the observations of LMM staining in the A band was not as satisfactory as that for the HMM staining. However, the observed changes in the staining pattern with sarcomere length were at least reasonably consistent with the sliding-filament model and with the fact that the interaction of the LMM portion of the myosin molecules to form the core of the filament would make this portion of the molecule least likely to have antigenic determinants, which are available for antibody binding on the surface of the filament.

The next steps in studies of antimyosin staining of the A band were made in electron microscopy. Pepe (119, 121) used unlabeled antimyosin, and the introduction of antibody protein produced an observable change in the organized structure of the unstained A band. Samosudova et al. (148) used ferritin-labeled antimyosin. The ferritin-labeled antibody did not penetrate the region of the A band where the myosin and actin filaments overlap. Only the nonoverlap region of the A band (the H band) was stained by the ferritin-labeled antibody. This is most likely due to the large size of the ferritin-antibody conjugate and the small surface-to-surface distance between the actin and myosin filaments. Pepe and Huxley (136) stained separated myosin filaments on grids with antimyosin and then negative stained them with uranyl acetate. The specific binding of the antimyosin to the myosin filaments was observed as protein visible on the surface of the myosin filaments with nothing adhering to the actin filaments on the grid. Pepe (119, 121) found that after staining muscle fibers with unlabeled antimyosin, seven narrow dense bands spaced 43 nm apart appeared in the middle of each half of the A band in electron microscopy (Fig. 6*A*). These bands did not change with change in sarcomere length and remained intact even when the muscle was stretched so that the actin filaments did not overlap the areas of the A band in which the bands were found. Therefore they were clearly related to the myosin filaments. There was also some increase in density in the A band near each A-I junction, but this was not periodic as was the staining in the middle of each half of the A band. At this point, there was reason to believe that these observations might be related to antimyosin staining and therefore an attempt was made to relate the patterns observed in electron microscopy (119, 121) and fluorescence microscopy (122). In addition a more detailed study of the fluorescent antimyosin-staining pattern of the A band was made by absorbing the antimyosin with LMM fragments obtained from myosin digested for different lengths of time. The corresponding electron microscopic studies were also done. The LMM obtained from extensively digested myosin (i.e., a shorter LMM fragment) did not absorb out the staining of the seven bands in each half of the A band observed in electron microscopy, but LMM obtained from myosin digested for a short time (i.e., a longer LMM fragment) did absorb out the staining of the seven bands in each half of the A band. Correspondingly, in fluorescence microscopy, absorption with the long LMM fragment (Fig. 5*C*) absorbed out a portion of the staining closer to the middle of the A band, which persisted in short myofibrils (1.7–1.8 μm) after absorption with the short LMM fragment (Fig. 5*D*). This fluorescent staining absorbed by the long LMM could be shown to correspond, in position, to the seven bands in each half of the A band observed in electron microscopy (Fig. 6*A*). The seven bands were considered to correspond to the staining of antigenic determinants on the trypsin-sensitive region of the myosin molecule and the periodicity was considered to represent a region of the filament in which the myosin molecules were much more highly organized than in the rest of the A band therefore giving the clearly defined periodic antibody density. The possibility that any parts of the A-band–staining patterns observed in either fluorescence or electron microscopy could be due to antibody to contaminants seemed unlikely because the entire staining pattern could be accounted for by absorption with the different fragments used. As was shown later (125, 133), however, antibodies to other proteins did contribute to the observed A-band–staining pattern.

Offer et al. (109) showed that myosin purified by

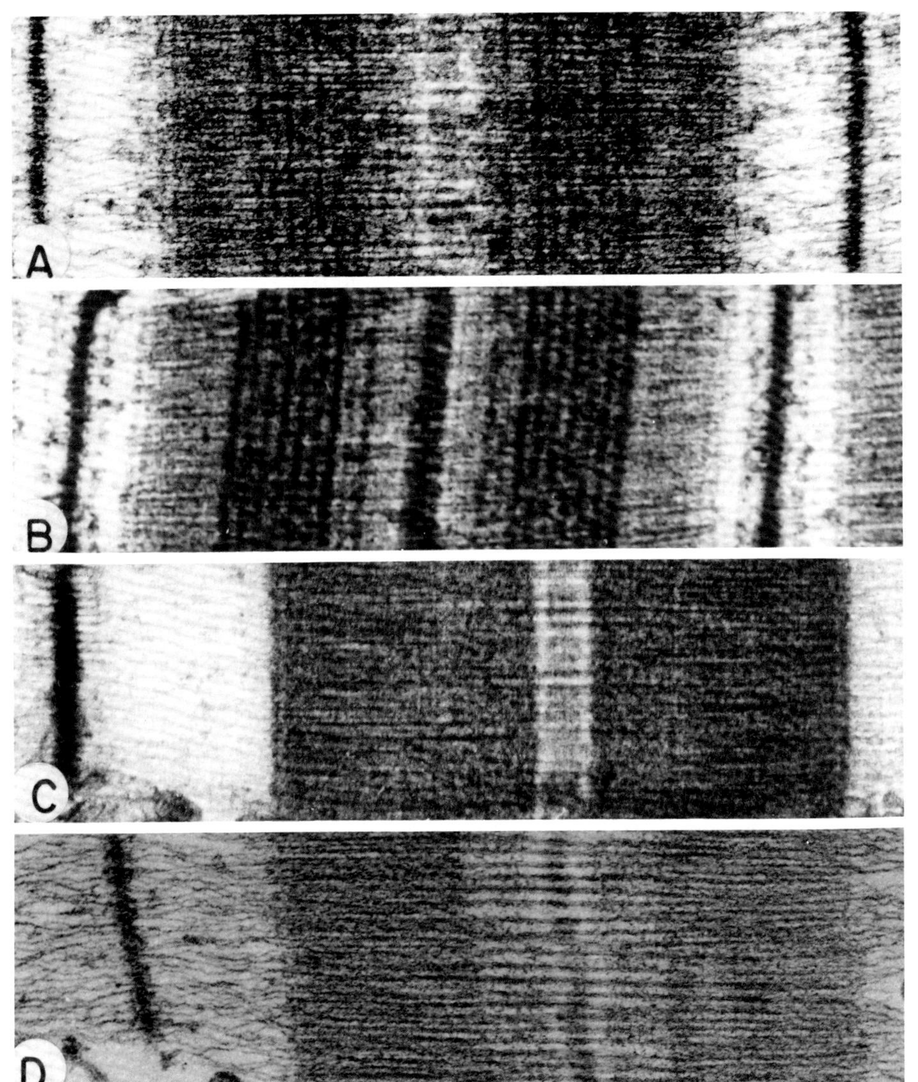

FIG. 6. *A*: antimyosin and anti–C-protein staining observed in electron microscopy. Antimyosin contaminated with anti–C protein. The 7 dense bands in middle third of each half of the A band are due to C protein (19, 107, 125, 133). C protein is present at intervals determined by myosin molecules to which it binds (13, 145). *B*: anti–C protein isolated by affinity purification from mixture of antimyosin and anti–C protein used in *A*. Note the 7 dense bands due to C protein. Weak 8th band and strong 9th band are due to 2 other proteins (see refs. 19, 133). *C*: antimyosin staining of A band. With heavy staining, normally less-dense nonoverlap region becomes indistinguishable from the rest of the A band because of the large amount of antibody protein introduced. *D*: unstained sarcomere. Note clearly less-dense nonoverlap region of the A band without heavy antimyosin staining.

column chromatography on diethylaminoethyl (DEAE)-Sephadex A-50 as described by Richards et al. (142) was free of the protein contaminants shown to be present in myosin purified by reprecipitation at low ionic strength (162). Pepe (125) put myosin, purified by reprecipitation, on a DEAE–Sephadex A-50 column as described by Richards et al. (142) and collected the peak of contaminants and the peak of column-purified myosin. He insolubilized each by coupling to resin and used the insolubilized proteins to isolate antibody to contaminants and specific antibodies to myosin from the antimyosin used in previous studies. Pepe (125) found that he could separate antibody that reacted only with myosin and antibodies that reacted only with contaminants on immunodiffusion. He further showed by immunodiffusion that a major constituent of the antibody to contaminants was antibody to C protein, which had been isolated from crude myosin preparations by Offer (107). The fluorescent antimyosin-staining pattern for the A band and its change with sarcomere length when using the highly specific antimyosin isolated by affinity binding was not significantly different from that previously observed (Fig. 5*A*). In electron microscopy, however, the seven bands spaced 43 nm apart in the middle of each half of the A band were not observed with the specific antimyosin (Fig. 6*C*), indicating that these were due to staining by antibody to one of the contaminants in conventionally purified myosin preparations. This protein turned out to be C protein (19, 107, 125–127, 133); e.g., see C PROTEIN, p. 125. With immunodiffusion, Pepe (125, 127) and Offer (107, 108) were able to show that anti–C protein is a major constitutent of the antimyosin preparations in previous studies (Fig. 7).

Although Pepe (125–127) and Pepe and Drucker (133) started with antiserum that contained antibodies to myosin and C protein and isolated specific antimyosin by affinity binding, Lowey and Steiner (83) prepared antibodies directly against column-purified myosin, as well as subfragment 1 (S1) and rod obtained from column-purified myosin. In this case, the immunoglobulin (IgG) fraction of antisera was used instead of isolated specific antibody. Lowey and Steiner (83) also did immunodiffusion and quantitative precipitin analysis to establish the specificity of their antibodies. Their antibody-staining studies were done in fluorescence microscopy but not in electron microscopy. The fluorescent antimyosin-staining pattern they observed was similar to that observed by Pepe (120, 122, 125). On absorption of the antimyosin with S1 they observed a diminution of the medial staining of the A band, whereas absorption with rod or its components LMM and S2 produced a diminution of the lateral staining of the A band. Staining of the A band with antirod closely resembled the pattern observed with antimyosin. They found that absorbing the antirod with either LMM or S2 removed most of the A-band staining, suggesting that the antirod is binding to antigenic determinants shared by both the LMM and S2 and that these are available throughout the A band. They warned that although the LMM and S2 may both share antigenic sites to which the antirod binds, "this does not mean that different portions of the rod actually have determinants in common." Absorption of the antirod with S1 did not change the staining pattern of the A band. Anti-S1 gave a pattern that was brightest in the region of the A band where the thin and thick filaments do not overlap and there was weaker staining along the rest of the A band. Absorption with LMM and S2 did not change the pattern. Absorption with S1 left a fine line of stain in the middle of the A band that could not be removed even by an excess of S1.

The results obtained by Lowey and Steiner (83) and by Pepe (120, 122, 125) are similar in that the antimyosin pattern consists of a nonuniform staining of the A band with medial and lateral bands and that HMM or S1 will absorb the medial staining preferentially and LMM will absorb the lateral staining preferentially. The difference between these two studies is that Lowey and Steiner (83) concluded from the anti-rod-staining pattern and its absorption with LMM and S2 that there are antigenic determinants on LMM and S2 that are available throughout the A band, whereas Pepe (120, 122) found that LMM determinants were only available in the A band along each A-I junction. It is possible that the difference in the two studies is due to differences in the antibody response to the same immunogen that can occur in different animals, and that in the case of Lowey and Steiner (83), antibodies were produced to different antigenic determinants on the LMM than were produced by Pepe (120, 122). This is possible because of the large size of the LMM rod. This means that if we are to truly understand the structural meaning of the staining patterns we observe, we should have some identification of the smallest region of the molecule possible to which the antibody specificity can be related. Ultimately we would like to be able to identify antibody specific for a single antigenic determinant, determine the position of that determinant in the molecule, and then correlate this information with the antibody-staining patterns obtained in fluorescence and electron microscopy under a variety of conditions. This would provide us with the potential for dissecting the structural organization of the myosin molecule and myosin filament in the myofibril under a variety of conditions. The technology that makes it possible to produce monoclonal antibodies (69) that are directed against a single antigenic determinant promises to make that a possibility. As we get finer and finer detail in the identification of antibodies to different antigenic determinants in different parts of the myosin molecule, we will have increasingly powerful tools for studying the structural organization of the myosin molecules in the myosin filament, as well as the structural changes involved in the interaction of myosin cross bridges with actin.

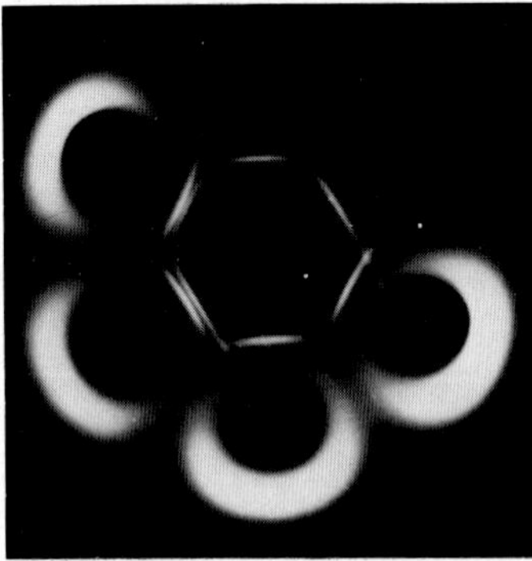

FIG. 7. Immunodiffusion of antimyosin and anti–C-protein mixture against purified myosin, purified C protein, and myosin contaminated with C protein. Mixture of antimyosin and anti–C protein is in *center well* (15 mg/ml IgG). The 2 wells at *top right* (not visible) contain C protein at 1 mg/ml. The 2 wells at *bottom right* contain column-purified myosin at 5 mg/ml. The 2 wells at *left* contain myosin contaminated with C protein at 6 mg/ml. Note the 2 lines with myosin contaminated with C protein and the fusion of 1 of these with the line formed with pure myosin and fusion of the other with the line formed with pure C protein.

With polyclonal antibodies, Pepe and Drucker (unpublished observations) defined different antibodies to the myosin fragments by sequential affinity binding to different myosin fragments that were insolubilized by coupling to CNBr-activated agarose. They started with antimyosin prepared with column-purified myosin as the immunogen. Although there was no antibody to contaminants detectable in the antimyosin by immunodiffusion, they found that if they passed the antimyosin over insolubilized contaminants, antibody to contaminants was removed. Then they isolated the specific antimyosin with insolubilized column-purified myosin. Specific antimyosin isolated in this way gave fluorescent antibody-staining patterns in the A band (Fig. 8*A*), similar to those described previously [Fig. 5*A*; (83, 120, 122)]. The next step was to pass the specific antimyosin over S1 and isolate all the antibody reacting with S1. This antibody reacted on immunodiffusion with both S1 and LMM. Therefore the anti-S1 was passed over insolubilized LMM, removing all of the anti-S1 that also reacted with LMM in immunodiffusion and leaving the antibody that reacts only with S1. This antibody showing a reaction with only S1 in immunodiffusion reacted with both S1 and S2 but not LMM when it was used to stain nitrocellulose sheets (169a) to which the fragments had been transferred (Fig. 8*C*). Recently, an antibody reacting only with the S1 fragment has been obtained (Pepe and Drucker, unpublished observations). The antimyosin from which the anti-S1 had been removed was now passed over insolubilized LMM and all the anti-LMM was removed. The LMM fragment was one produced by long (~ 40–60 min) trypsin digestion of myosin as described by Lowey and Cohen (81). The anti-LMM obtained in this way only reacted with LMM in immunodiffusion and on nitrocellulose sheets (Fig. 8*D*). The antimyosin from which both the anti-S1 and anti-LMM had been removed was finally passed over insolubilized S2, and all the anti-S2 was recovered. This was shown to react with both S1 and S2 in immunodiffusion. This anti-S2 was therefore put on insolubilized native S1. The antibody that did not bind reacted only with S2 in immunodiffusion and on nitrocellulose sheets (Fig. 8*B*).

MYOSIN (S1 PORTION). With polyclonal antibody that reacts with S1 and S2 on nitrocellulose sheets (Fig. 8*C*), the staining is essentially uniform throughout the A band regardless of the amount of overlap of the myosin and actin filaments. The staining pattern of the antibody that reacts only with S1 on nitrocellulose sheets has not been observed. Because the S1 and S2 make up the entire myosin cross bridges and because the bridges are present on the surface of the myosin filament, it is not surprising that staining is observed throughout the A band with the antibodies reacting with both S1 and S2.

MYOSIN (S2 PORTION). The staining pattern observed with specific anti-S2 and shown in Figure 8*B* is puzzling because the staining in the middle of the A band corresponds to the nonoverlap zone. It is present at long sarcomere lengths and absent at short sarcomere lengths. Therefore the interaction of S1 with actin appears to prevent staining of antigenic determinants on S2. An explanation for these observations might be plausible if the antigenic determinants are on a region of the S2 that undergoes a conformational change on interaction of the S1 with actin. This could be a region of the S2 that is involved in either the S1-S2 hinge or the S2-LMM hinge. I return to the staining observed with specific anti-S2 at each edge of the A band along the A-I junctions after a discussion of the staining patterns observed with specific anti-LMM.

MYOSIN (LMM PORTION). The staining is restricted to the lateral edges of the A band near each A-I junction at all sarcomere lengths (Fig. 8*D*). The antigenic determinants that bind the specific antibody are probably similar to those detected previously with anti-LMM staining [Fig. 5*B*; (120, 122)] because the staining patterns are indistinguishable. These LMM antigenic determinants do not correspond to those detected by Lowey and Steiner (83) with antirod because they observed a diminution in staining of all parts of the A band after absorption of the antirod with LMM. They may correspond to some of the determinants detected by Lowey and Steiner (83) with antimyosin because absorption of their antimyosin with LMM preferentially decreased the intensity of the lateral staining of the A band.

The restricted localization of specific anti-LMM to the edges of the A band near each A-I junction that does not change with sarcomere length does not lend itself easily to plausible explanations. There is considerable evidence that there are structural differences along the length of the myosin filament (129, 130) and it is conceivable that these structural differences may be responsible for the difference in availability along the filament for the antigenic determinants recognized by the specific anti-LMM. Evidence for structural differences along the filament comes from *1*) the bipolar structure of the filament (60); *2*) the binding characteristics of C protein (19, 107, 125, 133) and its restricted binding to only a portion of the filament (133); *3*) changes in the optical diffraction patterns observed from serial transverse sections of individual myosin filaments (130), and *4*) observations of the length of natural (172) and synthetic (129) myosin filaments as a function of KCl concentration.

Note that the staining in the A band along each A-I junction that is observed with specific anti-LMM is also observed with specific anti-S2 and that in both cases this staining does not change with sarcomere length (Fig. 8*B*, *D*). The fact that the LMM staining is not related to overlap and does not change with sarcomere length is consistent with the presence of the LMM in the backbone of the myosin filament, which is unaffected by change in sarcomere length. It is not clear why the S2 should have this portion of its staining pattern in common with LMM. A reasonable possibility for this observation presents itself on considering a number of different observations. First, in preparing LMM fragments to couple to CNBr-activated agarose for the affinity isolation of specific anti-LMM it was found that most LMM preparations (all obtained by 40–60 min of digestion of myosin with trypsin) in addition to binding anti-LMM also bound antibodies that reacted with S2 (ref. 126; F. A. Pepe and B. Drucker, unpublished observations). On only two occasions was an LMM preparation obtained that bound only the specific anti-LMM shown in Fig. 8*D*. There must be some antigenic determinants close to the end of the LMM rod that will bind the specific anti-S2 (Fig. 8*B*), and it is not easy to get them off by trypsin digestion. Therefore if the staining pattern is related to the packing of the myosin rods in the

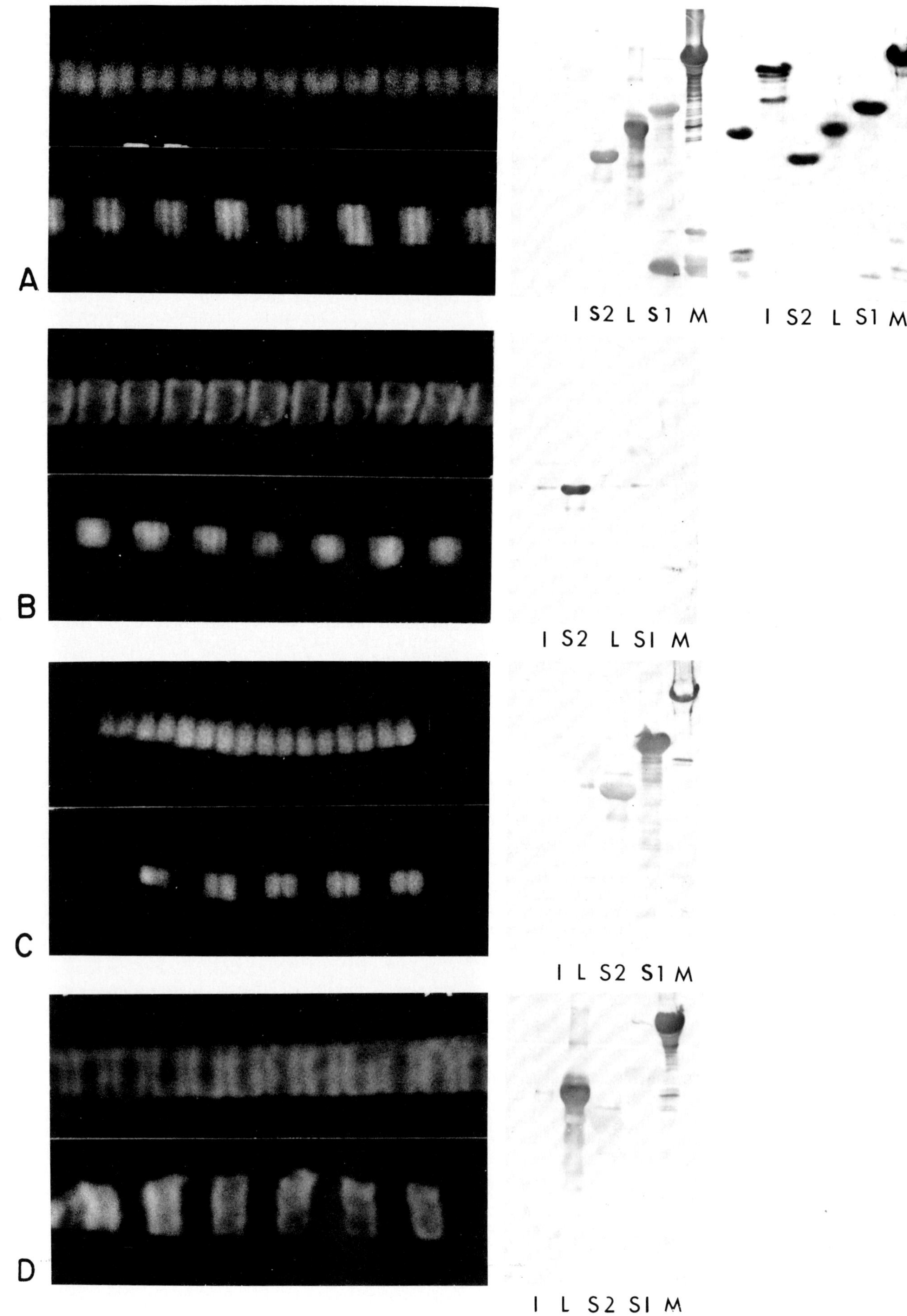
A
I S2 L S1 M
I S2 L S1 M
B
I S2 L S1 M
C
I L S2 S1 M
D
I L S2 S1 M

backbone of the filament it becomes more reasonable that these might stain in the A band in a pattern comparable to that for specific anti-LMM.

MYOSIN (LIGHT CHAINS). Lowey and Steiner (83) prepared antibodies against light chains and found that staining occurred in the A band giving a strong doublet in the nonoverlap region of the A band. This staining was eliminated by absorption with light chains or with HMM.

There are three light chains in fast-twitch skeletal muscle myosin. Two of these are the alkali light chains with molecular weights of 21,000 and 16,000, and the third is the 5′,5′-dithiobis(2-nitrobenzoate) (DTNB) light chain with a molecular weight of 18,000. Antibodies have been prepared against each of these (55–57, 82, 105). There is cross reactivity between the alkali light chains, but there is also a difference in antigenicity that can be accounted for by the NH_2-terminal portion on alkali light chain 1, which is unique to that light chain (57). There is no cross reactivity with the DTNB light chain. Antibodies specific for the alkali 1 and alkali 2 light chains can be obtained. Antibodies prepared against alkali 1 are absorbed with insolubilized alkali 2 to get antibodies specific for alkali 1 and vice versa to get antibodies specific for alkali 2. With fluorescent antibody staining, both alkali light chains were shown to be present in the myofibrils of the same muscle fiber. With separated myosin filaments, stained with the antibodies and negative stained for electron microscopy, both alkali light chains were also shown to be uniformly distributed in all myosin filaments (82, 157). This excludes the possibility that the myosins in a single filament all contain either alkali 1 or alkali 2 light chains. Monoclonal antibody has been prepared to the DTNB light chain of vertebrate skeletal myosin (155). This antibody did not react with native glycerinated myofibrils but it did stain the myofibrils strongly after acetone fixation.

C PROTEIN. Of the proteins identified by Starr and Offer (162) as being present in myosin preparations purified by repeated reprecipitation, C protein has been isolated and characterized (107, 109). Offer (107, 108) clearly showed from immunochemical studies, that C protein was not a degradation product of myosin, although the function of C protein on the myosin filaments in the A band is not known.

The characteristic localization of C protein in the A band along a portion of the length of the myosin filaments was determined by the application of immunological techniques in fluorescence microscopy (127, 133) and electron microscopy (19, 107, 125, 127, 133). The most puzzling characteristic of C-protein binding to myosin filaments is that it is restricted to the middle one-third of each half of the filament (133) and that it binds at intervals of 43 nm (19, 107, 125, 133) instead of binding at the 14.3-nm interval at which myosin cross bridges occur. In studies of C-protein localization with antibody to C protein in electron microscopy, unlabeled antibody has always been used and the most prominent feature of the A-band–staining pattern observed in electron micros-

FIG. 8. Fluorescent antibody staining of myofibrils with polyclonal antibodies isolated by sequential affinity binding. *A*: specific antimyosin isolated by binding to column-purified myosin coupled to agarose. A-band–staining patterns are shown for sarcomere lengths of 2.8 μm (*upper*) and 1.8 μm (*lower*). *Far right*, Coomassie blue–stained SDS gel containing protein controls in unlabeled lane. Controls were bovine serum albumin (68,000 daltons) and soybean trypsin inhibitor (22,000 daltons). Second lane contains protein contaminants (I) removed from myosin preparations on column purification on DEAE–Sephadex A-50. Other lanes contain heavy meromyosin S2 fragment of myosin (S2), light meromyosin fragment (L), heavy meromyosin S1 fragment of myosin (S1), and myosin (M), respectively. Similar gels were transferred to nitrocellulose sheets (169a), and bands were stained by immunoperoxidase techniques. This was done similarly for *B* through *D* where only immunoperoxidase-stained sheets are shown. Specific antimyosin clearly does not react with protein controls or contaminants (I) removed by column purification. However, it does react with S2, L, S1, and myosin. Fluorescent antimyosin-staining pattern is similar to that previously described for antimyosin contaiminated with anti–C protein (Fig. 5*A*). *B*: fluorescent antibody staining of myofibrils with antibody for an antigenic region specific to S2. Upper sarcomere length, 2.0 μm. Staining is restricted primarily to a band near each A-I junction. Lower sarcomere length, 2.6 μm. Staining in middle of A band corresponding to nonoverlap region of A band occurs in addition to staining near each A-I junction. Antibody binds only to the S2 fragment on nitrocellulose sheet. Occasionally the myosin, because of its high chain weight, does not transfer to the nitrocellulose sheet properly, as apparently happened here. This transfer difficulty was not encountered with other proteins. *C*: fluorescent antibody staining of myofibrils with antibody for antigenic determinants on S1 and S2. Upper sarcomere length, 1.8 μm. Total A-band staining with unstained gap in middle of A band corresponding to bare-zone region of myosin filaments. Lower sarcomere length, 2.7 μm. Essentially uniform staining throughout A band with unstained gap in middle of A band corresponding to bare-zone region of myosin filaments. There is a small increase in brightness corresponding to nonoverlap region of A band. This antibody gave a precipitin line only with S1 and myosin on immunodiffusion but clearly also shows a reaction with the S2 band on the nitrocellulose sheet. *D*: fluorescent antibody staining of myofibrils with antibody for an antigenic region specific to LMM. Upper sarcomere length, 1.7 μm; lower sarcomere length, 2.9 μm. In both, staining is restricted primarily in a single band near each A-I junction. This antibody stained only the LMM fragment of myosin and myosin on the nitrocellulose sheet. *A*–*D*: × 4,500.

copy is the seven dense bands in the middle of each half of the A band (Fig. 6). The pattern observed with antimyosin that contains contaminating antibodies to C protein (Fig. 6*A*) is not significantly different from that observed with anti–C protein alone (Fig. 6*B*), even though we know from fluorescence microscopy that the fluorescent staining pattern corresponding to Figure 6*A* covers the entire A band (Fig. 5*A*), whereas that corresponding to Figure 6*B* is restricted to a region of the A band corresponding to the seven bands in the middle of each half of the A band (Fig. 5*E*). This points out dramatically that unlabeled antibody may not be detectable in electron microscopy. Areas of the A band that are known to be stained from fluorescence microscopy (Fig. 5*A*) are not clearly evident as stained in electron microscopy (Fig. 6*A*). Therefore the restricted localization of C protein to the region of the A band showing bands spaced 43 nm apart can only be determined by comparison of the anti–C-protein staining in fluorescence microscopy (Fig. 5*E*) with anti–C-protein staining in electron microscopy (Fig. 6*B*) where it is clear that the fluorescent pattern corresponds in position to the bands spaced 43 nm apart observed in electron microscopy and there is no fluorescence anywhere else in the A band (133).

The 43-nm interval of C-protein binding to myosin filaments was first observed by Pepe (119, 121), although he did not realize he was observing C protein and not myosin. Pepe (119, 121) assumed that this 43-nm repeat represented the 43-nm axial repeat of myosin molecules that has been determined from X-ray–diffraction studies (61). Because C-protein binding to the myosin filament has been found to be determined by the underlying myosin molecules (13, 100, 101, 128, 145, 147), Pepe's assumption that this repeat represents the axial repeat of myosin molecules turned out to be correct even though the observed periodicity was from C protein rather than myosin. He used this repeat and its relation to the other structural characteristics of the A band and of individual myosin filaments to derive a model for the molecular packing of myosin molecules in myosin filaments (119, 121). The relationship of this model to recent data that are related to myosin filament structure and A-band structure has been reviewed (129).

The evidence that C-protein binding to the myosin filament is determined by the myosin molecules to which it binds and that it therefore does not have a slightly different periodicity than the myosin periodicity comes from a variety of sources. Rome et al. (145) stained glycerinated muscle fibers with anti–C protein and observed the change in the X-ray-diffraction pattern as a result of binding of the anti–C protein. They concluded that the periodicities of the myosin and C protein are most likely the same. Moos et al. (100, 101) observed the binding of C protein to LMM paracrystals and obtained an enhancement of the 43-nm repeat of the paracrystals as a result of C-protein binding. However, it was not possible to see both the LMM repeat and the C-protein repeat in the same paracrystals so that a small difference in periodicity between the two would not be detectable. Chowrashi and Pepe (13) were successful in getting C-protein binding to LMM paracrystal where the 43-nm repeat of the paracrystals and the repeat of the bound C protein were both visible and therefore established that the repeats were indeed the same. However, the use of LMM paracrystals, which have a 43-nm axial repeat and give C-protein binding with a 43-nm axial repeat, is not closely comparable to the myosin filament where, although the helical repeat of myosin cross bridges is 43 nm, the interval at which myosin cross bridges occur is 14.3 nm. An LMM paracrystal, which is more comparable to the myosin filament, is one with a 14.3-nm axial repeat. Safer and Pepe (147) found the C protein bound to such paracrystals at 43-nm intervals with the 14.3-nm interval of the paracrystal repeat also clearly visible. Although these studies provide strong evidence that the C-protein binding is determined by the underlying myosin molecules, the binding of C protein to only a restricted portion of the filament and binding at intervals of 43 nm instead of 14.3 nm, as has been determined by the application of immunological techniques in fluorescence and electron microscopy, is still puzzling. A possibility for explaining these puzzling observations based on the model for the myosin filament proposed by Pepe (119, 121) has been suggested (129).

Although the C-protein staining observed with antimyosin contaminated with anti–C protein (Fig. 6*A*) almost always gave seven bands spaced 43 nm apart in each half of the A band, occasionally a pattern of nine bands was observed (121). With antibody prepared with C protein purified as described by Offer et al. (109) as the immunogen, the pattern of nine bands in each half of the A band was almost always observed and therefore C protein was considered to be present at nine positions along each half of the myosin filament (107, 145). Further studies showed that only seven of the bands corresponding in position to those observed earlier (121) were specific for C protein, the other two bands (closest to the middle of the A band) were due to the presence of two other proteins (19, 133). Evidence that only seven of the bands were due to specific localization of C protein consisted of the following: *1*) consistent visibility of the seven bands and the variability in density of the other two depending on the amount of antibody accessible to the myofibrils (19, 133) suggested that the eighth and ninth bands were due to different antigens than the other seven, *2*) absorption of the anti–C protein with purified C protein resulted in eliminating the staining of eight of the bands, only the ninth band closest to the M band remaining (19), and *3*) affinity isolation of specific anti–C protein from antimyosin contaminated with anti–C protein resulted in an antibody that stained the seven bands and the ninth band but only stained the eighth band very faintly if at all (133). Together these observations provide strong evidence that only the seven bands consistently observed with anti–C protein are specific for C protein and that the eighth and ninth bands represent two other proteins associated with the myosin filament.

OTHER A-BAND PROTEINS. Although two proteins other than C protein have been detected as being present in the A band (19, 133) and being responsible for the eighth and ninth bands originally thought to also be C protein, they have not been identified. These proteins must represent a very small proportion of the A-band proteins of vertebrate skeletal muscle myofibrils. In addition to C protein and the eighth- and ninth-band antigens, other A-band proteins associated with the myosin filaments have been detected. These include α-component (80), I protein (113), and adenosine 5′-monophosphate (AMP) deaminase (5). Although these proteins have been identified, they have not been studied as thoroughly as C protein.

The α-component is a protein with a molecular weight of approximately 80,000 determined by gel filtration (80). Antiserum to α-component stains the A bands of vertebrate skeletal myofibrils, although the details of the staining pattern in the A band have not been described. The function of α-component has not been determined.

I protein has a molecular weight of 50,000 (110), is located in the A band of vertebrate skeletal muscle myofibrils (113), and inhibits the Mg-activated adenosine triphosphatase (ATPase) activity of actomyosin (91). I protein also has been shown to bind to myosin but not to actin (91). Fluorescent anti–I protein stained the A bands of myofibrils uniformly except for a narrow unstained region in the middle of the A band corresponding to the bare-zone region of the myosin filaments (113). Although the width of the A band seemed to be larger when measured from A bands stained with fluorescent antibody than from unstained A bands, it was not possible to determine if in fact this represented distribution of the I protein beyond the boundaries of the A band or whether it was an artifact of the fluorescent image. A curious change in the A-band–staining pattern was observed with time after staining. Myofibrils stained with anti–I protein for 2 h and observed 4 h later showed a decrease in fluorescence in the center of the A band with only the edges of the A band along each A-I junction remaining brightly stained. The reason for this change in staining pattern with time is not understood. The staining pattern for anti–I protein has not been observed in electron microscopy.

Adenosine 5′-monophosphate deaminase has long been known to be a contaminant of myosin preparations that have not been purified (149) by chromatography on DEAE–Sephadex A-50 (142). Recently, Ashby et al. (5) have prepared antibody to AMP deaminase and have shown by fluorescent antibody staining that it is localized in the A band along each A-I junction. This localization is similar to that for the LMM antigenic determinants to which LMM binds (Fig. 8*D*) as described above [see MYOSIN (LMM PORTION), p. 123]. Ashby and Frieden (4) have shown that AMP deaminase binds selectively to the S2 portion of the myosin molecule and does not bind to the LMM or S1 fragments of myosin. Therefore the localization of AMP deaminase to the edges of the A band along each A-I junction may be related to the staining of the A band obtained with A(S2) in this region. If the antigenic determinants stained in this region of the A band by A(S2) are closely related to the binding sites for AMP deaminase this would be expected. The A(S2) sites are also available in the nonoverlap zone (Fig. 8*C*) but there is no detectable AMP deaminase binding in this region of the A band. It is possible that because the A(S2) is a polyclonal antibody it may be directed against two different classes of antigenic sites, one class being available for antibody binding in the nonoverlap region of the A band and the other along each A-I junction. In this case, there would be no reason to expect both classes of antigenic determinants to have the same binding characteristics relative to AMP deaminase. The specificity of binding of the AMP deaminase to the A band along each A-I junction was dramatically demonstrated by its specific rebinding to myofibrils from which the AMP deaminase had been previously extracted and the demonstration of this specific rebinding by fluorescent antibody staining(5). The sensitivity of the fluorescent antibody-staining method attests to the highly specific restricted binding of the AMP deaminase in the A band.

M Band

The fine structure of the M band has been described in longitudinal sections. It is about 86 nm long and consists of five lines perpendicular to the long axis of the myosin filaments in the middle of the bare-zone region of the filaments. In transverse sections of the M band, M bridges are observed between neighboring myosin filaments (Fig. 1). Models for the structure of the M band have been proposed (71, 84, 126). The model proposed by Knappeis and Carlsen (71) consists of six M bridges at each M-line level of the M band. It also has an M filament parallel to the myosin filaments and perpendicular to the M bridges between two adjacent myosin filaments (Fig. 9*A*). This model was modified by Luther and Squire (84) to include a Y-shaped element between three adjacent myosin filaments with each of the three arms of the Y attached to one of the three myosin filaments (Fig. 9*B*). In the model proposed by Pepe (126) there are fewer than six M bridges at each M-line level, although in a transverse section, which includes the M band, there is at least one M bridge between all neighboring filaments (Fig. 9*C*).

Pepe (124, 126) has observed different patterns of lines in the M band (Fig. 10*A*) that correspond to what

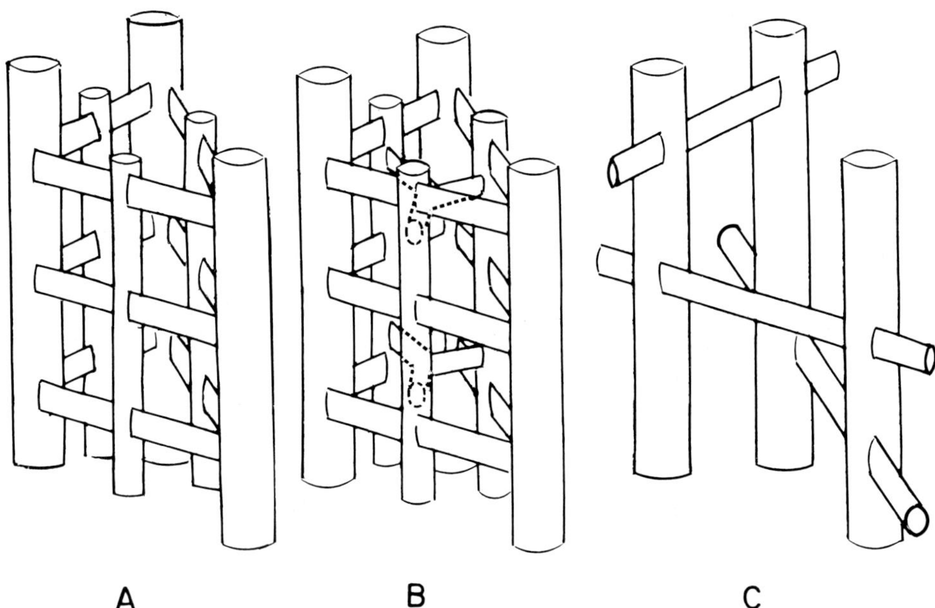

FIG. 9. Models for structure of M band. *A*: model proposed by Knappeis and Carlsen (71). There are 6 M bridges attached to each myosin filament at each level in M band where an M line is observed. Only middle 3 levels contributing to middle 3 M lines are shown here. An M filament parallel to myosin filaments attaches perpendicular to M bridges between any 2 myosin filaments. *B*: model proposed by Luther and Squire (84) is similar to that proposed by Knappeis and Carlsen (71) except that there is a Y-shaped element that attaches to each of 3 M filaments by 1 of 3 arms of Y as shown in diagram. This Y-shaped element is positioned relative to the 1st and 3rd M-line positions but a little closer to the center of the M band than the M lines themselves. *C*: model proposed by Pepe (126) is considerably different from the other 2 models in that there are no M filaments and M bridges at each level are all oriented similarly, but those at one level are oriented 60° relative to those at neighboring level. In transverse section 6 M bridges are observed on each filament, 1 bridging to each of neighboring filaments. In longitudinal section, depending on plane of section, M band consists of different patterns of M lines.

would be expected from his model for different planes of section parallel to the long axis of the myosin filament. These different M-line patterns were observed in different sarcomeres of the same fiber excluding the possibility that the different patterns come from different fiber types (Fig. 10*B*, *C*). In this model, the three central M lines arise from the arrangement of bridges shown in Figure 9*C*, and the other two M lines arise from more variable M-bridging patterns.

Sjöström and Squire (158) have evidence that patterns of three, four, or five lines in the M band may be related to fiber type. They have also described additional weaker lines in the M band from observations of longitudinal cryosections that were negatively stained (158, 159). Two of these additional lines are related to the position of the Y-shaped elements (84) in their model (Fig. 9*B*). Also, from transverse sections through the M band that they estimated to be about 200 Å thick, Luther and Squire (84) observed M bridges connecting all neighboring filaments and from this concluded that there are six M bridges at each level of the M band where a major M line is observed in longitudinal sections.

M PROTEINS: HISTORICAL BACKGROUND. From antibody staining and absorption studies, Pepe (120) concluded that the M band was made up of proteins other than myosin, actin, or tropomyosin. He showed that purified actin and tropomyosin, when used to absorb antibody that stained the M band strongly, did not affect the M-band staining and that purified myosin showed no reaction with the antibody. The first M protein to be isolated from skeletal muscle fibrils was termed "M-substance" by Masaki et al. (96). Antibody to this protein stained only the M band. Kundrat and Pepe (73) extracted myofibrils with 5 mM Tris at pH 8 and showed that the extracted protein could specifically absorb out M-band staining from an antibody preparation that stained both the M band and the I band. They also showed that removal of the M-band protein by this extraction procedure did not affect the antimyosin staining pattern of the A band, which suggests that the structure of the myosin filaments was not affected. This was consistent with the earlier finding by Stromer et al. (166) who showed that the protein extracted from the M band by low ionic strength buffer could be reintroduced into myofibrils from which the M band was previously extracted resulting in reconstitution of the M band. Therefore the binding sites for the M protein on the myosin filaments remain intact on extraction of the M-band protein. The next step in the identification of M-band proteins came from three laboratories all at about the same time. Eaton and Pepe (22) identified two proteins with chain weights of 100,000 and 40,000 as possible

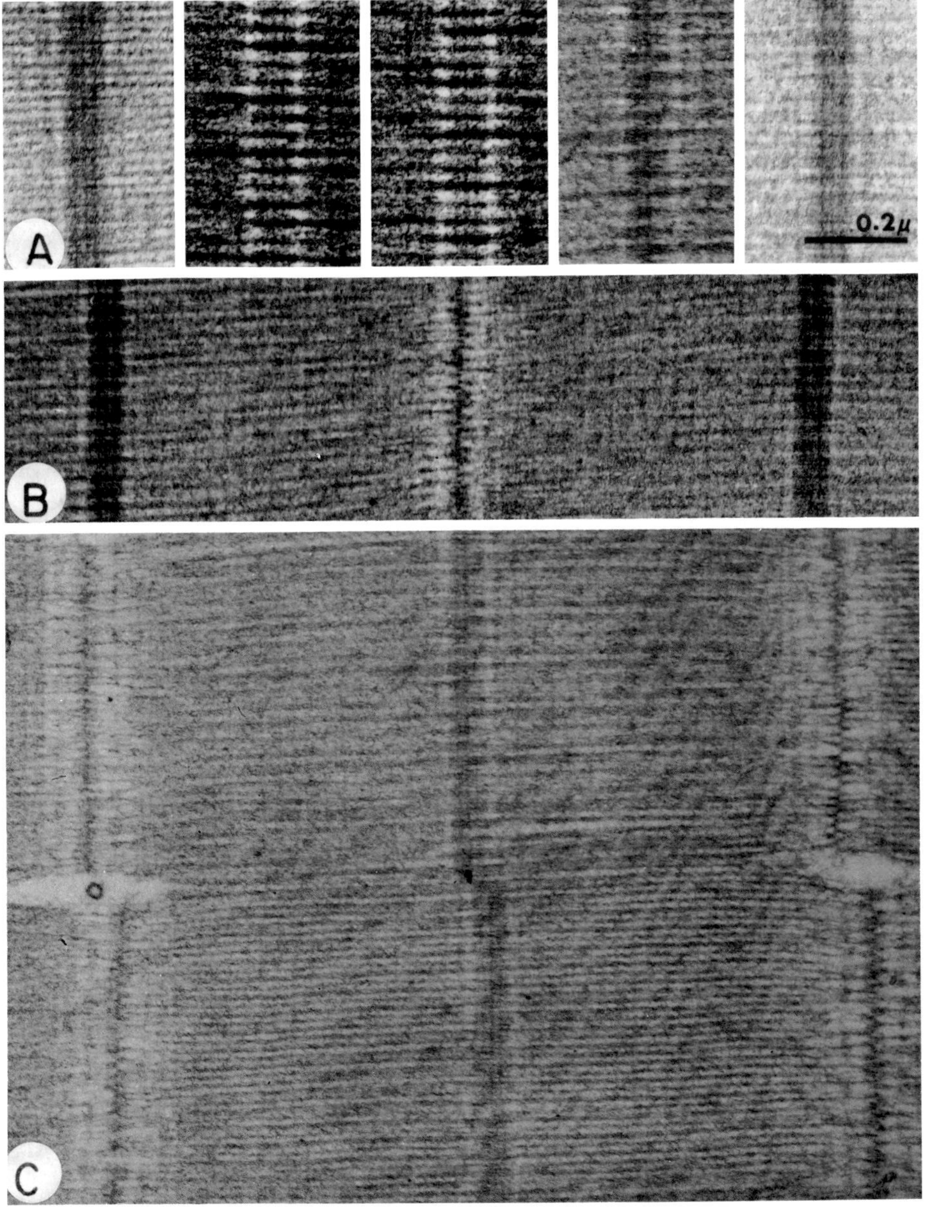

FIG. 10. M-band patterns observed in longitudinal sections. *A*: longitudinal sections through M band. Long axis of fibrils is horizontal. The most clearly observed patterns of lines in the M band are shown. From *left* to *right* these consist of 3 centrally placed lines, 5 lines generally with central 3 more distinct, 4 lines, 2 lines 1 of which is centrally placed, and 2 distinct lines placed 1 on each side of less distinct (or absent) central line. Lateral muscle of freshwater killifish (*Fundulus diaphanus*). *B*: different M-band patterns can be observed in sarcomeres of same myofibril. Note pattern of 3 lines in M band of sarcomere on *left* and pattern of 2 lines in M band of sarcomere on *right*. *C*: different patterns can also be observed in M bands of neighboring sarcomeres of different myofibrils in same cell. Note 2 neighboring lines are observed in sarcomere of myofibril at *top*, 1 of 2 lines being to *left* of central line. In neighboring sarcomere of myofibril on *bottom*, again 2 lines are observed in M band; however, 1 line is to *right* of central line of M band. These differences in pattern of lines in M band are what would be expected for M-band model proposed by Pepe (126).

M-band proteins; Morimoto and Harrington (102) identified a protein with a chain weight of 42,000; and Masaki and Takaiti (94) identified a protein with a chain weight of 155,000. All three studies involved antibody-staining methods to confirm localization of the proteins to the M band. The approximately 40,000 protein was shown to have creatine kinase activity (21, 176) and the 100,000 protein was shown to have phosphorylase activity (51, 126, 171, 173). Of the three proteins, the creatine kinase (102, 176) and the high-chain-weight (155,000–170,000) protein (86, 95, 173) have been clearly identified as M-band proteins. How these proteins are related to the structural components of the M band has not been clearly demonstrated.

CREATINE KINASE. Once Turner et al. (176) identified the 43,000 M-band protein isolated by Morimoto and Harrington (102) as creatine kinase, attention was given to whether or not the creatine kinase that binds to the filaments in the M band is different in any way from the cytoplasmic creatine kinase. The identity of all meromyosin (MM)–creatine kinase whether bound or unbound was confirmed by comparison of CNBr-peptide fragments and specific activity, in addition to immunologic cross reactivity (176, 179). Wallimann et al. (179) argued that the amount of creatine kinase bound to myofibrils is reasonably consistent with the possibility that creatine kinase may be the structural material of the M bridges. An observation that favors considering creatine kinase as the structural protein of the M band was made with the Fab′ fragment of anti-creatine kinase. When the normal bivalent antibody is used for staining the M band, a heavy accumulation of antibody protein is observed in the M band in electron microscopy; but treatment of the myofibrils with the Fab′ fragment of the antibody results in extraction of the M band (177, 178). Therefore, if interaction of the monovalent antibody (Fab′) with creatine kinase results in the removal of the M bridges perhaps the structural component of the M bridges is creatine kinase.

HIGH-MOLECULAR-WEIGHT COMPONENT. This component of the M band, originally described by Masaki and Takaiti (94, 95) as having a chain weight of 155,000, was further studied by Trinick and Lowey (173) who reported a chain weight of 170,000 and Mani and Kay (86) who reported a chain weight of 165,000. Trinick and Lowey (173) and Mani and Kay (86) also found that the protein consisted of a single polypeptide chain. Mani and Kay (86) further found that the 165,000-chain-weight M-band protein, when mixed with creatine kinase, could inhibit the creatine kinase activity with 30% inhibition obtained with a 2:1 molar ratio. Low-speed equilibrium ultracentrifuge studies also showed that a complex is formed between creatine kinase and the high-molecular-weight protein with the two proteins present in a 1:1 molar ratio in the complex. From electron-microscope studies of shadowed preparations of the 165,000 M protein, Woodhead and Lowey (187) have reported that it has a length of about 360 Å and a diameter of about 41 Å.

Chowrashi and Pepe (14) speculate that the 165,000-chain-weight protein is responsible for the structure of the M bridges. Speculation was based on observations of the reconstruction of the M band in myofibrils from which the M band had previously been extracted. They had a protein fraction of crude M-band extract that contained both the 165,000 component and creatine kinase in addition to other proteins. This mixture was capable of reconstructing the M band. They split the mixture into a high-molecular-weight fraction containing the 165,000 component and a low-molecular-weight fraction containing the creatine kinase. These, individually, did not reconstruct the M band. The low-molecular-weight fraction, however, did give some increase in density in the M-band region but no evidence of M bridges. On recombining the two fractions the M bridges were again reconstructed. This suggests that the creatine kinase is binding to the filaments and that the 165,000 component is bridging between them. One must be cautious about this interpretation, however. Chowrashi and Pepe (14) noted that purified creatine kinase or the 165,000 component alone did not reconstruct the M band; nor did a mixture of the two proteins. Therefore one of the other proteins in the fraction of crude M-band extract capable of reconstructing the M band may be involved in assembling the structure of the M band in addition to the creatine kinase and the 165,000 component. Mani and Kay (87), on the basis of the interaction of the 165,000 component with creatine kinase, suggest that it may be the M-filament protein in the model for the M band proposed by Knappeis and Carlsen (71). Woodhead and Lowey (187) also suggested this as a possibility based on about a 360-Å length and about a 41-Å diameter they found for the molecule observed in electron microscopy. Eppenberger et al. (35) have suggested the name "myomesin" for this high-molecular-weight component of the M band.

INTERACTION OF M PROTEIN WITH MYOSIN. Very little is known about how creatine kinase or the 165,000 protein interact with myosin. Some contradictory findings have been reported. Morimoto and Harrington (102) showed that creatine kinase could cause the aggregation of synthetic myosin filaments but they did not try to distinguish where on the myosin molecules the creatine kinase binds. Studies have been reported with circular dichroism measurements (85), electron paramagnetic resonance, and nanosecond fluorescence depolarization (10), which indicate that the creatine kinase binds to the S1 portion of the myosin molecule but not to the rod or LMM portion. Similarly, Woodhead and Lowey (187) found that the presence of creatine kinase did not significantly alter the banding pattern of LMM paracrystals and anti–creatine kinase staining gave no improvement, which indicates that creatine kinase binds weakly, if at all, to the LMM rod under in vitro conditions. In contrast to these findings

Houk and Putnam (58) found that with fluorescence-depolarization methods and creatine kinase labeled with an SH-specific dye, creatine kinase binds to the rod portion of the myosin and not to the S1. Similarly, Koons and Zobel (72) have found that the presence of creatine kinase induces the aggregation of LMM, which suggests that it binds to the LMM portion of the molecule. Mani and Kay (87) showed that the 165,000 component and a chymotryptic fragment of it with a chain weight of 100,000 bind specifically to the S2 portion of the myosin molecule. Binding to the S2 fragment occurred in a molar ratio of 1:1, but no binding was observed with LMM or S1. In contrast Masaki et al. (96) found that the 165,000 component promoted the aggregation of LMM but not HMM. Woodhead and Lowey (187) found that although they could not obtain significant alteration of the banding pattern of LMM paracrystals in the presence of the 165,000 component, if they stained the paracrystal with anti-165,000 component they did get an enhancement of the banding pattern suggesting that binding of the 165,000 M component to LMM did in fact occur.

As is evident from the contradictory evidence in the literature concerning the binding characteristics of creatine kinase or the 165,000 M-band protein to the myosin molecule, we are still far from understanding the true composition of the M band and how the M-band proteins are put together to give the structural characteristics of the M band. Although two proteins have been identified as M-band components primarily from antibody-staining techniques in fluorescence and electron microscopy (94, 102, 173, 176), it is clearly possible that there are other additional protein components involved in the structure of the M band (14, 187).

I Band

The I band is characterized by the presence of the thin filaments (e.g., see Fig. 1). These thin filaments are attached to the Z band at one end and interdigitate with the thick filaments of the A band. The interaction between the actin of the thin filaments and the myosin of the thick filaments shortens the sarcomeres. The thin filaments also contain the proteins tropomyosin and troponin that regulate the interaction between actin and myosin through the action of Ca^{2+}. A very nice review of the regulation of muscle contraction is given by Ebashi (24).

The actin monomers are arranged in the thin filament in two strands that are wound around one another with a crossover repeat of about 38 nm (48). It has been suggested that tropomyosin molecules, which are α-helical rods, are arranged end to end along each groove of the actin helix with one troponin molecule and seven actins related to each tropomyosin rod. This model is shown diagrammatically in Figures 11*A* and *B*. The troponin molecule that has a molecular weight of about 80,000 (26–28) was found to be made up of subunits (20, 23, 31, 43, 150, 151) that have been labeled troponin T (TN-T), troponin I (TN-I), and troponin C (TN-C) according to their function. Troponin T is involved in tropomyosin binding, TN-I is involved in the inhibition of actin-myosin interaction, and TN-C is involved in Ca^{2+} binding (16, 29, 31, 43, 44, 49, 151). A model for how these subunits are related to the tropomyosin molecule is shown diagrammatically in Figure 11*C* (24). In this model TN-T is shown as two fragments, TN-T1 and TN-T2. These are the fragments of TN-T obtained by chymotryptic digestion (116) and with antibody-staining specific for each fragment, the differential localization of these two portions of the TN-T subunit was determined (e.g., see TROPONIN, p. 132).

Models for the relations between the proteins of the thin filament have also been derived from structural studies in electron microscopy (99, 160, 169). A diagrammatic representation of the most recent model, a transverse section of the thin filament, is shown in Figure 13*C* in the chapter by Haselgrove in this *Handbook*. Positions of the tropomyosin (TM) relative to actin are shown for two different states of the filament (169).

ACTIN AND TROPOMYOSIN. Preparation of antiactin has presented problems because of its poor antigenicity. Antibodies obtained in response to actin injection in the early work were shown by Wilson and Finck (184) to be against the other thin filament proteins and not actin. More recently, antibodies have been obtained that are directed against actin and these have been produced with actin denatured by high pH (53) or by SDS (79) as the immunogen. Antiactin has also been obtained when the immunogen was *1*) actin bound to gel beads, *2*) actin made insoluble after ammonium sulfate precipitation (46), *3*) actin adsorbed to an alum precipitate (64), or *4*) glutaraldehyde-fixed actin (52). Although Groschel-Stewart et al. (46) report that one animal out of seven injected with native soluble actin did produce antiactin, a response with soluble actin is not generally obtained. Fluorescent antiactin has been shown to stain the I band of skeletal myofibrils without staining the Z band (46, 52, 64). In general, the staining appeared to be restricted to the I band and did not extend into the region of overlap between myosin and actin filaments. Observations of antiactin staining of myofibrils have been restricted to fluorescence microscopy and have generally been used as one example of the specificity of the antibody rather than for studying actin in the myofibril. Antiactin has primarily been used to study actin distribution in nonmuscle cells.

Fluorescent antitropomyosin has been shown to stain the I band of skeletal muscle myofibrils (34, 120). Although Pepe (120) did not see staining of the Z band, Endo et al. (34) sometimes did. Also, Pepe (120) did not observe staining of the overlap region of the actin and myosin filaments, whereas Endo et al. (34) did although in the overlap region the staining intensity was reduced. It is not clear what these differences

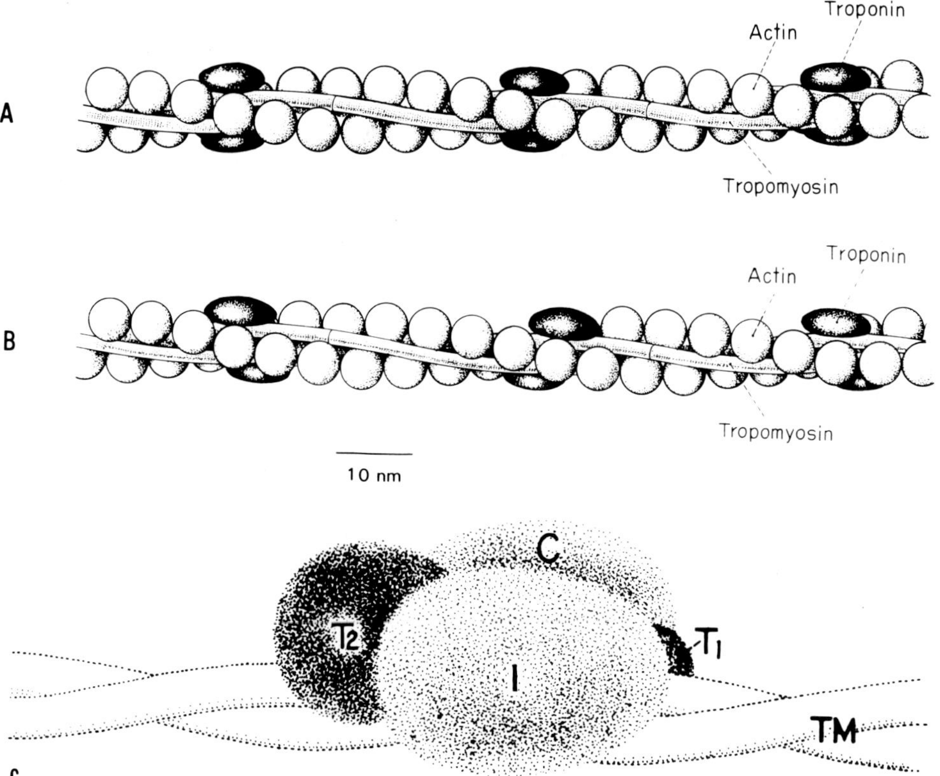

FIG. 11. Models for fine structure of thin filament. *A*: model proposed by Ebashi et al. (25). *B*: model amended by Ohtsuki (114) indicating position of joint between 2 adjacent tropomyosin molecules and bestowing helical symmetry on troponin molecules, so that 2 troponin molecules opposite each other are apart by a distance equal to diameter of actin molecule. *C*: model for fine location of troponin subunits proposed by Ohtsuki (I and C, troponin I and troponin C; T1 and T2, portions of troponin T corresponding to T1 and T2 fragments, respectively) in relation to tropomyosin (TM). (There remains a possibility that positions of troponin C and troponin I would be interchanged.) Z and H bands exist on far *right* and *left* sides, respectively. [From Ebashi (24).]

in observation are due to. Pepe (120) also observed an increase in density of the I band in electron microscopy after antitropomyosin staining. This increased density was observed in sectioned muscle fibers. Recently, Matsumara and Lin (96a) have obtained monoclonal antibodies to tropomyosin which, when bound to thin filaments, show a periodicity of about 38 nm along the length of the filament. This periodicity shows up because the monoclonal antibody recognizes a single antigenic determinant. The polyclonal antibody used by Pepe (120) recognizes many different antigenic determinants and the periodicity is obscured.

TROPONIN. The localization of fluorescent antitroponin in the I band of skeletal muscle myofibrils was first shown by Endo et al. (34). They concluded that the staining occurred along the entire length of the thin filament including the portion of the filaments overlapping with the thick filaments of the A band. The Z band remained unstained. Ebashi et al. (29) found that fluorescent antibody specific for each of the separate troponin components stained the sarcomere similarly to antibody to the total complex. Perry et al. (137) obtained fluorescent staining patterns for antitroponin and for anti–Tn-I, which were similar to those found by Endo et al. (34) and Ebashi et al. (29) except that the fluorescence in the filament overlap zone was not as intense as it was in the I band. They pointed out that in shortened sarcomeres a bright staining region appeared in the middle of the A band, which they related to the bare-zone region of the myosin filaments. In shortened sarcomeres the thin filaments pass through this region and presumably staining of the thin filaments is not inhibited in the bare-zone region because of the absence of myosin cross bridges.

Probably the most effective use of immunoelectron microscopy to obtain information about structure has been made with antitroponin. Major contributions in the use of these techniques have been made by Ohtsuki et al. (114–118).

Antitroponin staining of myofibrils and separated filaments was first observed by Ohtsuki et al. (118) in electron microscopy. The staining pattern observed consisted of narrow bands spaced 40 nm apart along the entire length of the thin filaments. The antitroponin used was tagged with ferritin and ferritin was clearly visible in the I band. In the region of overlap of the thin and thick filaments, however, ferritin was not visible although the periodicity was clearly visible. They concluded that the staining of the overlap region was probably due to untagged antibody and that the larger size of the tagged antibody probably prevented its diffusion into the overlap region where the surface-to-surface distance between filaments is considerably smaller than in the I band. The unlabeled antibody, however, was able to penetrate the overlap region. Ohtsuki et al. (118) also observed these bands in negatively stained separated filaments that had been stained with the antitroponin. In both the sectioned and the negatively stained material there were 24 bands along the length of the actin filaments. Because troponin binds to tropomyosin but not to actin, the repeat observed is probably determined by the tropomyosin bound along the actin filament and to which the troponin binds. Based on these observations, Ebashi et al. (25) proposed the model for the relation between actin, tropomyosin, and troponin shown in Figure 11*A*. From X-ray-diffraction studies of anti–TN-C stained glycerinated muscle fibers, Rome et al. (144) showed that the 38.5-nm reflection observed with unstained muscle was enhanced by the antibody staining. This is consistent with the model in Figure 11*A* where the repeat corresponds to seven actin monomers along a single strand of the actin helix.

Ebashi et al. (29, 30) and Ohtsuki (114) compared tropomyosin paracrystals that were formed in the presence and absence of troponin. They found that the ferritin-labeled troponin binds to the middle of the wide band of the tropomyosin paracrystals showing alternating wide (26.5-nm) light bands and narrow (13.5-nm) darker bands as shown in Figures 12*C* and *D*. From the way that the tropomyosin paracrystals terminate (Fig. 12*A*), or break (Fig. 12*B*), the position of the end of the tropomyosin rods can be identified and therefore it can be concluded that the troponin is binding about 27 nm from one end of the tropomyosin rod. More careful observations of antitroponin-stained thin filaments in electron microscopy showed that the first band observed from the free end of the actin filament was about 27 nm from the free end, which is consistent with the findings of troponin binding in tropomyosin paracrystals (29, 30, 114). As a result, the ends of the tropomyosin molecules could be indicated in the model shown in Figure 11*B*. The shift between the positions of the troponin at the same level on the two sides of the filament as shown in Figure 11*B* results from relating the tropomyosin on one side to one of the actin strands and the tropomyosin on the other side to the other actin strand.

The troponin molecule consists of three components (20, 23, 43). The distribution of these three components along the thin filaments has been studied in detail by Ohtsuki (115). The tropomyosin-binding component (TN-T), the Ca^{2+}-binding component (TN-C), and the inhibitory component (TN-I) are all distributed along the thin filament with a periodicity of 38 nm. Anti–TN-I and anti–TN-C form narrow dense bands along the filament with the first band from the free end of the thin filament occurring at 26 nm. Anti–TN-T gives wider dense bands 14–20 nm wide. These can also be observed to split into two bands. The near side of the first band closest to the free end of the filament corresponds with the edge of bands observed with anti–Tn-I or anti–TN-C, i.e., about 26 nm from the free end of the filament. The far side of the first band is about 40 nm from the free end of the filament. This extra width of staining is not generally seen with antibody to the total troponin complex, anti-TN. Using fluorescent anti–TN-I, anti–Tn-T, and anti–TN-C, Ebashi et al. (29) showed that staining by one of these antibodies blocked staining by either of the other two. Therefore depending on which antibody to the total troponin complex was bound, it would prevent staining of the same region by the other two. Occasionally wide bands were observed with anti-TN as would be expected.

Ohtsuki (116) further dissected the troponin complex. He produced chymotryptic fragments of TN-T, with chain weights of 26,000 (TN-T1) and 13,000 (TN-T2). The TN-T1 binds to tropomyosin and represents the NH_2-terminal portion of the molecule and the short TN-T2 fragment does not bind to tropomyosin and represents the COOH-terminal portion of the molecule. He prepared antibodies to these fragments and both the anti–TN-T1 and anti–TN-T2 gave a 38-nm repeat along the thin filament. However, the first band from the free end of the filament was 40 nm from the free end with anti–TN-T1 and 27 nm from the free end with anti–TN-T2. The anti–TN-T2 therefore corresponds to patterns obtained with anti–TN-I and anti–TN-C. These observations are summarized in Figure 13 and contribute to construction of the model shown in Figure 11*C* for how the troponin components are related to the tropomyosin molecule in the thin filament.

Antitroponin staining has been applied to both diseased (183, 185) and developing (106, 117, 154) skeletal muscle myofibrils and observed in both fluorescence and electron microscopy.

OTHER I-BAND PROTEINS. Other proteins have been identified as being associated with the I band of skeletal muscle myofibrils and have been reported as being associated with the actin filaments. Of these β-actinin has been localized specifically to the free ends of the thin filaments by Maruyama et al. (90) and to the I band by Heizmann et al. (50). Aldolase, glycogen phosphorylase, parvalbumin, calcium-binding protein, and arginine kinase have all been localized throughout the I band (3, 8, 50, 138). In addition, the 10*S* component of α-actinin has been localized to the I band by Sugita et al. (167).

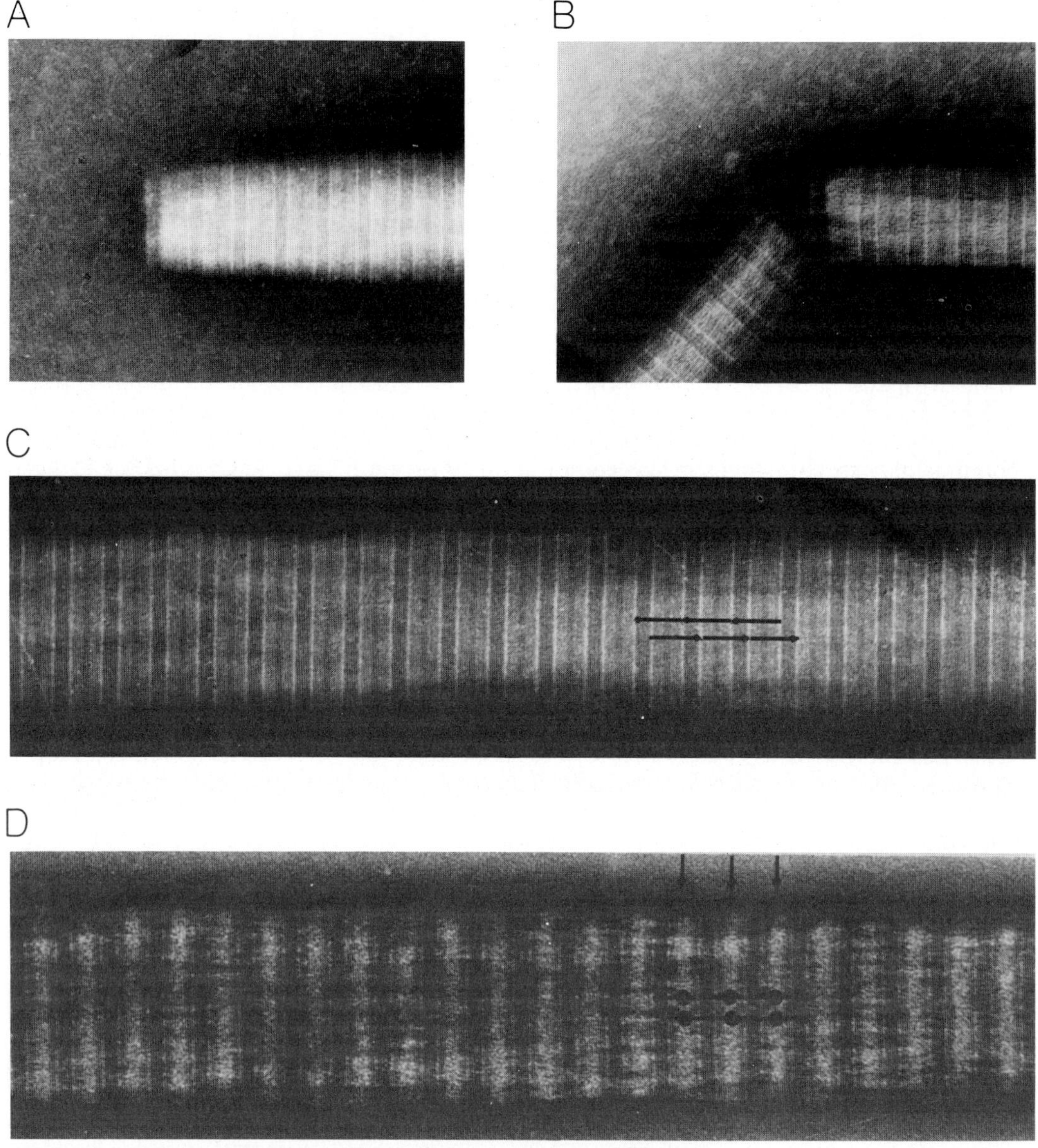

FIG. 12. Troponin binding in tropomyosin paracrystals. *A*: edge of tropomyosin paracrystal; paracrystal terminates at extreme edge of narrow dark band. × 121,000. *B*: broken portion of tropomyosin paracrystal. × 153,000. *C*: tropomyosin paracrystal; arrangement of tropomyosin molecules, represented as *bars* with *arrowheads*, shown schematically. × 160,000. *D*: troponin-tropomyosin paracrystal; troponin is localized in middle of wide bright band (indicated by *arrows*). × 160,000. [From Ebashi et al. (29).]

Although the glycolytic enzyme, aldolase, has been stained with fluorescent labeled antialdolase in muscle cultures (175), separated myofibrils were not stained. However, the association of aldolase with actin filaments has been demonstrated by studies of the binding of aldolase to isolated F-actin filaments (3, 138). The glycolytic enzyme, glycogen phosphorylase, has been shown to be localized in the I band of sarcomeres in the same way as actin with fluorescent antibody staining of myofibrils (8, 50, 138). Heizmann et al. (50) showed that glycogen phosphorylase could be washed off the myofibril by extraction with 5 mM Tris-HCl at pH 7.7.

In sections, it was found that although calcium-binding protein (9) and glycogen phosphorylase as well as many other glycolytic enzymes are localized in the I band along with actin, arginine kinase and parvalbumin were distributed throughout the cell (9). Fluorescent antibody staining of isolated myofibrils, however, showed that arginine kinase (8) and parvalbumin (50) are bound specifically to the I band (8) in addition to being present throughout the sarcoplasm. Parvalbumin could be washed out of the myofibrils with 5 mM Tris-HCl at pH 7.7 (8) as determined by fluorescent antibody staining. The β-actinin, like actin, could not be extracted from the I band under the same conditions.

Z Band

The Z band is made up of Z filaments that bridge between the thin filaments of adjacent sarcomeres, and there is unstructured dense material present between the Z filaments. There are four Z filaments attached to each thin filament on one side of the Z band, and these form a tetragon, with one actin attaching to the other end of each of the four Z filaments on the other side of the Z band (70). Z bands that are wider than the simple Z band will have more than one layer of Z filaments (146). These are probably arranged similarly to those in the one layer of the simple Z band (37). The actin filaments are thought to penetrate into the Z band in these wider bands, whereas in the simple Z band they do not.

A primary protein identified with the Z band is α-actinin and this was first localized in the Z band by Masaki et al. (93) with fluorescent antibody staining. The anti–α-actinin they obtained stained both the M band and the Z band, and they were able to show by absorption that antibody to the 6*S* component of the α-actinin was responsible for the specific staining of the Z band and that antibody to a protein contaminant of the α-actinin was responsible for the M-band staining. Therefore α-actinin is present only in the Z band of the myofibril.

In addition to the use of fluorescent antibody staining, α-actinin has been implicated as a component of the Z band from a number of different studies, although it has not been clear what structural features of the Z band are related to the α-actinin. A number of different treatments of the myofibrils have specific effects on the Z band and these effects can be related to the presence of α-actinin. For instance, a calcium-activated factor that specifically removes the Z bands of myofibrils (12) has been shown to effect the loss of α-actinin from the myofibril in parallel to the loss of the Z band (140). Studies of the binding of α-actinin to F actin have also suggested that α-actinin may be involved in the end-to-end linking of actin filaments in the Z band (1, 11, 39, 54, 143, 165). The binding of α-actinin to F actin was found to be dependent on temperature (39, 165). At 0°C the binding of α-actinin to F actin occurred along the entire length of the F actin and was strong enough to dislodge tropomyosin from the F-actin filament. At 37°C there was very limited binding of α-actinin to F actin. When tropomyosin was present at 37°C, two molecules of α-actinin were bound per F-actin filament 1 μm in length. These findings are consistent with the possibility that the two molecules of α-actinin are present at one end of the polar F-actin filament (one binding to each of the two strands of the actin polymer) and therefore with the possibility that α-actinin is present at the end that binds to the Z band, implicating α-actinin as the possible cross-linker of F-actin filaments at the Z band. The presence of α-actinin in isolated Z bands has also been shown by fluorescent antibody staining (40, 41, 77). The α-actinin is present throughout the Z band whereas the localization of desmin and vimentin corresponds to the surface of the myofibril, i.e., around

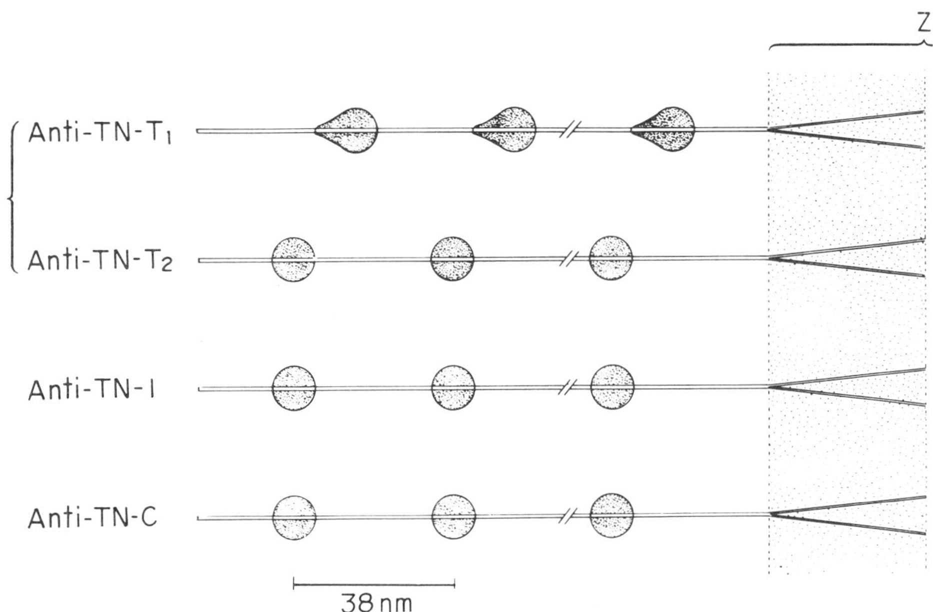

FIG. 13. Schematic illustration of antibody distribution of troponin components along thin filament. [From Ohtsuki (116).]

the periphery of the Z band. Therefore α-actinin is not present in the region of the Z band where desmin and vimentin are localized. From these studies the presence of α-actinin in the Z band of vertebrate skeletal muscles (40, 41, 76, 77, 93, 140, 152, 153) is now generally accepted although the structural feature of the Z band with which the α-actinin is associated could not be determined.

Chowrashi and Pepe (15) have recently studied two proteins of the Z band and related these to the structural characteristics of the Z band with a combination of sequential extraction, SDS-polyacrylamide gel electrophoresis, and fluorescent antibody staining in chicken pectoralis muscle myofibrils. They studied α-actinin and a protein with a chain weight of 85,000 that they called amorphin. Both of these proteins were localized specifically to the Z band by fluorescent antibody staining. They showed that the Z filaments are α-actinin and the amorphin is present as an unstructured material between the Z filaments. With these studies, it was not possible to exclude the possibility that proteins other than these are also present in the Z band. Using various extraction procedures, Etlinger et al. (36) identified a protein doublet in SDS gels that they labeled Z1 and Z2 as being related to the Z band. The chain weights of the Z1 and Z2 are approximately the same as that of α-actinin.

Other Z-band proteins such as 55,000-chain-weight protein (111, 112) and Eu-actinin, which has a chain weight of 42,000 (74), have been localized to the Z band. Antibody prepared against these proteins stains the Z band of skeletal muscle myofibrils specifically. The Eu-actinin has the same chain weight as actin; however, it can be separated from actin by isoelectric focusing. Whereas fluorescent antiactin stains the I band, fluorescent anti-eu-actinin staining is confined to the Z band verifying that they are different proteins. The function and structural relationship of these proteins in the Z band remains to be determined.

NONMYOFIBRILLAR PROTEINS

Most of the nonmyofibrillar proteins that have been localized by fluorescent antibody are related to the myofibril in some way. For instance, desmin, vimentin, synemin, and filamin are all peripherally located around the outside of the Z bands of myofibrils (6, 40–42, 77, 78). With fluorescent antibody staining other nonmyofibrillar proteins have also been localized such as calsequestrin and membrane ATPase protein, which have been localized to the sarcomplasmic reticulum (65–67), as well as glyceraldehyde-3-phosphate dehydrogenase, which has been localized to the mitochondria (33) of skeletal muscle cells.

With fluorescent antibody to desmin, which is a protein with a chain weight of 55,000, its localization with respect to the Z bands of mature myofibrils can be shown (7, 42). In preparations of isolated Z band stained with fluorescent specific antibody the desmin can be seen to stain around the periphery of the Z band whereas the localization of α-actinin is within the Z band. Therefore the localizations of desmin and α-actinin are completely separated and desmin is not included within the Z band itself. Likewise, vimentin, an intermediate filament protein with a chain weight of about 58,000, is localized in the same place as desmin (41). Although both desmin and vimentin are associated with mature skeletal muscle myofibrils, the ratio of desmin to vimentin in skeletal muscles is very high. Vimentin is found primarily in nonmuscle cells and in development of skeletal muscle myofibrils. The ratio of desmin to vimentin increases with the development of the muscle (7, 42).

Synemin, a protein with a chain weight of 230,000 that tends to copurify with the intermediate filament proteins desmin and vimentin, also localizes at the periphery of the Z bands as do desmin and vimentin (42). Filamin, with a chain weight of about 250,000, has a similar localization to desmin, vimentin, and synemin (6, 42). Filamin is an actin-binding protein that was originally isolated from chicken gizzard muscle (156, 178).

The Ca^{2+}-ATPase and Mg^{2+}-ATPase as well as calsequestrin have been localized to the sarcomplasmic reticulum (65–67). Calsequestrin is the extrinsic protein of the sarcoplasmic reticulum, whereas Ca^{2+}-ATPase and Mg^{2+}-ATPase are the intrinsic proteins. Both the ATPase and calsequestrin are present in relatively high amounts in fast-twitch muscles, whereas slow-twitch muscles have very low amounts of ATPase and moderate amounts of calsequestrin. Calsequestrin localization as observed with fluorescent specific antibody is related to the I band and is concentrated along the A-I junction. The ATPase is found related to the entire I band as well as to the center of the A band. These observations suggest that calsequestrin is located primarily in the terminal cisternae of the sarcoplasmic reticulum, whereas ATPase is distributed uniformly along the sarcoplasmic reticulum. This interpretation is consistent with the findings of Meissner (97), who separated the sarcoplasmic reticulum vesicles into light and heavy fractions. He found that the ATPase was present in both fractions but calsequestrin was present only in the heavy fraction. This difference in localization both by antibody staining and by the isolation of membrane fractions suggests that different portions of the system of sarcoplasmic reticulum have different functions. Winegrad (186), from physiological studies in frog fast-twitch skeletal muscles, suggested that Ca^{2+} was stored in and released from the terminal cisternae of the sarcoplasmic reticulum, whereas uptake occurred along the entire surface of the sarcoplasmic reticulum. This again suggests different functions for different parts of the sarcoplasmic reticulum. Similar localizations for calsequestrin as were found by Jorgensen et al. (65) were also found by Junker and Sommer (66,

67) with specific antibody to calsequestrin, except that Junker and Sommer (67) claim fluorescent antibody localization of calsequestrin along the entire length of the sarcoplasmic reticulum with stronger staining occurring at the terminal cisternae. They have also observed the distribution in electron microscopy with the unlabeled immunoperoxidase technique for localization (67).

Research was supported by a grant from the Public Health Service (HL-15835) to the Pennsylvania Muscle Institute.

REFERENCES

1. Arakawa, N., R. M. Robson, and D. E. Goll. An improved method for the preparation of alpha-actinin from rabbit striated muscle. *Biochim. Biophys. Acta* 200: 284–295, 1970.
2. Arndt, I., and F. A. Pepe. Antigenic specificity of red and white muscle myosin. *J. Histochem. Cytochem.* 23: 159–168, 1975.
3. Arnold H., and D. Pette. Binding of glycolytic enzymes to structure proteins of the muscle. *Eur. J. Biochem.* 6: 163–171, 1968.
4. Ashby, B., and C. Frieden. Interaction of AMP-aminohydrolase with myosin and its subfragments. *J. Biol. Chem.* 252: 1869–1872, 1977.
5. Ashby, B., C. Frieden, and R. Bischoff. Immunofluorescent and histochemical localization of AMP deaminase in skeletal muscle. *J. Cell Biol.* 81: 361–373, 1979.
6. Bechtel, P. J. Identification of a high molecular weight actin-binding protein in skeletal muscle. *J. Biol. Chem.* 254: 1755–1758, 1979.
7. Bennett, G. S., S. A. Fellini, Y. Toyama, and H. Holtzer. Redistribution of intermediate filament subunits during skeletal myogenesis and maturation *in vitro*. *J. Cell Biol.* 82: 577–584, 1979.
8. Benzonana, G., and G. Gabbiani. Immunofluorescent subcellular localization of some muscle proteins: a comparison between tissue sections and isolated myofibrils. *Histochemistry* 57: 61–76, 1978.
9. Benzonana, G., W. Wnuk, J. A. Cox, and G. Gabbiani. Cellular distribution of sarcoplasmic calcium-binding proteins by immunofluorescence. *Histochemistry* 51: 335–341, 1977.
10. Botts, J., D. B. Stone, A. T. L. Wang, and R. A. Mendelson. Electron paramagnetic resonance and nanosecond fluorescence depolarization studies on creatine phosphokinase interaction with myosin and its fragments. *J. Supramol. Struct.* 3: 141–145, 1975.
11. Briskey, E. J., K. Seraydarian, and W. F. Mommaerts. The modification of actomyosin by alpha-actinin. III. The interaction between alpha-actinin and actin. *Biochim. Biophys. Acta* 133: 424–434, 1967.
12. Busch, W. A., M. H. Stromer, D. E. Goll, and A. Suzuki. Ca^{2+}-specific removal of Z lines from rabbit skeletal muscle. *J. Cell Biol.* 52: 367–381, 1972.
13. Chowrashi, P. K., and F. A. Pepe. Light meromysin paracrystal formation. *J. Cell Biol.* 74: 136–152, 1977.
14. Chowrashi, P. K., and F. A. Pepe. M-band proteins: evidence for more than two components. In: *Motility in Cell Function*, edited by F. A. Pepe, J. W. Sanger, and V. T. Nachmias. New York: Academic, 1979, p. 419–422.
15. Chowrashi, P. K., and F. A. Pepe. The Z-band: amorphin and alpha-actinin and their relation to structure. *J. Cell Biol.* 94: 565–573, 1982.
16. Cohen, C., D. L. D. Caspar, J. P. Johnson, K. Nauss, S. S. Margossian, and D. A. D. Parry. Tropomyosin-troponin assembly. *Cold Spring Harbor Symp. Quant. Biol.* 37: 286–297, 1972.
17. Colowick, S. P., and N. O. Kaplan. *Methods in Enzymology. Immunochemical Techniques. Part A*, edited by H. V. Vunakis and J. J. Langone. New York: Academic, 1980, vol. 70.
18. Craig, R. Structure of A-segments from frog and rabbit skeletal muscle. *J. Mol. Biol.* 109: 69–81, 1977.
19. Craig, R., and G. Offer. The location of C-protein in rabbit skeletal muscle. *Proc. R. Soc. London Ser. B* 192: 451–461, 1976.
20. Drabikowski, W., R. Dabrowska, and B. Barylko. Separation and characterization of the constituents of troponin. *FEBS Lett.* 12: 148–152, 1971.
21. Eaton, B. L., and B. Mochan. The M-band: a structural protein plus creatine kinase. *J. Cell Biol.* 59: 86a, 1973.
22. Eaton, B. L., and F. A. Pepe. M-band protein: two components isolated from chicken breast muscle. *J. Cell Biol.* 55: 681–695, 1972.
23. Ebashi, S. Separation of troponin into three components. *J. Biochem. Tokyo* 72: 787–790, 1972.
24. Ebashi, S. Regulation of muscle contraction. *Proc. R. Soc. London Ser. B* 207: 259–286, 1980.
25. Ebashi, S., M. Endo, and I. Ohtsuki. Control of muscle contraction. *Q. Rev. Biophys.* 2: 351–384, 1969.
26. Ebashi, S., and A. Kodama. A new protein factor promoting aggregation of tropomyosin. *J. Biochem. Tokyo* 58: 107–108, 1965.
27. Ebashi, S., and A. Kodama. Interaction of troponin with F-actin in the presence of tropomyosin. *J. Biochem. Tokyo* 59: 425–426, 1966.
28. Ebashi, S., A. Kodama, and F. Ebashi. Troponin. I. Preparation and physiological function. *J. Biochem. Tokyo* 64: 465–477, 1968.
29. Ebashi, S., I. Ohtsuki, and K. Mihashi. Regulatory proteins of muscle with special reference to troponin. *Cold Spring Harbor Symp. Quant. Biol.* 37: 215–223, 1972.
30. Ebashi, S., I. Ohtsuki, R. Tsukui, and T. Fujii. The role of regulatory proteins in contractile mechanism. In: *Exploratory Concepts in Muscular Dystrophy II*. Amsterdam: Excerpta Med. Found., 1974, vol. II, p. 419–429. (Int. Congr. Ser. 333.)
31. Ebashi, S., T. Wakabayashi, and F. Ebashi. Troponin and its components. *J. Biochem. Tokyo* 69: 441–445, 1971.
32. Emes, C. H., and A. J. Rowe. Frictional properties and molecular weight of native and synthetic myosin filaments from vertebrate skeletal muscle. *Biochim. Biophys. Acta* 537: 125–144, 1978.
33. Emmart, E. W., D. R. Kominz, and J. Miquel. The localization and distribution of glyceraldehyde-3-phosphate dehydrogenase in myoblasts and developing muscle fibers growing in culture. *J. Histochem. Cytochem.* 11: 207–217, 1963.
34. Endo, M., Y. Nonomura, T. Masaki, I. Ohtsuki, and S. Ebashi. Localization of native tropomyosin in relation to striation patterns. *J. Biochem. Tokyo* 60: 605–608, 1966.
35. Eppenberger, H. M., J. Perriard, U. B. Rosenberg, and E. E. Strehler. The M_r 165,000 M-protein myomesin: a specific protein of cross-striated muscle cells. *J. Cell Biol.* 89: 185–193, 1981.
36. Etlinger, J. D., R. Zak, and D. Fischman. Compositional studies of myofibrils from rabbit striated muscle. *J. Cell Biol.* 68: 123–141, 1976.
37. Franzini-Armstrong, C. The structure of a simple Z line. *J. Cell Biol.* 58: 630–642, 1973.
38. Gauthier, G. F., and S. Lowey. Polymorphism of myosin among skeletal muscle fiber types. *J. Cell Biol.* 74: 760–779, 1977.
39. Goll, D. E., A. Suzuki, J. Temple, and G. R. Holmes. Studies on purified alpha-actinin. I. Effect of temperature and tropomyosin on the alpha-actinin/F-actin interaction. *J. Mol. Biol.* 67: 469–488, 1972.
40. Granger, B. L., and E. Lazarides. The existence of an insoluble Z disc scaffold in chicken skeletal muscle. *Cell* 15: 1253–1268, 1978.

41. GRANGER, B. L., AND E. LAZARIDES. Desmin and vimentin coexist at the periphery of myofibril Z disc. *Cell* 18: 1053–1063, 1979.
42. GRANGER, B. L., AND E. LAZARIDES. Synemin: a new high molecular weight protein associated with desmin and vimentin filaments in muscle. *Cell* 22: 727–738, 1980.
43. GREASER, M. L., AND J. GERGELY. Reconstitution of troponin activity from three protein components. *J. Biol. Chem.* 246: 4226–4233, 1971.
44. GREASER, M. L., M. YAMAGUCHI, AND C. BREKKE. Troponin subunits and their interactions. *Cold Spring Harbor Symp. Quant. Biol.* 37: 235–244, 1972.
45. GROSCHEL-STEWART, U. Comparative studies of human smooth and striated muscle myosins. *Biochim. Biophys. Acta* 229: 322–334, 1971.
46. GROSCHEL-STEWART, U., S. CEURREMANS, I. LEHR, C. MAHLMEISTER, AND E. PAAR. Production of specific antibodies to contractile proteins, and their use in immunofluorescence microscopy. II. Species-specific and species non-specific antibodies to smooth and striated chicken muscle actin. *Histochemistry* 50: 271–279, 1977.
47. GROSCHEL-STEWART, U., AND D. DONIACH. Immunological evidence for human myosin isoenzymes. *Immunology* 17: 991–994, 1969.
48. HANSON, J. Recent X-ray diffraction studies of muscle. *Q. Rev. Biophys.* 1: 177–216, 1968.
49. HARTSHORNE, D. J., AND A. MUELLER. Fractionation of troponin into two distinct proteins. *Biochem. Biophys. Res. Commun.* 31: 647–653, 1968.
50. HEIZMANN, C. W., I. E. BLAUENSTEIN, AND H. M. EPPENBERGER. Comparison of the localization of several muscle proteins in relaxed and contracted myofibrils. *Experientia* 34: 38–40, 1977.
51. HEIZMANN, C. W., AND H. M. EPPENBERGER. M-line proteins from chicken muscle. *Experientia* 32: 770, 1976.
52. HERMAN, I. M., AND T. D. POLLARD. Comparison of purified anti-actin and fluorescent-heavy meromyosin staining patterns in dividing cells. *J. Cell Biol.* 80: 509–520, 1979.
53. HIRABAYASHI, T., AND Y. HAYASHI. Antibody specific for actin from frog skeletal muscle. *J. Biochem. Tokyo* 71: 153–156, 1972.
54. HOLMES, G. R., D. GOLL, AND A. SUZUKI. Effect of alpha-actinin on actin viscosity. *Biochim. Biophys. Acta* 253: 240–253, 1971.
55. HOLT, J. C., AND S. LOWEY. An immunological approach to the role of the low molecular weight subunits in myosin. I. Physical—chemical and immunological characterization of the light chains. *Biochemistry* 14: 4600–4609, 1975.
56. HOLT, J. C., AND S. LOWEY. An immunological approach to the role of the low molecular weight subunits in myosin. II. Interaction of myosin and its subfragments with antibodies to the light chains. *Biochemistry* 14: 4609–4620, 1975.
57. HOLT, J. C., AND S. LOWEY. Distribution of alkali light chains in myosin: isolation of isoenzymes. *Biochemistry* 16: 4398–4408, 1977.
58. HOUK, T. W., AND S. V. PUTNAM. Location of the creatine phosphokinase binding site of myosin. *Biochem. Biophys. Res. Commun.* 55: 1271–1277, 1973.
59. HUXLEY, H. E. The double array of filaments in cross-striated muscle. *J. Biophys. Biochem. Cytol.* 3: 631–648, 1957.
60. HUXLEY, H. E. Electron microscopic studies on the structure of natural and synthetic protein filaments from striated muscle. *J. Mol. Biol.* 7: 281–308, 1963.
61. HUXLEY, H. E., AND W. BROWN. The low angle X-ray diagram of vertebrate striated muscle and its behavior during contraction and rigor. *J. Mol. Biol.* 30: 383–434, 1967.
62. HUXLEY, H. E., AND J. HANSON. Changes in the cross-striations of muscle during contraction and stretch and their structural interpretation. *Nature London* 173: 973–976, 1954.
63. HUXLEY, H. E., AND R. NIEDERGERKE. Interference microscopy of living muscle fibers. *Nature London* 173: 971–973, 1954.
64. JOCKUSCH, B. M., K. H. KELLEY, R. K. MEYER, AND M. M. BURGER. An efficient method to produce specific anti-actin. *Histochemistry* 55: 177–184, 1978.
65. JORGENSEN, A. O., V. KALNINS, AND D. H. MACLENNAN. Localization of sarcoplasmic reticulum proteins in rat skeletal muscle by immunofluorescence. *J. Cell Biol.* 80: 372–384, 1979.
66. JUNKER, J., AND J. R. SOMMER. Calsequestrin localization in rabbit and frog skeletal muscle by immunofluorescence. *J. Cell Biol.* 83: 384a, 1979.
67. JUNKER, J., AND J. R. SOMMER. Ultrastructural localization of calsequestrin by immunoperoxidase. *Federation Proc.* 39: 643, 1980.
68. KATSURA, I., AND H. NODA. Assembly of myosin molecules into the structure of thick filaments of muscle. *Adv. Biophys.* 5: 177–202, 1973.
69. KENNETT, R. H., T. J. MCKEARN, AND K. B. BECHTOL (editors). *Monoclonal Antibodies.* New York: Plenum, 1980.
70. KNAPPEIS, G. G., AND F. CARLSEN. The ultrastructure of the Z disc in skeletal muscle. *J. Cell Biol.* 13: 323–335, 1962.
71. KNAPPEIS, G. G., AND F. CARLSEN. The ultrastructure of the M-line in skeletal muscle. *J. Cell Biol.* 38: 202–211, 1968.
72. KOONS, S. J., AND C. R. ZOBEL. Aggregation of myosin and light meromyosin in the presence of creatine kinase. *Biophys. J.* 25: 246a, 1979.
73. KUNDRAT, E., AND F. A. PEPE. The M-band: studies with fluorescent antibody staining. *J. Cell Biol.* 48: 340–347, 1971.
74. KURODA, M., AND T. MASAKI. On the 42,000 dalton proteins in vertebrate skeletal muscle: actin and eu-actinin. In: *Muscle Contraction: Its Regulatory Mechanisms*, edited by S. Ebashi, K. Maruyama, and M. Endo. Berlin: Springer-Verlag, 1980, p. 507–514.
75. LAMVIK, M. K. Muscle thick filament mass measured by electron scattering. *J. Mol. Biol.* 122: 55–68, 1978.
76. LANGER, B., AND F. A. PEPE. New, rapid methods for purifying alpha-actinin from chicken gizzard and chicken pectoralis muscle. *J. Biol. Chem.* 255: 5429–5434, 1980.
77. LAZARIDES, E., AND B. L. GRANGER. Fluorescent localization of membrane sites in glycerinated chicken skeletal muscle fibers and the relationship of these sites to the protein composition of the Z-disc. *Proc. Natl. Acad. Sci. USA* 75: 3683–3687, 1978.
78. LAZARIDES, E., AND B. D. HUBBARD. Immunological characterization of the subunit of the 100 A filaments from muscle cells. *Proc. Natl. Acad. Sci. USA* 73: 4344–4348, 1976.
79. LAZARIDES, E., AND K. WEBER. Actin antibody: the specific visualization of actin filaments in non-muscle cells. *Proc. Natl. Acad. Sci. USA* 71: 2268–2272, 1974.
80. LEE, L., AND S. WATANABE. Gamma-component, a new myofibrillar protein of skeletal muscle. *J. Biol. Chem.* 245: 3004–3007, 1970.
81. LOWEY, S., AND C. COHEN. Studies on the structure of myosin. *J. Mol. Biol.* 4: 293–308, 1962.
82. LOWEY, S., L. SILBERSTEIN, G. F. GAUTHIER, AND J. C. HOLT. Isolation and distribution of myosin isoenzymes. In: *Motility in Cell Function*, edited by F. A. Pepe, J. W. Sanger, and V. T. Nachmias. New York: Academic, 1979, p. 53–67.
83. LOWEY, S., AND L. A. STEINER. An immunochemical approach to the structure of myosin and the thick filament. *J. Mol. Biol.* 65: 111–126, 1972.
84. LUTHER, P., AND J. SQUIRE. Three-dimensional structure of the vertebrate muscle M-region. *J. Mol. Biol.* 125: 313–324, 1978.
85. MANI, R. S., AND C. M. KAY. Physicochemical studies on the creatine kinase M-line protein and its interaction with myosin and myosin fragments. *Biochim. Biophys. Acta* 453: 391–399, 1976.
86. MANI, R. S., AND C. M. KAY. Isolation and characterization of the 165,000 dalton protein component of the M-line of rabbit skeletal muscle and its interaction with creatine kinase. *Biochim. Biophys. Acta* 533: 248–256, 1978.
87. MANI, R. S., AND C. M. KAY. Interaction of a 100,000 dalton chymotryptic fragment of rabbit skeletal M-line protein with

the S2 subfragment of myosin. *J. Biochem. Tokyo* 86: 1817–1820, 1979.

88. MARSHALL, J. M., H. HOLTZER, H. FINCK, AND F. PEPE. The distribution of protein antigens in striated myofibrils. *Exp. Cell Res. Suppl.* 7: 219–233, 1959.
89. MARSTON, S. B., AND R. T. TREGEAR. Evidence for a complex between myosin and ADP in relaxed muscle fibers. *Nature London New Biol.* 235: 23–24, 1972.
90. MARUYAMA, K., S. KIMURA, T. ISHI, M. KURODA, K. OHASHI, AND S. MURAMATSU. Beta-actinin, a regulatory protein of muscle. Purification, characterization, and function. *J. Biochem. Tokyo* 81: 215–232, 1977.
91. MARUYAMA, K., S. KUNITOMO, S. KIMURA, AND K. OHASHI. I-protein, a new regulatory protein from vertebrate skeletal muscle. III. Function. *J. Biochem. Tokyo* 81: 243–247, 1977.
92. MARUYAMA, K., AND A. WEBER. Binding of adenosine triphosphate to myofibrils during contraction and relaxation. *Biochemistry* 11: 2990–2998, 1972.
93. MASAKI, T., M. ENDO, AND S. EBASHI. Localization of 6S component of alpha-actinin at Z-band. *J. Biochem. Tokyo* 62: 630–632, 1967.
94. MASAKI, T., AND O. TAKAITI. Purification of M-protein. *J. Biochem. Tokyo* 71: 355–357, 1972.
95. MASAKI, T., AND O. TAKAITI. M-protein. *J. Biochem. Tokyo* 75: 367–380, 1974.
96. MASAKI, T., O. TAKAITI, AND S. EBASHI. "M-substance," a new protein constituting the M-line of myofibrils. *J. Biochem. Tokyo* 64: 909–910, 1968.

96a. MATSUMARA, F., AND J. J.-C. LIN. Visualization of monoclonal antibody binding to tropomyosin on native smooth muscle thin filaments by electron microscopy. *J. Mol. Biol.* 157: 163–172, 1982.

97. MEISSNER, G. Isolation and characterization of two types of sarcoplasmic reticulum vesicles. *Biochim. Biophys. Acta* 389: 51–68, 1975.
98. MILLMAN, B. M. X-ray diffraction from chicken skeletal muscle. In: *Motility in Cell Function*, edited by F. A. Pepe, J. W. Sanger, and V. T. Nachmias. New York: Academic, 1979, p. 351–354.
99. MOORE, P. B., H. E. HUXLEY, AND D. J. DEROSIER. Three dimensional reconstruction of F-actin, thin filaments and decorated thin filaments. *J. Mol. Biol.* 50: 279–295, 1970.
100. MOOS, C. Discussion: interaction of C-protein with myosin and light meromyosin. *Cold Spring Harbor Symp. Quant. Biol.* 37: 93–95, 1972.
101. MOOS, C., G. OFFER, R. STARR, AND P. BENNETT. Interaction of C-protein with myosin, myosin rod and light meromyosin. *J. Mol. Biol.* 97: 1–9, 1975.
102. MORIMOTO, K., AND W. F. HARRINGTON. Isolation and physical chemical properties of an M-line protein from skeletal muscle. *J. Biol. Chem.* 247: 3052–3061, 1972.
103. MORIMOTO, K., AND W. F. HARRINGTON. Isolation and composition of thick filaments from rabbit skeletal muscle. *J. Mol. Biol.* 77: 165–175, 1973.
104. MORIMOTO, K., AND W. F. HARRINGTON. Substructure of the thick filament of vertebrate striated muscle. *J. Mol. Biol.* 83: 83–97, 1974.
105. OBINATA, T., T. MASAKI, AND H. TAKANO. Immunochemical comparison of myosin light chains from chicken fast white, slow red, and cardiac muscle. *J. Biochem. Tokyo* 86: 131–137, 1979.
106. OBINATA, T., Y. SHIMADA, AND R. MATSUDA. Troponin in embryonic chick skeletal muscle cells in vitro. An immunoelectron microscopic study. *J. Cell Biol.* 81: 59–66, 1979.
107. OFFER, G. C-protein and the periodicity in the thick filaments of vertebrate skeletal muscle. *Cold Spring Harbor Symp. Quant. Biol.* 37: 87–93, 1972.
108. OFFER, G. The antigenicity of myosin and C-protein. *Proc. R. Soc. London Ser. B* 192: 439–449, 1976.
109. OFFER, G., C. MOOS, AND R. STARR. A new protein of the thick filaments of vertebrate skeletal myofibrils. Extraction, purification and characterization. *J. Mol. Biol.* 74: 653–676, 1973.
110. OHASHI, K., S. KIMURA, K. DEGUCHI, AND K. MARUYAMA. I-protein, a new regulatory protein from vertebrate skeletal muscle. I. Purification and characterization. *J. Biochem. Tokyo* 81: 233–236, 1977.
111. OHASHI, K., AND K. MARUYAMA. A new structural protein located in the Z lines of chicken skeletal muscle. *J. Biochem. Tokyo* 85: 1103–1105, 1979.
112. OHASHI, K., AND K. MARUYAMA. A new structural protein located in the Z line of chicken skeletal muscle. In: *Muscle Contraction: Its Regulatory Mechanisms*, edited by S. Ebashi, K. Maruyama, and M. Endo. Berlin: Springer–Verlag, 1980, p. 497–505.
113. OHASHI, K., T. MASAKI, AND K. MARUYAMA. I-protein, a new regulatory protein from vertebrate skeletal muscle. II. Localization. *J. Biochem. Tokyo* 81: 237–242, 1977.
114. OHTSUKI, I. Localization of troponin in thin filament and tropomyosin paracrystal. *J. Biochem. Tokyo* 75: 753–765, 1974.
115. OHTSUKI, I. Distribution of troponin components in the thin filament studied by immunoelectron microscopy. *J. Biochem. Tokyo* 77: 633–639, 1975.
116. OHTSUKI, I. Molecular arrangement of troponin-T in the thin filament. *J. Biochem. Tokyo* 86: 491–497, 1979.
117. OHTSUKI, I. Number of anti-troponin striations along the thin filament of chick embryonic breast muscle. *J. Biochem. Tokyo* 85: 1377–1378, 1979.
118. OHTSUKI, I., T. MASAKI, Y. NONOMURA, AND S. EBASHI. Periodic distribution of troponin along the thin filament. *J. Biochem. Tokyo* 61: 817–819, 1967.
119. PEPE, F. A. Organization of myosin molecules in the thick filament of striated muscle as revealed by antibody staining in electron microscopy. *Electron Microsc.* 2: 53–54, 1966.
120. PEPE, F. A. Some aspects of the structural organization of the myofibril as revealed by antibody-staining methods. *J. Cell Biol.* 28: 505–525, 1966.
121. PEPE, F. A. The myosin filament. I. Structural organization from antibody staining observed in electron microscopy. *J. Mol. Biol.* 27: 203–225, 1967.
122. PEPE, F. A. The myosin filament. II. Interaction between myosin and actin filaments observed using antibody staining in fluorescent and electron microscopy. *J. Mol. Biol.* 27: 227–236, 1967.
123. PEPE, F. A. Analysis of antibody-staining patterns obtained with striated myofibrils in fluorescent microscopy and electron microscopy. In: *International Review of Cytology*, edited by G. H. Bourne and J. F. Danielli. New York: Academic, 1968, vol. 24, p. 193–231.

123a. PEPE, F. A. Structural components of the striated muscle fibril. In: *Subunits in Biological Systems*, edited by S. Timasheff and G. Fasman. New York: Dekker, 1971, vol. 5, pt. A. (Biological Macromolecules Ser.)

124. PEPE, F. A. Structure of the myosin filament of striated muscle. *Prog. Biophys. Mol. Biol.* 22: 75–96, 1971.
125. PEPE, F. A. The myosin filament: immunochemical and ultrastructural approaches to molecular organization. *Cold Spring Harbor Symp. Quant. Biol.* 37: 97–108, 1972.
126. PEPE, F. A. Structure of muscle filaments from immunohistochemical and ultrastructural studies. *J. Histochem. Cytochem.* 23: 543–562, 1975.
127. PEPE, F. A. Detectability of antibody in fluorescence and electron microscopy. In: *Cell Motility*, edited by R. Goldman, T. Pollard, and J. Rosenbaum. New York: Cold Spring Harbor, 1976, vol. 3, p. 337–346. (Cold Spring Harbor Conf. Cell Proliferation.)
128. PEPE, F. A. The myosin filament: molecular structure. In: *Motility in Cell Function*, edited by F. A. Pepe, J. W. Sanger, and V. T. Nachmias. New York: Academic, 1979, p. 103–116.
129. PEPE, F. A. The structure of vertebrate skeletal muscle myosin filaments. In: *Cell and Muscle Motility,* edited by R. M. Dowben and J. W. Shay. New York: Plenum, 1982, vol. 2.
130. PEPE, F. A., F. T. ASHTON, P. DOWBEN, AND M. STEWART.

The myosin filament. VII. Changes in internal structure along the length of the filament. *J. Mol. Biol.* 145: 421–440, 1981.

131. PEPE, F. A., AND P. DOWBEN. The myosin filament. V. Intermediate voltage electron microscopy and optical diffraction studies of the substructure. *J. Mol. Biol.* 113: 199–218, 1977.
132. PEPE, F. A., AND B. DRUCKER. The myosin filament. IV. Observations of the internal structural arrangement. *J. Cell Biol.* 52: 255–260, 1972.
133. PEPE, F. A., AND B. DRUCKER. The myosin filament. III. C-protein. *J. Mol. Biol.* 99: 609–617, 1975.
134. PEPE, F. A., AND B. DRUCKER. The myosin filament. VI. Myosin content. *J. Mol. Biol.* 130: 379–393, 1979.
135. PEPE, F. A., H. FINCK, AND H. HOLTZER. The use of specific antibody in electron microscopy. III. Localization of antigens by the use of unmodified antibody. *J. Biophys. Biochem. Cytol.* 11: 533–547, 1961.
136. PEPE, F. A., AND H. E. HUXLEY. Antibody staining of separated thin and thick filaments of striated muscle. In: *Biochemistry of Muscle Contraction*, edited by J. Gergely. Boston, MA: Little, Brown, 1964, p. 320–329.
137. PERRY, S. V., H. A. COLE, J. F. HEAD, AND F. J. WILSON. Localization and mode of action of the inhibitory protein component of the troponin complex. *Cold Spring Harbor Symp. Quant. Biol.* 37: 251–262, 1972.
138. PETTE, D. Some aspects of supramolecular organization of glycolenolytic and glycolytic enzymes in muscle. *Acta Histochem. Suppl.* 14: 47–68, 1975.
139. POTTER, J. The content of troponin, tropomyosin, actin and myosin in rabbit skeletal muscle myofibrils. *Arch. Biochem. Biophys.* 162: 436–441, 1974.
140. REDDY, M. K., J. D. ETLINGER, M. RABINOWITZ, D. A. FISCHMAN, AND R. ZAK. Removal of Z-lines and alpha-actinin from isolated myofibrils by a calcium-activated neutral protease. *J. Biol. Chem.* 250: 4278–4284, 1975.
141. REEDY, M. K., K. R. LEONARD, R. FREEMAN, AND T. ARAD. Thick myofilament mass determination by electron scattering measurements with the scanning transmission electron microscope. *J. Muscle Res. Cell Motil.* 2: 45–64, 1981.
142. RICHARDS, E. G., C. S. CHUNG, D. B. MENZEL, AND H. S. OLCOTT. Chromatography of myosin on diethylaminoethyl-Sephadex A-50. *Biochemistry* 6: 528–540, 1967.
143. ROBSON, R. M., D. E. GOLL, N. ARAKAWA, AND M. H. STROMER. Purification and properties of alpha-actinin from rabbit skeletal muscle. *Biochim. Biophys. Acta* 200: 296–318, 1970.
144. ROME, E., T. HIRABAYASHI, AND S. V. PERRY. X-ray diffraction of muscle labeled with antibody to troponin-C. *Nature London New Biol.* 244: 154–155, 1973.
145. ROME, E., G. OFFER, AND F. A. PEPE. X-ray diffraction of muscle labeled with antibody to C-protein. *Nature London New Biol.* 244: 152–154, 1973.
146. ROWE, R. W. D. The ultrastructure of Z discs from white, intermediate and red fibers of mammalian striated muscles. *J. Cell Biol.* 57: 261–277, 1973.
147. SAFER, D., AND F. A. PEPE. Axial packing in light meromysin paracrystals. *J. Mol. Biol.* 136: 343–358, 1980.
148. SAMOSUDOVA, N. V., M. M. OGREVETSKAYA, M. V. KALAMKAROVA, AND G. M. FRANK. Use of ferritin antibodies for the electron microscopic study of myosin. III. Localization of ferritin antimyosin in the sarcomere. *Biofizika* 13: 877–880, 1968.
149. SAMUELS, A. The immuno-enzymology of muscle proteins. I. General features of myosin and 5′-adenylic acid deaminase. *Arch. Biochem. Biophys.* 92: 497–506, 1961.
150. SCHAUB, M. C., AND S. V. PERRY. The relaxing protein system of striated muscle. Resolution of the troponin complex into inhibitory and calcium-ion sensitizing factors and their relationship to tropomyosin. *Biochem. J.* 115: 993–1104, 1969.
151. SCHAUB, M. C., AND S. V. PERRY. The regulatory proteins of the myofibril. Characterization and properties of the inhibitory factor (troponin B). *Biochem. J.* 123: 367–377, 1971.
152. SCHOLLMEYER, J. E., D. E. GOLL, R. M. ROBSON, AND M. H. STROMER. Localization of alpha-actinin and tropomyosin in different muscles. *J. Cell Biol.* 59: 306a, 1973.
153. SCHOLLMEYER, J. E., M. H. STROMER, AND D. E. GOLL. Alpha-actinin and tropomyosin localization in normal and diseased muscle. *Biophys. J.* 12: 280a, 1972.
154. SHIMADA, Y., AND T. OBINATA. Troponin in embryonic chick skeletal muscle cells *in vitro*: an immunoelectron microscopic study. *Electron Microsc.* 2: 162–163, 1978.
155. SHIMIZU, T., T. MASAKI, AND D. A. FISCHMAN. Monoclonal antibodies to light chain 2 of breast myosin from adult chicken. *Biophys. J.* 33: 242a, 1981.
156. SHIZUTA, Y., H. SHIZUTA, M. GALLO, P. DAVIS, I. PASTAN, AND M. LEWIS. Purification and properties of filamin, an actin binding protein from chicken gizzard. *J. Biol. Chem.* 251: 6562–6567, 1976.
157. SILBERSTEIN, L., AND S. LOWEY. Isolation and distribution of myosin isoenzymes in chicken pectoralis muscle. *J. Mol. Biol.* 148: 153–190, 1981.
158. SJÖSTRÖM, M., AND J. M. SQUIRE. Cryo-ultramicrotomy and myofibrillar fine structure: a review. *J. Microsc. Oxford* 3: 239–278, 1977.
159. SJÖSTRÖM, M., AND J. M. SQUIRE. Fine structure of the A-band in cryo-sections. The structure of the A-band of human skeletal muscle fibers from ultra-thin cryo-sections negatively stained. *J. Mol. Biol.* 109: 49–68, 1977.
160. SPUDICH, J. A., H. E. HUXLEY, AND J. T. FINCH. Regulation of skeletal muscle contraction. II. Structural studies of the interaction of the tropomyosin-troponin complex with actin. *J. Mol. Biol.* 72: 619–632, 1972.
161. SQUIRE, J. M. General model of myosin filament structure. III. Molecular packing arrangement in myosin filaments. *J. Mol. Biol.* 77: 291–323, 1973.
162. STARR, R., AND G. OFFER. Polypeptide chains of intermediate molecular weight in myosin preparations. *FEBS Lett.* 15: 40–43, 1971.
163. STERNBERGER, L. A. *Immunochemistry.* New York: Wiley, 1979.
164. STEWART, M., F. T. ASHTON, R. LIEBERSON, AND F. A. PEPE. The myosin filament. IX. Determination of subfilament positions by computer processing of electron micrographs. *J. Mol. Biol.* 153: 381–392, 1981.
165. STROMER, M. H., AND D. E. GOLL. Studies on purified alpha-actinin. II. Electron microscopic studies on the competitive binding of alpha-actinin and tropomyosin to Z line extracted myofibrils. *J. Mol. Biol.* 67: 489–494, 1972.
166. STROMER, M. H., D. J. HARTSHORNE, H. MUELLER, AND R. V. RICE. The effect of various protein fractions on Z- and M-line reconstitution. *J. Cell Biol.* 40: 167–178, 1969.
167. SUGITA, H., T. MASAKI, AND S. EBASHI. Staining of myofibrils with fluorescent antibody against the 10S component of the original alpha-actinin preparation. *J. Biochem. Tokyo* 75: 671–673, 1974.
168. SZENT-GYORGYI, A. G., AND H. HOLTZER. Fixation of muscle proteins with antibodies. *Biochim. Biophys. Acta* 41: 14–19, 1960.
169. TAYLOR, K. A., AND L. A. AMOS. A new model for the geometry of the binding of myosin crossbridges to muscle thin filaments. *J. Mol. Biol.* 147: 297–324, 1981.

169a. TOWBIN, H., T. STAEHELIN, AND J. GORDON. Electrophoretic transfer of proteins from polyacrylamide gels to nitrocellulose sheets: procedure and some applications. *Proc. Natl. Acad. Sci. USA* 76: 4350–4354, 1979.

170. TREGEAR, R. T., AND J. M. SQUIRE. Myosin content and filament structure in smooth and striated muscle. *J. Mol. Biol.* 77: 279–290, 1973.
171. TRINICK, J. A. Identity of the 90,000 dalton M-protein from chicken muscle (Abstract). *Federation Proc.* 33: 1580, 1974.
172. TRINICK, J., AND J. COOPER. Sequential disassembly of vertebrate muscle thick filaments. *J. Mol. Biol.* 141: 315–321, 1980.
173. TRINICK, J., AND S. LOWEY. M-protein from chicken pectoralis muscle: isolation and characterization. *J. Mol. Biol.* 113: 343–368, 1977.
174. TUNIK, B., AND H. HOLTZER. The distribution of muscle anti-

gens in contracted myofibrils determined by fluorescein-labeled antibodies. *J. Biophys. Biochem. Cytol.* 11: 67–74, 1961.

175. TURNER, D. C., G. RUDOLF, H. G. LEBHERZ, M. SIEGRIST, T. WALLIMANN, AND H. M. EPPENBERGER. Differentiation in cultures derived from embryonic chicken muscle. II. Phosphorylase histochemistry and fluorescent antibody staining for creatine kinase and aldolase. *Dev. Biol.* 48: 284–307, 1976.
176. TURNER, D. C., T. WALLIMANN, AND H. M. EPPENBERGER. A protein that binds specifically to the M-line of skeletal muscle is identified as the muscle form of creatine kinase. *Proc. Natl. Acad. Sci. USA* 70: 702–705, 1973.
177. WALLIMANN, T., G. PELLONI, D. C. TURNER, AND H. M. EPPENBERGER. Monovalent antibodies against MM-creatine kinase remove the M-line from myofibrils. *Proc. Natl. Acad. Sci. USA* 75: 4297–4300, 1978.
178. WALLIMANN, T., G. PELLONI, D. C. TURNER, AND H. M. EPPENBERGER. Removal of the M-line by treatment with Fab′ fragments of antibodies against MM-creatine kinase. In: *Motility in Cell Function*, edited by F. A. Pepe, J. W. Sanger, and V. T. Nachmias. New York: Academic, 1979. p. 415–417.
179. WALLIMANN, T., D. C. TURNER, AND H. M. EPPENBERGER. Localization of creatine kinase isoenzymes in myofibrils. I. Chicken skeletal muscle. *J. Cell Biol.* 75: 297–317, 1977.
180. WANG, K., J. F. ASH, AND S. J. SINGER. Filamin, a new high-molecular-weight protein found in smooth muscle and non-muscle cells. *Proc. Natl. Acad. Sci. USA* 72: 4483–4486, 1975.
181. WEBER, A., R. HEIZ, AND I. REISS. The role of magnesium in the relaxation of myofibrils. *Biochemistry* 8: 2266–2271, 1969.
182. WEIR, D. M. (editor). *Handbook of Experimental Immunology. Immunochemistry.* Oxford, UK: Blackwell, 1979, vol. 1.
183. WILSON, F. J., D. CAMISCOLI, M. J. IRISH, AND T. HIRABAYASHI. Immunohistochemical and ultrastructural distribution of antibodies to troponin-C and troponin-I in normal and dystrophic chicken skeletal muscle. *J. Histochem. Cytochem.* 26: 258–266, 1978.
184. WILSON, F. J., AND H. FINCK. Actin: immunochemical and immunofluorescence studies. *J. Biochem. Tokyo* 70: 143–148, 1971.
185. WILSON, F. J., T. HIRABAYASHI, AND M. J. IRISH. Ultrastructure location of antibodies to troponin components in dystrophic skeletal muscle. In: *Motility in Cell Function*, edited by F. A. Pepe, J. W. Sanger, and V. T. Nachmias. New York: Academic, 1979, p. 377–380.
186. WINEGRAD, S. The intracellular site of calcium activation of contraction in frog skeletal muscle. *J. Gen. Physiol.* 55: 77–88, 1970.
187. WOODHEAD, J. L., AND S. LOWEY. Size and shape of skeletal muscle M-protein. *J. Mol. Biol.* 157: 149–154, 1982.
188. WRAY, J. Structure of the backbone in myosin filaments of muscle. *Nature London* 270: 37–40, 1979.
189. WRAY, J. X-ray diffraction studies of myosin filament structures in crustacean muscles. In: *Motility in Cell Function*, edited by F. A. Pepe, J. W. Sanger, and V. T. Nachmias. New York: Academic, 1979, p. 347–350.

CHAPTER 5

Structure of vertebrate striated muscle as determined by X-ray–diffraction studies

JOHN C. HASELGROVE | *Johnson Research Foundation, Department of Biochemistry and Biophysics, University of Pennsylvania, Philadelphia, Pennsylvania*

CHAPTER CONTENTS

THE REGULAR ARRANGEMENT of basic muscle proteins into helical filaments packed into a lattice makes muscle a suitable subject for X-ray–diffraction study. Both X-ray diffraction and electron microscopy have played major roles in the understanding of muscle contraction. Electron microscopy is a convenient technique since it yields a picture of the objects studied, but fixation and preparation for the microscope destroy the high-resolution information and may induce structural artifacts. In contrast X-ray diffraction may be performed on an untreated specimen when it is relaxed or generating tension without affecting the state of the muscle, although the data do not directly indicate the structure and require sophisticated interpretation.

The muscle diffraction pattern exhibits many different crystallographic features: high- and low-angle reflections, helical symmetry, rotational averaging, Bragg sampling by pseudoperfect lattices, and disordered arrays. Muscles act as very weak diffractors of X rays; therefore advances in X-ray–diffraction studies of muscle have been closely linked to technical developments in X-ray sources, cameras, and detectors (51).

Bernal and Fankuchen (14) in the 1920s and Astbury (9) in the 1940s took high-angle X-ray patterns of relaxed and contracting muscles. By studying the X-ray reflections from the α-helical backbone of the myosin molecule, they were able to correlate the structure of myosin with that of keratin and fibrinogen. Because they were unable to find any change in the diffraction pattern when the muscle contracted, further studies were discouraged. It has been confirmed that there is indeed little change in the helical content of the myosin molecules when a muscle contracts and thus the lack of change in the high-angle pattern has been explained.

In the early 1950s H. E. Huxley (62, 63), using a slit camera, pioneered the study of the low-angle diffraction patterns of vertebrate skeletal muscle (VSM). He studied the equatorial and meridional X-ray reflections arising from periodicities in the 10- to 40-nm region and found that the axial spacings did not change with sarcomere length. This observation, together with the constancy of the pattern during contraction, supports the idea that muscle shortens by the sliding of filaments (59, 73) that maintain a constant length. In the later 1950s and early 1960s, when it was possible to obtain patterns with some degree of resolution in two dimensions, Elliott (27) identified a series of layer lines as arising from a helical arrangement of projections on the myosin helix (64). Bear (12) and Selby and Bear (143) investigated a series of reflections arising from the actin content of muscle (see also ref. 17). Huxley (64) suggested that equatorial reflections arose from a hexagonal lattice with myosin filaments at the lattice points and actin filaments at the interstitial spaces.

A recording time of several hours for each X-ray pattern, however, was a major drawback in the study of contracting muscle because this is much longer than a skeletal muscle contraction can be maintained. Nonetheless the basic low-angle pattern of relaxed muscle had been characterized, and by the middle of the 1960s more intense X-ray sources were coupled to cameras that focus the X-rays, thereby increasing the available flux. Investigators could observe many minutes of integrated contraction by summing the patterns from many short tetani or twitches (29, 30, 70, 71). Different aspects of X-ray-diffraction studies on a variety of muscles have been reviewed (41, 51, 97, 108).

MUSCLE STRUCTURE: AN OVERVIEW

Vertebrate striated muscle is named for the transverse striations seen when the muscle fibers are viewed by a polarizing or interference light microscope. Band patterns are composed of dark A bands alternating with lighter I bands. The sarcomere is the repeating muscle unit and is defined from the dark Z line in the middle of each I band. The A bands thus sit in the middle of each sarcomere, and in the center of each A band there is a lighter region called the H zone. Fiber structure is described in detail in the chapter by B. R. Eisenberg in this *Handbook*.

The concept that muscles operate by the sliding of two sets of filaments past each other is based on observations in the light microscope that the H zone and I band shorten when the muscle shortens (59, 73). These filaments may now be seen in the electron microscope (Fig. 1). Thick myosin-containing filaments, 1.65 μm long and about 12 nm in diameter, extend the length of the A band and align transversely in a hexagonal lattice. Thinner actin-containing filaments (8 nm diam) extend 1.05 μm on each side of the Z line as far as the H zone, and within the A band they occupy the trigonal positions of the myosin-filament lattice. High-resolution electron micrographs show projections from the myosin filaments that are able to bridge the gap to the actin filaments (65) and thus are called cross bridges. The active site for ATPase in the myosin molecule rests in the cross bridge (see the chapter by Webb and Trentham in this *Handbook*). It is currently thought that the cross bridges, acting cyclically to pull the actin and myosin filaments past each other (57, 67), produce tension and shortening of the muscle. The polarity of the molecular packing at the ends of the myosin filaments and in the actin filaments is such that the interaction produces a force in only one direction—that which increases filament overlap (65).

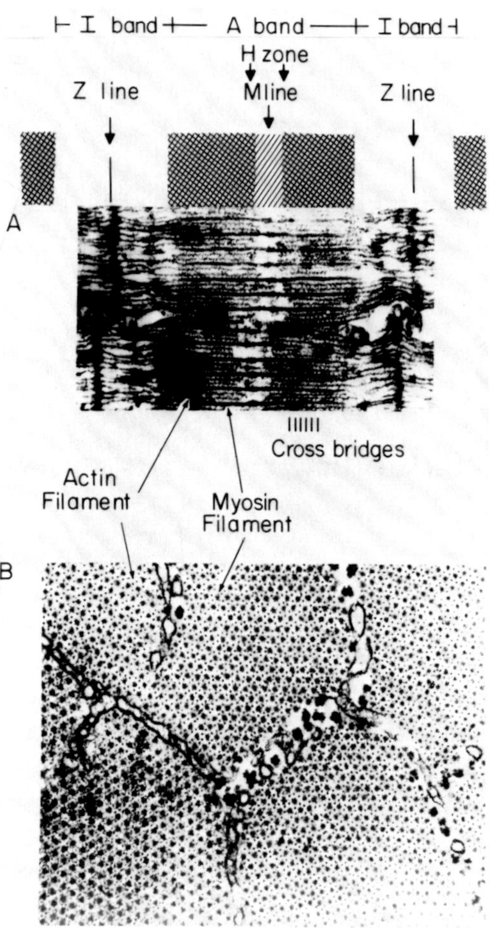

FIG. 1. Electron micrographs of the filament lattice in vertebrate striated muscle. *A*: longitudinal section parallel to the 1.1 plane (see also Fig. 5). Thick myosin-containing filaments lie in longitudinal register and thinner actin-containing filaments extend on either side of the Z line and interdigitate with myosin filaments. Cross bridges project from the thick filaments. Different zones are marked. *B*: transverse section through A bands of several myofibrils. Thick filaments are located at lattice points of a hexagonal lattice with actin filaments at trigonal positions, equidistant from 3 myosin filaments (see Fig. 5). [From H. E. Huxley, unpublished observations.]

The mechanism by which the cross bridges cycle and generate force has attracted considerable research effort. Structural and biochemical studies have led to a model of the cross-bridge cycle that correlates biochemical reactions with mechanical processes (58, 88). A currently useful model has four steps, shown in Figure 2. *1*) The cross bridge, with the products of ATP hydrolysis still bound to it, binds to actin at an angle approximately 90° to the filament axis (*A*→*B*). *2*) The attached cross bridge tilts 45°, pulling the actin and myosin filaments past each other (*B*→*C*), resulting in a cross-bridge orientation like that of rigor muscle. Release of bound nucleotide products occurs during this step. *3*) Adenosine triphosphate binds to the actin-myosin complex and causes dissociation of the myosin from the actin (*C*→*D*). *4*) This nucleotide is then cleaved to form the reactants of step *1* and the cycle repeats, except that the cross bridge binds to a

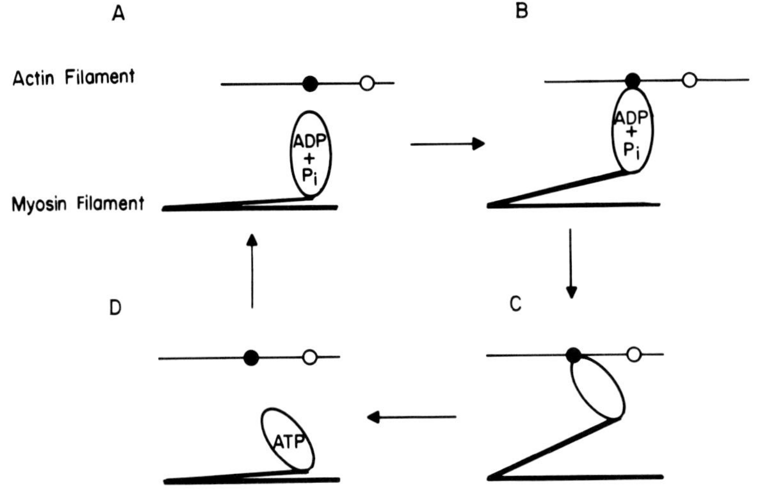

FIG. 2. A 4-step, 4-state model of cross-bridge action showing mechanical states with corresponding predominant biochemical species. Cross-bridge orientations in states *C* and *D* are often depicted as 45° angles; both *A* and *B* are shown as 90° angles. Although states *A* and *D* can be distinguished biochemically, differences in physical orientation are still unclear. The hinge region between head and tail of the myosin molecule is thought to be very flexible. *A*: myosin cross bridge, with cleaved ATP-hydrolysis products still bound to it, is not yet attached to actin. *B*: cross bridge attaches to actin monomer at approximate 90° angle. *C*: cross bridge–actin angle changes to 45°, pulling the filaments past each other while the cleaved nucleotide products dissociate from myosin. Resultant state is the rigor cross-link. *D*: ATP binds to rigor cross-link causing myosin cross bridge to dissociate from actin filament. Subsequent hydrolysis of ATP leaves the cross bridge in original state (*A*), ready to bind to the next available actin monomer.

different actin monomer. (The biochemical steps of the cycle are described in detail in the chapter by Webb and Trentham in this *Handbook.*) The interaction of the cross bridge with the actin in living muscle is obviously controlled not only by the availability of ATP but also by the relative positions and orientations of myosin and actin (see Fig. 10). The structural aspects are amenable to study by X-ray diffraction because both the actin and myosin filaments are helical and therefore give well-defined X-ray patterns.

Description of Low-Angle Diffraction Patterns

Low-angle X-ray-diffraction patterns from VSM and a schematic representation of the patterns are shown in Figures 3 and 4, respectively. The axial positions of the principal reflections are listed in Tables 1 and 2. It is technically impossible to take a single picture allowing simultaneous study of all the patterns' features; in practice one studies each region of the pattern by using a slightly different experimental setup. The muscle pattern is conventionally displayed as though it were taken with the muscle axis vertical. It consists of a series of spots called reflections and it is symmetrical about the vertical and horizontal axes, typical of fiber diffraction patterns from helical objects. The center of the pattern, the origin, usually appears white because a small lead backstop is placed in front of the film to prevent the undiffracted beam from striking it. It is convenient to distinguish three distinct regions of the X-ray pattern, each arising from different structural features of the intact muscle.

MERIDIAN. The axis of the pattern corresponding to the muscle axis is called the meridian. In the illustrations in this chapter it is always the vertical axis. The meridional reflections provide information about axial periodicities along the structure regardless of the lateral positions of the units in the filament helices. The

TABLE 1. *Principal Reflections in Low-Angle Diffraction Patterns of Living, Relaxed Frog Sartorius Muscle at Rest Length*

Meridian[a]		Myosin Layer Lines		Actin Layer Lines[b]	
Protein source	Axial spacing, nm	nm	Order of 42.9 nm	nm	Order of 77.3 nm
Actin	2.73				
				5.1	
				5.9	
Myosin	7.15	7.18	6		
	8.60	8.64	5		
	9.07				
	10.6	10.7	4		
	11.0				
				12.2	6
	12.8				
	14.11[c] } 14.31[d] }	143	3	18.2	4
	20.9 } 21.39 }	21.5	2	36.5[e]	2
Troponin	38.22 } 39.41 }				
C protein	41.76 } 44.09 }	42.9	1		

Data laid out to simulate top right-hand quadrant of Fig. 3*A*. Not all reflections are listed here–only those frequently discussed. See refs. 46, 70 for complete listing. [a] Meridional reflections have components from both the cross-bridge array and the backbone. A simple helix of cross bridges should have meridional reflections only at 14.3 and 7.15 nm. The other myosin meridional reflections are "forbidden." [b] Only high-order reflections (5.1 and 5.9 nm) can be seen in Fig. 3*A*. Intermediate reflections (12.2 and 18.2 nm) are very weak and lie outside the frame of Fig. 3*A* but can be seen in Fig. 12. [c] Doublets, coupled with a bracket, are thought to be reflections split because of interference effects between opposite halves of a sarcomere (118, 70). [d] The very sharp, strong reflection at 14.31 nm is usually used to calibrate film spacings. [e] This actin reflection is never seen by itself in relaxed muscle. A broad reflection with a spacing of about 40.0 nm is thought to be the superposition of the outer part of the 1st myosin layer line and the 1st actin layer line. The spacing of the 1st actin line is inferred from other measurements. Note that the first 3 actin layer lines are indexed as 2nd, 4th, and 6th order of 77 nm.

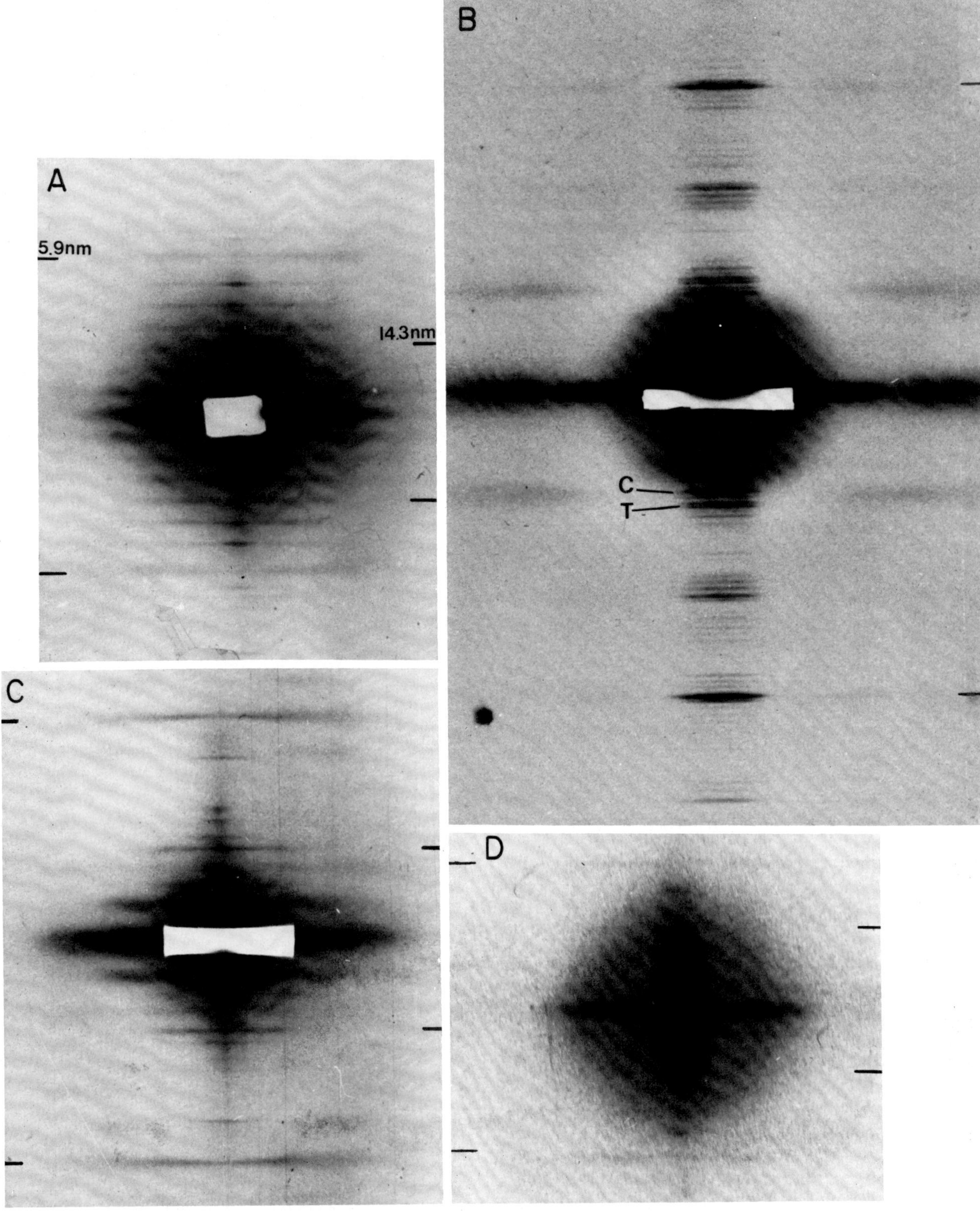

FIG. 3. Low-angle X-ray–diffraction patterns of frog sartorius muscles at rest length, displayed as if taken with muscle axis vertical. The vertical axis of symmetry is called the meridian; the horizontal axis is the equator. *Right* (in each picture), axial position of myosin meridional reflections (14.3 nm); *left*, axial position of actin layer line (5.9 nm). *A*: relaxed muscle. Pattern is dominated by layer lines arising from helical arrangement of cross bridges around myosin filament. *B*: relaxed muscle, meridional region (very low angle pattern). *T*, doublet near 38.5 nm arising from troponin repeat; *C*, doublet near 43.0 nm arising from C protein. *C*: rigor muscle. Relaxed myosin layer lines have disappeared, replaced by a new series of layer lines arising from cross bridges attached to actin. *D*: contracting muscle. The layer lines arising from myosin cross bridges are extremely weak and the pattern is dominated by layer lines from actin filament. [With permission from Haselgrove (46). Copyright by Academic Press Inc. (London) Ltd.]

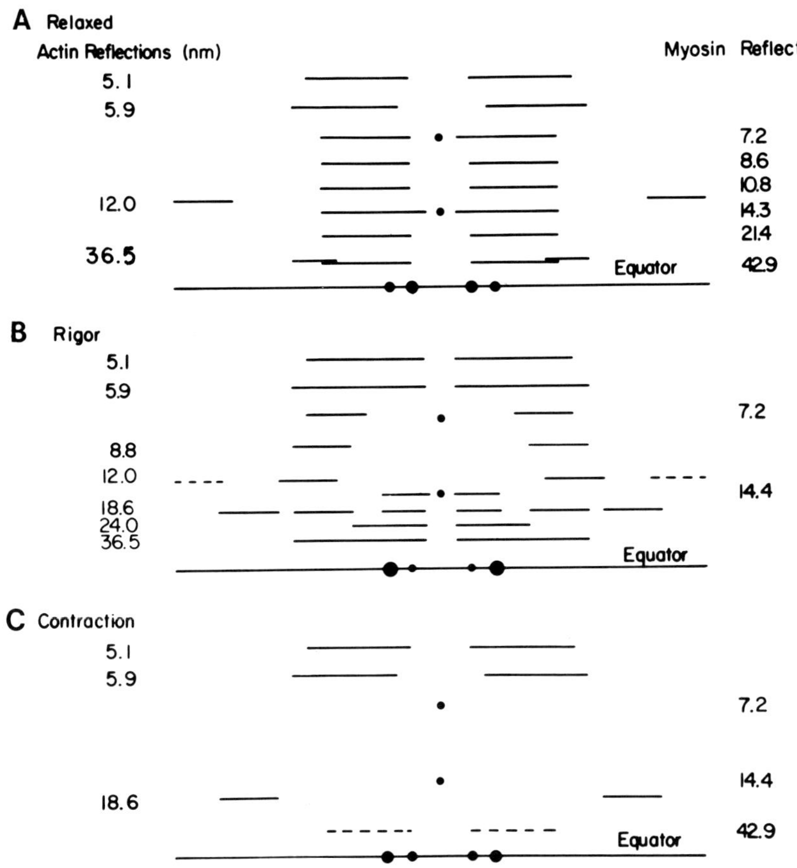

FIG. 4. Schematic representation of principal X-ray reflections from rest-length VSM. *Right*, spacings of myosin reflections; *left*, spacing of actin reflections. [From Haselgrove and Rodger (51).]

TABLE 2. *Principal Reflections in Low-Angle Diffraction Patterns of Rigor Frog Sartorius Muscle at Rest Length*

Meridian		Cross-Bridge Layer Lines*, nm	Actin Layer Lines†, nm
Protein source	Axial spacing, nm		
			5.1
			5.9
		6.9	
Myosin	7.2‡		
		8.8	
	10.18		
	11.08		
		12.2	12.2
Actin	12.75§		
Myosin/actin	14.45‡	14.45	
		18.6	18.6
Actin	19.2		
	21.2		
	22.7		
		24.18	
		36.5	36.5
Troponin	38.5		

Data laid out to simulate top right-hand quadrant of Fig. 3*C*. * These layer lines, visible in Fig. 3*C*, occur relatively close to the meridian and arise from cross bridges attached to the actin filament. † These layer lines occur farther from the meridian and also occur in live muscle. Low-angle reflections (12.2, 18.6, and 36.5 nm) are influenced by tropomyosin and troponin. They do not appear in Fig. 3*C* but can be seen in Fig. 12. ‡ Spacings of these reflections are both slightly but significantly greater than the corresponding ones in relaxed muscle. The 14.45-nm reflection is 0.85% ± 0.2% greater than the 14.31-nm reflection in relaxed muscle. The 7.2-nm reflection is 1.11% ± 0.3% greater than the corresponding 7.15-nm relaxed muscle reflection (46). § This reflection occurs even when cross bridges do not attach to actin, although in IFM it is interpreted as arising from the regularity of cross bridge–actin attachment.

reflections are usually identified by the periodicity in the muscle with which they correlate; thus the 14.3-nm meridional reflection arises from an axial period of 14.3 nm within the muscle.

EQUATOR. The horizontal axis of the pattern is termed the equator, and the equatorial reflections give information about the distribution of mass across the sarcomere. The positions of the distinct reflections are related to the type of lattice and the interfilament spacing, whereas the intensity depends on the distribution of mass between the filaments. Crystallographic nomenclature (Miller indices) is used to identify reflections, and each reflection is correlated with a series of repeating planes in the muscle, as shown schematically in Figure 5. For a hexagonal lattice, like that in VSM, the first three reflections are termed 1,0, 1.1, and 2.0, and they have relative spacings of 1, $\sqrt{3}$, and 2, respectively. Relative intensities from a rest-length live muscle are listed in Table 3.

LAYER LINES. The series of horizontal lines termed layer lines arise from the helical structure of the actin

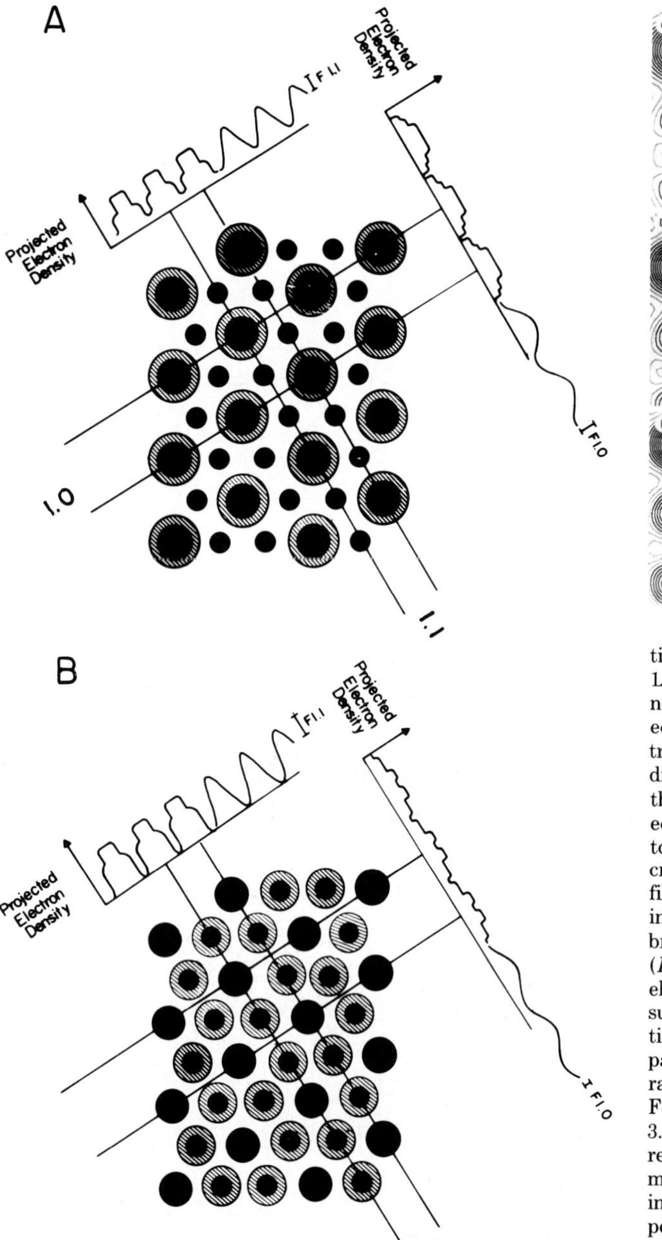

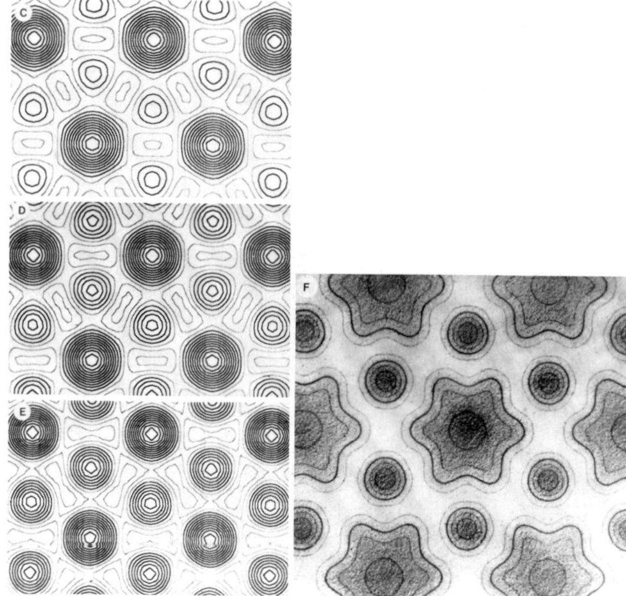

FIG. 5. Hexagonal filament lattice with myosin filaments at lattice positions, actin filaments at trigonal positions. (See also Fig. 1*A*.) *A* and *B*: different sets of planes have different crystallographic notations and their spacing determines the spacing of corresponding equatorial reflections. When the sarcomere's electron-density distribution is projected along the lattice planes, the resulting one-dimensional distribution can be described in terms of sine waves. the amplitude (F) of the fundamental sine wave (with a wavelength equal to the separation of the planes) controls and is proportional to the equatorial reflection amplitude for those planes. Transferring cross-bridge mass from the vicinity of thick filaments to that of thin filaments decreases intensity F^2 of the 1.0 reflection and increases intensity of the 1.1 reflection. Relaxed muscle (*A*): myosin cross bridges (*hatched area*) lie close to myosin filaments. Rigor muscle (*B*): myosin cross bridges lie close to actin filaments. *C, D, E*: radial electron-density maps for rest-length muscle constructed by Fourier summation from the amplitudes of the 1.0 and 1.1 equatorial reflections with phases of 0° for both reflections. Amplitudes taken from patterns of relaxed (*C*), contracting (*D*), and rigor (*E*) muscle. *F*: radial electron-density distribution of relaxed muscle calculated by Fourier summation; amplitudes calculated from intensities in Table 3. The 1.0, 1.1, and 3.0 reflections had phases of 0°; the 2.0 and 2.1 reflections had phases of 180°. Calculations assuming 6-fold symmetry gave rise to 6 projections, but no fine details can be usefully interpreted in terms of cross-bridge shape and postion. [*C–E* with permission from Haselgrove and Huxley (49). Copyright by Academic Press Inc. (London) Ltd.; *F* from Haselgrove et al. (52).]

and myosin filaments. The axial and radial positions of the layer lines are determined by the axial and radial parameters of the helix, whereas the intensity is governed both by the helix parameters and by the shape and position of the subunits. Since the actin and myosin helices have different parameters, the actin and myosin layer lines generally do not overlap and may often be distinguished by indexing. Two systems are currently in use for naming layer lines: in the first, one simply counts the observed lines starting at zero on the equator and in the second, one refers to the layer-line index based on the crystalline structure of the muscle. (Thus in insect rigor muscle, reflections on the first layer line have indices h, k, 3.) Note that the layer lines may have finite intensity on the meridian, and consequently the meridional component may be interpreted either as a layer-line component or as a meridional component; both interpretations are equivalent. Similarly the equator is technically the zero layer line and may be interpreted as such.

INTERPRETATION OF X-RAY PATTERNS

Theoretical Aspects

Any diffraction pattern can be interpreted analytically to yield the unique structure giving rise to the pattern only if both the amplitudes and the phases of each diffraction spot can be determined. Unfortunately one cannot measure the phases of the diffracted

TABLE 3. *Relative Intensities of Equatorial Reflections of Frog Sartorius Muscles*

Reflection	Intensity*
1.0	100
1.1	44
2.0	9
2.1, 1.2	9
3.0	12
2.2	20
3.1, 1.3	

* Values are for sarcomere length of 2.2 μm. Relative intensities of the 1.0 and 1.1 reflections are extremely sensitive to sarcomere length and muscle state (see Fig. 9). Higher-order reflections are very weak and close together; even mild amounts of lattice disorder cause them to merge and be invisible as in contracting and rigor muscle. It cannot be assumed therefore that their intensity decreases because of cross-bridge movement. [Data from Lymn (84).]

beams directly; this is the classic "phase problem" of X-ray crystallography. The techniques used by protein crystallographers for solution of the problem cannot yet be applied to muscle, and so one is forced to interpret the pattern inductively. Thus some prior knowledge of the structure of muscle derived from other sources is required, as well as a knowledge of the way the diffraction arises from different types of structures. It is sometimes possible to make a qualitative interpretation by inspection, although it is becoming increasingly necessary to perform quantitative model calculations by computer. The latter method must take into account all of the structural features affecting the pattern. [Vainshtein (165) provides a complete discussion of fiber diffraction, although Holmes and Blow (54) have written a simpler introduction.] An extended analysis of the structural features that affect the pattern is outside the scope of this chapter, but a list of some general relations between structure and X-ray patterns may be helpful.

1. Only structures organized as part of regular arrays contribute to the discrete reflections.
2. The dimensions and symmetry of the structural lattice govern the positions of the X-ray reflections, which can sometimes be measured with high accuracy. These reflections give information about the relative separation of the subunits in the muscle, although they do not directly give information about the absolute subunit positions within the muscle.
3. The intensities of the reflections are determined largely by the shape, size, and orientation of the subunits. Note that if the subunits at different parts of the array are not identical, then the X-ray–diffraction pattern depends on the average structure. If the structure changes with time, as in the moving cross bridges during contraction, the X-ray pattern gives the average structure over the recording time. Therefore the pattern corresponds to a space- and time-averaged picture. The intensity of the reflection is also affected by many other factors, including the number of subunits, the helix parameters, details of the type of lattice structure, and the amount of disorder.
4. Knowledge that a certain set of reflections comes from a helix with defined parameters does not necessarily indicate the identity of the helix or its function in the muscle. This information about the muscle must come from knowledge derived from other sources.

Low-angle equatorial reflections constitute a special case in the interpretation of the diffraction pattern. It has been argued that the phases of the low-angle equatorial reflections must be real (i.e., a phase angle of 0° or 180°) because the structure is probably centrosymmetric in projections (49, 52, 66, 84). Thus with a choice of only two possible phases for each equatorial reflection, it is easy to compute the transverse electron-density profiles in the muscle by Fourier summation with measured amplitudes and all possible phase combinations. Comparison of the Fourier maps with the electron-microscope pictures of transverse sections indicates that the phases of both the 1.0 and the 1.1 reflections must be 0° (see Fig. 5*C*). Inclusion of the higher-order reflections (Fig. 5*F*) brings more detail to the map but still not enough to allow identification of the shape or position of the cross bridges. From a theoretical standpoint it is not possible to investigate the detailed movement of cross bridges with diffraction data having, for the 3.0 reflection, a maximum resolution of only about 12 nm. At present, however, the equatorial reflections provide the best possible indication of the radial position of the cross bridges. By making assumptions about the absolute levels of electron density in the maps of Figure 5, it is possible to estimate the relative total electron-density mass associated with each filament. Changes in density coinciding with changes in muscle state may then be attributed to the transference of cross bridges between the region of myosin filaments and that of actin filaments. The investigator must then interpret the data in terms of attachment or detachment of cross bridges to actin.

Experimental Approaches

Extra information, derived principally from one of three sources, is required to interpret the X-ray–diffraction patterns: *1*) other techniques, such as electron microscopy, *2*) perturbing the muscle and watching the changes in the diffraction pattern, and *3*) comparative studies of different muscles .

OTHER TECHNIQUES. Electron microscopy and X-ray diffraction serve complementary functions in muscle structure studies. Electron micrographs are able to provide a general picture of the structure showing the filaments and their relative orientations. This information is then used in conjunction with the X-ray pattern, which is often able to give us accurate in vivo distance measurements of the filament fine structure, although the X-ray pattern itself does not unequivocally reveal the length and distribution of the filament in the muscle.

PERTURBATION. Perturbations of the muscle cause changes in the diffraction pattern. The most important physiological perturbation one can impart to the muscle is to change its state, causing alternation among the relaxed, contracting, and rigor modes. This can be somewhat of a bootstrap technique: it is necessary to perturb the muscle to confirm what one is looking at, and then by identifying what is seen, it is possible to interpret what was happening during perturbation. Changes in the main features of the diffraction pattern accompanying changes in muscle state, as well as a summary of interpretations of the changes, are shown in Table 4.

The living relaxed muscle is easily extended and generates no active force. Biochemically the sarcoplasm has a high level of ATP (approx. 5 mM), but no calcium. Thus cross bridges are inhibited from interacting with actin and no force develops. However, any treatment causing the release of Ca^{2+} into the sarcoplasm can induce contraction. Such treatments might include electrical stimulation or an increase in external potassium. The cross bridges, it is thought, then cyclically interact with actin, pulling the actin and myosin filaments past each other.

Three types of contraction are studied by X-ray diffraction. *1*) During isometric contraction the muscle generates tension without shortening. It is almost impossible experimentally to stimulate a whole muscle to contract without any length change unless sophisticated length-control systems are used (39); therefore a slight shortening of about 5% in X-ray studies has usually been considered isometric (49). *2*) In isotonic contraction the muscle shortens, usually with constant velocity, while pulling against a constant load. *3*) Insect flight muscle (IFM) operates in an oscillatory mode in which the muscle undergoes a maximum length change of about 5% but shortens and lengthens rapidly at frequencies of up to about 100 Hz (131).

Early X-ray studies of VSM (30, 49, 70) suffered from the problem that the muscles, fatigued during the experiments, gave patterns that contained reflections from both the relaxed and contracting parts of the muscle. Recent technical developments, however, have allowed patterns to be recorded rapidly from nonfatigued muscles, and quantitative results differed somewhat from those of earlier studies. Faruqi and H. E. Huxley (33) review recent technical developments, and this chapter also emphasizes later investigations.

The rigor state can be induced by a variety of techniques (49, 91, 138), including treatment with glycerol or Triton X-100, all of which deplete the muscle of ATP. In the absence of ATP all the cross bridges

TABLE 4. *Principal Features of X-Ray-Diffraction Patterns of Vertebrate Striated Muscles*

Feature of Pattern	State of Muscle			Interpretation of Pattern Change
	Relaxed	Contracting*	Rigor	
Intensity of myosin layer lines	Strong, 100%†	10%	Absent	Strong relaxed layer lines indicate helical ordering of xbs; xbs move on contraction and going into rigor
Intensity of 14.3-nm meridional reflection	Strong	Weak (varies)	Weak	Xbs and filaments well aligned in relaxed muscle; disorder weakens the reflection
Spacing of 14.3-nm reflection, nm	14.3	14.4	14.4	Increase in filament length or change in interference of diffraction from backbone and xb array
Intensity of 5.9- and 5.1-nm actin layer lines	100%†	120% ± 20%	Strong close to meridian	Xbs attach to actin during contraction and in rigor
Outer actin layer	2nd very weak 3rd weak	2nd strong 3rd very weak	2nd strong 3rd very weak	Change of position of tropomyosin in thin filament
Rigor layer lines	0%	≈0%	100%†	Xbs attach to actin and take up actin-helix positions in rigor
Equatorial ratio I1.0/I1.1 $s = 2.3$	2.93	0.45	0.31	Xbs move closer to actin-filament positions during contraction and rigor
Lattice spacing, nm	40	40	44	Contraction occurs with no change in lattice spacing; destruction of membrane allows expansion in rigor
Interpretation of pattern	Xbs well ordered on myosin filaments	Xbs move away from myosin-filament backbone and closer to actin; xb movement asynchronous; no direct evidence for attachment of xbs to actin	All xbs attached to actin filament in pseudocrystalline array	

Xbs, cross bridges; *s*, sarcomere length. * Steady state during peak tension development of tetanus. † Percentage figures refer to change of each reflection with state change. Different reflections have very different intensities.

that are sterically able to do so attach to the actin filaments, forming an extensive cross-linked structure. Thus the rigor muscle is inextensible, although it may be stretched about 1%–2% without breaking and made to sustain a tension. Those cross bridges that attach to actin in rigor are thought to attach all with the same orientation, corresponding to that at the end of the pulling stroke in the contraction cycle (88, 134). The rigor muscle is therefore an exceedingly useful tool in the interpretation of one state of the contraction cycle.

Scientists have recently produced biochemical analogues of ATP that cause all (or most) of the cross bridges to form steady-state complexes different from those of rigor. If most or all the cross bridges have the same configuration within a crystalline lattice, then the structure is suitable for X-ray-diffraction studies. Consequently there is much current interest in correlating the mechanical and biochemical states induced by these analogues.

One of the easiest perturbations to induce is a change in the sarcomere length (s) of the muscle. This enables investigators to study those features of the pattern that depend on the interaction of the cross bridges with adjacent actin filaments. Two reference lengths are frequently used. Rest length is the length of muscle in the living animal, which for a sartorius muscle is 2.2–2.3 μm. At this length all the cross bridges are able to interact with adjacent actin filaments (123). Nonoverlap length refers to any length above that at which the actin filaments stop just short of entering the A band (about 3.7 μm) so that none of the cross bridges are able to interact with actin filaments. Although one can gain much useful information by varying the value of s, the effects of sarcomere length on the equatorial reflections are so pronounced (Fig. 6; see also Fig. 9) that they can often mask the effects due to a change of state unless care is taken to record the muscle s value and the X-ray-diffraction pattern simultaneously. It is impossible to hold a whole muscle completely stationary during generation of isometric contraction, and small decreases in length contribute to changes in the equatorial pattern. The sarcomere lengths of the muscle can be measured with a high degree of accuracy by using a laser-diffraction system (44, 136). Light-diffraction patterns from muscles have attracted attention in the last few years, and investigators can apply X-ray-diffraction theories to light-diffraction patterns (142). Mechanical studies in which the muscle is stretched or allowed to shorten rapidly in periods of about 0.1 ms have proven enormously powerful in revealing certain details of cross-bridge action, but only very recently has experimental technology reached a state where X-ray data can be recorded with millisecond time resolution. (75).

COMPARATIVE STUDIES. Initially the mainstream of X-ray-diffraction studies concentrated on VSM because much complementary biochemical, structural, and mechanical work has been performed with these muscles. The rabbit psoas muscle is the typical striated muscle for biochemical work, but the muscle is difficult to keep alive in a form suitable for X-ray studies. Frog sartorius and semitendinosus muscles, used extensively for mechanical studies, are excellent for X-ray work, however. Since there appear to be no major differences in the structure of rabbit and frog muscles, the latter is usually considered to be a typical VSM from a structural viewpoint. Only the equatorial patterns (see Fig. 9) differ, and the variance probably

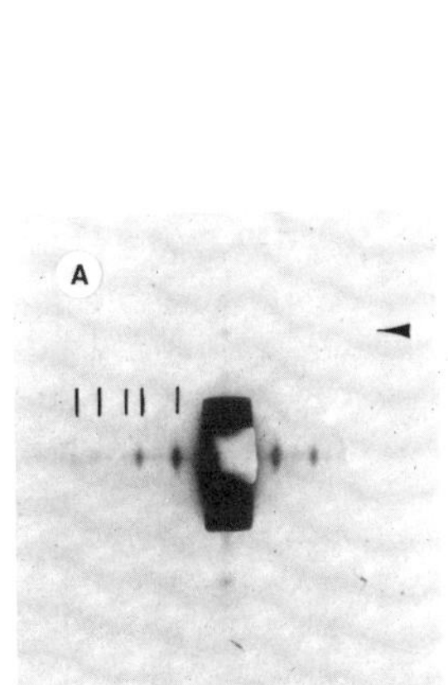

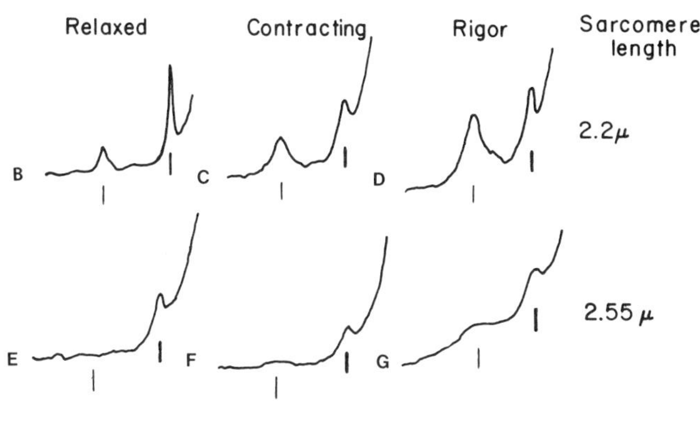

FIG. 6. *A*: equatorial diffraction pattern of relaxed frog sartorius muscle at rest length, showing the first 5 equatorial reflections arising from the filament lattice. From *right* to *left* from the origin, they are 1.0, 1.1, 2.0, 2.1, 3.0. A weak reflection lying between 1.0 and 1.1 is attributed to the Z line (183). Relative reflection intensities are shown in Table 3. *Center*, meridional reflection at 14.3 nm is indicated. To *right* of backstop, higher-order reflections obscured by part of the camera. *B–G*: densitometer tracings from equator of relaxed, contracting, and rigor muscles at different sarcomere lengths. *Thick line*, 1.0 reflection; *thin line*, 1.1 reflection. Tracings are not all to the same vertical scale. [*A* from Haselgrove et al. (48), © 1977 by The Institute of Physics. *B–G* with permission from Haselgrove and Huxley (49). Copyright by Academic Press Inc. (London) Ltd.]

arises solely from a difference in muscle filament lengths. The oscillatory, asynchronous mode of operation of IFM is very different from that of VSM and has proven useful for mechanical and structural studies (160). At present it is the system of choice for X-ray–diffraction studies of the action of ATP analogues because the muscle structure is so highly crystalline.

Many other muscle types from a variety of animal species have been studied by X-ray diffraction. This chapter explicitly describes the use of the VSM structure and refers without comment to studies of different muscle types in which results were the same as those for VSM. Often an understanding of the VSM system occurred as a result of research on other systems. Cases where different muscle types give different X-ray–diffraction data are discussed separately, however, so that both differences and similarities between these and VSM may be seen. Cardiac muscle X-ray–diffraction studies are discussed in a recent review by Matsubara (97).

FILAMENT LATTICE

In striated muscles the myosin filaments are ordered laterally at the points of a hexagonal lattice, and the actin filaments are positioned at the trigonal positions of the lattice between three myosin filaments (see Figs. 1 and 5). The spacing of the filaments in the lattices gives rise to Bragg lattice sampling of the X-ray pattern along the equator (see Fig. 6) and in some cases along the layer lines too [see Fig. 8; (70)]. Three features of the lattice may be distinguished by X-ray diffraction: *1*) the lattice spacing, *2*) the rotational orientation of the filaments about their own axes, and *3*) the radial distribution of electron density between the filaments.

Lattice Spacing

Although the hexagonal symmetry of the lattice may be seen directly in electron micrographs, its confirmation in vivo comes from the relative spacings of the equatorial reflections. The reflections have relative spacings from the origin of 1, $\sqrt{3}$, and 2, corresponding to those for a hexagonal lattice (62). The spacing of the first reflection (1.0) can be measured with an accuracy of about 1%; thus the average myosin-to-myosin filament separation (lattice spacing) can be calculated accurately also. Lattice spacing (d) can vary between about 20 and 50 nm and depends on a variety of parameters, some of which are described here.

It is often convenient and instructive to calculate the cross-sectional area ($\sqrt{3/2}d^2$) and the volume ($\sqrt{3/2}d^2s$) of the lattice unit cell bounded by four adjacent myosin filaments and their projections to the Z lines. The filament lattice behaves like a colloidal system in which the total volume is restricted by an external bounding membrane. The interplay of all the parameters affecting the lattice volume is being extensively studied, and the general effect of each of the following parameters is known.

FIBER VOLUME. The lattice spacing of an intact fiber is about 15% smaller than the equilibrium spacing of a skinned fiber in equivalent ionic conditions [Fig. 7; (2, 5)]. The lattice in the intact fiber is constrained by the fiber membrane to a volume about 30% less than the intrinsic value, and the lattice expands to fill the available space. The fiber membrane, the sarcolemma, behaves like an elastic, semipermeable membrane: fiber volume, and hence lattice volume, is decreased in hyperosmotic media and increased by about 20% in hyposmotic media (15, 34). Similar effects can be produced in skinned muscle fibers by use of solutions with high osmotic strengths containing large polymers that do not enter the filament lattice (91, 113).

SARCOMERE LENGTH. When VSM is stretched to lengths not normally achieved in vivo the lattice becomes increasingly disordered, although the order recovers again with time (46, 68). In a living intact fiber, the lattice volume, like the volume of the whole fiber, is independent of sarcomere length (2, 3, 31, 62, 98). Lattice spacing decreases, however, as sarcomere length increases so that d^2s = constant (see Fig. 7*A*). When the cell membrane is removed, d again varies inversely with s, but the lattice volume is generally not independent of sarcomere length (6, 98). The exact form of the relationship between d and s depends on the ionic conditions of the bathing medium.

IONIC CONDITIONS. Theoretical analysis of colloidal filament lattices indicates that the separation of the filaments in a nonbounded (skinned) fiber is governed by a balance of electrostatic repulsive forces between filaments and van der Waals attractive forces (28, 110). Filament separation thus depends on factors that influence the effects of the charges on the filaments. Lattice spacing possesses a complex dependence on pH and ionic strength [see Fig. 7*B*; (5, 136, 137)].

STATE OF THE MUSCLE. There is no significant change in the lattice spacing of muscles upon contraction. Early studies reported a slight decrease in spacing, but such decreases have since been shown to be experimental artifacts (30, 49). The force generated by each cross bridge seems to be independent of the filament separation, at least in the range of separations experienced in muscle (4). Muscles in rigor have lattice spacings about 10% greater than those in live muscles (44, 66), but this may be because the fiber membranes are no longer intact in rigor muscle.

The inverse relationship between sarcomere length and lattice spacing has given rise to many theories suggesting that the contraction force is not caused by axial force along the filaments per se but rather by a lateral expanding force that is transformed into an axial shortening force by the inherent constancy of the lattice volume (32, 145, 164). However, it seems nec-

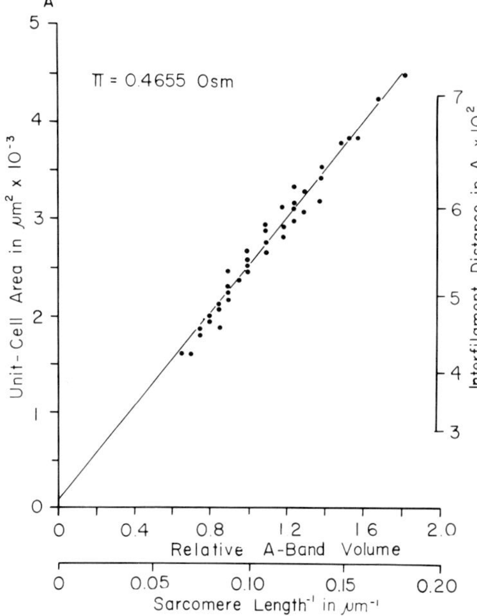

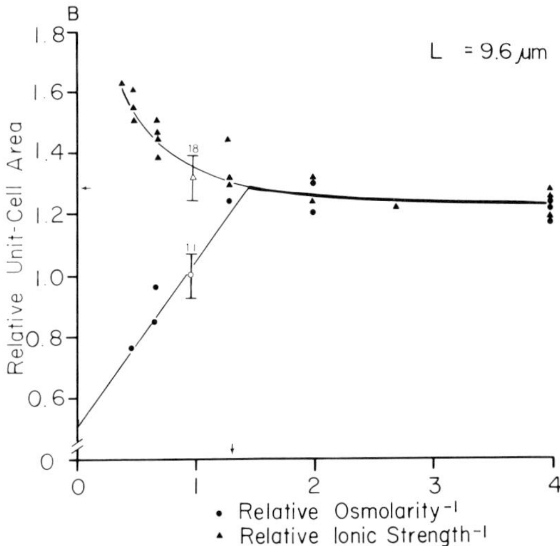

FIG. 7. *A*: relation between myosin-filament spacing (d) and sarcomere length (s) in intact living muscle fiber. Data fit a line of the form $d^2 \propto 1/s$. Thus lattice volume is independent of sarcomere length. *B*: comparison of filament lattice behavior of intact and skinned fibers. The lattice is constrained by the membrane in intact living fiber. *Filled circles*, relative unit cell areas of living intact fibers plotted against the inverse of the osmolarity of the bathing medium; *filled triangles*, area of skinned fibers plotted against the inverse of the corresponding ionic strength. *Open symbols*, mean values for muscles in normal physiological conditions. [*A* from April (3); *B* from April (2).]

essary that the lattice not be subject to external lateral constraints so that a lateral force can cause the lattice to expand transversely and simultaneously decrease in length. However, these theories are difficult to reconcile with the observation that the lattice is restricted by the surface membrane.

The positions occupied by the actin filaments in the myosin lattice vary from muscle to muscle and correlate with the ratio of the number of actin and myosin filaments. Vertebrate striated muscle has two actin filaments per myosin (see Figs. 1 and 5). In IFM, which has three actin filaments per myosin, the actin filaments are located at the diad positions of the lattice between two myosin filaments (see Fig. 16), whereas in certain invertebrate striated muscles there are sufficient actin filaments to form rings around the myosins. The lattice spacing varies considerably from muscle to muscle, but a common lattice feature is that the distance from the surface of the myosin-filament backbone to the surface of adjacent actin filaments is approximately the same in all muscles, i.e., about 8–15 nm. This presumably reflects the range of distances from myosin to actin over which the cross bridge can reach and still generate tension. In many smooth muscles the actin filaments pack together in square arrays containing no myosin filaments but giving a single strong equatorial reflection (80, 166). The actin-to-actin separation is about 12 nm and is independent of the length of the muscle.

Filament Orientations

The Bragg sampling of the layer lines in relaxed VSM indicates that the filaments have well-defined axial and azimuthal orientations (64). In relaxed VSM the radial positions at which layer lines are sampled are different from those of the equator, indicating that myosin filaments are not all aligned equivalently (Fig. 8). Two types of lattice have been described that would account for such sampling. One is a superlattice in which adjacent myosin filaments are rotated azimuthally by a value of $2\pi/3N$ (N = the rotational symmetry of the filament) with respect to each other so that no two adjacent myosin filaments are similarly oriented (70). Luther and Squire (83) deduced the second lattice from the observed orientations of the triangular profiles of the myosin filament seen in electron micrographs of transverse sections. In this model the myosin filaments can be in one or two orientations 180° apart, forming a pseudosuperlattice.

There is no evidence that actin filaments in VSM have any specific orientation. Indeed, compared with the myosin filaments, they seem poorly oriented (30, 49). The effect of sarcomere length on equatorial intensities of relaxed muscle shows that the actin filaments are very poorly ordered in the I band of the sarcomere and are only positioned at the trigonal positions of the myosin-filament lattice within the A band (31). In contrast, when actin filaments pack in the actin–filament lattice of smooth muscles, they sometimes do so with a high degree of axial and azimuthal correlation between filaments. This causes the 5.9-nm actin layer line to be well sampled (80, 166). The actin and myosin filaments in IFM are highly ordered translationally and rotationally; therefore at low resolution the whole lattice can be assigned a crystallographic space group—$P6_4$ or $P6_2$ (56), or $P6_1$ or $P6_5$ (176).

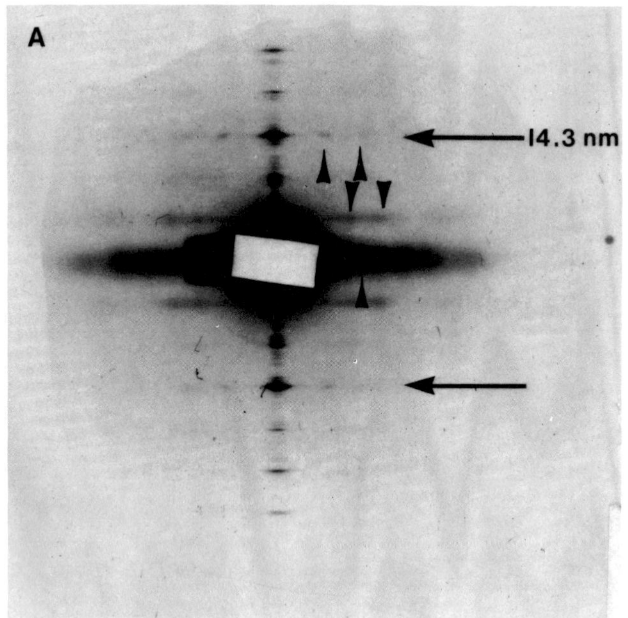

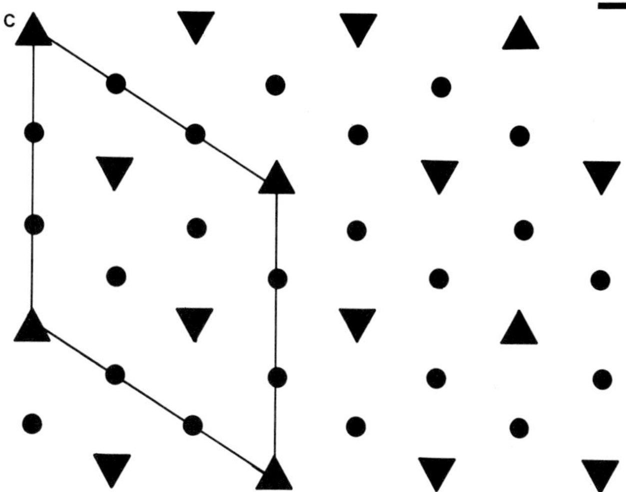

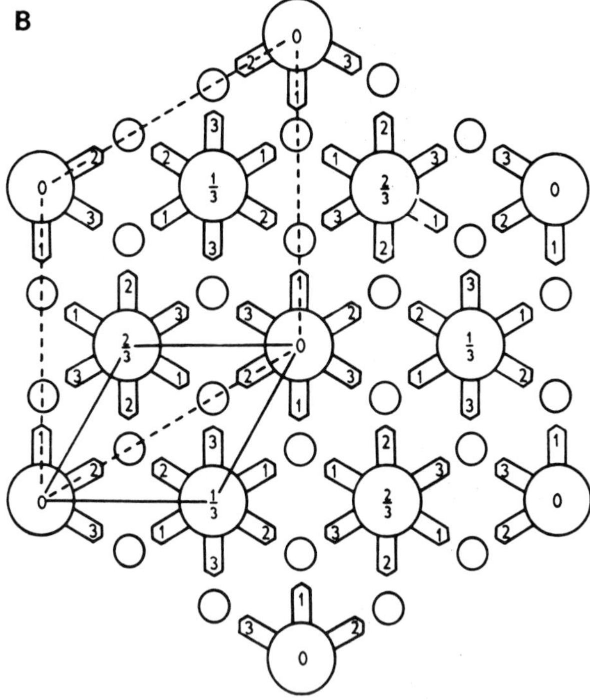

FIG. 8. *A*: X-ray pattern showing myosin layer lines in relaxed muscle sampled by Bragg reflections, *arrows*, from the myosin-filament lattice. Sampling on 1st and 2nd layer lines occurs at different radial positions from the equator and 3rd layer line, indicating that the lattice is not a simple one with all myosin filaments having the same orientation. *B*: superlattice proposed by H.E. Huxley and Brown to explain the X-ray sampling. (This illustration is for a 2-stranded filament, but the logic may be applied to filaments of any symmetry.) Numbers on the cross bridges represent the level (in steps of 14.3 nm) along the filament at which the cross bridges project in the direction shown. Nearest neighbors are rotated through ⅓ or ⅔ revolution with respect to each other. Superlattice, *broken line*, links adjacent filaments with the same orientation. In cross section, myosin filaments have triangular profiles and on such a superlattice all triangles would point in the same direction. *C*: Squire's superlattice in which filaments face in only 2 directions. [*A* from Haselgrove et al. (48); *B* with permission from Huxley and Brown (70). Copyright by Academic Press Inc. (London) Ltd.; *C* adapted from Luther and Squire (83).]

Radial Electron-Density Distribution

The intensities of the equatorial reflections are determined by the electron-density distribution of the sarcomere when projected along the muscle filament axis. The dominant features of the sarcomere contributing to the transverse distribution of electron density are the length and position of the myosin filament backbone, the position of the actin filament in the lattice, and the distribution of the cross bridges in the space between the filament backbones. At the level of resolution of the first two reflections (1.0 and 1.1), one observes that whenever the amount of electron-dense material around the positions of the actin filaments rises with respect to that around the myosin filament, the 1.0 reflection's intensity decreases as that of the 1.1 reflection increases (see Fig. 5). As the sarcomere length of the muscle decreases, the relative intensities of the 1.0 and the 1.1 reflections (I1.0/I1.1) decrease as shown in Figure 9 (see also Fig. 6). This is true for all muscle states, and it indicates that the actin filaments are ordered at the trigonal positions of the lattice within the A band but are disordered within the I band (31, 49, 66). Distribution of the cross bridges across the sarcomere is described under CROSS BRIDGES, p. 160.

The varying positions of actin filaments in the lattices of different muscles give a wide range of equatorial reflection densities. In IFM the actin filaments occupy diad positions between two myosin filaments. The 1.1 reflection is almost absent, although the 2.0 reflection is strong (36, 107, 109).

ACTIN-CONTAINING FILAMENTS

The structure of the thin, actin-containing filaments is remarkably well conserved in all muscles. The G-actin monomers are arranged to form a right-handed,

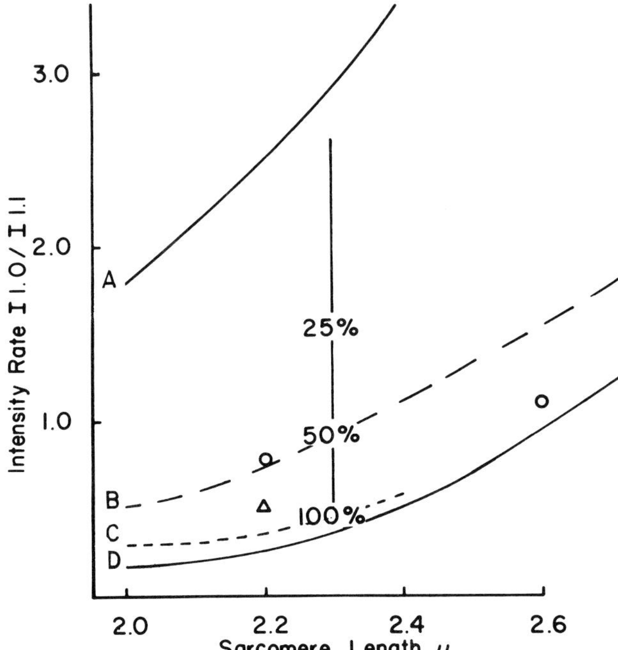

FIG. 9. Plot of equatorial intensity ratio I1.0/I1.1 for different muscle states. All data are for frog striated muscle except the *open circles* for live relaxed rabbit psoas muscle. [From Huxley (66).] *A*, relaxed living muscle; *B* and *C*, isometrically contracting muscle; *D*, rigor muscle. *Vertical line*, ratios depend on tension for muscles that, although contracting isometrically, generate only a fraction of the maximum isometric tension. Tensions of 0%, 25%, 50%, and 100% are shown (182). *Open triangle*, isometric contraction (105). Two reflections arise from lattice planes across the muscle (see Fig. 5). Ratio I1.0/I1.1 falls when electron density at actin position relative to myosin position rises. This occurs *1*) if actin filaments are more ordered at short as opposed to long sarcomere lengths or *2*) if cross bridges move from the myosin-filament region to that of actin when the muscle contracts or passes into rigor. [Data for *A*, *B*, *D* from Haselgrove and Huxley (49); data for *C* from Podolsky et al. (129).]

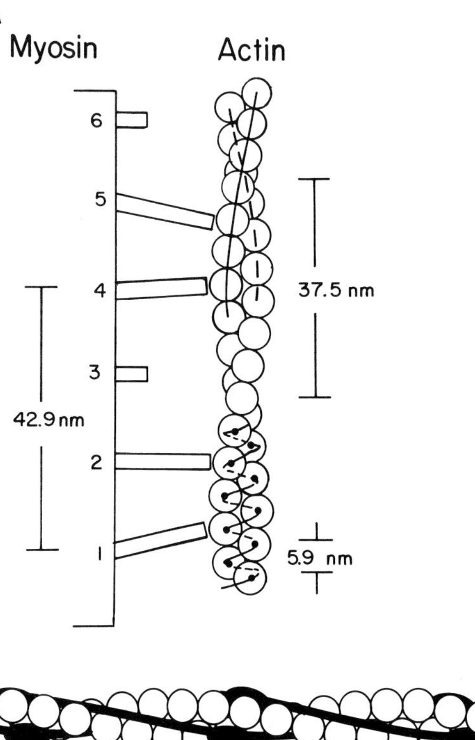

FIG. 10. *A*: the actin helix may be considered either a two-stranded structure with a half-pitch of about 37.5 nm (*top* part of helix) or a single-stranded genetic helix with a pitch of about 5.9 nm (*lower* part). Because the pitches of the actin and myosin helices are different in VSM, actin-myosin interaction does not repeat exactly; note the difference in attachment geometry between the 1st and 4th cross bridges. Here only the helical structure of the actin filament is emphasized, although attachment positions of myosin cross bridges to actin are determined by the helical structures of both filaments. *B*: structure of the actin filament with tropomyosin and troponin. [*A* adapted from Haselgrove and Reedy (50).]

two-stranded, helical filament of F actin that has a pitch of about 77 nm and a diameter of about 8 nm [Fig. 10; (22, 43)]. Because the structure is two-stranded, the whole filament has an apparent repeat of one-half the helix pitch of each strand. Thus one may say that an actin helix has a pitch of 77.0 nm or a pitch of 2 × 38.5 nm. Tropomyosin binds to actin in the groove of the actin double helix (43, 114). One troponin molecule binds to each tropomyosin molecule, and the binding of calcium to each troponin molecule is responsible for regulating the interaction of all the actin molecules of that section of the helix with myosin (24, 170). Conventionally the term *actin filament* describes the filament containing only actin, whereas the term *thin filament* is used for the structure containing actin, tropomyosin, and troponin.

Helix Parameters

Although the actin filament is conveniently described as a two-stranded structure, it may also be described as a single-stranded genetic helix (see Fig. 10). The latter is more convenient for the mathematical prediction of the diffraction pattern. Conceptually, however, it is not as useful for investigating the positions at which the cross bridges can attach to actin. Therefore the two-stranded description is more common and is used here.

The diffraction pattern from such a filament is shown schematically in Figure 11, and some low-angle layer lines are visible in patterns from VSM (see Fig. 12). A strong meridional reflection at 2.73 nm, outside the fields of Figures 3 and 12, represents the axial spacing of the G-actin monomers (70). A distance of 5.46 nm separates the monomers axially along each strand of the filament, and the monomers on each strand are displaced axially by half that value, 2.73 nm, with respect to the other strand. One can derive the long double-helix pitch by measuring the separation of the layer lines near 5.1 and 5.9 nm or from the spacing of the first low-angle line of the series [see Fig. 11; (70, 112, 143, 171)]. Because all these lines are diffuse, accurate measurement of the helix pitch is impossible, but the best estimates from X-ray patterns indicate that the pitch of VSM lies between 36.5 and 37.5 nm (70). The actin-filament pitch measured by

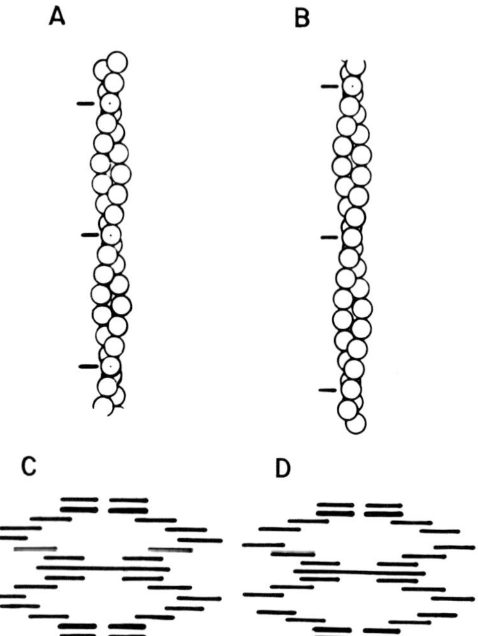

FIG. 11. *A* and *B*: diagrams of two actin filaments with different axial repeats. *A* repeats after 2 × 35.5 nm whereas *B* repeats after 2 × 40.9 nm. Superficially the filaments appear very similar, but differences are clear if one holds the page at eye level and sights from *left* to *right*. *C* and *D*: low-angle diffraction patterns anticipated from the structures of *A* and *B*, respectively. By sighting across the page one can see that changes in the long helix pitch make only very slight changes in layer-line positions. Since layer lines tend to be broad parallel to the meridian it is impossible to measure their axial spacing with any accuracy or, therefore, to obtain a reliable measure of the long helix pitch to an accuracy of better than ~3% (2 × 1 nm in 2 × 38.5 nm).

electron microscope is sensitive to the method of filament preparation and can vary between 35 and 40 nm (40).

The biochemical binding stoichiometry of troponin and tropomyosin to actin indicates that there is one troponin and one tropomyosin for every seven actin monomers, i.e., every 7 × 5.46 nm [see Fig. 10; (149, 150, 170)]. Electron-microscope evidence that troponin has an axial spacing of about 38.5 nm was confirmed for VSM by direct demonstration that antibodies to troponin enhance the intensity of an X-ray-pattern meridional doublet having a spacing of about 38.5 nm [see Fig. 3*B*; (122, 140)]. Therefore the axial repeat of the troponin-tropomyosin complex is not the same as the half-pitch of the helix (36.5 nm). In some invertebrate muscles the troponin complex affects the X-ray layer lines in a detectable way (89, 176), and the half-pitch of 38.5 nm in the actin filament exactly matched that of the troponin-tropomyosin repeat. Unlike those in VSM, these actin filaments probably have a true crystallographic repeat equal to the actin pitch: a period consists of exactly 14 G-actin subunits along each strand, and the genetic helix is thus an integral 28/15 helix (108, 176).

Thin-Filament Regulation of Contraction

The second actin layer line in patterns from relaxed muscle is somewhat weaker than predicted from the helix of actin monomers alone, and the effect is due to the presence of tropomyosin, which is positioned much closer to one chain of actin monomers than to the other [see Fig. 13; (45, 68, 114, 124, 149)]. The actin

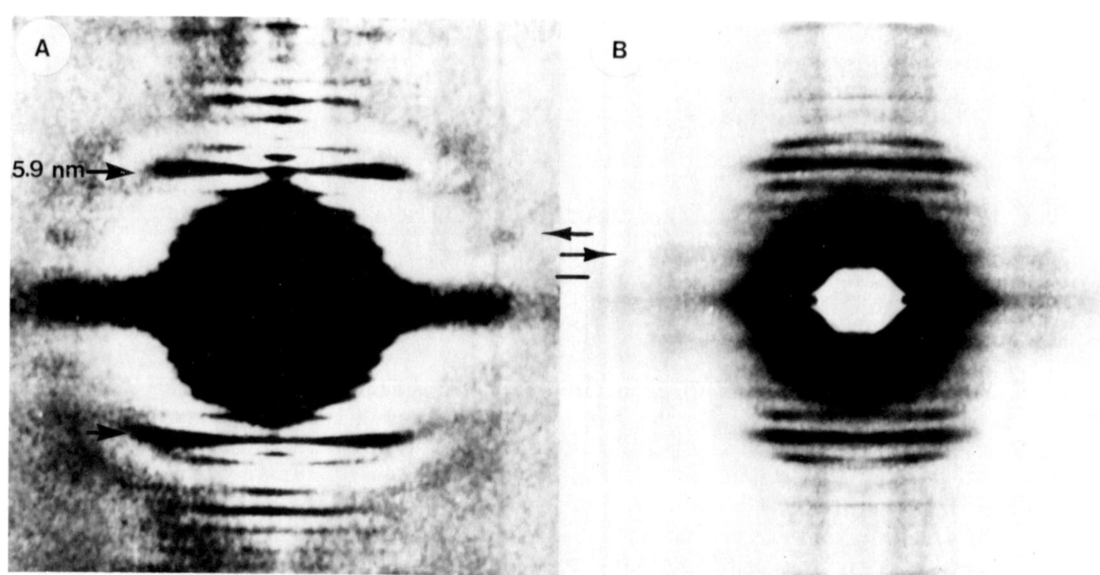

FIG. 12. X-ray patterns printed by enhancement technique [see (166)] to show actin-filament layer lines (cf. Fig. 11). Positions of first 3 layer lines, influenced by tropomyosin, are marked between the 2 patterns. *A*: relaxed muscle; 3rd layer line is stronger than 2nd because tropomyosin molecule is positioned near the edge of the actin groove (see also Fig. 13). *B*: rigor muscle; 2nd layer line is stronger than 3rd because tropomyosin has moved nearer to center of groove. [From Vibert et al. (166). Copyright by Academic Press Inc. (London) Ltd.]

layer lines are so weak and diffuse that it is impossible to make accurate quantitative intensity measurements of the intensity changes that occur when the muscle contracts or passes into rigor (Fig. 12). The second layer line, barely visible in relaxed muscle, becomes more intense than the third layer line in a contracting or rigor muscle (45, 68, 166, 167). Similar changes are seen at nonoverlap sarcomere lengths as well as in many different muscle types (45, 81, 166, 167). Furthermore, X-ray-diffraction studies of actin–filament gels show that in the absence of tropomyosin the pattern resembles the actin layer line of relaxed muscle but that in the presence of tropomyosin the pattern resembles the contracting pattern (42). The latter led researchers to relate the changes in the X-ray pattern to the presence of tropomyosin in the filament, whereas computer-modeling studies indicated that the changes in the intensity of the layer lines could be produced just by moving the tropomyosin molecules from the edge to the center of the helix groove (45, 68, 124).

Optical diffraction and image analysis of electron micrographs of thin filaments confirmed the X-ray interpretation. In conditions corresponding to relaxed muscle the tropomyosin is close to one strand of actin monomers, whereas in conditions correlating with active muscle it is near the center of the groove [see Fig. 13; (169)]. Low-angle layer lines in optical-diffraction patterns of actin paracrystals formed with or without calcium showed qualitative changes similar to those in X-ray patterns (35).

Between 1970 and 1972, when the movement of tropomyosin was first recognized, electron-microscope techniques were unable to image both the myosin subfragment 1 (S1) and the tropomyosin on actin simultaneously or to determine their relative positions from the X-ray patterns. By assuming that the tropomyosin and S1 both bind to sites on the same side of the actin monomers, however, investigators developed the attractively simple steric-block model for actin-filament activation (45, 68, 124). In this model tropomyosin in relaxed muscle covers the site on actin to which myosin S1 binds, and on activation of the filament the tropomyosin is moved out of the way—presumably by troponin when it binds Ca^{2+}. The model offers a simple explanation for how the binding of calcium to a single troponin molecule can regulate the action of seven actin monomers. Although activation of the filaments undoubtedly results in a shift in the position of tropomyosin, the validity of the steric-blocking mechanism in its simple formulation is uncertain; similar X-ray changes are seen during the contraction of muscles that are myosin regulated and contain little troponin (81, 166). It is therefore quite possible that the tropomyosin sits on the opposite side of the actin groove from the S1 binding site and that regulation is an allosteric effect (Fig. 13*B*). Recent electron-microscope studies have attempted to resolve this problem. They indicate that both the tropomyosin and the S1 are positioned on the opposite side of the filament from where they were originally thought to be; therefore the S1 does reach around to meet the tropomyosin [Fig. 13*C*; (157)]. Researchers believe that a steric effect operating between the cross bridge and tropomyosin may be involved in the control of actin-myosin interaction, but the details of the mechanism are not yet fully understood.

The X-ray data for VSM indicate that there is no change in the helix pitch when the muscle is activated and enters the rigor state (46, 70). Calcium causes a slight increase in pitch in paracrystalline specimens observed in the electron microscope (35), but the helix pitch measured by microscopy is known to depend on ionic conditions (40). X-ray studies of crab striated muscles, however, indicate that at the onset of rigor the actin-helix pitch increases from 36.5 to 38.5 nm (90).

MYOSIN-FILAMENT BACKBONE

The gross structure of the thick myosin-containing filaments differs significantly from muscle to muscle, although the surface lattice of the backbone from which cross bridges project is very similar in different muscles. This suggests that there are probably some general principles controlling how all myosin molecules pack when forming filaments (151–153). A common feature seems to be that the heads of the molecules project from the filament in a surface lattice to form cross bridges that project every 14.3 nm axially and are separated by about 10.0 nm transversely. The chapter by Pepe in this *Handbook* describes the structure of the myosin filament, and although the details of packing are not yet known, several schemes have been proposed (125, 126, 153). Basic features, however, such as the exact number of myosin heads projecting every 14.3 nm at each "crown," need further investigation. Myosin is not the only constituent of thick filaments—VSM contains C protein as well (119, 121). The myosin of invertebrate muscles is packed around a core of paramyosin.

Axial Packing of Myosin

The strong meridional reflections with spacings of 14.3 and 7.2 nm [see Fig. 3; (27, 62)] have been positively identified as myosin reflections because they appear in diffraction patterns from light meromyosin filaments (156). Cross bridges also contribute to this reflection because the axial positions of the cross bridges are governed by the backbone structure. Although the 14.3-nm reflection is a general indication of a regular subunit axial spacing of 14.3 nm, there is some evidence that the cross bridges are grouped so that the true axial repeat is 42.9 nm (111, 180). In VSM there is a slight increase of about 1% in the spacing of these two meridional reflections at 14.3 and 7.2 nm when the muscle contracts or passes into rigor

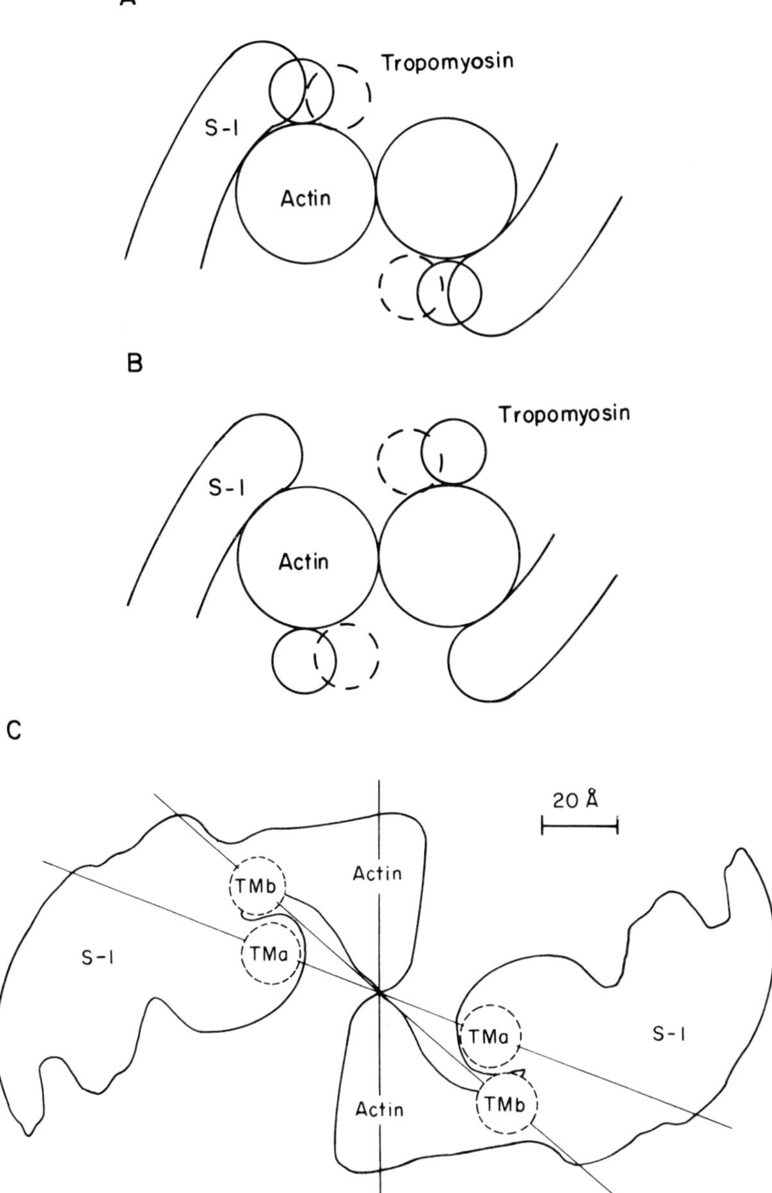

FIG. 13. Schematic diagrams illustrating movement of tropomyosin when thin filaments are activated, and possible correlation to myosin S1–actin binding. All diagrams drawn as if looking along the filament from M line to Z line. *A* and *B*: the 3-D reconstruction data of Moore et al. indicate that myosin S1 binds on each filament strand approximately as shown. X-ray data show that tropomyosin moves toward the center of the helix groove when the relaxed filament (*solid circle* position) is activated (*broken circle* position); X-ray data, however, cannot be used to determine on which side of the filament tropomyosin sits. One is, therefore, unable to distinguish between 2 possible geometries, *A* and *B*. *A*, original steric-blocking mechanism; *B*, tropomyosin position as deduced by Seymour and O'Brien. In the latter model, tropomyosin position cannot control S1. *C*: recent data indicating that S1 probably extends to a position where tropomyosin can physically prevent attachment. TMa, position of tropomyosin in activated muscle; TMb, position in relaxed muscle. [*C* with permission from Taylor and Amos (157). Copyright by Academic Press Inc. (London) Ltd.]

[see Tables 1 and 2; (44, 46, 70, 100)]. In rigor the change occurs whether or not the cross bridges are able to interact with actin, and H.E. Huxley (69) reports that during contraction the change precedes the development of tension. It is not yet known, however, whether this change in spacing is due to a real increase in filament length preceding tension development—with possible implications about the myosin-filament activation (44)—or whether it is an artifact caused by interference effects between the X rays diffracted from the filament backbone and those diffracted by the cross bridges (139). In the latter case, cross-bridge movement might affect the apparent spacing despite no real spacing change in the filament.

Meridional reflections near 14.4 and 72.2 nm in the myosin-filament diffraction pattern are a universal muscle feature (70, 79, 82, 109, 111, 146, 151, 172, 175). The exact spacing varies slightly from muscle to muscle but is always in the range of 14.3–14.6 nm, and this reflection has been used as a diagnostic indicator of the presence of myosin filaments in smooth muscles where they cannot always be detected by electron microscopy. Vertebrate cardiac muscle is the only other muscle in which a change in the spacing of this reflection has been reported (100).

Helical Packing of Myosin

A large part of what is known about the helical packing of myosin molecules in the backbone of the filament is suggested by the distribution of cross bridges on the filament surface. These cross bridges give rise to the series of layer lines, shown in Figure 14, that index as orders of 42.9 nm (see also Fig. 3*A*) and have the strongest meridional reflection at 14.3 nm (27, 70). Thus one can immediately determine two features of the cross-bridge surface lattice. *1*) The mean axial spacing between subunits is given by the meridional spacing, 14.3 nm, and *2*) the axial repeat of the whole structure is that of the layer lines, 42.9 nm. A whole family of surface lattices, each with a different rotational symmetry, fits these conditions (152, 154); three such lattices are shown in Figure 14. Note that the axial repeat (A) of the whole structure is related to its rotational symmetry (N) and to the pitch of one strand of the helix (P) by the relationship A = P/N. It is important in the function of striated muscle that the subunit repeat and the helix repeat are not rational fractions of the actin-helix parameters; therefore at any sarcomere length there are always some cross bridges that interact optimally with actin, while others do not (70).

The rotational symmetry of the filament is unknown. Evidence from a variety of biochemical and biophysical techniques indicates that there are either three (23, 78, 94, 106, 130, 163) or four (76, 96, 116, 127) myosin molecules for each crown of cross bridges, every 14.3 nm along the filament. It is not yet possible to choose unambiguously among models proposing two-, three-, or fourfold symmetry; the X-ray pattern may be satisfactorily interpreted by using any of these models (47, 154).

Simple surface lattices like those in Figure 14*B–D* would only give meridional reflections at orders of 14.3 nm, and thus the presence of forbidden reflections on the meridian with spacing near 42.9, 21.6, and 11.0 nm, etc. (see Tables 1 and 2) indicates that the surface cross-bridge lattice cannot be a simple lattice like those shown in any of the diagrams (see Fig. 14). Indeed the lattice is not unmodified from the H zone to the end of the filament: one of the cross-bridge crowns is missing where the filament tapers at the end (18, 19). This absence cannot account for the forbidden reflections, however, and some researchers have suggested that the axial cross-bridge repeat is not a regular 14.3 nm but rather that successive periods are 16.1, 16.1, and 10.7 nm (111, 180), thus retaining the axial periodicity of 42.3 nm (see Fig. 14*E–F*).

The shape and size of myosin filaments vary greatly between different muscle types, but the myosin molecules always pack so that the cross bridges project from the backbone to form lattices basically similar to the VSM lattice (151). In certain invertebrate muscles, backbone reflections may be distinguished from cross-bridge reflections, and intensity distributions along the layer lines indicate that the myosin molecules are packed into cables that are then wrapped together to form the filament backbone (173). In crustacean muscles the cables are wrapped to form a cylinder with a hollow core, although in vertebrate muscle the filament backbone is solid. The thick-filament core in arthropod catch muscles is made of the protein paramyosin. Myosin packs on the surface of these paramyosin-filament cores in a well-defined Bear-Selby surface lattice (13) in which the successive nodes occur

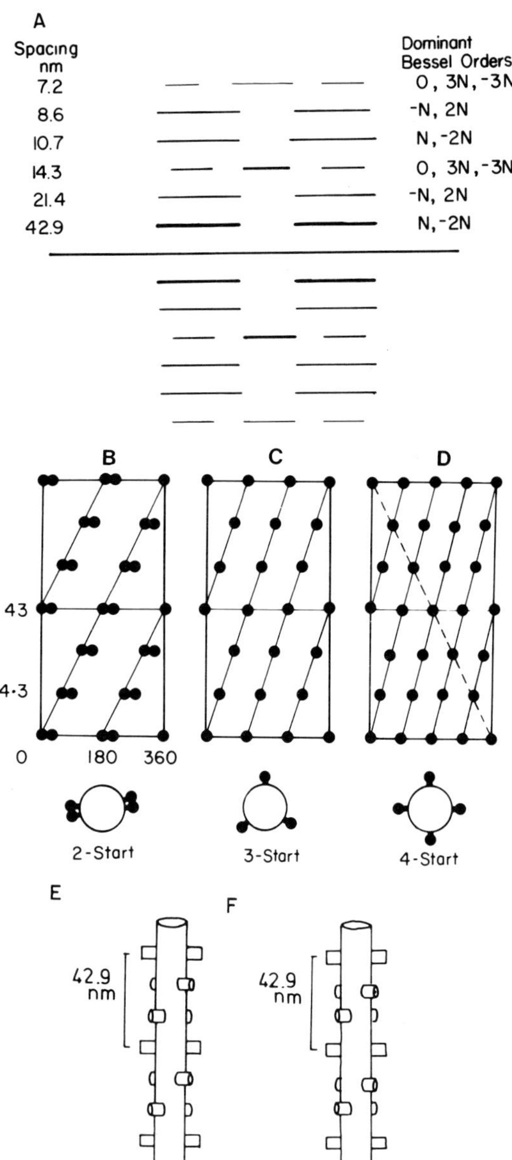

FIG. 14. *A*: schematic representation of layer lines from myosin cross-bridge array. Layer lines are indexed on a helix with a subunit pitch of 14.3 nm and a helix pitch of N × 14.3 where N = rotational symmetry of the filament. *B, C, D*: nets of surface lattices that can give rise to layer lines. The N values of myosin VSM filament are thought to be 2, 3, or 4. Note that each lattice has an axial repeat subunit of 14.3 nm and repeats exactly after 42.9 nm, although the basic helical strand, *thin line*, has a pitch of N × 42.9 nm. Perfect lattices like those in *B, C*, and *D* would give meridional reflections at orders of 14.3 nm only; the presence of forbidden reflections (see Tables 1 and 2; Fig. 3) indicates that the lattice is not perfect. A possible perturbation might be for the axial subunit repeat to be nonuniform. *E*: a 2-stranded filament with regular repeat of 14.3 nm between cross bridges. *F*: sequence of 16, 11, and 16 nm. Note that since the filament's rotational symmetry is not known, any suitable symmetry may be used for illustrating general structural features. [*B–D* with permission from Luther and Squire (83). Copyright by Academic Press Inc. (London) Ltd.; *E* and *F* from Yagi et al. (180).]

with an axial repeat of 14.5 nm as in VSM but the whole structure has an axial repeat of 72.5 nm rather than 43 nm (25).

Axial Repeat of C Protein

There has long been speculation about how the myosin-filament length is regulated so precisely. One possibility is that a vernier mechanism is operative: the myosin-filament backbone has two separate components with slightly different spacings and the filament grows until the two components are out of register by a predetermined amount (70). The C protein is thought to be a possible length-determining protein; it is present in each half of the thick filament in seven bands separated by about 43 nm (18). Whether the C-band spacing is identical to that of the myosin-filament repeat of 42.9 nm or is fractionally different is still unclear. The C protein has been identified as the source of a pair of meridional reflections at 44.1 and 41.8 nm [see Fig. 3*B*; (139, 141)]. The doublet is thought to arise from interference effects between the two halves of the A band on a peak with a unique spacing, but it is a matter of interpretation whether the spacing of the C protein is about 44 nm and therefore different from the myosin repeat (70) or whether it is 42.9 nm, the same as the myosin repeat (139, 140). In addition some electron-microscope studies of myosin A-band structure suggest that the C-band spacing is indistinguishable from that of the myosin structure (18), but another study indicates that the C-protein bands may have a spacing of 44 nm (147). The C protein is known to affect the packing of myosin molecules into filaments (77, 115), but the details of the interaction have yet to be elucidated. Estimates of the quantity of C protein are between two and four molecules per band, and it is likely that the number of molecules equals the rotational symmetry of the filament (20).

CROSS BRIDGES

The regions of the X-ray pattern arising from cross bridges are in many cases the most intense parts of the pattern and undergo the most pronounced changes when the muscle contracts. In the relaxed pattern six layer lines, which index as successive orders of a 42.9-nm helix repeat, are clearly visible (see Figs. 3 and 14; Tables 1 and 2). Since the cross bridges are thought to be the sites at which force is generated in the muscle (57, 67), this region of the pattern has received considerable attention.

Relaxed Muscle

Cross bridges can be seen projecting from the myosin filament in electron micrographs (Fig. 1), but little detail of the shape and orientation can be discerned. Electron micrographs of individual molecules (26, 148) and studies of S1 fragments bound to actin (114, 157) have provided most information. Electron-micrograph studies of isolated myosin (26) indicate that each head (S1) of the molecule is pear shaped and is about 18.0 nm long and at most 9.0 nm wide. Reconstructed images of S1 bound to actin filaments, however, indicate that S1 is a curved cylinder about 12.0 nm long and 5.5 nm in diameter (114, 157). Thus there is still doubt about the exact shape and size of the myosin S1. Because they have already been well interpreted by straight S1 models, X-ray patterns yield no further details about the shape and size of cross bridges. The intensity distribution along the myosin layer lines, however, does indicate the cross-bridge orientation on the filament in vivo.

Model-building studies indicate that in VSM the cross-bridge axis is not normal to the surface of the filament but rather lies close to the plane of the surface, tilted about 30° along the axis [Fig. 15; (47, 154)]. The two parts of the cross bridges are tilted in opposite directions, and the radial position of the peak intensity along the layer lines depends on both the rotational symmetry, unknown at present, and on the radial position of the cross bridge. If the filament has two-, three-, or fourfold symmetry, then the cross bridges' center of mass lies at 9.5, 12.5, or 15.5 nm from the filament axis, respectively.

The way the myosin molecules pack into the backbone of the filament presumably governs the regular lattice of cross bridges on the filament surface. The regular positioning of the cross bridges at the lattice positions is not affected by muscle motion as long as the muscle remains inactivated (44, 46). Passive muscle stretching to long sarcomere lengths, however, does cause a change in the pattern similar to that seen during contraction. Muscle stretching causes all the cross bridges to move from the lattice positions, but the layer-line pattern recovers again if the muscle is

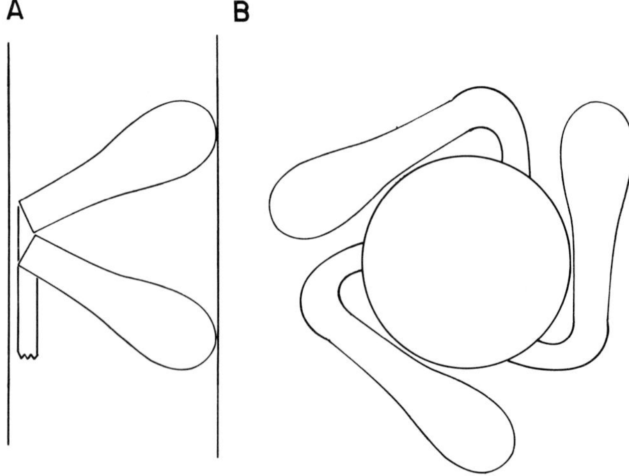

FIG. 15. Possible cross-bridge orientations on backbone of relaxed muscle. Cross-bridge shape is described by Elliott and Offer (26). *A*: view perpendicular to filament axis. Two parts of the cross bridges, perhaps representing 2 S1 heads, are tilted slightly along the axis. *B*: view looking down on one crown of a 3-stranded model. Heads lie close to filament surface, and one head of each molecule lies behind the other in this view. [Adapted from Haselgrove (47).]

left stretched for a day (46, 68). The cause of this effect is not yet known.

The study of invertebrate striated muscles is yielding much information both about the myosin filament structure per se and about the way VSM patterns should be interpreted. The shape of the third layer line in invertebrate muscles can sometimes be used to determine the radial positions of the cross bridges; the other layer lines then indicate the rotational symmetry of the filament (175, 176). For VSM such a correlation cannot yet be made with confidence, and it cannot be made at all for IFM. Insect flight muscle was originally thought to be two-stranded (132), and then six-stranded (133, 152). Now there is increasing evidence for a four-stranded structure (172, 173).

Relaxed muscle preparations in which the membranes have been removed mechanically or chemically are often important for biochemical and mechanical measurements because substrates can be infused freely into the filament lattice without hindrance by the membrane. Glycerinated fiber bundles may be relaxed by treatment with pyrophosphate or ATP in the absence of calcium. After this the muscle is relaxed from a mechanical viewpoint, but the relaxed X-ray pattern recovers relatively poorly (85, 87, 138). It may be concluded, therefore, that the positioning of the cross bridges against the myosin filament in a well-ordered array is not a requirement for mechanical relaxation (44). A better relaxed preparation, from the X-ray standpoint, may be made by combining the relaxing ingredients ATP and ethylene glycol-bis(β-aminoethylether)-*N*,*N*′-tetraacetic acid (EGTA) with a detergent skinning bath (91).

Rigor Muscle

In the electron micrographs of rigor muscle, cross bridges appear to be attached to the actin filament at an angle of about 45° to the filament axis; IFM demonstrates this much more clearly, however, than VSM [Fig. 16; (132)]. Although detailed image analysis of the cross bridges attached to actin in intact muscle has not yet been achieved, current belief is that attached cross bridges all bind with the same conformation with which free myosin S1 binds to F actin in vitro (109, 114, 134, 135, 157). In the latter the subfragments attach at an angle of about 45° to the muscle axis and twist azimuthally so that the subunit axis makes an angle of about 60° to a radial line through the attachment point. Caution is warranted, however, because recently two different rigor structures have been identified for a myosin-regulated invertebrate muscle; the presence or absence of one of the light chains affects the orientation of the bound cross bridge and hence the X-ray pattern (168). The two heads of each myosin molecule may bind to adjacent G-actin monomers along one strand of F-actin filament (21) or may extend to attach to different actin filaments (120). Because most or all the cross bridges in a rigor muscle probably have a configuration corresponding to one of the steps of the cross-bridge cycle (88), the interpretation of the axial X-ray pattern from rigor muscle is of considerable importance as a reference for interpretation of the pattern from contracting muscle.

When a muscle of any length is put into rigor, the relaxed myosin layer-line pattern disappears completely, indicating unambiguously that all the cross bridges have moved from their resting positions whether or not they are able to attach to actin [see Fig. 3; (45, 46, 68, 70)]. Since this change occurs even when calcium has been chelated, it is evident that the cross-bridge positions are influenced by other factors besides the presence of calcium (45). In muscles at rest length the myosin layer lines are replaced by a new series of rigor layer lines, much weaker and more diffuse, that index as reflections from an actinlike lattice. The new layer lines do not appear when a muscle is stretched to nonoverlap length before entering the rigor state [Fig. 17; (46, 70)], and this indicates that the layer lines arise from those cross bridges attached to the actin filament. At rest length the intensity of the actin layer lines at 5.1 nm and 5.9 nm increases near the meridian, as expected with cross bridges that are attached to actin and thereby increase the average radius of the filament structure (70, 81, 166).

The ratio of the two equatorial reflections I1.0/I1.1 (sometimes quoted as the reciprocal I1.1/I1.0) decreases when VSM passes into rigor (31, 49, 66). Similar effects are seen in IFM (109), and several investigators have interpreted these changes to mean that the cross bridges have moved laterally from the vicinity of the myosin filament to that of the actin filament (49, 66). The movement certainly has a radial component away from the axis of the myosin filament and probably has an azimuthal component around the myosin filament as well (52, 84). The spatial resolution of the highest observable reflection in rigor (1.1) is about 20 nm; this part of the pattern, therefore, cannot be used as evidence that the cross bridges attach to actin (49). In addition present attempts to use the rigor layer-line pattern to estimate the number of attached cross bridges are impractical because of the large number of unknown parameters affecting the intensity of that part of the pattern. Conservative estimates based on the probable steric freedom of cross-bridge motion suggest that only about two-thirds of all myosin heads can attach to actin at any one time (152). Direct measurement of cross-bridge orientation by electron spin resonance, however, suggests that 100% of the cross bridges are instantaneously attached to actin (158, 159). Fourier analysis of X-ray equatorial intensities indicates that the mass transferred from the region of the thick filaments to the thin is about 50% of the original mass of the thick filaments; this mass corresponds to the total cross-bridge mass (49, 66).

The positions along the actin filament at which the cross bridges attach to actin presumably depend on the structure of the actin and myosin filaments and

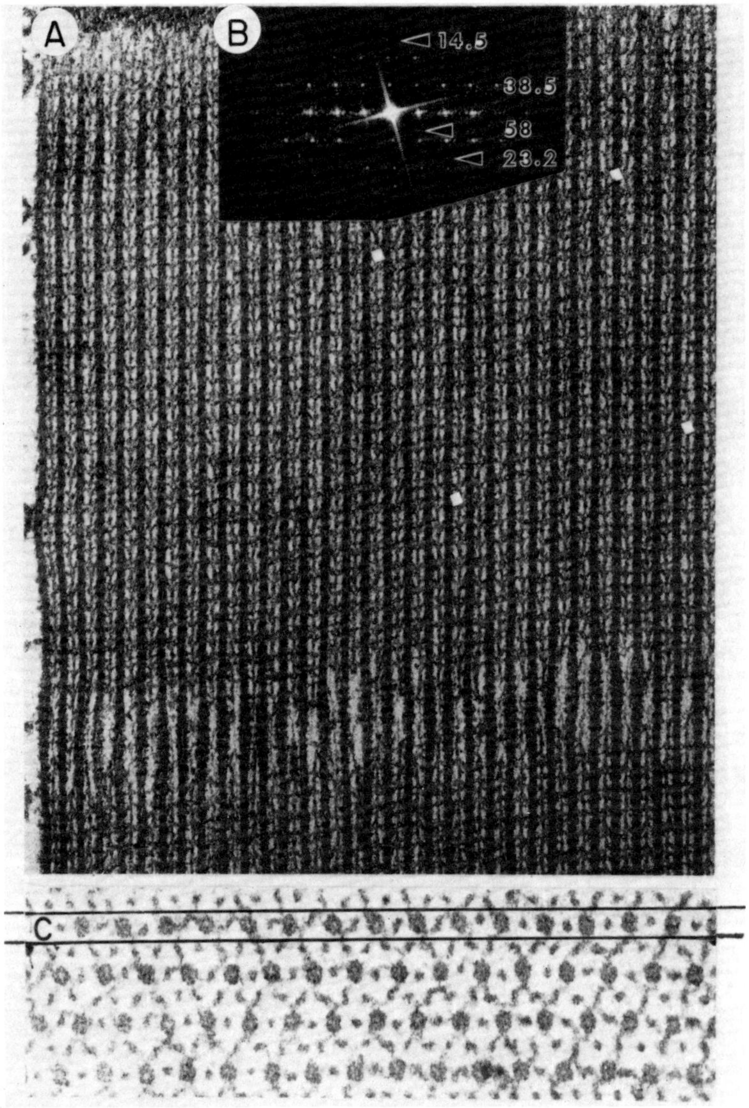

FIG. 16. Electron micrographs of insect flight muscle, IFM, in rigor (cf. Fig. 1.). *A*: longitudinal section, 2 cross bridges attach to actin every 38.5 nm along all filaments throughout the fibril. *B*: *insert*, optical-diffraction pattern of longitudinal section. *C*: transverse section, 4 cross bridges connect each myosin filament to 4 of the adjacent actin filaments. Because this section is cut at a slight angle, the axial level of sectioning changes across the picture: flared X made by the cross bridges rotates clockwise by about 60° from *left* to *right*. Note that IFM actin filaments are in different lattice positions than those in VSM. [From Haselgrove and Reedy (50).]

on the freedom of motion of individual cross bridges. The spatial distribution of cross bridges bound to actin in VSM has not yet been investigated in detail but is believed to be influenced by the same parameters that affect IFM, which has been studied more extensively (50, 120, 132, 152; see also ref. 160). Insect flight muscle forms a crystalline structure because the pitches of the actin and myosin helices have a common repeat period of 232 nm (10, 109, 132). Insect muscle cross bridges attach to actin only at target zones every 38.5 nm, where the actin monomer orientation is appropriate for cross-bridge attachment from an adjacent myosin filament (132). Researchers have observed two cross bridges attached to actin on each target zone and a crown of four cross bridges every 14.6 nm connecting each myosin filament to four of the six adjacent actin filaments. This flared X formed by the cross bridges rotates through about 60° every 14 nm along the filament [see Fig. 16; (132, 152)]. There are, however, important structural differences between IFM and VSM that affect the positions in the lattice at which the cross bridges attach. For example the myosin filaments have different rotational symmetries (4- or 6-fold in IFM, 2- or 3-fold in VSM), and the actin filaments are at different lattice positions, with different lattice symmetries.

Recently it has been recognized that the intensities of some of the rigor layer lines are influenced by the positions at which the cross bridges attach to actin, as well as by the shape of the attached cross bridges (10, 56, 89). When free S1 is infused into a rigor muscle to bind to the actin filaments, the outer layer lines increase in intensity while the inner ones decrease (10, 139). This could mean that the outer layer lines arise solely from the cross-bridge–actin attachment, whereas the inner ones arise as a "beat" effect due to labeling every 14.3 nm or so, with free S1 filling in the unlabeled monomers (56). This interpretation, how-

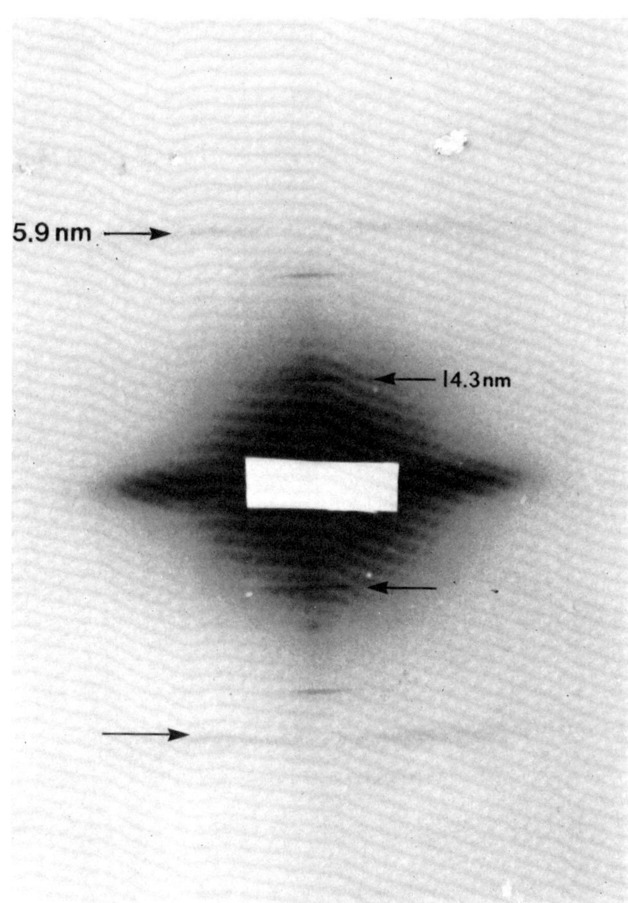

FIG. 17. X-ray pattern of semitendinosus muscle in rigor at nonoverlap length (cf. Fig. 3*C*). Myosin layer lines have disappeared, but because the actin filaments have been withdrawn from the A band, cross bridges do not attach to actin and no rigor layer lines are seen. [With permission from Haselgrove (46). Copyright by Academic Press Inc. (London) Ltd.]

ever, was not recognized at the time that the experiment was first reported (139).

The influence of cross bridges binding only every 38.5 nm is thus evident in the relative strength of the inner, low-order layer lines as compared with the outer ones near 5.9 nm. X-ray analysis of insect diffraction patterns indicated that the target zone every 38.5 nm extends axially for about 13 nm (56), although a real-space analysis of electron micrographs yields a higher value of about 18 nm (50). The discrepancy is significant but as yet unexplained. Interpretive techniques being developed for IFM with much success are sure to be applied to VSM in the near future.

Contracting Muscle

During contraction cross bridges interact with actin cyclically and independently of each other. Because the X-ray pattern gives information about the space-averaged structure, which is also averaged over the recording time, the patterns so far do not provide much detailed information about the individual cross-bridge cycles. However, a great deal of useful knowledge has been obtained about the bulk cross-bridge responses to activation.

ISOMETRIC CONTRACTION. When a rest-length muscle contracts, the myosin layer-line pattern almost disappears (see Fig. 3), indicating that most of the cross bridges have moved from their resting positions (30, 46, 69, 70, 72). The distances moved are relatively large (about 10.0 nm) because all the layer lines show a similar decrease (46). The 1.0 equatorial reflection decreases while the 1.1 reflection increases in intensity so that the ratio 1.0/1.1 approaches that of rigor [see Fig. 9; (49, 105, 129)]. Most if not all cross bridges are now in the vicinity of the actin filaments. The cross bridges move radially and azimuthally to reach the actin filaments as they do in rigor (52).

Although there is considerable indirect evidence for cross-bridge attachments to actin from tension and stiffness measurements (58), there is no direct evidence for attachment from the equatorial patterns per se. When muscles are partially activated by caffeine, however, the intensities of the equatorial reflections do vary with the tetanic tension produced, demonstrating an empirical relationship between the number of attached cross bridges and the equatorial intensities (182). Experiments with cardiac muscle also show a direct correlation between the ratio I1.0/I1.1 and tension: as tension rises the ratio falls, indicating more cross bridges in the vicinity of the actin filament (97, 99, 104). Amemiya et al. (1), however, have found no change in the equatorial ratio when the isometric tension is increased by slowly stretching an active VSM. Rigor layer lines, which indicate that cross bridges are attaching to actin filaments, are not visible at all in patterns from contracting muscle, and therefore cross bridges do not attach with the same crystalline regularity in contraction as in rigor (46, 70, 72, 75). The slight increase in intensity of the actin layer lines at 5.9 nm and 5.1 nm may be caused by cross bridges attaching to actin filaments (124), although the measurement reliability (20% ± 20%) is not high.

Early experiments indicated that cross-bridge motion following muscle activation occurred independently of cross-bridge interaction with actin (44, 46, 68). These results suggested that the myosin filament per se responds to muscle activation in VSM just as it does in IFM where, in the latter, the myosin filament is sensitive to calcium (8, 107). More recent experiments with VSM, however, show that the movement of cross bridges during contraction does seem to depend on their ability to interact with actin (unlike the case in rigor): the myosin layer-line pattern changes very little if muscles are activated at nonoverlap lengths (72, 178, 179), and the equatorial pattern doesn't change at all (69). Nevertheless, when the filaments partially overlap, the loss of the layer-line pattern seems to be greater than that expected from the degree of overlap alone (68). There is no explanation for the phenomenon yet, but positive cooperativity between cross bridges on a filament may be a possibility.

Measurements of the kinetic changes in the pattern have now been made with time resolution of about 10 ms or less [Fig. 18; (72, 103)]. These results provide excellent support for the concept that cross bridges that move from the myosin filament and attach to the actin filament generate tension. The onset of the intensity change in the 1.0 reflection correlates closely with the initial development of tension, but later the

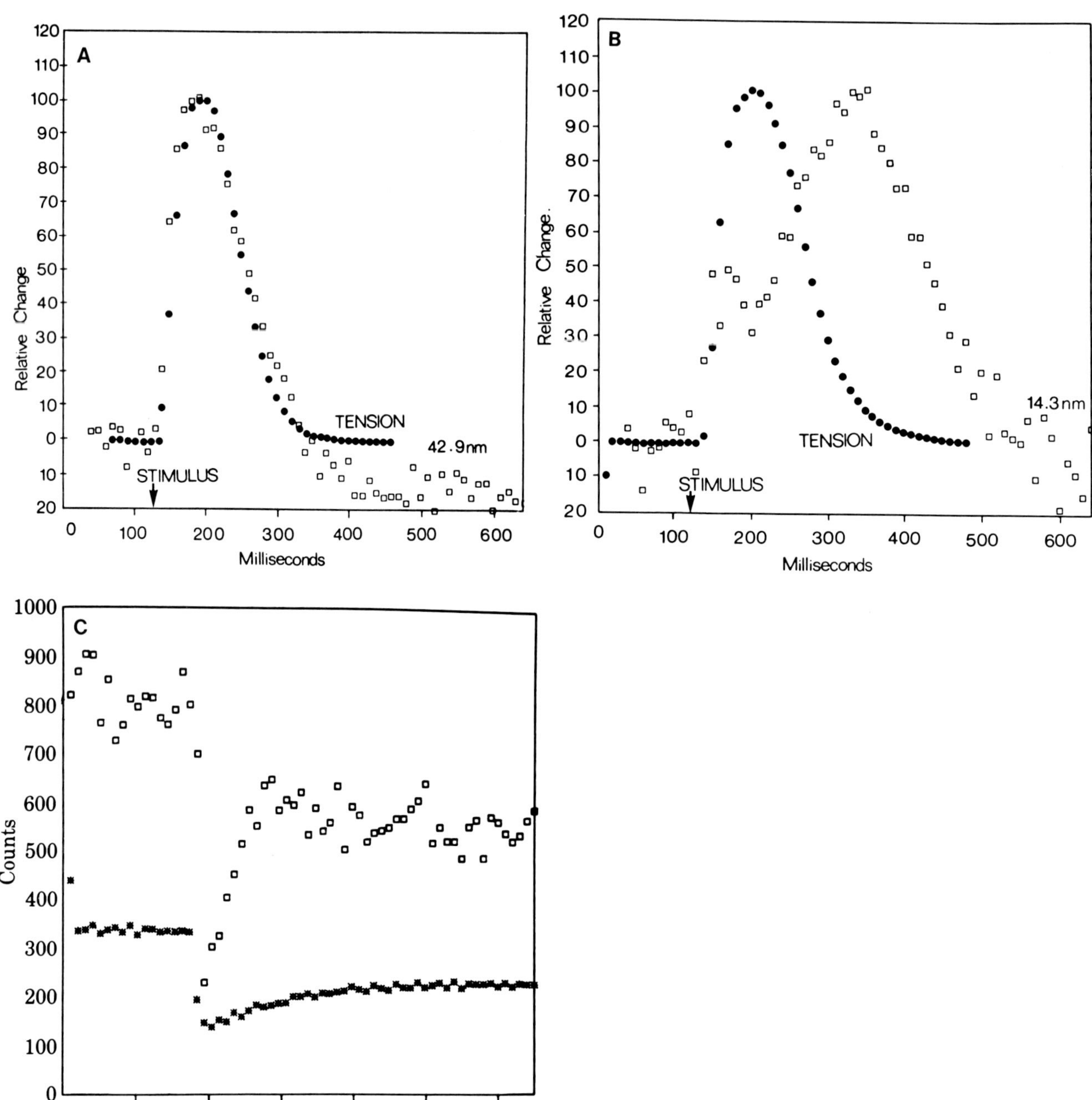

FIG. 18. Kinetic data following time course of changing X-ray reflections during tension development and relaxation. *Open squares*, intensity; *filled circles*, tension. *A* and *B*: curves plotted as percentage of maximal change. *A*: 42.9-nm layer line during a single twitch. Three hundred separate twitches were summed for a total integrated time of 3 s for each 10-ms time interval. Note that intensity decreased by 90%. *B*: 14.3-nm meridional reflection and tension during a twitch at 10°C. Total exposure is 1.5 s in each 10-ms time slot. *C*: time course of change in intensity of the 14.3-nm reflection during a quick release in a tetanus. Release was 1.3% of initial length. [*A* and *B* from Huxley et al. (72); *C* from Huxley et al. (75).]

X-ray reflection intensity changes faster than tension; the total change in the 1.0 intensity is half completed about 10 ms before the tension reaches half its peak value (69, 74). The 1.1 reflection changes much faster than tension partly because it is more sensitive than the 1.0 reflection to the slight sarcomere length shortening that occurs rapidly even in isometric contractions. The decrease in intensity of the 42.9-nm layer line is probably a better index of the number of cross bridges that move and is very closely correlated with the increase in tension produced by the muscle (72). The 14.3-nm meridional reflection shows a biphasic response (75, 178); it rapidly decreases in intensity during the onset of tension, recovers again while full tension is generated, and decreases again during relaxation. The intensity is lowest when the layer-line pattern has almost completely recovered. The two times of lowest intensity during both activation and relaxation coincide with the periods when muscle sarcomeres show considerable motion (16); therefore longitudinal filament disorder in the moving muscle as well as specific cross-bridge motions may govern the intensity of reflection (75).

During the relaxation phase of a twitch or tetanus, the X-ray reflections return to their resting values milliseconds to seconds later than when the tension has returned to zero (68, 69, 72, 102, 177). By the time the tension has fallen to zero the myosin layer lines have recovered their resting values, although the equatorial reflections are still not fully recovered and the 14.3-nm meridional reflection is very far from its resting level.

It is now possible to obtain X-ray information with 1-ms time resolution (75) and thus to follow mechanical transients while a large fraction of the cross bridges are presumably working in phase. The X-ray pattern should give information on individual cross-bridge cycles. Transient releases and stretches of about 10 nm per half sarcomere both result in a 50% or greater decrease in the intensity of the 14.3-nm meridional reflection. The reflection intensity recovers again, however, within 5–6 ms, indicating close coupling between longitudinal cross-bridge movement and axial displacements of the filaments [Fig. 18; (75)]. These data are so far the most direct X-ray evidence of physical attachment of VSM cross bridges to actin during contraction. Transient length changes do not seem to have a significant effect on the equatorial or layer-line reflections.

ISOTONIC CONTRACTION. As expected from the sliding-filament model for contraction, the X-ray pattern of an isometric contracting muscle is independent of the muscle's precontraction length (49). Although scientists are unable to use X-ray patterns to demonstrate attachment of cross bridges, they are greatly interested in the equatorial patterns of contracting muscles: different mechanical models for the action of cross bridges have been proposed based on the relative numbers of cross bridges attached to actin at different velocities of shortening (58). One model (128) predicts that more cross bridges attach during shortening, whereas another, more generally accepted model (60, 61) proposes that fewer cross bridges attach during shortening. Empirical correlation of isometric tension with equatorial intensities does encourage such X-ray experiments (182), although it is theoretically clear that determination of the exact number of attached cross bridges is not possible by this means.

When a muscle shortens under a load of about 30% of maximal isometric tension, both equatorial reflections increase slightly. The ratio I1.0/I1.1, however, remains approximately the same as in the isometric case (129). When the muscle is loaded more lightly so that it shortens faster, the ratio I1.0/I1.1 is about 30% of the way toward reaching the relaxed value (69, 155). The simplest interpretation of these data (but not the only one) is that during shortening the average center of mass of the cross bridges lies at the same distance from the actin filament, or closer to the myosin filament, than it does during isometric contraction. It is thus thought that fewer cross bridges are attached when the muscle shortens rapidly. The number of heads (70%) still in the vicinity of the actin filament greatly exceeds the 10% tension.

Difficulty in interpreting the equatorial pattern is compounded by the many parameters affecting the reflection intensity (31, 49, 66). For example merely changing the configuration of the cross bridges from a 90° to a 45° angle—without changing the number of attached cross bridges—brings the cross bridges close to the actin-filament axis and affects the pattern in a manner similar to that of an increase in the number of cross bridges (86). Thus changing the number of attached cross bridges while changing the orientation may not affect the pattern.

INSECT FLIGHT MUSCLE. There are two distinct steps in the activation of IFM (8, 107). *1)* In the absence of any applied length change, calcium ions cause a radial cross-bridge movement. Mass transfer between the myosin and actin filaments corresponds to about 20% of the total cross-bridge mass. At this stage the muscle generates no tension. *2)* An increase in length results in tension production, and an oscillatory length change results in an oscillatory tension production in which the tension output lags behind the length so that the muscle performs net work on the surroundings. The intensity of the 14.6-nm meridional reflection varies 180° out of phase with the tension as though the cross bridges were cycling between a 90° angle when the tension is low and a 45° angle when the tension is high (162). Tilted cross bridges correspond to the generation of tension.

ANALOGUES OF ATP

The desire to work with muscle cross bridges all preserved at the same step of the cross-bridge cycle (as in rigor) has encouraged muscle studies with ATP analogues. The analogues are either cleaved very slowly by myosin or not cleaved at all; thus all the myosin molecules that bind ATP are trapped at the same step of the biochemical cycle. The four analogues listed in Table 5 have been infused into muscle fiber bundles that have been treated wih Triton X-100 or glycerol to remove the membrane.

Two analogues, α,β-methylene ATP ($ATP\alpha\beta CH_2$) and adenosine 5′-*O*-(3-thiotriphosphate), i.e., $ATP\gamma S$, are cleaved by myosin and actomyosin (38, 92). Both analogues also serve to relax the muscle. The most useful analogue so far is β-γ-imido ATP (AMPPNP), which, although it is not hydrolyzed at all and remains bound to myosin, also relaxes the muscle (36, 181). Adenosine diphosphate (ADP) has also been investigated as an ATP analogue (135).

Because of its intrinsically well-defined pattern, IFM is more useful than VSM for studying the effects of ATP analogues. The following observations have, however, been made on VSM. When a rigor VSM is treated with ATP in the absence of calcium, the rigor-like layer lines disappear and the relaxed myosin layer lines reappear, but the pattern is generally not as clear as in a living, relaxed muscle (138). By contrast, AMPPNP does not lower the stiffness of VSM—indicating that the bridges do not detach—although the equatorial intensity ratio is shifted toward the relaxed value (85, 87). The interpretation of VSM experiments is the same as that for the IFM studies described here.

Details of IFM X-ray patterns from muscles in different states are summarized in Table 5. In rigor the first two layer lines are relatively intense, with the innermost reflection on the first layer line, $10\bar{1}3$, stronger than the corresponding reflection on the second layer line, $10\bar{1}6$ (38, 53, 55). The 14.5-nm reflection, 009, is weaker than the 12.9-nm reflection, 008, and the ratio of the equatorial intensities I1.0/I2.0 is low. The pattern is interpreted in terms of cross bridges attached at 45° angles and at regular 38.5-nm intervals along the actin filaments. The rigor pattern is not influenced by the absence or presence of ADP even though the ADP does bind to the attached cross bridges (135).

Muscle relaxation by addition of ATP in the absence of calcium causes changes in the patterns that repre-

TABLE 5. *Principal Features of X-Ray–Diffraction Pattern of Insect Flight Muscle*

	Bound Nucleotide					Interpretation of Muscle and Pattern Features in Terms of Cross Bridges
	None	ATP, absence of Ca^{2+}	$ATP\alpha\beta CH_2$	$ATP\gamma S$	AMPPNP, 4°C	
Muscle features						
Hydrolysis of nucleotide		No	Slow	Fast	No	
Tension	High	Low	Low	Low	Low	
Stiffness	High	Low	Low	Low	High	High stiffness due to xb attachment to actin
Pattern features						
Equatorial ratio (r = I1.0/I2.0)	0.8	2.2	1.7–2.2	2.2	1.6	Low ratio due to closeness of xbs to actin
First layer line, 38.8 nm						Strong 38.8- and 19.4-nm layer lines, as well as the 12.7-nm meridian results from attached xbs
$10\bar{1}3$	Strong	Very weak	Very weak	Very weak	Weak	
$20\bar{2}3$	Weak				Strong	
$11\bar{2}3$	Strong				Weak	
Second layer line, 19.4 nm						
$10\bar{1}6$	Weak	Very weak	Very weak	Very weak	Strong	
Meridian						
14.5 nm	Weak	Strong and narrow	Strong	Strong	Strong and broad	Strong 14.5-nm lines may be due to regular spacing of xbs every 14.5 nm and/or xbs perpendicular to axis
12.9 nm	Weak	Very weak	Very weak	Very weak	Medium	Strong 12.9-nm line arises from xb attachment to actin
Pattern interpretations	All xbs attached to actin at specific sites (rigor)	All xbs detached from actin (relaxed)	Relaxed pattern	Relaxed pattern	Xbs still attached to actin but in new positions and at different angle	

Xbs, cross bridges. * Compare $10\bar{1}3$ values in different states with those for the $10\bar{1}6$ reflection on the 2nd layer line.

sent the cross bridges detaching from the actin, moving radially back to the myosin filaments, and tilting back to 90° angles. The intensity of the first two layer lines decreases and the equatorial ratio increases. The 14.3-nm meridional reflection increases in intensity as well, while the 12.7-nm meridional reflection decreases (53). Both ATP$\alpha\beta CH_2$ and ATPγS give X-ray patterns that are very similar to the relaxed pattern (38, 53), and the mechanical stiffness of the muscle decreases to the level of the relaxed muscle.

Studies with AMPPNP have provided the most informative results to date. The effects of this analogue depend on the temperature at which it is added. Muscles treated with AMPPNP at 4°C maintain a high degree of stiffness (93); this signifies that the cross bridges are still attached to actin even though there are distinct changes in the X-ray pattern (11, 53, 161). The pattern is not simply a mixture of the rigor and relaxed patterns: layer lines and meridional reflections have values indicative of attached rigor cross bridges, although the equatorial ratio suggests that the cross-bridge center of mass is now closer to the myosin filament than in rigor (Table 5). The pattern can be interpreted with a model in which the cross bridges are still attached to actin but rotated to a 90° angle (53); this would account for the slight increase in sarcomere length occurring with the addition of the analogue (95). Rotation may occur while the cross bridges are still attached to actin, or they may detach and reattach at the 90° angle. The latter seems likely, since the X-ray pattern indicates that the cross bridges are attached at positions along the actin filaments that differ from those in rigor (10, 56, 161). Thus the analogue seems to affect the myosin so as to impose different binding constraints on the actin. When the experiment is performed at room temperature, the pattern is similar to the rigor pattern (38), but this observation has yet to be correlated with the effect of temperature on the steady state of the myosin-nucleotide complex.

REFERENCES

1. Amemiya, Y., H. Sugi, and H. Hashizume. Effect of slow stretch on the cross-bridges in active frog skeletal muscle. In: *Proc. Int. Symp. Biophys., 4th, Ibaraki, 1978.* Ibaraki, Japan: Taniguchi Found., 1978, p. 152–163.
2. April, E. W. Liquid-crystalline characteristics of the thick filament lattice of striated muscle. *Nature London* 257: 139–141, 1975.
3. April, E. W. The myofilament lattice: studies on isolated fibers. IV. Lattice equilibria in striated muscle. *J. Mechanochem. Cell Motil.* 3: 111–121, 1975.
4. April, E. W., and P. W. Brandt. The myofilament lattice: studies on isolated fibers. 3. The effect of myofilament spacing upon tension. *J. Gen. Physiol.* 61: 490–508. 1973.
5. April, E. W., P. W. Brandt, and G. F. Elliott. The myofilament lattice: studies on isolated fibers. II. The effects of osmotic strength, ionic concentration, and pH upon the unit-cell volume. *J. Cell Biol.* 53: 53–65, 1972.
6. April, E. W., and D. Wong. Non-isovolumetric behavior of the unit cell of skinned striated muscle fibers. *J. Mol. Biol.* 101: 107–114, 1976.
7. Armitage, P., A. Miller, C. D. Rodger, and R. T. Tregear. The structure and function of insect muscle. *Cold Spring Harbor Symp. Quant. Biol.* 37: 379–387, 1972.
8. Armitage, P. M., R. T. Tregear, and A. Miller. Effect of activation on the X-ray diffraction pattern from insect flight muscle. *J. Mol. Biol.* 92: 39–53, 1975.
9. Astbury, W. T. On the structure of biological fibres and the problem of muscle. *Proc. R. Soc. London* 134: 303–328, 1947.
10. Barrington-Leigh, J., R. S. Goody, W. Hofman, K. Holmes, H. G. Mannhertz, G. Rosenbaum, and R. T. Tregear. The interpretation of X-ray diffraction from glycerinated flight muscle fibre bundles: new theoretical and experimental approaches. In: *Insect Flight Muscle,* edited by R. T. Tregear. Amsterdam: Elsevier/North-Holland, 1977, p. 137–146.
11. Barrington-Leigh, J., K. C. Holmes, H. G. Mannhertz, F. Eckstein, and R. Goody. Effects of ATP analogues on the low-angle X-ray diffraction pattern of insect flight muscle. *Cold Spring Harbor Symp. Quant. Biol.* 37: 443–448, 1972.
12. Bear, R. S. Small-angle X-ray diffraction studies on muscle. *J. Am. Chem. Soc.* 67: 1625, 1945.
13. Bear, R. S., and C. C. Selby. The structure of paramyosin fibrils according to X-ray diffraction. *J. Biophys. Biochem. Cytol.* 2: 55–69, 1956.
14. Bernal, J. D., and I. Fankuchen. X-ray and crystallographic studies of plant virus preparations. *J. Gen. Physiol.* 25: 111–146, 1941.
15. Blinks, J. R. Influence of osmotic strength on cross section and volume of isolated single muscle fibres. *J. Physiol. London* 177: 42–47, 1965.
16. Carlson, F. D., R. Bonner, and A. Fraser. Intensity fluctuation autocorrelation studies of contracting frog sartorius muscle. *Cold Spring Harbor Symp. Quant. Biol.* 37: 389–396, 1972.
17. Cohen, C., and J. Hanson. An X-ray diffraction study of F actin. *Biochim. Biophys. Acta* 21: 177–178, 1956.
18. Craig, R. Structure of A-segments from frog and rabbit skeletal muscle. *J. Mol. Biol.* 109: 69–81, 1977.
19. Craig, R., and G. Offer. Axial arrangement of crossbridges in thick filaments of vertebrate skeletal muscle. *J. Mol. Biol.* 102: 325–332, 1976.
20. Craig, R., and G. Offer. The location of C-protein in rabbit skeletal muscle. *Proc. R. Soc. London Ser. B* 192: 451–461, 1976.
21. Craig, R., A. G. Szent-Gyorgyi, L. Beese, P. Flicker, P. Vibert, and C. Cohen. Electron microscopy of thin filaments decorated with a Ca^{2+}-regulated myosin. *J. Mol. Biol.* 140: 35–55, 1980.
22. Depue, R. H., and R. Rice. F-actin is a right-handed helix. *J. Mol. Biol.* 12: 302–303, 1965.
23. Eames, C. H., and A. J. Rowe. Frictional properties and molecular weight of native and synthetic myosin filaments from vertebrate skeletal muscle. *Biochim. Biophys. Acta* 537: 125–144, 1978.
24. Ebashi, S., M. Endo, and I. Ohtsuki. Control of muscle contraction. *Q. Rev. Biophys.* 2: 351–384, 1969.
25. Elliott, A., and J. Lowy. A model for the coarse structure of paramyosin filaments. *J. Mol. Biol.* 53: 181–203, 1970.
26. Elliott, A., and G. Offer. The shape and flexibility of the myosin molecule. *J. Mol. Biol.* 123: 505–519, 1978.
27. Elliott, G. F. X-ray diffraction studies on striated and smooth muscles. *Proc. R. Soc. London Ser. B* 160: 467–472, 1964.
28. Elliott, G. F. Force-balances and stability in hexagonally-packed polyelectrolyte systems. *J. Theor. Biol.* 21: 71–87, 1968.
29. Elliott, G. F., J. Lowy, and B. M. Millman. X-ray diffraction from living striated muscle during contraction. *Nature London* 206: 1357–1358, 1965.
30. Elliott, G. F., J. Lowy, and B. M. Millman. Low-angle x-

ray diffraction studies of living striated muscle during contraction. *J. Mol. Biol.* 25: 31–45, 1967.

31. Elliott, G. F., J. Lowy, and C. R. Worthington. An x-ray and light diffraction study of the filament lattice of striated muscle in the living state and in rigor. *J. Mol. Biol.* 6: 295–305, 1963.
32. Elliott, G. F., E. M. Rome, and M. Spencer. A type of contraction hypothesis applicable to all muscles. *Nature London* 226: 417–420, 1970.
33. Faruqi, A. R., and H. E. Huxley. A review of techniques for time-resolved X-ray studies on muscle. In: *Scattering Techniques Applied to Supramolecular and Nonequilibrium Systems*, edited by S. H. Chem, B. Chu, and R. Nossall. New York: Plenum, 1981. (Nato Adv. Study Inst. Ser. B Phys.)
34. Gayton, D. C., and G. F. Elliott. Structural and osmotic studies of single giant fibres of barnacle muscle. *J. Muscle Res. Cell Motil.* 1: 391–407, 1980.
35. Gillis, J. M., and E. J. O'Brien. The effect of calcium on the structure of reconstituted muscle thin filaments. *J. Mol. Biol.* 99: 445–459, 1975.
36. Goody, R. S., J. Barrington-Leigh, H. G. Mannhertz, R. T. Tregear, and G. Rosenbaum. X-ray titration of binding of beta, gamma-imido-ATP to myosin in insect flight muscle. *Nature London* 262: 613–615, 1976.
37. Goody, R. S., and F. Eckstein. Thiophosphate analogues of nucleoside di- and tri-phosphates. *J. Am. Chem. Soc.* 93: 6252, 1971.
38. Goody, R. S., K. C. Holmes, H. G. Mannhertz, J. Barrington-Leigh, and G. Rosenbaum. Cross bridge conformation as revealed by X-ray diffraction studies of insect flight muscles with ATP analogues. *Biophys. J.* 15: 687–705, 1975.
39. Gordon, A. M., A. F. Huxley, and F. J. Julian. Tension development in highly stretched vertebrate muscle fibres. *J. Physiol. London* 184: 143–169, 1966.
40. Hanson, J. Axial period of actin filaments. *Nature London* 213: 353–356, 1967.
41. Hanson, J. Recent X-ray diffraction studies of muscle. *Q. Rev. Biophys.* 1: 177–216, 1968.
42. Hanson, J., V. Lednev, E. J. O'Brien, and P. M. Bennett. Structure of the actin-containing filaments in vertebrate skeletal muscle. *Cold Spring Harbor Symp. Quant. Biol.* 37: 311–318, 1972.
43. Hanson, J., and J. Lowy. The structure of F-actin and of actin filaments isolated from muscle. *J. Mol. Biol.* 6: 46–60, 1963.
44. Haselgrove, J. C. X-ray diffraction studies on muscle. Cambridge, UK: Univ. of Cambridge, 1970. Dissertation.
45. Haselgrove, J. C. X-ray evidence for a conformational change in the actin-containing filaments of vertebrate striated muscles. *Cold Spring Harbor Symp. Quant. Biol.* 37: 341–352, 1972.
46. Haselgrove, J. C. X-ray evidence for conformational changes in the myosin filaments of vertebrate striated muscle. *J. Mol. Biol.* 92: 113–143, 1975.
47. Haselgrove, J. C. A model of myosin cross-bridge structure consistent with the low-angle X-ray diffraction pattern from vertebrate muscle. *J. Muscle Res. Cell Motil.* 2: 177–191, 1980.
48. Haselgrove, J. C., A. R. Faruqi, H. E. Huxley, and V. W. Arndt. The design and use of a camera for low-angle x-ray diffraction experiments with synchrotron radiation. *J. Phys. E* 10: 1035–1046, 1977.
49. Haselgrove, J. C., and H. E. Huxley. X-ray evidence for radial cross-bridge movement and for the sliding filament model in actively contracting muscle. *J. Mol. Biol.* 77: 549–568, 1973.
50. Haselgrove, J. C., and M. K. Reedy. Modeling rigor cross-bridge patterns in muscle: initial studies of the rigor lattice of insect flight muscle. *Biophys. J.* 24: 713–728, 1978.
51. Haselgrove, J. C., and C. Rodger. The interpretation of X-ray diffraction patterns from vertebrate striated muscle. *J. Muscle Res. Cell Motil.* 1: 371–390, 1980.
52. Haselgrove, J. C., M. Stewart, and H. E. Huxley. Cross-bridge movement during muscle contraction. *Nature London* 261: 606–608, 1976.
53. Holmes, K. C. The myosin cross-bridge as revealed by structure studies. In: *Myocardial Failure*, edited by G. Reiker, A. Weber, and J. Goodwin. New York: Springer-Verlag, 1977, p. 16–27.
54. Holmes, K. C., and D. M. Blow. *The Use of X-Ray Diffraction in the Study of Protein and Nucleic Acid Structure.* New York: Wiley, 1966.
55. Holmes, K. C., R. S. Goody, H. G. Mannhertz, J. Barrington-Leigh, and G. Rosenbaum. An investigation of the cross-bridge cycle using ATP analogues and low-angle X-ray diffraction from glycerinated fibres of insect flight muscle. In: *Molecular Basis of Motility*, edited by L. Heilmeyer, J. C. Ruegg, and T. H. Wieland. Heidelberg: Springer-Verlag, 1976, p. 26–41. (Ges. Biol. Chem., 26th, Mosbach, Germany, April 10–12, 1975.)
56. Holmes, K. C., R. T. Tregear, and J. Barrington-Leigh. Interpretation of the low-angle diffraction from insect flight muscle. *Proc. R. Soc. London Ser. B* 207: 13–33, 1980.
57. Huxley, A. F. Muscle structure and theories of contraction. *Prog. Biophys. Biophys. Chem.* 7: 255–318, 1957.
58. Huxley, A. F. Muscular contraction. *J. Physiol. London* 243: 1–43, 1974.
59. Huxley, A. F., and R. Niedergeerke. Structural changes in muscle during contraction. *Nature London* 173: 171–173, 1954.
60. Huxley, A. F., and R. M. Simmons. Proposed mechanism of force generation in striated muscle. *Nature London* 233: 533–538, 1971.
61. Huxley, A. F., and R. M. Simmons. Mechanical transients and the origin of muscular force. *Cold Spring Harbor Symp. Quant. Biol.* 37: 669–680, 1972.
62. Huxley, H. E. X-Ray Diffraction Studies on Muscle. Cambridge, UK: Univ. of Cambridge, 1952. Dissertation.
63. Huxley, H. E. X-ray analysis and the problem of muscle. *Proc. R. Soc. London Ser. B* 141: 59–62, 1953.
64. Huxley, H. E. The double array of filaments in cross-striated muscle. *J. Biophys. Biochem. Cytol.* 3: 631–647, 1957.
65. Huxley, H. E. Electron microscope studies of the structure of natural and synthetic protein filaments from striated muscle. *J. Mol. Biol.* 7: 281–308, 1963.
66. Huxley, H. E. Structural difference between resting and rigor muscle: evidence from intensity changes in the low-angle equatorial X-ray diagram. *J. Mol. Biol.* 37: 507–520, 1968.
67. Huxley, H. E. The mechanism of muscle contraction. *Science* 164: 1356–1366, 1969.
68. Huxley, H. E. Structural changes in the actin- and myosin-containing filaments during contraction. *Cold Spring Harbor Symp. Quant. Biol.* 37: 361–376, 1972.
69. Huxley, H. E. Time resolved X-ray diffraction studies on muscle. In: *Cross-Bridge Mechanism in Muscle Contraction*, edited by H. Sugi and G.H. Pollack. Tokyo: Univ. of Tokyo Press, 1979, p. 391–401.
70. Huxley, H. E., and W. Brown. The low-angle x-ray diagram of vertebrate striated muscle and its behaviour during contraction and rigor. *J. Mol. Biol.* 30: 383–434, 1967.
71. Huxley, H. E., W. Brown, and K. C. Holmes. Constancy of axial spacings in frog sartorius muscle during contraction. *Nature London* 206: 1358, 1965.
72. Huxley, H. E., A. R. Faruqi, J. Bordas, M. H. J. Koch, and J. R. Milch. The use of synchrotron radiation in time-resolved X-ray diffraction studies of myosin layer-line reflections during muscle contraction. *Nature London* 284: 140–143, 1980.
73. Huxley, H. E., and J. Hanson. Changes in the cross-striations of muscle during contraction and stretch and their structural interpretation. *Nature London* 173: 973–974, 1954.
74. Huxley, H. E., and J. C. Haselgrove. The structural basis of contraction in muscle and its study by rapid X-ray diffraction methods. In: *Myocardial Failure*, edited by G. Reiker, A. Weber, and J. Goodwin. New York: Springer-Verlag, 1977, p. 4–15.

75. HUXLEY, H. E., R. M. SIMMONS, A. R. FARUQI, M. KRESS, AND J. BORDAS. Millisecond time-resolved changes in X-ray reflections from contracting muscle during rapid mechanical transients, recorded using synchrotron radiation. *Proc. Natl. Acad. Sci. USA* 78: 2297–2301, 1981.
76. KATSURA, I., AND H. NODA. Assembly of myosin molecules into the structure of thick filaments of muscle. *Adv. Biophys.* 5: 177–202, 1973.
77. KORETZ, J. F. Effects of C-protein on synthetic myosin filament structure. *Biophys. J.* 27: 433–446, 1979.
78. LAMVIK, M. K. Muscle thick filament mass measured by electron scattering. *J. Mol. Biol.* 122: 55–68, 1978.
79. LOWY, J., F. R. POULSEN, AND P. J. VIBERT. Myosin filaments in vertebrate smooth muscle. *Nature London* 225: 1053–1054, 1970.
80. LOWY, J., AND P. J. VIBERT. Structure and organisation of actin in a molluscan smooth muscle. *Nature London* 215: 1254–1255, 1967.
81. LOWY, J., AND P. J. VIBERT. Studies of the low-angle X-ray diffraction patterns of a molluscan smooth muscle during tonic contraction and rigor. *Cold Spring Harbor Symp. Quant. Biol.* 37: 353–359, 1972.
82. LOWY, J., P. J. VIBERT, J. C. HASELGROVE, AND F. R. POULSEN. The structure of the myosin elements in vertebrate smooth muscles. *Philos. Trans. R. Soc. London Ser. B* 265: 191–196, 1973.
83. LUTHER, P. K., AND J. SQUIRE. Three-dimensional structure of the vertebrate muscle A band. *J. Mol. Biol.* 141: 409–439, 1980.
84. LYMN, R. W. Equatorial X-ray reflections and cross arm movement in skeletal muscle. *Nature London* 258: 770–772, 1975.
85. LYMN, R. W. Low-angle x-ray diagrams from skeletal muscle: the effect of AMP-PNP, a non-hydrolyzed analogue of ATP. *J. Mol. Biol.* 99: 567–582, 1975.
86. LYMN, R. W. Myosin subfragment-1 attachment to actin. Expected effect on equatorial reflections. *Biophys. J.* 21: 92–98, 1978.
87. LYMN, R. W., AND H. E. HUXLEY. X-ray diagrams from skeletal muscle in the presence of ATP analogues. *Cold Spring Harbor Symp. Quant. Biol.* 37: 449–453, 1972.
88. LYMN, R. W., AND E. W. TAYLOR. Mechanism of adenosine triphosphate hydrolysis by actomyosin. *Biochemistry* 10: 4617–4624, 1971.
89. MAEDA, Y. X-ray diffraction patterns from molecular arrangements with 38-nm periodicities around muscle thin filaments. *Nature London* 277: 670–672, 1979.
90. MAEDA, Y., I. MATSUBARA, AND N. YAGI. Structural changes in thin filaments of crab striated muscle. *J. Mol. Biol.* 127: 191–201, 1979.
91. MAGID, A., AND M. K. REEDY. X-ray diffraction observations of chemically skinned frog skeletal muscle processed by an improved method. *Biophys. J.* 30: 27–40, 1980.
92. MANNHERTZ, H. G., J. BARRINGTON-LEIGH, K. HOLMES, AND G. ROSENBAUM. Identification of the transitory complex myosin-ATP by the use of α, β-methylene-ATP. *Nature London New Biol.* 241: 226, 1973.
93. MARSTON, S. B., C. D. RODGER, AND R. T. TREGEAR. Changes in muscle crossbridges when beta, gamma-imido-ATP binds to myosin. *J. Mol. Biol.* 104: 263–276, 1976.
94. MARSTON, S. B., AND R. T. TREGEAR. Evidence for a complex between myosin and ADP in relaxed muscle fibres. *Nature London New Biol.* 235: 23–24, 1972.
95. MARSTON, S. B., R. T. TREGEAR, C. D. RODGER, AND M. L. CLARKE. Coupling between the enzymatic site of myosin and the mechanical output of muscle. *J. Mol. Biol.* 28: 111–126, 1979.
96. MARUYAMA, K., AND A. WEBER. Binding of ATP to myofibrils during contraction and relaxation. *Biochemistry* 11: 2990–2998, 1972.
97. MATSUBARA, I. X-ray diffraction studies of the heart. *Annu. Rev. Biophys. Bioeng.* 9: 81–105, 1980.
98. MATSUBARA, I., AND G. F. ELLIOTT. X-ray diffraction studies on skinned single fibres of frog skeletal muscle. *J. Mol. Biol.* 72: 657–669, 1972.
99. MATSUBARA, I., A. KAMIYAMA, AND H. SUGA. X-ray diffraction study of contracting heart muscle. *J. Mol. Biol.* 111: 121–128, 1977.
100. MATSUBARA, I., AND B. M. MILLMAN. X-ray diffraction patterns from mammalian heart muscle. *J. Mol. Biol.* 82: 527–536, 1974.
101. MATSUBARA, I., H. SUGA, AND N. YAGI. An X-ray diffraction study of the cross-circulated canine heart. *J. Physiol. London* 270: 311–320, 1977.
102. MATSUBARA, I., AND N. YAGI. A time-resolved X-ray diffraction study of muscle during twitch. *J. Physiol. London* 278: 297–307, 1978.
103. MATSUBARA, I., N. YAGI, AND M. ENDOH. Behaviour of myosin projections during the staircase phenomenon of heart muscle. *Nature London* 273: 67, 1978.
104. MATSUBARA, I., N. YAGI, AND M. ENDOH. Movement of myosin heads during a heart beat. *Nature London* 278: 474–476, 1979.
105. MATSUBARA, I., N. YAGI, AND H. HASHIZUME. Use of an X-ray television for diffraction of the frog striated muscle. *Nature London* 255: 728–729, 1975.
106. MAW, M. C., AND A. ROWE. Fraying of A-filaments into three subfilaments. *Nature London* 286: 412–414, 1980.
107. MILLER, A., AND R. T. TREGEAR. Evidence concerning crossbridge attachment during muscle contraction. *Nature London* 226: 1060–1061, 1970.
108. MILLER, A., AND R. T. TREGEAR. X-ray studies on the structure and function of invertebrate muscle. In: *Contractility of Muscle Cells and Related Processes*, edited by R. J. Podolsky. London: Prentice-Hall, 1971.
109. MILLER, A., AND R. T. TREGEAR. Structure of insect fibrillar flight muscle in the presence and absence of ATP. *J. Mol. Biol.* 70: 85–104, 1972.
110. MILLER, A., AND J. WOODHEAD-GALLOWAY. Long range forces in muscle. *Nature London* 229: 470–473, 1971.
111. MILLMAN, B., AND P. M. BENNETT. Structure of the cross-striated adducter muscle of the scallop. *J. Mol. Biol.* 103: 439–467, 1976.
112. MILLMAN, B. M., G. F. ELLIOTT, AND J. LOWY., Axial period of actin filaments: X-ray diffraction studies. *Nature London* 213: 356–358, 1967.
113. MILLMAN, B. M., T. J. RACEY, AND I. MATSUBARA. Effects of hyperosmotic solutions on the filament lattice of intact frog skeletal muscle. *Biophys. J.* 33: 189–202, 1981.
114. MOORE, P. B., H. E. HUXLEY, AND D. J. DEROSIER. Three-dimensional reconstruction of F-actin, thin filaments and decorated thin filaments. *J. Mol. Biol.* 50: 279–295, 1970.
115. MOOS, C., G. OFFER, R. STARR, AND P. BENNETT. Interaction of C-protein with myosin, myosin rod and light meromyosin. *J. Mol. Biol.* 97: 1–9, 1975.
116. MORIMOTO, K., AND W. F. HARRINGTON. Substructure of the thick filament of vertebrate striated muscle. *J. Mol. Biol.* 83: 83–97, 1974.
117. NAMBA, K., K. WAKABAYASHI, AND T. MITSUI. X-ray structure analysis of the thin filament of crab striated muscle in the rigor state. *J. Mol. Biol.* 138: 1–26, 1980.
118. O'BRIEN, E. J., P. M. BENNETT, AND J. HANSON. Optical diffraction studies of myofibrillar structure. *J. Mol. Biol.* 83: 83–97, 1971.
119. OFFER, G. C-protein and periodicity in the thick filaments of vertebrate skeletal muscle. *Cold Spring Harbor Symp. Quant. Biol.* 37: 87–95, 1972.
120. OFFER, G., AND A. ELLIOTT. Can a myosin molecule bind to two actin filaments? *Nature London* 271: 325–329, 1978.
121. OFFER, G., C. MOSS, AND R. STARR. A new protein of the thick filaments of vertebrate skeletal myofibrils. *J. Mol. Biol.* 74: 653–676, 1973.
122. OHTSUKI, I. T., Y. MASAKI, Y. NONOMURA, AND S. EBASHI. Periodic distribution of troponin along the thin filament. *J. Biochem. Tokyo* 61: 817–819, 1967.

123. PAGE, S., AND H. E. HUXLEY. Filament lengths in striated muscle. *J. Cell Biol.* 19: 369–370, 1963.
124. PARRY, D. A. D., AND J. M. SQUIRE. Structural role of tropomyosin in muscle regulation: analysis of the X-ray diffraction patterns from relaxed and contracting muscles. *J. Mol. Biol.* 75: 33–55, 1973.
125. PEPE, F. A. The myosin filament. I. Structural organization from antibody staining observed in electron microscopy. *J. Mol. Biol.* 27: 203–225, 1967.
126. PEPE, F. A., F. T. ASHTON, P. DOWBEN, AND M. STEWART. The myosin filament. VII. Changes in internal structure along the length of the filament. *J. Mol. Biol.* 145: 421–440, 1981.
127. PEPE, F. A., AND B. DRUKER. The myosin filament. *J. Mol. Biol.* 130: 379–393, 1979.
128. PODOLSKY, R. J., AND A. C. NOLAN. Muscle contraction transients, cross-bridge kinetics and the Fenn effect. *Cold Spring Harbor Symp. Quant. Biol.* 37: 661–668, 1972.
129. PODOLSKY, R. J., H. ST. ONGE, L. YU, AND R. W. LYMN. X-ray diffraction of actively shortening muscle. *Proc. Natl. Acad. Sci. USA* 73: 813–817, 1976.
130. POTTER, J. The content of troponin, tropomyosin, actin and myosin in rabbit skeletal muscle myofibrils. *Arch. Biochem. Biophys.* 162: 436–441, 1974.
131. PRINGLE, J. W. S. The mechanical characteristics of insect fibrillar muscle. In: *Insect Flight Muscle*, edited by R. T. Tregear. Amsterdam: Elsevier/North-Holland, 1977, p. 177–196.
132. REEDY, M. K. Ultrastructure of insect flight muscle. *J. Mol. Biol.* 31: 155–176, 1968.
133. REEDY, M. K., G. F. BAHR, AND D. A. FISCHMAN. How many myosins per cross bridge? I. Flight muscle myofibrils from the blowfly. *Cold Spring Harbor Symp. Quant. Biol.* 37: 397–422, 1972.
134. REEDY, M. K., K. C. HOLMES, AND R. T. TREGEAR. Induced changes in orientation of the cross-bridges of glycerinated insect flight muscle. *Nature London* 207: 1276–1280, 1965.
135. RODGER, C. D., AND R. T. TREGEAR. Crossbridge angle when ADP is bound to myosin. *J. Mol. Biol.* 86: 495–497, 1974.
136. ROME, E. Light and X-ray diffraction studies of the filament lattice of glycerol-extracted rabbit psoas muscle. *J. Mol. Biol.* 27: 591–602, 1967.
137. ROME, E. X-ray diffraction studies of the filament lattice of striated muscle in various bathing media. *J. Mol. Biol.* 37: 331–344, 1968.
138. ROME, E. Relaxation of glycerinated muscles: low-angle X-ray diffraction studies. *J. Mol. Biol.* 65: 331–345, 1972.
139. ROME, E. Structural studies by X-ray diffraction of striated muscle permeated with certain ions and proteins. *Cold Spring Harbor Symp. Quant. Biol.* 37: 331–339, 1972.
140. ROME, E. M., T. HIRABAYASHI, AND S. V. PERRY. X-ray diffraction of muscle labelled with antibody to troponin-C. *Nature London New Biol.* 244: 154–155, 1973.
141. ROME, E. M., G. OFFER, AND F. A. PEPE. X-ray diffraction of muscle labelled with antibody to C-protein. *Nature London New Biol.* 244: 152–154, 1973.
142. RÜDEL, R., AND F. ZITE-FERENCZY. Interpretation of light diffraction by cross-striated muscle as Bragg reflection of light by the lattice of contractile proteins. *J. Physiol. London* 290: 317–330, 1979.
143. SELBY, C., AND R. S. BEAR. The structure of actin-rich filaments of muscles according to X-ray diffraction. *J. Biophys. Biochem. Cytol.* 2: 71–85, 1956.
144. SEYMOUR, J., AND E. J. O'BRIEN. The position of tropomyosin in muscle thin filaments. *Nature London* 283: 680–681, 1980.
145. SHEAR, D. B. Electrostatic forces in muscle contraction. *J. Theor. Biol.* 28: 531–546, 1970.
146. SHOENBERG, C. F., AND J. C. HASELGROVE. Filaments and ribbons in vertebrate smooth muscle. *Nature London* 249: 152–154, 1974.
147. SJÖSTRÖM, M., AND J. M. SQUIRE. Fine structure of the A-band in cryo-sections. The structure of the A-band of human skeletal muscle fibres from ultra-thin cryo-sections negatively stained. *J. Mol. Biol.* 109: 49–68, 1977.
148. SLAYTER, H. S., AND S. LOWEY. Substructure of the myosin molecule as visualized by electron microscopy. *Proc. Natl. Acad. Sci. USA* 58: 1611–1618, 1967.
149. SPUDICH, J. A., H. E. HUXLEY, AND J. T. FINCH. Regulation of skeletal muscle contraction. II. Structural studies of the interaction of the tropomyosin-troponin complex with actin. *J. Mol. Biol.* 72: 619–632, 1972.
150. SPUDICH, J. A., AND S. WATT. The regulation of rabbit skeletal muscle contraction. *J. Biol. Chem.* 246: 4866–4871, 1971.
151. SQUIRE, J. M. General model for the structure of all myosin-containing filaments. *Nature London* 233: 457–462, 1971.
152. SQUIRE, J. M. General model of myosin filament structure. II. Myosin filaments and cross-bridge interactions in vertebrate striated and insect flight muscles. *J. Mol. Biol.* 72: 125–138, 1972.
153. SQUIRE, J. M. General model of myosin filament structure. III. Molecular packing arrangements in myosin filaments. *J. Mol. Biol.* 77: 291–323, 1973.
154. SQUIRE, J. M. Muscle filament structure and muscle contraction. *Annu. Rev. Biophys. Bioeng.* 4: 137–163, 1975.
155. SUGI, H., Y. AMEMIYA, AND H. HASHIZUME. Time-resolved X-ray diffraction from skeletal muscle during the course of an after-loaded isotonic twitch. In: *Proc. Int. Symp. Biophys., 4th, Ibaraki, 1978.* Ibaraki, Japan: Taniguchi Found., 1978, p. 164–176.
156. SZENT-GYORGYI, A. G., C. COHEN, AND D. E. PHILPOTT. Light meromyosin fraction I: a helical molecule from myosin. *J. Mol. Biol.* 2: 133–142, 1960.
157. TAYLOR, K. A., AND L. A. AMOS. A new model for the geometry of the binding of the myosin crossbridges to muscle thin filaments. *J. Mol. Biol.* 147: 297–324, 1981.
158. THOMAS, D. D., AND R. COOKE. The measurement of myosin head orientation in muscle fibers using nitroxide spin labels. *Biophys. J.* 25: 19a, 1979.
159. THOMAS, D. D., AND R. COOKE. Orientation of spin labelled myosin heads in glycerinated muscle fibers. *Biophys. J.* 32: 891–906, 1980.
160. TREGEAR, R. T. (editor). *Insect Flight Muscle.* Amsterdam: Elsevier/North-Holland, 1977.
161. TREGEAR, R. T., J. R. MILCH, R. S. GOODY, K. C. HOLMES, AND C. D. RODGER. The use of some novel X-ray diffraction techniques to study the effect of nucleotides on cross-bridges in insect flight muscle. In: *Cross-Bridge Mechanism in Muscle Contraction*, edited by H. Sugi and G. H. Pollack. Tokyo: Univ. of Tokyo Press, 1979, p. 391–401.
162. TREGEAR, R. T., AND A. MILLER. Evidence of crossbridge movement during contraction of insect flight muscle. *Nature London* 222: 1184–1185, 1969.
163. TREGEAR, R. T., AND J. M. SQUIRE. Myosin content and filament structure in smooth and striated muscle. *J. Mol. Biol.* 77: 279–290, 1973.
164. ULLRICK, W. A theory of contraction for striated muscle. *J. Theor. Biol.* 15: 53–69, 1976.
165. VAINSHTEIN, B. K. *Diffraction of X-Rays by Chain Molecules.* Amsterdam: Elsevier, 1966.
166. VIBERT, P. J., J. C. HASELGROVE, J. LOWY, AND F. R. POULSEN. Structural changes in actin-containing filaments of muscle. *J. Mol. Biol.* 71: 757–767, 1972.
167. VIBERT, P. J., J. LOWY, J. C. HASELGROVE, AND F. R. POULSEN. Structural changes in actin filaments of muscle. *Nature London New Biol.* 236: 182–183, 1972.
168. VIBERT, P., A. G. SZENT-GYORGYI, R. CRAIG, J. WRAY, AND C. COHEN. Changes in crossbridge attachment in a myosin-regulated muscle. *Nature London* 273: 64–66, 1978.
169. WAKABAYASHI, T., H. E. HUXLEY, L. A. AMOS, AND A. KLUG. Three-dimensional image reconstruction of actin-tropomyosin complex and actin-tropomyosin-troponin T-troponin I complex. *J. Mol. Biol.* 93: 477–497, 1975.
170. WEBER, A., AND R. D. BREMEL. Regulation of contraction and

relaxation in the myofibril. In: *Contractility of Muscle Cells and Related Processes*, edited by R.J. Podolsky. London: Prentice-Hall, 1971, p. 37–53.
171. WORTHINGTON, C. R. Large axial spacings in striated muscle. *J. Mol. Biol.* 1: 398–401, 1959.
172. WRAY, J. S. Structure of the backbone in myosin filaments of muscle. *Nature London* 277: 37–40, 1979.
173. WRAY, J. S. Filament geometry and the activation of flight muscles. *Nature London* 280: 325–326, 1980.
174. WRAY, J. S., P. J. VIBERT, AND C. COHEN. Cross-bridge arrangements in *Limulus* muscle. *J. Mol. Biol.* 88: 343–348, 1974.
175. WRAY, J. S., P. J. VIBERT, AND C. COHEN. Diversity of cross-bridge configurations in invertebrate muscles. *Nature London* 257: 561–564, 1975.
176. WRAY, J., P. J. VIBERT, AND C. COHEN. Actin filaments in muscle: pattern of myosin and tropomyosin/troponin attachments. *J. Mol. Biol.* 124: 501–521, 1978.
177. YAGI, N., M. H. ITO, H. NAKAJIMA, T. IZUMI, AND I. MATSUBARA. Return of myosin heads to thick filaments after muscle contraction. *Science* 197: 685–687, 1977.
178. YAGI, N., AND I. MATSUBARA. Recent progress in fast X-ray diffraction of muscle. In: *Proc. Int. Symp. Biophys., 4th, Ibaraki, 1978.* Ibaraki, Japan: Taniguchi Found., 1978, p. 142–151.
179. YAGI, N., AND I. MATSUBARA. Myosin heads do not move on activation in highly stretched vertebrate striated muscle. *Science* 207: 307–308, 1980.
180. YAGI, N., E. J. O'BRIEN, AND I. MATSUBARA. Changes of thick filament structure during contraction of frog striated muscle. *Biophys. J.* 33: 121–138, 1981.
181. YOUNT, R. G., D. OJALA, AND D. BABCOCK. Interaction of P-N-P and P-C-P analogues of adenosine triphosphate with heavy meromyosin, myosin and actomyosin. *Biochemistry* 10: 2490–2496, 1971.
182. YU, L. C., J. E. HARTT, AND R. J. PODOLSKY. Equatorial X-ray intensities and isometric force levels in frog sartorius muscle. *J. Mol. Biol.* 132: 53–67, 1979.
183. YU, L. C., R. W. LYMN, AND R. J. PODOLSKY. Characterization of a non-indexable equatorial X-ray reflection from frog sartorius muscle. *J. Mol. Biol.* 115: 455–464, 1977.

CHAPTER 6

Force generation and shortening in skeletal muscle

RICHARD J. PODOLSKY
MARK SCHOENBERG
Laboratory of Physical Biology, National Institute of Arthritis, Diabetes, and Digestive and Kidney Diseases, National Institutes of Health, Bethesda, Maryland

CHAPTER CONTENTS

IN THIS CHAPTER we review a number of experiments that have influenced our ideas about the contraction mechanism in striated muscle cells. Most of the physiological data we discuss comes from work with frog skeletal muscle preparations, although some is taken from work with rabbit and insect muscles. The biochemical data are mainly from experiments with rabbit preparations. The assumption is often made that the same basic mechanisms are involved in rabbit, frog, and insect muscles. This is most likely to be true in frog and rabbit muscles; however, insect muscles have some unique physiological properties, such as the ability to oscillate, and special mechanisms may have evolved to carry these out.

EXPERIMENTAL PREPARATIONS

The contraction mechanism of the skeletal muscle cell has been studied in whole muscles as well as in simpler preparations. Whole muscles are easily dissected out of the animal and attached to force and displacement transducers. They consist of a large number of long cells, or fibers, which are terminated at each end by tendinous material connecting with the bone. The length of the cell is of the order of 10^{-2}–10^{-1} m, and the diameter is in the range of 10^{-5}–10^{-4} m (10–100 μm). Normally the cell membrane is electrically polarized, and the relaxed cell is activated physiologically by a wave of depolarization that is triggered by a nerve impulse at the neuromuscular junction. This depolarization stimulates the release of calcium from the sarcoplasmic reticulum (SR) throughout the muscle cell. A single nerve impulse elicits a single force impulse, or twitch, from the cell. A train of nerve impulses elicits a train of force impulses, which in some muscles can fuse to develop a steady tension, or tetanus. It is also possible to activate the muscle fibers by passing current from external electrodes across the cell membrane, by changing the ionic composition of the bathing solution so that the cell membrane depolarizes, or by adding certain drugs such as caffeine. The first technique is generally used when the mechanical properties of the cell are being studied. More finely controlled experiments can be made with single fibers, which are obtained by dissecting all but one of the fibers away from a muscle.

Another useful preparation is the skinned muscle fiber, in which the outer membrane has been either dissected away mechanically from a fiber segment (50), or made permeable by treatment with glycerin (61), glycerin and a detergent (42), or a chelating agent (6). In all cases the interior of the cell becomes chemically accessible and is under direct experimental control. This type of preparation is generally activated by raising the concentration of ionized calcium in the bathing medium.

The protein constituents of the contraction mechanism, primarily actin and myosin (the major components of the thin and thick filaments) and troponin and tropomyosin (which interact with calcium to regulate activation), can be extracted from the cell. In the absence of calcium, troponin-tropomyosin inhibits the ability of actin and myosin to hydrolyze adenosine triphosphate (ATP). Calcium binding to troponin releases this inhibition.

STATES OF THE FIBER

A muscle fiber can exist in three qualitatively different states: relaxed, activated, and rigor. These states may be characterized in terms of their tension and stiffness. Stiffness is defined as the change in force produced by a small change in length. Active force is operationally defined as force that disappears with a quick 1% decrease in muscle length but subsequently redevelops without further change of length. It is believed to be due to cross bridges between the myosin-containing and actin-containing filaments. Passive tension is more or less constant and depends only on the length of the muscle. Its origin is uncertain. [In whole muscle a large portion of the passive resting tension is due to connective tissue in parallel with the muscle cells, although some of this tension may be related to cross bridges (28).]

In the relaxed state the muscle does not generate active force and is not very stiff. It may show a small amount of passive resting tension. In the activated state, however, the fiber is several orders of magnitude stiffer than a resting muscle, develops active force, and has the ability to shorten extensively. The rigor state can be induced in intact fibers by depleting the intracellular ATP. This can be done by adding a reagent (such as iodoacetic acid) that interferes with ATP synthesis and by stimulating the muscle. In rigor the fiber is about as stiff as in the activated state (18), but it does not generate active tension and is unable to shorten extensively, even though its great stiffness enables it to bear almost as much tension as an active muscle.

In skinned fibers it is possible to change states reversibly. Under conditions of normal ionic strength, the relaxed state requires that MgATP be present at about 10^{-3} M and the $[Ca^{2+}]$ be kept below 10^{-7} M. The fiber becomes fully activated when $[Ca^{2+}]$ is above 10^{-6} M (7, 24). Rigor occurs when ATP is removed from the bathing solution.

PROPERTIES OF ACTIVATED FIBERS

Force-Velocity Relation

When the length of the fiber is held constant, the mechanical condition is isometric. When the external force applied to the muscle, called the load, is constant, the mechanical condition is isotonic. The earliest quantitative studies of the contraction mechanism dealt with the relation between the contraction velocity and the load. After a fiber is activated and a steady isometric force, P_0, is established, it will shorten if the load is reduced to a level $P < P_0$. In many types of fiber, the shortening velocity becomes nearly steady shortly after the load is changed. The relation between shortening velocity and the load is hyperbolic, the contraction velocity being greater the lighter the load (see Fig. 8). A commonly used expression describing the force-velocity relation is $(P + a)V = b(P_0 - P)$ where V is the contraction velocity and a and b are experimental parameters; this is generally known as the A. V. Hill force-velocity relation (27).

Viscoelastic Theory

The force-velocity relation was explained initially by supposing that contractile force was developed by a continuous springlike, elastic structure immersed in a viscous medium (26). The force at the ends of the fiber would then be the difference between the force in the elastic structure and the induced viscous force A steady speed would be established when the net contractile force just balanced the force of the load: the greater the speed, the greater the viscous force and the smaller the net force.

Fenn Effect

Although the viscoelastic theory provided a qualitative explanation for the force-velocity relation, it failed to account for the energetic changes that accompany contraction. In particular the energy output (heat + work) for a given amount of shortening does not remain constant, as required by the viscoelastic theory, but rather increases with load and therefore decreases with velocity (13, 14). The most likely explanation of the Fenn effect is that energy liberation is due to chemical processes during contraction rather than changes in the internal energy of a strained elastic structure.

Quick Releases

The maximum steady velocity of unloaded shortening in terms of the Hill relation is $V_{max} = bP_0/a$. When a muscle is released much more quickly than V_{max}, the force falls to zero after a displacement of about 1% of the fiber length (41). In many cases a muscle can be adequately represented by a contractile element, characterized by the force-velocity relation, in series with an elastic element whose force falls to zero after a 1% decrease in length (27, 41). A more detailed understanding of muscle contraction, however, requires a knowledge of the fine structure of the muscle cell.

Discovery of Sliding Filaments and Cross Bridges

Although the bands, or striations, that mark the length of striated muscle fibers had been objects of study for many years (e.g., ref. 33), and muscle was known to be composed of repeating sarcomeres, each composed of an A band (anisotropic in the polarizing microscope) and an I band (isotropic in the polarizing microscope), the relation of the bands to the contraction mechanism was not at all understood before important observations by H. E. Huxley and Hanson (40) on contracting glycerinated myofibrils with the phase-

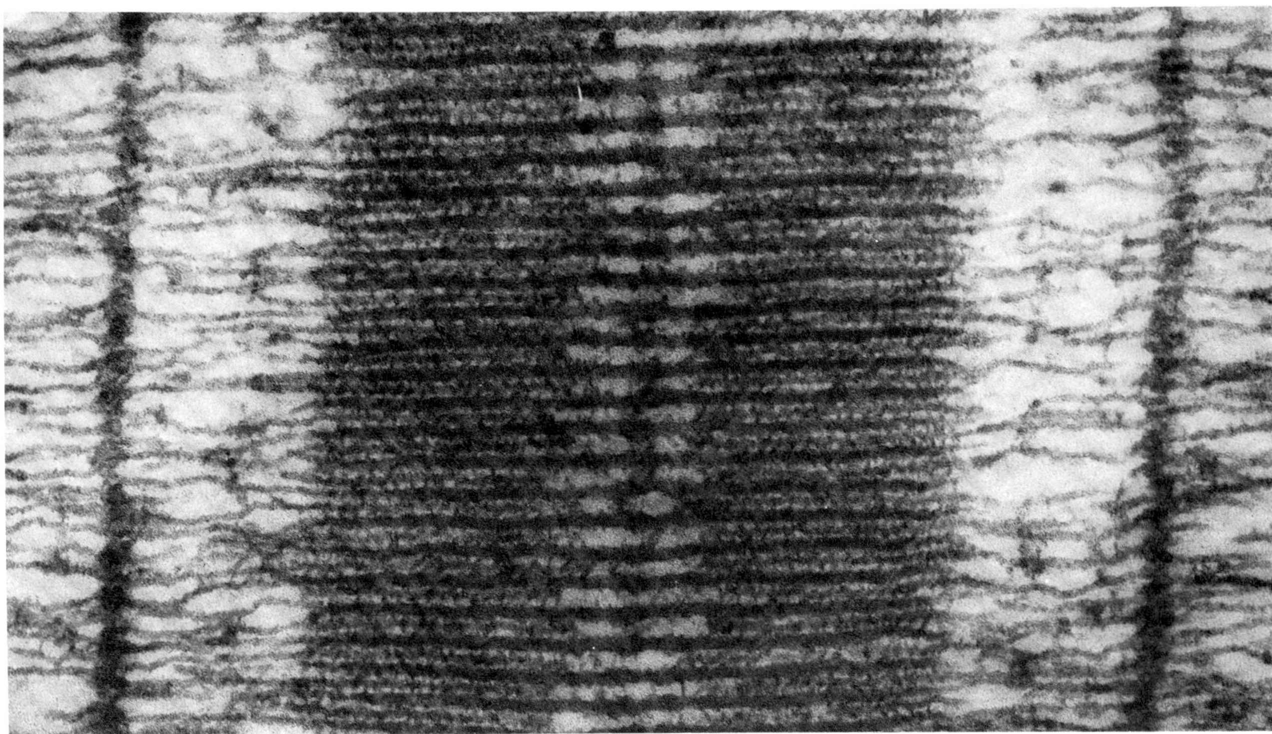

FIG. 1. Double array of myofilaments in a sarcomere. Array of thick filaments in center of sarcomere forms the A band. Thin filaments extend into the thick-filament array from the dense Z line. The part of the thin-filament array that does not interdigitate with thick filaments forms the I band. The part of the thick-filament array that does not interdigitate with thin filaments forms the H zone. × 67,000. [From Huxley (37).]

contrast microscope, and A. F. Huxley and Niedergerke (34) on shortening intact muscle fibers with the interference microscope. These studies showed that sarcomere shortening in both active and relaxed fibers results in a decrease in the axial I-band width, and that the A band remains constant in width. Correlated studies with the electron microscope (37) showed that the band patterns were produced by two sets of interdigitating filaments: thick, myosin-containing filaments, generally tethered transversely at their midpoints by interfilamentary M connections, and thin, actin-containing filaments, joined at their midpoints by connections that form the Z disk (Fig. 1). The thick filaments form the A band, whereas the thin filaments extend from the Z disk into the A band where they interdigitate with the thick filaments. The noninterdigitating part of the thin filaments forms the I band. The fact that the length of the filaments appeared to remain constant during both active and passive shortening, and during stretch, indicated that the generation of force was due to interaction *between* the filaments rather than to an axial dimensional change in one or both of them. This interpretation was strongly supported by the demonstration that, as fibers were stretched, the ability of intact fibers to shorten after electrical activation (35) and skinned fibers to shorten after calcium application (52) was lost at the sarcomere length where the two sets of filaments were pulled just out of overlap.

Electron micrographs of a rigor muscle revealed the existence of short (about 10-nm) lateral connections between the thick and thin filaments in the region of overlap (Fig. 1). It was suggested that these cross bridges were the force-generating structures (31, 37). X-ray–diffraction studies of muscle fibers in the relaxed and activated states, which showed that with activation mass moved from the thick filaments toward the thin filaments, provided additional evidence that force development was associated with some kind of lateral interaction between the two types of filament (23).

Force-Length Relation

The discovery of two sets of filaments in muscle fibers, and the realization that there were simple relations between sarcomere length and filament configuration, provided the impetus for a reinvestigation of the force-length relation (57) with finer definition of the force associated with a given sarcomere length. This was achieved through the use of a feedback device with which the length of a defined segment of a single fiber could be set at a certain value in the relaxed fiber and then maintained at that value in the

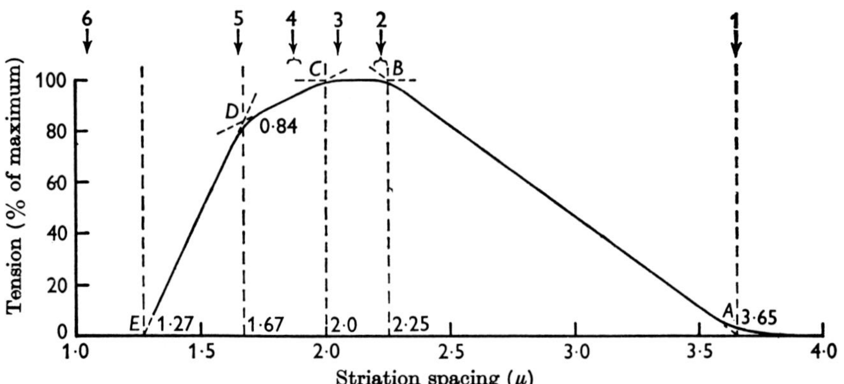

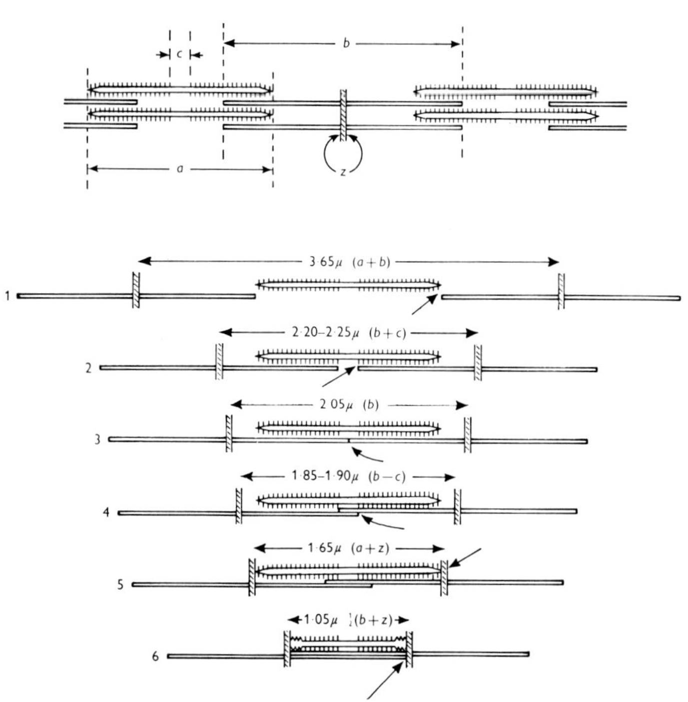

FIG. 2. Length-tension relation and filament dispositions at various sarcomere lengths. *Upper diagram*: length-tension relation for frog muscle. *Middle diagram*: sarcomere—*a*, thick-filament length; *b*, thin-filament length; *c*, length of central bare region of thick filament; *Z*, width of the Z band. *Lower diagrams*: filament dispositions at various striation spacings. Number at left of each diagram corresponds to numbered parts of length-tension relation. Note that *1*, *2*, *3*, and *5* are close to discontinuities in length-tension relation. [From Gordon et al. (19).]

activated state (19). The results are shown in the *upper part* of Figure 2, which should be compared with the filament configurations shown in the *lower part* of the figure. The key experimental points are *1*) the plateau of force at sarcomere lengths between 2.05 and 2.25 μm, *2*) the linear decline in force between 2.25 and 3.65 μm, and *3*) the loss of the ability to develop force at a sarcomere length close to 3.65 μm. The force plateau appears to be related to the fact that the central region of the thick filament does not contain myosin projections; thus increasing the sarcomere length from 2.05 to 2.25 μm does not change the number of potential sites at which cross bridges can be formed. The linear drop in force at longer sarcomere lengths is associated with the decrease in filament overlap, and the loss in force-generating ability at 3.65 μm corresponds to the complete loss of overlap at this sarcomere length. These features of the force-length relation can be simply explained if the force-generating structures are the projections from the myosin filament and these projections interact laterally with a site on the actin-containing filament to produce force.

The discontinuities in the force-length relation at sarcomere lengths of 1.7 and 2.0 μm appear to be related to axial dimensions of filaments rather than to cross bridges. At a sarcomere length close to 2.0 μm the ends of the thin filament make contact with each other, and at about 1.7 μm the ends of the thick filament make contact with the Z disk. These axial filament interactions seem to perturb the cross-bridge system so that less force is produced than at 2.0 μm. Another factor that may affect the force-length relation below 2.0 μm is an effect on the inward spread of electrical activation. At short sarcomere lengths the core of the fiber is inactive (62).

Kinetic Properties of Cross Bridges

In addition to producing force, cross bridges generate motion when the load on the sarcomere is less than P_0. According to electron microscopy, the length of the cross bridge is about 10 nm; therefore cross bridges must turn over many times during an activity cycle to produce the displacements of more than 100 nm per half sarcomere that are seen experimentally.

Do cross bridges act independently or cooperatively? One indication that they act independently is that the force-length relation falls linearly when the sarcomere length is increased from 2.25 to 3.65 μm, which is a range where the number of cross bridges also falls linearly (Fig. 2). Another relevant observation is that when a sarcomere in an electrically activated fiber is extended to 3.0 μm and then allowed to shorten under a very light load down to 2.0 μm, the velocity is nearly constant over the entire contraction (8, 19). Because the amount of filament overlap, and presumably the number of interacting cross bridges, increases during the course of the motion, the constancy of the velocity throughout the motion implies that the kinetic properties of each cross bridge are independent of their number.

Additional evidence comes from a comparison of the contraction kinetics of fully activated and partially activated skinned muscle fibers. The isometric force produced by a skinned muscle fiber increases when the calcium ion concentration in the bathing solution is increased above 10^{-7} M, and reaches a plateau at about 10^{-6} M [Fig. 3; (24)]. The increase in force in this range appears to be due to the increase in the number of force-generating cross bridges (25, 63). Therefore the axial distance between adjacent attached cross bridges in the overlap region would be expected to decrease at the higher calcium levels. Under appropriate experimental conditions (21, 22, 55), the contraction velocity at a given relative load is the same at different degrees of activation (Fig. 4). This result indicates that the cross bridges act independently and that cooperative effects of cross bridges attaching to the thin filament (20) do not affect the contraction kinetics under these conditions.

Cross-Bridge Model of A. F. Huxley

When the sliding-filament mechanism of muscle contraction was introduced, A. F. Huxley (31) in 1957 worked out a quantitative model for explaining the

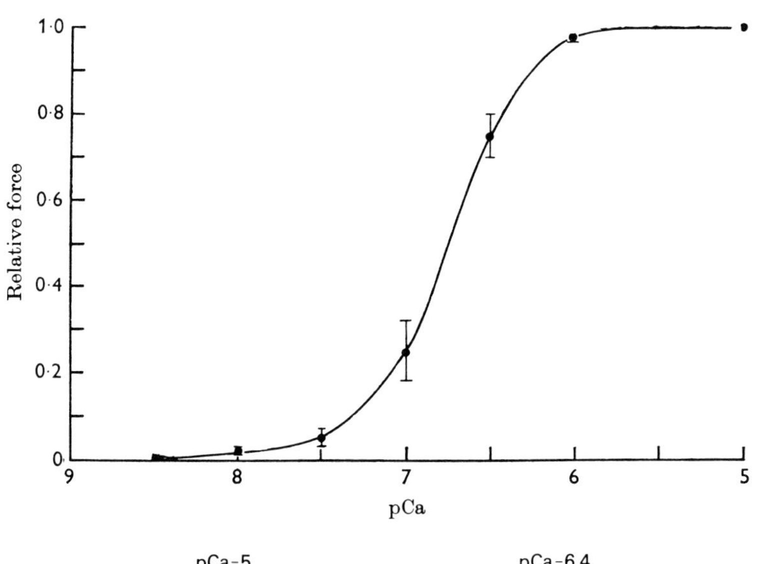

FIG. 3. Force-pCa relation for skinned frog muscle fiber. [From Hellam and Podolsky (24).]

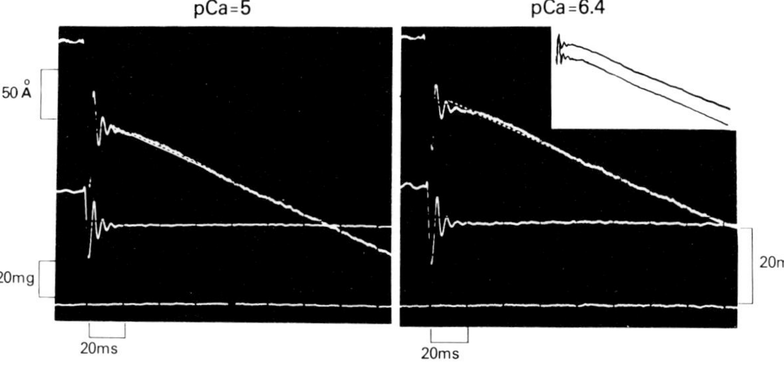

FIG. 4. Contraction kinetics of a skinned frog muscle fiber at different free-calcium concentrations. *Top trace*, displacement; *middle trace*, force; *bottom trace*, zero force. Fiber is fully activated at pCa 5 and half-activated at pCa 6.4. *Dashed line* on displacement trace is back extrapolation of steady motion. The 2 displacement traces, which are juxtaposed in *inset*, are almost the same. [From Gulati and Podolsky (21).]

mechanical and chemical properties of a population of independent cross bridges. The general features of the model are described briefly; the reader is referred to the original article (31) for a more detailed exposition.

The model assumes that a site on a projection from the myosin filament can interact with a site on the actin filament over a relatively wide range of distances (± ca. 10 nm) and considers the events that take place as the actin site moves past the myosin site with velocity v. If one end of the muscle fiber is fixed, v is related to the velocity V of the moving end by the expression $v = sV/2L$, where s is the sarcomere length and L is the fiber length. When myosin attaches to actin [forming the state actomyosin (AM)] the cross bridge develops force $k(x)x$ where x is the axial distance between the actual position of the actin site and the actin site position at which the cross bridge exerts zero force. The stiffness of the cross bridge is $k(x)$. Because the myosin site is either unattached (M) or in a single attached state (AM), this is a two-state model.

The rate constants for the reactions that make and break the cross bridge are $f(x)$ and $g(x)$, respectively. The functions used by Huxley are shown in Figure 5. The value of h, the reach of the cross bridge, was 15 nm, and the stiffness was assumed to be independent of x, so that $k(x) = k$. This set of rate and force constants generates force and produces motion because the probability for making a cross bridge is higher when the force of the cross bridge is positive, whereas the probability for breaking the bridge is higher when the force is negative. This is the essential feature of most cross-bridge models.

The cross-bridge distributions during steady motion depend on the relative velocity of the filaments as well as the rate constants $f(x)$ and $g(x)$. Figure 6 shows the distributions for several different velocities for the set of rate constants given in Figure 5. The fraction of available myosin projections that bind to actin at a

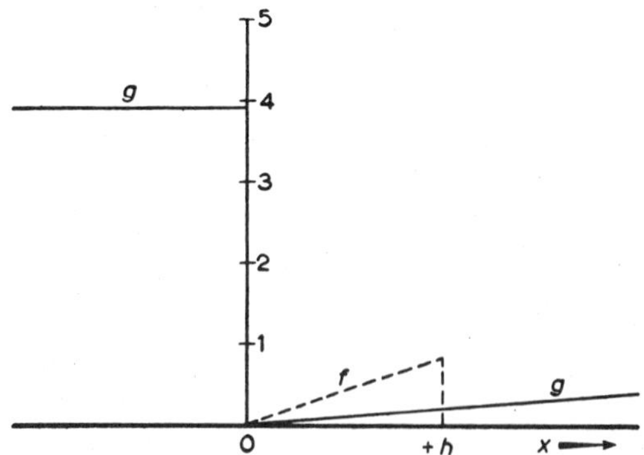

FIG. 5. Rate functions for cross-bridge interaction in the 1957 model of A. F. Huxley. Here f is the rate function for cross-bridge formation, g is the rate function for cross-bridge dissociation, x is the distance between the actual position of the actin site and the actin position at which the cross bridge exerts zero force, and h is the value of x at which f reaches a maximum value. [From Huxley (31), © 1957, with permission from Pergamon Press, Ltd.]

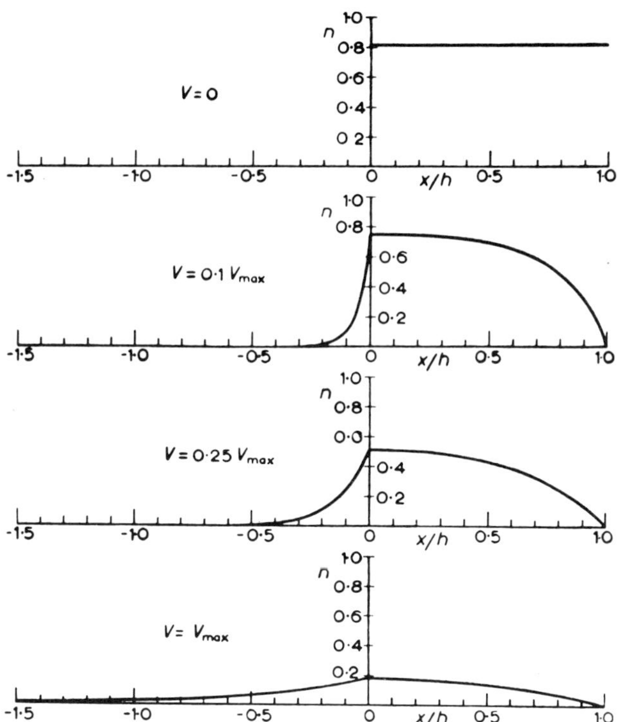

FIG. 6. Cross-bridge distributions at different steady speeds. Note that area of distribution function (and therefore instantaneous number of cross bridges) decreases as contraction speed increases. [From Huxley (31), © 1957, with permission from Pergamon Press, Ltd.]

given x is n. When $v = 0$, AM cross bridges are present only for $x > 0$. The parameters of the model imply that the rate of reaction of myosin with actin is relatively slow in the region of positive x. Therefore as the contraction velocity increases, the probability that the actin site passes a myosin site without forming a cross bridge increases, and the total number of cross bridges, $\int n(x)dx$, decreases. In addition, the force, which is proportional to $\int n(x)k(x)xdx = k\int xn(x)dx$, also decreases. At $v = v_{max}$, the force of the positive-force bridges is exactly balanced by that of the negative-force bridges and the net force is zero. The relation between force and velocity in the model can be made similar to the A. V. Hill force-velocity relation by appropriate choice of model parameters. The relation between energy output and velocity can also be approximately matched (see *Fenn Effect*, p. 174) if it is assumed that one ATP molecule is split each time a cross bridge turns over.

An important feature of this model is that cross-bridge force is determined as a single-valued function of x. In the original version (31) this was the case because force came from the kinetic energy of the projection and was exerted as soon as the myosin projection attached to the actin filament. It should be noted that the mathematical formalism of the model can be used with other force-generating mechanisms as long as the force function remains single valued. An example in which force is generated by a very rapid irreversible configurational change in the cross bridge is shown in Figure 7. If the configurational change occurs on a time scale that is slow relative to that of the observation, or is not irreversible, the force function is no longer single valued and a more elaborate treatment is needed to describe the operation of the model.

High-Time-Resolution Mechanical Measurements

In recent years several new techniques have been developed for making high-time-resolution mechanical measurements on activated muscles. Three particularly useful techniques have been used: isotonic quick release (51), isometric quick release (36), and sinusoidal analysis (44, 45). In the first technique, the load on the muscle is suddenly changed and the resulting isotonic velocity transient recorded. In the second technique, the length of the muscle is suddenly changed to a new value and the isometric force transient recorded. With the third technique, the length of the muscle is oscillated sinusoidally and the force change is recorded. The first technique has the advantage that during the transient phase any series compliance is kept at constant length (due to the constant force). The second technique has the advantage that it may be easier to interpret (because the sarcomere is held fixed after the initial change) and also that the length change can be made more rapidly than force changes. The third technique has the advantage that the apparent rate constants that describe the data are readily extracted from it.

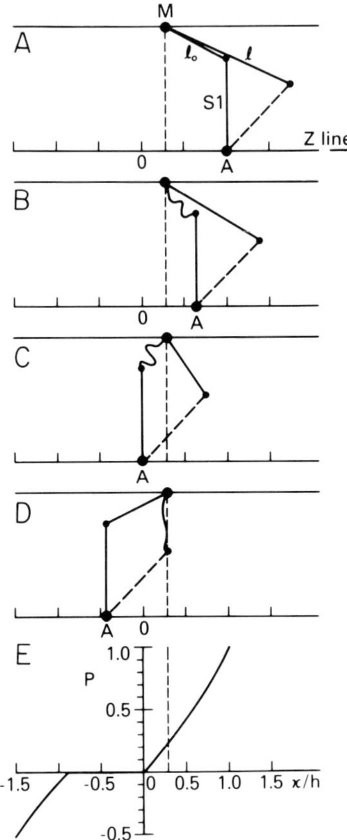

FIG. 7. Cross-bridge mechanism in which force is generated by a very rapid configurational change. The S1 moiety of the myosin molecule is attached to the thick filament at M through a flexible region that can be extended to length l_0 by thermal energy. It is assumed that S1 attaches to an actin site A in one configuration (*solid line*) and then very rapidly and irreversibly changes to another configuration (*broken line*) that can stretch the flexible region beyond l_0 and produce force. *A*: change in state stretches the flexible region to length l and force is proportional to $l - l_0$. *B*: flexible region is not completely extended when S1 attached to A, and stretched length of flexible region is less than l. *C*: stretched length of flexible region is l_0 and force is zero. *D*: change in configuration of S1 moiety does not stretch flexible region beyond l_0 and force is zero. If S1 remains attached to A, flexible region can be stretched by motion of the thin filament; negative force is produced when $x/h < -0.8$. *E*: force function for this mechanism. Note that stiffness is not a measure of number of attached cross bridges in this mechanism, because cross bridges in flat region of force curve do not show stiffness.

These techniques have revealed that events occur in muscle on at least three time scales. Fast rate constants, from 300 s^{-1} to greater than 1,000 s^{-1}, are necessary to describe the early responses (see Fig. 11). Slow rate constants, believed to correspond to the steady-state rate through one cross-bridge cycle, are on the order of 1–10 s^{-1}. In addition, there appear to be interesting rate processes occurring on the time scale of 50–200 s^{-1} (3, 45). When one oscillates a skeletal muscle at these intermediate frequencies, the muscle performs oscillatory work (45). An understanding of the origin of each of these rate processes would greatly enhance our understanding of the molecular basis of contraction.

Force Steps

When Podolsky (51) and Civan and Podolsky (3) reexamined the isotonic quick-release experiment (27, 41) with improved time resolution, they discovered that the steady velocity of shortening took 10–40 ms to be established at 3°C (Fig. 8). During this time, the velocity exhibited large deviations from its final behavior. Civan and Podolsky showed that the initial motions of the muscle after a quick reduction in force to a value less than P_0 were similar to the kinds of motion one would expect from a cross-bridge model. By changing the rate constants in the 1957 Huxley cross-bridge scheme (31), it was possible to closely match the actual velocity transients (53). Whereas in the Huxley scheme the maximum value of f was small compared with the maximum value of g, Podolsky and Nolan (53) found they had to make f large compared with g (Fig. 9) to match the transients. This led them to suggest that the initial rapid phase of the isotonic velocity transient might be due to the attachment of additional cross bridges and that during shortening the number of cross bridges was greater than that present during isometric contraction (Fig. 10). To account for the Fenn effect, they suggested that during

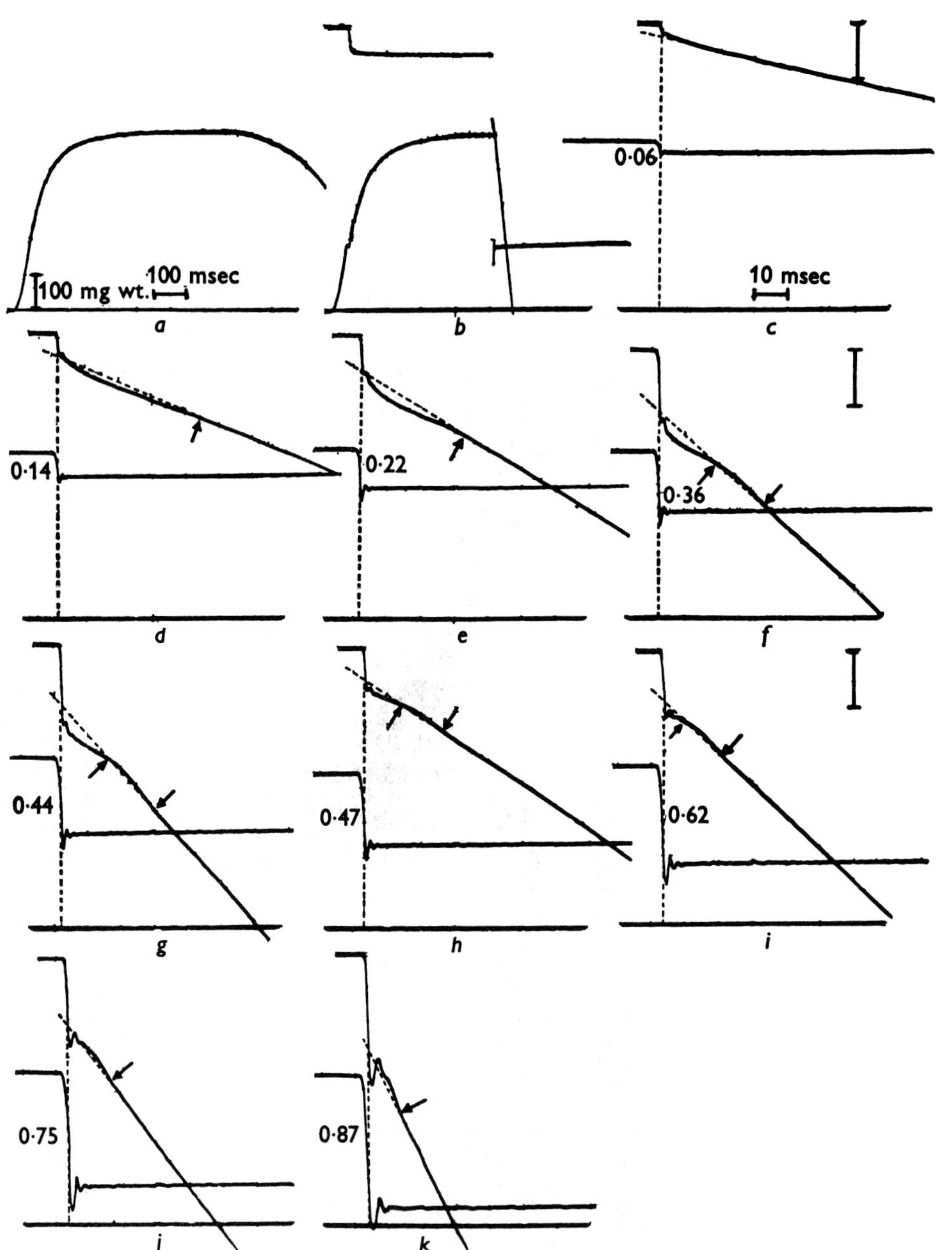

FIG. 8. Response of frog muscle fibers to sudden changes in load at 3°C. *Lower traces,* force records; *upper traces,* displacement. *a,* Isometric tension; *b,* record after sudden change in load, slow time scale; *c–k,* changes in load, rapid time scale. Force step as fraction of P_0 is given along side force trace. *Arrows* mark points at which actual motion intersects back extrapolation of steady motion. Note that force is steady ~2–6 ms after force step, but displacement transient lasts 10–40 ms. Displacement scale bar is 4 nm per half sarcomere in *panels c* through *g* and 8 nm per half sarcomere in the other panels. [From Civan and Podolsky (3).]

motion at high velocity some myosin cross bridges might dissociate from actin without splitting ATP, simply by reversal of the step A + M → AM. This seemed to agree with the findings of Curtin and Davies (5) that with constant-velocity stretching of active muscle much force is exerted but ATP usage is quite low, suggesting that cross bridges can detach without ATP being split.

Length Steps

Huxley and Simmons (36) were able to obtain transient data on a faster time scale than Civan and Podolsky by rapidly changing the length of an activated muscle fiber and recording the resulting isometric force transient. To make certain that a length of the muscle was held constant during the force tran-

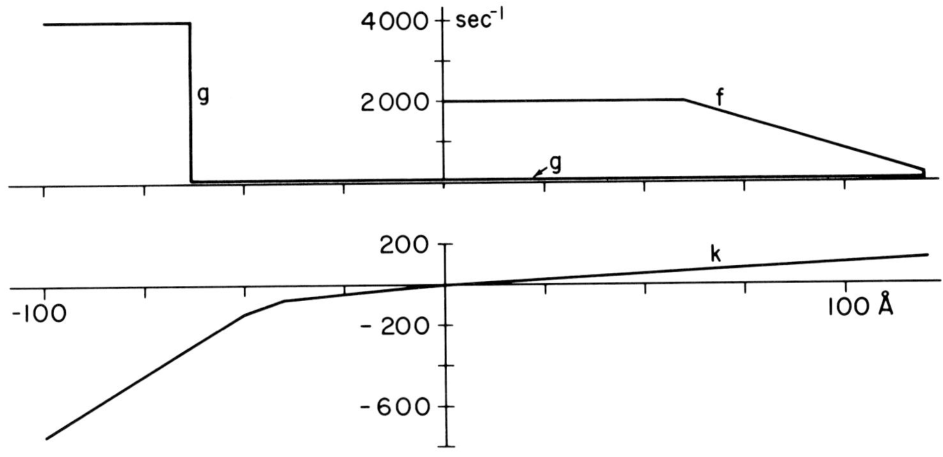

FIG. 9. Rate functions for cross-bridge interaction in the model of Podolsky and Nolan. *Upper panel*: f is rate function for cross-bridge formation; g is rate function for cross-bridge dissociation. *Lower panel*: k is force function for cross bridge. [From Podolsky and Nolan (53), © 1971, reprinted by permission of Prentice-Hall, Inc., Englewood Cliffs, NJ.]

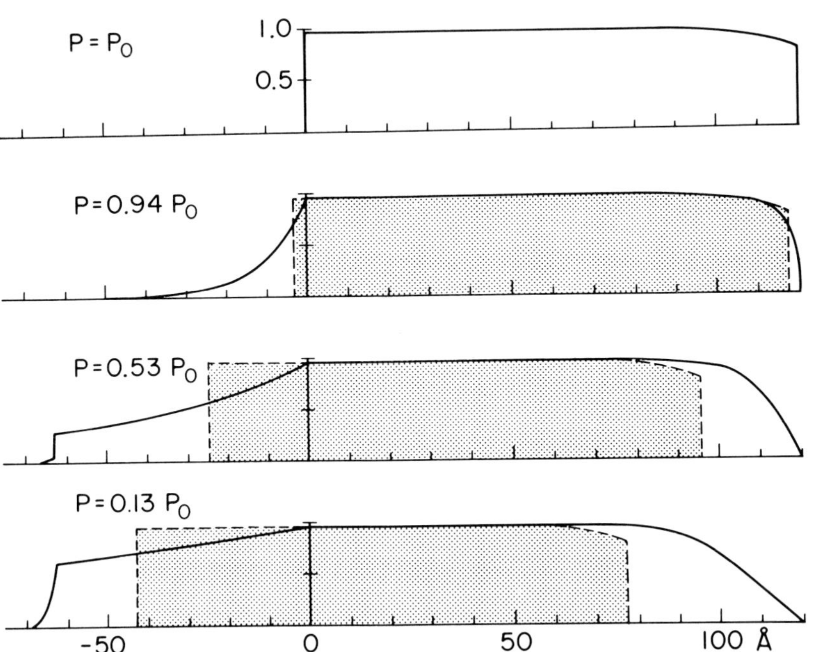

FIG. 10. Cross-bridge distributions in force-step experiments. *Top panel* shows distribution during isometric contraction. When load is suddenly changed to $P < P_0$, isometric distribution shifts to the left as shown in *lower panels*. Steady-state distribution for each load is given by *solid line*. Note that area of steady-state distribution function (and therefore instantaneous number of cross bridges) increases as load decreases and contraction speed increases. [From Podolsky and Nolan (53), © 1971, reprinted by permission of Prentice-Hall, Inc., Englewood Cliffs, NJ.]

sient, they used the same type of motorized feedback device that had been used in the muscle-length tension studies e.g., see *Force-Length Relation*, p. 175. As can be seen from Figure 11, they discovered that a muscle exhibits transient behavior even on the submillisecond time scale. For small steps, force redevelops to nearly the full isometric value. The time course of force redevelopment depends on the size of the force step: the rate increases when the magnitude of the force step is increased.

Figure 12 shows the force transient on a slower time scale and the corresponding velocity transient. After the step both transients contain a rapid phase, followed by a much slower phase, and finally an approach to steady state. It seems likely that corresponding phases of both transients reflect the same underlying cross-bridge processes.

To explain the rapid force changes during the initial portion of the isometric force transient, Ford, Huxley, and Simmons (16, 17, 36) suggested that the attached cross bridge might exist in two or more states, each having a different configuration, and that the initial part of the force transient might be due to changes in cross-bridge configuration.

Huxley and Simmons (36) pointed out that their description of the cross bridge would fit nicely with a model of the cross bridge in which the cross-bridge head attached to the actin filament at 90° and then rotated toward 45° (38, 56). It was necessary, however, to assume that part of the cross bridge was elastic. For

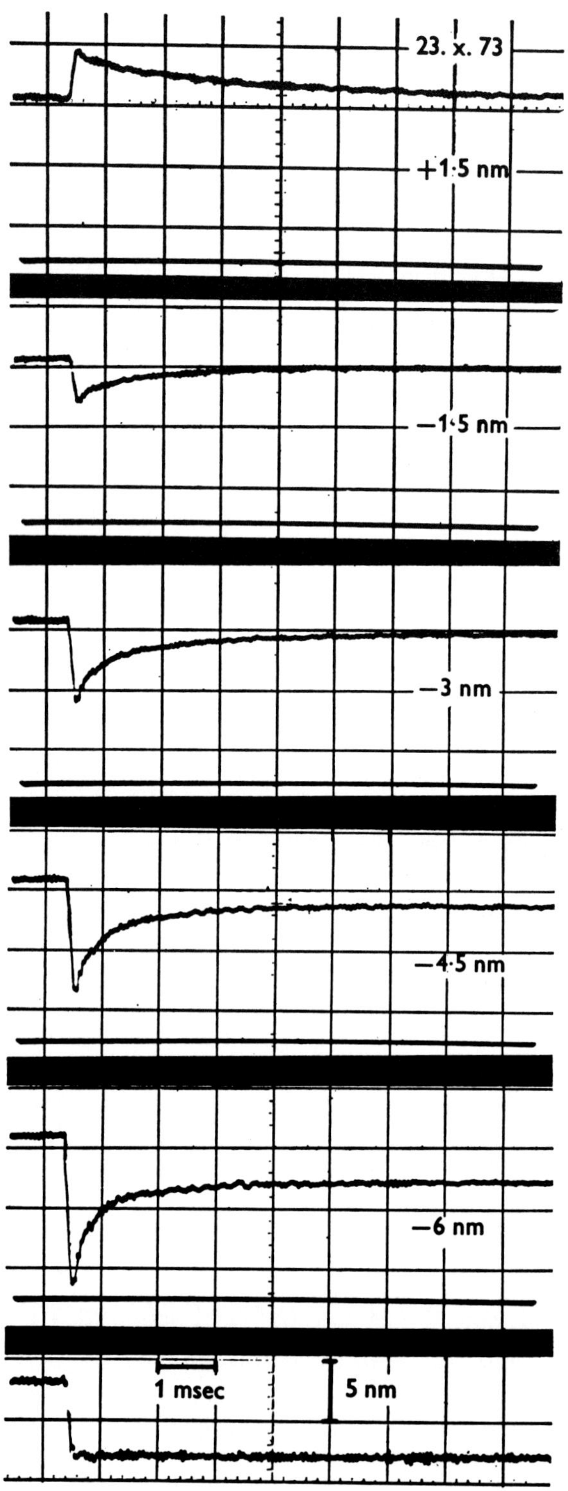

FIG. 11. Transient changes in tension exerted by a stimulated frog muscle fiber when suddenly stretched (*top panel*) or shortened (*middle panels*). *Bottom panel* shows typical release. Number next to each record shows size of corresponding length change per half sarcomere (in nm). [From Huxley (32).]

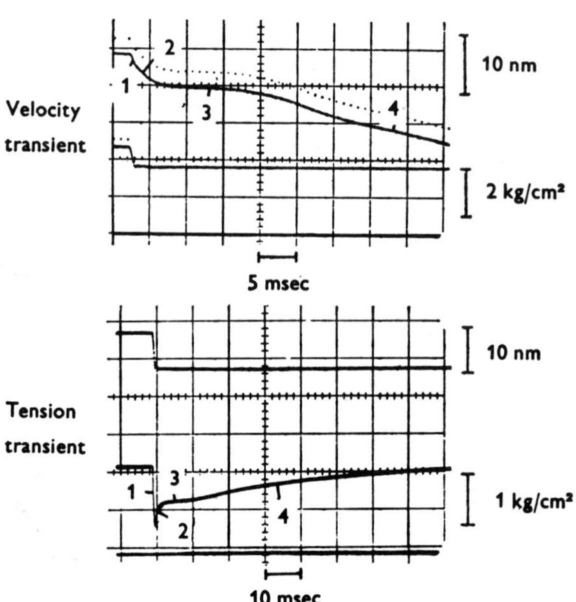

FIG. 12. Relation between velocity transient and tension transient. Phase 1 represents an instantaneous elasticity. Phase 2 is a rapid shortening in velocity transient or a rapid tension recovery in tension transient. Phase 3 is a marked reduction of either shortening speed or tension recovery. Phase 4 is steady shortening in the velocity transient or a very slow recovery of tension in the tension transient. Note that duration of phases is not the same in the two types of transient. Phases 1 and 2 of the tension transient are shown on a faster time scale in Figure 11. [From Huxley (32).]

simplicity, they assumed this elasticity resided in the subfragment-2 region of the cross bridge. The cross bridge consists of the globular head region of the myosin molecule, about 12 nm in length, called subfragment 1 (S1), and a region linking S1 to the myosin filament. This link was assumed to be the long (60 nm) largely α-helical portion of the myosin molecule known as subfragment 2 (S2).

The scheme of Huxley and Simmons is illustrated in Figure 13. The cross bridge attaching in the "90°" state (state 1) is illustrated by *A*. In this state the spring in S2 is not very stretched and only a small amount of force is exerted by the cross bridge. Force then quickly develops to a value, T_o, as many of the cross bridges rock to state 2, accompanied by a stretching of the spring, as in *B*, and some even rotate to state 3. This accounts for the development of isometric tension. As filaments are rapidly displaced relative to one another, as at the initiation of the isometric transient, the tension in the S2 spring is immediately reduced (*C*). This drops the tension exerted by the cross bridge to a value that Huxley and Simmons referred to as T_1. Huxley and Simmons proposed that the tension in the cross-bridge spring might control the equilibrium between states. Therefore the fall in tension would shift the equilibrium between states so that cross bridges still in state 1 would rock to state 2 and cross bridges in state 2 would rotate to state 3, the "45°" state (*D*). Restretching of the cross-bridge spring as in *D* leads to redevelopment of force to a value, T_2. After some time, cross bridges in state 3 detach, *E*, restarting the cycle. In the case of the isometric transient this last step would slowly bring the force back to the isometric level, T_o. Huxley and Simmons' model thus offered an explanation for the development of

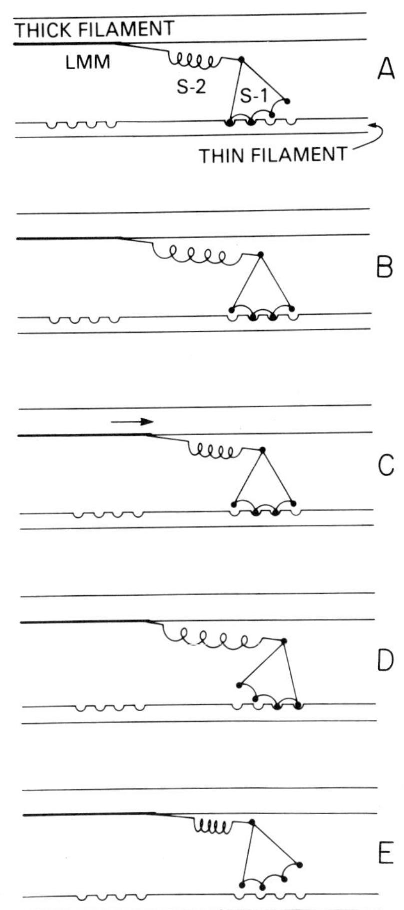

FIG. 13. Behavior of the cross-bridge head and compliance (spring) in the model of Huxley and Simmons during tension development and during an isometric transient. There are 3 attached states: state 1 (*A*), state 2(*B* and *C*), and state 3(*D*). Step length change of muscle occurs between *B* and *C*. [Adapted from Huxley and Simmons (36).]

isometric tension, *A* going to *B*; the instantaneous elasticity, *B* going to *C*; the rapid phase of the isometric transient, *C* going to *D*; and the slow redevelopment of isometric tension, *D* going to *E*, *A*, and to *B* again. The values of T_1 and T_2 as a function of the amount the filaments are moved past one another are shown in Figure 14. By doing these experiments at different sarcomere lengths, thereby changing the total number of cross bridges, Ford, Huxley, and Simmons (17) were able to show that most of the measured instantaneous elasticity, 4–6 nm of compliance per half sarcomere (see intercept of T_1 curve in Fig. 14), resides in the cross bridges.

In the Huxley 1957 model (31) the force of an attached cross bridge was determined by the kinetic energy of the cross bridge prior to attachment. In the Huxley-Simmons 1971 model (36), force is generated shortly after attachment as thermal energy stretches the cross-bridge elasticity and the cross bridge passes into more stable configurational states. An important feature of this model is that the rate at which the cross bridge goes into a more stable configuration depends on the activation energy going from the less stable to the more stable state and the strain energy stored in the cross-bridge elasticity. The back rate constant depends only on the activation energy going from the more stable to the less stable configuration. This model did not make any assumptions about the specific biochemical entities that might exist in any of the configurational states, although it assumed that ATP was responsible for the dissociation from stable state 3.

MUSCLE BIOCHEMISTRY

About the time the model of Huxley and Simmons was introduced, a scheme for the hydrolysis of ATP

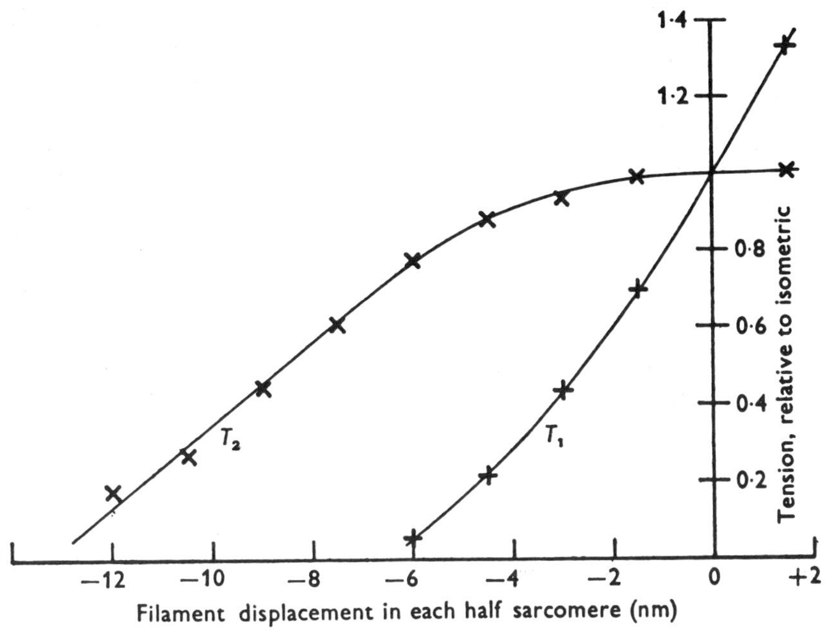

FIG. 14. Effect of step amplitude size on T_1 (extreme tension) and T_2 (tension approached during rapid recovery phase), both as a fraction of T_o, which is isometric tension immediately before the step. [From Huxley (32).]

by actomyosin was proposed by Lymn and Taylor (47). Their kinetic scheme was

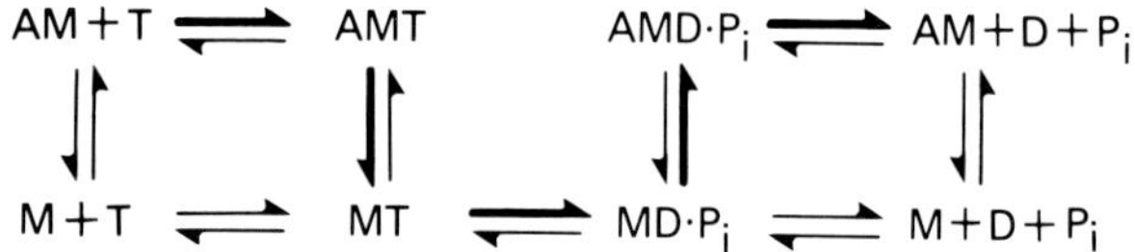

where T stands for ATP (adenosine triphosphate), D for ADP (adenosine diphosphate), and P_i for inorganic phosphate. The major pathway when ATP is added to actomyosin is shown by the darkened arrows. In this model, hydrolysis of ATP occurs when actin and myosin are dissociated but release of products occurs after reassociation. This kinetic scheme suggested the following possible cycle for the functioning cross bridge

$$\begin{array}{ccc} AM & \xleftarrow{\;D+P_i\;} & AMD\cdot P_i \\ {\scriptstyle T}\downarrow & & \uparrow \\ MT & \longrightarrow & MD\cdot P_i \end{array}$$

It was proposed that AMD·P_i and AM might correspond to different attached cross-bridge states. It seemed reasonable to associate the state AM with the 45° state because electron micrographs of cross bridges in muscles depleted of ATP appear to show the cross bridges oriented near 45° (58).

The hydrolysis scheme of Lymn and Taylor was attractive because it suggested a biochemical mechanism whereby actin and myosin might cyclically attach and detach in the course of ATP hydrolysis. In the Lymn-Taylor scheme, attachment (MT → MD·P_i → AMD·P_i) was faster than detachment (AMD·P_i → AM → MT), because the rate-limiting step was product release, AMD·P_i → AM. This agreed with the cross-bridge model of Podolsky and Nolan (53) for the organized system. Eisenberg and Kielley (12) presented evidence, however, that there might be two forms of MD·P_i: one, MD·P_{iN}, that seemed to bind strongly to actin and one, MD·P_{iR}, that did not. This suggested the following possible cycle

$$\begin{array}{ccccc} AM & \xleftarrow{\;D+P_i\;} & & & AMD\cdot P_i \\ {\scriptstyle T}\downarrow & & & & \uparrow \\ MT & \longrightarrow & MD\cdot P_{iR} & \longrightarrow & MD\cdot P_{iN} \end{array}$$

in which the rate-limiting step is MD·P_{iR} → MD·P_{iN}. In this case attachment would be the rate-limiting biochemical step as in the 1957 Huxley scheme.

It seemed possible that these relatively simple biochemical schemes might be able to fit with the existing cross-bridge models. They appeared to offer a way of deciding on the relative magnitude of f and g, and it even seemed, based on one early attempt (10, 11), that it might be possible to explain the isometric transient in terms of the transition between known biochemical states that had been measured in vitro.

Other Experiments: Some Puzzling Results

It did not take long to find evidence that did not fit in with the above picture. With skinned fiber preparations, Abbott and Steiger (1) and Kawai (44) found that the fast rate constant in activated muscle appeared to change with ATP concentration in the millimolar range. This did not fit with the idea that ATP merely caused dissociation and that the fast transient was either independent of ATP or depended solely on the reaction AMD·P_i → AM.

Another problem arose with regard to the biochemical cycles. These schemes had been proposed on the basis of experiments with low concentrations of actin and suggested that hydrolysis of ATP does not occur when actin and myosin are associated (i.e., the step AMT → AMD·P_i occurs very slowly). If this is correct, then in experiments done at higher concentrations of actin the hydrolysis rate should be significantly slower. When experiments were done with higher concentrations of actin, however, this was not the case (60). The hydrolysis of ATP was hardly inhibited at all at high concentrations of actin. Thus hydrolysis can occur equally well in both the associated and the dissociated states.

Another problem that arose with the way cross bridges were thought to behave in the early 1970s was that many of the rate constants initially thought to be more or less unidirectional were found, in solution, to be reversible (59, 60).

Recent Biochemical Studies

Recent studies (59, 60) suggest that it may be necessary to consider many more cross-bridge states. For example, the minimum number of steps necessary for myosin to hydrolyze ATP are

$$M \overset{+T}{\rightleftharpoons} MT \rightleftharpoons MD\cdot P_i \overset{-P_i}{\rightleftharpoons} MD \overset{-D}{\rightleftharpoons} M$$

and for actomyosin

$$AM \overset{+T}{\rightleftharpoons} AMT \rightleftharpoons AMD\cdot P_i \overset{-P_i}{\rightleftharpoons} AMD \overset{-D}{\rightleftharpoons} AM$$

Drawing these schemes in parallel and including possible cross steps we have

$$\begin{array}{ccccccccc} M & \rightleftharpoons & MT & \rightleftharpoons & MD\cdot P_i & \rightleftharpoons & MD & \rightleftharpoons & M \\ \updownarrows & & \updownarrows & & \updownarrows & & \updownarrows & & \updownarrows \\ AM & \rightleftharpoons & AMT & \rightleftharpoons & AMD\cdot P_i & \rightleftharpoons & AMD & \rightleftharpoons & AM \end{array}$$

as a minimal scheme. Evidence indicates that there may even be additional biochemical states important in ATP hydrolysis (12, 60). Exactly how many of these states are of importance in a contracting muscle is not yet known.

Hill Formalism

At the same time that the biochemical schemes were getting more complicated, T. L. Hill (29, 30) developed a formalism that made it possible to describe each cross-bridge state in a way that was useful for cross-bridge modeling, was thermodynamically self-consistent, and made it possible to relate muscle biochemistry to proposed cross-bridge cycles (10). He pointed out that each biochemical state could be characterized in terms of its free energy. For an unattached state, this is straightforward. For an attached state, it is only slightly more complicated. As discussed above, cross bridges appear to have elasticity, i.e., springlike behavior. Springs are described by a stiffness constant, k, which gives the ratio of the increment in force to the increment in length above zero-tension length [Huxley (31) used this same notation]. If x is the length increment, kx is the force increment, and $\frac{1}{2} kx^2$ is the energy stored in the spring. For an attached cross-bridge state having a linear elasticity, Hill pointed out that one can write the total basic free energy, A, as the sum of the minimum free energy, A_o, plus the strain energy, $\frac{1}{2} kx^2$.

One reason this way of looking at cross-bridge states is useful is that the rate constants for transition between any two states must be related to their difference in free energy, ΔA, according to the relation $r_+/r_- = \exp(-\Delta A/kT)$ where r_+ is the forward rate constant; r_-, the reverse rate constant; k, Boltzmann's constant; and T, temperature. Therefore, as long as a model follows this rather simple constraint, it will be thermodynamically self-consistent.

Application of Hill Formalism

In the cross-bridge model of Huxley and Simmons (36) the rate of transition between various cross-bridge configurations depended only on the minimum free energy of each state and the strain in a springlike region of the cross bridge (situated in the S2 moiety of the myosin molecule in the example in *Length Steps*, p. 180). The rates of transition between attached configurations were therefore possibly independent of any particular biochemical rate constant and constrained by the strain in the spring. An alternative class of models is one in which each cross-bridge configuration corresponds to a particular biochemical state and the rates of transition between configurations depend on the rate of a specific biochemical step. Although the Hill formalism applies for either class of models, it is particularly useful in the latter case because it suggests a way of relating specific biochemical information to the cross-bridge model.

As an example of how the formalism may be applied to the latter class of models, consider Figure 15, which shows a possible free-energy diagram for the following simplified biochemical cross-bridge model

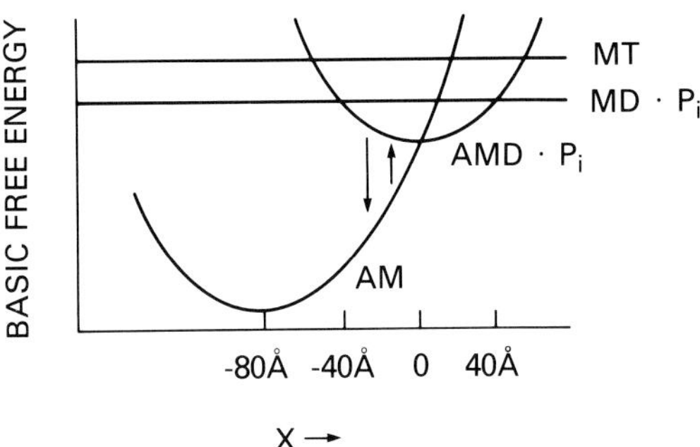

FIG. 15. One possible free-energy diagram corresponding to the biochemical cycle AMD·P_i ⇌ AM ⇌ MT ⇌ MD·P_i ⇌ AMD·P_i shown in text. Free-energy levels of unattached states are independent of x, a measure of strain in an attached cross bridge, more rigorously defined in *Cross-Bridge Model of A. F. Huxley*, p. 177. Free-energy curves of attached states are parabolas. Minimum free energy of AM state is to left of that for state AMD·P_i under the assumption that equilibrium configuration for AM state is more acutely angled than that for AMD·P_i (i.e., equilibrium configuration for AMD·P_i looks like Fig. 13*B* and AM more like Fig. 13*D*). Other states, such as M and AMT, are considered unimportant in this simple model. [Adapted from Eisenberg and Hill (10).]

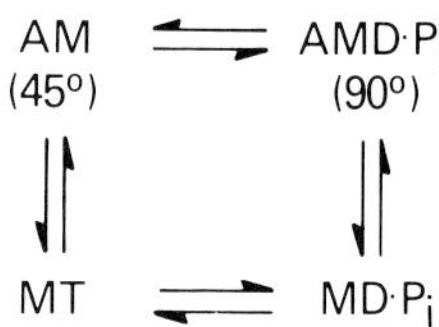

The cross bridge in state AMD·P_i is assumed to have its minimum free energy corresponding to a configuration angled at 90°; the state AM, at 45°. The free energy of the unattached states is independent of x. If the cross-bridge elasticity is assumed linear, the free-energy diagrams of the attached states are parabolas. The two attached states in Figure 15 have their parabolas shifted along x because their difference in angular configuration causes the minimum strain position (point of minimum free energy) to occur at different relative positions between actin and myosin sites.

To relate the biochemistry to the cross-bridge mechanism the approximation is made that at the point of minimum free energy, a given attached state behaves in muscle just as it would in solution because in each case the cross-bridge moiety is unstrained. (The validity of this approximation is discussed in ref. 11.) Therefore one can assume that the difference in minimum free energy between any two attached cross-bridge states (or any two unattached cross-bridge states) is similar to the difference in free energy between the corresponding biochemical states in solution. Therefore the relative vertical position of some of the lines and curves in Figure 15 can be obtained from biochemical equilibrium constants when these are known.

Some of the rate constants may also be obtained by

assuming that the biochemical rate constants in solution correspond to the muscle rate constants at minimum free energy (11). Solution biochemistry studies, however, cannot tell us how the rate constants vary with strain (x), nor can they tell us the relative horizontal position between states on the free-energy diagrams. Some of this information can be deduced from physiological experiments. For example, the stiffness of muscle (from T_1 curves as in Fig. 14) tell us something about the shape (width) of the free-energy parabolas because the width of any parabola depends on the stiffness of that particular cross-bridge state. Also the dependence of the rate constant for force redevelopment with relative filament displacement tells us something about how the rate constants of transition between states might vary with x. Furthermore, experiments by Marston, Tregear, and others (48, 49) have shown that insect muscle (and rabbit muscle to a lesser extent), starting from the rigor condition, appears to lengthen when AMPPNP (an analogue of ATP that binds to the myosin active site but is not hydrolyzed) is added. This suggests that the state AM·AMPPNP may lie to the right of the state AM in the free-energy diagram. If this is correct, it may be an analogue of the 90° state assumed to exist in the simple model of Figure 15.

This discussion is meant to illustrate how the Hill formalism may be used to relate various experimental findings to a cross-bridge model. The interested reader is referred to references 9 and 11 for more detailed attempts at this.

CURRENT FRONTIERS

Although a general outline of how muscle works is beginning to emerge, many of the details remain to be discovered. It is not known, for example, whether the rate constants for transitions between cross-bridge states are controlled by a single springlike element, as in the model of Huxley and Simmons (36), or whether they depend on biochemical transitions, as in the models of Eisenberg, Hill, and Chen (10, 11). The location of the cross-bridge elasticity remains uncertain, although recent structural evidence suggests some of it may be located in the region of the myosin S1-S2 junction (4). Currently much work is being devoted to learning the details of possible cross-bridge configurations. The use of molecular probes, resonance spectroscopy, and time-resolved X-ray diffraction all promise to be informative.

CONCLUSION

In this chapter we outline the development of models of muscle contraction. We show how the simple viscoelastic model for muscle gave way to a contractile-element model and eventually to cross-bridge models of muscle contraction. We show how simpler models having only a few states and unidirectional rate constants were modified to include more states and reversible rate constants.

Muscle force is probably generated by a myosin cross bridge attaching to actin in one state and then undergoing a change to a new state whose minimum free energy is lower and shifted in the direction of lower strain compared to the original state. During steady-state shortening, the cross-bridge elastic element is constantly shortened, which leads to a reduction in the cross-bridge tension. This allows further changes in state, facilitating completion of the cross-bridge cycle, and allowing cross-bridge detachment and subsequent reattachment. It appears that stiffness during muscle shortening may be reduced relative to the isometric state (43), which suggests either that the number of cross bridges is reduced during shortening or that the cross bridges appear less stiff in a shortening muscle. Limits to the possible change in cross-bridge number are given by X-ray–diffraction patterns of shortening muscle, which show that the strong equatorial reflections are considerably less sensitive to steady shortening than is contractile force (39, 54). It also seems possible that the rapid phase of the isometric and isotonic transients, once argued to be due either to cross-bridge conformational change or attachment, may need to be explained by a combination of the two. Clearly much interesting work remains to be done in the area of muscle contraction.

REFERENCES

1. Abbott, R. H., and G. J. Steiger. Temperature and amplitude dependence of tension transients in glycerinated skeletal and insect fibrillar muscle. *J. Physiol. London* 266: 13–42, 1977.
2. Chock, S. P., P. B. Chock, and E. Eisenberg. Pre-steady state kinetic evidence for a cyclic interaction of myosin subfragment-1 with actin during the hydrolysis of ATP. *Biochemistry* 15: 3224–3253, 1976.
3. Civan, M. M., and R. J. Podolsky. Contraction kinetics of striated muscle fibres following quick changes in load. *J. Physiol. London* 184: 511–534, 1966.
4. Craig, R., A. G. Szent-Gyorgyi, L. Beese, P. Flicker, P. Vibert, and C. Cohen. Electron microscopy of thin filaments decorated with a Ca^{2+}-regulated myosin. *J. Mol. Biol.* 140: 35–55, 1980.
5. Curtin, N. A., and R. E. Davies. Chemical and mechanical changes during stretching of activated frog skeletal muscle. *Cold Spring Harbor Symp. Quant. Biol.* 37: 619–626, 1972.
6. Eastwood, A. B., D. S. Wood, K. L. Bock, and M. M. Sorenson. Chemically skinned mammalian skeletal muscle. I. The structure of skinned rabbit psoas. *Tissue Cell* 11: 553–566, 1979.
7. Ebashi, S., and M. Endo. Calcium ion and muscle contraction. *Prog. Biophys. Mol. Biol.* 18: 123–183, 1968.
8. Edman, K. A. P. The velocity of unloaded shortening and its relation to sarcomere length and isometric force in vertebrate muscle fibres. *J. Physiol. London* 291: 143–159, 1979.
9. Eisenberg, E., and L. E. Greene. The relation of muscle biochemistry to muscle physiology. *Annu. Rev. Physiol.* 42: 293–309, 1980.
10. Eisenberg, E., and T. L. Hill. A cross-bridge model of muscle contraction. *Prog. Biophys. Mol. Biol.* 33: 55–82, 1978.
11. Eisenberg, E., T. L. Hill, and Y. Chen. Cross-bridge model of muscle contraction. Quantitative analysis. *Biophys. J.* 29: 195–227, 1980.
12. Eisenberg, E., and W. W. Kielley. Evidence for a refractory

state of heavy meromyosin and subfragment-1 unable to bind to actin in the presence of ATP. *Cold Spring Harbor Symp. Quant. Biol.* 37: 145–152, 1972.

13. FENN, W. O. A quantitative comparison between the energy liberated and the work performed by the isolated sartorius muscle of the frog. *J. Physiol. London* 58: 175–203, 1923.
14. FENN, W. O. The relation between the work performed and the energy liberated in muscular contraction. *J. Physiol. London* 58: 373–395, 1924.
16. FORD, L. E., A. F. HUXLEY, AND R. M. SIMMONS. Tension responses to sudden length change in stimulated frog muscle fibres near slack length. *J. Physiol. London* 269: 441–515, 1977.
17. FORD, L. E., A. F. HUXLEY, AND R. M. SIMMONS. The relation between stiffness and filament overlap in stimulated frog muscle fibres. *J. Physiol. London* 311: 219–249, 1981.
18. GOLDMAN, Y., AND R. M. SIMMONS. Active and rigor muscle stiffness. *J. Physiol. London* 269: 55P–57P, 1977.
19. GORDON, A. M., A. F. HUXLEY, AND F. J. JULIAN. The variation in isometric tension with sarcomere length in vertebrate muscle fibres. *J. Physiol. London* 184: 170–192, 1966.
20. GREENE, L. E., AND E. EISENBERG. Cooperative binding of myosin subfragment-1 to the actin-troponin-tropomyosin complex. *Proc. Natl. Acad. Sci. USA* 77: 2616–2620, 1980.
21. GULATI, J., AND R. J. PODOLSKY. Contraction transients of skinned muscle fibers: effects of calcium and ionic strength. *J. Gen. Physiol.* 72: 701–716, 1978.
22. GULATI, J., AND R. J. PODOLSKY. Isotonic contraction of skinned muscle fibers on a slow time base. Effects of ionic strength and calcium. *J. Gen. Physiol.* 78: 233–257, 1981.
23. HASELGROVE, J. C., AND H. E. HUXLEY. X-ray evidence for radial cross-bridge movement and for the sliding filament model in actively contracting muscle. *J. Mol. Biol.* 77: 549–568, 1973.
24. HELLAM, D. C., AND R. J. PODOLSKY. Force measurements in skinned muscle fibres. *J. Physiol. London* 200: 807–819, 1969.
25. HERZIG, J. W., T. YAMAMOTO, AND J. C. RUEGG. Dependence of force and immediate stiffness on sarcomere length and Ca^{2+} activation in frog muscle fibres. *Pfluegers Arch.* 389: 97–103, 1981.
26. HILL, A. V. The maximum work and mechanical efficiency of human muscles and their most economical speed. *J. Physiol. London* 56: 19–41, 1922.
27. HILL, A. V. The heat of shortening and the dynamic constants of muscle. *Proc. R. Soc. London Ser. B* 126: 136–195, 1938.
28. HILL, D. K. Tension due to interaction between the sliding filaments in resting striated muscle: the effect of stimulation. *J. Physiol. London* 199: 637–684, 1968.
29. HILL, T. L. Theoretical formalism for the sliding filament model of contraction of striated muscle. Part I. *Prog. Biophys. Mol. Biol.* 28: 267–340, 1974.
30. HILL, T. L. Theoretical formalism for the sliding filament model of contraction of striated muscle. Part II. *Prog. Biophys. Mol. Biol.* 29: 105–159, 1974.
31. HUXLEY, A. F. Muscle structure and theories of contraction. *Prog. Biophys. Biophys. Chem.* 7: 255–318, 1957.
32. HUXLEY, A. F. Muscular contraction. *J. Physiol. London* 243: 1–43, 1974.
33. HUXLEY, A. F. *Reflections on Muscle.* Princeton, NJ: Princeton Univ. Press, 1980.
34. HUXLEY, A. F., AND R. NIEDERGERKE. Interference microscopy of living muscle fibres. *Nature London* 173: 971–973, 1954.
35. HUXLEY, A. F., AND L. D. PEACHEY. The maximum length for contraction in vertebrate striated muscle. *J. Physiol. London* 156: 150–165, 1961.
36. HUXLEY, A. F., AND R. M. SIMMONS. Proposed mechanism of force generation in striated muscle. *Nature London* 233: 533–538, 1971.
37. HUXLEY, H. E. The double array of filaments in cross-striated muscle. *J. Biophys. Biochem. Cytol.* 3: 631–648, 1957.
38. HUXLEY, H. E. The mechanism of muscular contraction. *Science* 164: 1356–1366, 1969.
39. HUXLEY, H. E. Time resolved X-ray diffraction studies on muscle. In: *Cross-Bridge Mechanism in Muscle Contraction*, edited by H. Sugi and G. H. Pollack. Tokyo: Univ. of Tokyo Press, 1979, p. 391–401.
40. HUXLEY, H. E., AND J. HANSON. Changes in the cross-striations of muscle during contraction and stretch and their structural interpretation. *Nature London* 173: 973, 1954.
41. JEWELL, B. R., AND D. R. WILKIE. An analysis of the mechanical components in frog's striated muscle. *J. Physiol. London* 143: 515–540, 1958.
42. JULIAN, F. J. The effect of calcium on the force-velocity relation of briefly glycerinated frog muscle fibres. *J. Physiol. London* 218: 117–145, 1971.
43. JULIAN, F. J., AND M. R. SOLLINS. Variation of muscle stiffness with force at increasing speeds of shortening. *J. Gen. Physiol.* 66: 287–302, 1975.
44. KAWAI, M. Head rotation or dissociation? A study of exponential rate processes in chemically skinned rabbit muscle fibers when MgATP concentration is changed. *Biophys. J.* 22: 97–103, 1978.
45. KAWAI, M., AND P. W. BRANDT. Sinusoidal analysis: a high resolution method for correlating biochemical reactions with physiological processes in activated skeletal muscles of rabbit, frog, and crayfish. *J. Muscle Res. Cell Motil.* 1: 279–303, 1980.
46. LOWEY, S., H. S. SLAYTER, A. G. WEEDS, AND H. BAKER. Substructure of the myosin molecule. *J. Mol. Biol.* 43: 1–29, 1969.
47. LYMN, R. W., AND E. W. TAYLOR. Mechanism of adenosine triphosphate hydrolysis by actomyosin. *Biochemistry* 10: 4617–4624, 1971.
48. MARSTON, S. B., C. D. RODGER, AND R. T. TREGEAR. Changes in muscle cross bridges when β, γ-imido-ATP binds to myosin. *J. Mol. Biol.* 104: 263–276, 1976.
49. MARSTON, S. B., R. T. TREGEAR, C. D. RODGER, AND M. L. CLARK. Coupling between the enzymatic site of myosin and the mechanical output of muscle. *J. Mol. Biol.* 128: 111–126, 1979.
50. NATORI, R. The property and contraction process of isolated myofibrils. *Jikeikai Med. J.* 1: 119–126, 1954.
51. PODOLSKY, R. J. Kinetics of muscular contraction: the approach to the steady state. *Nature London* 188: 666–668, 1960.
52. PODOLSKY, R. J. The maximum sarcomere length for contraction of isolated myofibrils. *J. Physiol. London* 170: 110–123, 1964.
53. PODOLSKY, R. J., AND A. C. NOLAN. Cross-bridge properties derived from physiological studies of frog muscle fibers. In: *Contractility of Muscle Cells*, edited by R. J. Podolsky. Englewood Cliffs, NJ: Prentice-Hall, 1971, p. 247–260.
54. PODOLSKY, R. J., R. ST. ONGE, L. YU, AND R. W. LYMN. X-ray diffraction of actively shortening muscle. *Proc. Natl. Acad. Sci. USA* 73: 813–817, 1976.
55. PODOLSKY, R. J., AND L. E. TEICHHOLZ. The relation between calcium and contraction in skinned muscle fibres. *J. Physiol. London* 211: 19–35, 1970.
56. PRINGLE, J. W. S. The contractile mechanism of insect fibrillar muscle. *Prog. Biophys. Biophys. Chem.* 17: 1–60, 1967.
57. RAMSEY, R. W., AND S. F. STREET. The isometric length-tension diagram of isolated skeletal muscle fibers of the frog. *J. Cell. Comp. Physiol.* 15: 11–34, 1940.
58. REEDY, M. K., K. C. HOLMES, AND R. T. TREGEAR. Induced changes in orientation of the cross bridges of glycerinated insect flight muscle. *Nature London* 207: 1276–1280, 1965.
59. SLEEP, J. A., AND R. L. HUTTON. Actin mediated release of ATP from a myosin-ATP complex. *Biochemistry* 17: 5423–5430, 1978.
60. STEIN, L. A., R. P. SCHWARZ, P. B. CHOCK, AND E. EISENBERG. The mechanism of actomyosin ATPase: evidence that ATP hydrolysis can occur without dissociation of the actomyosin complex. *Biochemistry* 18: 3894–3909, 1979.
61. SZENT-GYORGYI, A. Free-energy relations and contractions of actomyosin. *Biol. Bull. Woods Hole Mass.* 96: 140–161, 1949.
62. TAYLOR, S. R., AND R. RUDEL. Striated muscle fibers: inactivation of contraction induced by shortening. *Science* 167: 882–884, 1970.
63. YU, L. C., J. E. HARTT, AND R. J. PODOLSKY. Equatorial X-ray intensities and isometric force levels in frog sartorius muscle. *J. Mol. Biol.* 132: 53–67, 1979.

CHAPTER 7

Energetics of muscle contraction

MARTIN J. KUSHMERICK | *Department of Physiology, Harvard Medical School, Boston, Massachusetts*

CHAPTER CONTENTS

THE PRIMARY FUNCTION of skeletal muscle is generation of force. Organization into motor units with appropriate neural control and connections to the skeleton allow the developed force to cause movements useful to the animal. The energy for this muscular activity is ultimately derived from metabolic oxidation of substrates stored in the animal or ingested from the environment like the energy supply available to any other cell type. Secondarily, skeletal muscle provides heat to the animal by shivering and possibly by nonshivering mechanisms of thermogenesis and supplies gluconeogenic precursors by net protein degradation during fasting.

Muscle is characteristically a chemomechanical converter that can be studied from two viewpoints. The first focus is on the chemical energy demands of actomyosin interactions and of mechanisms for electrical and osmotic work. The second concerns the integrated operation of aerobic and anaerobic metabolic pathways, providing chemical potential energy for those energy-requiring mechanisms. The subject of energetics includes both foci and encompasses the enumeration, description, and quantitation of the processes involved in all cellular energy transformations. The results of these descriptive studies provide necessary, but not sufficient, information for determining the energy costs of specific muscular functions and eventually the thermodynamic efficiency of specific conversions. This information permits a more analytical approach that aims to define the operating rules for integrating and regulating energy transformations. Thus muscle energetics quantifies integrative molecular and cellular physiology. In concert with information derived from muscle structure, from biochemical characteristics of contractile proteins, and from mechanical events, energetics becomes an essential tool for testing specific hypotheses of actomyosin interaction. This is so precisely because muscle is a chemomechanical converter and because the kinetics of actomyosin interactions must depend, in ways not yet known, on the presence of a mechanical stress on the proteins. Unfortunately such tests have not been adequately pursued, not for lack of interest or imagination, but because of the requirement for descriptive information.

All cells are organized as outlined by Lipmann (151): oxidative metabolism supplies effective concentrations of relatively few intermediates, which supply chemical potential energy to cellular functions. He coined the phrase "energy-rich phosphate compounds," adenosine 5′-triphosphate (ATP) and phosphocreatine (PCr) being the most ubiquitous examples, to focus on their role as readily convertible forms of chemical potential energy necessary to provide the driving force for all cellular processes that do not proceed spontaneously. Cells have evolved a wide variety of mechanisms by which the free energy of hydrolysis of ATP to adenosine 5′-diphosphate (ADP) and inorganic phosphate (P_i), for example, is mechanistically coupled to a nonspontaneous process useful to the cell. The coupling mechanism allows the second process to occur. Examples include formation of solute and electrical potential gradients, macromolecular biosyntheses, and cell movements.

Muscle tissue and cells are unique for carrying out energetic studies largely because they are differentiated. The metabolic rate of muscles increases many times in transition from a resting state to a contracting state. For example, the basal oxygen consumption of resting frog sartorius muscles at 0°C (for more than one-half century the physiologists' favored preparation) accounts for more than 90% of the total energy requirements and amounts to approximately 7 nmol$\cdot g^{-1}$ wet wt$\cdot min^{-1}$ (141). This value corresponds to a steady-state turnover of approximately 0.8 nmol ATP$\cdot g^{-1}$ wet wt$\cdot s^{-1}$. During the first few seconds of an isometric tetanus, the rate of ATP turnover is nearly 10^3 higher, and this higher rate of metabolism declines to the base line in relaxation. There are, therefore, obvious experimental advantages to measuring energetic parameters during and after contractile activity. In addition the large difference in rates of energy transformation between resting and contracting muscle allows study of the kinetics of metabolic pathways when muscle contraction causes a transient perturbation in levels of energy-rich phosphate compounds from the resting steady state. A detailed investigation of the time course of recovery metabolism after a step depletion of the pools of high-energy phosphate compounds is feasible since the metabolic time scale is measured in minutes and the contraction time scale is measured in seconds or fractions thereof. Since available methods for the study of energetics use whole muscle tissues, an experimenter can correlate a specific cellular function, mechanical output, with measurable extents of chemical reactions and associated heat production.

HISTORICAL PERSPECTIVES

Nature of the Muscle Machine

It was appreciated for centuries that muscle was some kind of living mechanical device. In contraction muscles became palpably stiffer than at rest; they developed force and could shorten. Strenuous exercise was associated with the liberation of body heat at a rate much above that in the resting condition. It was assumed that muscular activity was the source of this additional body heat, so most observers deduced that there was a mechanistic link between the mechanical changes in muscle and the heat liberated. What kind of machine is muscle? One obvious possibility evolved from the development of thermodynamics. Muscle might be a heat machine. Since it seemed obvious that a certain amount of heat was liberated during muscular activity, the contractile machine might somehow be similar to other known and well-described devices transforming temperature gradients into useful mechanical work. Another view, that muscle was a chemical machine, began to emerge and was catapulted to the forefront by the meticulous quantitative investigations of chemical changes in living cells by Fletcher and Hopkins (69, 70). In Hopkins' view neural or direct electrical excitation of muscles somehow allowed one or more chemical reactions to proceed spontaneously; these reactions caused muscle contraction and in the process liberated heat. However, biochemical and metabolic investigation of cells was at its infancy, so very little was known about chemical compounds present in cells or the reactions in which they might participate.

At the beginning of this century thermodynamics provided a basis for thinking about all machines, including living cells, because devices for measuring mechanical work, temperature change, and therefore heat production were available and could, in principle, be applied to living cells, including contracting muscles. The synthetic and predictive power of thermodynamics was well appreciated for two well-known machines: heat engines, in which changes in the volume of a working substance are employed and electromagnetic engines, in which useful work is done by electrical currents. It was widely assumed that the muscle machine was more akin to heat engines than to electromagnetic motors. Except for batteries, chemical machines such as chemomechanical threads (214) were unknown.

Experimenters in the last part of the nineteenth century were able to detect temperature increases in muscles and deduced there was net heat production. The repeatability and resolution of the methods were not sufficiently developed to begin quantitative studies. Chemical investigations of muscular contraction were unfortunately even less advanced. In this context one may imagine the eagerness and enthusiasm with which a dedicated experimentalist used the thermogalvanometer made by Blix (12) to measure temperature changes in muscle. Thus Langely introduced A. V. Hill to the problem of muscle energetics by offering him Blix's device. Hill's early work developed this device to measure and describe, albeit in a crude and inaccurate manner by today's standard, the basic characteristics of heat production associated with isometric tetanus of frog muscle. Figure 1 is one of his and Hartree's earliest sets of data from an isometric contraction (88) and shows that the rate of heat production is initially greater than decreases in rate; at any corresponding condition, muscle heat production rate increases with temperature. His early experiments also demonstrated how technical advances often open up entire vistas. Hill made major improvements in Blix's thermogalvanometer that increased its sensitivity and temporal resolution. With the aid of Hartree, Hill analyzed the behavior of galvanometers until they transformed them into sensitive and reliable instruments for measuring muscle temperature during and after contraction in ways not possible in the original.

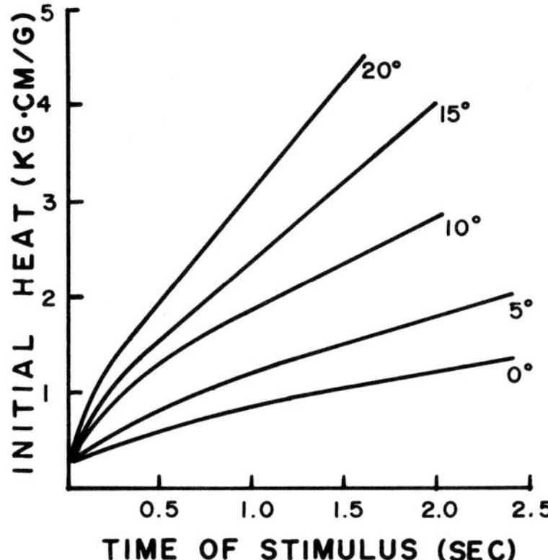

FIG. 1. Time course of heat production during a maintained isometric tetanus of frog muscle at various temperatures. [Redrawn from Hartree and Hill (88).]

For example, the records that Blix (12) published showed at best temperature oscillations from which he could only conclude that muscle contraction was associated with transient evolution of heat. The conceptual weakness now apparent from reading the beginnings of muscle energetics is the assumption that the hypothetical chemical reactions associated with contraction were all exothermic. It was therefore thought that evolution of heat indicated the occurrence of a chemical reaction. It was not explicitly supposed that relevant chemical reactions could be thermally neutral or endothermic.

Chemical Discoveries

Obviously discovery of the existence of certain chemical compounds and reliable analytical tools must precede measurement of changes in composition of those chemical compounds because of muscular activity. A pattern is often repeated: discovery of compound Y, deduction of a reaction X → Y, and formulation of a hypothetical model for muscle contraction such as X → Y + heat + energy for muscular contraction. Fletcher and Hopkins (69, 70) clearly showed the formation of lactate as a consequence of muscle activity and thereby launched the experimental basis for the lactic acid theory of muscle contraction, that synthesis of lactate from an unknown precursor caused muscle contraction. In Meyerhof's laboratory, as well as in other biochemical centers, the foundations of intermediary metabolism were being laid (176). The discovery that the formation of lactate in the fermentation process is exothermic fitted nicely with the prevailing lactic acid theory of muscle contraction. Thus the increasingly refined measurements of heat production during muscle contraction from Hill's laboratory tied in with the known chemical basis for muscular contraction.

The existence of a variety of hexose phosphates, first shown in investigations of yeast fermentation, was recognized in muscle as was their ubiquitous role in intermediary metabolism in many types of cells. Chemical reactions involving sugar phosphates dominated views of muscle energetics. For example, the Eggletons (52, 53) at University College London showed the existence of a labile phosphate-containing compound in muscle, which they termed "phosphagen." Consistent with the prevailing concepts, they considered phosphagen to be a novel and labile form of one of the hexose phosphates. Work of Fiske and his assistant SubbaRow at Harvard led to a dramatically different view. A reliable and accurate analysis of P_i was first developed and became an essential tool (66). Indeed Fiske and SubbaRow (66, 67) confirmed that P_i is liberated during muscular contraction, but the parent compound is not a sugar phosphate but a new compound, phosphocreatine. Soon in Meyerhof's laboratory calorimetric studies showed the hydrolysis of PCr liberates approximately 45 kJ/mol of heat, an unusually large amount and certainly more than expected for the hydrolysis of any hexose phosphate (175). In a real sense, therefore, the work of Fiske and SubbaRow began the chemical energetics of muscle contraction in terms of energy-rich phosphate compounds. The central role of PCr in muscular contraction was clearly shown by Lundsgaard (159, 160), who blocked the production of lactate with the inhibitor iodoacetate and showed that muscle contraction still occurred. He also showed that depletion of PCr and the resultant formation of P_i accompanied muscular contraction. The 30-yr-old theory about lactic acid was disproven.

Additional careful analytical work in Berlin and Boston led to the discovery of another phosphagen, ATP. Its role was initially not understood until Lohmann (152) showed the existence of an enzyme that catalyzes the reversible transphosphorylation between ATP and creatine that forms ADP and PCr. The final basic piece of information came unexpectedly from investigations of the characteristics of fibrous proteins from muscle. The major protein present in muscle was then called myosin, now known to be a combination of actin and myosin. Actomyosin is clearly a structural protein, but it also catalyzes the hydrolysis of ATP (57). Therefore the basic descriptive outline of chemical reactions associated with muscular contraction was already in place before the experimental, intellectual, and social disruptions of World War II. The primary fuel for muscular contraction is ATP. Phosphocreatine is a storage form of energy-rich phosphate that readily regenerates ATP during contractile activity. Finally, the heat production accompanying contraction is proportional to the observed net splitting of PCr. The scheme appeared to be established but quantitative tests of these ideas would have to await the development of better chemical tools.

Energetics as an Analytical Tool

Work in A.V. Hill's laboratory had advanced sufficiently that the time course of heat evolution during and after muscle contraction could be described. In 1920, Hill and Hartree (99) were able to divide muscle heat production into four phases: initial heat, maintenance heat, relaxation heat, and recovery heat. These phases of a continuum were devised to correspond with the four phases of an isometric contraction-relaxation cycle. *Initial heat* was evolved at a diminishing rate during a continued isometric tetanus (Fig. 1). The initial heat rate declined until a smaller constant rate of heat production, *maintenance heat*, was reached. This heat rate was continuous as long as the stimulation continued, and it ended soon after the end of the stimulus. The time course of heat evolution during the first few seconds of stimulation of frog sartorius muscle at 0°C was found to be independent of the presence of oxygen, so it was deduced that the underlying chemical reactions were entirely nonoxidative. The magnitude of the maintenance heat rate increased with temperature (Fig. 1); in frog muscle the isometric force changes little with increasing temperature. *Relaxation heat* describes a rather sudden release of heat that occurs in mechanical relaxation and is now understood to be largely a thermoelastic effect when force changes rapidly. *Recovery heat* was a prolonged and slow rate of heat production after relaxation, which in total amount approximately equaled the sum of the other heats. At 0°C the recovery heat was at the limit of detection in these early experiments, but at 20°C it was clearly evident and paralleled oxidative metabolic changes. Recovery heat clearly required the presence of oxygen.

It is useful here to consider the several additional subdivisions of muscle heat production commonly distinguished, their modern definitions, and interpretation. [The review by Abbott and Howarth (1) should be consulted for additional details.] Unstimulated or resting frog sartorius muscle at 20°C consumes O_2 at a rate of 59 nmol $O_2 \cdot g^{-1} \cdot min^{-1}$ (163, 164), which at 475 kJ/mol O_2 consumed metabolically yields a value of 28 $mJ \cdot g^{-1} \cdot min^{-1}$ for resting heat production; at 0°C the value would be 3 $mJ \cdot g^{-1} \cdot min^{-1}$. This value, while small, is subject to substantial increases by exposing the muscle to increased [K^+] [the Solandt effect (211)] or by subjecting the muscle to a passive stretch [the Feng effect (61)]. The initial heat production is distinguished from the recovery heat production by a basic concept in energetics that is developed in ENERGY BALANCE, p. 210. Initial heat is operationally divided into three components. This plausible division has not been proved mechanistically significant.

1. *Activation heat* is that amount of heat that is produced at a very rapid rate early in a tetanus or twitch and that is independent of tension maintenance (96). To measure activation heat the total heat production in an isometric twitch or brief isometric tetanus is measured as a function of increasing muscle length and therefore of decreasing force development. Extrapolation to zero force yields the activation heat (113, 210), which can also be defined by its time course (196). In an isometric twitch at 0°C activation heat is 3–4 mJ/g. Its magnitude increases little with temperature (196). Because of all these properties activation heat is thought to be the net result of Ca^{2+} movements associated with activation of the contractile mechanism.

2. *Maintenance heat* is the steady-state rate of heat production during an isometric tetanus. It is a function of the developed force and therefore of muscle length. It is produced as long as the muscle is stimulated. Therefore maintenance heat is thought to represent the net heat caused by steady-state actomyosin interactions, steady turnover of Ca^{2+}, and reuptake by the sarcoplasmic reticulum (SR). In frog sartorii at 0°C its rate is approximately 8–12 $mJ \cdot g^{-1} \cdot s^{-1}$ (109). Its value increases with temperature with a Q_{10} of approximately 2.5, and its magnitude varies greatly from muscle to muscle presumably in proportion to actomyosin ATPase rate and the content and specific activity of the SR.

3. *Shortening heat* originally was defined as that heat rate produced above the isometric heat rate (maintenance heat) when the muscle shortens (94, 98). Hill considered the amount of shortening heat to be proportional to the distance shortened and its rate to be proportional to the velocity of shortening. A reinvestigation of shortening heat shows that its magnitude also depends on the actual force developed during shortening (112, 114). One possible interpretation is that shortening heat results from a higher rate of turnover of actomyosin interactions during shortening than in the isometric state. This may be incorrect, and a more detailed explanation in terms of a redistribution of myosin states during shortening compared to the isometric state is more likely.

Experimental work in Hill's laboratory provided tools to ask basic questions concerning the nature of the muscle chemomechanical machine. Is muscle really a heat machine like some other known converters of energy into useful mechanical work? It was believed by some that microscopic temperature gradients of more than 100°C existed and that the contractile mechanism was able to convert heat directly into force and muscular work. Fick (65) argued for many years that muscle was definitely not a heat machine because of the improbability of significant temperature gradients within muscle, but experimental evidence was lacking. He argued further that if muscle were a heat machine, the thermodynamic efficiency would be improbably low. Again quantitative measurements of efficiency were lacking, but the argument is sound because in a Carnot cycle the thermodynamic efficiency decreases as the temperature gradients decrease.

The work of Fenn in Hill's laboratory (more precisely in the basement of Hill's home) forced a return to basic questions regarding the nature of the muscle machine. When Fenn was given the best available equipment to work with, he focused on ways to get at fundamental questions rather than to confirm accepted dogma by achieving higher accuracy in the prevailing measurements. If one assumes that muscle is a chemomechanical converter and that electrical excitation allows a set of chemical reactions to proceed, one must still distinguish between two fundamentally different models. In the first, a fixed amount of chemical potential energy is made available for contraction by the excitatory stimulus. Depending on the details of the chemomechanical generator and external connections, a variable fraction of work is obtained, and the remainder of the potential energy is dissipated as heat. Thus this model states that the total energy released during contraction is constant. This is the basic concept embodied in the "viscoelastic theory" of muscle contraction. The alternative model is that the extent of the chemical reaction(s) is coupled to the performance of work such that a variable amount of chemical potential energy is able to be converted into useful work. Depending on the duration of the contraction and the arrangement of the mechanical apparatus, the muscle does more or less work and expends more or less total energy. Thus a clear experimental prediction is made provided efficiency does not change. If the second model were correct, there would be more energy utilization when more mechanical work was performed, whereas the first model predicts a constant amount of energy utilization independent of work performance.

Fenn's experimental approach to this issue was to measure the heat production in a muscle that shortens various distances against various loads (62, 63). The external work done was thus manipulated by varying independently the distance moved and the load. The heat production from working muscles was compared with that of isometric controls. What Fenn found was that however he made the experiment the muscle released more total energy in an isotonic working contraction than in an isometric one. Figure 2 reproduces one of his first experiments. The muscle was arranged on an afterloaded isotonic lever and stretched with a preload of between 25 and 50 g. The muscle was tetanized for less than 1 s; it raised the load and the load reextended the muscle during relaxation. The heat produced under isometric conditions in the same muscle, 1.9 mJ, is the base line and defines the origin of the graph. At the point of maximum work (with the 50-g load) 0.6 mJ of additional heat was produced over and above the isometric amount. This additional heat includes 0.39 mJ of external mechanical work. Notice that the muscle was reextended by the weight so the potential energy of the weight was dissipated as heat within the muscle in relaxation. In Fenn's words (62, p. 180–181):

> The important points to be noted are, (i) less heat is liberated in the isometric contraction than in any of those where shortening is allowed, (ii) that the increase in heat (above the isometric heat) is roughly parallel to the work done, and (iii) that the process in muscle which causes this extra liberation of energy takes place after the stimulus is over . . . and hence after the number of fibers brought into activity is presumably completely determined.

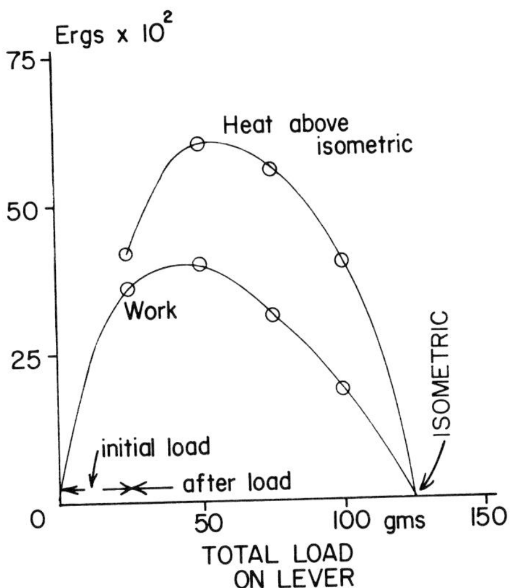

FIG. 2. Variations of external mechanical work and heat in excess of isometric heat as a function of load in isotonic afterloaded contractions; 1 J = 10^7 ergs. [From Fenn (62).]

The evidence was thus decisively against the viscoelastic concept of muscle energetics. Quite clearly, in some unknown manner, the chemomechanical mechanism of muscle is able to adjust its rate and total amount of energy transformation according to the load and extent of contraction.

An important logical point, which Fenn did not discuss and which appears to be a flaw in all work up to that time, was that it was assumed that there was a fixed stoichiometric ratio between the underlying chemical reactions and the measured heat output, independent of conditions and duration of stimulation. This question is not yet answered satisfactorily (e.g., see RESULTS OF ENERGY BALANCE EXPERIMENTS, p. 212).

The important question is what is the appropriate isometric control in Fenn's experiments? One answer a priori is to average the data obtained at the long and short lengths, since the muscle shortens from one to the other and isometric contractions at the long and the short lengths clearly define the extremes. Alternatively arranging that contractions occur at comparable forces during both isometric and isotonic conditions might be appropriate. Fenn set up the isometric controls at the initial and final lengths of the isotonic contraction. The difference in the isometric heat liberated at the two lengths was reasonably small and certainly not enough to confuse the primary observation.

Fenn's important conclusions can be criticized because they are not universally observed. For example, Blix (12) with data of lower quality was adamant that the isometric condition always was associated with a greater heat production than isotonic ones. Blix's belief was in fact confirmed by Hill (93) using gastrocnemius or semimembranosus muscles. In those experiments muscle length appeared to be the important determinant of the amount of energy released. The objection that Fenn's results are not universally true is periodically raised even in the contemporary literature. However, it seems unwise to conclude that certain striated muscles have fundamentally a different type of chemomechanical mechanism from others. Thus part of the significance of Fenn's results is that he fortunately chose a preparation (frog sartorius) and experimental conditions (moderately stretched and at relatively low temperatures) that were particularly favorable to demonstrate an important property of chemomechanical conversions. Woledge (236) summarized the available data (Fig. 3), which show clearly that results different from Fenn's results can actually be obtained.

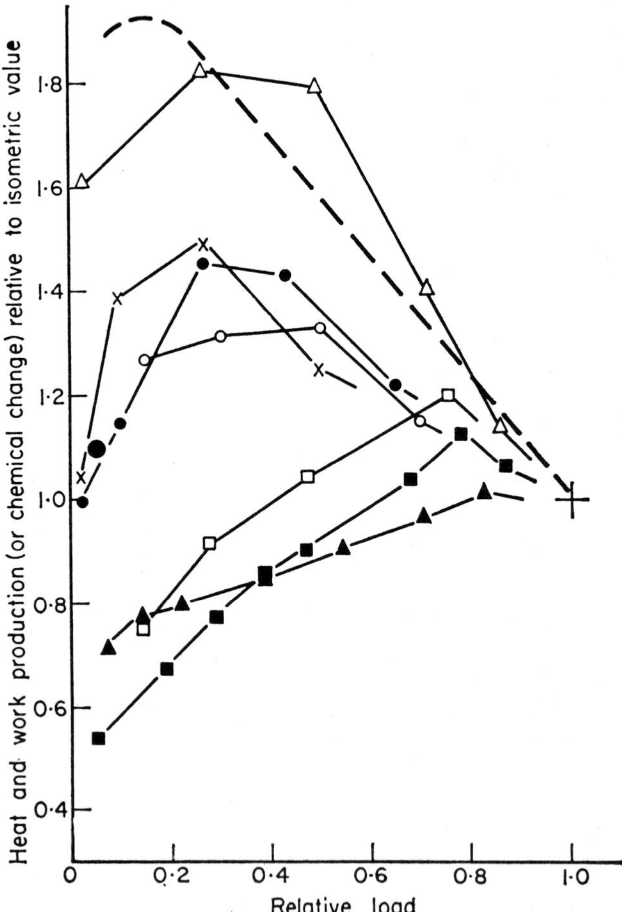

FIG. 3. Measurements of total energy output or chemical change as a function of load in working contractions studied by different investigators. All values are relative to a reference isometric contraction (+). ▲, ■, □, Experiments made above 10°C; ●, ×, △, experiments made near 0°C. *Interrupted line* depicts expected energy output as the sum of activation heat, shortening heat, and external work done. [From Woledge (236), © 1971, with permission from Pergamon Press, Ltd.]

The generality of the Fenn effect is clearly demonstrated by the analysis of Homsher et al. (112) shown schematically in Figure 4. These authors redefined the appropriate isometric reference as that isometric contraction that gives the same force as the load on the muscle during the isotonic working contraction. On the *left* side of Figure 4 is an experiment much like Fenn's original one shown in Figure 2. The experiment on the *right* was done at 20°C, the temperature at which the Fenn effect is minimal or absent. The external work done during a twitch is plotted as a function of the load by the lowest curve, labeled w; w varies in a way predictable from the force-velocity curve with the maximum at about 0.3–0.5 P_0, depending on the temperature. The maximum isometric twitch force, P_0, was 96 g at 0°C and 62 g at 20°C. The uppermost curve, labeled $h + w$, defines the total energy released during the isotonic twitches as a function of load. Clearly at 0°C, but not at 20°C, the total energy liberated exceeds that produced in the standard isometric twitch. Remember that Fenn's original experiments showed that the excess energy above isometric was always equal to or greater than the work done. The curves labeled $h - w$ plot this algebraic difference as a function of the load. Whereas one could claim Fenn's results are obtained at 0°C, clearly at 20°C all values for $h - w$ are well below the isometric energy cost. Why should the isometric reference contraction be that which gives the maximum force when the muscle undergoing isotonic twitches is bearing a substantially lighter load? The value of the experimental analysis of Homsher et al. (112) is that they posed this question and also that they measured the isometric twitch heat in muscles stretched beyond optimal overlap of the thin and thick filaments. They

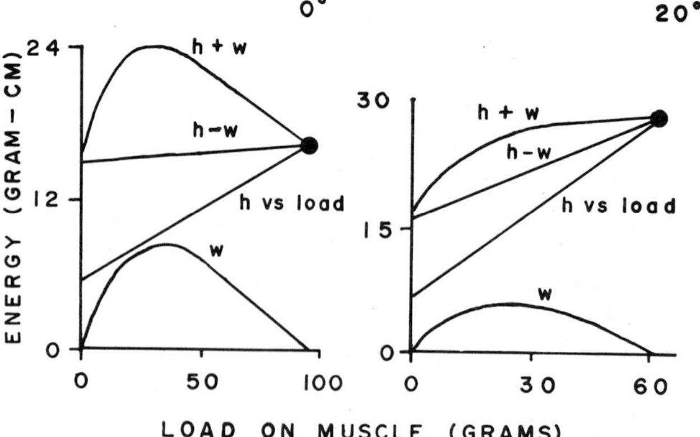

FIG. 4. Energy output in single isotonic twitches of frog sartorius muscles as a function of load. *Filled circle*, heat output in an isometric twitch; curve w, represents external work done; curve $h + w$, total energy released; line h vs. load, isometric twitch heat measured at increasingly long lengths and therefore at decreasing isometric forces; line $h - w$ is the difference between uppermost and lowermost curve. [Adapted from Homsher et al. (112).]

thus obtained total heat production as a function of decreasing twitch force. These data are illustrated by the line labeled h vs. load and show the predicted decrease in the total energy cost for an isometric twitch as the length increases and therefore as force decreases. There is therefore always an increase in the total energy released during the working contraction above an isometric reference at the same force development. Thus Fenn's remarkably insightful result is substantiated. Note also that the difference between the lines $h - w$ and h vs. load defines the shortening heat: the extra energy released in addition to the work done above that in an appropriate isometric reference contraction.

The most important conclusion to draw from this discussion is that continued debates over the magnitude of the Fenn effect or even its presence in a certain muscle or in a certain set of conditions is not likely to be productive because the molecular basis for increased energy utilization during working contractions is not understood quantitatively. Furthermore, because interpretation of muscle heat measurements in terms of the underlying chemical reactions remains incompletely defined and since measurements of heat production on whole muscle do not necessarily or uniquely correlate with actomyosin interactions, the most valid interpretation of Fenn's experiments clearly is the original one, which excludes decisively a viscoelastic concept of chemomechanical transduction as the dominant mechanism.

Direct Measurements of Chemical Change

The discovery of PCr and of ATP in muscles and of enzymes catalyzing reactions in which they participate (discussed in detail in CHEMICAL REACTIONS AND METABOLIC PRINCIPLES, p. 196) leads to the conclusion that ATP is the primary and PCr the secondary source of chemical energy for muscular contraction. Those facts plus the interpretation put on energetics by Fenn's experiments made a straightforward prediction: there is significant splitting of ATP and/or PCr continuously during a maintained contraction, and the rate of splitting increases when the muscle shortens against a load to perform work. The verification of this prediction was not easy to make experimentally. The problem was not merely to show that muscles could split ATP and PCr. That fact thas been repeatedly demonstrated in a variety of studies of prolonged contractions or fatigued muscle. The issue is whether there is a demonstrable decrease in ATP or PCr in the muscle during the development of force in a single twitch or brief tetanus. If an experimental result clearly excluded a splitting of ATP and PCr during the initial phase of a contraction, the conclusion would have to be that another chemical reaction provided the necessary energy for contraction. The conclusions from the detailed discussion (e.g., see RESULTS OF ENERGY BALANCE EXPERIMENTS, p. 212) are that some still-unknown reaction releases part of the initial heat, but that in any contraction where net external mechanical work is done there is measurable ATP and PCr splitting, and this splitting accounts for the work done.

Initial efforts to make experimental measurements of decreases in ATP and PCr led to inconsistent data and, in fact, failed to show decisively any chemical change of a magnitude sufficient to account for the force developed or the work done (145, 161, 179, 181, 224). Reactions involving changes in a variety of other compounds were also examined because of the urgent necessity to identify which compound or compounds provided the primary energy source for muscular contraction (42, 178). In retrospect, the sources of these difficulties were first, inadequate freezing technologies that did not allow the temporal resolution initially attributed to them, and second, the freezing methods activated muscles to various degrees so that the so-called unstimulated or resting controls were not actually obtained. The reader may wish to consult an account of an experiment described by Mommaerts (178) showing that in the process of immersing a heart in liquid nitrogen with the goal of freezing it rapidly, "5 or 10 quite normal electrocardiograms could be recorded." Other chilled liquids were clearly superior to liquid nitrogen, which readily forms a gaseous insulating layer, but it was not until the mid-1960s that Kretzschmar (taking his doctoral studies in Wilkie's laboratory) satisfactorily worked out the conditions necessary to freeze muscles sufficiently rapidly to achieve a time resolution of approximately 0.1s. His rapid-freezing hammer apparatus (133) and the Wollenberger clamp (238) are the prototypes of all rapid-freezing apparatus used today. Eventually with improved analytical methods and sufficiently rapid freezing techniques, it was possible to show decisively a decrease in PCr content of muscle during contraction (122). Finally, the last piece of the puzzle was put into place in 1962. Cain and Davies (18) showed that creatine kinase could be inhibited, and in that situation muscle contraction is accompanied by a decrease in ATP content without change in PCr content. At last the challenge issued to biochemists by A.V. Hill (95, 97) to show that splitting of ATP occurs in muscle contraction was met.

Summary

A complete description of the basic energetic phenomena of muscular contraction appeared to be in place, and the opportunity to apply muscle energetics to analyze critically ideas concerning the mechanism of muscle contraction seemed at hand in the early 1960s (41). The sliding-filament mechanism had been put forward (119, 120) as well as an outline of a cross-bridge mechanism (118). However real this potential appeared, not much quantitative analysis was done of the contractile mechanism based on energetic data, because important quantitative problems emerged concerning the relationship between chemical reactions occurring during contraction and the amounts of heat and mechanical energy liberated. Much of the early myothermic experimentation tacitly assumed a fixed relationship between the extent of chemical reactions and the heat production in contraction; however, this was not experimentally tested until the late 1950s. A necessary and sufficient basis for further analyses of muscle energetics was affirmative experimental answer to the following question: does the total energy output of muscle during a contraction-relaxation cycle and portions thereof agree quantitatively with the decrease in chemical potential energy? Obviously, in principle, an affirmative answer exists, otherwise at least one or both of the following principles must be violated: muscle converts some form of energy, other than chemical, into both mechanical work and heat and conservation of energy does not apply to muscle contraction. To appreciate the experimental work of the past two decades on this question of energy balance it is necessary to examine in detail first, the chemical reactions that occur in muscle and metabolic principles governing them and second, chemical thermodynamics as applied to muscle.

CHEMICAL REACTIONS AND METABOLIC PRINCIPLES

All cells extract energy necessary for their internal functions from components available in their environment. By highly integrated sequences of chemical reactions, metabolic pathways convert these substrates into cellular components, chemical and osmotic gradients, and storage of chemical potential energy. In aerobic cells, the net metabolic strategy is the controlled oxidation of substrates. Oxygen is the ultimate electron acceptor. Energy made available by metabolic sequences is stored by accumulation of *1*) ATP and other so-called energy-rich phosphate compounds to provide the driving force for most cellular processes, *2*) other compounds such as reduced nicotinamide-adenine dinucleotide phosphate (NADPH), which provides reducing power for biosynthesis of cellular components, and *3*) acetyl-CoA, which is the carrier of "activated" acyl groups. The strategy is simple. Many processes necessary for cell and organism survival do not proceed spontaneously. This type of process is called *endergonic*; $\Delta G'$ (change in free energy) is positive (e.g., see THERMODYNAMICS, p. 207). Examples are maintenance of intracellular ionic gradients, protein synthesis, and muscle force development. For an endergonic process to proceed, chemical energy must be provided. Hydrolysis of ATP to ADP and P_i is thermodynamically spontaneous; in the cell the concentration ratio of products to substrate is such that the free energy is very favorable (see THERMODYNAMICS, p. 207). This latter type of process is called *exergonic*; $\Delta G'$ is negative. Nature has evolved a large variety of endergonic processes necessary for cellular survival and a limited number of exergonic metabolic reactions that can provide the required energy. A specific chemical mechanism must also have evolved that enables a coupling between the exergonic and the endergonic reactions such that there is a net extent of reaction for both. If the coupling mechanism does not exist, only the exergonic reaction occurs spontaneously. It is important to realize that the chemical nature of these compounds, the energetics of their interconversions, and the stoichiometry of the coupled metabolic processes are not predictable from chemical and thermodynamic principles. The molecular bases of the coupling mechanisms and the quantitative details of integrated metabolic processes are central issues in contemporary cell physiology.

The central role of ATP in cellular energetics as clearly elaborated by Lipmann (151) is embodied by the phrase energy-rich phosphate compounds. This phrase does not refer to any physical-chemical characteristics of the phosphorus atomic bonds, but to the biological facts of *1*) the ubiquity of ATP and related compounds in cellular energy interconversions, *2*) the arrangement of metabolic reactions that act to maintain the ratio $[ATP]/[ADP][P_i]$ sufficiently large so that the hydrolysis of ATP is very favorable, and *3*) the specific coupling requirement of many cellular processes for ATP and related compounds. Therefore the experimental focus of chemical energetics of muscle is on ATP consumption and generation during the contraction-recovery cycle.

One might be tempted to extrapolate from the hypothesis that all interconversions of energy are linked to energy-rich phosphate compounds, but this view is not valid. Most transformations are, but the example of respiration-dependent Ca^{2+} uptake by mitochondria is one well-documented exception. The primary physiological source of energy is certainly ATP for actomyosin interactions and Ca^{2+}, Na^+, and K^+ movements across the cell and SR membranes. Phosphocreatine is not a direct substrate for any of these processes. There are seven reactions and metabolic sequences that bear importantly on muscle energetics examined in detail here.

Adenosine Triphosphatases

The hydrolysis of ATP is written

$$ATP + H_2O \rightarrow ADP + P_i + \alpha H^+ + \text{work} \qquad (1)$$

The work term is explicitly included to emphasize that chemical hydrolysis of ATP per se does not occur to any appreciable extent under normal cellular conditions. The reaction is always coupled, for example, by actomyosin to the performance of mechanical work, by Ca^{2+}-transport protein within the membrane of SR to achieve a Ca^{2+}-activity gradient across its membrane, and by Na^+-K^+-transport proteins in the sarcolemmal and T-system membranes to achieve gradients of Na^+ and K^+ activities and of electrical potential. At the pH of the sarcoplasm, 7.0–7.2, less than one equivalent of proton is liberated ($\alpha = 0.6$) because of differences in pK_a values of P_i and of the terminal phosphates of ADP and ATP (78).

In a contraction-relaxation cycle there are three major endergonic mechanisms coupled to the splitting of ATP.

1. Actomyosin ATPase is the most active of these. The content of myosin catalytic sites is 0.3 μmol/g wet wt of muscle in frog muscle (49). The maximal enzymatic turnover rate (K_{cat}) for actin-activated frog myosin subfragment 1 at 0°C, pH 7, and 10 mM KCl (64) is 4.5 s^{-1}. From these data the predicted maximal rate of ATP splitting is 1.4 $\mu mol \cdot g^{-1} \cdot s^{-1}$, a value that compares favorably with the observed rate of ATP utilization during maximally working frog sartorius muscles, 1.4 $\mu mol \cdot g^{-1} \cdot s^{-1}$ (139), and with the steady utilization rate during an isometric tetanus, approximately 0.3–0.4 $\mu mol \cdot g^{-1} \cdot s^{-1}$ (33, 142). These values are expected to vary among different muscle types more or less proportionally to the specific myosin ATPase activity (8).

2. The cellular amount and activity of Ca^{2+}-transport ATPase are greater in pale muscle fibers than in more oxidative ones (15, 213). Frog muscle contains about 15% vol/vol of SR (193), which contains up to 2–3 μmol Ca^{2+}/g muscle when maximally loaded. Under normal conditions the SR may contain only 0.5–1 μmol Ca^{2+}/g, and only a fraction of this is released in a twitch, perhaps 0.2 μmol/g. This estimate takes into account the Ca^{2+} required to saturate myofibrillar and cytoplasmic binding sites and to raise $[Ca^{2+}]$ from 10^{-7} M to 10^{-5} M during contraction (56, 165). These amounts may be underestimated for frog muscle, which contains up to 0.4 μmol Ca^{2+}-binding site/g muscle in parvalbumin, a soluble Ca^{2+}-binding protein of unknown function. These data indicate up to 0.2–0.6 μmol Ca^{2+}/g muscle is taken up after a twitch. The energy requirement would be 0.1–0.3 μmol/g ATP, taking a fixed stoichiometry of two Ca^{2+} transported per ATP hydrolyzed (162, 168, 225). It is not proven, but there is likely to be a continuous release and reuptake of Ca^{2+} during a maintained tetanus because *1)* cytoplasmic levels of free Ca^{2+} remain elevated near 10^{-5} M although the levels may not be steady (11), and *2)* in vitro fragmented SR demonstrates saturation kinetics for Ca^{2+} transport and ATPase in the Ca^{2+} range of 10^{-7}–10^{-5} M. Although there remain some uncertainties concerning the ability of the SR to accumulate Ca^{2+} rapidly enough to explain the rate of relaxation (15, 56), it is possible to estimate the maximal velocity of Ca^{2+} transport in frog muscle at 0°C for physiological levels of Ca^{2+} loading. From data obtained on skinned fibers (5, 72) for a gram muscle it is about 0.1–0.2 $\mu mol\ Ca^{2+} \cdot g^{-1} \cdot s^{-1}$, which would require the splitting of about 0.1 $\mu mol\ ATP \cdot g^{-1} \cdot s^{-1}$.

3. Sodium ions enter and potassium ions leave the muscle cells during each action potential; the original ionic intracellular environment is restored by the action of an electrogenic Na^+-K^+-ATP–driven pump for some minutes after the stimulation. The amount of ions flowing can be estimated from electrophysiological measurements. The capacitance of the surface membrane is approximately 1×10^{-3} F/g and in the T tubules is approximately 5×10^{-3} F/g, so that the total membrane capacitance in frog fibers is approximately 6×10^{-3} F/g (2). For a single action potential of 100 mV, the amount of charge necessary to discharge this capacitance is 6×10^{-4} C/g, which is equivalent to 6 nmol/g of monovalent ion. With the stoichiometry of Na^+-K^+-ATPase equal to 3 Na^+:2 K^+:1 ATP (85, 219), the energy cost to restore the initial conditions during recovery is therefore equivalent to approximately 2 nmol of energy-rich phosphate (~P) per gram for each depolarization. Notice that this is only a few percent of the total energy cost for an isometric or isotonic twitch. Obviously the energy cost would be greater in tetanic stimulation. For example, for each second of an isometric tetanus at 20 Hz, the energy requirement would be 0.04 μmol/g. The measured Na^+ influx as a consequence of electrical stimulation (22) was several times higher and was independent of the frequency of stimulation. Therefore the estimated energy cost for sodium pump activity for each second of tetanic stimulation is not likely to be greater than 0.1–0.2 μmol/g.

Creatine Phosphokinase

The enzyme catalyzing this near-equilibrium reaction is ATP:creatine phosphokinase (CPK)

$$ATP + Cr \rightleftarrows PCr + ADP + \alpha H^+ \qquad (2)$$

Notice the position of equilibrium is a function of cytoplasmic pH; $\alpha \approx 0.8$. There is an absolute requirement for divalent metal cations for enzymatic activity: Mg^{2+}, Mn^{2+}, and Ca^{2+} (135, 136, 187, 188). The enzyme is inhibited by Cl^-, SO_4^{2-}, and other inorganic anions. Activity can be completely abolished by sulfhydryl reagents as was done in vivo in the frog sartorius by Cain and Davies (18) with 2,4-fluorodinitrobenzene (FDNB). The work of Lundsgaard (160, 161) and Lohmann (152) and others assigned to this enzyme the role of maintaining access to a second pool of energy-rich phosphate compounds that effectively buffers ATP levels during contractile activity; a similar role has been assigned for it in brain metabolism (27). For this function of CPK the following conditions must be obtained: *1)* Creatine kinase, its reactants, and its products must be located in the same volume without diffusion barriers. *2)* The activity of CPK must be greater than the rate of ATP utilization during contraction. *3*) The reaction must be at or near equilibrium so that the extent of the reaction in the forward direction (PCr synthesis) is energetically as favorable as the reverse (ATP synthesis).

The enzyme is found at three strategic locations in the muscle cell (206): on the myofibril as a component of the M line, in the outer membrane of the mitochondria, and in the cytoplasm. These facts may indicate nature's efforts to minimize the diffusion distance between reagents and enzyme. Although evidence was presented that ^{14}C-labeled creatine and ATP are localized to specific portions of the myofibril (102, 103), direct measurements of ATP diffusivity (144) and the quantitative agreements among PCr, ATP, and P_i content that are measured by direct chemical assay and by ^{31}P nuclear magnetic resonance (NMR) spectrometry (43, 138) provide evidence against any substantial amount of binding or compartmentation of substrates and products in skeletal muscle.

The standard method for assessing the activity of CPK in muscle is to perform assays on aliquots of homogenates; these assays are made at optimal pH, substrate, and activator concentrations. As the results require an uncertain extrapolation to intracellular conditions, methods have been developed to measure directly the forward and reverse chemical fluxes in intact frog sartorius (77) and in perfused cat biceps and soleus muscles (138). The available data indicate that the measured forward and reverse rates in resting muscle are on the order of 2–5 times the ATP turnover rate during contraction (Table 1). The fluxes through CPK are just sufficient to support the widely believed notion that CPK functions as a high-energy phosphate buffer.

TABLE 1. *Chemical Energetic Characteristics of Isolated Frog and Mouse Muscles*

	Frog		Mouse	
	Sartorius, 0°C	Sartorius, 20°C	Extensor digitorum longus, 20°C	Soleus, 20°C
Metabolite content in resting muscle, μmol/g wet wt				
PCr	30	26	24	13
ATP	4	3	6	5
P_i	3	7	9	7
Total creatine	35	35	30	20
Metabolic rate of resting muscle, $nmol \cdot g^{-1} \cdot min^{-1}$				
O_2 consumption rate	7	50	150	150
Aerobic lactate production rate	2	22*	9	5
Tetanic rate of ~P consumption, $\mu mol \cdot g^{-1} \cdot s^{-1}$	0.3	2	4	1.3
Rate constant for recovery O_2 consumption, min^{-1}	0.07	0.2	0.4	1.7

* Anaerobic rate.

Phosphocreatine is a reactant that participates in only one metabolic reaction. The CPK reaction can therefore be called a dead-end reaction. Because of this fact and the experimental observation that the level of PCr in muscle is constant under resting conditions, it must be true that the forward and backward fluxes are identical in resting muscle. This means CPK catalyzes a reaction near equilibrium in the steady metabolic state characterizing resting muscle, which only limits the size of the fluxes in that they must exceed the resting net ATPase rate. Measurements of the mass-action ratios (the observed ratios of concentration of products to the concentration of reactants) are the same as equilibrium mixtures in vitro at appropriate pH and Mg^{2+} concentrations (20, 23, 147, 220). However, lack of accurate knowledge of the true sarcoplasmic MgADP concentration limits this experimental approach. Indeed with existing information we can proceed logically without assumptions to calculate the free-ADP concentration, since the CPK reaction is close to equilibrium. The cytosolic pH is close to 7 (3, 17, 200, 201), and the apparent equilibrium constant is close to 5×10^{-10} M (169, 220, 223); the free-ADP concentration can be obtained by inserting appropriate metabolite levels

$$[ADP] = \frac{K'_{eq}\,[ATP]\,[Cr]}{[PCr]\,[H]^{\alpha}} \tag{3}$$

$$= \frac{(5 \times 10^{-10}\ M)\ (4 \times 10^{-3}\ M)\ (6 \times 10^{-3}\ M)}{(30 \times 10^{-3}\ M)\ (10^{-7}\ M)^{0.8}}$$

$$= 1.6 \times 10^{-7}\ M$$

Typically measured ADP content of freeze-clamped muscle is approximately 5×10^{-4} M (0.5–1 μmol/g wet wt). Clearly the difference between the calculated and observed values means much of the total ADP content measured is bound to actin, mitochondria, and enzymes. Although the large amount of actin-bound ADP is well known, Veech et al. (220) made a good case that the dominant factor influencing low cytosolic ADP levels is the tissue content of mitochondria. In summary, in skeletal muscle the evidence indicates that CPK catalyzes a reversible reaction near equilibrium with ADP and ATP, so that PCr and CPK can function as an effective and reversible buffer of ATP levels. The capacity of this buffer approaches 10 times the size of the ATP pool in some pale skeletal muscles (Table 1).

In cardiac muscle, evidence suggests that there is some degree of compartmentation of the components of the CPK reaction. The mitochondrial content is much greater than in skeletal muscle, up to 40% by volume in cardiac and less than 5% in fast-twitch skeletal muscle. Thus the mitochondrial CPK activity may be a significant fraction of the total; cell fractionation studies indicate it is about 10% of total cell activity. Respiring cardiac muscle mitochondria can readily phosphorylate creatine with only endogenous nucleotides (4, 9, 203, 222). The hypothesis currently under investigation (10, 124, 125) is that the energy-rich compounds actually diffusing between the mitochondria and the myofibrils are a Cr-PCr pair instead of an ATP-ADP pair. However, the supporting data are incomplete; it is not even established that there are poorly exchanging pools of substrates and products. Also the functional significance of distinguishing between PCr and ATP fluxes is not clear. If there were some sort of compartmentation, then the free energy available would be reduced by the amount of chemical work necessary to maintain the segregated components, which is given by

$$RT \ln\left(\frac{\Gamma}{K'_{eq}}\right) \tag{4}$$

where Γ is the actual mass-action ratio of products and reactants in some compartment, K'_{eq} is the apparent equilibrium constant for the reaction in the cellular environment in the absence of compartmentation, R is the gas constant, 8.31 $J \cdot mol^{-1} \cdot {}^{\circ}K^{-1}$, and T is in degrees Kelvin. To maintain a 10-fold increase in Γ over K'_{eq}, 5.6 kJ/mol is required.

Adenylate Kinase

This reaction is catalyzed by ATP:AMP phosphoryltransferase, known by both of its trivial names, adenylate kinase and myokinase

$$2\ ADP \rightleftharpoons ATP + AMP \tag{5}$$

For enzymatic activity Mg^{2+} is absolutely required.

Maximal rates of ATP formation by adenylate kinase reaction, based on enzyme content of rabbit muscle and activity under optimal assay conditions, are about one-third of the maximal velocity of ATP formation by CPK reaction (186), but measurements of the unidirectional fluxes of the adenylate kinase reaction in the sarcoplasm have not yet been attempted. The reaction is also thought to be an equilibrium in skeletal muscle (14, 23, 52, 202). Thus with rising ADP levels during contraction, ATP can also be generated this way with equimolar production of AMP. Adenylate kinase is notoriously stable to acid and heat denaturation, the practical consequence of which is that the composition of improperly prepared muscle extracts may be altered during storage by the activity of this enzyme.

The behavior of relevant cytosolic metabolites as a function of net splitting of PCr has been modeled (147, 169, 223) with appropriate apparent equilibrium constants for the CPK and adenylate kinase reactions. The important form of the adenine nucleotides is their Mg^{2+} complexes. As a first approximation it is safe to consider that the adenine nucleotides in muscle are present as Mg^{2+} complexes; however, the nucleotides have different association constants and the free-Mg^{2+} level is not large enough (~1×10^{-3} M) to ensure complete complex formation (17, 83). The results of one set of calculations are reproduced in Figure 5, which shows the expected result: as PCr levels fall, H^+ falls, and P_i and creatine levels rise, but ATP and ADP levels change little until PCr depletion is well advanced. Although it is obviously not possible to review exhaustively how these changes in energetically important compounds might influence metabolic reactions, several important points emerge. *1*) pH changes could be sufficiently large to remove any H^+ inhibitory effect on phosphofructokinase. *2*) Changes in PCr and Cr levels relative to resting values are not as large as the relative changes in P_i levels. *3*) For the small extents of PCr utilization (ξ~P) the [ATP]/[ADP] [P_i] ratio changes are almost entirely due to changes in P_i. The large changes in free-creatine content were thought to be an important metabolic signal (123), but subsequent more careful experiments could not reproduce the results (76). High PCr levels do inhibit glyceraldehyde-3-phosphate dehydrogenase, phosphofructokinase, and pyruvate kinase, but almost complete loss of PCr levels is necessary to remove the inhibition of the last two enzymes (169). The resting level of P_i in muscle cells is probably overestimated at least in part because of the extreme lability of PCr during the freezing and extraction procedures. Evidence is presented in NEW DIRECTIONS, p. 229, that in cat fast-twitch muscles the resting level of P_i may be below 5 $\times 10^{-4}$ M. If in unstimulated muscle P_i levels were so low, then P_i should be reconsidered as regulatory for metabolic pathways, oxidative phosphorylation, and even for actomyosin interactions. Note that the very low levels of ADP set by the CPK reaction limits adenylate kinase activity until PCr levels fall substantially to allow ADP to increase (Fig. 5).

Adenylate Deaminase and the Purine Nucleotide Cycle

This irreversible reaction is the direct source of ammonia production in muscle and is catalyzed by

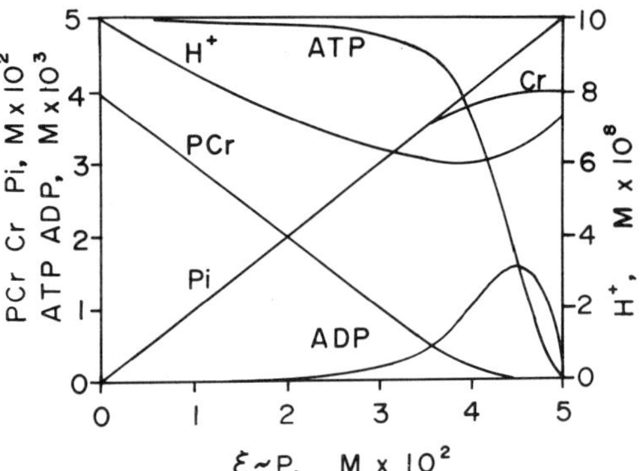

FIG. 5. Model of behavior of energy-rich phosphate compounds as a function of extent of PCr splitting, $\xi \sim P$, for coupled equilibria of creatine phosphokinase and adenylate kinase reactions. Conditions for resting muscle are plotted at the origin. [Adapted from Vincent and Blair (223).]

adenosine 5′-monophosphate (AMP) deaminase, which is present in substantial amounts in pale, skeletal muscle (148, 172)

$$AMP + H_2O + H^+ \rightarrow IMP + NH_4^+ \quad (6a)$$

The AMP deaminase reaction proceeds to a very significant extent in prolonged contractions and in muscle fatigue (191), conditions associated with decreased intracellular pH, markedly decreased content of energy-rich phosphate compounds, and elevated levels of P_i, AMP, and ADP. Although the reaction is irreversible, inosine 5′-monophosphate (IMP) can be reaminated by the following reaction sequences involving guanosine tri- and diphosphate

$$IMP + aspartate + GTP \rightarrow adenylosuccinate + GDP + P_i \quad (6b)$$

$$adenylosuccinate \rightarrow AMP + fumarate \quad (6c)$$

These three reactions together constitute the purine nucleotide cycle (153). Although several functions have been attributed to this cycle, recent evidence shows that in rat muscle the complete cycle does not operate during moderate to intense contractile activity (173, 174). Modest amounts of IMP are formed during the contraction phase, but restoration of the normal level of adenine nucleotide occurs slowly during recovery.

The function of AMP deaminase is not clearly established, but there are several possibilities.

1. It may reduce AMP levels so that in concert with creatine phosphokinase and adenylate kinase, ATP/ADP ratios are kept high.

2. AMP deaminase may supply NH_4^+, which activates flux through glycolysis by activation of phosphofructokinase (215), and in a more complex manner it may regulate glycolysis by a sustained oscillation of AMP, IMP, adenylosuccinate, and reduced nicotinamide-adenine dinucleotide (NADH) levels (153). Such oscillations have not been shown in intact muscle.

3. AMP deaminase may increase the content of Krebs cycle intermediates, that is, fumarate synthesis, during recovery or during increased steady-state work loads.

Glycogenolysis and Glycolysis

A detailed discussion of glycolysis and the activation of the enzyme cascade leading to the activation of glycogen phosphorylase is not presented. My purpose does require some discussion of a few points.

Activation of glycogen phosphorylase involves a Ca^{2+}-activated kinase and phosphorylation of the phosphorylase molecule in the presence of calcium ions in the range of 10^{-5} M. Thus it is a reaction to take into account at the onset of contractile activity. Is the process significant in energy terms? Glycogen, glycogen phosphorylase, glycogen synthetase, regulatory kinases, phosphatases, and other enzymes exist as a protein-glycogen complex, the "glycogen particle" (91). Calcium directly activates phosphorylase kinase, which catalyzes the conversion of phosphorylase *b* to phosphorylase *a* by ATP-dependent phosphorylation of a serine residue, 1 mol/mol phosphorylase subunit. A phosphatase catalyzes the inactivation and liberates 1 mol P_i/mol subunit (40). The phosphatase activity does not change during contraction, nor is it very dependent on temperature. Thus the level of phosphorylase *a* activity is regulated by calcium activation of phosphorylase *b* kinase. During contraction the rate of phosphorylase activation exceeds the rate of its inactivation by a factor of about 10, and during recovery the reverse is true. The rate constant for conversion of phosphorylase *b* to phosphorylase *a* in electrically stimulated frog sartorius is 0.9 s^{-1} at 30°C, 0.08 s^{-1} at 10°C, and 0.008 s^{-1} at 0°C [(40); Kushmerick, unpublished observations]. The rate constant of inactivation ranged from 0.001 to 0.06 s^{-1} over the stated temperature range, results that confirm in living muscle the lack of influence of temperature and Ca^{2+} on the phosphatase activity. All of the above information suggests a simple model in which glycogen phosphorylase is activated with the onset of contractile activity following approximately first-order kinetics to a level of activity governed by experimental conditions. The extent of phosphorylase activation appears to reach a maximum as a function of stimulus duration. However, it appears the situation is not so simple because there is an interesting and unexplained correlation of the extent of phosphorylase activation with the total energy consumed in a series of twitches (180) or in a maintained tetanus with the extent of energy-rich phosphate utilization (Fig. 6). Both measures of the cost of contractile energy are not proportional to stimulus duration. In view of the evidence presented in Figure 6 the factors regulating activation of glycogen phosphorylase should be further evaluated quantitatively.

The amount of phosphorylase in muscle is approximately 1–3 mg enzyme/g muscle wet wt, which is equivalent to 0.02 μmol subunit/g. The energy cost for activation of this enzyme in units of ATP utilization is thus small. In a maintained contraction with the ratio of rate constants of formation to breakdown approximately equal to 10, a steady rate in muscle of 0.003 $\mu mol\ ATP \cdot g^{-1} \cdot s^{-1}$ would be consumed in maintaining the degree of activation of phosphorylase. In terms of total energy-rich phosphate utilization and also in terms of muscle heat production, these values for energy use are negligible unless it turns out that the enthalpy of phosphorylase activation in the glycogen particle is very large, much greater than 100 kJ/mol.

The second issue concerns the fact that phosphorolysis of glycogen produces glucose 1-phosphate and consumes P_i. It has been shown repeatedly that in prolonged tetanic contractions there is a rise in hexose phosphate in muscle, but the P_i levels are below that

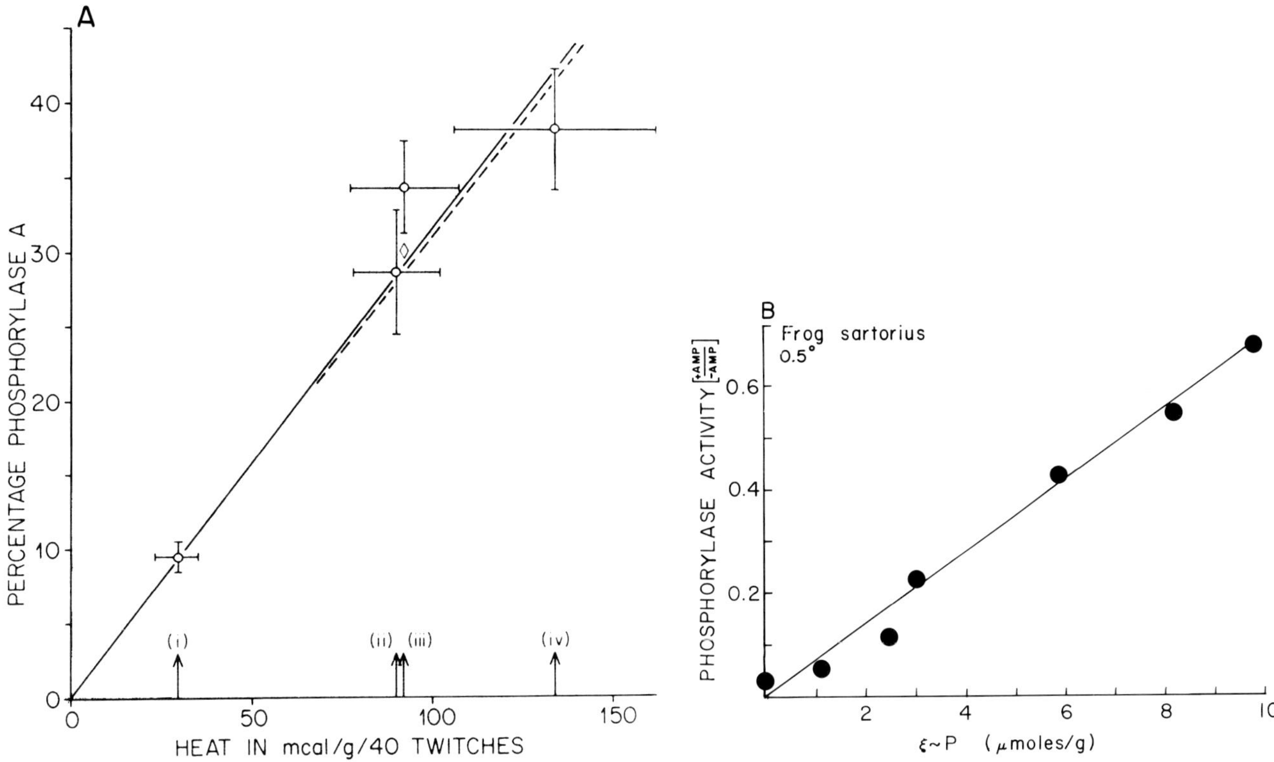

FIG. 6. *A*: activation of glycogen phosphorylase during contractile activity of aerobic frog muscle. *B*: fractional phosphorylase activity as a function of the extent of high-energy phosphate splitting ($\xi \sim$ P) during a single isometric tetanus. [*A* from Mommaerts et al. (180); *B* data from M. J. Kushmerick, unpublished observations.]

expected from the net breakdown of PCr (79, 139). The reason this issue is raised is that formation of hexose phosphates leads to the apparent lack of stoichiometry between the breakdown of PCr and the increase in its products (creatine and P_i) if hexose phosphates are not measured. In contraction of short duration this problem does not arise.

In regulation of phosphorylase activation, the last point is that glycolysis and the formation of lactate maintaining a steady redox of NAD/NADH lead to the formation of ATP from ADP, which is called substrate level phosphorylation. From glycogen the net stoichiometry is 1 glucosyl unit + 3 ADP + 3 P_i $\rightarrow$ 3 ATP + 2 lactate. If the substrate were glucose, one ATP would be used by the hexokinase reaction to form glucose 6-phosphate, which enters glycolysis; then the net stoichiometry is 1 glucose + 2 ADP + 2 $P_i \rightarrow$ 2 ATP + 2 lactate. To the extent that substrate level phosphorylation occurs during contraction, the true breakdown of high-energy phosphate compounds during contraction will be underestimated. The extent of glycolysis depends inter alia on the duration of stimulation, temperature, and intracellular pH. In frog muscles at 0°C, stimulation must continue for more than 20 s before any lactate production is detectable during the tetanus (142). Transient lactate production is detected during the recovery period in muscles tetanized for more than 10 s (142). Importantly in aerobic conditions there is a proportionality between recovery oxygen consumption and recovery lactate production, approximately 1 mol lactate being produced for each 4 mol O_2 being consumed. Thus lactate formation does not necessarily indicate anaerobiosis. Glycolysis can be blocked at the glyceraldehyde-phosphate dehydrogenase step by iodoacetate (23).

Oxidative Metabolism

This class of reactions includes those of aerobic metabolism in the mitochondria, namely the reduction of oxygen coupled to the oxidation of substrates and the generation of ATP. Only the description of the overall time course of those reactions and an outline of the mechanisms controlling the rate of O_2 consumption are presented. The basic plan of oxidative phosphorylation is outlined in Figure 7.

TIME COURSE OF RECOVERY EVENTS. By a spectrophotometric method applied to a perfused cat soleus muscle near body temperature, Millikan (177) showed a decrease in oxyhemoglobin saturation of blood in the muscle capillaries within 200 ms of the onset of the tetanic activity, a time near the limit of the response times of his apparatus. Because local blood flow changes more slowly than muscle activation, this response was taken to indicate the rapid reduction of O_2

in mitochondria. A maximal response was reached within 1 s of the onset of a tetanic contraction. After the end of a tetanus a few seconds in duration, return to base-line levels of hemoglobin oxygenation required about 10 s, a delay due to O_2 diffusion and to the response time of the microcirculation to increased capillary blood flow. This return to base line should not be confused with the return to basal levels of O_2 consumption.

D. K. Hill measured the time course of recovery O_2 consumption directly by a differential volumetric technique (102) such that O_2 consumption associated with a contraction was measured above the base line of an unstimulated control muscle. He used frog sartorius muscles at 0°C. Oxygen consumption could only be detected after contractile activity ceased. After a tetanus, O_2 consumption persists for tens of minutes and approximates the time course of aerobic recovery heat. Millikan's and Hill's results obviously do not contradict each other because they measured different parameters, because of the large difference in aerobic respiratory capacity in the muscles used, and because of the strong temperature dependence of respiration rate. There is a great range of mitochondrial content and of maximal aerobic capacity in different muscles (116, 146). In a comparative study of a large number of skeletal muscles in wild animals (116), mitochondrial volume fraction (volume to volume of whole muscle) ranged from 2% to 10% vol/vol. Romanul (199) showed a correspondence between aerobic capacity and capillary density, both of which increase adaptively with endurance training (71). There is also a wide range in amount of ATPase during contraction relative to the volume fraction of the muscle occupied by mitochondria. In frog sartorius the mitochondrial volume fraction is approximately 1%, whereas in cat soleus it is approximately 15%; also, at the same temperature the ATPase activity in the frog muscle is several times higher. The significance of these data is that in a muscle with high ATPase rates and low aerobic capacity, such as amphibian muscles at 0°C, there can be a complete temporal separation between ATP utilization during a brief contraction and later ATP regeneration. On the other hand, for muscles with relatively low ATPase rates and large aerobic capacities [examples are pigeon breast muscle, mammalian soleus muscle, and cardiac muscle (190)] it is easy to achieve a temporal overlap between contractile and recovery processes. It is even possible to approach a quasi steady state in which the time average of ATP utilization is balanced by the time average of oxidative ATP regeneration. This last possibility is illustrated by normally functioning cardiac muscle and has been achieved in a maintained isometric tetanus of mouse soleus (30). In both examples contractile activity continues in a steady state with steady average cellular contents of ATP, PCr, P_i, and other metabolites, provided a steady supply of O_2 and oxidizable substrate is available, and CO_2 and other metabolic products are removed.

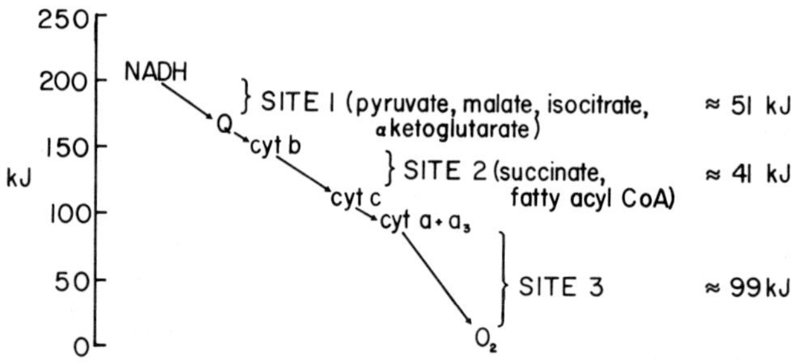

FIG. 7. Scheme of steps in mitochondrial oxidative phosphorylation omitting mechanisms of generating proton gradients. Each site is a mechanism for formation of one ATP from ADP and P_i coupled to the proton motive force generated by the stepwise oxidation of one reducing equivalent by one-half O_2. Some substrates enter the chain distal to site 1 and bypass first ATP-generating site.

Other signals related to recovery metabolism can also be measured. The work of Jöbsis (126, 127) set forth the basis for interpretation of intrinsic fluorescent signals in muscle associated with contraction-recovery cycle in terms of changes in the redox status of mitochondrial NAD/NADH. Mitochondria in aerobic muscle are usually considered to be saturated with O_2 and oxidizable substrate, and respiration could be regulated by the availability of ADP. This conclusion follows from the original work of Chance and Williams (25), who described various metabolic states of mitochondria (Table 2). In that view mitochondria in resting muscle are considered to be in state 4, in which the rate-limiting step is the availability of substrates for ATP synthesis, either ADP or P_i. Because measured P_i levels (ca. 10^{-3} M) in cytoplasm greatly exceed ADP (ca. 10^{-6} M) levels with respect to their apparent

TABLE 2. *Metabolic States of Isolated Mitochondria*

State	Characteristics					Percentage Reduction in Steady State	
	$[O_2]$	[ADP]	[Substrate]	Respiration rate	Rate-limiting substance	NADH	Cytochrome *a*
1	>0	Low	Low	Slow	ADP	90	0
2	>0	High	Low	Slow	Substrate	0	0
3	>0	High	High	Maximal	Respiratory chain	53	<4
4	>0	Low	High	Slow	ADP	>99	0
5	0	High	High	0	O_2	100	100

K_m values for mitochondria, respiration is thought to be controlled by ADP availability (24). Thus from resting state to contracting state, the mitochondria are thought to change from state 4 to state 3 respiration at the start of contractile activity, returning to state 4 at the end of the recovery cycle. This type of kinetic control of respiration conveniently explained the observed decrease in fluorescence and hence decrease in mitochondrial NADH levels that occur after a twitch (Fig. 8). These experiments were done in toad muscle, which has about twice the aerobic capacity of a frog sartorius. Godfraind-de Becker (80) also found the correlation between the time course of fluorescent change and aerobic recovery heat. Furthermore she showed that the earliest fluorescent change was a quick reduction of NAD^+ (that is, an increase in NADH levels) followed by a more oxidized level characteristic of state 3 mitochondrial respiration. Using anaerobic muscles and muscles poisoned with iodoacetate as controls, she concluded that the fluorescent signals were not entirely due to mitochondrial NADH, as was the conclusion of Jöbsis, but represented a significant contribution of cytoplasmic NADH levels as well. In conclusion the fluorescent signals obtained from muscle during the contraction recovery cycle may not represent entirely mitochondrial redox state of the NAD/NADH couple.

The following argument indicates that physical dif-

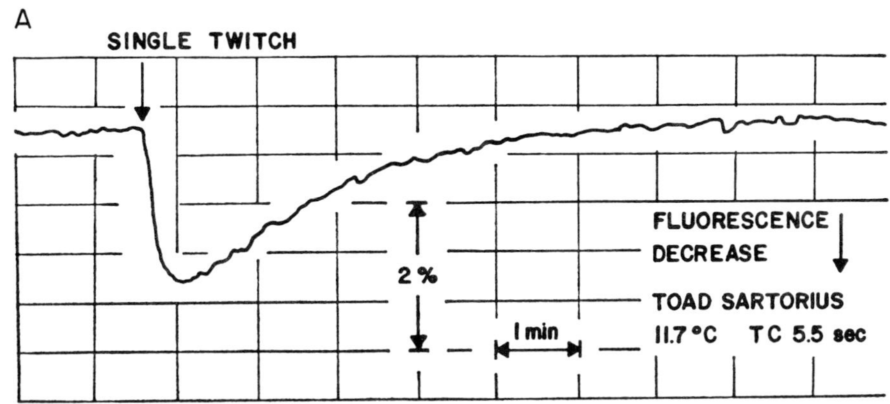

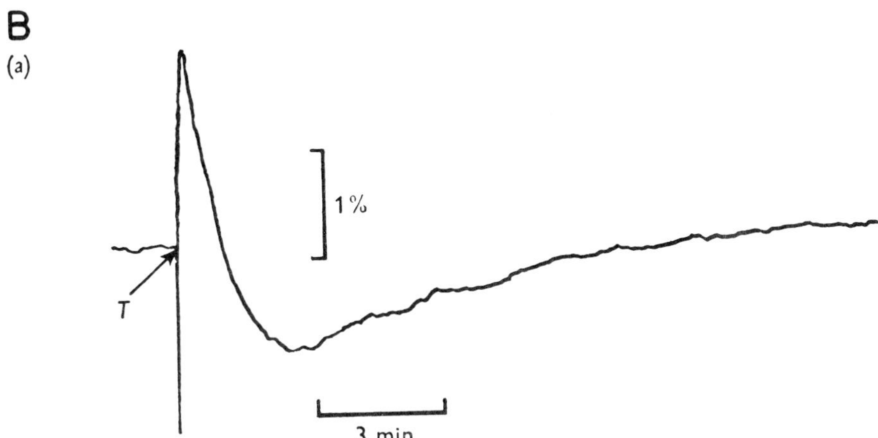

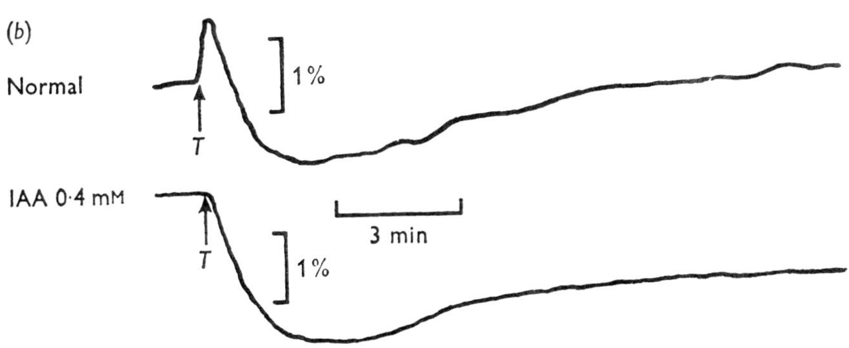

FIG. 8. Fluorescent signals obtained from intact anuran muscles. *A*: record of a decrease in fluorescence after a twitch at 12°C, which indicates a transient decrease (or oxidation) of NADH. *B*: records of fluorescence changes after a 0.5-s tetanus at 20°C showing a transient increase in fluorescence or increase in NADH, which in *A* is partly obscured by a movement artifact. In *B* this artifact has been subtracted, and the fast transient increase in NADH is blocked by iodoacetate, which indicates that a portion of the response can be attributed to glycolytic redox transients in the cytosol. [*A* from Jöbsis and Duffield (127); *B* from Godfraind-de Becker (80).]

fusion of a chemical signal is probably not the rate-limiting step for the control of oxidative phosphorylation. Diffusion distances from myofibrils to mitochondria are about 1–10 μm, depending on the type of muscle under consideration. The diffusion coefficient in muscle of ADP could not be measured, but is probably not far from the measured diffusivity of MgATP, $2 \times 10^{-6}\ cm^2 \cdot s^{-1}$ (144). The time for 50% of the concentration change of ADP in the myofibril to diffuse 10 μm is 60 ms; if the diffusion distance were 1 μm, as is the case in mitochondria-rich muscles, the time would be 100 times less. This calculation is based on assumptions for planar diffusion and a maintained gradient (28). Thus even the earliest events of the onset of increased respiratory activity are not likely to be limited by chemical diffusion within the myofibrillar space.

CONTROL OF OXIDATIVE PHOSPHORYLATION. The concept of ADP-controlled respiration is no doubt valid for suspensions of mitochondria in vitro in solutions containing saturating concentrations of P_i, substrate, and O_2 (Fig. 9). However, despite the superficial resemblance of the time course of recovery O_2 consumption after a contraction (Fig. 9) to that of ADP-stimulated mitochondrial respiration, current evidence is against the kinetic control of respiration by low ADP levels per se and is in favor of a control near equilibrium

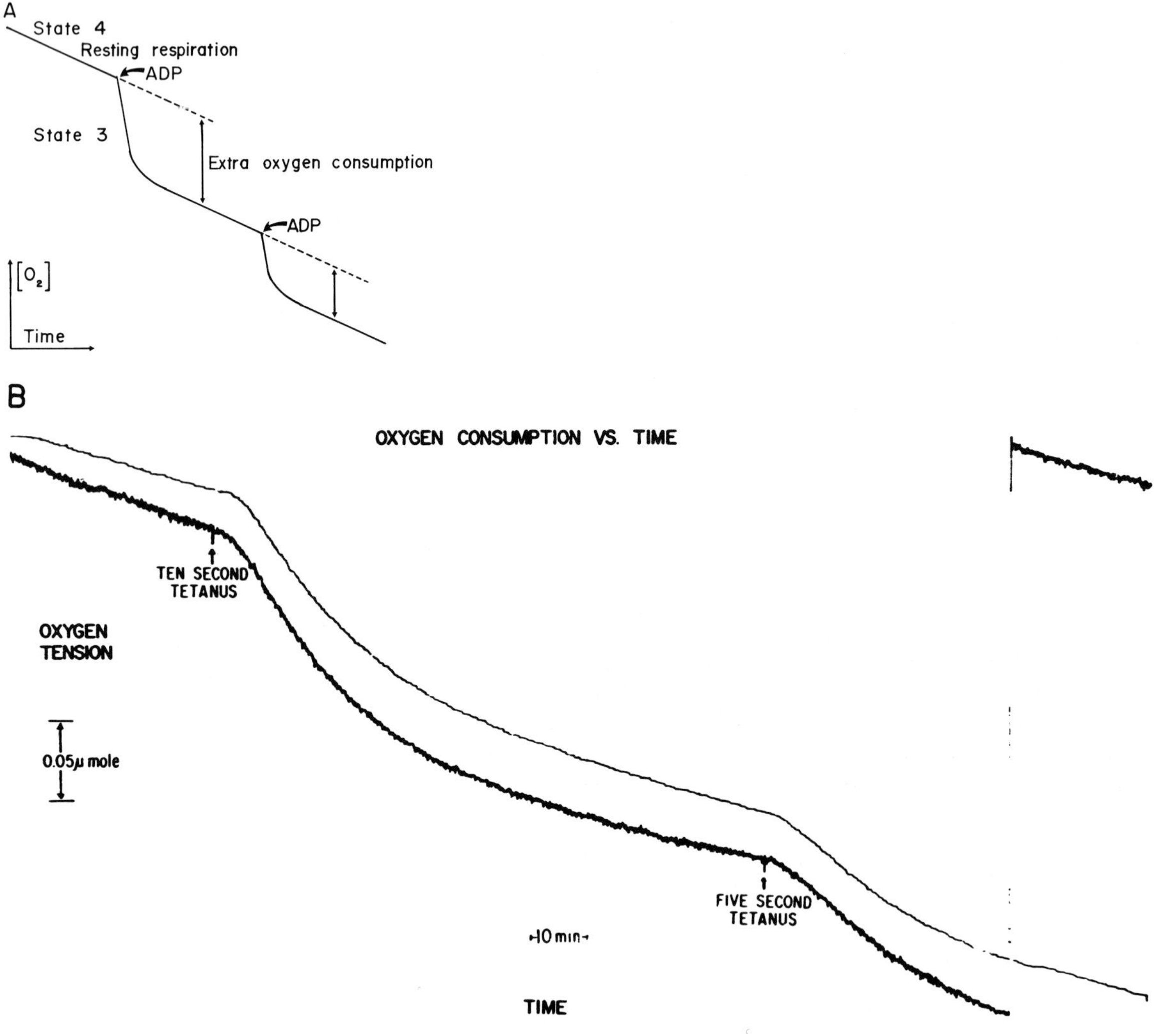

FIG. 9. Oxygen consumption as a function of time in a mitochondrial suspension (*A*) and in intact frog sartorius muscle at 0°C (*B*). After addition of ADP to a mitochondrial suspension, respiration rate becomes maximal, characteristic of state 3, and returns to state 4 when added ADP is completely phosphorylated. The first addition of ADP is about twice the amount of the second. Two recovery O_2 consumption records are presented in *B*, one from each member of a pair of sartorius muscles from 1 animal. There is a diffusional delay between tetanus and first sign of increased O_2 consumption. Rate of O_2 consumption after a single contraction is always much less (here about ⅓) than the maximal respiratory capability of the muscle (141). [*B* from Paul and Kushmerick (192).]

achieved by varying ratios of adenine nucleotide substrates and products. The earliest evidence for this latter view was based on the findings of Chance and Williams (25) that the substrates and products of the first phosphorylation site were close to equilibrium. That is, the following reaction of site 1 was observed to be reversible

$$\text{NADH} + \text{flavoprotein } 1_{\text{oxidized}} + \text{ADP} + \text{P}_i \rightleftarrows \text{NAD}^+ + \text{ATP} + \text{flavoprotein } 1_{\text{reduced}} \quad (7)$$

Thus with a suitably large $NADH/NAD^+$ ratio the reaction could be driven in the direction of ATP synthesis; conversely by large $ATP/(ADP \cdot P_i)$ ratios, the reaction can be driven to the left. It is now known that in suspensions of mitochondria in state 4 (58), in cell suspensions (230, 231), and in perfused hearts and livers (89, 231) near-equilibrium conditions exist for the sequence of reactions in mitochondria from NADH to cytochrome *c*, that is, sites 1 and 2. Thus the overall reaction is near equilibrium

$$\text{NADH} + 2 \text{ cyt } c^{3+} + 2 \text{ ADP} + 2 \text{ P}_i \rightleftarrows \text{NAD} + 2 \text{ cyt } c^{2+} + 2 \text{ ATP} \quad (8)$$

As discussed there is also near equilibrium among cytoplasmic adenine nucleotides, creatine, PCr, H^+, and Mg^{2+} concentrations via creatine kinase and adenylate kinase reactions. In addition Veech et al. (220) provided substantial evidence for near-equilibrium conditions for the reactions catalyzed by glyceraldehyde-3-phosphate dehydrogenase, 3-phosphoglycerate kinase, and lactate dehydrogenase in liver, erythrocyte, brain, and muscle. Thus lactate, pyruvate, NAD, NADH, and P_i as well as other metabolic intermediates are clearly interconnected by near-equilibrium enzymatic reactions. The general conclusion, clearly put forward by Krebs and Veech (132), is that there is a network of near-equilibrium reactions involving metabolites of energetic interest, so that changes in the ratios of products to reactants of one of the component reactions are necessarily coupled to the same changes in other component reactions. An important exception, of course, occurs if there is any kinetic compartmentation. Measurement of actual chemical fluxes through these reactions in living cells is needed for a quantitative understanding of cellular energetics; a new approach is discussed in NEW DIRECTIONS, p. 229.

The process of recovery O_2 consumption is thus the response of a near-equilibrium network of cytoplasmic and mitochondrial reactions to a step perturbation induced by contractile activity in the ratios of adenine nucleotides, PCr, and P_i levels away from equilibrium. The network subsequently relaxes from this position to its initial near-equilibrium position, and the kinetics of the process is observed to be pseudo–first order (Fig. 9). The rate constant so measured is the rate constant of the whole network with the probable rate-limiting step at cytochrome *a*. Because near-equilibrium conditions are maintained by relatively small changes in metabolites that are easily achieved experimentally, the observed rate constant applies to the flux through each of the component reactions. Since it is possible to vary the intracellular pH, for example, by varying the external partial pressure of CO_2 (P_{CO_2}), and since the cellular metabolite levels are likely to depend on the nutritional and endocrine status of the animal, it is possible to study the kinetics of recovery O_2 consumption as a function of those parameters to test the stated model of aerobic metabolism. This aspect of muscle energetics deserves further experimental study.

It is well known that cellular respiration decreases at P_{O_2} less than several Torr (24, 226). At a partial pressure of O_2 (P_{O_2}) above a certain "critical P_{O_2}," respiration is independent of O_2 levels; that is, respiration shows zero-order kinetics with respect to O_2 concentration once a certain level of O_2 is attained. Below the critical P_{O_2}, respiration rate shows first-order kinetics with respect to O_2, but the apparent K_m depends on the metabolic status of the cell and in particular on the level of the reduction of cytochrome a_3 (24). Thus it is possible to write an equation for the respiration rate, v, in the region of a linear response both to O_2 and cytochrome a_3 redox state

$$\text{v} = k_{\text{rate}} [\text{cyt } a_3^{2+}] [\text{O}_2] \quad (9)$$

The evidence leading to the conclusion that cytoplasmic phosphorylation state, $ATP/ADP \cdot P_i$, intramitochondrial NAD/NADH ratio, and (cytochrome c^{3+})/(cytochrome c^{2+}) ratio are close to equilibrium has been presented. Owen and Wilson (189) modeled cellular respiration on the assumption that all three phosphorylation sites are at equilibrium; thus one can write

$$K_{\text{eq}} = \frac{[\text{NAD}]}{[\text{NADH}]} \cdot \frac{\text{cyt } a_3^{2+}]^2}{[\text{cyt } a_3^{3+}]^2} \cdot \frac{[\text{ATP}]^3}{[\text{ADP}]^3 [\text{P}_i]^3} \quad (10)$$

By rearranging, one obtains

$$[\text{cyt } a_3^{2+}] = \left(K_{\text{eq}} \cdot \frac{[\text{NADH}]}{[\text{NAD}]}\right)^{1/2} \cdot [\text{cyt } a_3^{3+}] \cdot \left(\frac{[\text{ATP}]}{[\text{ADP}] \cdot [\text{P}_i]}\right)^{-3/2} \quad (11)$$

The concentration of oxidized cytochrome a_3, [cyt a_3^{3+}], can be considered a constant, since cytochrome a_3 is usually more than 99% oxidized in tissues until nearly anoxic conditions are obtained. Thus [cyt a_3^{3+}] = C for any particular cell, realizing that the magnitude of C has a wide range depending on the mitochondrial volume fraction in the cell. With the combined expression for the kinetics of the respiration rate, v, and the equilibrium conditions for the three phosphorylation sites

$$v = (k_{rate}\, C\, [O_2]) \cdot \left(K_{eq} \frac{[NADH]}{[NAD]} \right)^{1/2} \cdot \left(\frac{[ATP]}{[ADP]\,[P_i]} \right)^{-3/2} \quad (12)$$

The first term on the right of the equation represents the dependence of respiration on the partial pressure of O_2, which is not normally limiting. The second term reflects the redox state. The third term shows the contribution of the phosphorylation potential. Note that this equation assumes a constant intracellular pH: H^+ is a product of ATP hydrolysis (see *Adenosine Triphosphatases*, p. 196). Thus the respiration rate at falling concentrations of O_2 can be maintained by appropriate adjustments of (cyt a^{3+})/(cyt a^{2+}), of NAD/NADH, and of the cytoplasmic phosphorylation state (59, 189, 229, 230). The practical result is that it is incorrect to conclude from a constant respiration rate that O_2 levels are well above saturating levels at the mitochondria in tissues.

All of the discussion has tacitly assumed there are no diffusional or permeability barriers for cellular substrates in oxidative phosphorylation. There is a carrier on the inner mitochondrial membrane for adenine nucleotides, the translocase (195). It is not yet known to what extent translocation may place kinetic limits on the rate of oxidation phosphorylation. Matters are more involved: translocation involves a difference in charge of the transported species, ATP^{4-} versus ADP^{3-}, and is electrogenic (130). The uptake of P_i appears to be electrically neutral (26), so the net uptake of P_i and ADP requires the equivalent uptake of one proton against an energy gradient (the proton motive force is greater in the mitochondrial matrix than outside). Thus transport across the inner mitochondrial membrane may place a limit on O_2 consumption and oxidative phosphorylation rates, but this possibility has not been evaluated yet (84).

BASIC ENERGETIC MODEL

A general scheme of muscle energetics synthesizes the information in previous sections.

1. The primary source of chemical energy during contraction is the coupled hydrolysis of ATP, but this is not directly observable without suitable inhibition of CPK.

2. The reaction catalyzed by CPK is sufficiently near equilibrium that utilization of ATP is observed as a net breakdown of PCr. The Lohmann reaction buffers the ATP levels as follows

$$ATP \rightarrow ADP + P_i \quad (13)$$

$$ADP + PCr \leftrightharpoons Cr + ATP \quad (14)$$

$$\text{Net:} \quad PCr \rightarrow Cr + P_i \quad (15)$$

3. With appropriately brief durations of contraction and with only small depletions of PCr, the number of reactions to be considered in drawing up a description of a contraction-recovery cycle can be reduced to a consideration of net PCr breakdown and subsequent recovery O_2 consumption. It must always be remembered, however, that because of the near-equilibrium condition of the cytoplasmic and mitochondrial reactions, all of the reactions in the equilibrium network shift their mass-action ratios appropriately even though some of these changes in concentrations (i.e., changes in ADP levels) may not be measurable by current techniques.

The energetics model is expanded with reference to Figure 10 to focus on two aspects of the basic paradigm of energetics: *1)* there is a net decrease in chemical potential energy during muscle activity measured as the breakdown of PCr; *2)* there exists a recovery period after mechanical relaxation during which oxidative metabolism utilizes substrate to regenerate the initial precontraction steady-state composition of high-energy phosphate compounds. At least under certain experimental conditions it is possible to separate completely processes occurring during the contraction phase (PCr splitting) from those occurring during the recovery phase (O_2 consumption). The basis for the separability into two phases in most muscles lies in the greatly differing time constants of the relevant chemical processes. For example, in amphibian skeletal muscle at 0°C the rate constant for utilization of PCr is approximately 0.02 s^{-2} during tetanic contractions, whereas the rate constant for oxidative resynthesis of energy-rich phosphate compounds is on the order of 0.001 s^{-1}. For mouse skeletal muscles at 20°C the rates are each about 5- to 10-fold higher. For slow-twitch, oxidative, skeletal muscle fibers and for cardiac muscle there is a closer correspondence between the rate of energy-rich phosphate utilization, which is lower than in fast-twitch fibers, and resynthesis, which is higher than in fast-twitch fibers because of the large content of mitochondria. Therefore there is some degree of overlap of the contractile and recovery processes in these more oxidative types of muscles.

The contractile phase is on the *left* in Figure 10. The progression from left to right indicates the time course of a contraction-recovery cycle; note the different time scale. Panel *A* shows the development of isometric force on stimulation. During the recovery period on the *right* there is no mechanical activity. In panel *B* the actual ATPase rate is plotted to define the energy utilization rate. Before stimulation it has a small positive value equivalent to the basal rate of energy metabolism, indicated by a dashed line. With the onset of stimulation the ATPase rate rapidly rises. Current evidence suggests that ATPase rate is initially high, and it decreases to a steady rate during a maintained tetanus very much higher than the basal rate. As a consequence of this increased rate of ATP turnover and maintenance near equilibrium of CPK, PCr levels

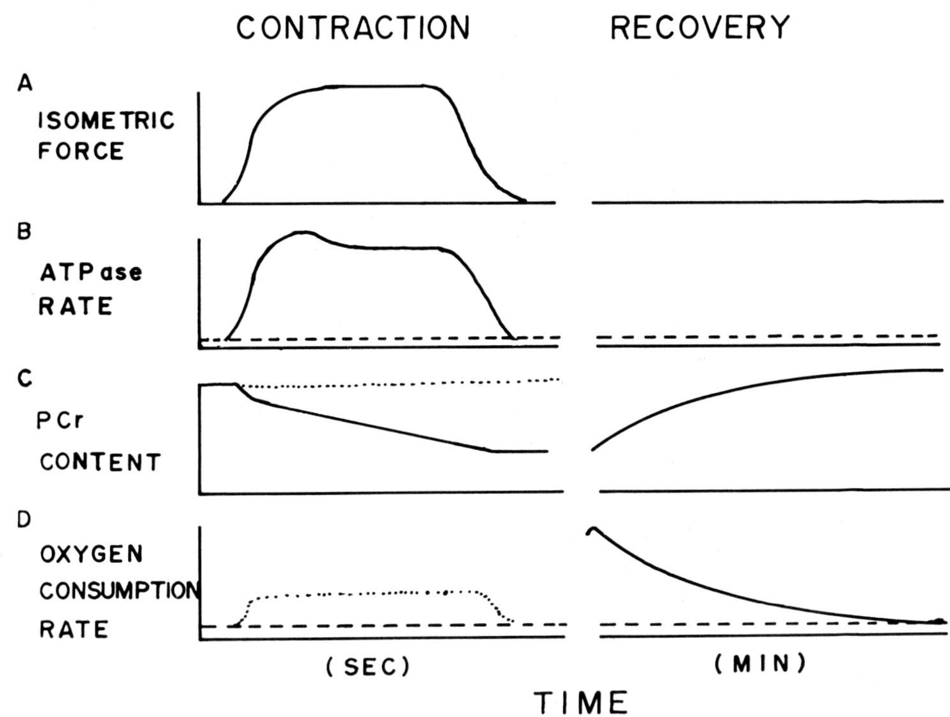

FIG. 10. Chemical changes during contraction and subsequent recovery during which initial steady-state conditions are restored.

follow the time course indicated by panel *C*; the rate of decrease is proportional to ATP turnover. Thus PCr levels rapidly decrease during the initial part of the tetanus and thereafter fall at a steady rate. Notice that additional reactions shown in Figure 5 also occur. Panel *D* shows the condition where O_2 consumption remains at basal resting levels throughout the brief contraction (panel *D*, *left*, dashed line). After a brief contraction or at later times during a prolonged contraction, the O_2-consumption rate increases (panel *D*, *right*) to a rate proportional to the deviation from the near-equilibrium condition characteristic of resting muscles. The rate of O_2 consumption declines exponentially from this value to basal values. The apparent rate constant, *k*, is defined by the equations in CHEMICAL REACTIONS AND METABOLIC PRINCIPLES, p. 196. The return of O_2 consumption to basal values marks the end of the recovery period. The increased rate of O_2 consumption above basal during recovery and the very low basal ATP rates during the recovery period (dashed line, panel *B*, *right*) result in net synthesis of energy-rich phosphate and the return of PCr levels to precontractile state (panel *C*, *right*). The rate of net PCr synthesis is directly proportional to the O_2-consumption rate above the base line.

The diagram in Figure 10 also shows a second energetic model. Consider the possibility that rates of ATP utilization and the rates of ATP synthesis can be made equal both at rest and during contraction; that is, assume that the rates of oxidative phosphorylation match the rate of energy-rich phosphate utilization. Such a possibility appears to be the case for smooth muscle in which the ATPase rates during contraction are only 2–3 times above the basal rate and aerobic capacity is sufficient to maintain ATP levels constant in this new steady state. In this situation there would be an increased ATPase rate associated with contraction and a simultaneous increase in O_2 consumption proportional to the ATPase rate (dots, panel *D*, *left*). Thus PCr levels remain constant or fall only slightly during the contraction (dots, panel *C*, *left*). Obviously the division between contractile phase and recovery energetic phase is meaningless in this second type of energetic model. The first mentioned model can be applied to single contractions of skeletal muscle.

THERMODYNAMICS

The problem of understanding the relationship between measurements of heat production and the underlying chemical reactions is one of applying chemical thermodynamics to muscle. This topic has been discussed in considerable detail by several authors (178, 228, 236).

An isolated muscle is a closed thermodynamic system exchanging heat and work with the environment but not matter, if a sufficiently brief contraction-relaxation cycle is considered. For a complete contraction-relaxation cycle the muscle is an open system, and exchanges of matter must be explicitly considered. As a closed system the chemical composition of the muscle must not change by exchange of substrate or end products with the environment, but of course the muscle may undergo a change in internal composition by one or more of the reactions previously described. For a closed system or for an open system in a steady state, the following discussion is valid; for closed systems near equilibrium the arguments are simpler. The first law of thermodynamics or the conservation of energy demands that the difference in total energy between two states be given by

$$\Delta U = q + w \quad (16)$$

ΔU is the increase in internal energy of the muscle gained from the quantity of heat absorbed (q) and the work done (w) on the system by the surroundings. For a muscle going from the state of rest to the state of contraction, the quantity ΔU decreases because heat is released into the environment and external work may also be done on the surroundings. Note that any internal mechanical work done by stretching series elastic elements and any chemical or electrical work done by establishing ionic and osmotic gradients within the muscle remains within the muscle and will appear as heat when dissipated because it is not performed against the surroundings.

Pressure-volume work is negligible because most muscles operate at constant atmospheric pressure, because volume changes are less than 1 part in 10^5, and because muscle contains no rigid walls to withstand pressure gradients. Thus under conditions of constant pressure it is valid to write

$$-\Delta U = -\Delta H \quad (17)$$

where ΔH is the enthalpy change. This useful thermodynamic quantity, ΔH, is conveniently accessible to experimental measurement (236) by writing

$$-\Delta H = h + w \quad (18)$$

where h is the heat released by muscle. The symbol q is used in thermodynamic texts to indicate the quantity of heat exchanged, whereas in the muscle literature it is conventional to use the symbol h. The quantity h can be conveniently measured with a good time resolution by a suitable thermopile. Temperature changes are actually measured. Net heat equals $C_p\Delta T$, where C_p is the heat capacity, assumed to be constant, and ΔT is the temperature change. The quantity w is the extent of mechanical energy output, which is measured by the total force produced by the muscle times the distance moved.

For any chemical reaction that occurs, the actual enthalpy change is given by

$$-\Delta H = \xi_i \Delta H_i \quad (19)$$

where ξ_i is the molar extent of the reaction and ΔH_i is the molar enthalpy change. Measurement of ξ_i is by analytical chemical procedures, and measurement of ΔH_i requires a calorimeter. The value and sign of the enthalpy of a reaction is a specific property of each reaction and is equal to the energy content of the product minus the energy content of the reactants. For the number of reactions that might occur, and by substituting from the above equations

$$h + w = \Sigma \xi_i \Delta H_i \quad (20)$$

This relationship is valuable and very powerful. The heat liberated by muscle and mechanical work done can be calibrated with great accuracy and can be measured with good time resolution. Thus in terms of energy units the magnitude of the sum ($\Sigma \xi_i \Delta H_i$) can be totally and correctly defined by physical measurements of $h + w$.

The following data are required for application of this relationship to muscle contraction.

1. $h + w$. The temporal resolution of currently available thermopiles and mechanical apparatus allows this quantity to be measured at any interval throughout a contraction-relaxation cycle with a time resolution 1–10 ms. Since a thermopile measures temperature accurately, it is necessary to know the total thermal capacity of the apparatus, which includes the muscle and all adhering solution. The use and calibration of thermopiles were critically evaluated by Hill and Woledge (101). More recently a better calibration method with the muscle and adhering fluid in place can be made by taking advantage of the Peltier effect of the thermojunctions (134).

2. ξ_i. The extent of all identified reactions must be measured during the period that the measurements of $h + w$ are made. The introduction of the rapid-freezing hammer apparatus by Kretzschmar and Wilkie (133) allows the experimenter to stop metabolic reactions with a temporal precision greater than 0.1 s. The formation of stable extracts that are suitable for chemical analyses and that validly represent the composition of muscle at the time of freezing complete the experimental requirements. Quite good results are obtained by pulverizing tissues in liquid nitrogen, mechanically mixing a pulverized frozen solution of a protein denaturant, usually perchloric acid, and slowly warming the mixture with continuous agitation until all portions are completely thawed (154–156). The use of contractions of brief duration and of inhibitors when required allows a considerable reduction in the potential number of reactions to consider. For example, treatment with O_2-free nitrogen and iodoacetate blocks glycolysis and oxidative phosphorylation.

3. ΔH_i. For each identified reaction, the molar enthalpy must be measured in a calorimeter. This measurement often includes accounting of the uptake or release of H^+, so enthalpies of buffer reactions must also be known. Woledge (237) measured the enthalpy of PCr and ATP splitting over a range of pH and magnesium ion concentrations that bracket the physiological range. Even with the uncertainties of defining the intracellular cytoplasmic environment exactly, it

is believed these quantities are in error by less than 10% because the enthalpy values are not strong functions of the independent variables.

With the required information one can test whether the fundamental relationship, Equation 20, is satisfied experimentally during contraction. If the results of any set of measurements do not satisfy this equation, then one or more of the component values used in the equation is in error or there is another energetically significant reaction occurring that was not on the original list. This fundamental relationship is the basis of myothermal energy balance experiments that test whether the known reactions and their measured extents adequately account for the total energy liberated. The value of this approach resides in its rigorous definition. It should be obvious that the one question not being asked by using this fundamental relation is whether the first law of thermodynamics applies to living muscle!

Note that the relationship makes no statement regarding the partition of the total enthalpy change between h and w. Another thermodynamic quantity, the free energy, and the second law of thermodynamics are required to make such a statement. The maximum amount of work obtainable by any working mechanism from a reaction of 1 mol of the substance is called the molar free energy. The change in free energy between two thermodynamic states, ΔG, is defined

$$\Delta G = w_{\max} = \Delta H - T\Delta S \tag{21}$$

One statement of the second law of thermodynamics is that for all spontaneous processes $\Delta S \geqslant 0$. If $\Delta S = 0$, the process is reversible and $\Delta G = w_{\max} = \Delta H$. If $\Delta S > 0$, then there is a reversible heat production

$$h_{\text{reversible}} = T\Delta S = \Delta H - w_{\max} \tag{22}$$

$\Delta G = w_{\max}$ only for thermodynamically reversible processes. For actual processes occurring at finite rates, only a fraction of $w_{\max}$ is obtained, and a portion of ΔG is always irreversibly degraded to heat. Thus the total heat in a reaction is derived from two terms

$$\text{total heat} = T\Delta S + (\Delta G - \text{actual } w) \tag{23}$$

or

$$\text{total heat} = h_{\text{reversible}} + (w_{\max} - w) \tag{24}$$

Because for spontaneous processes $S > 0$, and because $T > 0$, the quantity of reversible heat ($T\Delta S$) is positive. It may be negative only for one element of a coupled process, that part that is not spontaneous. For such a pair of coupled reactions, it must be true that the overall entropy change is greater than zero for the coupled processes to occur.

The irreversible heat, $w_{\max} - w$, is the heat that results from the fact that reactions occur at a finite velocity. It decreases inversely with the thermodynamic efficiency of the process.

An example will illustrate these principles. Consider ATP hydrolysis occurring in the cytoplasm under two hypothetical conditions. *1*) The hydrolysis is not coupled to the performance of useful work by any energy converter so that no work is performed. *2*) The hydrolysis is coupled reversibly by suitable means so that $w = w_{\max}$; that is, at 100% efficiency.

The standard free energy of ATP hydrolysis (ΔG^0) at 20°C, pH 7, and ionic strength 0.25 is −29.9 kJ/mol (220). The actual free energy available in the cytoplasm is calculated by

$$\Delta G' = \Delta G^0 - RT \ln \frac{[\text{ATP}]}{[\text{ADP}][\text{P}_i]} \tag{25}$$

The appropriate values for the concentration terms (see CHEMICAL REACTIONS AND METABOLIC PRINCIPLES, p. 196) are by direct analysis: [ATP] = 4×10^{-3} M and [P_i] = 2×10^{-3} M and by calculation: [ADP] = 1.6×10^{-7} M. A lower value of P_i than is listed in Table 1 is used because of recent reevaluations (see NEW DIRECTIONS, p. 229) of its sarcoplasmic levels. Thus, $\Delta G'$ = −29.9 kJ/mol − 39.8 kJ/mol = −69.7 kJ/mol. This is also the initial driving force for the net reaction, PCr splitting. The appropriate enthalpy change is that of PCr hydrolysis, ΔHPCr = −34 kJ/mol (37, 236). If CPK is blocked by FDNB, the appropriate enthalpy change is that for net ATP hydrolysis, ΔHATP = −46 kJ/mol. Therefore for the reactions shown on p. 206, Equation 13 occurs mechanistically and governs the overall free energy of the coupled reactions, but ξATP ≈ 0 because of advancement of Equation 14. The extent of net reaction (Eq. 15) determines the enthalpy change. Therefore the following thermodynamic quantities apply for resting muscle $\Delta H'$ = −34 kJ/mol (refs. 37, 236); $\Delta G'$ = −70 kJ/mol (by calculation); $T\Delta S'$ = +36 kJ/mol (by subtraction).

Example 1: If $w = 0$, heat produced per mole is equal to ΔH_{PCr} = −34 kJ/mol. The muscle gives heat to the surroundings.

Example 2: If $w = w_{\max}$, heat produced is only the reversible heat

$$h_{\text{reversible}} = T\Delta S' = 36 \text{ kJ/mol} \tag{26}$$

Since $T\Delta S'$ is positive, the muscle takes up heat from the surroundings in this example, i.e., it cools.

Consider these thermodynamic quantities when ξPCr = 5×10^{-3} M (about 5 μmol/g, neglecting the fraction of solvent water). This means PCr content falls, and Cr and P_i content rises. Recalculation of the free ADP yields a new value of about 1×10^{-5} M. Recalculation of $\Delta G'$ with the appropriate values: [ATP] = 4×10^{-3} M; [ADP] = 1×10^{-5} M; [P_i] = 7×10^{-3} M yields the lower value, $\Delta G'$ = −56.6 kJ/mol. So long as the pH-buffering and ion-binding reactions are still valid, as appears to be the case, the enthalpy value remains at −34 kJ/mol.

The free energy ($\Delta G' = w_{\max}$) is a function of the actual substrate and product concentrations, and of course, these change continuously during a contraction. Therefore the correct method to assess the actual free-energy change is to integrate the change in free energy with respect to the advancement of the reaction

$$\Delta G' = \int (dG'/d\xi)d\xi \quad (27)$$

For the remainder of this chapter, external work, efficiency, and the like are not discussed, but the discussion concentrates on the total energy change, $\Delta H' = h + w$.

ENERGY BALANCE

Myothermic Method

The first objective in an analysis of chemical energetics in muscular contraction is to ascertain whether all energetic parameters and extents of reactions are accurately measured. All forms of energy transformation are detected by making measurements of $h + w$, for reversible and irreversible reactions, whether the reactions are linked to energy-rich phosphate compounds or not. The unique value of the myothermic method is thus its generality. Heat measurements are of mechanistic use only if they are traceable to identified reactions. Although the enthalpy of a reaction is a specific property of that reaction, the identity of a chemical reaction in muscle cannot be deduced from heat measurements. The reaction may be significant mechanistically, but because it happens to have a small molar enthalpy value, it contributes little to the total enthalpy production. Conversely, a reaction may have a very large enthalpy and be of little mechanistic significance. Nonetheless the myothermic method is the foundation for quantitative studies of muscle energetics.

As outlined in THERMODYNAMICS, p. 207, the basis of a test of myothermic energy balance is given by the conservation equation $h + w = \Sigma\xi_i\Delta H_i$ (Eq. 20). The quantities to be measured experimentally are $h + w$, ξ_i, and ΔH_i, and it is possible to arrange experimental conditions where there is expected to be only one net reaction $PCr \rightarrow P_i + Cr$ (Eq. 15). Energy conservation applied to this hypothesis states

$$h + w = \xi PCr\Delta HPCr \quad (28)$$

If equality is obtained within experimental error, then the hypothesis is supported or, more correctly, it cannot be excluded. If the quantity $(h + w) \neq (\xi PCr\Delta HPCr)$, then another reaction exists or some mistake was made. In the analysis of a finding that $(h + w) > (\xi PCr\Delta HPCr)$, it will prove convenient to divide the total enthalpy into the explained enthalpy $(\xi PCr\Delta HPCr)$ and the unexplained enthalpy, which is the remainder, $(h + w) - (\xi PCr\Delta HPCr)$ (37). There should be no confusion concerning the meaning of the explained enthalpy: if the measured extent of net PCr decrease (ξPCr) and the molar enthalpy ($\Delta HPCr$) are measured accurately and precisely, then the product surely is a defined portion of the total observed enthalpy. The meaning of the difference, called the unexplained enthalpy, is also clear. It must be caused by the net advancement of some known or unknown reaction that was not added in the initial sum $(\xi PCr\Delta HPCr)$ and that may be exothermic or endothermic.

Biochemical Method

Muscles in the animal and in vitro continuously dissipate free energy to remain in a steady state with respect to their initial energy content and chemical composition, which is different from their environment. Each therefore operates as an open system taking up substrate and O_2 and releasing CO_2, water, and other metabolites as required by the moment to moment demands of oxidative metabolism. I have discussed in detail the energetically significant metabolic reactions (see CHEMICAL REACTIONS AND METABOLIC PRINCIPLES, p. 196) and the fact that a near-equilibrium metabolic network exists and involves adenine nucleotides, PCr, cytoplasmic NAD and NADH, and H^+ in the regulation of oxidative phosphorylation and recovery O_2 consumption. To establish a biochemically based energy balance scheme, the stoichiometries of the reactions must be known, and they must be constant at least within the range of conditions achieved experimentally.

The strategy and details of metabolic sequences are the products of evolution and are not the result of deductions from first principles as is the case for the basic myothermic conservation equation. There is no a priori chemical or thermodynamic necessity for any particular set of metabolic reactions. Evolution has maintained a highly conserved series of metabolic reactions on which a systematic view of energetics can be based. A biochemical energy balance technique therefore focuses on pathways of recovery metabolism that return the muscle's chemical state to a precontracting resting level and specifically on the relationship observed between measures of recovery and measures of the extent of energy-yielding reactions during contraction. Provided that the initial chemical, osmotic, electrical, and mechanical changes arising from activation and contraction are reversed during the recovery period, the muscle returns to a definable state indistinguishable from the state preceding contraction. The net difference is that some substrate (endogenous or exogenous) and O_2 have been consumed, and CO_2 and H_2O are liberated. It is common experience that living cells and organisms behave in this way, and thus on an experimental level these concepts have the same level of generality as did observations on heat and mechanical change over two centuries ago when the experimental foundations of thermodynamics were laid.

The advantage of a biochemical energy balance technique is twofold. *1*) It identifies and measures individual reactions and thus specifies the results of the myothermic technique. *2*) It is able to define more accurately any suspected source of an observed discrepancy because it relies on assumptions about the actual chemical pathways. Its disadvantage is obvious: the biochemical technique is only able to detect those transformations defined by standard chemical pathways, measurable by available techniques, and linked to recovery oxidations. However, when an energy imbalance is found, these techniques complement each other and aid interpretation and experimental design.

Restricting the discussion to recovery measurements involving the recovery oxygen (ξO_2) or lactate production (ξlac) is practical because experimentally muscles can be constrained to metabolize carbohydrate. From considerations of metabolic homeostasis for oxidative recovery

$$\xi \sim P = k\xi O_2 \tag{29}$$

where $\xi \sim P$ is the utilization of energy-rich phosphate compounds from the onset of contraction to the moment of mechanical relaxation; ξO_2 is the total recovery O_2 consumption, which in suitable experimental conditions and according to this model of energetics occurs after relaxation. The stoichiometric factor, k, is derived from known metabolic pathways. For oxidative recovery, $k = 6.3$ (a dimensionless number relating the moles of energy-rich phosphate synthesized per mole of O_2 consumed, $\xi \sim P/\xi O_2$). The equation states the conditions for chemical energy balance: the initial utilization of energy-rich phosphate compounds equals the amount resynthesized by oxidative recovery metabolism. What is tested is the hypothesis that the experimentally measured quantities satisfy the stated stoichiometric relationship.

For completely anaerobic recovery via the Embden-Meyerhof pathway of glycogenolysis and glycolysis

$$\xi \sim P = l\xi\text{lac} \tag{30}$$

where $\xi \sim P$ has the same meaning as above; ξlac is the total lactate production during the recovery; and l is the stoichiometric coupling factor, $l = 1.5$ (a dimensionless number relating the moles of energy-rich phosphate resynthesized per mole of lactate produced, $\xi \sim P/\xi\text{lac}$). If glucose is available, taken up by the hexokinase reaction, and completely substitutes for glycogenolysis, the factor l has a value of 1.0.

Finally, as recovery may be partially aerobic and partially anaerobic

$$\xi \sim P = k\xi O_2 + l\xi\text{lac} \tag{31}$$

because the metabolic sequences are mechanistically and stoichiometrically independent, because a priori it is not known what fraction of energy-rich phosphate resynthesis occurs by glycolytic, substrate-level phosphorylation alone or by oxidative phosphorylation, and because there are no other pathways for the restoration of initial levels of metabolites in vertebrate muscles studied so far.

What evidence is there that the values of the factors k and l are constant, that is independent of metabolic and physiological conditions? Second, how accurately are the coupling coefficients known? The important characteristic of enzymes is their specificity, both of the binding of substrate and in the formation of product. However, the specificity is not absolute, and in principle, side reactions can occur, especially with multifunctional enzymes under specific conditions. For example, in the glyceraldehyde-3-phosphate dehydrogenase reaction an acyl enzyme is an obligatory intermediate. Its formation is not limited to the normal substrate, glyceraldehyde 3-phosphate, for acetaldehyde and other aldehydes are also substrates (74, 87), especially when the enzyme is chemically modified. Normally an energy-rich acylphosphate is the product (1,3-diphosphoglycerate), but the enzyme also catalyzes the formation of acylarsenates, which are extremely unstable in water, and the formation of acetyl phosphate from acetaldehyde. Although these unphysiological substrates are normally absent, the demonstrated nonspecificity raises the possibility of variable metabolic coupling coefficients. Fortunately side reactions do not appear to occur under physiological conditions. Scopes (207, 208) reconstituted the enzymes for glycogenolysis and glycolysis in vitro in conditions thought to mimic the cytosol and observed the orthodox stoichiometry for the entire pathway. There was no evidence for a stoichiometry different from $l = 1.5$.

The possibility of uncoupling mitochondrial oxidative phosphorylation exists. The stoichiometric parameter of interest is the number of atoms of energy-rich phosphate synthesized per atom of oxygen reduced; this is called the P/O ratio in the mitochondria literature. Because practical measurements in tissues are normally calibrated in molar units of O_2, in this chapter the term $\sim P/O_2$ is used and the relationship is simply: $2(P/O) = \sim P/O_2$. Common techniques for measuring the quantity P/O use manometric measurements of the O_2 consumption by mitochondria suspended in solution and a chemical measure of the ATP synthesized. The latter is conveniently measured by reacting glucose with ATP by hexokinase. A second method takes advantage of the phenomenon of respiratory control. A measured amount of ADP is added to the mitochondrial suspension provided with an adequate amount of P_i and substrate; the O_2 content of the mixture is monitored. There is a burst of O_2 consumption (Fig. 9) until the ADP is phosphorylated completely. The quantity, ADP/O, is identical to the quantity P/O only if all extraneous ATPases are controlled for and if all the ADP is phosphorylated. For NADH-coupled oxidative phosphorylation many experimental values of P/O are close to 3 but usually somewhat lower. Thermodynamic calculations and evidence for three coupling sites (Fig. 7) have led to the view that the experimentally observed values of P/O contain certain unavoidable losses of energy, and so it is deduced that the correct physiologically relevant value for mitochondrial oxidative phosphorylation is an integer and is 3; $P/O_2 = 6$. In intact cells there is a small additional energy-rich phosphate resynthesis by substrate level phosphorylation.

However, one should not accept this value of P/O_2 uncritically. The precise relationship between the number of protons transported across the inner mitochondrial membrane for each molecule of O_2 reduced and for each molecule of ATP synthesized is not yet adequately defined. It remains a possibility, therefore, that the stoichiometric factor is neither constant nor independent of conditions; it may even be fractional. It is known that the proton motive force generated ultimately by the reduction of O_2 can be coupled to the transport of calcium and other ions into the mitochondrial matrix (170). In that circumstance the apparent stoichiometric relationship P/O would be different with the simultaneous ion transport than without. Hinkle and Yu (107) have presented evidence that the experimentally observed P/O values are lower than currently accepted ones and are not necessarily integers. Whatever the explanation, Hinkle and Yu did observe in liver mitochondria that P/O for NADH-coupled β-hydroxybutyrate oxidation is 2 and for flavin nucleotide–coupled succinate oxidation the value is 1.3 instead of the conventionally accepted values of 3 and 2, respectively. Only in mitochondria isolated from brown adipose tissue is there evidence, however, that a physiological and regulated uncoupling of proton motive force from energy-rich phosphate generation occurs (106, 183, 184) where it is a mechanism for heat generation. The following questions concerning the coupling of the proton motive force to ~P synthesis can be clearly formulated and require quantitative data under a variety of conditions before the value for P/O anticipated in intact cells can be definitively established. *1*) Is the H^+/O ratio a fixed quantity (226) and is its value 9 or 12, which is sufficient to allow for P/O value of 3 at moderate thermodynamic efficiency? *2*) What is the stoichiometry of the ATPase? A value of 2 H^+ for each ATP molecule synthesized (218) may be correct. *3*) What are the actual energy requirements for ATP, ADP, and P_i transport across the inner mitochondrial membrane? Energy is required for the exchange of ADP and P_i for ATP over and above that required for ATP synthesis. Energized uptake of Ca^{2+} by mitochondria (29, 170, 205) does not appear to occur during a contraction-relaxation cycle (212).

Although certain important problems in mitochondrial energetics and mechanism remain, there are whole cell and tissue preparations in which it is possible to observe a P/O_2 ratio close to 6; these experiments were made in mouse skeletal muscles (RESULTS OF ENERGY BALANCE EXPERIMENTS, p. 212) and in renal tubules (86). Although such large-scale measurements do not specifically answer the questions about the mechanism of coupling, these macroscopic measurements certainly limit the integration of those mechanisms. Therefore this discussion of muscle energetics assumes the conventional view that oxidative phosphorylation in mitochondria in cells is normally fully coupled, and the complete oxidation of 1 mol glucosyl unit of glycogen yields 37 or 39 mol ATP. The uncertainty is due to the fact that the mechanism of transporting reducing equivalents into the mitochondria is not yet settled. If the carrier of cytoplasmic reducing equivalents into the mitochondria is the α-glycerol phosphate–dihydroxyacetone phosphate shuttle, 37 mol ATP are produced per mole of glucosyl unit oxidized, because this shuttle transfers electrons to flavoproteins (Fig. 7, site 2). If malate-oxaloacetate shuttle is the carrier mechanism, 39 mol ATP are produced, because this carrier is linked to site 1. In the absence of a decisive answer, a coupling coefficient, $k = 6.3$, will be used. The uncertainty is about 5%.

RESULTS OF ENERGY BALANCE EXPERIMENTS

The focus of experimental work in the past two decades has been testing whether an energy balance exists during muscle contraction. Is it experimentally demonstrable that known chemical changes can be accurately measured and account quantitatively for the energetics of the contractile events? Ironically the initial studies led to a false sense of security. The experimental design is to measure the total energy associated with a contraction and to compare that quantity with one predicted from the measured extent of known chemical reactions. If the two quantities agree, then an energy balance is said to occur; or more precisely, the possibility cannot be excluded that all pertinent reactions involved in the contraction are identified and measured. Both the biochemical and myothermic techniques relate some measure of the total energy change to the chemical changes involving energy-rich phosphate compounds that occur during the contraction. Recall that total enthalpy change is related to the measured chemical reactions and their molar enthalpies by Equation 20, p. 208. Total recovery ~P synthesis is related to the measured chemical reactions by Equation 31, p. 211. Lack of equality in either relationship means that at least one of the following must be true: *1*) the conversion factors (ΔH_i, k,l) are incorrect; *2*) the extent of chemical reactions (ξ_i, $\xi \sim P$, ξO_2, ξlac) are incorrectly measured; *3*) there is at least one unidentified chemical reaction or thermally important process not included on the balance sheet.

It may be possible to use the information gathered from each technique to define the nature of any observed discrepancy. For example, if the time course of an initial discrepancy measured by a myothermic technique parallels the time course of a discrepancy measured by recovery biochemical reactions, then the excess recovery metabolism may represent the reversal of a process that resulted in the initial unexplained enthalpy. The extent of the extra energy utilization needed to reverse the missing reaction can be estimated from the quantitative measurements of the recovery metabolism. If it is assumed that the discrepancy results from a single reaction and that a precise stoichiometry exists between the extent of that reaction and the energy-rich phosphate needed for its reversal, then it is further possible to obtain a value for the extent of that initial unknown reaction in units of $\xi \sim P$. Despite the temptation toward minimalism, it must be emphasized that any imbalance detected by both methods may not be the same imbalance because the methods are based on independent observations.

Carlson, Hardy, and Wilkie (21, 22) applied myothermic methods to assess energy balance with anaerobic frog sartorius muscles at 0°C, poisoned with iodoacetate. For a series of twitches or for a 10-s tetanus, the observed relationship between enthalpy production and PCr splitting $[(h + w) \div \xi\text{PCr})]$ was constant, −42 kJ/mol. In an extensive series of experiments with frog sartorius under similar conditions and a newly designed integrating thermopile, Wilkie (228) also found a constant relationship of −46.4 kJ/mol for isometric twitches and for working tetanic contractions. These values agreed quite well with the accepted value of $\Delta H\text{PCr} = -46$ kJ/mol obtained earlier by Meyerhof and Schulz (175). The question of a myothermic energy balance thus appeared to be answered in the affirmative.

A mistake was made, however. A careful reevaluation of the enthalpy of PCr hydrolysis and of other relevant reactions (37, 237) resulted in a significant downward revision of the magnitude of $\Delta H\text{PC}$ to a value of −34 kJ/mol. Thus all the conclusions based on prior work must be altered in light of this new information: energy imbalance is well outside of any experimental error. To illustrate the magnitude of the imbalance consider Curtin and Woledge's (37, 236) reanalysis of the data of Carlson et al. (22) for a 10-s tetanus: the enthalpy change and PCr breakdown are normalized to the total creatine content as a measure of total muscle cell mass

observed enthalpy = 5.99 ± 0.22 mJ/mol total creatine

observed chemical change = 0.117 ± 0.007 mol PCr/mol total creatine

explained enthalpy = 3.98 ± 0.23 MJ/mol total creatine

unexplained enthalpy = 2.01 ± 0.14 mJ/mol total creatine

The unexplained enthalpy fraction is ⅓(2.01/5.99). The conclusion is inescapable that a major energy imbalance exists. This is true not only for frog sartorius, but [as reviewed by Curtin and Woledge (37) and by Homsher and Kean (109)] there are no data for which a myothermic energy balance has been demonstrated, including data for frog, tortoise (235), and rat muscles (82). Furthermore a biochemical energy imbalance was also shown in frog sartorii (142) because $\xi \sim P < k\xi O_2$.

Because of the logical necessity of being able to identify and measure all chemical reactions before any further analysis of muscle energetics can proceed and because study of this problem has dominated experimental work in the field since the late 1950s, the experimental results for the several preparations used are taken up in detail.

Energy Balance Studies in Rana temporaria

MYOTHERMIC STUDIES. In the experiments of Carlson, Hardy, and Wilkie (21, 22, 228), all measurements were made on the same pair of muscles. A value for heat + work in the stimulated muscle was first obtained with the use of a thermopile; the other muscle was an unstimulated control. The apparatus was opened and the pair of muscles removed and frozen rapidly by immersion into a heat-conducting liquid cooled to about −70°C. A period of about 30 s elapsed between the contraction and the moment of freezing. The associated chemical change was measured by the difference in the chemical composition of the experimental muscle minus the control. The improved hammer-freezing apparatus (133) required a change in the experimental design: separate pairs of muscles were used for thermal and for chemical measurements. Comparison between the two sets of data was made possible by suitable controls (228). Most of the data obtained at that time are expressed as energy production or chemical change per micromole total creatine, which is a good measure of muscle mass. To convert these quantities to units of muscle weight, a value of about 35 μmol total creatine per gram blotted wet weight can be used, but it should be remembered that the total creatine content fluctuates between different batches of frogs and with the season of the year [e.g., see Table 2 in ref. 115 and (166)].

Since there is clearly an energy imbalance over a full contraction-relaxation cycle, the next question is: is there an energy imbalance throughout the course of an isometric tetanus? Kretzschmar developed the tools to make these experiments possible (79). The data showed an approximately constant PCr-splitting rate with tetanic duration, but the rate of liberation of total energy was substantially greater during the first few seconds than afterwards, a result consistent with most other heat measurements (for example, see Fig. 1). The results were therefore decisive: at no time was there an energy balance and, further, for no duration of contraction (0.5 s–15 s) was there a constant relationship between the total energy liberated (heat + work) and the amount of PCr split.

One possible explanation for the unexplained enthalpy was that an additional unknown process was stoichiometrically coupled to PCr splitting. The results of Gilbert et al. (79) were inconsistent with this view, but they were not decisive. The problem was specifically tested by Curtin and Woledge (35), and a significant unexplained enthalpy fraction was found in muscles with and without FDNB-poisoning, a reagent that blocks the creatine kinase reaction (see *Creatine Phosphokinase*, p. 197). The use of the inhibitor may introduce secondary effects. Unexpectedly for short tetanic durations the unexplained enthalpy fraction was reduced, and for longer tetanic durations the unexplained energy fraction was increased compared with unpoisoned muscles. Nonetheless the major results are clear: the unexplained energy could not be understood simply in terms of an unknown reaction stoichiometrically linked to the extent of creating phosphate hydrolysis.

What properties then does the hypothetical reaction have? The experiments of Gilbert et al. (79) and of Curtin and Woledge (35) imply that the missing reaction is independent of oxidative or glycolytic recovery. This inference is not strong because of the differences in total enthalpy production between poisoned and unpoisoned muscles but is supported by the known lack of significant advancement of aerobic or anaerobic recovery metabolism during very brief tetanuses (see BIOCHEMICAL STUDIES, p. 218). Oxidative phosphorylation and ATP synthesis during the contraction could not have contributed more than 10% of the unexplained enthalpy even if it is assumed that recovery O_2 consumption begins with the onset of the stimulus. The missing reaction does not appear to involve proton buffer reactions since the phenomenon of unexplained energy is found in two sorts of muscles: unpoisoned muscles in which net PCr breakdown is accompanied by net uptake of H^+ (Fig. 5) and in FDNB-treated muscles in which net ATP breakdown is accompanied by release of H^+. These results also exclude a substantial error in estimates of the buffer heats. The glycolytic reactions distal to glyceraldehyde-3-phosphate dehydrogenase are excluded because iodoacetate blocks this enzyme, and in that circumstance there is still a significant unexplained enthalpy.

Examination of the time course of evolution of the unexplained energy fraction by two laboratories (38, 111) revealed an important property. It is now clear that the production of unexplained enthalpy (presumbly, but not necessarily, a single reaction) goes to completion over a period of about 5–10 s at 0°C. Heat and chemical changes were carefully compared for tetanic durations 0.75 s to 20 s independently in two labs (38, 100). As the results show (Fig. 11) the data from both labs are very similar (panels *A* and *B*). All those data therefore lead to the conclusion illustrated in panel *C* of Figure 11: that an unidentified reaction begins at the onset of contractile activity, that its extent is limited, and that the reaction goes to completion by 10 s or so of a continued stimulation in the experimental conditions studied. However, it may prove too simplistic to assert that there is a single unidentified reaction.

The time course and magnitude of the unexplained enthalpy correspond well to the previously described phenomenon of "labile heat" as defined by Aubert's experiments (6). He quantitated the curvilinear heat production in a maintained isometric tetanus and used this equation to fit his data

$$H_t = h_A(1 - e^{-at}) + h_B t \tag{32}$$

where H_t is the heat produced at any time t; h_A, h_B, and a are constants. The first term on the right defines the labile heat with a rate constant, a, approximately 1/s. The second term on the right is the stable maintenance heat. The property of labile heat most relevant in our present context is that its evolution is complete within about 5 s. To indicate the magnitude of these quantities, in a 10-s tetanus the total energy released $(h + w)$ was 961 mJ/g dry wt in the experiments of Curtin and Woledge (38) (Fig. 11*B*), and of this total, labile heat amounted to 240 mJ/g dry wt. Curtin and Woledge made a quantitative examination of the time course of unexplained and explained enthalpy and of labile heat. They found the unexplained enthalpy appears to be evolved at a slower rate than the labile heat, but at 10 s the magnitudes of each were not significantly different. If one assumes the labile heat is caused by only one reaction, then their data exclude the possibility that the unexplained enthalpy and labile heat originate from the same chemical reaction. Homsher et al. (110) did related experiments and came to the same conclusion. However, it is possible that the unexplained enthalpy represents two or perhaps more reactions, one of which is manifested by labile heat. Clearly the testing of these hypotheses requires additional experimentation.

Another characteristic of unexplained enthalpy and labile heat shows their close linkage despite the evidence for their lack of identity. Aubert and Maréchal (7) showed that the amount of labile heat is substantially reduced in the second of two tetanuses closely spaced in time. Curtin and Woledge (36) found that the unexplained enthalpy in the second of two 5-s tetanuses separated by 3 s was decreased to 0.39 of the unexplained enthalpy observed in the first tetanus. Other important characteristics of labile heat are *1)* its magnitude increases with temperature with a $Q_{10} \approx 1$ in contrast to the stable maintenance heat rate that has a $Q_{10} \approx 3$. *2)* The replacement of Cl^- by I^- in Ringer's solution potentiates twitch tension and increases labile heat and its rate constant. *3)* With decreased overlap of the thick and thin filaments achieved by stretching a muscle beyond a sarcomere length of 2 μm, tetanic force and stable maintenance heat rate (h_B) decrease, but the magnitude of labile heat remains approximately constant (109). It is, therefore, a plausible working hypothesis that reactions manifested as labile heat and unexplained enthalpy have more to do with events of muscle activation and early stages of contraction rather than with

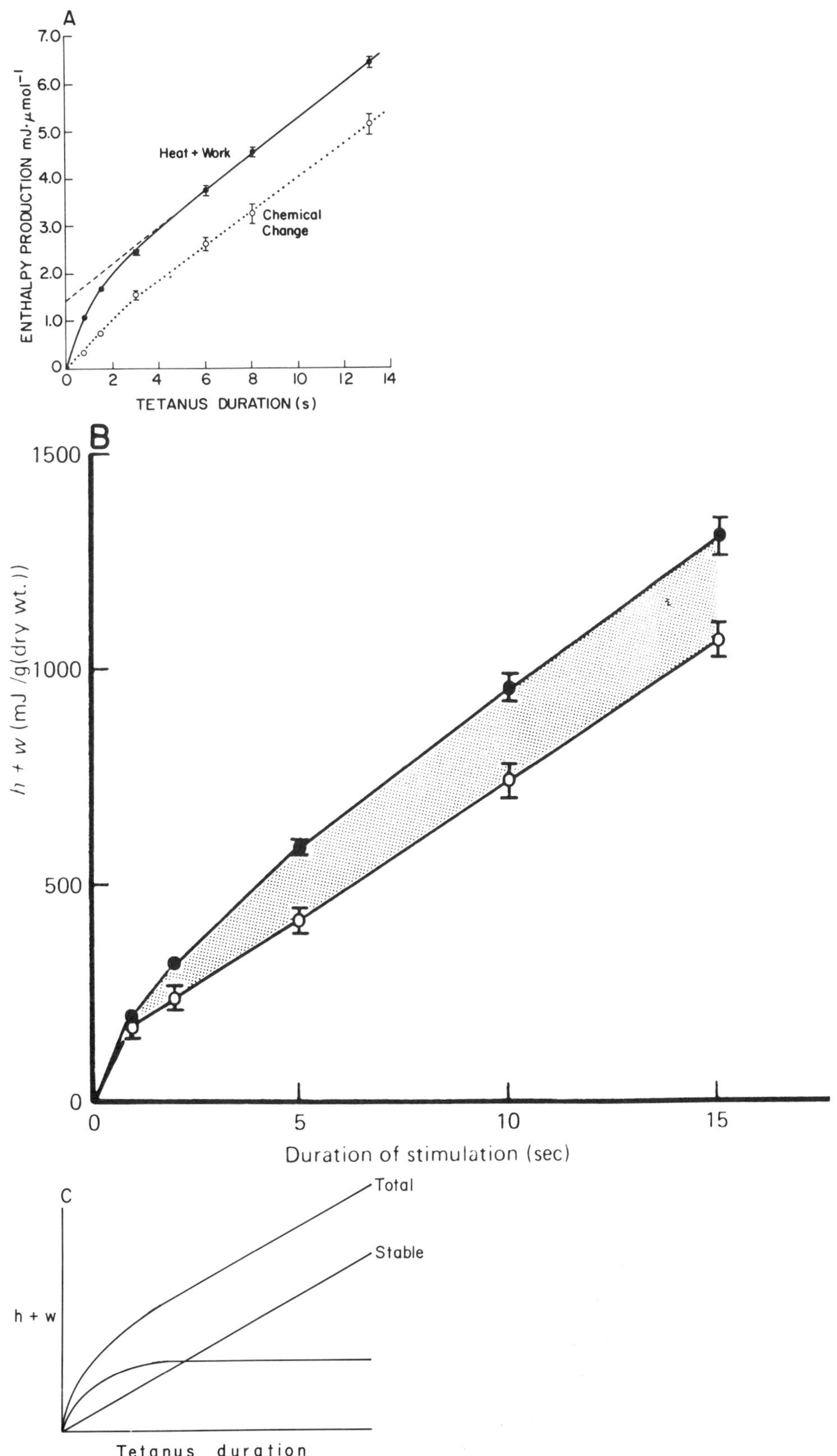

FIG. 11. Relationship between total enthalpy production ($h + w$) and explained enthalpy during isometric tetanuses of various durations. *A* and *B*: explained enthalpy (○) and $h + w$ (●). *C*: a scheme in which it is imagined that the unknown reaction goes to completion and is added linearly to the stable rate of enthalpy production to give observed total enthalpy production. [*A* from Homsher et al. (110); *B* from Curtin and Woledge (38).]

the development and maintenance of force caused by actomyosin interactions. If the mechanisms underlying labile heat and unexplained enthalpy are not identical, they are certainly phenomenologically linked.

Three classes of events occur at the onset of contractile activity and therefore are candidate mechanisms for labile heat and unexplained enthalpy: *1)* membrane depolarization and the release of calcium ions from the SR that bind subsequently to troponin, parvalbumin, and possibly other proteins as well—that is, all the processes of excitation-contraction coupling; *2)* redistribution of myosin kinetic states from those in a relaxed muscle to those in contracting muscle; *3)* an acceleration of one or more of the reactions that occur at a steady rate during a maintained contraction during the beginning of a tetanus.

The third possibility is the most easily excluded because the myothermic evidence discussed shows that the unexplained enthalpy cannot be stoichiometrically linked to PCr or ATP splitting directly.

The first and second possibility may be conceptually described as the occurrence of only one portion of a cyclic reaction. The concept is illustrated

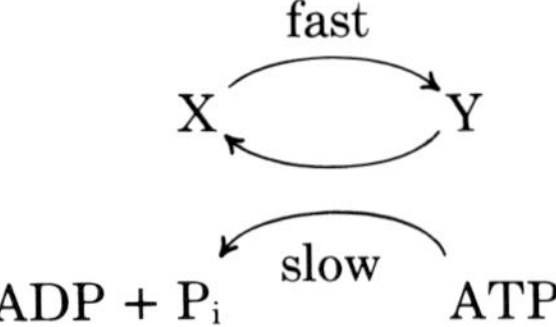

The first reaction (X → Y) is unknown and not yet measured. It occurs rapidly at the onset of contraction with a molar enthalpy, ΔHX. The extent of the reaction ξX is given by

$$\xi X = [X]_0 - [X]_t \qquad (33)$$

where $[X]_0$ is the initial content, and $[X]_t$ is the content at some later time, *t*. The second reaction is assumed to be slower and is stoichiometrically coupled to reverse the direction of the first reaction. The molar enthalpy of the second reaction is ΔHATP and the extent of the reaction, ξATP, is similarly given by

$$\xi ATP = [ATP]_0 - [ATP]_t \qquad (34)$$

The conservation equation applies for all times; therefore

$$h + w = \xi X \Delta H X + \xi ATP \Delta H ATP \qquad (35)$$

Consider two special conditions. For very short times when ζATP = 0

$$h + w = \xi X \Delta H X \qquad (36)$$

When the second reaction reverses reaction 1 completely, of course, ξX = 0 and

$$h + w = \xi ATP \Delta H ATP \qquad (37)$$

After a time ξX reaches some value, and the forward and reverse fluxes through reaction 1 eventually become equal in a steady state; thereafter there is no more advancement. In the final steady state, total ξX may be small, but in general it will not be zero. Thus in this model some of the total enthalpy production must be attributed to the net advancement of the hypothetical reaction ξX, that is, by the advancement of only a portion of a cyclic reaction. An equivalent statement of the advancement of a portion of a reaction cycle is that the corresponding thermodynamic cycle is incomplete. This notion further requires a reversal of reaction 1 after the end of contraction and the accompanying reversal of its enthalpy change. Indeed there is a net uptake of heat by muscle after relaxation (75), a phenomenon that is usually overshadowed by exothermic recovery reactions and the thermoelastic effect. The list of possible candidates for reaction 1 is very large: conformation or structural changes of actin, myosin, or of larger order structures; calcium and correlated ion movements; phosphorylation and other covalent modification of enzymes and contractile proteins; and metabolic reactions that occur predominantly in recovery but might occur to a significant extent during contraction.

With this conceptual reaction scheme in mind, the suggestion of Curtin and Woledge (37) is appealing. Of all the cyclical events of the contraction-relaxation cycle actomyosin interactions are surely central to force development and shortening. Rall et al. (197) showed that more unexplained enthalpy was produced within the first second of contraction by muscle shortening rapidly than by isometric contractions. One interpretation of those results is that unexplained enthalpy production is closely linked to actomyosin interactions rather than to other events associated with excitation-contraction coupling. Kinetic analyses of the myosin and actomyosin ATPase indicate a multistep cycle (55). In relaxed muscle, the predominant form of myosin is in the form of myosin-product complex (167) and the cross bridges are in a detached state. In contracting muscle then there is certainly an increase in the content of attached states and a redistribution among the unattached states. The maximal extent of any transition is given by the total content of myosin, which is 0.3 μmol actin-binding and ATPase sites per gram of muscle (see *Adenosine Triphosphatases*, p. 196). Kodama and Woledge (131) used purified subfragment 1 to measure the enthalpy changes associated with some of the steps in the myosin kinetic cycle. The cleavage of ATP on subfragment 1 was actually endothermic (ΔH = +83 kJ/mol), whereas ATP hydrolysis in solution is exothermic (see THERMODYNAMICS, p. 207). The binding of ATP to subfragment 1 was highly exothermic (ΔH = −90 kJ/mol). The enthalpies of product release were also interesting. Release of P_i is strongly exothermic (ΔH = −88 kJ/mol), whereas release of ADP is strongly endothermic (ΔH = +72 kJ/mol). The concept that emerges from this data is that large enthalpy changes, both positive and negative, are associated with individual steps in the myosin kinetic cycle and largely cancel each other in completed cycles in the steady state. However, when there is a major redistribution of kinetic states as certainly occurs with the onset of contraction and during transient length or force steps, the occurrence of partial kinetic cycles and therefore partial thermodynamic cycles will make important contributions to the total observed enthalpy change. The relation of these partial cycles to the problem of unexplained enthalpy has been discussed in detail by Curtin and Woledge (37). To proceed with this type of analysis the following information must be obtained experimentally: *1*) enthalpy of the formation of the various actomyosin force-generating states, which cannot be obtained by studying only solutions of proteins; *2*) identification of force-generating actomyosin steps and the fraction of myosin in those states as a function of time; *3*) the total number of myosin molecules undergoing cyclic interactions with actin in a steady isometric contraction as well as in other modes of contraction; *4*) which of several kinetic pathways actually occurs during contraction (55).

The other class of candidates for the unexplained enthalpy is all the processes of excitation-contraction coupling; of central importance are Ca^{2+} movements. There is a substantial redistribution of intracellular calcium during and after contraction (212, 232). Experimentally the frog semitendinosus muscles have the useful property that they can be reversibly stretched to an average sarcomere length greater than 3.6 μm; because of denser collagen fiber network the sartorius cannot be stretched that much without substantial damage. No force is generated in stimulated muscles without filament overlap (81). Homsher and Kean (111) measured the explained and unexplained enthalpy at normal and stretched lengths. In a 5-s tetanus at 0°C and at an average sarcomere length of 2.3 μm, the total enthalpy was 59.8 ± 1.0 mJ/g and the unexplained enthalpy was 11.5 ± 3.8 mJ/g. The total enthalpy production in a 5-s tetanus at the long length (3.8 μm) was 20.1 ± 0.7 mJ/g. The significant new finding was that the unexplained enthalpy at 3.8 μm was 9.8 ± 1.8 mJ/g, that is, the same value as observed at 2.3 μm within experimental error. A further experiment confirmed this result. A pair of semitendinosus muscles were mounted, one at an average sarcomere length of 2.3 μm and the other at an average sarcomere length of 3.7 μm. Both muscles were stimulated for 5 s and the energy balance was tested. The predicted outcome is that the difference in production of enthalpy in the two conditions would be completely explained by the difference in chemical energy utilization, since presumably the same amount of unexplained enthalpy is produced in both and cancels in the subtraction of experimental minus control muscle. The observed enthalpy was 31.3 ± 1.7 mJ/g, and the explained enthalpy was 32.1 ± 2.3 mJ/g. Since there was no unexplained enthalpy (−0.8 ± 2.9 mJ/g), in excellent agreement with the first experiment, the clear conclusion is that the events associated with excitation-contraction coupling are sufficient to be the source of the unexplained enthalpy and that the amount of unexplained enthalpy is independent of filament overlap and tension generation.

This conclusion is based on three assumptions. First, there are no actomyosin interactions in muscles stretched to an average sarcomere length of 3.7 μm. This is reasonable since little force (about 0.07 P_0) was developed in the stretched muscles used for energy balance. Second, there is no redistribution among the myosin kinetic states in highly stretched muscles. This assumption is also reasonable because there is no change in the intensity of the 43-nm myosin reflection in the X-ray–diffraction pattern (239), there is no change in attitude of fluorescently labeled myosin in glycerinated rabbit psoas fibers (185), and there is no detectable change in the confirmation of fluorescently labeled subfragment 1 in isolated synthetic thick filaments on the addition of calcium (171). Third, the mechanisms of excitation-contraction coupling are not quantitatively or qualitatively altered by stretch. This assumption is supported by the following evidence: the size of the action potential is not altered by stretch (204), the mechanical threshold (defined as the degree of depolarization by external potassium necessary to develop force) was not changed from 25 mM K^+ by moderate stretches (113), and the twitch:tetanus ratio is independent of muscle length above the rest length (210). However, the light output, reflecting in a nonlinear fashion the sarcoplasmic Ca^{2+} levels, in aequorin-injected fibers (11) in twitches and tetanuses is dependent on muscle length. Light output increases slightly from rest length to a maximal value between an average sarcomere length of 2.4–3.0 μm and then decreases dramatically with progressive stretch to 30% at an average sarcomere length of 3.6 μm. There may be no contradiction between the aequorin experiments and the others since the aequorin response only reflects the sarcoplasmic free-calcium concentrations that, in a twitch and brief tetanus, are not necessarily in equilibrium with the bound calcium responsible for activation mechanisms on the thin filament. Indeed, as mentioned in *Adenosine Triphosphatases*, p. 196, most of the calcium released by the SR is bound during contraction, and thus for kinetic reasons rapid variations in cytoplasmic free-calcium concentrations are compatible with negligibly small changes in the calcium actually bound to regulatory sites on the myofibrils. Curtin and Woledge (37) summarize the existing data for enthalpies of binding of calcium to various proteins. Unfortunately no experiments were made with proteins derived from frog muscle or with calmodulin. Calcium binding to troponin C can be significantly exothermic, and calcium binding to whole troponin is even more exothermic. However, the magnitude and sign of the enthalpy change are very dependent on temperature. Calcium binding to parvalbumin is also exothermic, although the enthalpy change per mole of protein is smaller than for troponin. Thus mechanisms of calcium release and binding are able to contribute very substantially to the unexplained enthalpy. To settle these matters, however, additional quantitative calorimetric studies are required as well as a detailed time course of the extent and rate of calcium-binding reactions in muscle cells rather than sarcoplasmic free-Ca^{2+} levels. In any event, during the recovery period, the Ca^{2+} is reaccumulated into the terminal cisternae of the SR by an ATP-driven pump.

Robertson et al. (198) developed a calculation for the time-dependent occupancy of calcium-binding sites that assumes a constant sarcoplasmic Mg^{2+} level of 2.5×10^{-3} M, a value consistent with chemical shift of ATP measured by phosphorus NMR (17, 43, 83). The calculation uses measured or calculated rate constants for binding and release of Ca^{2+}. They then calculated the amount of calcium bound to troponin, parvalbumin, calmodulin, and myosin during a transient rise in sarcoplasmic Ca^{2+} thought to mimic a twitch and under conditions of constant sarcoplasmic Ca^{2+} thought to mimic a tetanus. This model shows that only the calcium-specific sites on troponin and the binding to calmodulin undergo a significant change in saturation during a transient rise in sarcoplasmic Ca^{2+}. The other calcium-binding sites, namely myosin, parvalbumin, and the nonspecific Ca^{2+}-Mg^{2+}-binding sites on troponin, exchange too slowly to have their low degree of saturation altered much during a twitch. The sluggishness of exchange in this class of sites is due largely to the slow release of previously bound Mg^{2+}. When Ca^{2+} levels were maintained at 6×10^{-6} M (that is, a calculation for a tetanus) or when a steady-state series of twitchlike transients of calcium levels were modeled, the slowly exchanging sites also became appreciably saturated with Ca^{2+}. If the unexplained enthalpy and labile heat are to be explained in terms of Ca^{2+}-binding reactions, their kinetics could correspond only with Ca^{2+} binding to the slowly exchanging Ca^{2+}-Mg^{2+}-binding sites. However, the available data discussed previously suggest labile heat and unexplained enthalpy are not the same phenomenon. The calculations of Robertson et al. also influence the interpretation of activation heat (see *Energetics as an Analytical Tool*, p. 191). Activation heat is defined for a tetanus, and it is generally believed that twitch activation heat summates as stimulus frequency increases to produce tetanus activation heat. Hill (96) originally used the term for twitch to represent "presumably a triggered reaction setting the muscle in a state in which it can shorten and do work." Thus twitch activation heat is also thought to be due to Ca^{2+} movements (196). Although twitch and tetanic activation heat may be related, tetanic activation heat does not correspond quantitatively with unexplained enthalpy because *1*) tetanic activation heat is 25 mJ/g when measured in a 10-s isometric tetanus as a function of muscle length (113); *2*) the unexplained enthalpy, which is completely released by 5 s, is less than one-half as large, 10 mJ/g; and *3*) their time courses differ. If tetanus activation heat is the sum-

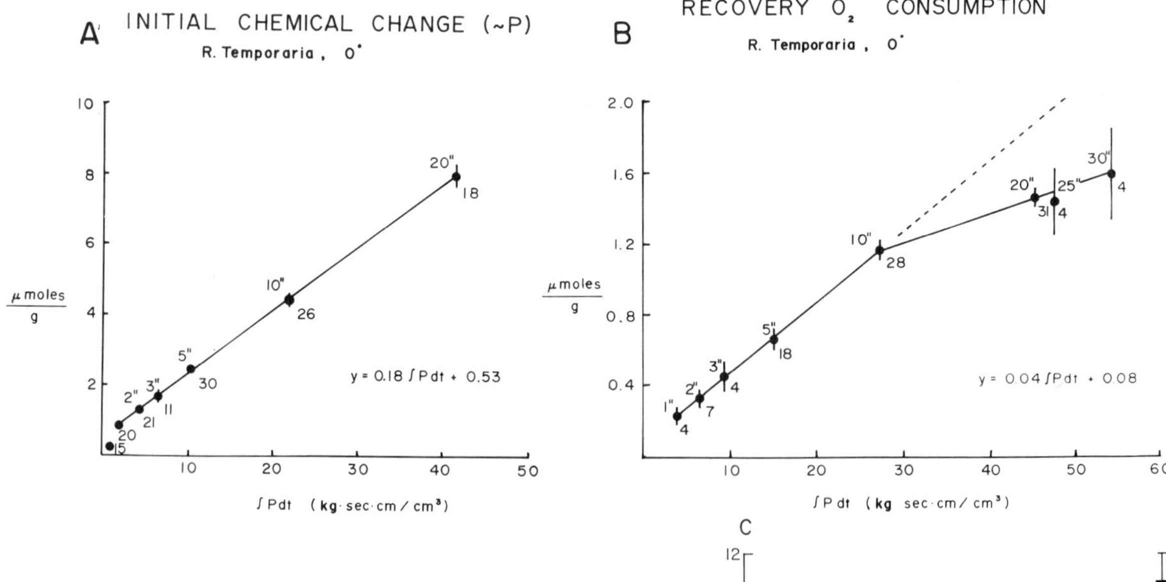

FIG. 12. Utilization of chemical energy during contraction as a function of tension-time integral for isometric tetanuses up to 20 s in duration. *A*: initial chemical changes (initial $\xi \sim$ P); *B*: recovery O_2 consumption (recovery $\xi \sim$ P). Sartorii from *Rana temporaria* were studied at 0°C. In *A* and *B* $\xi \sim P$ and ξ_{O_2} are plotted separately. *C*: $\xi \sim$ P is replotted (●); $\xi_{O_2} \times 6.3$ is plotted on the same graph (■). Break in *upper curve* in *C* occurs between 5 and 10 s of stimulation. Tension-time integral for each second of stimulation is approximately 2.1 kg·cm^{-1}·s^{-1}·g^{-1}. (M. J. Kushmerick, unpublished observations.)

mation of twitch activation heat, Ca^{2+} binding to slowly exchanging sites on troponin and parvalbumin is excluded on kinetic grounds as its mechanism. Finally, if labile heat and unexplained enthalpy are of similar magnitude but have different kinetics and underlying mechanisms, only one may be correlated with slow Ca^{2+} binding. Therefore if there are really three phenomenologically distinguishable heats, activation heat, labile heat, and unexplained enthalpy, only one can be mechanistically associated with slow Ca^{2+} binding to troponin and parvalbumin and none may be associated with rapid Ca^{2+} binding to troponin and calmodulin. Only if twitch activation heat is mechanistically divorced from tetanus activation heat can it be associated with rapid Ca^{2+} binding. What is sorely needed and will be difficult to achieve is a direct test of these hypotheses.

BIOCHEMICAL STUDIES. The basic approach described in *Biochemical Method*, p. 210, is based on testing the equality of the following relationship

$$(\xi \sim \text{P})_{\text{contraction}} = k\xi\text{O}_2 + l\xi\text{lac} \qquad (38)$$

The experimental protocol and methods of Kushmerick and Paul (141, 142) were used to study isometric tetanic durations of 1–30 s in sartorius muscles of *R. temporaria*. Net lactate production and thus the amount of energy-rich phosphate resynthesis by net glycolysis is negligible in these conditions. The practical result is that the predicted relationship to be tested is

$$\xi \sim \text{P} = 6.3\ \xi\text{O}_2 \qquad (39)$$

However, the data for tetanic durations up to 10 s were only explainable with a value of $k = 4.5$ (Fig. 12). Thus an energy imbalance is clearly detected by the biochemical method as well as by the myothermic method. For tetanic durations longer than 10 s, the extent of recovery O_2 consumption falls below the interrupted line (Fig. 12*B*) that gives the predicted O_2 consumption if the same stoichiometric coefficient ($k = 4.5$) were applied to all tetanic durations. It is thus quite clear from Figure 12*C* that a biochemical energy balance is attained after about 10 s of continued stimulation. Hence the data are consistent with a fairly simple and unified picture: the basic pattern of an energy imbalance during the first several seconds of a tetanus is transformed to an energy balance 10 s later, and this result is observed by both myothermic and biochemical energy balance techniques. The possible partial thermodynamic cycles discussed earlier are certainly plausible mechanisms to explain these biochemical data.

SUMMARY. The major energy imbalance that became increasingly obvious during the late 1950s is detected both by myothermic and biochemical techniques. The reaction(s) that causes this imbalance occurs early in an isometric tetanus and appears to go to completion between 5 and 10 s of continued stimulation. Defined and testable hypotheses are now formulated, but evidence to support them will be difficult to obtain because several types of simultaneous measurements are required for quantitative conclusions. Cross correlations among heat production, extent of chemical reactions, mechanical response, state of myosin in its kinetic cycle, and cytoplasmic calcium levels, to name the most obvious ones, are necessary.

Energy Balance Studies in Rana pipiens

MYOTHERMIC STUDIES. The myothermic evidence for an energy imbalance exists in muscles from this species studied at 0°C. However, the evidence (Fig. 13) is not nearly so well developed as for *R. temporaria*, and the amount of unexplained enthalpy is less. In a 5-s tetanus there is about twice the amount of unexplained enthalpy in *R. temporaria* as in *R. pipiens* (cf. Figs. 11 and 13). In the experiments of Homsher et al. (115), which show an energy imbalance in isometric tetanuses ranging from 0.6 to 5 s duration, the unexplained enthalpy fraction is 0.26 and appears to be constant over the range of tetanic durations studied; that is, the amount of unexplained enthalpy appears to increase as stimulation continues. Dawson et al. (45) directly compared sartorii from both frog species. Although there is some significant disagreement in the actual

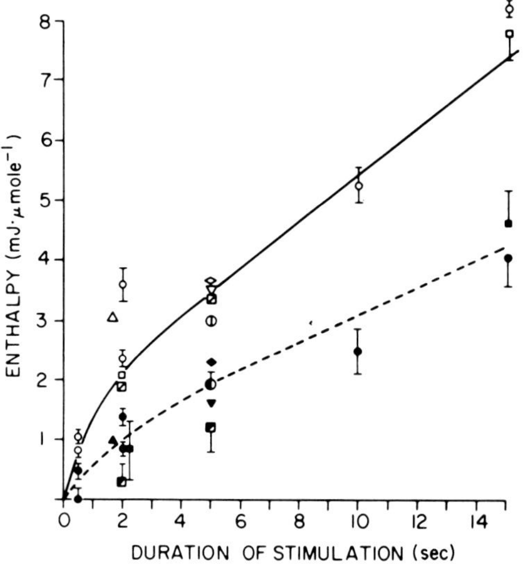

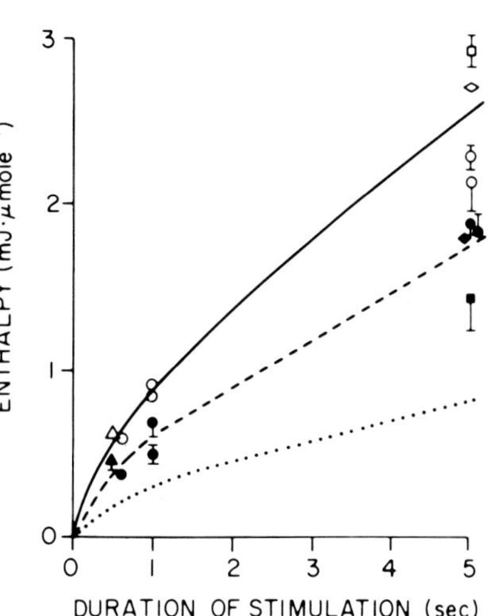

FIG. 13. Energy imbalance in *Rana temporaria* (*left*) and *Rana pipiens* (*right*). *Open symbols* and *full line*, *h* + *w*; *closed symbols* and *dashed line*, explained enthalpy. *Dotted curve* on *right* is the unexplained enthalpy. [From Homsher and Kean (109). Reproduced, with permission, from *Annu. Rev. Physiol.*, vol. 40, © 1978 by Annual Reviews, Inc.]

quantities, the three sets of data consistently show an energy imbalance in muscles from both species. Unfortunately myothermic energy balance in *R. pipiens* has not been studied for stimulations longer than 5 s, so it is not known whether the production of unexplained enthalpy halts after 5 s as is the case for *R. temporaria* or continues to increase as the data in Figure 13 suggests. For reasons that are made clear in the subsequent paragraphs, it is important to settle this issue.

Two additional quantitative differences to be noted are first, maintenance heat rate is about 11 $mJ \cdot g^{-1} \cdot s^{-1}$ and 15 $mJ \cdot g^{-1} \cdot s^{-1}$ for sartorii of *R. pipiens* and *R. temporaria*, respectively [see Homsher and Kean (109) for a complete tabulation of existing data]. Second, the steady isometric rate of turnover of energy-rich phosphate is correspondingly lower in *R. pipiens*, namely 0.3 $\mu mol \cdot g^{-1} \cdot s^{-1}$ and 0.4 $\mu mol \cdot g^{-1} \cdot s^{-1}$ for sartorii from *R. pipiens* and *R. temporaria*, respectively. There are presently no data to prove the energetic pattern or the phenomenon of energy imbalance is substantially different in the two species, but, equally, there is insufficient evidence to prove the pattern is identical.

BIOCHEMICAL STUDIES. Kushmerick and Paul (141, 142) reinvestigated recovery metabolism and sought to establish quantitative relationships among the parameters: force development, energy-rich phosphate splitting, lactate production, and O_2 consumption. The kinetics of recovery O_2 consumption in sartorii in *R. pipiens* at 0°C is clearly exponential (Fig. 9). This pseudo-first-order rate paralleled the time course of resynthesis of PCr with an average time constant of 14 min. There was a measurable lactate production in both resting and contracting muscle that averaged 0.27 mol lactate produced per mol of O_2 consumed so long as the muscle remained well oxygenated. As expected much more lactate production and therefore a much larger amount of glycolitic recovery occurred if the muscles became hypoxic. Recall from the section *Biochemical Method*, p. 210, that the expected stoichiometric coupling factors for an energy balance are $k = 6.3$ and $l = 1.5$ with glycogen as the substrate. Thus the relative fraction of energy-rich phosphate resynthesized by net glycolysis is about 0.06 of the total resynthesized by oxidative metabolism. In their data analysis, Kushmerick and Paul have not included this fraction because it was of similar size to the experimental error. Thus in practice the basic biochemical relationship to be tested reduces to $\xi \sim P = k\xi O_2$. The experiment was designed to measure $\xi \sim P$ and ξO_2 on similar pairs of muscles. In some cases measurements of ξO_2 were made and then a measurement of $\xi \sim P$ was made on the same pair of muscles, thereby providing internal controls. The condition for an energy balance is that both sides of the basic equation are equal. If $\xi \sim P$ is less than $k\xi O_2$, the total amount of energy-rich phosphate resynthesized exceeds that actually utilized during the contraction. If the reverse were true and not accounted for by ξlac then there is an unknown mode of energy-rich phosphate synthesis. Thus an unexplained amount of recovery metabolism is compatible with the thermodynamic energy imbalance on the assumption that the exothermic reaction(s) responsible for the initial unexplained enthalpy is reversed after relaxation by net utilization of ATP, which in turn is regenerated by recovery metabolism. Note that if $\xi \sim P < k\xi O_2$ an equivalent statement is that measurements of net energy-rich phosphate utilization during contraction do not provide a measure of the total energy cost for that contraction.

For isometric tetanuses of 1-s to 30-s durations, there is a consistent relationship between tetanic duration and $\xi \sim P$ or ξO_2 (Fig. 14). If the independent variable is expressed as a tension-time integral (61) to take into account both the fatigue of isometric force in prolonged tetanization and uncontrolled variations in force development among the muscles, the relationship between the $\xi \sim P$ and ξO_2 and the tension-time integral is a linear one in the form: $y = mx + b$. In this form the data for initial and recovery chemical changes are most easily seen to be superimposable (142) by multiplying by an appropriate constant. Figure 15 shows a direct comparison of $\xi \sim P$ and $4 \times \xi O_2$; clearly this stoichiometric factor describes the data. The important conclusion is $\xi \sim P$ and ξO_2 are related by a constant stoichiometric coefficient. However, the measured coefficient k had a value of 4, which is only ⅔ of the predicted value, $k = 6.3$.

These biochemical energy balance data may be interpreted independently of any myothermic results. One possibility is that in frog muscle mitochondria or in mitochondria in general at 0°C oxidative phosphorylation may have a different stoichiometry than it does in mitochondria at more commonly studied temperatures. There is positive evidence against this possibility, however. I found (137) a typical P/O ratio of 3 using the same apparatus and calibrations as were used for studying frog muscle metabolism. In a more detailed study Skoog et al. (209) reported standard values for P/O and respiratory control ratios. Another possibility is that mitochondria isolated and studied in vitro have different stoichiometric coefficients than do mitochondria in the sarcoplasm. This possibility is tantamount to a hypothesis that oxidative phosphorylation is partly uncoupled under normal physiological conditions as discussed in *Biochemical Method*, p. 210. This possibility cannot be excluded but the evidence to be presented in *Mammalian Muscles*, p. 224, renders it highly unlikely.

A more likely possibility to explain the lower observed value for k is that a significant energy-rich phosphate utilization occurs some time after relaxation. The obvious candidates for this energy expenditure are the ATP-dependent transport of Ca^{2+} into the SR or ATP hydrolysis to detach myosin, possibilities already discussed in *Energy Balance Studies in Rana temporaria*, p. 213. However, no burst of PCr breakdown was found up to 200 s after the end of a tetanus

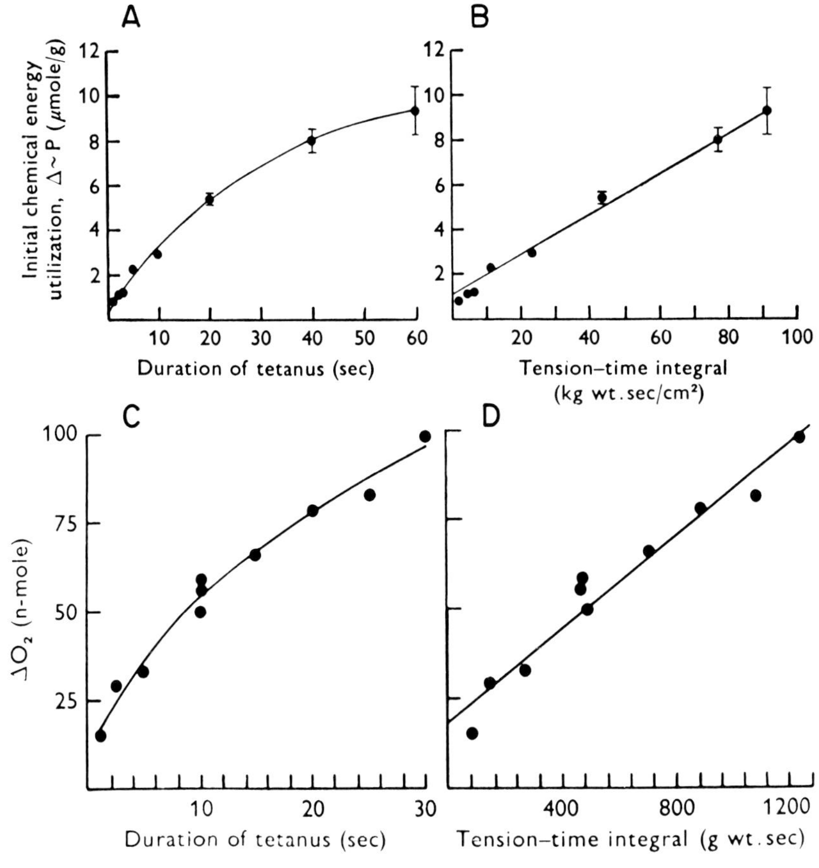

FIG. 14. Relationships between initial changes in high-energy phosphate compounds [Δ ~ P/g, (ξ ~ P)] and stimulus duration (*A*) and tension-time integral (*B*). Mean values ± SE are shown. Relationships between recovery O_2 consumption [ΔO_2/g, (ξ_{O_2})] and tetanus duration (*C*) and tension-time integral (*D*) are shown for data obtained in 1 muscle. [From Kushmerick and Paul (142).]

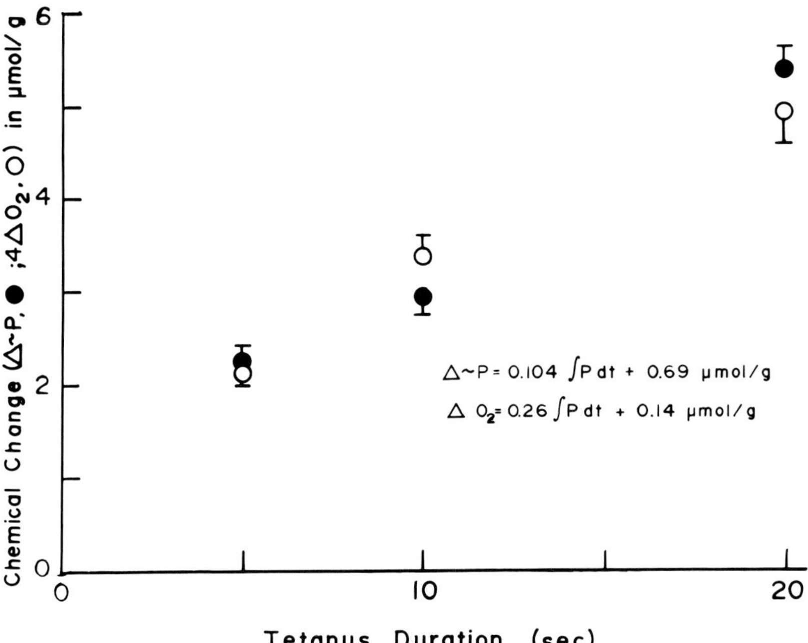

FIG. 15. Initial and recovery chemical changes as a function of duration of isometric tetanus. ●, Direct measurements of ξ ~ P; ○, measurements of ξ_{O_2} multiplied by a factor of 4 to scale with ξ ~ P. Regression equations given in *insert*. Aerobic sartorii of *Rana pipiens* at 0°C. [Data from Kushmerick and Paul (142).]

(34, 142). Curtin and Woledge (34) found some additional enthalpy production and PCr splitting during the relaxation period and shortly thereafter in *R. temporaria*. All of the enthalpy production during relaxation could not be explained by the measured chemical change, and thus the amount of unexplained enthalpy was not reversed during relaxation and even increased.

Despite these negative results, there must be a substantial utilization of energy-rich phosphate some time after mechanical relaxation. Because the time course of recovery O_2 consumption is pseudo–first order, this postulated utilization of energy-rich phosphate must occur slowly and be spread out during the entire recovery period. By modifying the model of a separable contraction phase and a recovery phase (BASIC ENERGETIC MODEL, p. 206) and by taking account of the lack of evidence for additional splitting of PCr shortly after mechanical relaxation, the biochemical energy balance equation can be rewritten to indicate explicitly a utilization of energy-rich compounds sometime during the recovery period

$$(\xi \sim P)_{contraction} + (\xi \sim P)_{recovery} = k\xi O_2 \qquad (40)$$

Because k is observed to be approximately equal to 4, it is clear that $(\xi \sim P)_{recovery}$ is about 0.5 $(\xi \sim P)_{contraction}$. This explanation is consistent with the model of partial reactions and incomplete thermodynamic cycles discussed in *Myothermic Method*, p. 210.

An important unresolved problem remains, however. The current understanding of unexplained enthalpy in *R. temporaria* (see *Energy Balance Studies in Rana temporaria*, p. 213) is that the causal reaction(s) goes to completion with a time course of 5–10 s. This fact and the assumption that the unknown reaction is reversed during recovery by ATP utilization demand that the ratio $\xi \sim P/\xi O_2$ increase as a function of tetanic duration and approach the value k = 6.3. Homsher and Kean (109) have argued that our data [Kushmerick and Paul (141, 142)] cannot exclude this possibility. Despite the significant experimental error, the experimentally determined values of the ratio $\xi \sim P/\xi O_2$ certainly did not increase in any systematic manner with tetanic duration. Thus this interpretation is unwarranted without further experimental justification. Furthermore it is not yet settled whether or not the energy balance patterns in *R. temporaria* and *R. pipiens* are identical (see *Energy Balance Studies in Rana pipiens*, p. 219). The issue still unsettled is that the temporal pattern of energy balance and of explained enthalpy production may be different in the two species of frogs!

Other experiments provide valuable additional information. The total energy cost measured as ξO_2 for an isometric tetanus depends on the contractile history of the muscle in a manner similar to the phenomenon of labile heat. If the interval between successive tetanuses is approximately several seconds, the total recovery O_2 consumption is less than for a series of contractions in which the interval between individual tetanuses is larger, 200 s. One set of data illustrates this point (143). For a series of six 3-s tetanuses, spaced at 5-s intervals, the total recovery O_2 consumption is 1.31 ± 0.13 μmol/g wet wt, a value not different from the energy requirement (1.29 ± 0.14 μmol/g) of a single 20-s isometric tetanus, which developed the same tension-time integral as the sum of the series of six individual tetanuses. However, when the six 3-s tetanuses were spaced at 200-s intervals, the total energy cost was substantially larger, 1.81 ± 0.17 μmol/g wet wt. These data as well as other data for various tetanic durations and intervals between tetanuses were readily fit by an equation of the following form

$$\xi O_2 = I(1 - e^{-\alpha t}) + kl_0\int P dt \qquad (41)$$

The term $I(1 - e^{-\alpha t})$ represents a postulated time-dependent process that goes to completion during a maintained tetanus with a rate constant $\alpha = 0.7\ s^{-1}$. Note that both α and t refer to times during the contraction, whereas the actual measurement of recovery O_2 consumption occurs long afterward. The term $kl_0\int P dt/g$ is the tension-dependent energy utilization, determined previously in a single prolonged tetanus (142). There is thus an obvious similarity among these data for recovery O_2 consumption and the phenomena of labile heat and maintenance heat. Both labile heat (see *Energy Balance Studies in Rana temporaria*, p. 213) and the term $I(1 - e^{-\alpha t})$, which we might tentatively call "labile O_2 consumption," indicate the energy cost repaid during recovery from a tension-independent process that goes to completion during a maintained tetanus of several seconds duration. This labile O_2 consumption is linearly added to the steady energy cost, which is directly proportional to the isometric force and the duration of tetanus; of course, recovery O_2 consumption occurs after the tetanus. Once the process underlying the labile recovery O_2 consumption goes to completion, a period of several minutes is necessary for its repriming (143).

The magnitude of this labile O_2 consumption can be estimated in various ways (142, 143) and amounts to approximately 0.29 μmol O_2/g or 1.1 μmol ~P/g, for measurements of recovery O_2 consumption and initial chemical change, respectively. These amounts are more than sufficient to account for the labile heat that in *R. pipiens* is 26 mJ/g (109). Because the experiments just discussed were made on muscles obtained from batches of animals different from the ones used for heat measurements and because different experimental conditions were used, the quantitative comparisons just made cannot be taken as settled. They do provide sufficient evidence, however, to put forward a hypothesis that the labile heat in *R. pipiens* seems to be accounted for by the additional utilization of high-energy phosphate during recovery and thus by an extra amount of O_2 consumption. The evidence for a biochemical equivalent for a labile heat argues strongly that the mechanisms responsible for unexplained enthalpy and labile heat are different.

SUMMARY. The following points summarize the major features of the biochemical energetics of muscles from *R. pipiens*. *1*) The observed rate of PCr splitting decreases during an isometric tetanus; this fact remains true when the data are normalized to the average developed tension. *2*) The same pattern of energy utilization is obtained when the total recovery O_2

consumption is the measure of the energy cost. *3*) The observed stoichiometric constant that scales $\xi \sim P$ and $\xi\ O_2$ is clearly less than the standard value, $k = 6.3$, and thus there is a substantial amount of unexplained recovery O_2 consumption. *4*) The fraction of unexplained O_2 consumption appears to be independent of the duration of tetanus up to 20 s at 0°. *5*) Myothermic data for the unexplained enthalpy are not available over a sufficiently wide range of contraction durations to settle the question whether the myothermic energy imbalance follows qualitatively the pattern obtained from the biochemical energy imbalance or the pattern of unexplained enthalpy found in *R. temporaria*. *6*) There is sufficient labile energy-rich phosphate splitting or labile O_2 consumption to account for the labile heat in *R. pipiens*.

Amphibian Muscles

Employing muscles from *R. temporaria* at 20°C, Canfield, Lebacq, and Maréchal (19) found a large unexplained enthalpy fraction during isometric tetanuses of various durations at 20°C. The result showed the phenomenon of energy imbalance was not an artifact of studying muscles near 0°C. Is there a biochemical energy imbalance both in aerobic and anaerobic conditions? The question is important. If there were an unexplained recovery O_2 consumption in aerobic muscles but a stoichiometrically predicted amount of recovery lactate production in anaerobic muscles, the conclusion would be that the mechanism giving rise to the biochemical imbalance was related to oxidative metabolism and probably localized in the mitochondria. If, on the other hand, an energy imbalance were found under both conditions (the result predicted from the myothermic studies), then specific mechanisms residing in pathways of oxidative metabolism are excluded.

Three measurements are required. First is $\xi \sim P$ for aerobic and anaerobic muscles under similar isometric conditions. The expectation is that the energy utilization is independent of O_2 supply. The second measurement is of ξO_2 for which techniques are readily available. The measurement of ξ lactate required that the following conditions be satisfied. *1*) The muscle could actually recover anaerobically. *2*) The muscle was truly anaerobic and all recovery metabolism was glycolytic. *3*) Metabolism of 1 mol glycogen produces 2 mol lactate. *4*) The lactate produced was the only end product of metabolism and left the muscle cells, so that the initial content of metabolites before contraction was restored completely at the end of the anaerobic recovery cycle. Fortunately all of these conditions were satisfied (46). The rate of anaerobic recovery is too slow at 0°C to make experimentation practical, so it was done at 20°C. Anaerobic frog sartorius muscles are able to recover completely from contractile activity. Time course is several hours. The results clearly indicate a chemical energy imbalance aerobically and anaerobically. The data for isometric tetanic durations of 0.5–5 s are illustrated in Figure 16. The utilization of energy-rich phosphate compounds as a function of tension-time integral is not different in aerobic and anaerobic muscles as was expected. Both measures of recovery metabolism, $l \times (\xi\text{lac})$ and $k \times (\xi O_2)$ were larger than predicted from the initial energy-rich phosphate utilization. Thus for anaerobic and aerobic muscles, there is a substantial fraction of recovery metabolism not explained by initial high-energy phosphate utilization. These results confirm and extend the pattern of energy imbalance that was observed at 0°C in sartorii from *R. pipiens*. Notice that the amount of unexplained recovery metabolism increases with tetanic duration and does not show an indication of diminishing with continued tetanic stimulation. This result again suggests that the pattern of unexplained energy may be different in *R. pipiens* from that in *R. temporaria*. Finally, the results clearly exclude the possibility that any aspect of mitochondrial oxidative phosphorylation is responsible for the unexplained recovery metabolism; ATP-driven ion or substrate transport into mitochondria is not excluded, however.

Aerobic biochemical energy balance experiments were also made by Mahler (163, 164). He finds the predicted stoichiometry between $\xi \sim P$ and ξO_2 for aerobic tetanuses up to 1-s duration to be $\xi \sim P = 6.3 \times \xi O_2$. The method used for measuring ξO_2 is a good one for observing the kinetics of recovery O_2 consumption but may be inaccurate. The method is designed to indicate faithfully time-dependent changes in tissue P_{O_2}, but the time course of P_{O_2} changes must be integrated to measure ξO_2, and the integration requires knowledge of the solubility of oxygen and the

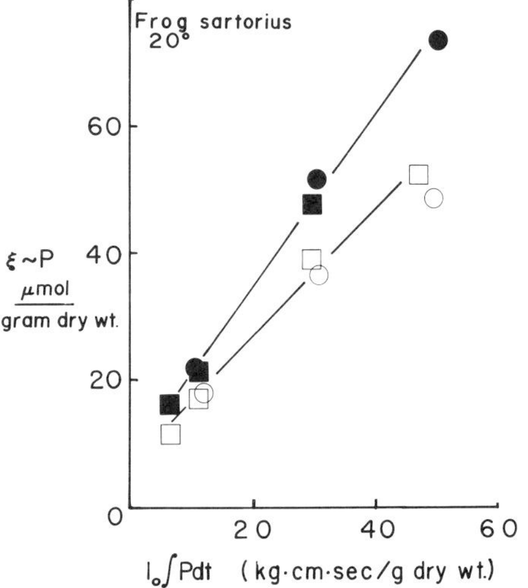

FIG. 16. Relationship between initial changes in high-energy phosphates, $\xi \sim P$ (*open symbols*) and high-energy phosphate resynthesis by recovery metabolism (*closed symbols*) as a function of tension-time integral. Contraction durations were 0.5, 1, 3, and 5 s. *Circles*, aerobic muscles; *squares*, anaerobic muscles; *filled circles*, $6.3 \times \xi_{O_2}$; *filled squares*, $1.5 \times \xi$ lactate. Aerobic and anaerobic sartorii of *Rana pipiens* at 20°C. [Data replotted from DeFuria and Kushmerick (46).]

diffusion coefficient for O_2 in muscle. Second, the magnitude of the unexplained enthalpy and of the unexplained recovery metabolism is smaller in brief tetanuses of *R. pipiens* than in similar contractions of *R. temporaria* (Fig. 13), and thus an imbalance is more difficult to detect by any method. To settle the matter completely a side-by-side comparison of both methods is needed. Energy balance issues aside, Mahler's experiments show very clearly the kinetics of recovery O_2 consumption above the base line similar to the energetic model given in BASIC ENERGETIC MODEL, p. 206. A comparison of the kinetics of O_2 consumption obtained by this technique with the fluorescent measurements of cellular NADH/NAD^+ discussed in *Oxidative Metabolism*, p. 201, has not yet been made, and it would be expected to yield valuable data on the kinetics, control, and integration of oxidative metabolism.

Mammalian Muscles

An important reason for studying energetics in mammalian muscles is that a range of metabolic and contractile properties can be studied by comparing predominantly fast-twitch muscles with slow-twitch types. The use of differing types of muscles offers the experimenter a chance to capitalize on variations of important properties achieved by nature (194). Manipulations of these parameters are very difficult to achieve experimentally and are slow to occur as the cross-innervation experiments have demonstrated. The second advantage is purely an experimental one. For the most part workers in the field appear to assume implicitly that the constituent muscle fibers in sartorius or semitendinosus muscles of amphibians are similar in metabolic and mechanical properties if not even homogeneous. This is not true for it is certainly known that there is a threefold range in twitch times in individual motor units in amphibian sartorii (158). Also important quantitative differences among the different batches of animals probably reflect uncontrolled seasonal, nutritional, and age variations. In contrast inbred strains of rodents maintained under constant conditions are available at specific age ranges.

A detailed study was made of chemical energetics of mouse extensor digitorum longus (EDL), a fast-twitch muscle, and of mouse soleus, a slow-twitch muscle (30). In vitro at 20°C in the absence of added substrate, the muscles are capable of a number of isometric tetanic contraction-recovery cycles without any diffusional lack of oxygen and without significant fatigue. Larger muscles obtained from rats are probably hypoxic and, in our pilot experiments, did not give reproducible results. The mouse muscles are as stable as amphibian muscles and show significantly lower variation in any measured parameter than is usually obtained in comparable studies of frog sartorii. Crucial features in handling the muscles are maintaining high O_2 tensions during dissection, maintaining in vivo muscle length, and stimulating near fusion frequency. High-frequency stimulation (greater than 150 Hz) uniformly led to muscle damage, easy fatiguability, and lack of reproducibility. Thus the extent of recovery metabolism, ξO_2, and ξlac were easily measured. In the more aerobic soleus, lactate production is much lower than in the EDL. The length of individual muscle fibers and their axial orientation with respect to the long axis of the muscle are known. Although both muscles are pennate, the fiber arrangement is sufficiently parallel to the whole muscle axis and the fiber length is sufficiently uniform that comparisons between muscles can be based reliably on developed tension per cross-sectional fiber area. In the absence of added substrate, the respiratory quotient is near unity, supporting the assumption that muscles utilize their endogenous glycogen stores. The data clearly showed three major points (Table 3). *1*) There was a biochemical energy balance because

$$(\xi - \text{P})_{\text{contraction}} = 6.3\ \xi O_2 \qquad (41a)$$

2) The energy cost for a maintained tetanus of soleus per unit cross-sectional area was independent of a stimulus duration. *3*) However, the energy cost of maintaining a steady isometric force per cross-sectional area in the EDL fell from a value about 2.7 times that of soleus to a final value only 1.1 times larger. Thus the commonly held view that slow-twitch fibers are very much more economical in holding isometric attention depends on experimental conditions and is only true for very brief contractions.

Perhaps the most important aspect of this work in the context of this chapter is that chemical energy balance is observed in mouse hindlimb muscle. Therefore the energetics of these muscles differs importantly from that observed in *R. temporaria* where the data clearly indicate a large imbalance at the beginning of contractile activity with the emergence of an energy

TABLE 3. *Comparison of Initial Chemical Change and Recovery Synthesis in Mammalian Muscle*

Tetanus Interval, s	Soleus		EDL	
	$(\xi \sim \text{P})_{\text{initial}}$*	$(\xi \sim \text{P})_{\text{recovery}}$†	$(\xi \sim \text{P})_{\text{initial}}$	$(\xi \sim \text{P})_{\text{recovery}}$
0–3	9.1 ± 1.8	8.9 ± 0.4	24.1 ± 3.6	22.1 ± 1.1
3–6	8.4 ± 1.4	8.6 ± 0.5	19.4 ± 2.1	19.1 ± 1.3
6–9	8.9 ± 1.9	8.7 ± 0.3	14.8 ± 3.9	14.5 ± 1.9
9–12	8.6 ± 1.0	8.6 ± 0.2	11.8 ± 3.3	10.5 ± 1.2
12–15	8.8 ± 2.5	8.8 ± 0.3	10.0 ± 1.2	11.4 ± 1.4

Values are means ± SE in $\mu\text{mol}\cdot\text{N}^{-1}\cdot\text{cm}^{-1}\cdot\text{s}^{-1}$. * $(\xi \sim \text{P})_{\text{initial}}$ are direct measurements of changes in relevant energy-rich phosphate compounds. † $(\xi \sim \text{P})_{\text{recovery}}$ are derived from direct measurements of recovery O_2 consumption and recovery lactate production by the use of the formula: $(\xi \sim \text{P})_{\text{recovery}} = 6.3\ \xi O_2 + 1.5\ \xi\text{lac}$. All values are normalized to the tension-time integral, which is about $0.2\ \text{N}\cdot\text{m}^{-1}\cdot\text{s}^{-1}\cdot\text{g}^{-1}$ for a 1-s tetanus. The reported chemical changes given are the differences over 3-s intervals during a maintained isometric tetanic contraction at optimal muscle length. [Data from Crow and Kushmerick (30).]

balance only after some 5–10 s continued activity. That pattern also differs from that obtained in *R. pipiens* where the available data indicate that the extent of imbalance is smaller than in *R. temporaria* and that the imbalance may continue to grow.

Gower and Kretzschmar (82) reported the unexplained enthalpy in rat soleus is 39 mJ/g, a large value inconsistent with the predictions from the mouse muscle data. These authors studied myothermic energy balance in anaerobic and iodoacetate-poisoned muscles at 18°C. The only tetanus duration studied was a 10-s isometric contraction, so there were no data on the time course of chemical change or of enthalpy production. Furthermore the reported $\xi \sim$ P was only 16% of the comparable data on mouse muscles obtained in this laboratory (30). It seems clear that differences of this magnitude cannot be explained by relatively small differences in temperature of the experiment; however, many other experimental conditions differed. For the present time Crow and I have an extensive biochemical energy balance study (30), which indicates complete energy balance in mouse fast- and slow-twitch muscle, whereas Gower and Kretzchmer have a myothermic energy balance study (82), which shows a large unexplained enthalpy production in a 10-s tetanus of rat soleus. A complete myothermic energy balance study is clearly feasible and would shed valuable light on the general problem of energy balance in muscle. This is especially true since mammalian muscles contain much less parvalbumin than amphibian muscles (13).

ENERGETICS OF MUSCLES THAT SHORTEN OR ARE STRETCHED

Perhaps the first question to ask is whether there is an energy imbalance in muscles that perform substantial amounts of external work. A tentative answer in the affirmative is given by the experiments of Carlson, Hardy, and Wilkie (21, 228), already referred to in RESULTS OF ENERGY BALANCE EXPERIMENTS, p. 212. Curtin et al. (33) made a study with an improved experimental design and settled this issue decisively. Muscles were arranged so that the total enthalpy production was approximately equal in two modes of contraction. In the first mode, the muscle was stimulated isometrically for approximately 1.7 s; the total enthalpy released was 71 mJ/g. A small amount of work was performed in the isometric muscles against series compliances and measured 10% of the total enthalpy change. In the other mode of contraction, the muscle was stimulated for about 1.1 s and contracted at a constant velocity thereby performing a substantial amount of external work; about one-third of the total energy released was in the form of work. The total enthalpy in this case was 79 mJ/g. A portion of these data is reproduced in Table 4. The following are the major features to be derived from the data: *1*)

TABLE 4. *Total Energy and Work Balance*

Energy Parameter	Isometric Contraction	Working Contraction
1. $h + w$, mJ/g	70.8	79.0
2. w, mJ/g	7.3	25.8
3. ξPCr, μmol/g	0.71	1.16
4. Explained enthalpy, mJ/g	24	39
5. Unexplained enthalpy	0.66	0.51
6. W_{max} available, mJ/g	38	63

Rows 1, 2, and 3 are direct measurements. Row 4 is obtained by ΔHPCr $\times$ ξPCr, where ΔHPCr = −34 kJ/mol. Row 5 is calculated from values given in rows 1 and 4. Row 5 is obtained by $\Delta G' \times \xi$PCr, where $\Delta G'$ is the value given in ref. 33 and not the larger value discussed in THERMODYNAMICS, p. 207. [From Curtin et al. (33).]

There was a substantial amount of unexplained enthalpy in both the isometric and working contractions. *2*) For approximately the same total energy released, the utilization of high-energy phosphate ($\xi \sim$ P) is greater when work is done; for an 11% greater total energy output, the working muscles hydrolyzed 63% more PCr. *3*) The maximum amount of work that could be obtained ($\Delta G' \times \xi \sim$ P) was greater then the actual work obtained, which means that the work performed was adequately explained by the measured utilization of PCr. There is no evidence to support the notion that the process giving rise to the unexplained enthalpy also provided energy for the performance of work. This last point is extremely important because it means that in addition to all the other properties of the reaction or reactions underlying the unexplained enthalpy discussed in ENERGY BALANCE, p. 210, the same process or processes do not drive actomyosin interactions in the performance of muscular work.

An earlier and more extensive experimental series studied related questions by means of measurements of chemical change during working contractions (139). These data provide additional information on the relationships between external work done, velocity of shortening, and $\xi \sim$ P. While heat measurements were not made, the data obtained by Kushmerick and Davies (139) were used to predict a significant amount of unexplained enthalpy. To avoid problems of anaerobic or glycolytic resynthesis of $\xi \sim$ P, the muscles were inhibited by incubation in FDNB and strict anaerobic conditions. Thus ATP was directly measured. The experiments were designed so that the muscles produced the maximal amount of work possible per unit distance shortened. This was achieved by prestretching the muscle to about 1.3 l_0, releasing the stimulated muscle at constant velocity, and recording the force produced during the shortening. The force record traced out a force-length curve, scaled down appropriately from the isometric curve according to the force-velocity curve. In this way it was possible to extract significantly greater amounts of external work during the contraction than is possible in isotonic contractions. The main findings are shown in Figure 17. *1*) The rate of work performance and the rate of ATP

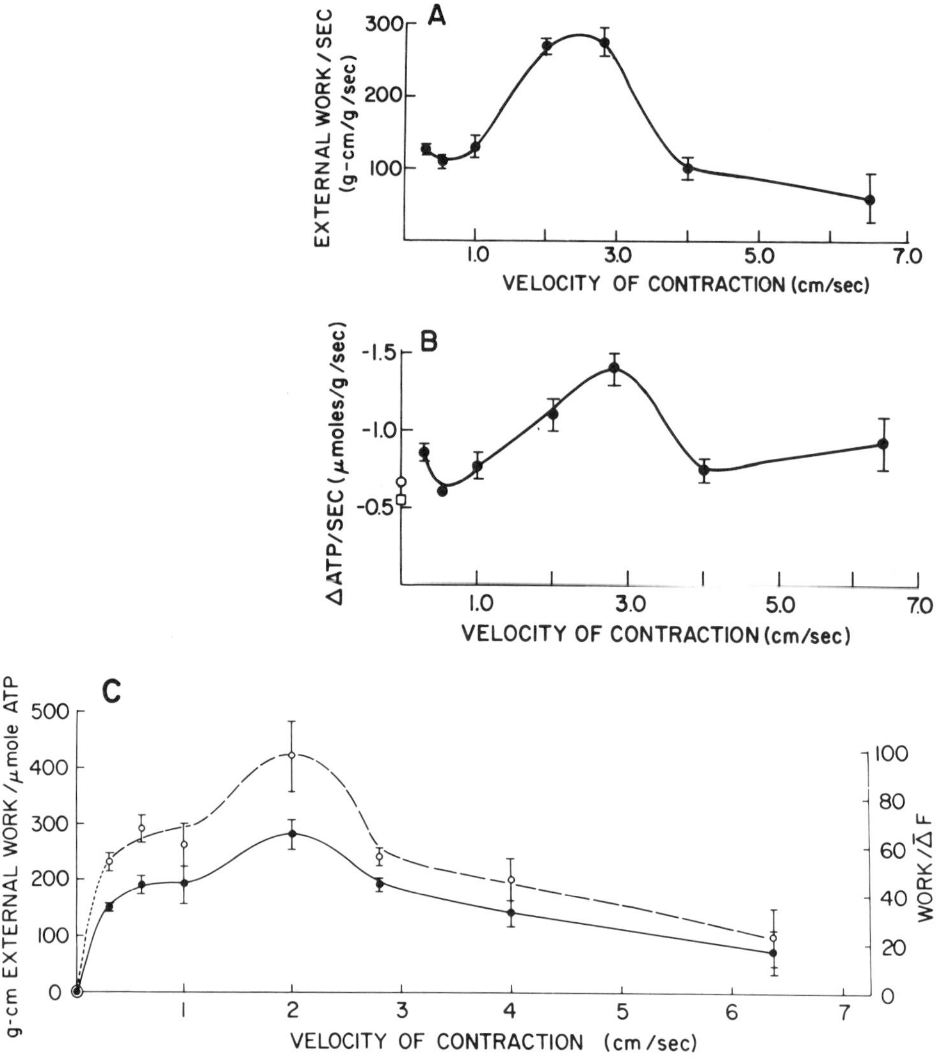

FIG. 17. Mechanical power, chemical power, and efficiency of muscular work as a function of velocity of shortening. Muscles were constrained to shorten at constant velocities. *A*: rate of mechanical work–mechanical power. *B*: rate of utilization of high-energy phosphates or chemical power input, measured directly as ATP splitting in fluorodinitrobenzene-treated muscles (creatine phosphokinase blocked). *C*: efficiency of work performance derived from the data in *A* and *B* (*solid line*). *Interrupted line* is efficiency after subtracting an estimated amount of ATP splitting thought to represent nonactomyosin energy costs. [From Kushmerick and Davies (139).]

splitting as functions of the velocity of shortening agreed quite well. *2*) When external work was done, the rate of ATP splitting was generally greater than the isometric rate, a result that is the biochemical equivalent of the Fenn effect. *3*) The chemical efficiency of work performance, a quantity given by the actual work done divided by ξATP, was a curvilinear function of the velocity of shortening. The efficiency reached a maximum of 24 kJ/mol at 0.3 V_{max} (323 g-cm work/g, and 1.32 mol/g of ATP splitting at 2 cm/s shortening velocity) or about 0.6 of the calculated thermodynamic efficiency. An effort was made to estimate the tension-independent energy cost. When this estimated amount was subtracted from the total, the efficiency values for work performance rose to nearly 100% at the velocity of maximal mechanical power. Despite the inaccuracy of the estimates, the data show that the contractile mechanism operates at very high efficiency, which is a function of velocity of shortening.

My experiments with Davies may be criticized because of their use of inhibitors that might have altered the muscle in unknown ways beyond the blocking of CPK, glycolysis, and respiration. This was directly tested; for muscles that were untreated and oxygenated, that were poisoned by iodoacetate alone, and that were treated by FDNB in anaerobic conditions, none of the following parameters were altered: total external work done, $\xi \sim$ P, or the chemical efficiency, $w/\xi \sim$ P (Table 5, ref. 139). Another criticism that arises from the results of subsequent experiments and that cannot be answered without additional experimentation is that all of the contraction durations were sufficiently brief (0.45–4.2 s) that they were made precisely at the time that in the isometric condition is associated with a nonsteady-state rate of high-energy phosphate splitting and over the interval when the rate of unexplained enthalpy production is the greatest. Steady-state conditions for the rate of ATP splitting can be achieved in amphibian muscles by prestimulating under isometric conditions for several seconds. If muscles from *R. temporaria* are used, the problem of unexplained enthalpy can be avoided entirely by tetanizing the muscle for about 8 s (Fig. 11). Then the muscles can be released to perform work; the control muscle would then be stimulated identically up to the moment of release. In mammalian muscles this practical difficulty is mitigated since there is no energy imbalance. These kinds of experiments are urgently needed because they provide the only experimental approach now possible to measure energetic parameters that set limits on or test models of muscle contraction. For example, in the model of Eisenberg, Hill, and Chen (55) and Figure 18 the calculated maximal efficiency is 0.55, and this value compares very favorably with that observed in my experiments with Davies (139). The predicted shape of the efficiency as a function of velocity of shortening (cf. Fig. 17 with Fig. 18) is roughly similar in form. However, the predicted ATPase rate in the working contraction normalized to the observed ATPase rate in the isometric contraction is considerably different. The data shown in Figure 17 provide some evidence against the fivefold decrease predicted by the model, as do the data of Infante et al. (122), who studied isotonic contractions at various loads and therefore velocities of shortening. Finally the parameter $\bar{r}$, which is the mean number of ATP molecules hydrolyzed per unit distance shortened, has never been systematically evaluated as a function of velocity of shortening. It is therefore timely that additional experiments of improved design be made to measure functionally significant energetic parameters and to provide valuable additional tests of models of muscle contraction.

When muscles are forcibly extended during contraction they develop a force greater than the isometric force. The mode of contraction of these muscles is sometimes described as negatively working contractions; that is, work is put into the muscle. The notion that the muscles developing larger forces liberate more energy and have a greater $\xi \sim P$ was proven wrong by the first set of experiments. At slow to moderate rates of stretch, the enthalpy production is reduced, and in some cases, is totally supressed (100). The rate of ATP splitting is also substantially reduced compared to the isometric rate (31, 32, 121). This mode of contraction has another interesting and unexplained feature: the enhanced tension developed by stretching an active muscle persists for some time after the stretch (50, 105). These stretch-activation effects increase with sarcomere length up to about 3 μm, whereas normal isometric force decreases over this range of sarcomere lengths. It is entirely unknown how these phenomena come about. Curtin and Woledge (39) recently suggested that a forcible stretch of an active muscle induces a long-lasting state of actomyosin different from that in muscles contracting isotonically or isometrically. Unfortunately doing experiments of this type is difficult since often a forcible stretch also causes irreversible changes in mechanical and energetic parameters. Nonetheless it should be emphasized that this mode of contraction is not an experimental curiosity because it is well known from studies of animal locomotion that active muscles are in fact stretched physiologically during ordinary limb movements.

In addition to the performance of work, muscles that shorten also produce heat at a rate greater than in isometric contractions (94), so-called shortening heat, as explained in HISTORICAL PERSPECTIVES, p. 190. Taken together Hill's work indicates that the total energy produced, E, can be written (114, 236)

$$E = A + f(l, t) + a_f x + w \tag{42}$$

where, as defined in ENERGETICS AS AN ANALYTICAL

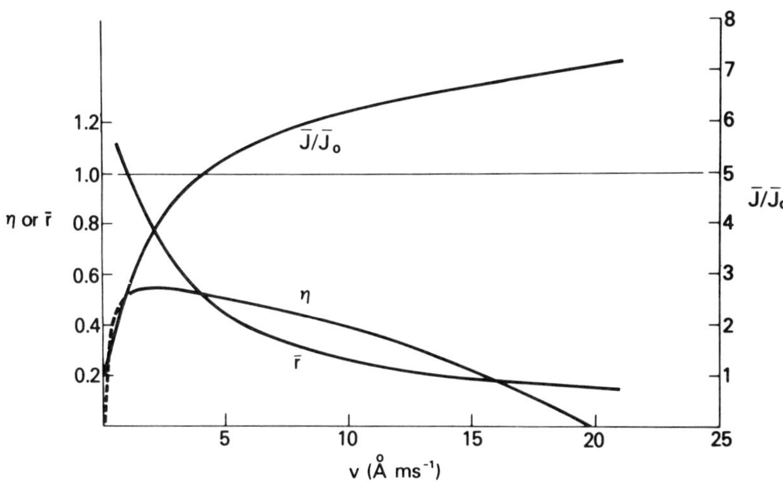

FIG. 18. Calculations based on the cross-bridge model of Eisenberg, Hill, and Chen (55). $\bar{J}/\bar{J}_o$, rate of high-energy phosphate splitting normalized to the isometric rate. η, Efficiency of chemomechanical coupling; $\bar{r}$, number of ATP molecules hydrolyzed per unit distance shortened. All parameters graphed as a function of steady-state velocity of shortening. [From Eisenberg et al. (55).]

TOOL, p. 191, A is the activation heat; f(l, t) is the maintenance heat, which is a function of muscle length, l, and duration of contraction, t; $a_f x$ is the shortening heat; and w is the mechanical work done. The question is whether these energy terms are really independent and linearly additive. Fundamentally the real question is what is the mechanism and $\xi \sim$ P associated with each term? Analyses of the energetics of shortening muscle must take into account the following. The phenomenon of unexplained enthalpy production first observed in isometric contractions is also observed in isotonic ones, although the unexplained enthalpy fraction is lower in muscles that do work (33). Second, there is little or no correlation of the extent of shortening per se with $\xi \sim$ P. That is, a biochemical equivalent of shortening heat has not been demonstrated, although there is a good correlation of $\xi \sim$ P with the amount of work done. For example, in my work with Larson and Davies (140), there was a very small energy cost ($\xi \sim$ P) in muscles shortening rapidly, although the calculated heat rate was very large. These issues remained dormant until recently.

In 1976, Rall et al. (197) reported that the unexplained enthalpy fraction was much greater (about 0.6–0.85) during a 0.5- to 0.75-s tetanus of a rapidly shortening muscle, whereas at 3 s when the muscle had relaxed, the unexplained fraction was much smaller (about 0.3). What appeared to be happening is this: during the first moments (about 0.6 s) of a contraction of a lightly loaded muscle there was considerable heat produced with relatively little chemical change, whereas thereafter there was additional PCr splitting with relatively little heat production. Therefore the working hypothesis is that rapid shortening induces a phase shift between heat production and $\xi \sim$ P. Very likely this involves important aspects of cross-bridge cycling, because the amount of shortening heat per unit distance shortened is a function of a sarcomere length. Recent work from Homsher's lab (111) has tested this hypothesis, and they interpret their new data in the light of incomplete chemical and thermodynamic cross-bridge cycles outlined in RESULTS OF ENERGY BALANCE EXPERIMENTS, p. 212. In the new experiments all muscles were stimulated isometrically at an average sarcomere length of 2.6 μm for 2 s and thereafter divided into two groups. In the first, an ordinary isometric contraction continued for one additional second. In that 1-s period, as expected from all other data, there was a significant unexplained enthalpy fraction (0.18). Muscles of the second group were allowed to shorten rapidly to 1.8 μm for 0.3 s and subsequently redeveloped tension isometrically from 2.3 to 3.0 s. As expected from the properties of shortening heat and the absence of an equivalent chemical change, there was a very large average rate of heat output and a small average rate of PCr splitting during the period of rapid shortening (2.0–2.3 s). The explained enthalpy fraction during that period was 0.58. Now the new and exciting finding is that in the postshortening period (2.3 to 3.0 s) $\xi \sim$ P was much greater than the heat production, so much so that the imbalance was in the opposite direction—too little enthalpy production for the observed $\xi \sim$ P. Thus the large amount of unexplained enthalpy produced during rapid shortening is nicely balanced by $\xi \sim$ P with little heat production during the redevelopment of the isometric state. Overall in the 1-s interval (from 2 to 3 s) for both groups there is a net energy balance. Notice the remarkable difference in the energetic pattern when a muscle redevelops the isometric state after rapid shortening (too little enthalpy for the measured $\xi \sim$ P) and in the development of the isometric state in the previously relaxed muscle (too much enthalpy produced for the measured $\xi \sim$ P). Also the occurrence of a myothermic energy balance between the second and third second of contraction of sartorii from *R. pipiens* is not consistent with the possibility that the amount of unexplained enthalpy increases during a maintained contraction (Fig. 13; see *Energy Balance Studies in Rana pipiens*, p. 219) nor with the result that the amount of unexplained recovery O_2 consumption increases in proportion to tetanus duration (Fig. 15).

These phase shifts between enthalpy production and $\xi \sim$ P can be interpreted qualitatively in terms of a cross-bridge interaction in which the relative distribution of myosin states in its kinetic cycle changes abruptly during rapid shortening: additional ATP splitting is apparently necessary immediately after rapid shortening to restore the initial isometric distribution. During the shortening period, the extent of production of creatine and of P_i matched. The P_i may or may not have been bound to the myosin since the perchloric acid extraction procedure used removes bound P_i and nucleotides from myosin. The increase in free creatine means that there was release of ADP provided the CPK reaction is sufficiently rapid to maintain near-equilibrium conditions. Because the net enthalpy production was so low during this period, either there was no ATP splitting, or as the high rate of product release shows, the ATP splitting occurred concomitant with the endothermic portion of the myosin kinetic cycle (RESULTS OF ENERGY BALANCE EXPERIMENTS, p. 212). By inference an exothermic part of the actomyosin cycle occurs predominantly during the rapid shortening phase. During the rapid shortening phase itself, which amounted to 0.4 μm per one-half sarcomere, there is a measurable $\xi \sim$ P at a rate equal to 0.48 ± 0.24 $\mu mol \cdot g^{-1} \cdot s^{-1}$ or approximately 1.6 turnovers of myosin per second. Since the force was low during rapid shortening, it was quite likely that not all the myosins interacted, and so the turnover rate per myosin is elevated by an unknown factor, perhaps 4- to 6-fold. Although the interpretation of this energetic data is limited, these are precisely the sort of quantitative data that are necessary to test current and future cross-bridge cycling models. This information is uniquely available from studies of energetics.

NEW DIRECTIONS

The readers who have persisted to this point already realize that there are plenty of painstaking experiments to be done if experimenters only use existing approaches. Indeed it is a propitious time for extensive investigations of muscle performing work. The calorimeter is being used to measure the enthalpies of calcium binding to regulatory proteins and the change in enthalpy content between myosin and actomyosin kinetic states. All of these experiments will yield important and, it is to be hoped, clarifying results. In addition there are two approaches to problems in muscle energetics that have been recently introduced and that deserve some discussion.

Phosphorus Nuclear Magnetic Resonance Spectroscopy

The phenomenon of NMR was first observed in 1946. The nuclei of certain chemical elements have quantized spin states when placed in a strong magnetic field, and these states absorb energy in the megahertz frequency range. The technique is relatively insensitive so that relatively large amounts of compounds must be present to be detectable. Furthermore different nuclei have different sensitivities; for the same magnetic field the relative sensitivity of ^{31}P is only 6.6% of that of ^{1}H. Recent advances in spectrometer design, which allow larger sample sizes, and the use of signal-averaging techniques now make it possible to detect and quantify the amounts of ^{31}P, the naturally abundant isotope, present in compounds in living cells. For example, by averaging more than 20 spectra, it is possible to detect approximately 10^{-7} mol in a volume of about 1 ml, or a concentration of 10^{-4} M. The value of ^{31}P NMR as an analytical tool is that despite its relative insensitivity, the spectra obtained are extremely sensitive to variations in the local electronic environment of the phosphorus atoms that it detects. Thus the location of ^{31}P among inorganic phosphates, sugar phosphates, PCr, and the individual phosphoryl groups of adenine nucleotides gives resonances at different frequencies. Thus the different phosphorus atoms in constitutent compounds can be distinguished and quantified. For muscle studies this is fortunate, for these are precisely the compounds of greatest interest energetically. Other compounds no less interesting or important for their regulation of metabolism—for example, cyclic AMP—are present in concentrations too low to be detectable.

Because of the relatively low sensitivity, the experimenter works to optimize conditions by increasing the sample size and using long signal-averaging periods; for example, in the study of frog sartorii (43) a number of them were suspended in oxygenated Ringer's solution, and at least several hundred spectra were averaged. Another approach, which has been taken in my lab, has involved the development of larger muscle preparations, 2–4 g, which because of their size require perfusion of oxygen- and substrate-carrying solutions through their vasculature (138). Figure 19 illustrates the analytical and temporal resolution now available. In the *upper portion*, one single spectrum of a perfused, cat biceps muscle weighing 3 g is shown. Obviously the signal-to-noise ratio can be greatly improved, as illustrated in the *lower portion* by appropriate signal averaging. Tissue content of the various phosphorus-containing compounds can be made directly proportional to the area under the peaks. Absolute calibration is possible but is not readily achieved by NMR data alone; relative concentrations by ratios of peak areas can be made quite accurately. From ratios of areas in NMR spectra and accurate measurements of one of the constituent compounds by standard chemical or enzymatic reactions, for example of ATP, PCr, or P_i, the spectral areas can be directly scaled into chemical amounts per muscle weight. The use of ^{31}P NMR for muscle studies was pioneered by Hoult et al. (117), and it has been applied to a variety of tissues and cell suspensions. Skeletal muscle, however, appears to provide the best physio-

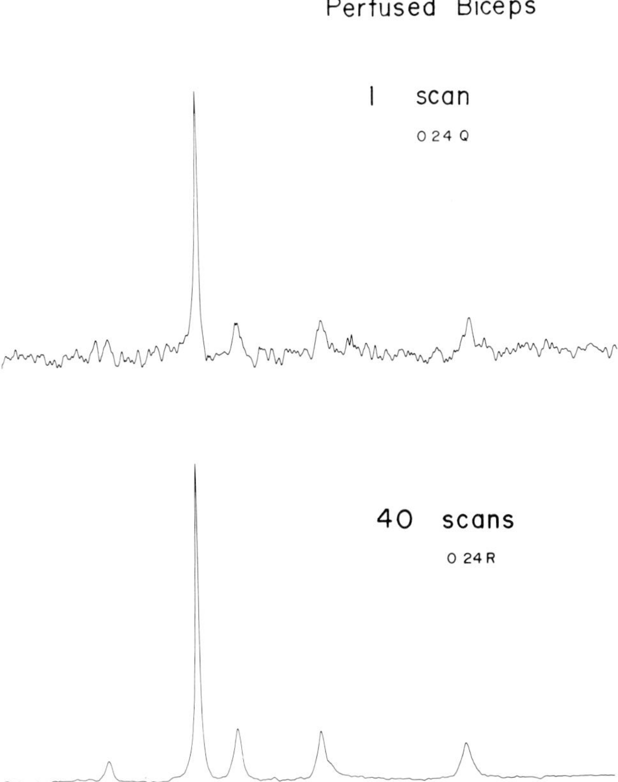

FIG. 19. ^{31}P NMR spectra of cat biceps muscle (138). Muscle was perfused in vitro through branches of capillary artery with an oxygenated synthetic commercial fluorocarbon suspension (Fluosol-43) containing papaverine at 30 μg/ml; flow was 0.2 ml/min for this 3-g muscle. *Upper curve* is spectrum obtained with a single NMR scan; *lower curve* is spectrum obtained by averaging 40 scans, each taken at 15-s intervals. Identification of the peaks from *left* to *right*: P_i; PCr; γ-, α-, and β-phosphorus of ATP. Shoulder on α-ATP is probably NAD/NADH.

logical preparations for energetic and metabolic studies because of its favorable size and shape, stability, and probably most importantly because of its range of physiological conditions into which it can easily be put, for example the resting state versus a steady-state contraction.

Intracellular pH and the extent of MgATP complex formation can be measured by ^{31}P NMR, and substantial amounts of glycerol 3-phosphorylcholine and other phosphorus-containing compounds not commonly identified or measured can be identified (17, 43, 83). Dawson et al. (43, 44) studied sartorii and gastrocnemii superfused with Ringer's solution so that the muscles were approximately in a steady state. They were able to correlate increase in PCr with decreases in P_i content during recovery from a contraction. An important quantitative finding relevant to the problem of unexplained enthalpy and possible missing reactions was that NMR methods and chemical methods give the same measurements of phosphorus-containing compounds. In their second paper (44) the potential of the method as an analytical tool for studying complex physiological phenomena such as fatigue of anaerobic muscles was demonstrated. Unfortunately the mechanism or mechanisms underlying fatigue of force and causing slowing of relaxation was not clearly identified. The use of ^{31}P NMR as a quantitative analytical tool is established.

However, there is an additional use of NMR that provides unique information: chemical exchanges between suitable metabolites can be measured by following the kinetics of magnetic energy transfer. Simply described this method puts a temporary magnetic label onto a specific phosphorus resonance. In the saturation-transfer method the magnetic label destroys the normal Boltzmann energy distribution so that there is no net magnetization between possible spin states; in the inversion-transfer technique the population of spin states is inverted so that their magnitude is algebraically the negative of the normal Boltzmann distribution. In the absence of any chemical exchange the individual nucleus relaxes to the appropriate Boltzmann distribution with characteristic time constants, which is approximately 2–4 s for the phosphorus compounds of interest. The chemical exchange rates at times faster than this may be detected by observing changes in the rate of loss of magnetization (inversion transfer) or change in steady-state magnetization (saturation transfer). Using the saturation-transfer kinetic method it is possible to show that the CPK reaction in frog muscle at 4°C is near equilibrium (77), since the unidirectional flux in the forward direction, PCr → ATP, is 1.7×10^{-3} M/s and in the reverse direction is 1.2×10^{-3} M/s. In perfused, cat biceps inversion transfer was used to measure the same exchanges (138), which were found to be approximately 5×10^{-3} M/s in both directions, data indicating that the CPK reaction is close to equilibrium in mammalian muscle as well. Thus these data provide direct evidence that CPK reaction is near equilibrium in resting muscle (see *Creatine Phosphokinase*, p. 197). The potential for kinetic NMR measurements is clearly enormous and is only now beginning to be exploited.

Use of Single Fibers

Heilbrunn and Wiercinski (90) injected small amounts of various cations into single muscle cells to observe their effects on contraction and relaxation. Natori (182) showed how to surgically remove the sarcolemma thereby exposing the interior of the cell to a bathing solution of controlled composition. The Natori preparation is commonly called a mechanically skinned segment of a muscle fiber. Alternate methods for rendering the surface membrane permeable to solutes up to the size of small globular proteins involve the use of glycerol, divalent ion chelators, and nonionic detergents, and these produce what are called chemically skinned segments of muscle fibers. Isometric studies have been made (92) that established the calcium requirements for development of steady-state isometric force. Julian (128) and others (217) used permeabilized segments to study force-velocity curves as a function of calcium concentration. Levy, Umazume, and I (150) developed methods for simultaneous measurements of steady-state ATPase rates during an isometric contraction of mechanically and chemically skinned segments. By choosing suitable solution conditions, we showed the observed ATPase was due to actomyosin interactions and so, in principle, the problem of multiple ATPases contributing to the total energy cost (see *Adenosine Triphosphatases*, p. 196) in chemical measurements of whole muscle can be avoided with these preparations. A related problem has also been studied by Applegate and Homsher (5), who showed that SR remains functional after myosin extraction in solutions of high-ionic strength. They were thus able to study calcium uptake and simultaneous SR ATPase. Their results showed that the SR can function quite normally in these preparations and that the stoichiometry of calcium transport is $2Ca^{2+}$/ATP. The major limitation for energetic experiments with fiber segments at the present time is that long time periods are required for ATPase measurements, typically several minutes. This is several powers of 10 too slow for detecting any transients in ATPase rate during rapid mechanical transitions. Improvement in the time resolution is possible by using coupled enzymatic indicator reactions (157, 216) to monitor optically the extent of ATP hydrolysis. The potential of these approaches is clear, especially since the composition of the filament-lattice space can be well controlled and varied so as to study the influence on mechanics and ATPase of activators, inhibitors, substrate-to-product ratios (i.e., free energy), ionic strength, pH, Mg^{2+}, and Ca^{2+}, to mention the most obvious ones.

REFERENCES

1. ABBOTT, B. C., AND J. V. HOWARTH. Heat studies in excitable tissues. *Physiol. Rev.* 53: 120–158, 1973.
2. ADRIAN, R. H., W. K. CHANDLER, AND A. L. HODGKIN. The kinetics of mechanical activation in frog muscle. *J. Physiol. London* 204: 207–231, 1969.
3. AICKIN, C. C., AND R. C. THOMAS. Micro-electrode measurement of the intracellular pH and buffering power of mouse soleus muscle fibres. *J. Physiol. London* 267: 791–810, 1977.
4. ALTSCHULD, R. A., AND G. P. BRIERLEY. Interaction between the creatine kinase of heat mitochondria and oxidative phosphorylation. *J. Mol. Cell. Cardiol.* 9: 875–893, 1977.
5. APPLEGATE, D. E., AND E. HOMSHER. Calcium transport and ATPase activity in intact sarcoplasmic reticulum (Abstract). *Federation Proc.* 39: 294, 1980.
6. AUBERT, X. *Le Couplage energetique de la contraction musculaire.* Brussels: Arscia, 1956.
7. AUBERT, X., AND G. MARÉCHAL. La fraction labile de la thermogenese associée au maintien de la contraction isometrique. *Arch. Int. Physiol. Biochim.* 71: 282–283, 1963.
8. BÁRÁNY, M. ATPase activity of myosin correlated with speed of muscle shortening. *J. Gen. Physiol.* 50: 197–216, 1967.
9. BESSMAN, S. P., AND A. FONYO. The possible role of the mitochondrial bound creatine kinase in regulation of mitochondrial respiration. *Biochem. Biophys. Res. Commun.* 22: 597–602, 1966.
10. BESSMAN, S. P., AND P. J. GEIGER. Transport of energy in muscle: the phosphorylcreatine shuttle. *Science* 211: 448–452, 1981.
11. BLINKS, J. R., R. RUDEL, AND S. R. TAYLOR. Calcium transients in isolated amphibian skeletal muscle fibres: detection with aequorin. *J. Physiol. London* 277: 291–323, 1978.
12. BLIX, M. Studien über Muskelwärme. *Skand. Arch. Physiol.* 12: 52–126, 1902.
13. BLUM, H. E., P. LEHKY, L. KOHLER, E. A. STEIN, AND E. H. FISCHER. Comparative properties of vertebrate parvalbumin. *J. Biol. Chem.* 252: 2834–2838, 1977.
14. BOWEN, W. J., AND T. D. KERWIN. The kinetics of myokinase. III. Studies of heat denaturation, the effects of salts and the state of equilibrium. *Arch. Biochem. Biophys.* 64: 278–284, 1956.
15. BRIGGS, F. N., J. L. POLAND, AND R. J. SOLARO. Relative capabilities of sarcoplasmic reticulum in fast and slow mammalian skeletal muscles. *J. Physiol. London* 266: 587–594, 1977.
16. BROSTROM, C. O., F. L. HUNKELER, AND E. G. KREBS. The regulation of skeletal muscle phosphorylase kinase by Ca^{++}. *J. Biol. Chem.* 246: 1961–1967, 1971.
17. BURT, C. T., T. GLONEK, AND M. BÁRÁNY. Analysis of phosphate metabolites, the intracellular pH and the state of adenosine triphosphate in intact muscle by phosphorus nuclear magnetic resonance. *J. Biol. Chem.* 251: 2584–2591, 1976.
18. CAIN, D. F., AND R. E. DAVIES. Breakdown of adenosine triphosphate during a single contraction of working muscle. *Biochem. Biophys. Res. Commun.* 8: 361–366, 1962.
19. CANFIELD, P., J. LEBACQ, AND G. MARÉCHAL. Energy balance in frog sartorius muscle during an isometric tetanus at 20°C. *J. Physiol. London* 232: 467–483, 1973.
20. CANFIELD, P., AND G. MARÉCHAL. Equilibrium of nucleotides in frog sartorius muscle during an isometric tetanus at 20°C. *J. Physiol. London* 232: 453–466, 1973.
21. CARLSON, F. D., D. J. HARDY, AND D. R. WILKIE. Total energy production and phosphocreatine hydrolysis in the isotonic twitch. *J. Gen. Physiol.* 46: 851–882, 1963.
22. CARLSON, F. D., D. HARDY, AND D. R. WILKIE. The relation between heat produced and phosphorylcreatine split during isometric contraction of frog's muscle. *J. Physiol. London* 189: 209–235, 1967.
23. CARLSON, F. D., AND A. SIGER. The mechanochemistry of muscular contraction. I. The isometric twitch. *J. Gen. Physiol.* 44: 33–60, 1960.
24. CHANCE, B. Reaction of oxygen with the respiratory chain in cells and tissues. *J. Gen. Physiol.* 49, Suppl.: 163–188, 1965.
25. CHANCE, B., AND C. R. WILLIAMS. The respiratory chain and oxidative phosphorylation. *Adv. Enzymol. Relat. Areas Mol. Biol.* 17: 65–134, 1956.
26. CHAPELL, J. B. Systems used for the transport of substrates into mitochondria. *Br. Med. Bull.* 24: 150–157, 1968.
27. COLLINS, R. C., J. B. POSNER, AND F. PLUM. Cerebral energy metabolism during electroshock seizures in mice. *Am. J. Physiol.* 218: 943–950, 1970.
28. CRANK, J. *The Mathematics of Diffusion.* London: Oxford Univ. Press, 1956.
29. CROMPTON, M., M. CAPANO, AND E. CARAFOLI. Respiration-dependent efflux of magnesium ions from heart mitochondria. *Biochem. J.* 154: 735–742, 1976.
30. CROW, M. T., AND M. J. KUSHMERICK. The relationship between initial chemical change and recovery chemical input in isolated hindlimb muscles of the mouse. *J. Gen. Physiol.* 79: 147–166, 1982.
31. CURTIN, N. A., AND R. E. DAVIES. Chemical and mechanical changes during stretching of activated frog skeletal muscle. *Cold Spring Harbor Symp. Quant. Biol.* 37: 619–626, 1973.
32. CURTIN, N. A., AND R. E. DAVIES. Very high tension with very little ATP breakdown by active skeletal muscle. *J. Mechanochem. Cell Motil.* 3: 147–154, 1975.
33. CURTIN, N. A., C. GILBERT, D. M. KRETZSCHMAR, AND D. R. WILKIE. The effect of the performance of work on total energy output and metabolism during muscular contraction. *J. Physiol. London* 238: 455–472, 1974.
34. CURTIN, N. A., AND R. C. WOLEDGE. Energetics of relaxation in frog muscle. *J. Physiol. London* 238: 437–446, 1974.
35. CURTIN, N. A., AND R. C. WOLEDGE. Energy balance in DNFB-treated and untreated frog muscle. *J. Physiol. London* 246: 737–752, 1975.
36. CURTIN, N. A., AND R. C. WOLEDGE. A comparison of the energy balance in two successive isometric tetani of frog muscle. *J. Physiol. London* 270: 455–471, 1977.
37. CURTIN, N. A., AND R. C. WOLEDGE. Energy changes and muscular contraction. *Physiol. Rev.* 58: 690–761, 1978.
38. CURTIN, N. A., AND R. C. WOLEDGE. Chemical change and energy production during contraction of frog muscle: how are their time courses related? *J. Physiol. London* 288: 353–366, 1979.
39. CURTIN, N. A., AND R. C. WOLEDGE. Chemical change, production of tension and energy following stretch of active muscle of frog. *J. Physiol. London* 297: 539–550, 1979.
40. DANFORTH, W. H., E. HELMREICH, AND C. F. CORI. The effect of contraction and of epinephrine on the phosphorylase activity of frog sartorius muscle. *Proc. Natl. Acad. Sci. USA* 48: 1191–1199, 1962.
41. DAVIES, R. E. Molecular theory of muscle contraction: calcium-dependent contractions with hydrogen bond formation plus ATP-dependent extensions of part of the myosin-actin cross-bridges. *Nature London* 199: 1068–1074, 1963.
42. DAVIES, R. E., D. CAIN, AND A. M. DELLUVA. The energy supply for muscular contraction. *Ann. NY Acad. Sci.* 81: 468–476, 1959.
43. DAWSON, M. J., D. G. GADIAN, AND D. R. WILKIE. Contraction and recovery of living muscles studied by ^{31}P nuclear magnetic resonance. *J. Physiol. London* 267: 703–735, 1977.
44. DAWSON, M. J., D. G. GADIAN, AND D. R. WILKIE. Mechanical relaxation rate and metabolism studied in fatiguing muscle by phosphorus nuclear magnetic resonance. *J. Physiol. London* 299: 465–485, 1980.
45. DAWSON, J., D. GOWER, K. M. KRETZSCHMAR, AND D. R. WILKIE. Heat production and chemical change in frog sartorius: a comparison of *R. pipiens* with *R. temporaria*. *J. Physiol. London* 254: 41P–42P, 1975.
46. DEFURIA, R. R., AND M. J. KUSHMERICK. ATP utilization associated with recovery metabolism in anaerobic frog muscle. *Am. J. Physiol.* 232 (*Cell Physiol.* 1): C30–C36, 1977.

47. DeWeer, P., and A. G. Lowe. Myokinase equilibrium. *J. Biol. Chem.* 248: 2829–2835, 1973.
48. Dixon, M., and E. C. Webb. *Enzymes.* New York: Academic, 1964, p. 274–275.
49. Ebashi, S. E., and M. Endo. Calcium ion and muscle contraction. *Prog. Biophys. Mol. Biol.* 18: 123–183, 1968.
50. Edman, K. A. P., G. Elzinga, and M. I. M. Noble. Enhancement of mechanical performance by stretch during tetanic contractions of vertebrate skeletal muscle fibres. *J. Physiol. London* 281: 139–155, 1978.
51. Eggleston, L. V., and R. Hems. Separation of adenosine phosphates by paper chromatography and the equilibrium constant of the myokinase system. *Biochem. J.* 52: 156–160, 1952.
52. Eggleton, G. P., and P. Eggleton. A method of estimating phosphagen and some other phosphorus compounds in muscle tissue. *J. Physiol. London* 68: 193, 1929–30.
53. Eggleton, P., and G. P. Eggleton. The inorganic phosphate and a labile form of organic phosphate in the gastrocnemius of the frog. *Biochem. J.* 21: 190–195, 1927.
54. Eisenberg, E., and L. E. Greene. The relation of muscle biochemistry to muscle physiology. *Annu. Rev. Physiol.* 42: 293–309, 1980.
55. Eisenberg, E., T. Hill, and Y. Chen. Cross-bridge model of muscle contraction. *Biophys. J.* 29: 195–226, 1980.
56. Endo, M. Calcium release from the sarcoplasmic reticulum. *Physiol. Rev.* 57: 71–108, 1977.
57. Engelhardt, V. A., and M. N. Lyubimova. Myosin and adenosinetriphosphatase. *Nature London* 144: 668, 1939.
58. Erecińska, M., R. L. Veech, and D. F. Wilson. Thermodynamic relationships between the oxidation-reduction reactions and the ATP synthesis in suspensions of isolated pigeon heart mitochondria. *Arch. Biochem. Biophys.* 160: 412–421, 1974.
59. Erecińska, M., D. F. Wilson, and K. Nishiki. Homeostatic regulation of cellular energy metabolism: experimental characterization in vivo and fit to a model. *Am. J. Physiol.* 234(*Cell Physiol.* 3): C82–C89, 1978.
60. Feng, T. P. The heat tension ratio in prolonged tetanic contractions. *Proc. R. Soc. London Ser. B* 108: 522–537, 1931.
61. Feng, T. P. The effect of length on the resting metabolism of muscle. *J. Physiol. London* 74: 441–454, 1932.
62. Fenn, W. O. A quantitative comparison between the energy liberated and the work performed by the isolated sartorius muscle of the frog. *J. Physiol. London* 58: 175–203, 1923.
63. Fenn, W. O. The relation between the work performed and the energy liberated in muscular contraction. *J. Physiol. London* 58: 373–395, 1924.
64. Ferenczi, M. A., E. Homsher, R. M. Simmons, and D. R. Trentham. Reaction mechanism of the magnesium ion-dependent adenosine triphosphatase of frog muscle myosin and subfragment 1. *Biochem. J.* 171: 165–175, 1978.
65. Fick, A. Einige Bemerkungen zu Englemann's Abhandlung über den Ursprung der Muskelkraft. *Pfluegers Arch. Gesamte Physiol. Menschen Tiere* 53: 606–615, 1893.
66. Fiske, C. H., and Y. SubbaRow. The nature of inorganic phosphate in voluntary muscle. *Science* 65: 401–403, 1927.
67. Fiske, C. H., and Y. SubbaRow. The isolation and function of phosphocreatine. *Science* 67: 169–170, 1928.
69. Fletcher, W. M., and F. G. Hopkins. Lactic acid in amphibian muscle. *J. Physiol. London* 35: 247–309, 1907.
70. Fletcher, W. M., and F. G. Hopkins. The respiratory process in muscle and the nature of muscular motion. *Proc. R. Soc. London Ser. B* 89: 444–467, 1917.
71. Folkow, B., and H. D. Halicka. A comparison between "red" and "white" muscle with respect to blood supply, capillary surface area and oxygen uptake during rest and exercise. *Microvasc. Res.* 1: 1–14, 1968.
72. Ford, L. E., and R. J. Podolsky. Calcium uptake and force development by skinned muscle fibres in EGTA buffered solutions. *J. Physiol. London* 223: 1–19, 1972.
73. Foster, D. O., and M. L. Frydman. Tissue distribution of cold-induced thermogenesis in conscious warm- or cold-acclimated rats re-evaluated from changes in tissue blood flow: the dominant role of brown adipose tissue in the replacement of shivering by nonshivering thermogenesis. *Can. J. Physiol. Pharmacol.* 57: 257–270, 1979.
74. Francis, S. H., B. P. Meriwether, and J. H. Park. Effects of photooxidation of Histidine-38 on the various catalytic activities of glyceraldehyde-3-phosphate dehydrogenase. *Biochemistry* 12: 346–355, 1973.
75. Frazer, A., and F. D. Carlson. Initial heat production in isometric frog muscles at 15°C. *J. Gen. Physiol.* 62: 271–285, 1973.
76. Fry, D. M., and M. F. Morales. A reexamination of the effects of creatine on muscle protein synthesis in tissue culture. *J. Cell Biol.* 84: 204–297, 1980.
77. Gadian, D. G., G. K. Radda, T. R. Brown, E. M. Chance, M. J. Dawson, and D. R. Wilkie. The activity of creatine kinase in frog skeletal muscle studied by saturation-transfer nuclear magnetic resonance. *Biochem. J.* 195: 1–14, 1981.
78. George, P., and R. J. Rutman. The "high energy phosphate bond" concept. *Prog. Biophys. Biophys. Chem.* 10: 2–53, 1960.
79. Gilbert, C., K. M. Kretzschmar, D. R. Wilkie, and R. C. Woledge. Chemical change and energy output during muscular contraction. *J. Physiol. London* 218: 163–193, 1971.
80. Godfraind-de Becker, A. Heat production and fluorescence changes of toad sartorius muscle during aerobic recovery after a short tetanus. *J. Physiol. London* 223: 719–734, 1972.
81. Gordon, A. M., A. F. Huxley, and F. J. Julian. The variation in isometric tension with sarcomere length in vertebrate muscle fibres. *J. Physiol. London* 184: 170–192, 1966.
82. Gower, D., and K. M. Kretzschmar. Heat production and chemical change during isometric contraction of rat soleus muscle. *J. Physiol. London* 258: 659–671, 1976.
83. Gupta, R. K., and R. D. Moore. ^{31}P NMR studies of intracellular free Mg^{++} in intact frog skeletal muscle. *J. Biol. Chem.* 255: 3987–3992, 1980.
84. Hansford, R. G. Control of mitochondrial substrate oxidation. *Curr. Top. in Bioenerg.* 10: 217–278, 1980.
85. Harris, E. J. The stoichiometry of sodium ion movement from frog muscle. *J. Physiol London* 193: 455–458, 1967.
86. Harris, S. I., R. S. Balaban, and L. J. Mandel. Oxygen consumption and cellular ion transport: evidence for adenosine triphosphate to O_2 ratio near 6 in intact cell. *Science* 208: 1148–1150, 1980.
87. Harting, J., and S. F. Velick. Acetyl phosphate formation catalyzed by glyceraldehyde-3-phosphate dehydrogenase. *J. Biol. Chem.* 207: 857–865, 1954.
88. Hartree, W., and A. V. Hill. The regulation of the supply of energy in muscular contraction. *J. Physiol. London* 55: 133–158, 1921.
89. Hassinen, I. C. Respiratory control in isolated perfused rat heart: role of the equilibrium relations between the mitochondrial electron carriers and the adenylate system. *Biochim. Biophys. Acta* 408: 319–330, 1975.
90. Heilbrunn, L. V., and F. J. Wiercinski. The action of various cations on muscle protoplasm. *J. Cell. Comp. Physiol.* 29: 15–32, 1947.
91. Heilmeyer, L. M. G., F. Meyer, R. H. Haschke, and E. H. Fischer. Control of phosphorylase activity in a muscle glycogen particle II. Activation by calcium. *J. Biol. Chem.* 245: 6649–6656, 1970.
92. Hellam, D. C., and R. J. Podolsky. Force measurements in skinned muscle fibres. *J. Physiol. London* 200: 807–819, 1969.
93. Hill, A. V. The absolute mechanical efficiency of the contraction of an isolated muscle. *J. Physiol. London* 46: 435–469, 1913.
94. Hill, A. V. The heat of shortening and the dynamic constants of muscle. *Proc. R. Soc. London Ser. B* 126: 136–195, 1938.
95. Hill, A. V. Adenosine triphosphate and muscular contraction. *Nature London* 163: 320, 1949.
96. Hill, A. V. The heat of activation and the heat of shortening

in a muscle twitch. *Proc. R. Soc. London Ser. B* 136: 195–211, 1949.

97. HILL, A. V. A challenge to biochemists. *Biochim. Biophys. Acta* 4: 4–11, 1950.
98. HILL, A. V. The effect of load on the heat of shortening of muscle. *Proc. R. Soc. London Ser. B* 159: 297–318, 1964.
99. HILL, A. V., AND W. HARTREE. The four phases of heat production of muscle. *J. Physiol. London* 54: 84–128, 1920.
100. HILL, A. V., AND J. V. HOWARTH. The reversal of chemical reactions in contracting muscle during an applied stretch. *Proc. R. Soc. London Ser. B* 151: 169–193, 1959.
101. HILL, A. V., AND R. C. WOLEDGE. An examination of absolute values in myothermic measurements. *J. Physiol. London* 162: 311–333, 1962.
102. HILL, D. K. The time course of the oxygen consumption of stimulated frog's muscle. *J. Physiol. London* 98: 207–227, 1940.
103. HILL, D. K. The location of creatine phosphate in frog's striated muscle. *J. Physiol. London* 164: 31, 1962.
104. HILL, D. K. The location of adenine nucleotide in the striated muscle of the toad. *J. Cell Biol.* 20: 435–458, 1964.
105. HILL, L. A-band length, striation spacing and tension change on stretch of active muscle. *J. Physiol. London* 266: 677–685, 1977.
106. HIMMS-HAGEN, J. Cellular thermogenesis. *Annu. Rev. Physiol.* 38: 315–351, 1976.
107. HINKLE, P. C., AND M. L. YU. The phosphorus/oxygen ratio of mitochondrial oxidative phosphorylation. *J. Biol. Chem.* 254: 2450–2455, 1979.
108. HOMSHER, E., M. IRVING, AND A. WALLNER. High-energy phosphate metabolism and energy liberation associated with rapid shortening in frog skeletal muscle. *J. Physiol. London* 321: 423–436, 1981.
109. HOMSHER, E., AND C. J. KEAN. Skeletal muscle energetics and metabolism. *Annu. Rev. Physiol.* 40: 93–131, 1978.
110. HOMSHER, E., C. J. KEAN, A. WALLNER, AND V. GARIBIAN-SARIAN. The time-course of energy balance in an isometric tetanus. *J. Gen. Physiol.* 73: 553–567, 1979.
111. HOMSHER, E., AND C. J. C. KEAN. Unexplained enthalpy production in isometric contractions and its relation to intracellular calcium movements. In: *The Regulation of Muscle Contraction: Excitation-Contraction Coupling.* New York: Academic, 1980, pp. 337–347.
112. HOMSHER, E., W. F. H. M. MOMMAERTS, AND N. V. RICCHIUTI. Energetics of shortening muscles in twitches and tetanic contractions. *J. Gen. Physiol.* 62: 677–692, 1973.
113. HOMSHER, E., W. F. H. M. MOMMAERTS, N. V. RICCHIUTI, AND A. WALLNER. Activation heat, activation metabolism and tension-related heat in frog semitendinosus muscles. *J. Physiol. London* 220: 601–625, 1972.
114. HOMSHER, E., AND J. A. RALL. Energetics of shortening muscles in twitches and tetani contractions. I. A reinvestigation of Hill's concept of shortening heat. *J. Gen. Physiol.* 62: 663–676, 1973.
115. HOMSHER, E., J. A. RALL, A. WALLNER, AND N. V. RICCHIUTI. Energy liberation and chemical change in frog skeletal muscle during single isometric tetanic contractions. *J. Gen. Physiol.* 65: 1–21, 1975.
116. HOPPELER, H., D. MATHIEU, R. KRAUER, H. CLOASEN, R. B. ARMSTRONG, AND E. R. WEIBEL. Distribution of mitochondria and capillaries in various muscles. *Respir. Physiol.* 44: 87–111, 1981.
117. HOULT, D. I., S. J. W. BUSBY, D. G. GADIAN, G. K. RADDA, R. E. RICHARDS, AND P. J. SEELEY. Observation of tissue metabolites using ^{31}P nuclear magnetic resonance. *Nature London* 252: 285–287, 1974.
118. HUXLEY, A. F. Muscle structure and theories of contraction. *Prog. Biophys. Biophys. Chem.* 7: 255–318, 1957.
119. HUXLEY, A. F., AND R. NIEDERGERKE. Structural changes in muscle during contraction. *Nature London* 173: 971–973, 1954.
120. HUXLEY, H., AND J. HANSON. Changes in the cross-striations of muscle during contraction and stretch and their structural interpretation. *Nature London* 173: 973–976, 1954.
121. INFANTE, A. A., D. KLAUPIKS, AND R. E. DAVIES. Adenosine triphosphate: changes in muscles doing negative work. *Science* 144: 1577–1578, 1964.
122. INFANTE, A. A., D. KLAUPIKS, AND R. E. DAVIES. Phosphorylcreatine consumption during single working contractions of isolated muscle. *Biochim. Biophys. Acta* 94: 504–515, 1965.
123. INGWALL, J. S., C. D. WEINER, M. F. MORALES, E. S. DAVIS, AND F. E. STOCKDALE. Specificity of creatine in the control of muscle protein synthesis. *J. Cell Biol.* 63: 145–151, 1974.
124. JACOBUS, W. E., AND J. S. INGWALL (editors). *Heart Creatine Kinase.* Baltimore, MD: Williams & Wilkins, 1980.
125. JACOBUS, W. E., AND A. L. LEHNINGER. Creatine kinase of rat heart mitochondria. *J. Biol. Chem.* 248: 4803–4810, 1973.
126. JÖBSIS, F. F. Spectrophotometric studies on intact muscle. I. Components of the respiratory chain. *J. Gen. Physiol.* 46: 905–928, 1963.
127. JÖBSIS, F. F., AND J. C. DUFFIELD. Oxidative and glycolytic recovery metabolism in muscle. *J. Gen. Physiol.* 50: 1009–1047, 1967.
128. JULIAN, F. J. The effect of calcium on the force-velocity relation of briefly glycerinated frog muscle fibres. *J. Physiol. London* 218: 117–145, 1971.
129. KENNEDY, B. G., AND P. DEWEER. Strophanthidin-sensitive sodium fluxes in metabolically poisoned frog skeletal muscle. *J. Gen. Physiol.* 68: 405–420, 1976.
130. KLINGENBERG, M., AND H. ROTTENBERG. Relation between the gradient of the ATP/ADP ratio and the membrane potential across the mitochondrial membrane. *Eur. J. Biochem.* 73: 125–130, 1977.
131. KODAMA, T., AND R. C. WOLEDGE. Enthalpy changes for intermediate steps of the ATP hydrolysis catalyzed by myosin subfragment-1. *J. Biol. Chem.* 254: 6382–6386, 1979.
132. KREBS, H. A., AND R. L. VEECH. Pyridine nucleotide control in Mitochondria. In: *The Energy Level and Metabolic Control in Mitochondria,* edited by S. Papa, J. M. Tager, E. Quagliariello, and E. C. Slater. Bari, Italy: Adriatica Editrice, 1969, p. 329–382.
133. KRETZSCHMAR, K. M., AND D. R. WILKIE. A new approach to freezing tissues rapidly. *J. Physiol. London* 202: 66P–67P, 1969.
134. KRETZSCHMAR, K. M., AND D. R. WILKIE. The use of the Peltier effect for simple and accurate calibration of thermoelectric devices. *Proc. R. Soc. London Ser. B* 190: 315–321, 1975.
135. KUBY, S. A., L. NODA, AND H. A. LARDY. Adenosinetriphosphate-creatine transphosphorylase. I. Isolation of the crystalline enzyme from rabbit muscle. *J. Biol. Chem.* 209: 191–201, 1954.
136. KUBY, S. A., L. NODA, AND H. A. LARDY. Adenosinetriphosphate-creatine transphosphorylase III. Kinetic studies. *J. Biol. Chem.* 210: 65–95, 1954.
137. KUSHMERICK, M. J. Energy balance in muscle contraction: a biochemical approach. *Curr. Top. Bioenerg.* 6: 1–37, 1977.
138. KUSHMERICK, M. J., T. BROWN, AND M. CROW. Rates of ATP: creatine phosphorytransferase reaction in skeletal muscle by ^{31}P nuclear resonance spectroscopy (Abstract). *Federation Proc.* 39: 1934, 1980.
139. KUSHMERICK, M. J., AND R. E. DAVIES. The chemical energetics of muscle contraction. II. The chemistry, efficiency and power of maximally working sartorius muscles. *Proc. R. Soc. London Ser. B* 1174: 315–353, 1969.
140. KUSHMERICK, M. J., R. E. LARSON, AND R. E. DAVIES. The chemical energetics of muscle contraction. I. Activation heat, heat of shortening and ATP utilization for activation-relaxation processes. *Proc. R. Soc. London Ser. B* 174: 293–313, 1969.
141. KUSHMERICK, M. J., AND R. J. PAUL. Aerobic recovery metabolism following a single isometric tetanus in frog sartorius muscle at 0°C. *J. Physiol. London* 254: 693–709, 1976.
142. KUSHMERICK, M. J., AND R. J. PAUL. Relationship between initial chemical reactions and oxidative recovery metabolism for single isometric contractions of frog sartorius at 0°C. *J. Physiol. London* 254: 711–727, 1976.

143. KUSHMERICK, M. J., AND R. J. PAUL. Chemical energetics in repeated contractions of frog sartorius muscle at 0°C. *J. Physiol. London* 267: 249–260, 1977.
144. KUSHMERICK, M. J., AND R. J. PODOLSKY. Ionic mobility in muscle cells. *Science* 166: 1297–1298, 1969.
145. LANGE, G. Über die Dephosphorylierung von Adenosinetriphosphat zu Adenosinediphosphat während der Kontraktionphase von Froschrectus-Muskel. *Biochem. Z.* 326: 172, 1955.
146. LAWRIE, R. A. The activity of the cytochrome system in muscles and its relation to myoglobin. *Biochem. J.* 55: 298–305, 1953.
147. LAWSON, J. W. R., AND R. L. VEECH. Effects of pH and free Mg^{2+} on the K_{eq} of the creatine kinase reaction and other phosphate hydrolyses and phosphate transfer reactions. *J. Biol. Chem.* 254: 6528–6537, 1979.
148. LEE, Y. P. 5′-Adenylic acid deaminase. III. Properties and kinetic studies. *J. Biol. Chem.* 227: 999–1007, 1957.
149. LEHNINGER, A. L., A. VERCESI, AND E. A. BABABUNMI. Regulation of Ca^{++} release from mitochondria by the oxidation-reduction state of pyridine nucleotides. *Proc. Natl. Acad. Sci. USA* 75: 1690–1694, 1978.
150. LEVY, R. M., Y. UMAZUME, AND M. J. KUSHMERICK. Ca^{2+} dependence of tension and ADP production in segments of chemically skinned muscle fibers. *Biochim. Biophys. Acta* 430: 352–365, 1976.
151. LIPMANN, F. Metabolic generation and utilization of phosphate band energy. *Adv. Enzymol. Relat. Areas Mol. Biol.* 1: 99–162, 1941.
152. LOHMANN, K. Über die enzymatische Aufspaltung der Kreatinephosphorsäure; zugleich ein Beitrag zum Chemismus der Muskelkontraktion. *Biochem. Z.* 271: 264–277, 1934.
153. LOWENSTEIN, J. M. Ammonia production in muscle and other tissues: the purine nucleotide cycle. *Physiol. Rev.* 52: 382–414, 1972.
154. LOWRY, O. H., AND J. V. PASSONNEAU. The relationships between substrates and enzymes of glycolysis in brain. *J. Biol. Chem.* 239: 31–42, 1964.
155. LOWRY, O. H., AND J. V. PASSONNEAU. *A Flexible System of Enzymatic Analysis.* New York: Academic, 1972.
156. LOWRY, O. H., J. V. PASSONNEAU, F. X. HASSELBERGER, AND D. W. SCHULZ. Effect of ischemia on known substrates and cofactors of the glycolytic pathway in brain. *J. Biol. Chem.* 239: 18–30, 1964.
157. LOXDALE, H. P. A method for the continuous assay of picomole quantities of ADP released from glycerol-extracted skeletal muscle fibres on MgATP activation. *J. Physiol. London* 247: 71–89, 1975.
158. LUFF, A. R., AND U. PROSKE. Properties of motor units of the frog sartorius muscle. *J. Physiol. London* 258: 673–685, 1976.
159. LUNDSGAARD, E. Untersuchungen uber Muskelkontraktion ohne Milchsaure. *Biochem. Z.* 217: 162–177, 1930.
160. LUNDSGAARD, E. The biochemistry of muscle. *Annu. Rev. Biochem.* 7: 377–398, 1938.
161. LUNDSGAARD, E. The ATP content of resting and active muscle. *Proc. R. Soc. London Ser. B* 137: 73–76, 1950.
162. MACLENNAN, D. H., AND P. C. HOLLAND. Calcium transport in sarcoplasmic reticulum. *Annu. Rev. Biophys. Bioeng.* 4: 377–404, 1975.
163. MAHLER, M. Diffusion and consumption of oxygen in the resting frog sartorius muscle. *J. Gen. Physiol.* 71: 533–557, 1978.
164. MAHLER, M. Kinetics of oxygen consumption after a single isometric tetanus of frog sartorius muscle at 20°C. *J. Gen. Physiol.* 71: 559–580, 1978.
165. MARBAN, E., T. J. RINK, R. W. TSIEN, AND R. Y. TSIEN. Free calcium in heart muscle at rest and during contraction measured with Ca^{++}-sensitive microelectrodes. *Nature London* 286: 845–850, 1980.
166. MARÉCHAL, G. *Le Metabolisme de la phosphorylcreatine et de l'adenosine triphosphate durant la contraction musculaire.* Brussels: Arscia, 1962.
167. MARSTON, S. B., AND R. T. TREGEAR. Evidence for a complex between myosin and ADP in relaxed muscle fibres. *Nature London New Biol.* 235: 23–24, 1972.
168. MARTONOSI, A., AND R. FERETOS. Sarcoplasmic reticulum. II. Correlation between adenosine triphosphatase activity and Ca^{++} uptake. *J. Biol. Chem.* 239: 659–668, 1964.
169. MCGILVERY, R. W., AND T. W. MURRAY. Calculated equilibria of phosphocreatine and adenosine phosphates during utilization of high energy phosphate by muscle. *J. Biol. Chem.* 249: 5845–5850, 1974.
170. MELA, L. Mechanism and physiological significance of calcium transport across mammalian mitochondrial membranes. In: *Current Topics in Membranes and Transport,* edited by F. Bronner and A. Kleinzeller. New York: Academic, 1977, vol. 9, p. 321–366.
171. MENDELSON, R. A., AND P. CHEUNG. Muscle crossbridges: absence of direct effect of calcium on movement away from the thick filaments. *Science* 194: 190–192, 1976.
172. MEYER, R. A., J. GILLOTEAUX, AND R. L. TERJUNG. Histochemical demonstration of differences in AMP deaminase activity in rat skeletal muscle fibers. *Experientia* 36: 676–677, 1980.
173. MEYER, R. A., AND R. L. TERJUNG. Differences in ammonia and adenylate metabolism in contracting fast and slow muscle. *Am. J. Physiol.* 237 (*Cell Physiol.* 6): C111–C118, 1979.
174. MEYER, R. A., AND R. L. TERJUNG. AMP deamination and IMP reamination in working skeletal muscle. *Am. J. Physiol.* 239 (*Cell Physiol.* 8): C32–C38, 1980.
175. MEYERHOF, O., AND W. SCHULZ. Über die Energieverhältnisse bei der enzymatischen Milchsäurebildung und der Synthese der Phosphagene. *Biochem. Z.* 281: 292–305, 1935.
176. MEYERHOF, O., W. SCHULZ, AND P. SCHUSTER. Über die enzymatische Synthese der Kreatinephosphosäure und die biologische Reaktionsform des Zuckers. *Biochem. Z.* 293: 309–337, 1937.
177. MILLIKAN, G. A. Experiments on muscle hemoglobin *in vivo*; the instantaneous measurement of muscle metabolism. *Proc. R. Soc. London Ser. B* 123: 218–241, 1939.
178. MOMMAERTS, W. F. H. M. Energetics of muscular contraction. *Physiol. Rev.* 49: 427–508, 1969.
179. MOMMAERTS, W. F. H. M., AND J. C. RUPP. Dephosphorylation of adenosinetriphosphate in muscular contraction. *Nature London* 158: 957, 1951.
180. MOMMAERTS, W. F. H. M., K. VEGH, AND E. HOMSHER. Activation of phosphorylase in frog muscle as determined by contractile activity. *J. Gen. Physiol.* 66: 657–669, 1975.
181. MUNCH-PETERSEN, A. Dephosphorylation of adenosinetriphosphate during the rising phase of a muscle twitch. *Acta Physiol. Scand.* 29: 202–219, 1953.
182. NATORI, R. The property and contraction process of isolated myofibrils. *Jikeikai Med. J.* 1: 119–126, 1954.
183. NICHOLS, D. G. The bioenergetics of brown adipose tissue mitochondria. *FEBS Lett.* 61: 103–110, 1976.
184. NICHOLS, D. G. Hamster brown adipose mitochondria. *Eur. J. Biochem.* 62: 223–228, 1976.
185. NIHEI, T., R. A. MENDELSON, AND J. BOTTS. The site of force generation in muscle contraction as deduced from fluorescence polarization studies. *Proc. Natl. Acad. Sci. USA* 71: 274–277, 1974.
186. NODA, L. Adenosine triphosphate-adenosine monophosphate transphosphorylase. III. Kinetic studies. *J. Biol. Chem.* 232: 237, 1958.
187. NODA, L., S. A. KUBY, AND H. A. LARDY. Adenosinetriphosphate-creatine transphosphorylase. II. Homogeneity and physiochemical properties. *J. Biol. Chem.* 209: 203–210, 1954.
188. NODA, L., S. A. KUBY, AND H. A. LARDY. Adenosinetriphosphate-creatine transphosphorylase. IV. Equilibrium studies. *J. Biol. Chem.* 210: 83–95, 1954.
189. OWEN, C. S., AND D. F. WILSON. Control of respiration by mitochondrial phosphorylation state. *Arch. Biochem. Biophys.* 161: 581–591, 1974.

190. PAGE, E. Quantitative ultrastructural analysis in cardiac membrane physiology. *Am. J. Physiol.* 235 (*Cell Physiol.* 4): C147-C158, 1978.
191. PARNAS, J. K., AND W. MOZOLOWSKI. Über die Ammoniakgehalt und die Ammoniakbildung in Muskel und deren Zusammenhang mit Funktion und Zustandsanderung. *Biochem. Z.* 184: 399-441, 1927.
192. PAUL, R. J., AND M. J. KUSHMERICK. Apparent P/O ratio and chemical energy balance in frog sartorius muscle in vitro. *Biochim. Biophys. Acta* 347: 483-490, 1974.
193. PEACHEY, L. D. The sarcoplasmic reticulum and transverse tubules of the frog's sartorius. *J. Cell Biol.* 25: 209-231, 1965.
194. PETER, J. B., R. J. BARNARD, V. R. EDGERTON, C. A. GILLESPIE, AND K. E. STENGEL. Metabolic profiles of three fiber types of skeletal muscle in guinea pigs and rabbits. *Biochemistry* 11: 2627-2633, 1972.
195. PFAFF, E., AND M. KLINGENBERG. Adenosine nucleotide translocation of mitochondria. *Eur. J. Biochem.* 6: 66-70, 1968.
196. RALL, J. A. Effects of temperature on tension, tension-dependent heat, and activation heat in twitches of frog skeletal muscle. *J. Physiol. London* 291: 265-275, 1979.
197. RALL, J. A., E. HOMSHER, A. WALLNER, AND W. F. H. M. MOMMAERTS. A temporal dissociation of energy liberation and high energy phosphate splitting during shortening in frog skeletal muscles. *J. Gen Physiol.* 68: 13-27, 1976.
198. ROBERTSON, S. P., J. D. JOHNSON, AND J. D. POTTER. The time course of Ca^{++} exchange with calmodulin, troponin, parvalbumin and myosin in response to transient increases in Ca^{++}. *Biophys. J.* 34: 559-569, 1981.
199. ROMANUL, F. C. A. Capillary supply and metabolism of muscle fibers. *Arch. Neurol.* 12: 497-509, 1965.
200. ROOS, A. Intracellular pH and buffering power of rat muscle. *Am. J. Physiol.* 221: 182-188, 1971.
201. ROOS, A. Intracellular pH and distribution of weak acids across cell membranes. A study of D- and L-lactate and of DMO in rat diaphragm. *J. Physiol. London* 249: 1-25, 1975.
202. ROSE, I. A. The state of magnesium in cells as estimated from the adenylate kinase equilibrium. *Proc. Natl. Acad. Sci. USA.* 61: 1079-1086, 1968.
203. SAKS, V. A., G. B. CHERNOUSOVA, R. VETTER, V. N. SMIRNOV, AND E. I. CHAZOV. Kinetic properties and the functional role of particulate mm-isoenzyme of creatine phosphokinase bound to heart muscle myofibrils. *FEBS Lett.* 62: 293-296, 1976.
204. SANDBERG, J. A., AND F. D. CARLSON. The length dependence of phosphorylcreatine hydrolysis during an isometric tetanus. *Biochem. Z.* 345: 212-231, 1966.
205. SARIS, N.-E., AND K. E. D. AKERMAN. Uptake and release of bivalent cations in mitochondria. *Curr. Top. in Bioenerg.* 10: 103-179, 1980.
206. SCHOLTE, H. R. On the triple localization of creatine kinase in heart and skeletal muscle cells of the rat: evidence for the existence of myofibrillar and mitochondrial isoenzymes. *Biochim. Biophys. Acta* 305: 413-427, 1973.
207. SCOPES, R. K. Studies with a reconstituted muscle glycolytic system. The rate and extent of creatine phosphorylation by anaerobic glycolysis. *Biochem. J.* 134: 197-208, 1973.
208. SCOPES, R. K. Studies with a reconstituted glycolytic system. The anaerobic glycolytic response to simulated tetani contraction. *Biochem. J.* 138: 119-123, 1974.
209. SKOOG, C., U. KROMER, R. W. MITCHELL, J. HOOGSTRATEN, AND N. L. STEPHENS. Characterization of frog muscle mitochondria. *Am. J. Physiol.* 234 (*Cell Physiol.* 3): C1-C6, 1978.
210. SMITH, I. C. H. Energetics of activation frog and toad muscle. *J. Physiol. London* 220: 583-599, 1972.
211. SOLANDT, D. Y. The effect of potassium on the excitability and resting metabolism of frog's muscle. *J. Physiol. London* 86: 162-170, 1936.
212. SOMLYO, A. V., H. GONZALEZ-SERRATOS, H. SHUMAN, G. MCCLELLAN, AND A. P. SOMLYO. Calcium release and ionic changes in the sarcoplasmic reticulum of tetanized muscle: an electron probe study. *J. Cell Biol.* 90: 577-594, 1981.
213. SRÉTER, F. A. Temperature, pH and seasonal dependence of Ca-uptake and ATPase activity of white and red muscle microsomes. *Arch. Biochem. Biophys.* 134: 25-33, 1969.
214. STEINBERG, I. Z., A. OPTALKA, AND A. KATCHALSKY. Mechanochemical engines. *Nature London* 210: 568-571, 1966.
215. SUGDEN, P. H., AND E. A. NEWSHOLME. The effects of ammonium, inorganic phosphate and potassium ions on the activity of phosphofructokinase from muscle and nervous tissue of vertebrates and invertebrates. *Biochem. J.* 150: 113-122, 1975.
216. TAKASHI, R., AND S. PUTNAM. A fluorimetric method for continuously assaying ATPase: application to small specimens of glycerol-extracted muscle fibers. *Anal. Biochem.* 92: 375-382, 1979.
217. THAMES, M. D., L. E. TEICHHOLZ, AND R. J. PODOLSKY. Ionic strength and the contraction kinetics of skinned muscle fibers. *J. Gen. Physiol.* 63: 509-530, 1974.
218. THAYER, W. S., AND P. C. HINKLE. Stoichiometry of adenosine triphosphate-driven proton translocation in bovine heart submitochondrial particles. *J. Biol. Chem.* 248: 5395-5402, 1973.
219. THOMAS, R. C. Electrogenic sodium pump in nerve and muscle cells. *Physiol. Rev.* 52: 563-594, 1972.
220. VEECH, R. L., J. W. R. LAWSON, N. W. CORNELL, AND H. A. KREBS. Cytosolic phosphorylation potential. *J. Biol. Chem.* 254: 6538-6547, 1979.
221. VENOSA, R. A. Inward movement of sodium ions in resting and stimulated frog's sartorius muscle. *J. Physiol. London* 241: 155-173, 1974.
222. VIAL, C., C. GODINOT, AND D. GAUTHERON. Creatine kinase (E.C.2.7.3.2.) in pig heart mitochondria. Properties and role in phosphate potential regulation. *Biochimie* 54: 843-852, 1972.
223. VINCENT, A., AND J. MCD. BLAIR. The coupling of the adenylate kinase and creatine kinase equilibria. Calculation of substrate and feedback signal levels in muscle. *FEBS Lett.* 7: 239-244, 1970.
224. WAJZER, J., R. WEBER, J. LERIQUE, AND J. NEKHOROCHIFF. Reversible degradation of adenosine triphosphate to inosine acid during a single muscle twitch. *Nature London* 178: 1287-1288, 1956.
225. WEBER, A. Regulatory mechanisms of the calcium transport system of fragmented rabbit sarcoplasmic reticulum. I. The effect of accumulated calcium on transport and adenosine triphosphate hydrolysis. *J. Gen. Physiol.* 57: 50-63, 1971.
226. WIKSTRÖM, M., AND K. KRAB. Respiration-linked H^+ translocation in mitochondria: stoichiometry and mechanism. *Curr. Top. Bioenerg.* 10: 51-101, 1980.
227. WILKIE, D. R. Thermodynamics and the interpretation of biological heat measurements. *Prog. Biophys. Biophys. Chem.* 10: 260-298, 1960.
228. WILKIE, D. R. Heat work and phosphorylcreatine breakdown in muscle. *J. Physiol. London* 195: 157-183, 1968.
229. WILSON, D. F., M. ERECIŃSKA, C. DROWN, AND I. A. SILVER. Effect of oxygen tension on cellular energetics. *Am. J. Physiol.* 233 (*Cell Physiol.* 2): C135-C140, 1977.
230. WILSON, D. F., M. STUBBS, N. OHSINO, AND M. ERECIŃSKA. Thermodynamic relationships between the mitochondrial oxidation-reduction reactions and cellular ATP levels in ascites tumor cells and perfused rat liver. *Biochemistry* 13: 5305-5311, 1974.
231. WILSON, D. F., M. STUBBS, R. L. VEECH, M. ERECIŃSKA, AND H. A. KREBS. Equilibrium relations between the oxidation-reduction reactions and the ATP triphosphate synthesis in suspensions of isolated liver cells. *Biochem. J.* 140: 57-64, 1974.
232. WINEGRAD, S. The intracellular site of calcium activation of contraction in frog skeletal muscle. *J. Gen. Physiol.* 55: 77-88, 1970.
233. WITTENBERG, J. B. Myoglobin-facilitated oxygen diffusion: role of myoglobin in oxygen entry into muscle. *Physiol. Rev.* 50: 559-636, 1970.
234. WOLEDGE, R. C. The thermoelastic effect of change of tension in active muscle. *J. Physiol. London* 155: 187-208, 1961.

235. WOLEDGE, R. C. The energetics of tortoise muscle. *J. Physiol. London* 197: 685–707, 1968.
236. WOLEDGE, R. C. Heat production and chemical change in muscle. In: *Progress in Biophysics and Molecular Biology*, edited by J.A.V. Butler and D. Noble. New York: Pergamon, 1971, vol. 22, p. 37–72.
237. WOLEDGE, R. C. *In vitro* calorimetric studies relating to the interpretation of muscle heat experiments. *Cold Spring Harbor Symp. Quant. Biol.* 37: 629–634, 1972.
238. WOLLENBERGER, E., G. KRAUSE, AND B. E. WAHLER. Orthophosphat und Phosphokreatingeholt des Herzmuskels. *Naturwissenschaften* 45: 294, 1958.
239. YAGI, N., AND I. MATSUBARA. Myosin heads do not move on activation in highly stretched vertebrate striated muscle. *Science* 207: 307–308, 1980.

CHAPTER 8

Chemical mechanism of myosin-catalyzed ATP hydrolysis

MARTIN R. WEBB
DAVID R. TRENTHAM
Department of Biochemistry and Biophysics, University of Pennsylvania School of Medicine, Philadelphia, Pennsylvania

CHAPTER CONTENTS

THIS CHAPTER DESCRIBES our present knowledge of the protein myosin adenosine triphosphatase (ATPase) and its catalytic function in the hydrolysis of adenosine triphosphate (ATP). What is of interest in this essentially chemical description to a physiologist? First, ATP hydrolysis is an intrinsic component of muscle contraction. Understanding ATP hydrolysis at the molecular level is therefore necessary for an overall understanding of contraction. Second, the energetics and kinetics of the chemical step involving ATP hydrolysis are integral components of the energetics and kinetics of muscle contraction. Third, there must be underlying structural constraints on the protein molecules accompanying ATP hydrolysis to ensure the vectorial motion inherent in muscle contraction. These constraints must be defined before the structural basis of energy transduction in muscle can be understood.

An overview of the energetics of muscle contraction is given in the chapter by Kushmerick in this *Handbook*, and so a brief summary suffices here. Hydrolysis of ATP provides the energy that is manifested in the mechanical work done by the muscle. The rate of ATP hydrolysis depends on the demands of the muscle: whether it is in a relaxed state or whether, when activated, it is shortening or isometric. During ATP hydrolysis, the concentrations of ATP and adenosine diphosphate (ADP) are fairly constant under most circumstances. This is because the reaction in Equation 1, catalyzed by creatine kinase, enables ATP to be replenished utilizing the large pool of phosphocreatine (26)

$$\text{phosphocreatine} + \text{ADP} \rightleftharpoons \text{creatine} + \text{ATP} \quad (1)$$

This means that the free energy (ΔG) of ATP hydrolysis in muscle is approximately constant because ΔG depends directly on the concentration ratio of ATP and ADP

$$\Delta G = \Delta G^0 + RT\ln[\text{ADP}][\text{P}_i]/[\text{ATP}] \quad (2)$$

where RT is the product of the gas constant and the absolute temperature. Curtin et al. (25) calculated that $\Delta G = -54$ kJ/mol in frog muscle at pH 6.9 and 0°C. Larger negative values of ΔG have been calculated based on more recent measurements of ATP, ADP, and P_i concentrations (see the chapter by Kushmerick in this *Handbook*).

Biochemical analysis of muscle contraction began with the discovery by Szent-Gyorgyi (107) that actin and myosin, the essential contractile proteins, can be dissociated by ATP. Hydrolysis of ATP in resting muscle has magnesium-dependent myosin ATPase activity as a counterpart in vitro. In contracting muscle, however, ATP hydrolysis is related to a magnesium-dependent actomyosin ATPase activity. Comparison of ATP hydrolysis rates in frog muscle with those of isolated proteins supports this hypothesis (38).

Proposal and general acceptance of the sliding-filament hypothesis (51–53) have led to the great challenge of correlating cross-bridge movement with the biochemistry of actomyosin ATPase. Numerous reviews and articles have been written and the following are representative references: 1, 35, 36, 48–50, 54, 60, 74, 103, 109, 128, 129. However, a complete description of the steps relating systems in vivo and in vitro does not exist and there is no general acceptance that any one of the proposed schemes is completely correct. The Lymn-Taylor scheme (76) shown in Figure 1 is reasonably simple and clear, incorporating several key features that are almost certainly correct.

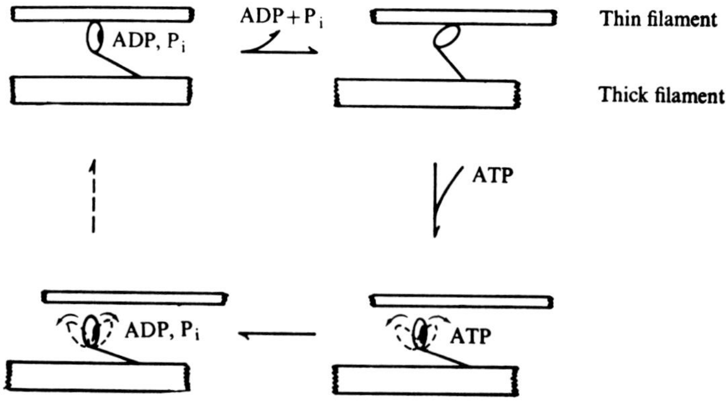

FIG. 1. Biochemical events of actomyosin ATPase linked to cross-bridge cycle. Scheme based on Lymn-Taylor model (76).

Myosin catalyzes ATP hydrolysis by a mechanism that involves several intermediates (115)

$$\begin{aligned} &M + ATP \rightleftharpoons M\cdot ATP \rightleftharpoons M^{*}\cdot ATP \rightleftharpoons M^{**}\cdot ADP\cdot P_i \\ &\rightleftharpoons M^{*}\cdot ADP\cdot P_i \rightleftharpoons M^{*}\cdot ADP + P_i \rightleftharpoons M + ADP + P_i \end{aligned} \tag{3}$$

Myosin or its active fragments, prepared by mild proteolysis (72), are represented by M. Asterisks designate different states of the protein-nucleotide complexes. Like the actomyosin mechanism, this scheme is undergoing continual refinement, but the simplified mechanism in Figure 2 suffices for our purposes. The intermediates $M^{*}\cdot ATP$ and $M^{**}\cdot ADP\cdot P_i$ in Figure 2 are shown with their Lymn-Taylor counterparts to highlight a key postulate of the Lymn-Taylor scheme—that the hydrolysis step is common to both myosin and actomyosin ATPases. However, it is likely that under appropriate conditions ATP hydrolysis also can occur when ATP is bound to an associated actomyosin complex (54, 83, 104, 105). In addition the pictorial representations of $M^{*}\cdot ATP$ and $M^{**}\cdot ADP\cdot P_i$ emphasize the multiplicity of conformations of the myosin heads: the attachment of $M^{**}\cdot ADP\cdot P_i$ to actin is at a different orientation from that preferred in the nucleotide-free complex. It should be recognized, however, that our knowledge about such orientations is at a very rudimentary stage.

Most of the kinetic studies that led to present hypotheses of the myosin ATPase mechanism were done with proteolytic myosin fragments that are soluble at physiological ionic strength. These fragments have practical advantages, especially in spectroscopic studies (61). The protein component subfragment 1 [M_r 115,000 (72)] is a single head of the myosin molecule containing both the ATPase catalytic site and the site on myosin that interacts with actin. Heavy meromyosin, on the other hand, contains both heads of the myosin molecule. Myosin ATPase activity appears to be relatively unaffected by proteolysis, but various kinetic parameters of actomyosin ATPase differ widely from those of the actin-activated ATPase of the proteolytic fragments, probably because of structural constraints imposed by the myosin filament (84, 112). Kinetic differences between actin–subfragment 1 ATPase and that of actin–heavy meromyosin are relatively small (109).

Rate constants and equilibrium constants for all steps shown in Figure 2 are listed in Table 1. In KINETICS OF ATP BINDING AND HYDROLYSIS, p. 238, we elaborate the principles behind the methods for determining these rate constants, which have generally been measured at an ionic strength of 0.15 M at pH 8 and 21°C. This choice of conditions probably has historical origins, since many steady-state kinetic measurements of ATPase activity utilize proton release—1.0 mol for each mole of ATP hydrolyzed at pH 8. Unfortunately there is no complete set of data from experiments at physiological pH, and some processes (such as the transformation of $M^{*}\cdot ATP$ to $M^{**}\cdot ADP\cdot P_i$), are most readily monitored at low ionic strength (16). The kinetics of most processes have significant dependence on pH, ionic strength, and temperature (54, 61, 108).

Step 3, the process that involves P_i release and is controlled by k_{+3}, determines the overall rate of the myosin ATPase reaction (see Table 1). This step is accelerated by actin and the acceleration leads to actin activation of the ATPase. Reversibility of ATP hydrolysis when the nucleotide is bound to myosin is remarkably different compared to that of hydrolysis in aqueous solution. The large difference in affinity to myosin between ATP and ADP reflects this (Table 2).

KINETICS OF ATP BINDING AND HYDROLYSIS

An important feature of myosin ATPase is that the cleavage step is much more rapid than overall ATP turnover. The most direct evidence for this comes from experiments in which radioactive ATP is mixed

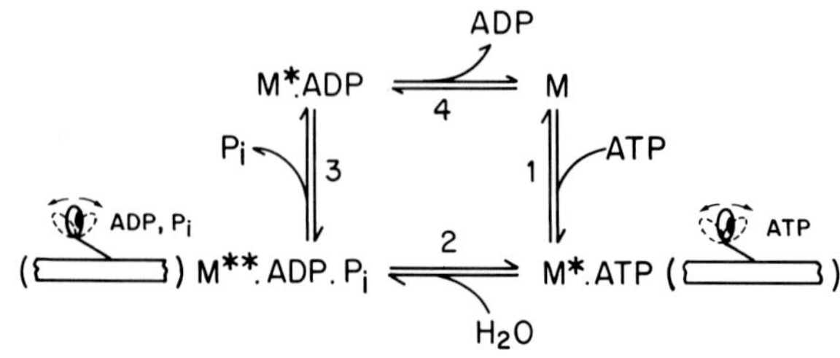

FIG. 2. Simplified mechanism of myosin ATPase. Numbers refer to sequential steps.

TABLE 1. *Rate Constants and Equilibrium Constants for Myosin ATPase Mechanism*

Step i	k_{+i}	k_{-i}*	K_i†
1	$1.8 \times 10^6\ M^{-1} \cdot s^{-1}$	$10^{-4}\ s^{-1}$	$3.4 \times 10^{11}\ M^{-1}$‡
2	$160\ s^{-1}$	$18\ s^{-1}$	9
3	$0.06\ s^{-1}$	$0.23\ M^{-1} \cdot s^{-1}$	0.26 M
4	$1.4\ s^{-1}$	$1.5 \times 10^6\ M^{-1} \cdot s^{-1}$	9.4×10^{-7} M

k_{+i}, k_{-i}, and K_i are forward and reverse rate constants and the equilibrium constant of the *i*th step in the myosin ATPase mechanism formulated in Fig. 2. Data with both heavy meromyosin and subfragment 1 were obtained at 21°C and pH 8.0 (except k_{-1} at pH 7.0). * Rate constants except for k_{-1} (13) and k_{-3} (122) are from Trentham et al. (115). Trentham et al. set the values for k_{+2} and k_{-2} as lower limits, but it now seems likely that they are close to actual values as given by Johnson and Taylor (61). † K_2, K_3, and K_4 are calculated from the rate constants; $K_1 = K/K_2K_3K_4$ where K, the overall equilibrium constant, is 7.5×10^5 M. ‡ k_{+1}/k_{-1} differs from K_1 by a factor of 19 (reasons for this discrepancy are discussed in ref. 13).

with myosin and the reaction is then terminated by quenching with acid at various times. A significant amount of P_i forms much more quickly than the steady-state rate of P_i production, and the amount of P_i formed in this pre-steady-state phase is such that 1 mol of nucleotide must have been bound per mole of subfragment 1 at the active site. Although this result comes from a number of laboratories, it was established most rigorously by Taylor and Weeds (110), who separated subfragment 1 from rabbit skeletal muscle into two active fractions differing in their alkali light-chain components. Their data are shown in Figure 3.

Inoue et al. (54) claim that an equal concentration of myosin heads exists that does not show this pre-steady-state P_i formation. It is difficult to reconcile this interpretation with results from other laboratories, however (17, 108, 110). Lymn and Taylor (75) and Taylor (108) have shown that significantly more than 50% of the heads in both myosin and heavy meromyosin bind nucleotide in the pre-steady-state phase. On structural grounds one would expect to see different amino acid sequences in each of the two heads of a myosin molecule if the important functional difference proposed by Inoue et al. (54) exists. Sequence heterogeneity arising from the two principal genotypes in fast-twitch rabbit skeletal muscle cannot, however, be the structural basis for the results of Inoue et al. This is because each of Taylor and Weeds' two subfragment-1 preparations (see Fig. 3) contained both heavy-chain isozymes; thus H_1A_1, H_1A_2, H_2A_1, and H_2A_2 are all active. (H represents the heavy chain, A represents the alkali light chain, and the subscripts distinguish the two isozymes.) Now that the amino acid sequences of all the myosin chains are being determined (63), whether or not the two myosin heads are mechanistically distinct in their catalysis of ATP hydrolysis should soon be known unambiguously.

TABLE 2. *Equilibrium Constants for Myosin ATPase Mechanism Showing Relative Affinity of ATP and ADP for Myosin*

	Equilibrium Expression	Equilibrium Constant
K_1	$\frac{[M^* \cdot ATP]}{[M][ATP]}$	$3.4 \times 10^{11}\ M^{-1}$
$1/K_4$	$\frac{[M^* \cdot ADP]}{[M][ADP]}$	$1.06 \times 10^6\ M^{-1}$
K_2	$\frac{[M^{**} \cdot ADP \cdot P_i]}{[M^* \cdot ATP]}$	9
K_2K_3	$\frac{[M^* \cdot ADP][P_i]}{[M^* \cdot ATP]}$	2.34 M
K	$\frac{[ADP][P_i]}{[ATP]}$	7.5×10^5 M

Values obtained with both heavy meromyosin and myosin subfragment 1 at 21°C and pH 8.0. They were calculated from rate constants provided by various investigations [(13, 115, 122); see Table 1].

The predominant intermediates of myosin ATPase, $M^* \cdot ATP$ and $M^{**} \cdot ADP \cdot P_i$, interconvert rapidly. Figure 4 shows the time course of $M^* \cdot ATP$ and $M^{**} \cdot ADP \cdot P_i$ formation when radioactive ATP was mixed with excess subfragment 1 and the reaction was terminated with acid at different times. Formation of P_i or ADP was measured to give the rate of $M^{**} \cdot ADP \cdot P_i$ formation, and total amount of bound nucleotide was measured by making use of the fact that once ATP is bound to the protein, it does not dissociate as ATP but is committed to be hydrolyzed. Thus radioactive ATP was mixed with the protein as before, and then a large pool of unlabeled ATP was added at various times. All the radioactive ATP bound to the protein was hydrolyzed, but the radioactive ATP present in the medium was prevented from being hydrolyzed because of the effective competition of the unlabeled ATP pool for the ATPase active site. This allowed measurement of the combined concentration of $M^* \cdot ATP$ plus $M^{**} \cdot ADP \cdot P_i$, and since the concentration of $M^{**} \cdot ADP \cdot P_i$ was already known, that of $M^* \cdot ATP$ could be calculated. Because the total nucleotide concentration was constant, the concentration of free ATP could also be calculated. Figure 4 displays these data.

Some rate and equilibrium constants in Figure 2 can be evaluated from this type of experiment as well. At concentrations of ATP and subfragment 1 less than 50 μM, the kinetics of ATP binding are first order in each component and therefore k_{+1} can be calculated. The value K_2 represents the ratio of the concentration of $M^{**} \cdot ADP \cdot P_i$ to that of $M^* \cdot ATP$ after a reaction time of 200 ms. Figure 4 describes how k_{+2} and hence k_{-2} are calculated by using a kinetic simulation procedure. Many variations on this experiment have enabled rate constants to be measured over a wide range of condi-

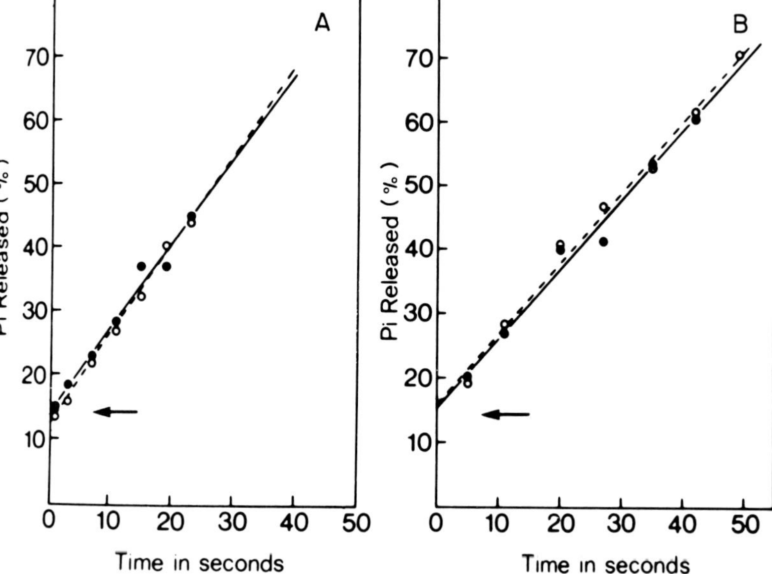

FIG. 3. Production of P_i from Mg^{2+}-ATP catalyzed by myosin subfragment 1 at pH 8.0 and 25°C. *A* and *B* result from use of different quenching techniques (110). Initial concentration of subfragment 1 was 4.8 μM and that of [γ-^{32}P]ATP was 28.4 μM. Measured mean equilibrium constant K_2 was 4.26. *Arrows*, theoretical P_i (13.7%) formed in pre-steady-state phase if 1 mol of nucleotide binds per mole of subfragment 1. Subfragment 1 contained either the alkali 1 light chains (*filled circles*) or alkali 2 light chains (*open circles*). [From Taylor and Weeds (110).]

tions (7, 16, 61, 108). The release of P_i from the protein is controlled by a process with rate constant k_{+3}, and ADP release occurs subsequent to P_i release (114). Since k_{+3} is only 0.06 s^{-1}, all P_i at 200 ms (in the experiment of Fig. 4) is present as M**·ADP·P_i; therefore the amount of M**·ADP·P_i can be determined for calculation of K_2. The reviews mentioned above give considerably more detail about the kinetics of nucleotide binding and about the subdivision of the process into discrete steps (see Eq. 3), but for our purposes it is unnecessary to introduce these complexities.

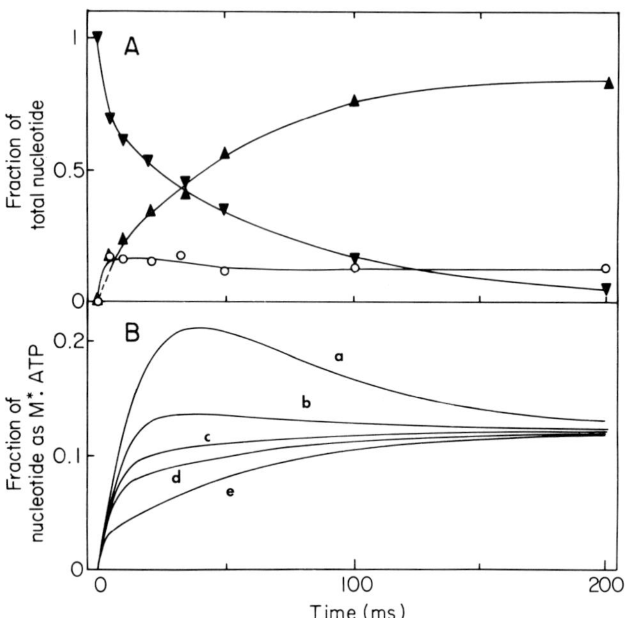

FIG. 4. Time course of M*·ATP and M**·ADP·P_i formation in a single turnover of subfragment 1 ATPase. *A*: 19 μM subfragment 1 mixed with 5 μM [γ-^{32}P]ATP in a solution of 50 mM KCl, 5 mM $MgCl_2$, and 50 mM Tris [tris(hydroxymethyl)aminomethane] adjusted to pH 8.0 with HCl at 20°C. *Inverted filled triangles*, fraction of nucleotide present as free ATP; *open circles*, M*·ATP; *upright filled triangles*, M**·ADP·P_i. *B*: computer simulation of fraction of nucleotide present as M*·ATP for various values of K_b in the scheme $X \xrightarrow{k_{+a}} Y \underset{k_{-b}}{\overset{k_{+b}}{\rightleftharpoons}} Z$, where X = ATP, Y = M*·ATP, and Z = M**·ADP·P_i. Values of k_{+a} = 17 s^{-1} and K_b (= k_{+b}/k_{-b}) = 7 determined from the time course of disappearance of free ATP and the ratio M**·ADP·P_i/M*·ATP at 200 ms. Simulations a, b, c, d, and e: K_{+b} takes values of 50, 100, 150, 200, and 500 s^{-1}, respectively. [Reproduced with permission from Geeves and Trentham (41). Copyright 1982, American Chemical Society.]

The first calculation of k_{-1}, the rate constant controlling ATP dissociation from subfragment 1, was the product of a series of experiments by Mannherz et al. (78). In a typical experiment, illustrated in Figure 5, ADP and P_i were added to a solution containing subfragment 1 to form a measurable quantity of ATP. The overall equilibrium constant *K* for ATP hydrolysis precluded significant ATP formation in the medium and therefore essentially all the ATP was protein bound. Determination of bound ATP concentration permitted calculation of K_1 and hence k_{-1} (see Table 2). An important prediction of the experiment is that ATP formation should occur as an exponential process with a rate constant essentially equal to the catalytic center activity of the ATPase (Fig. 5). Since this was observed within the sensitivity of the experiment, one is confident that ATP formation occurred at the active site. Four papers on this topic, the most recent discussing a direct measurement of k_{-1}, make interesting reading (13, 46, 78, 131).

NATURE OF ATP HYDROLYSIS STEP

Thus far we have outlined the kinetics of the myosin ATPase mechanism and presented evidence that during ATPase activity, predominant steady-state intermediates are M*·ATP and M**·ADP·P_i, effectively in equilibrium. The assumption is made here (and in Fig. 2) that the transformation of M*·ATP to M**·ADP·P_i is the hydrolysis step, and we now explore the

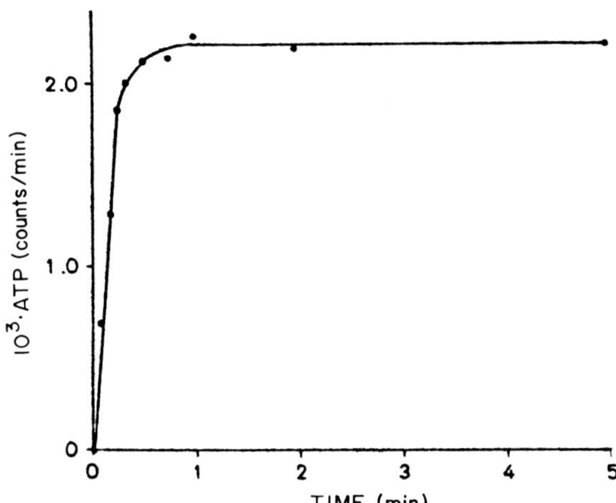

FIG. 5. Time course of ATP synthesis from ADP and P_i in the presence of myosin subfragment 1; 0.4 M [^{32}P]P_i and 50 μM Mg^{2+}-ADP were incubated with 100 μM subfragment 1 at pH 6.0 and 23°C. [From Mannherz et al. (78).]

validity of this assumption and elaborate on our present understanding of the hydrolysis mechanism. The main evidence for the chemical nature of $M^* \cdot ATP$ and $M^{**} \cdot ADP \cdot P_i$ comes from studies in which intermediates are trapped by quenching with acid and the nucleotides and P_i are isolated. It is possible, however, that the isolated species are not the same as those bound to myosin but rather are acid hydrolysis products of, for example, a pentacovalent phosphorus species.

Techniques used to determine the chemical mechanism of hydrolysis rely predominantly on the two stable heavy isotopes of oxygen, ^{17}O and ^{18}O, which are denoted in equations and figures as ⊗ and ●, respectively. Oxygen-18 is the more readily available and can be obtained as [^{18}O]water with greater than 99% isotopic enrichment. Oxygen-17 is more expensive and commercial [^{17}O]water contains 40%–60% enrichment; the rest is a combination of ^{16}O and ^{18}O. Substituting either of the heavy isotopes for ^{16}O in substrate, product, or water leaves the chemical and biochemical properties effectively the same because isotope effects due to mass differences are small.

When enzymes catalyze the hydrolysis of ATP to ADP and P_i, the extra oxygen atom derived from the solvent is invariably incorporated into P_i, and ATP is cleaved between the $\beta\gamma$-bridging oxygen atom and the γ-phosphorus (19). In Equation 4 and in subsequent molecular structures the protonation states, π-bonds, and negative charges are omitted for clarity

$$\mathrm{A{-}O{-}\overset{O}{\underset{O}{P}}{-}O{-}\overset{O}{\underset{O}{P}}{-}O{\wr}\overset{O}{\underset{O}{P}}{-}O + H_2O \longrightarrow A{-}O{-}\overset{O}{\underset{O}{P}}{-}O{-}\overset{O}{\underset{O}{P}}{-}O + O{-}\overset{O}{\underset{O}{P}}{-}O} \quad (4)$$

The group transferred from ATP is PO_3, the phosphoryl group. Although Equation 4 and most illustrations in this chapter show a two-dimensional representation of nucelotides and P_i, the phosphate moiety PO_4 is actually tetrahedral, with bond directions similar to those in methane.

The simplest mechanism for group transfer would involve direct displacement of ADP by a water molecule in a single step. Alternatively there could be a hydrolysis intermediate, and three possible intermediate species are shown in Figure 6. If an oxygen from water adds to the γ-phosphorus prior to ADP leaving, a pentacovalent species, *1*, forms as intermediate. Another possibility is transfer of the γ-phosphoryl group to a protein residue E to form a phosphoenzyme intermediate, *2*, which is then hydrolyzed to P_i. A third possibility is that ADP might be cleaved from the γ-phosphorus to give ADP and the intermediate metaphosphate, *3*. A water oxygen then adds to the metaphosphate to form P_i.

Five classes of experiments making use of oxygen isotopes are described in this chapter. They have enabled us to learn more about myosin-catalyzed ATP hydrolysis.

1. Oxygen exchange. Oxygen from water exchanges under appropriate conditions with oxygen atoms in P_i and the three nonbridging oxygen atoms attached to the γ-phosphorus atom of ATP. This allows us to explore the reversibility of steps in the myosin ATPase mechanism as well as the constraints on P_i mobility within the myosin molecule.
2. Oxygen isotope incorporation. One oxygen atom from water must be incorporated into P_i even if there is no oxygen exchange (see Eq. 4). Use of ^{18}O allows this to be investigated and to determine at which stage of ATP hydrolysis incorporation occurs.
3. Positional isotope exchange. This analysis explores exchange of oxygen isotopes within the ATP molecule as opposed to exchange with water oxygens. It provides an unambiguous test of whether any ATP that is isolated from a reaction mixture has undergone reversible cleavage.
4. Stereochemical course of phosphoryl group transfer. This provides evidence of whether or not there is a phosphoenzyme intermediate.
5. Structure of magnesium-nucleotide complexes. Several approaches have been used to investigate the role of metal ions in the catalysis of ATP hydrolysis.

Oxygen Exchange

Levy and Koshland (67) observed that when ATP was hydrolyzed in the presence of myosin and [^{18}O] water, each product P_i molecule contained more than one oxygen atom from the solvent water

$$M + ATP + H_2● \rightarrow M + ADP + P●_nO_{4-n} \quad (5)$$

where $1 < n \leqslant 4$. Had there been no exchange, only one oxygen atom in each product P_i molecule would be ^{18}O; this is the oxygen that must be incorporated from water during hydrolysis. Exchange accompanying ATP hydrolysis (Eq. 5) is termed intermediate exchange.

If P_i and ADP are incubated with myosin, oxygen exchange with water also occurs (27)

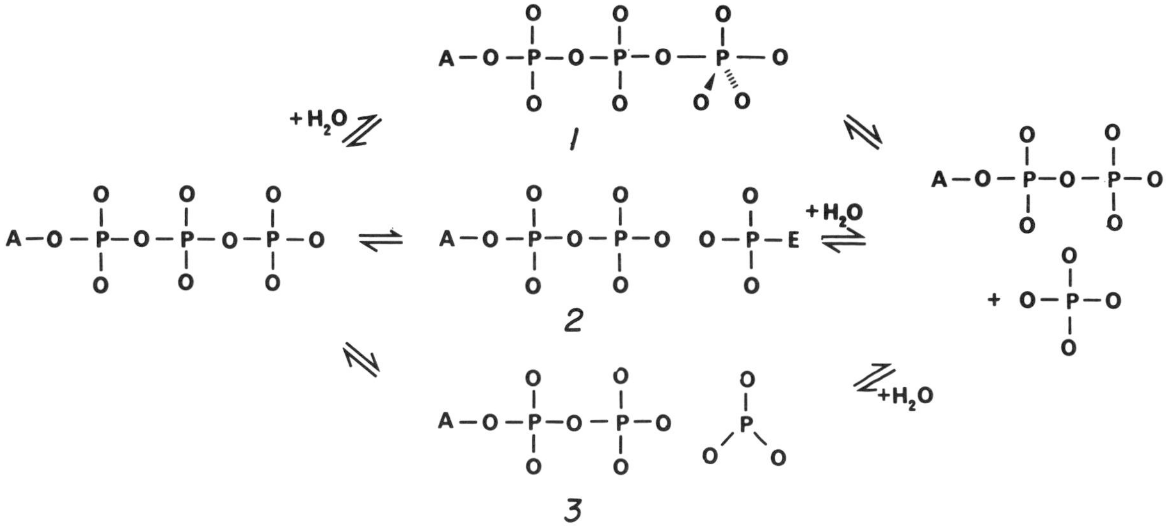

FIG. 6. Three possible intermediates in the myosin-catalyzed ATP hydrolysis step: *1*, pentacovalent species; *2*, phosphoenzyme; *3*, metaphosphate. E, protein residue.

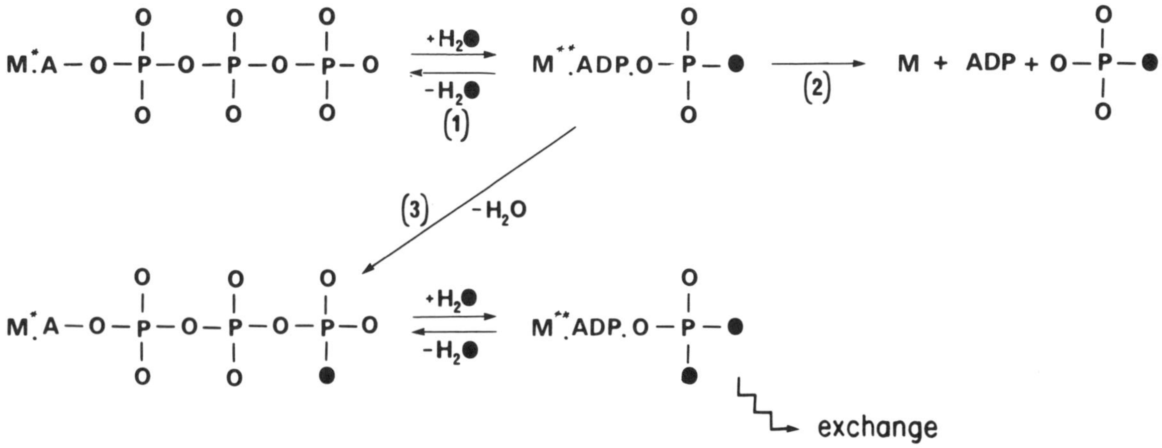

FIG. 7. Mechanism of oxygen exchange between phosphate and water during myosin-catalyzed ATP hydrolysis. *Filled circles*, ^{18}O originally present in water becomes incorporated in the intermediates and in phosphate.

$$M + ADP + PO_4 + H_2\bullet \rightarrow M + ADP + P\bullet_n O_{4-n} \quad (6)$$

where $0 < n < 4$. Here exchange requires no ATP hydrolysis and is called medium exchange. In contrast to intermediate exchange, it generally occurs slowly in a time-dependent manner.

The extent of each type of exchange is independent of whether heavy meromyosin or subfragment 1 is used (106) but does depend on other conditions, including the choice of the specific divalent metal ion used as cofactor (62, 69). In the presence of Mg^{2+} intermediate exchange is almost total—i.e., the product P_i derives its oxygens almost completely from water—and medium exchange is slow. On the other hand, Ca^{2+} produces no intermediate exchange, whereas medium exchange occurs approximately 6 times faster than with Mg^{2+} (106, 132). Extent of exchange depends on modification of either nucleotide (68, 106) or protein (66, 96), as well as on the concentration of actin (85, 93–96, 101). Oxygen-exchange studies carried out in the presence of Mg^{2+} are the concern of the remainder of this subsection.

Establishing a satisfactory mechanism for the exchange phenomena in general required extensive study of oxygen exchange. One proposed mechanism for oxygen exchange and supportive experimental evidence are presented here.

Irreversible binding of ATP to myosin to form $M^* \cdot ATP$ is followed by conversion of $M^* \cdot ATP$ to $M^{**} \cdot ADP \cdot P_i$ by reaction with water and subsequent incorporation of one oxygen atom from water (Fig. 7). The $M^{**} \cdot ADP \cdot P_i$ can then take one of three possible paths. *1*) It could lose the ^{18}O it gained and re-form as $M^* \cdot ATP$, containing all its original oxygens. *2*) It could release products to give P_i containing one solvent oxygen (i.e., no exchange). *3*) The P_i could rotate in the active site so that re-formation of $M^* \cdot ATP$ results in loss of a different oxygen—one that was originally on ATP. This M*·ATP would now contain one solvent oxygen atom, and when it again forms M**·ADP·P_i, it would gain a second solvent oxygen atom. One assumes here that water molecules have free access to the active site. The M**·ADP·P_i containing two solvent oxygens—one incorporated, one exchanged—can also undergo the three processes described. Eventually, therefore, P_i may contain four solvent oxygen atoms.

The comparative importance of the three pathways depends on their rate constants. Pathway 2 (product release) is controlled by k_{+3} (see Fig. 2), which has a value of 0.06 s^{-1} (pH 8.0, 20°C); re-formation of M*·ATP (pathways 1 and 3 together) is likely to have a rate constant of the order of 10 s^{-1} (109). Thus M*·ATP and M**·ADP·P_i can interconvert many times, on the average, before P_i is released. The relative importance of pathways 1 and 3 depends on how freely P_i rotates in the active site. If rotation is completely free, oxygen loss from P_i should be random, as is assumed in the reaction in Figure 7, so that pathways 1 and 3 have rate constants of $k_{-2}/4$ and $3k_{-2}/4$, respectively. The fact that myosin does promote extensive oxygen exchange supports the proposed mechanism, at least qualitatively.

A similar explanation can be provided for medium exchange. Free P_i binds slowly to M*·ADP to give M**·ADP·P_i. Once this intermediate forms, exchange can occur by partitioning between product release and M*·ATP formation as described above.

We now review the evidence for the exchange mechanism and describe further conclusions obtained from ^{18}O-exchange experiments. Some key features of intermediate exchange were established by Sartorelli et al. (90) and Bagshaw et al. (9). Sartorelli et al. showed that when ATP is hydrolyzed in the presence of myosin, both the P_i formed in the first turnover and all P_i formed subsequently contained an extensive amount of solvent oxygen. No solvent oxygen appeared in the unhydrolyzed ATP, however. This is consistent with the interpretation in Figure 7, since M*·ATP does not release ATP into the medium at a significant rate (13). Bagshaw et al. (9) carried out single turnover experiments with [γ-^{18}O]-ATP and unlabeled solvent water. This arrangement of isotopes has two advantages: only a small molar amount of ^{18}O is required and a higher isotopic enrichment is possible. Labeled ATP was mixed rapidly with excess myosin subfragment 1; M*·ATP and M**·ADP·P_i formed quickly and at time 2 s their isotopic content was analyzed after an acid quench. Both the isolated ATP and P_i had lost most of their isotope because M*·ATP and M**·ADP·P_i rapidly interconvert, reacting with a water molecule each time, so that both species exchange oxygen with the solvent (see Fig. 7).

The ^{18}O content of P_i and ATP was analyzed after transferring the oxygens of P_i to carbon. (P_i was formed as necessary from ATP.) The volatile CO_2 generated could be subjected to mass spectrometry (10). Although mass spectrometry is a sensitive procedure, it nevertheless provides information only on the amount of ^{18}O in P_i, not on its distribution. Recently two methods of analysis have been developed that permit determination of the distribution as well as the amount of ^{18}O in P_i. High-resolution ^{31}P nuclear magnetic resonance (NMR) spectroscopy is one method: ^{18}O attached to a phosphorus atom causes a small upfield shift in the ^{31}P resonance relative to ^{16}O (20, 71, 73), and the shift increases as the number of ^{18}O atoms attached to the phosphorus increases. This is illustrated for P_i in Figure 8*A* (122), which shows the spectrum of a mixture of 47% [$^{18}O_4$]P_i, 38% [$^{18}O_3$]P_i, 11% [$^{18}O_2$]P_i, 1% [$^{18}O_1$]-P_i, and 3% unlabeled P_i. Peak areas are proportional to the corresponding populations of molecules. Because NMR spectroscopy is nondestructive, one can use it to observe changes in ^{18}O during a reaction. Another advantage is that it can be used to determine the ^{18}O distribution in molecules other than P_i, such as ATP or its analogues. Relative

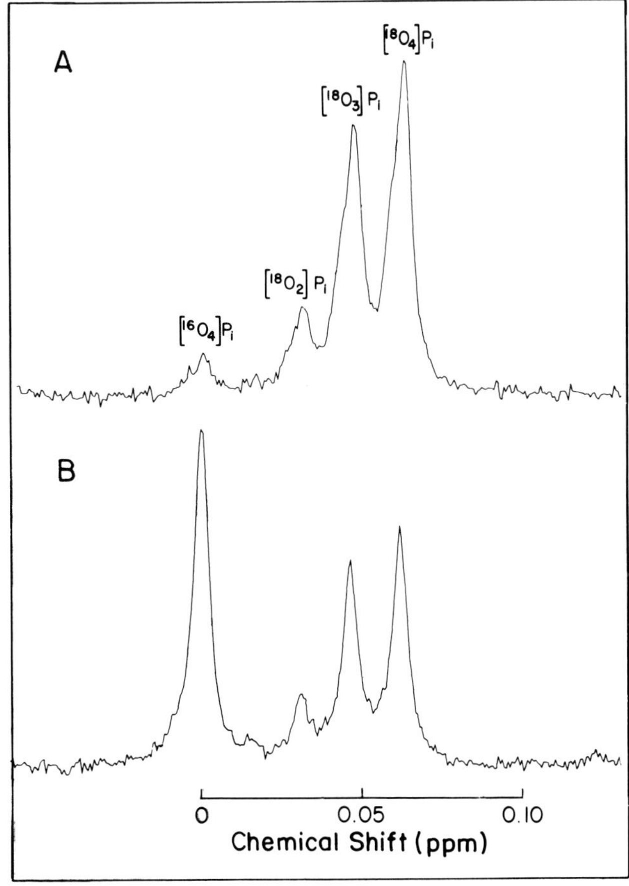

FIG. 8. ^{31}P NMR spectra of [^{18}O]P_i causes a small upfield shift in the ^{31}P resonance relative to ^{16}O (20, 69, 71); the shift increases as the number of ^{18}O attached to phosphorus increases. *A*: ^{31}P NMR spectrum of P_i consisting of 47% [$^{18}O_4$]P_i, 38% [$^{18}O_3$]P_i, 11% [$^{18}O_2$]P_i, 1% [$^{18}O_1$]P_i, and 3% unlabeled P_i. *B*: spectrum of same P_i (20 mM) after incubation at 22°C for 12 h with myosin subfragment 1 (43.5 μM). Solution also contained 100 mM Tris buffer (pH 8.0), 2.8 mM ADP, 3 mM $MgCl_2$, 0.5 mM EDTA (ethylenediamine tetraacetic acid), and 1.46 μM diadenosine pentaphosphate. The last of these inhibits any adenylate kinase impurity. [From Webb, McDonald, and Trentham (122).]

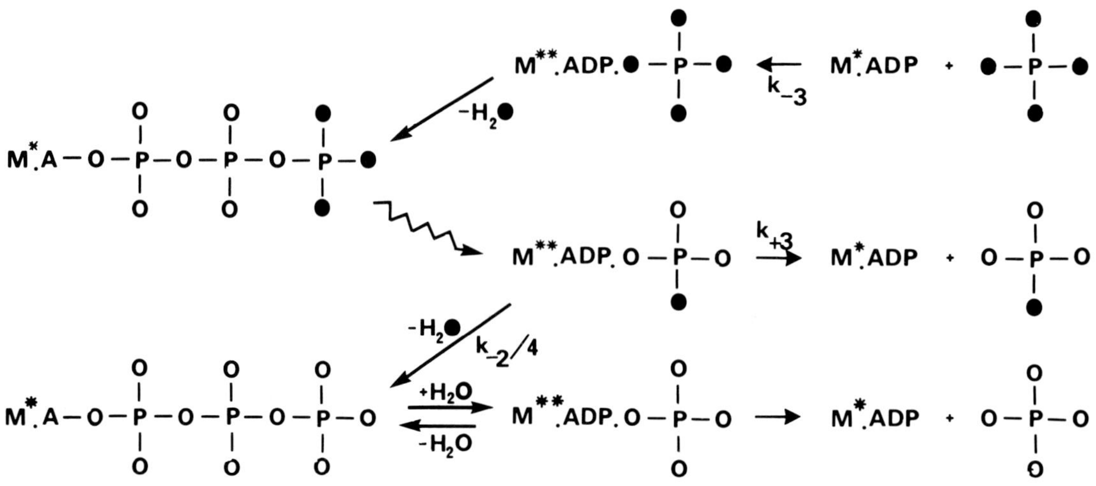

FIG. 9. Mechanism of myosin-catalyzed medium oxygen exchange between inorganic phosphate and water. *Filled circles,* ^{18}O.

to mass spectrometry, however, it is insensitive, requiring at least 1 μmol of material. Formation of a volatile derivative of P_i that can be subjected to mass spectrometry is a second method of determining the extent and distribution of ^{18}O in P_i. Two principal derivatives have been used: trimethyl phosphate (82) and tris(trimethylsilyl)phosphate (29). The PO_4 structure remains intact, and the mass spectrometer separates species depending on the number of ^{18}O atoms per molecule.

Use of these techniques has made it possible to further characterize the exchange reactions and to provide considerably more information about the ATPase reaction. Webb et al. (122) used ^{31}P NMR to study the medium exchange catalyzed by myosin subfragment 1 in situ. The P_i initially contained ^{18}O with a distribution as in Figure 8*A*, but it lost ^{18}O when it was incubated with MgADP and the protein. Only the unlabeled P_i peak increased in size; all other peaks decreased, although their sizes remained constant relative to each other (see Fig. 8*B*). Thus any molecule of $[^{18}O]P_i$ that underwent exchange lost all of its ^{18}O because ADP and P_i bind to myosin to form the equilibrium mixture of $M^* \cdot ATP$ and $M^{**} \cdot ADP \cdot P_i$ as in Figure 9. These species interconvert many times and undergo oxygen exchange before P_i is released.

Exchange was monitored as a function of time and the rate constant for P_i binding to $M^* \cdot ADP$ was determined. The rate constant could be obtained because binding is the rate-determining process in forming $M^{**} \cdot ADP \cdot P_i$ from M, ADP, and P_i (115) and hence in the overall exchange process. The reported rate constant is $0.23\ M^{-1} \cdot s^{-1}$, one that agrees with that calculated by Goody et al. (46) in studies of the formation of myosin-bound ATP from ADP and P_i. This type of experiment also proved that k_{-2} is much greater than k_{+3} because essentially no $[^{18}O_1]P_i$ is released into the medium: all $M^{**} \cdot ADP \cdot [^{18}O_1]P_i$ must partition to unlabeled $M^* \cdot ATP$ and so give unlabeled P_i (see Fig. 9).

Sleep et al. (100) performed a similar study of medium exchange by mass spectrometry of a volatile phosphate compound. They established conditions (pH 7.0, 0°C) in which only partial medium exchange occurred each time a P_i molecule bound to the protein. In their experiment P_i still contained some ^{18}O when it was released from the protein. Their data support previous experimental results and give $k_{-2}/k_{+3} = 17$, assuming free rotation of the P_i molecule in the active site. Observed distribution changes in $[^{18}O]P_i$ strongly suggest that exchange occurs by reversal of the reaction pathway as far as $M^* \cdot ATP$, as described in Figures 7 and 9.

Experimental results and subsequent interpretation of intermediate exchange have been less clear; different laboratories have obtained various extents of exchange for what seemed to be identical conditions. Determination of ^{18}O distribution, however, has now clarified the situation. Sleep et al. (101) showed that when $[\gamma\text{-}^{18}O]ATP$ was hydrolyzed in the presence of myosin subfragment 1, the P_i product contained almost no residual ^{18}O, and this was consistent with the known ratio of k_{-2}/k_{+3}. A similar result was obtained with myosin itself—except that a small, variable proportion of P_i was formed with little or no exchange. Sleep et al. (101) ascribed this variable proportion of P_i containing almost all its original ^{18}O to a contaminant ATPase; when the myosin was purified, such anomalous P_i was not formed. Other researchers observed a similar formation of anomalous P_i in reactions catalyzed by subfragment 1 as well as by myosin (126), in proportions that depended on the protein preparation.

Because there is almost total exchange with myosin alone, the final distribution of isotope in the product permits only limited insight into the rate constants of

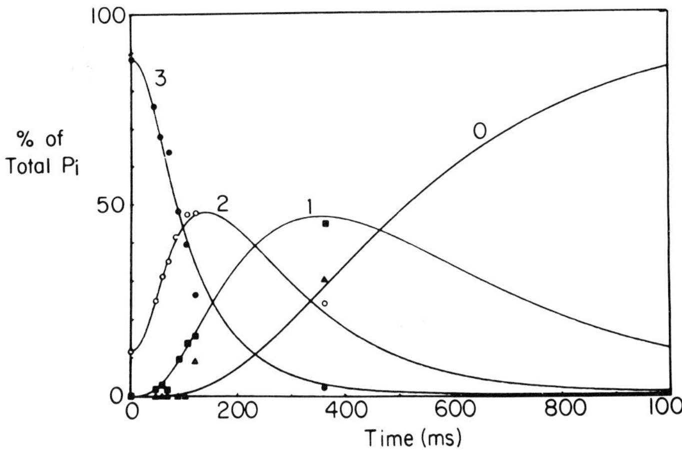

FIG. 10. ^{18}O exchange involving the P_i of $M^{**} \cdot ADP \cdot P_i$; 43 μM [γ-$^{18}O_3$]ATP and 86 μM myosin subfragment 1 were mixed in 10 mM Tris (pH 8.0, 20°C), and 2 mM $MgCl_2$. The mixture was acid quenched at various times. *Solid circles*, %P_i containing 3 ^{18}O atoms per molecule; *open circles*, 2 ^{18}O atoms; *solid squares*, 1 ^{18}O atom; *solid triangles*, no ^{18}O atoms. Curves calculated for $k_{+1} = 2 \times 10^6\ M^{-1} \cdot s^{-1}$, $k_{+2} = 80\ s^{-1}$, and $k_{-2} = 15\ s^{-1}$ and numbered according to the number of ^{18}O atoms per molecule. Curves are relatively insensitive to minor changes in k_{+1} and k_{+2}. [From Webb and Trentham (126).]

intermediate steps. A different type of experiment (126), however, provided more detail about the interaction of nucleotide with water in the active site. Rapid mixing of [γ-$^{18}O_3$]ATP with a molar excess of subfragment 1 resulted in the binding of all nucleotide to form $M^* \cdot ATP$ and $M^{**} \cdot ADP \cdot P_i$. The mixture was quenched with acid at reaction times of up to 0.4 s, and the protein-bound P_i and ATP were isolated. During this time these species underwent oxygen exchange as illustrated in Figure 10. Curves show the calculated distribution of species for an exchange mechanism like that in Figure 7. Close agreement between calculated and observed distributions implies that all P_i oxygens of $M^{**} \cdot ADP \cdot P_i$ are equivalent. Hence rotation of P_i in $M^{**} \cdot ADP \cdot P_i$ must be fast, indicating that the former is not tightly coordinated in the active site. Both ATP and P_i lose ^{18}O atoms at rates consistent with the scheme in Figure 7 and k_{-2}, with a value of 15 s^{-1}, agrees closely with the value obtained from other methods of measurement (41). This experiment provides strong evidence that exchange occurs on the reaction pathway by direct interconversion of $M^* \cdot ATP$ and $M^{**} \cdot ADP \cdot P_i$ rather than via a hitherto undetected, high-energy intermediate such as metaphosphate or pentacovalent species.

In the presence of actin the extent of intermediate exchange decreases with increasing actin concentration (85, 93–96, 99, 101). Qualitatively this is expected if the scheme in Figure 7 is correct. An increase in the rate of product release is the major pathway for actin activation. Actin, at least at low concentration (105), has no effect on the interconversion of $M^* \cdot ATP$ and $M^{**} \cdot ADP \cdot P_i$. Rather it interacts with the product complex in a bimolecular process so as to increase the rate of product release (99, 129).

Work in a number of laboratories has shown that myosin and subfragment 1 catalyze the intermediate exchange of all oxygens with equal probability in the presence of actin, as in its absence, and the extent of exchange is as described here. There can be a component of P_i that is variable in amount, however, and that is formed with little or no exchange (81, 97, 101, 126). The physiological significance of this effect is still unclear.

Oxygen Isotope Incorporation

Trentham (113) used a different approach to determine how the oxygen from water is added to ATP. The ATP was mixed rapidly with excess myosin subfragment 1 to give $M^* \cdot ATP$ and $M^{**} \cdot ADP \cdot P_i$, and the reaction was quenched with acid after a short enough time to ensure that little or no product had been released. With ^{18}O present either in the reaction solvent or in the quenching acid, the chemical state of $M^{**} \cdot ADP \cdot P_i$ could be investigated by determining how much ^{18}O was incorporated into the product as opposed to being exchanged.

When ^{18}O was in the reaction solvent, P_i, bound as $M^{**} \cdot ADP \cdot P_i$, contained an amount of ^{18}O equivalent to one solvent oxygen per molecule. This experiment was done in the presence of Ca^{2+} rather than Mg^{2+} to eliminate any intermediate oxygen exchange (106, 132). In the converse experiment with Mg^{2+} rather than Ca^{2+}, the reaction was performed in unlabeled water and quenched with [^{18}O]water. The fact that the P_i contained almost no ^{18}O showed that the extra oxygen from the solvent is added prior to the quench. Thus an oxygen from solvent water is added as $M^{**} \cdot ADP \cdot P_i$ forms

$$M + ATP + H_2\bullet \rightarrow M^{**} \cdot ADP \cdot PO_3\bullet \qquad (7)$$

Had $M^{**} \cdot ADP \cdot P_i$ contained an acylphosphate or metaphosphate, this would not have been the case because these species do not contain a solvent oxygen. However, the experiments do not rule out acylphosphate or metaphosphate as a transient intermediate prior to $M^{**} \cdot ADP \cdot P_i$ formation.

Positional Isotope Exchange

Oxygen-exchange and -incorporation experiments provide strong evidence that water adds to ATP during step 2 of the ATPase mechanism (see Fig. 2). This does not preclude the presence of an intermediate with a pentacovalent phosphorus, however. Korman and McLick (65) and Young et al. (135) pointed out that such species are indeed compatible with oxygen-exchange results. They postulated that water enters the reaction pathway prior to step 2, and the extra oxygen on the pentacovalent terminal phosphorus of M*·ATP (species *4*, Eq. 8) is derived from water. Step 2 is proposed to be a pseudorotation in which the pentacovalent structure changes to give species *5*, which is equivalent to M**·ADP·P_i

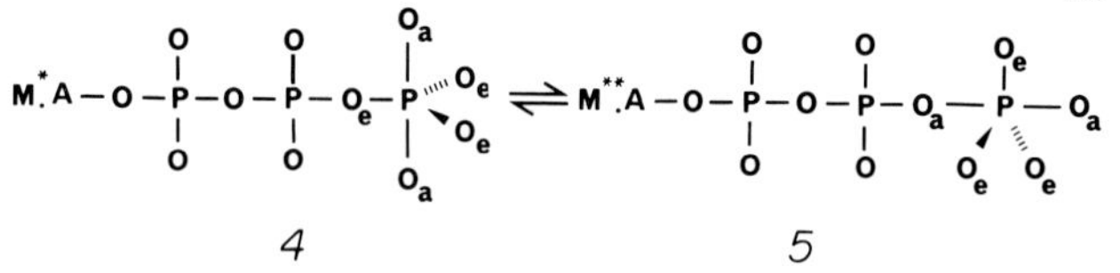

$$\underset{4}{M^*\cdot A{-}O{-}P(O)(O){-}O{-}P(O)(O){-}O_e{-}P(O_a)(O_a)(O_e)(O_e)} \rightleftharpoons \underset{5}{M^{**}\cdot A{-}O{-}P(O)(O){-}O{-}P(O)(O){-}O_a{-}P(O_e)(O_e)(O_e){-}O_a} \tag{8}$$

Orientation of the oxygen atoms about the pentacovalent phosphorus is trigonal bipyramidal with empirical rules governing which bonds take up apical (a) or equatorial (e) positions. The most important rule is that electron-withdrawing groups prefer apical positions (127). Bonds break and form at an apical position and therefore, when this equilibrium mixture is quenched with acid to isolate the nucleotides, it is these apical bonds that break. This causes species *4* to liberate ATP and *5* to liberate ADP and P_i.

According to the pseudorotation hypothesis, the $\beta\gamma$-oxygen–γ-phosphorus bond of ATP is not cleaved along the reaction pathway until the rate-determining, essentially irreversible step 3. This feature of the hypothesis can be tested by the positional isotope exchange method (82), which investigates the reversibility of ATP cleavage in a protein active site. This approach uses ^{18}O to distinguish the $\beta\gamma$-bridging oxygen from the β-nonbridging oxygens in ATP and analyzes oxygen exchange within the ATP molecule. The principle of the experiment is illustrated here

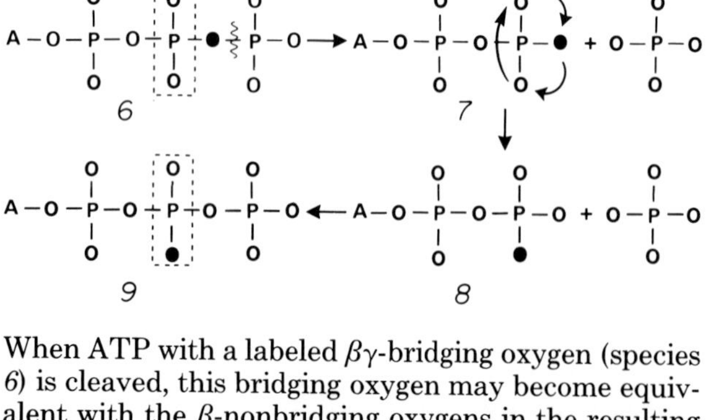

$$\underset{6}{A{-}O{-}P(O)(O){-}O{-}P(O)(O){-}\bullet{-}P(O)(O){-}O} \rightarrow \underset{7}{A{-}O{-}P(O)(O){-}O{-}P(O)(O){-}\bullet} + O{-}P(O)(O){-}O$$
$$\downarrow$$
$$\underset{9}{A{-}O{-}P(O)(O){-}O{-}P(O)(\bullet){-}O{-}P(O)(O){-}O} \leftarrow \underset{8}{A{-}O{-}P(O)(O){-}O{-}P(O)(\bullet){-}O} + O{-}P(O)(O){-}O \tag{9}$$

When ATP with a labeled $\beta\gamma$-bridging oxygen (species *6*) is cleaved, this bridging oxygen may become equivalent with the β-nonbridging oxygens in the resulting ADP (species *7*) because of the tetrahedral nature of phosphate. Assuming this occurs and that the β-phosphate of ADP can rotate, the ^{18}O becomes randomized so that ADP is a mixture of *7* and *8*. If ATP cleavage is reversed, some of the ATP formed would have nonbridging ^{18}O, as in species *9*. The ATP species *6* and *9* can be distinguished from each other by obtaining P_i that contains the β-nonbridging oxygen atoms and the β-phosphorus (enclosed by the *dashed line*) but does not contain the $\beta\gamma$-bridging oxygen

$$\underset{6}{A{-}O{-}P(O)(O){-}O{-}P(O)(O){-}\bullet{-}P(O)(O){-}O} \rightarrow O{-}P(O)(O){-}O$$
$$\underset{9}{A{-}O{-}P(O)(O){-}O{-}P(O)(\bullet){-}O{-}P(O)(O){-}O} \rightarrow O{-}P(O)(\bullet){-}O \tag{10}$$

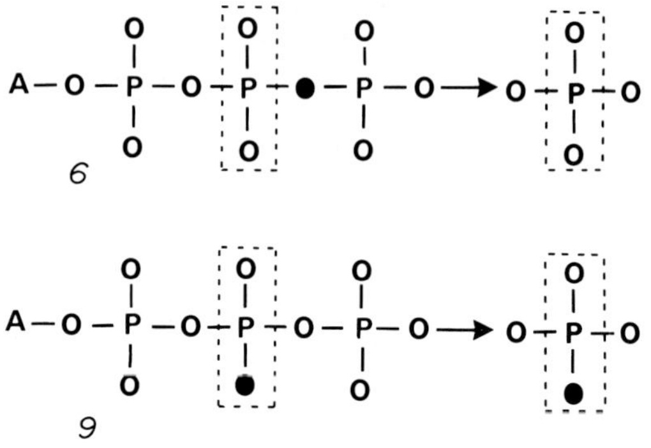

Extraction of this β-phosphate group is done by a series of enzymic (82) or chemical (119) reactions. Mass spectral analysis of P_i gives the extent to which ^{18}O has undergone positional isotope exchange.

This experiment was performed with myosin subfragment 1 (42). Here only the protein-bound ATP—not the ATP in the solvent—could possibly exhibit positional isotope exchange because no ATP is released from M*·ATP back into the medium. When [^{18}O]ATP was mixed with protein and allowed to react for 2 s before being quenched with acid, analysis of M*·ATP showed that positional isotope exchange had occurred; therefore ATP is cleaved reversibly during the myosin ATPase reaction. A pentacovalent phosphorus mechanism (135) in which the cleavage is irreversible is thus ruled out, and the evidence supports the previous conclusion that step 2 of Figure 2 is a straightforward interconversion of ATP and ADP + P_i.

It is interesting that positional isotope exchange was incomplete even though interconversion of ATP and ADP + P_i should have occurred many times in 2 s. A probable explanation is that the β-phosphate of ADP is not completely free to rotate in the active site when it exists as M**·ADP·P_i because of tight coordination between at least one β-oxygen and a group in the myosin active site. This is in contrast to the free rotation of P_i in M**·ADP·P_i as shown by oxygen-exchange experiments (101, 126). Evidence for coordination of a β-oxygen to Mg^{2+} is presented in *Structure of Magnesium-Nucleotide Complexes*, p. 248.

Stereochemistry of Phosphoryl Group Transfer

Determination of stereochemical course is a powerful technique to elucidate the chemical mechanism of phosphoryl group transfer. Because of the tetrahedral coordination of the phosphate species, transfer reactions can occur with either inversion or retention of configuration. Determining which pathway occurs, requires that each atom bound to the phosphorus be different. The atoms S, ^{16}O, ^{17}O, and ^{18}O are used in the reaction shown in the following equation. Since four positions must be uniquely labeled and only three oxygen isotopes are suitable, sulfur is used as an analogue of oxygen, giving ATPγS rather than ATP. Although the reaction kinetics are altered, it is likely that the chemical mechanism for ATPγS is the same as for ATP (5, 87). The possible phosphate species that can be formed are the two enantiomers of inorganic [^{16}O, ^{17}O, ^{18}O]thiophosphate

$$\text{A-O-P(O)(O)-O-P(O)(O)-O-P(S)(O)(\bullet)} + H_2\otimes \longrightarrow \text{ADP} + \otimes\text{-P(S)(O)(\bullet)} \quad \text{or} \quad \text{P(S)(O)(\bullet)-}\otimes \qquad \text{(II)}$$

10 *S* (retention) *R* (inversion)

Techniques used to study the stereochemistry of phosphoryl group transfer to species other than water (e.g., kinase-catalyzed transfer) have been developed recently and are reviewed by Knowles (64). Accumulated results suggest that when a phosphoryl group is transferred enzymically, each step occurs with inversion of configuration. If the reaction involves a single, direct transfer between substrates, the overall reaction shows inversion. If the reaction occurs in two steps (usually via a phosphoenzyme), the overall reaction shows retention of configuration. A one- or two-step mechanism is the simplest explanation of the results, but it is possible for overall inversion of configuration to be due to any odd number of transfer steps, each individual step itself occurring with inversion. Overall retention would result from any even number of such transfer steps, also singly occurring with inversion. For any of the ATPases that have been studied, though, a more complicated, multistep mechanism is unlikely.

In studies with myosin, the substrate used was ATPγS stereospecifically labeled with ^{18}O in the γ-position, species *10*. Because ATPγS does not give rise to any intermediate oxygen exchange, the product was either one of the enantiomers of inorganic thiophosphate or possibly a racemic mixture. A method for analysis of the configuration of such inorganic thiophosphate was developed by Webb and Trentham [(123); see also (120)] and requires the stereospecific incorporation of the inorganic thiophosphate into ATPβS by a series of enzymic reactions. These result in loss of one of the three original thiophosphate

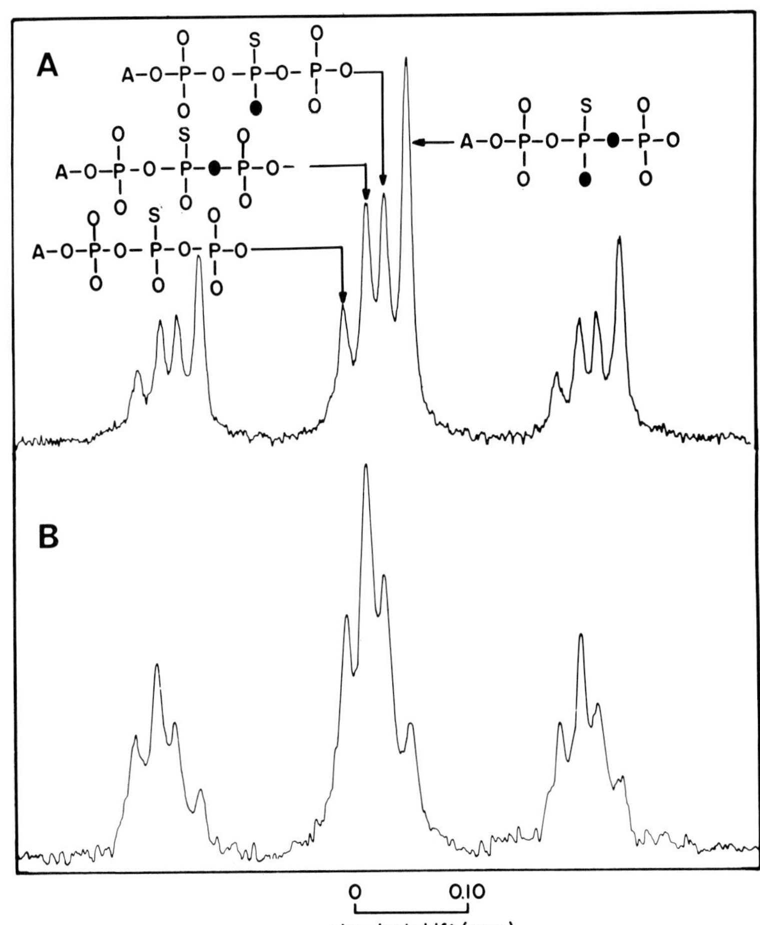

FIG. 11. ^{31}P NMR spectra of the β-phosphorus of ATPβS. *Filled circles*, ^{18}O. *A*: mixture of unlabeled ATPβS (9%), [βγ-^{18}O]ATPβS (21%), [β-^{18}O]ATPβS (21%), and [β-^{18}O; βγ-^{18}O]ATPβS (49%) arising from labeling of ATPβS with ^{18}O in the β- and βγ-positions, 70% extent. *B*: ATPβS derived from inorganic [^{16}O, ^{17}O, ^{18}O]thiophosphate product of myosin subfragment 1-catalyzed hydrolysis of (γ-*R*)[βγ-^{18}O; γ-^{18}O]ATPγS in ^{17}O-enriched water. [Adapted from Webb and Trentham (124).]

oxygens: a third of the molecules lose ^{16}O, another third lose ^{17}O, and the final third lose ^{18}O. When ^{17}O is lost

(12)

S → *11*

R → *12*

These ATPβS molecules can be distinguished by ^{31}P NMR because the extent of the ^{18}O upfield shift on the ^{31}P resonance depends on whether the ^{18}O is bridging or nonbridging (21, 70, 123). This is illustrated in Figure 11*A*, which shows the ^{31}P NMR spectrum of a mixture of unlabeled ATPβS (9%), [$\beta\gamma$-^{18}O]ATPβS (21%), [β-^{18}O]ATPβS (21%), and [β-^{18}O; $\beta\gamma$-^{18}O]-ATPβS (49%). Because these species are virtually identical in chemical terms, the population of molecules is proportional to the peak area.

Inorganic [^{16}O, ^{17}O, ^{18}O]thiophosphate also gives rise to ATPβS species in which ^{17}O is retained; β-^{31}P resonance is broadened and split due to the nuclear spin of ^{17}O (117). In effect, no peak is observed for these species—the major peak expected is that for species *11* or *12*. When this experiment was done with myosin and with [γ-$^{18}O_1$]ATPγS enriched to an extent of 75% in [^{17}O]water (45% enriched), the final ATPβS spectrum obtained is shown in Figure 11*B* (124). It indicates that there was an excess of ATPβS species *12* over *11* and that the myosin-catalyzed reaction proceeded with inversion of configuration at the transferred phosphorus atom. Because isotopic purities are well below 100%, other peaks are experimentally observed and one only expects to see excess ATPβS species *11* or *12*. Once the isotope enrichments are taken into account, the observed spectrum agrees well with that predicted for complete inversion (see Table 3).

The inversion observed for myosin ATPase is strong evidence for a direct in-line displacement of ADP by a water oxygen. By contrast the sarcoplasmic reticulum ATPase reaction—with a well-defined phosphoenzyme intermediate—inhibits retention of configuration at the transferred phosphoryl group (125). This also increases confidence in the interpretation of the myosin result.

Structure of Magnesium-Nucleotide Complexes

Myosin catalyzes ATP hydrolysis in the presence of a variety of metal ions (136), the Mg^{2+}-dependent

TABLE 3. *Estimated and Observed Peak Intensities for ^{31}P NMR Spectrum of β-Phosphorus of ATPβS*

	Relative Peak Intensities, %			
	Unlabeled	$^{18}O_1$, bridging	$^{18}O_1$, nonbridging	$^{18}O_2$
Estimated for retention*	40	22	34	4
Estimated for inversion*	40	34	22	4
Observed	39	34	22	5

NMR, nuclear magnetic resonance. ATPβS was derived from inorganic thiophosphate in a series of enzymic reactions. * Estimated values calculated from known isotopic enrichments of ^{18}O (75%) and of ^{17}O (45% ^{17}O, also containing 12% ^{18}O). It is assumed that there is 12% hydrolysis during the incorporation procedure (see ref. 124).

reaction being physiologically relevant. Both ADP and ATP form Mg^{2+} complexes that are kinetically labile, undergoing rapid ligand exchange with a rate constant of 10^3–10^4 s^{-1} (64). Uncomplexed divalent cations bind only negligibly in the myosin active site (6), but Mg^{2+} in conjunction with the nucleotide does bind to and dissociate from myosin (3, 8, 39, 77). Thus it is likely that the reacting species is a Mg^{2+}-nucleotide complex and that the metal ion may be important in the chemical mechanism of ATP cleavage. The nature of Mg^{2+}-nucleotide complexes during the ATPase reaction must first be understood before the detailed mechanism can be determined.

Knowles (64) discusses possible roles of Mg^{2+} in catalysis. He points out that Mg^{2+} coordination can stabilize negative charges on β-phosphate oxygens, thereby enhancing ADP as a leaving group. Coordination could also stabilize a particular triphosphate conformation and thus facilitate cleavage catalyzed by other groups in the active site. In the case of myosin, involvement in ATP cleavage is not the only possible function for the metal ion; control of product release is almost certainly influenced by Mg^{2+} coordination.

For the purpose of understanding which of these metal ion functions are operative, investigators are attempting to determine which phosphate oxygens are coordinated to Mg^{2+} and how this coordination changes during the course of the reaction. Because Mg^{2+}-nucleotides exchange ligands rapidly, direct study of these complexes is difficult. Three methods developed to answer these questions, however, have been successfully applied to myosin ATPase. The first, developed by Cleland and his co-workers (18, 23, 24, 28), uses metal-nucleotide complexes with kinetically stable metal-ligand bonds. The second uses thiophosphoryl nucleotides in which one particular phosphate oxygen atom is replaced by sulfur (32, 55, 57). The third, developed by Reed and Leyh (88), involves the detection of superhyperfine coupling between ^{17}O-labeled nucleotides and Mn^{2+} by electron paramagnetic resonance (EPR) spectroscopy.

In principle, Mg^{2+} can interact with any combination of oxygens from the three phosphates of ATP to give mono-, bi-, or tridentate complexes. Furthermore, the α- and β-phosphates are prochiral: if one of the two nonbridging oxygens on one phosphorus atom becomes coordinated to a metal ion, all four ligands on that phosphorus atom will be different and therefore the phosphate becomes chiral. This is illustrated in Figure 12*A* for the $\beta\gamma$-bidentate MgATP, where the two diastereoisomers are termed Λ and Δ (80). Since the active site of myosin is asymmetric—surrounded by L-amino acids—one expects the two configurations to behave very differently. Determination of the correct Mg^{2+}-nucleotide complex not only requires knowledge of which phosphates are coordinated but also which oxygen of those phosphates.

Cleland and co-workers (18, 23, 24, 28) have synthesized Cr^{3+} and Co^{3+} complexes of ATP and ADP that exchange metal ions some 10^{10} times more slowly than the Mg^{2+} complexes. Mono-, bi-, and tridentate complexes were prepared and some diastereoisomers could be separated to give a range of exchange-inert analogues of MgATP and MgADP. These have been tested on various enzymes and the relative specificity of each complex determined. In the case of myosin subfragment 1, Eccleston and Trentham (30) and Connolly and Eckstein (22) could not detect any interaction between such metal complexes and the protein. Yee and Eckstein (134) originally reported that the β-monodentate complex of Cr^{3+} with ADP inhibited myosin ATPase. Connolly and Eckstein (22) and Goody et al. (45), however, found that this inhibition was very weak and could be accounted for by traces of ADP in the CrADP.

Substitution of sulfur for an oxygen atom at either the α- or β-position of ATP, or the α-position of ADP, results in two diastereoisomers in each case (33, 56, 91). Absolute configurations of these thiophosphoryl nucleotides have been determined (11, 12, 55, 58, 89). Many enzymes show specificity toward one diastereoisomer (31); this may be caused either by the sulfur atom interacting adversely in one position in the active site but not in the other, or by preferred metal coordination.

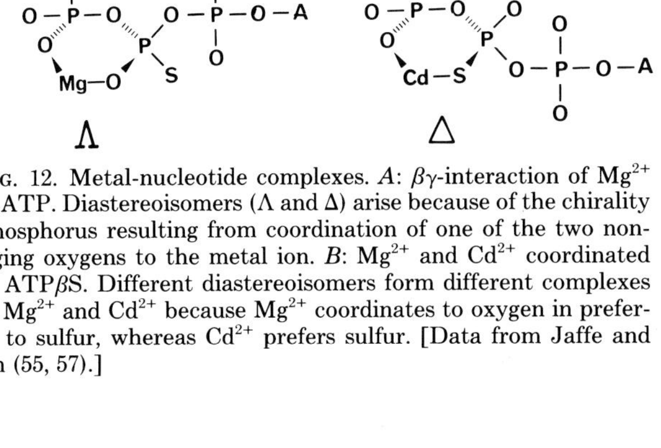

FIG. 12. Metal-nucleotide complexes. *A*: $\beta\gamma$-interaction of Mg^{2+} with ATP. Diastereoisomers (Λ and Δ) arise because of the chirality of phosphorus resulting from coordination of one of the two nonbridging oxygens to the metal ion. *B*: Mg^{2+} and Cd^{2+} coordinated with ATPβS. Different diastereoisomers form different complexes with Mg^{2+} and Cd^{2+} because Mg^{2+} coordinates to oxygen in preference to sulfur, whereas Cd^{2+} prefers sulfur. [Data from Jaffe and Cohn (55, 57).]

Jaffe and Cohn (55, 57) developed a method to test for metal coordination. Because Mg^{2+} coordinates to oxygen in preference to sulfur, whereas Cd^{2+} prefers sulfur, a given diastereoisomer of ATPβS would form different complexes with Mg^{2+} and Cd^{2+} (see Fig. 12*B*): Mg^{2+} gives the Λ complex with the β-*R* isomer of ATPβS, and Cd^{2+} gives the Δ complex. The configuration of the complexes would be reversed with the β-*S* isomer of ATPβS. If the enzyme is specific for one configuration of the complex, this should be reflected in specificity for one diastereoisomer of ATPβS with Mg^{2+} and for the other diastereoisomer of ATPβS with Cd^{2+}. If there is no such reversal of specificity, however, it is likely that the metal does not bind to the thiophosphate moiety of the nucleotide.

Connolly and Eckstein (22) used the thiophosphate method to investigate the ADP complex. Their studies with ADPαS in the presence of Mg^{2+} and Cd^{2+} showed that there was no reversal of metal specificity as measured by the inhibition constant of the nucleotide. Goody et al. (45) showed that each ADPαS diastereoisomer's rate constant for dissociation from subfragment 1 was similarly independent of which metal was used. Thus it is unlikely that the α-phosphate is bound to the metal.

This method still leaves some ambiguity about the nature of MgATP coordination (22, 44, 133), however. Connolly and Eckstein (22) studied the stereoselectivity of myosin for ATPαS and ATPβS in the presence of Mg^{2+} and Cd^{2+} and, based on the overall catalytic activity of myosin with these analogues, concluded that myosin uses the $\beta\gamma$-bidentate metal–nucleotide complex as substrate. Goody and Hofmann's work (44) on the thiophosphate analogues' rate constants for binding to myosin and for dissociation from actomyosin suggested an $\alpha\beta\gamma$-tridentate configuration for the active MgATP complex. Their experiments did not study the reversal of enzyme specificity with the change from Mg^{2+} to Cd^{2+}, however. Perhaps these two studies offer varying conclusions because different steps of the reaction pathway were being observed and, as noted, metal coordination is believed to change during the course of the reaction. This aspect of the mechanism awaits further work to fully clarify the role of Mg^{2+} in the myosin ATPase reaction.

A third approach compares two EPR spectra of the Mn^{2+}-nucleotide–myosin subfragment 1 complex—those for the nucleotide with and without ^{17}O labeling at a particular phosphate. The Mn^{2+} is used as an analogue of Mg^{2+} since it is paramagnetic and a reasonably good substitute for Mg^{2+} in many enzymes. Oxygen-17, unlike ^{16}O, has a nuclear spin of 5/2 that couples with the unpaired electron of Mn^{2+} when the two atoms are directly bonded (43). Because this superhyperfine coupling constant is less than the signal width, the coupling produces an inhomogeneous

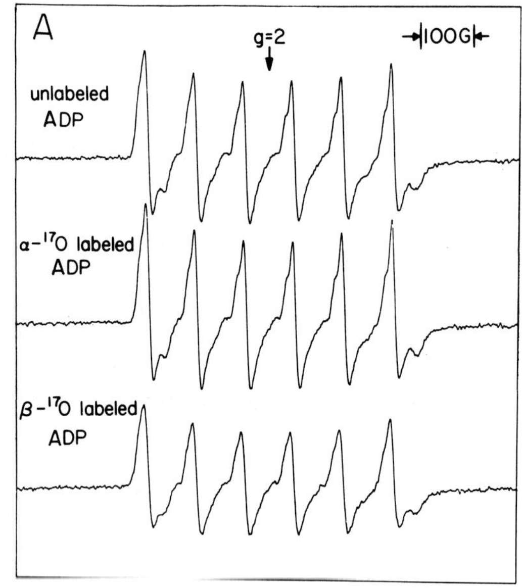

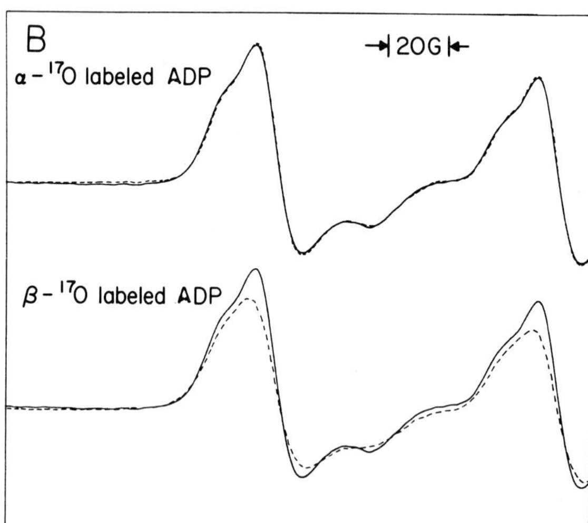

FIG. 13. Electron paramagnetic resonance spectra of ADP–Mn^{2+}–subfragment 1 complexes. Spectra, at 35 GHz, taken of a solution containing 1.0 mM myosin subfragment 1, 1.07 mM ADP, 0.50 mM $MnCl_2$, 10 μM diadenosine pentaphosphate in 50 mM Tris buffer (pH 8.0, 3°C). Under these conditions essentially all Mn^{2+} is in a protein-bound complex with ADP. *A*: unlabeled ADP, [α-^{17}O]-ADP and [β-^{17}O]ADP (40% enriched in each position). Peak broadening is observed for [β-^{17}O]ADP but not for [α-^{17}O]ADP. *B*: *broken lines*, expansion of the first transitions with labeled ADP; *solid line*, unlabeled ADP. [From Webb et al. (121).]

broadening of the EPR signal that can be used to determine which oxygen atoms of a nucleotide are bound to Mn^{2+} in the complex on a protein (88).

This approach has been used to study M*·ADP, the Mn^{2+}–ADP–myosin subfragment 1 complex (121). Figure 13 shows spectra of this complex with unsubstituted ADP, [α-^{17}O]ADP, and [β-^{17}O]ADP. Inhomogeneous broadening of the EPR signal is evident in the [β-^{17}O]ADP spectrum, meaning that a β-oxygen of ADP is bound to the metal. In contrast there is no effect observed for [α-^{17}O]ADP. One concludes, therefore, that these α-oxygens are not bound to the metal, in agreement with the thiophosphate experiments (22, 45). The EPR approach—by comparing the spectra from samples in [^{17}O]- and [^{16}O]water—also allows the number of water oxygens coordinated to Mn^{2+} in the M*·ADP complex to be determined. Results suggest that there are probably two water molecules in this complex, one of which exchanges rapidly with the solvent (6). The spectra account for three ligands on the metal, and since the EPR spectra are characteristic of a metal with six ligands in octahedral coordination, there are probably three protein ligands also bound to Mn^{2+}. Evidence that the metal is bound to the protein may explain the lack of binding of the Cr^{3+}- and Co^{3+}-nucleotide complexes because these complexes have all six coordination sites already filled.

PERSPECTIVES ON MECHANISM AND FUNCTION OF ATP HYDROLYSIS IN MUSCLE

In this chapter we have described various techniques used to elucidate the chemical mechanism by which ATP + H_2O and ADP + P_i are interconverted in the myosin catalytic site. Some aspects of the mechanism such as the role of metal ions and protons remain uncertain, but we do know that a proton must be released for each overall ATP hydrolysis cycle at pH 8.0. Measurements of the release and uptake of protons have been made at different stages of the overall catalytic cycle, and these were reviewed by Trentham et al. (115). Stoichiometric proton release from the myosin-nucleotide complex does not occur during the hydrolysis step, although a fraction of a proton is released under appropriate conditions (14). There is no information about proton movement between nucleotide and protein during the catalysis even though, as pointed out in discussing the role of Mg^{2+}, local charge neutralization by metal ions or protons would aid the catalysis.

Other aspects of ATP cleavage, however, are supported by direct evidence. Stereochemical inversion of configuration at the γ-phosphorus atom effectively rules out a phosphoenzyme intermediate; this is supported by evidence from other studies (113, 130). Oxygen-isotope-incorporation experiments, showing that a water oxygen is covalently bound to the transferring phosphorus atom at the same time that M**·ADP·P_i is formed, provide evidence against M**·ADP·P_i containing a metaphosphate. The occurrence of positional isotope exchange in M*·ATP means that ADP is cleaved from the transferring phosphoryl group in M**·ADP·P_i in a reversible reaction, thus precluding a pentacovalent phosphorus intermediate. In addition the kinetics and distribution of oxygen exchange provide evidence that ATP + H_2O and ADP + P_i are rapidly and directly interconverted without any characterizable intermediate between M*·ATP and M**·ADP·P_i. It is likely that the γ-phosphorus of ATP is transferred directly in an in-line process from ADP to an oxygen of water

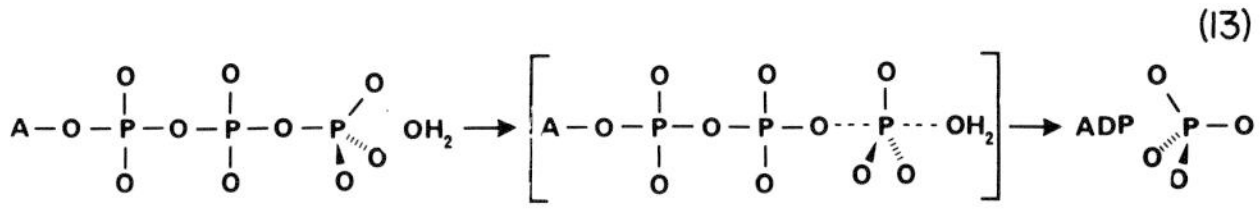

$$\mathrm{A{-}O{-}P(O)(O){-}O{-}P(O)(O){-}O{-}P(O)(O)(O)\quad OH_2 \longrightarrow \left[A{-}O{-}P(O)(O){-}O{-}P(O)(O){-}O\cdots P(O)(O)(O)\cdots OH_2\right] \longrightarrow ADP\quad P(O)(O)(O){-}O} \tag{13}$$

At the present time there is no strong evidence that transfer requires direct interaction of amino acids in the active site; rather the protein's role is to accelerate the hydrolysis step by stabilizing the transition state.

Clues about how this acceleration occurs are provided by studies of metal-nucleotide interaction and by the observed slow rate of positional isotope exchange, both indicating that a β-oxygen of ADP is coordinated to Mg^{2+}. This coordination could facilitate the cleavage of ADP from the γ-phosphorus by neutralizing negative charge on the β-phosphate moiety and by positioning the phosphate favorably. Almost total oxygen exchange led researchers to conclude that water must have free access to and from the catalytic site. Furthermore P_i molecules—at least in $M^{**}\cdot ADP\cdot P_i$—can rotate freely in the catalytic site. The very slow release of P_i from the active site determined by k_{+3}, however, suggests that a protein conformation change may be required for this process.

The energetics of the catalyzed reaction have been discussed by Jencks (59, 60), who proposed that the transition state species of the hydrolysis step should be tightly bound in the catalytic site in order to achieve a high rate of catalysis. Since $M^*\cdot ATP$ also exhibits tight binding, ATP and the transition state may share some common features of such binding including electrostatic interaction between protein and phosphate negative charges. For $M^{**}\cdot ADP\cdot P_i$ any such favorable interactions are counteracted by destabilization effects—the loss of the entropy possessed by ADP and P_i in aqueous solution and perhaps conformational strain. These destabilizing effects account for an equilibrium constant for the interconversion of $M^*\cdot ATP$ and $M^{**}\cdot ADP\cdot P_i$ that is close to unity. Albery and Knowles (2) discuss the influence of the tight binding of substrate and transition state, as well as differential binding between intermediates, on the effectiveness of catalysis.

The significance of the ready reversibility of the hydrolysis step to actomyosin ATPase and muscle contraction is now considered. Adenosine triphosphate binds to the actomyosin complex, which then dissociates. Although myosin binds tightly to both actin and ATP separately, each of the latter binds only weakly in the presence of the other—it is a negatively heterotropic interaction. According to the Lymn-Taylor model, the cross bridge is detached during hydrolysis. The equilibrium constant of the hydrolysis step is between 1 and 10 depending on experimental conditions, and this has important implications for the energetics of muscle contraction. No mechanical work can be done by $M^*\cdot ATP$ or $M^{**}\cdot ADP\cdot P_i$, and any free-energy change ΔG occurring during the transformation of $M^*\cdot ATP$ to $M^{**}\cdot ADP\cdot P_i$ is not available for mechanical work. For efficient transformation of chemical to mechanical energy this free-energy change must be small relative to the overall free-energy change of −54 kJ/mol associated with ATP hydrolysis in muscle (25). Relative concentrations of $M^*\cdot ATP$ and $M^{**}\cdot ADP\cdot P_i$ in actively contracting muscle are not known, but since their interconversion is not likely to be rate determining, they are probably not far from their equilibrium ratio. For this step ΔG^0 (i.e., $-RT\ln K_2$) is −5.5 kJ/mol, so that ΔG for this step is probably only a small fraction of the overall free-energy change of −54 kJ/mol because

$$\Delta G = \Delta G^0 + RT\ln\,[M^{**}\cdot ADP\cdot P_i]/[M^*\cdot ATP] \tag{14}$$

Is there any structural change occurring in the transformation of $M^*\cdot ATP$ to $M^{**}\cdot ADP\cdot P_i$ that is essential for the mechanical function of the myosin head in muscle contraction? Experiments analyzing the gross structure of myosin in either the isolated proteins or relaxed muscle suggest that there is very little difference between the two states. Fluorescence depolarization and EPR studies both show that there is extensive rotational mobility of the myosin head (79, 111). The large range of orientations in a fiber of the presumed $M^{**}\cdot ADP\cdot P_i$ state (84, 112) leads to the representation of the head shown in Figures 1 and 2.

The X-ray studies of Goody et al. (47) provided further information about cross-bridge orientation in relaxed muscle. The steady-state intermediate in the myosin-catalyzed ATPγS hydrolysis is $M^*\cdot ATP\gamma S$, which is probably a good structural analogue of $M^*\cdot ATP$. However, the major steady-state intermediate in relaxed fibers with ATP as substrate is probably $M^{**}\cdot ADP\cdot P_i$. It follows that muscle relaxation with ATP and ATPγS gives rise predominantly to the $M^{**}\cdot ADP\cdot P_i$ and $M^*\cdot ATP$ states, respectively. The X-ray data indicate that the intermediates are indistinguishable in gross structural terms. However, some distinctions are apparent at the molecular level. The reactivity of protein thiols in the myosin-nucleotide complex is different in $M^*\cdot ATP\gamma S$ (and thus presumably $M^*\cdot ATP$) as compared to $M^{**}\cdot ADP\cdot P_i$ (118). Intrinsic protein fluorescence increases in the transformation of $M^*\cdot ATP$ to $M^{**}\cdot ADP\cdot P_i$ (4, 61).

Even if there is no gross distinction between the detached states of $M^*\cdot ATP$ and $M^{**}\cdot ADP\cdot P_i$, structural changes during their transformation may define the attached states of the cross bridge. This arises from the fact that, in terms of the cross-bridge cycle in Figure 1, $M^*\cdot ATP$ must dissociate from an actin monomer different from the one to which $M^{**}\cdot ADP\cdot P_i$ reassociates in order for the filaments to move relative to each other. It is not clear whether this phenomenon is derived from differences between the two unassociated states $M^*\cdot ATP$ and $M^{**}\cdot ADP\cdot P_i$, or whether it is a property of the overall cross-bridge cycle. The possible importance of a structure change accompanying the ATP hydrolysis step has been considered by Jencks (60) in a general discussion of coupled vectorial processes. Most current models of the cross-bridge cycle do not propose a difference in preferred orientation of attachment between M*·ATP and M**·ADP·P_i but do suggest such a difference between the rigor (nucleotide-free) complex and the actomyosin·ADP·P_i complex.

Identifying the steps associated with myosin and actomyosin ATPase is still a very active research field, as exemplified by the abundance of recent literature (15, 34, 35, 37, 40, 92, 98, 99, 102, 116). Our short discussion of these processes has allowed us to concentrate on the chemical aspects of ATP hydrolysis, although another consideration was the uncertainty about the extent to which various transformations are physiologically significant. A recent important development was the discovery that the ATP hydrolysis step can occur in an undissociated actomyosin complex as well as by the dissociative pathway indicated in the Lymn-Taylor scheme in Figure 1 (83, 104, 105). Although a pathway including a nondissociative ATP hydrolysis step has yet to be established in active muscle, there is no a priori reason why it should not be physiologically significant (104). The relationship between the elementary steps of actomyosin ATPase and the mechanical events of contraction are discussed further in the chapter by Podolsky and Schoenberg in this *Handbook*.

Understanding the changes in protein structure during the transformation of M*·ATP to M**·ADP·P_i requires further study. The techniques described in this chapter promise to be valuable in formulating a chemical description of this transformation (and perhaps the actomyosin transformation of AM*·ATP to AM**·ADP·P_i), as well as of the relationship of the kinetics and energetics of this process to the overall cross-bridge cycle.

We are grateful for financial support from the National Institutes of Health (Grant AM-23030 to Dr. D.R. Trentham and HL-15835 to the Pennsylvania Muscle Institute), the Muscular Dystrophy Association of America, and the Whitehall Foundation.

REFERENCES

1. Adelstein, R. L., and E. Eisenberg. Regulation and kinetics of the actin-myosin-ATP interaction. *Annu. Rev. Biochem.* 49: 921–956, 1980.
2. Albery, W. J., and J. R. Knowles. Efficiency and evolution of enzyme catalysis. *Angew. Chem. Int. Ed. Engl.* 16: 285–293, 1977.
3. Bagshaw, C. R. The kinetic mechanism of the manganous ion-dependent adenosine triphosphatase of myosin subfragment 1. *FEBS Lett.* 58: 197–201, 1975.
4. Bagshaw, C. R., J. F. Eccleston, F. Eckstein, R. S. Goody, H. Gutfreund, and D. R. Trentham. The magnesium ion-dependent adenosine triphosphatase of myosin. Two-step processes of adenosine triphosphate association and adenosine diphosphate dissociation. *Biochem. J.* 141: 351–364, 1974.
5. Bagshaw, C. R., J. F. Eccleston, D. R. Trentham, D. W. Yates, and R. S. Goody. Transient kinetic studies of the Mg^{++}-dependent ATPase of myosin and its proteolytic subfragments. *Cold Spring Harbor Symp. Quant. Biol.* 37: 127–135, 1972.
6. Bagshaw, C. R., and G. H. Reed. Investigations of equilibrium complexes of myosin subfragment 1 with the manganous ion and adenosine diphosphate using magnetic resonance techniques. *J. Biol. Chem.* 251: 1975–1983, 1976.
7. Bagshaw, C. R., and D. R. Trentham. The reversibility of adenosine triphosphate cleavage by myosin. *Biochem. J.* 133: 323–328, 1973.
8. Bagshaw, C. R., and D. R. Trentham. The characterization of myosin-product complexes and of product-release steps during the magnesium ion-dependent adenosine triphosphatase reaction. *Biochem. J.* 141: 331–349, 1974.
9. Bagshaw, C. R., D. R. Trentham, R. G. Wolcott, and P. D. Boyer. Oxygen exchange in the γ-phosphoryl group of protein-bound ATP during Mg^{2+}-dependent adenosine triphosphatase activity of myosin. *Proc. Natl. Acad. Sci. USA* 72: 2592–2596, 1975.
10. Boyer, P. D., and D. M. Bryan. The application of ^{18}O methods to oxidative phosphorylation. *Methods Enzymol.* 10: 60–71, 1967.
11. Bryant, F. R., and S. J. Benkovic. Stereochemical course of the reaction catalyzed by 5′-nucleotide phosphodiesterase from snake venom. *Biochemistry* 18: 2825–2828, 1979.
12. Burgers, P. M. J., and F. Eckstein. Absolute configuration of the diastereomers of adenosine 5′-*O*-(1-thiotriphosphate): consequences for the stereochemistry of polymerization by DNA-dependent RNA polymerase from *Escherichia coli*. *Proc. Natl. Acad. Sci. USA* 75: 4798–4800, 1978.
13. Cardon, J. W., and P. D. Boyer. The rate of release of ATP from its complex with myosin. *Eur. J. Biochem.* 92: 443–448, 1978.
14. Chock, S. P. The mechanism of the skeletal muscle myosin ATPase. III. Relationship of the H^+ release and the protein absorbance change induced by ATP to the initial P_i burst. *J. Biol. Chem.* 254: 3244–3248, 1979.
15. Chock, S. P., P. B. Chock, and E. Eisenberg. Pre-steady-state kinetic evidence for a cyclic interaction of myosin subfragment one with actin during the hydrolysis of adenosine 5′-triphosphate. *Biochemistry* 15: 3244–3253, 1976.
16. Chock, S. P., P. B. Chock, and E. Eisenberg. The mechanism of the skeletal muscle myosin ATPase. II. Relationship between the fluorescence enhancement induced by ATP and the initial P_i burst. *J. Biol. Chem.* 254: 3236–3243, 1979.
17. Chock, S. P., and E. Eisenberg. The mechanism of the skeletal muscle myosin ATPase. I. Identity of the myosin active sites. *J. Biol. Chem.* 254: 3229–3235, 1979.
18. Cleland, W. W., and A. S. Mildvan. Chromium (III) and cobalt (III) nucleotides as biological probes. *Adv. Inorg. Chem.* 1: 163–191, 1979.
19. Cohn, M. Magnetic resonance studies of metal activation of enzymic reactions of nucleotides and other phosphate substrates. *Biochemistry* 2: 623–629, 1963.
20. Cohn, M., and A. Hu. Isotopic (^{18}O) shift in ^{31}P nuclear magnetic resonance applied to a study of enzyme-catalyzed phosphate-phosphate exchange and phosphate (oxygen)-water exchange reactions. *Proc. Natl. Acad. Sci. USA* 75: 200–203, 1978.
21. Cohn, M., and A. Hu. Isotopic ^{18}O shifts in ^{31}P NMR of adenine nucleotides synthesized with ^{18}O in various positions. *J. Am. Chem. Soc.* 102: 913–916, 1980.
22. Connolly, B. A., and F. Eckstein. Structures of the mono- and divalent metal nucleotide complexes in the myosin ATPase. *J. Biol. Chem.* 256: 9450–9456, 1981.
23. Cornelius, R. D., and W. W. Cleland. Substrate activity of (adenosine triphosphato)tetraamminecobalt(III) with yeast hexokinase and separation of diastereomers using the enzyme. *Biochemistry* 17: 3279–3286, 1978.
24. Cornelius, R. D., P. A. Hart, and W. W. Cleland. Phosphorus-31 NMR studies of complexes of adenosine triphosphate, adenosine diphosphate, tripolyphosphate, and pyrophosphate with cobalt(III) ammines. *Inorg. Chem.* 16: 2799–2805, 1977.
25. Curtin, N. A., C. Gilbert, K. M. Kretzchmar, and D. R. Wilkie. The effect of the performance of work on total energy

output and metabolism during muscular contraction. *J. Physiol. London* 238: 455–472, 1974.
26. DAWSON, M. J., D. G. GADIAN, AND D. R. WILKIE. Contraction and recovery of living muscle studied by ^{31}P nuclear magnetic resonance. *J. Physiol. London* 267: 703–735, 1972.
27. DEMPSEY, M. E., P. D. BOYER, AND E. S. BENSON. Characteristics of an orthophosphate oxygen exchange catalyzed by myosin, actomyosin and muscle fibers. *J. Biol. Chem.* 238: 2708–2715, 1963.
28. DUNAWAY-MARIANO, D., AND W. W. CLELAND. Investigations of substrate specificity and reaction mechanism of several kinases using chromium (III) adenosine 5′-triphosphate and chromium(III) adenosine 5′-diphosphate. *Biochemistry* 19: 1506–1515, 1980.
29. EARGLE, D. H., V. LICKO, AND G. L. KENYON. Kinetic studies of ^{18}O exchange of inorganic phosphate using mass spectral measurements on the tris-(trimethylsilyl) derivative. *Anal. Biochem.* 81: 186–195, 1977.
30. ECCLESTON, J. F., AND D. R. TRENTHAM. Studies of stable metal nucleotide complexes interacting with myosin subfragment 1. In: *Frontiers of Biological Energetics*, edited by P. L. Dutton, J. S. Leigh, and A. Scarpa. New York: Academic, 1978, p. 707–714.
31. ECKSTEIN, F. Phosphorothioate analogues of nucleotides. *Acc. Chem. Res.* 12: 204–210, 1979.
32. ECKSTEIN, F. Nucleotide analogues for the study of enzyme mechanism. *Trends Biochem. Sci.* 5: 157–159, 1980.
33. ECKSTEIN, F., AND R. S. GOODY. Synthesis and properties of diastereoisomers of adenosine 5′-*O*-(1-thiotriphosphate) and adenosine 5′-*O*-(2-thiotriphosphate). *Biochemistry* 15: 1685–1691, 1976.
34. EISENBERG, E., L. DOBKIN, AND W. W. KIELLEY. Heavy meromyosin: evidence for a refractory state unable to bind to actin in the presence of ATP. *Proc. Natl. Acad. Sci. USA* 69: 667–671, 1972.
35. EISENBERG, E., AND L. E. GREENE. The relation of muscle biochemistry to muscle physiology. *Annu. Rev. Physiol.* 42: 293–309, 1980.
36. EISENBERG, E., T. L. HILL, AND Y. CHEN. Cross-bridge model of muscle contraction. *Biophys. J.* 29: 195–227, 1980.
37. EISENBERG, E., AND W. W. KIELLEY. Evidence for a refractory state of heavy meromyosin and subfragment 1 unable to bind actin in the presence of ATP. *Cold Spring Harbor Symp. Quant. Biol.* 37: 145–152, 1972.
38. FERENCZI, M. A., E. HOMSHER, R. M. SIMMONS, AND D. R. TRENTHAM. Reaction mechanism of the magnesium ion-dependent adenosine triphosphatase of frog muscle myosin and subfragment 1. *Biochem. J.* 171: 165–175, 1978.
39. FINLAYSON, B., AND E. W. TAYLOR. Hydrolysis of nucleoside triphosphate by myosin during the transient state. *Biochemistry* 8: 802–810, 1969.
40. FRASER, A. B., E. EISENBERG, W. W. KIELLEY, AND F. D. CARSON. The interaction of heavy meromyosin and subfragment 1 with actin. Physical measurements in the presence and absence of adenosine triphosphate. *Biochemistry* 14: 2207–2214, 1975.
41. GEEVES, M. A., AND D. R. TRENTHAM. Protein-bound adenosine 5′-triphosphate: properties of a key intermediate of the magnesium-dependent subfragment 1 adenosinetriphosphatase from rabbit skeletal muscle. *Biochemistry* 21: 2782–2789, 1982.
42. GEEVES, M. A., M. R. WEBB, C. F. MIDELFORT, AND D. R. TRENTHAM. Mechanism of adenosine 5′-triphosphate cleavage by myosin: studies with oxygen 18-labeled adenosine 5′-triphosphate. *Biochemistry* 19: 4748–4754, 1980.
43. GOODMAN, B. A., AND J. B. RAYNOR. Electron spin resonance of transition metal complexes. *Adv. Inorg. Chem. Radiochem.* 13: 135–362, 1970.
44. GOODY, R. S., AND W. HOFMANN. Stereochemical aspects of the interaction of myosin and actomyosin with nucleotides. *J. Muscle Res. Cell Motil.* 1: 101–115, 1980.
45. GOODY, R. S., W. HOFMANN, AND M. KONRAD. On the structure of the myosin-ADP-Mg complex. *FEBS Lett.* 129: 169–172, 1981.
46. GOODY, R. S., W. HOFMANN, AND H. G. MANNHERZ. The binding constant of ATP to myosin S1 fragment. *Eur. J. Biochem.* 78: 317–324, 1977.
47. GOODY, R. S., K. C. HOLMES, H. G. MANNHERZ, J. BARRINGTON-LEIGH, AND G. ROSENBAUM. Cross-bridge conformation as revealed by X-ray diffraction studies of insect flight muscles with ATP analogues. *Biophys. J.* 15: 687–705, 1975.
48. HILL, T. L. Theoretical formalism for the sliding filament model of contraction of striated muscle. Part I. *Prog. Biophys. Mol. Biol.* 28: 267–340, 1974.
49. HILL, T. L. *Free Energy Transduction in Biology*. New York: Academic, 1977.
50. HUXLEY, A. F. Muscle structure and theories of contraction. *Prog. Biophys. Biophys. Chem.* 7: 255–318, 1957.
51. HUXLEY, A. F., AND R. NIEDERGERKE. Interference microscopy of living muscle fibres. *Nature London* 173: 971–973, 1954.
52. HUXLEY, H. E. The mechanism of muscular contraction. *Science* 164: 1356–1366, 1969.
53. HUXLEY, H. E., AND J. HANSON. Changes in the cross-striations of muscle during contraction and stretch and their structural interpretation. *Nature London* 173: 973–976, 1954.
54. INOUE, A., H. TAKENAKA, T. ARATA, AND Y. TONOMURA. Functional implications of the two-headed structure of myosin. *Adv. Biophys.* 13: 1–194, 1979.
55. JAFFE, E. K., AND M. COHN. Divalent cation-dependent stereospecificity of adenosine 5′-*O*-(2-thiotriphosphate) in the hexokinase and pyruvate kinase reactions. The absolute stereochemistry of the diastereoisomers of adenosine 5′-*O*-(2-thiotriphosphate). *J. Biol. Chem.* 253: 4823–4825, 1978.
56. JAFFE, E. K., AND M. COHN. ^{31}P nuclear magnetic resonance spectra of the thiophosphate analogues of adenine nucleotides; effects of pH and Mg^{2+} binding. *Biochemistry* 17: 652–657, 1978.
57. JAFFE, E. K., AND M. COHN. Diastereomers of the nucleoside phosphorothioates as probes of the structure of the metal nucleotide substrates and of the nucleotide binding site of yeast hexokinase. *J. Biol. Chem.* 254: 10839–10845, 1979.
58. JARVEST, R. L., AND G. LOWE. Synthesis of methyl (*R*)- and (*S*)-[^{18}O]phosphorothioates and determination of the absolute configuration at phosphorus of the diastereoisomers of adenosine 5′-(1-thiotriphosphate) *J. Chem. Soc. Chem. Commun.* 364–366, 1979.
59. JENCKS, W. P. Binding energy, specificity, and enzymic catalysis: the circe effect. *Adv. Enzymol.* 43: 219–410, 1975.
60. JENCKS, W. P. The utilization of binding energy in coupled vectorial processes. *Adv. Enzymol.* 51: 75–106, 1980.
61. JOHNSON, K. A., AND E. W. TAYLOR. The intermediate states of subfragment 1 and actosubfragment 1 ATPase—a reevaluation of the mechanism. *Biochemistry* 17: 3432–3442, 1978.
62. KARANDASHOV, E. A., N. A. BIRO, AND N. S. PANTELEEVA. ^{18}O-exchange reactions catalyzed by subfragment 1 of myosin molecule. *Biochemistry USSR* 41: 1185–1191, 1976.
63. KARN, J., L. BARNETT, AND A. D. MCLACHLAN. *Unc* 54 myosin heavy chain gene; genetic sequence structure. In: *The Molecular Control of Muscle Development*, edited by M. Pearson. Cold Spring Harbor, NY: Cold Spring Harbor, in press.
64. KNOWLES, J. R. Enzyme-catalyzed phosphoryl transfer reactions. *Annu. Rev. Biochem.* 49: 877–919, 1980.
65. KORMAN, E. F., AND J. MCLICK. Stereochemical reaction mechanism formulation for enzyme-catalyzed pyrophosphate hydrolysis, ATP hydrolysis, and ATP synthesis. *Bioorg. Chem.* 2: 179–190, 1973.
66. KULEVA, N. V., E. A. KARANDASHOV, AND N. S. PANTALEEVA. Effect of trinitrophenylation of myosin on the isotopic exchange reaction of oxygen in the myosin-ATP-H_2O^{18} system. *Biochemistry USSR* 35: 33–37, 1970.
67. LEVY, H. M., AND D. E. KOSHLAND. Mechanism of hydrolysis of adenosine triphosphate by muscle proteins. *J. Biol. Chem.* 234: 1102–1107, 1959.
68. LEVY, H. M., E. M. RYAN, S. S. SPRINGHORN, AND D. E. KOSHLAND. Further evidence for oxygen exchange at an inter-

mediate stage in myosin hydrolysis. *J. Biol. Chem.* 237: 1730–1731, 1962.

69. LEVY, H. M., N. SHARON, E. LINDEMANN, AND D. E. KOSHLAND. Properties of the active site in myosin hydrolysis of adenosine triphosphate as indicated by the O^{18}-exchange reaction. *J. Biol. Chem.* 235: 2628–2632, 1960.
70. LOWE, G., B. V. L. POTTER, B. S. SPROAT, AND W. E. HULL. The effect of ^{17}O and the magnitude of ^{18}O-isotope shift in ^{31}P nuclear magnetic resonance spectroscopy. *J. Chem. Soc. Chem. Commun.* 733–735, 1979.
71. LOWE, G., AND B. S. SPROAT. ^{18}O-isotope shifts on the ^{31}P nuclear magnetic resonance of adenosine 5′-phosphate and inorganic phosphate. *J. Chem. Soc. Chem. Commun.* 565–566, 1978.
72. LOWEY, S., H. S. SLAYTER, A. G. WEEDS, AND H. BAKER. Substructure of the myosin molecule. Subfragments of myosin by enzymatic degradation. *J. Mol. Biol.* 42: 1–29, 1969.
73. LUTZ, O., A. NOLLE, AND D. STASCHEWSKI. Oxygen isotope effect on ^{31}P NMR spectra in the phosphate ion. *Z. Naturforsch.* 33a: 380–382, 1978.
74. LYMN, R. W. Kinetic analysis of myosin and actomyosin ATPase. *Annu. Rev. Biophys. Bioeng.* 8: 145–163, 1979.
75. LYMN, R. W., AND E. W. TAYLOR. Transient state phosphate production in the hydrolysis of nucleoside triphosphates by myosin. *Biochemistry* 9: 2975–2983, 1970.
76. LYMN, R. W., AND E. W. TAYLOR. Mechanism of adenosine triphosphate hydrolysis by actomyosin. *Biochemistry* 10: 4617–4624, 1971.
77. MANDELKOW, E. M., AND E. MANDELKOW. Fluorometric studies on the influence of metal ions and chelators on the interaction between myosin and ATP. *FEBS Lett.* 33: 161–166, 1973.
78. MANNHERZ, H. G., H. SCHENCK, AND R. S. GOODY. Synthesis of ATP from ADP and inorganic phosphate at the myosin-subfragment 1 active site. *Eur. J. Biochem.* 48: 287–295, 1974.
79. MENDELSON, R. A., M. F. MORALES, AND J. BOTTS. Segmental flexibility of the S-1 moiety of myosin. *Biochemistry* 12: 2250–2255, 1973.
80. MERRITT, E. A., M. SUNDARALINGAM, R. D. CORNELIUS, AND W. W. CLELAND. X-ray crystal and molecular structure and absolute configuration of (dihydrogen tripolyphosphato)-tetraamminecobalt(III) monohydrate, $Co(NH_3)_4H_2P_3O_{10}\cdot H_2O$. A model for a metal-nucleoside polyphosphate complex. *Biochemistry* 17: 3274–3278, 1978.
81. MIDELFORT, C. F. On the mechanism of actomyosin ATPase from fast muscle. *Proc. Natl. Acad. Sci. USA* 78: 2067–2071, 1981.
82. MIDELFORT, C. F., AND I. A. ROSE. A stereochemical method for detection of ATP terminal phosphate transfer in enzymatic reactions. Glutamine synthetase. *J. Biol. Chem.* 251: 5881–5887, 1976.
83. MORNET, D., R. BERTRAND, P. PANTEL, E. AUDERMARD, AND R. KASSAB. Structure of the actin-myosin interface. *Nature London* 292: 301–306, 1981.
84. NIHEI, T., A. MENDELSON, AND J. BOTTS. Use of fluorescence polarization to observe changes in attitude of S-1 moieties in muscle fibers. *Biophys. J.* 14: 236–242, 1974.
85. PANTALEEVA, N. S., N. A. BIRO, E. A. KARANDASHOV, F. FABIAN, I. E. KRASOVSKAYA, N. V. KULEVA, AND E. G. SKVORTSEVICH. ^{18}O-exchange catalyzed by myosin, heavy meromyosin, heavy meromyosin subfragment 1 and their complexes with actin. *Acta Biochim. Biophys. Acad. Sci. Hung.* 12: 37–44, 1977.
86. PHILLIPS, R. Adenosine and the adenine nucleotides. Ionization, metal complex formation and conformation in solution. *Chem. Rev.* 66: 501–527, 1966.
87. PLIURA, D. H., D. SCHOMBURG, J. P. RICHARD, P. A. FREY, AND J. R. KNOWLES. Stereochemical course of a phosphokinase using a chiral [^{18}O]phosphorothioate. Comparison with the transfer of a chiral [$^{16}O,^{17}O,^{18}O$]phosphoryl group. *Biochemistry* 19: 325–329, 1980.
88. REED, G. H., AND T. S. LEYH. Identification of the six ligands to manganese(II) in transition-state-analogue complexes of creatine kinase: oxygen-17 superhyperfine coupling from selectively labeled ligands. *Biochemistry* 19: 5472–5480, 1980.
89. RICHARD, J. P., H.-T. HO, AND P. A. FREY. Synthesis of nucleoside [^{18}O]pyrophosphorothioates with chiral [^{18}O]phosphorothioate groups of known configuration. Stereochemical orientations of enzymatic phosphorylations of chiral [^{18}O]phosphorothioates. *J. Am. Chem. Soc.* 100: 7756–7757, 1978.
90. SARTORELLI, L., H. J. FROMM, R. W. BENSON, AND P. D. BOYER. Direct and ^{18}O-exchange measurements relevant to possible activated or phosphorylated states of myosin. *Biochemistry* 5: 2877–2884, 1966.
91. SHEU, K.-F. R., AND P. A. FREY. Enzymatic and ^{31}P nuclear magnetic resonance study of adenylate kinase-catalyzed stereospecific phosphorylation of adenosine 5′-phosphorothioate. *J. Biol. Chem.* 252: 4445–4448, 1977.
92. SHRIVER, J. W., AND B. D. SYKES. Phosphorus-31 nuclear magnetic resonance evidence for two conformations of myosin subfragment 1 nucleotide complex. *Biochemistry* 20: 2004–2012, 1981.
93. SHUKLA, K. K., AND H. M. LEVY. Comparative studies of oxygen exchange catalyzed by myosin, heavy meromyosin, and subfragment 1. Evidence that the γ-phosphoryl group of adenosine triphosphate binds to myosin in the region of the (subfragment 1)-(subfragment 2) hinge. *Biochemistry* 16: 5199–5206, 1977.
94. SHUKLA, K. K., AND H. M. LEVY. Evidence from oxygen exchange measurements for a cooperative interaction between the two heads of myosin. *Nature London* 266: 190–191, 1977.
95. SHUKLA, K. K., AND H. M. LEVY. Mechanism of oxygen exchange in actin-activated hydrolysis of adenosine triphosphate by myosin subfragment 1. *Biochemistry* 16: 132–136, 1977.
96. SHUKLA, K. K., AND H. M. LEVY. Oxygen exchange by single-headed myosin. *J. Biol. Chem.* 253: 8362–8365, 1978.
97. SHUKLA, K. K., H. M. LEVY, F. RAMIREZ, J. F. MARECEK, S. MEYERSON, AND E. S. KUHN. Distribution of [^{18}O]P_i species from [γ-^{18}O]ATP hydrolysis by myosin and heavy meromyosin. *J. Biol. Chem.* 255: 11344–11350, 1980.
98. SLEEP, J. A. Single turnovers of ATP by myofibrils and actomyosin subfragment 1. *Biochemistry* 20: 5043–5051, 1981.
99. SLEEP, J. A., AND P. D. BOYER. Effect of actin concentration on the intermediate oxygen exchange of myosin: relation to the refractory state and the mechanism of exchange. *Biochemistry* 17: 5417–5422, 1978.
100. SLEEP, J. A., D. D. HACKNEY, AND P. D. BOYER. Characterization of phosphate oxygen exchange reactions catalyzed by myosin through measurement of the distribution of ^{18}O-labeled species. *J. Biol. Chem.* 253: 5235–5238, 1978.
101. SLEEP, J. A., D. D. HACKNEY, AND P. D. BOYER. The equivalence of phosphate oxygens for exchange and the hydrolysis characteristics revealed by the distribution of [^{18}O]P_i species formed by myosin and actomyosin ATPase. *J. Biol. Chem.* 255: 4094–4099, 1980.
102. SLEEP, J. A., AND R. L. HUTTON. Actin mediated release of ATP from a myosin-ATP complex. *Biochemistry* 17: 5423–5430, 1978.
103. SLEEP, J. A., AND S. J. SMITH. Actomyosin ATPase and muscle contraction. *Curr. Top. Bioenerg.* 11: 239–286, 1981.
104. STEIN, L. A., P. B. CHOCK, AND E. EISENBERG. Mechanism of the actomyosin ATPase: effect of actin on the ATP hydrolysis step. *Proc. Natl. Acad. Sci. USA* 78: 1346–1350, 1981.
105. STEIN, L. A., R. P. SCHWARZ, P. B. CHOCK, AND E. EISENBERG. Mechanism of actomyosin adenosine triphosphatase. Evidence that adenosine 5′-triphosphate hydrolysis can occur without dissociation of the actomyosin complex. *Biochemistry* 18: 3895–3909, 1979.
106. SWANSON, J. R., AND R. G. YOUNT. The properties of heavy meromyosin and myosin catalyzed "medium" and "intermediate" ^{18}O-phosphate exchange. *Biochem. Z.* 345: 395–409, 1966.

107. SZENT-GYORGYI, A. Discussion. *Stud. Inst. Med. Chem. Univ. Szeged. (1941–42)*, 1: 67–71, 1943.
108. TAYLOR, E. W. Transient phase of adenosine triphosphate hydrolysis by myosin, heavy meromyosin, and subfragment 1. *Biochemistry* 16: 732–740, 1977.
109. TAYLOR, E. W. Mechanism of actomyosin ATPase and the problem of muscle contraction. *Crit. Rev. Biochem.* 6: 103–164, 1979.
110. TAYLOR, R. S., AND A. G. WEEDS. Transient-phase of ATP hydrolysis by myosin subfragment 1 isoenzymes. *FEBS Lett.* 75: 55–60, 1977.
111. THOMAS, D. D., J. C. SEIDEL, J. S. HYDE, AND J. GERGELY. Motion of subfragment-1 in myosin and its supramolecular complexes: saturation transfer electron paramagnetic resonance. *Proc. Natl. Acad. Sci. USA* 72: 1729–1733, 1975.
112. THOMAS, D. D., S. I. SHIWATA, J. C. SEIDEL, AND J. GERGELY. Submillisecond rotational dynamics of spin-labeled myosin heads in myofibrils. *Biophys. J.* 32: 873–890, 1980.
113. TRENTHAM, D. R. The adenosine triphosphatase reactions of myosin and actomyosin and their relation to energy transduction in muscle. *Biochem. Soc. Trans.* 5: 5–22, 1977.
114. TRENTHAM, D. R., R. G. BARDSLEY, J. F. ECCLESTON, AND A. G. WEEDS. Elementary processes of the magnesium ion-dependent adenosine triphosphatase activity of heavy meromyosin. *Biochem. J.* 126: 635–644, 1972.
115. TRENTHAM, D. R., J. F. ECCLESTON, AND C. R. BAGSHAW. Kinetic analysis of ATPase mechanisms. *Q. Rev. Biophys.* 9: 217–281, 1976.
116. TRYBUS, K. M., AND E. W. TAYLOR. Kinetics of ADP and AMP-PNP binding to SF-1. *Biophys. J.* 25: 21a, 1979.
117. TSAI, M.-D. Use of phosphorus-31 nuclear magnetic resonance to distinguish bridge and nonbridge oxygens of oxygen-17-enriched nucleoside triphosphates. Stereochemistry of acetate activation by acetyl coenzyme A synthetase. *Biochemistry* 18: 1468–1472, 1979.
118. WATTERSON, J. G., AND M. C. SCHAUB. Conformational differences in myosin. II. Evidence for differences in the conformation induced by bound or hydrolyzed adenosine triphosphate. *Hoppe-Seyler's Z. Physiol. Chem.* 354: 1619–1625, 1973.
119. WEBB, M. R. A method for determining the positional isotope exchange in a nucleoside triphosphate: cyclization of nucleoside triphosphate by dicyclohexylcarbodiimide. *Biochemistry* 19: 4744–4748, 1980.
120. WEBB, M.R. The stereochemical course of nucleoside triphosphatase reactions. *Methods Enzymol.* In press.
121. WEBB, M. R., D. E. ASH, T. S. LEYH, D. R. TRENTHAM, AND G. H. REED. Electron paramagnetic resonance studies of Mn(II) complexes with myosin subfragment 1 and oxygen-17 labeled ligands. *J. Biol. Chem.* 257: 3068–3072, 1982.
122. WEBB, M. R., G. G. MCDONALD, AND D. R. TRENTHAM. Kinetics of oxygen-18 exchange between inorganic phosphate and water catalyzed by myosin subfragment 1, using the ^{18}O shift in ^{31}P NMR. *J. Biol. Chem.* 253: 2908–2911, 1978.
123. WEBB, M. R., AND D. R. TRENTHAM. Analysis of chiral inorganic [^{16}O, ^{17}O, ^{18}O]thiophosphate and the stereochemistry of the 3-phosphoglycerate kinase reaction. *J. Biol. Chem.* 255: 1775–1779, 1980.
124. WEBB, M. R., AND D. R. TRENTHAM. The stereochemical course of phosphoric residue transfer during the myosin ATPase reaction. *J. Biol. Chem.* 255: 8629–8632, 1980.
125. WEBB, M. R., AND D. R. TRENTHAM. The stereochemical course of phosphoric residue transfer catalyzed by sarcoplasmic reticulum ATPase. *J. Biol. Chem.* 256: 4884–4887, 1981.
126. WEBB, M. R., AND D. R. TRENTHAM. The mechanism of ATP hydrolysis catalyzed by myosin and actomyosin using rapid reaction techniques to study oxygen exchange. *J. Biol. Chem.* 256: 10910–10916, 1981.
127. WESTHEIMER, F. H. Pseudorotation in the hydrolysis of phosphate esters. *Acc. Chem. Res.* 1: 70–78, 1968.
128. WHITE, D. C. S., AND J. THORSON. The kinetics of muscle contraction. *Prog. Biophys. Mol. Biol.* 27: 175–255, 1973.
129. WHITE, H. D., AND E. W. TAYLOR. Energetics and mechanism of actomyosin adenosine triphosphatase. *Biochemistry* 15: 5818–5826, 1976.
130. WOLCOTT, R. G., AND P. D. BOYER. On the nature of *p*-nitrothiophenylated myosin. *Biochim. Biophys. Acta* 303: 292–297, 1973.
131. WOLCOTT, R. G., AND P. D. BOYER. The reversal of the myosin and actomyosin ATPase reactions and the free energy of ATP binding to myosin. *Biochem. Biophys. Res. Commun.* 57: 709–716, 1974.
132. WOLCOTT, R. G., AND P. D. BOYER. Isotopic probes of catalytic steps of myosin adenosine triphosphatase. *J. Supramol. Struct.* 3: 154–161, 1975.
133. YEE, D., AND F. ECKSTEIN. Phosphorothioate analogues of ATP as substrates for myosin ATPase. *Hoppe-Seyler's Z. Physiol. Chem.* 361: 353–354, 1980.
134. YEE, D., AND F. ECKSTEIN. Structure of the metal-nucleotide chelate in the myosin-product complex. *FEBS Lett.* 112: 10–12, 1980.
135. YOUNG, J. J., M. MCLICK, AND E. F. KORMAN. Pseudorotation mechanism of ATP hydrolysis in muscle contraction. *Nature London* 249: 474–476, 1974.
136. YOUNT, R. G., AND D. E. KOSHLAND. Properties of O^{18} exchange reaction catalyzed by heavy meromyosin. *J. Biol. Chem.* 238: 1708–1713, 1963.

CHAPTER 9

Conformational changes and molecular dynamics of myosin

JOHN GERGELY
JOHN C. SEIDEL

Department of Muscle Research, Boston Biomedical Research Institute; Department of Neurology, Massachusetts General Hospital; and Departments of Neurology and Biological Chemistry, Harvard Medical School, Boston, Massachusetts

CHAPTER CONTENTS

BEFORE REVIEWING THE ROLE of conformational changes in the dynamics of myosin and muscle contraction, conformation and conformational changes must be clarified. A. F. Huxley (58), echoing the feelings of many, suggests the word *conformational* has little meaning, indicating only that the word *change* will follow. Nevertheless, following current practice, we use *conformation* and *conformational* in a sense roughly equivalent to *structure* and *structural.* Changes that occur on interaction of two or more molecules can range from a shift in the position of a few atoms only a few angstroms to a structural rearrangement that changes the shape and length of the molecule. Such major changes occur in the transition from the α-helix to a random coil in proteins, the transition of a polymer from a stretched to a randomly coiled state, or in the melting of the double helix of deoxyribonucleic acid (DNA). The latter illustrates a further complexity, viz., the change in the quaternary structure, involving changes in subunit-subunit interactions, which also take place in multichain proteins.

Early theories of muscle contraction relied on concepts developed by polymer chemists and involved large changes in structure, such as a transition between an extended and a coiled form. On the basis of X-ray–diffraction studies, Astbury (6), who dealt with muscle before the development of the sliding-filament model (59, 65), proposed that such extensive rearrangements of structure do not occur in muscle contraction.

Engelhardt and Lyubimova (36) preceded the sliding-filament model with the discovery that what was then considered myosin catalyzes the hydrolysis of adenosine 5′-triphosphate (ATP), and the free energy from this reaction is converted to mechanical work. Straub (151) and Szent-Györgyi (155) and their colleagues showed that what Engelhardt and Lyubimova had regarded as myosin was myosin-actin complex. Some 10 years later myosin and actin were recognized as the chief components of the two sets of filaments.

The sliding-filament model presupposes a cyclic interaction between myosin and actin accompanied by ATP hydrolysis and resulting in a changed overlap between the myosin and actin filaments (see the chapters by Haselgrove and Pepe in this *Handbook*) without permanent changes in the shape and size of the myosin and actin molecules. Changes attributed earlier to shape changes in myosin (123) are now recognized as changes in the myosin-actin association (42, 177).

Transient conformational changes of interest involve changes in the relative position of parts within the myosin molecule and changes in the relation of parts within the myosin molecule and the actin filament. Changes that occur on a smaller scale within the myosin structure because of its interaction with actin and with small molecules such as ATP and metal ions are also of interest. The cyclic changes in myosin and actin and in their interaction occur on a millisecond and submillisecond time scale and are in essence motions. The relation of such inter- and intramolecular motions to the physiological phenomena of contraction and tension development poses some exciting problems.

As techniques have been refined and new methods developed, researchers have studied changes in submolecular and supramolecular structures with optical techniques, nuclear magnetic resonance (NMR), electron paramagnetic resonance (EPR), and refined electron-microscopic and X-ray methods.

In current models (theories) of muscle contraction, myosin is the more dynamic moiety. We first discuss some of the structural and functional features of myosin and then its interaction with ATP and actin. One important current concern is the site of force generation; although considerable evidence places it in the region of actin-myosin interaction, recent evidence favors a force-generating mechanism based on structural changes wholly within the myosin molecule.

Another unresolved problem is the relation, on the molecular level, of the elastic element and the force generator. Are the two functions localized in the same part of the myosin molecule, are they found in structurally distinct elements of myosin, or are they not found in the same molecule but distributed between myosin and actin?

MYOSIN STRUCTURE

Subunits

Myosin (M_r 480,000) consists of six polypeptide chains. Two heavy chains (M_r 200,000) form a coiled-coil helical tail region with a length of ~150 nm and separate into two globular heads that contain the adenosine triphosphatase (ATPase) and actin-binding sites. (39, 44, 85, 88). In rabbit skeletal muscle myosin each head contains one 18,000-M_r light chain referred to as LC_2 or the DTNB light chain [removed by 5,5′-dithiobis(2-nitrobenzoate)] and one alkali light chain (removed at alkaline pH). In fast-twitch muscle the latter is the 25,000-M_r LC_1, referred to as A1, or the 16,000-M_r LC_3, A2 (87, 134, 178). The quoted M_r of LC_1 is only an apparent value, which is based on electrophoretic mobility on sodium dodecyl sulfate–containing gels. The true M_r deduced from the amino acid sequence is 21,000 (177a).

PROTEOLYTIC FRAGMENTS. Proteolytic enzymes cleave myosin without destroying its enzymatic activity and produce well-defined fragments: heavy meromyosin (HMM), light meromyosin (LMM), subfragment 1 (S1), subfragment 2 (S2), or myosin rod (40, 41, 43, 105, 130, 156). Papain cleaves the molecule at the junction between the tail and head regions, which forms two S1s, each corresponding to a single head, and the coiled-coil myosin rod (81, 88), corresponding to the tail (Fig. 1). Cleavage with trypsin (156) or chymotrypsin (43) produces HMM (M_r 350,000), consisting of the two heads attached to a short piece of the rod, and LMM (M_r 120,000), representing the remainder of the tail (88). The latter makes up the backbone of the myosin filament in vivo. Subfragment 1 is also obtainable by tryptic digestion of HMM (119). Subfragment 2 corresponds to that part of rod that in situ connects the head and core of the myosin filament (84). Recently researchers have shown that, depending on the conditions of digestion, a shorter and longer form of S2 is obtained (89, 152, 179), the two differing at their COOH-terminal end.

With further tryptic or chymotryptic digestion that portion of the heavy chain that is in the head gives rise to smaller well-characterized fragments. Starting at the NH_2-terminal end these fragments have been referred to as the 25,000-, 50,000-, and 20,000-M_r peptides (11, 114, 115, 185–187). Some uncertainty exists with regard to the precise molecular weight of these fragments; some authors refer to the first two fragments as 27,000- or 51,000-M_r fragments and to the 20,000-M_r fragment as 21,000- or 22,000-M_r fragments. Researchers have also shown that the 27,000- (25,000) and 20,000-M_r fragments are formed by the breakdown of the slightly larger 29,000- (27,000-) and 27,000-M_r peptides, respectively [Fig. 2; (56, 114, 115)]. Important functions of myosin and preferentially reacting residues have been identified in the fragments. We discuss these in more detail next.

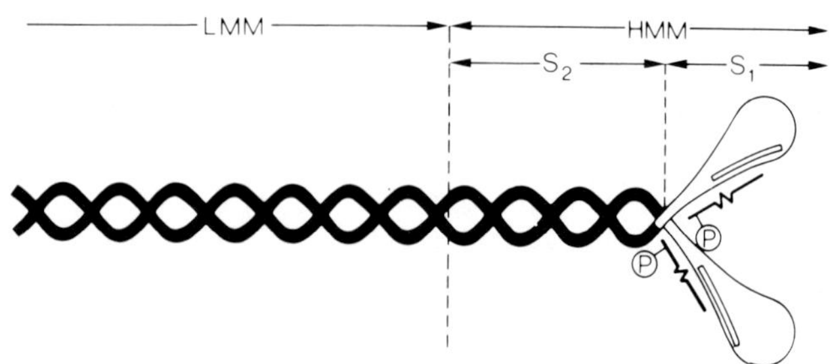

FIG. 1. Myosin molecule showing points (*broken lines*) at which limited proteolysis results in formation of stable fragments. Elongated light chain subunits possibly interact with region of S1-S2 junction. Phosphorylatable light chain Ⓟ is LC_2 of skeletal muscle or LC_1 of smooth muscle. Hinge regions postulated at S1-S2 junction and S2-LMM junction. Intertwined heavy chains, α-helical regions. Not drawn to scale. [From Kendrick-Jones and Scholey (79).]

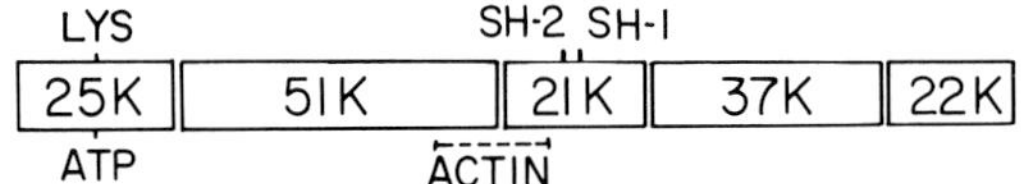

FIG. 2. Alignment of proteolytic fragments of heavy chain in S1 region and adjacent rod portion. Putative localization of ATP- and actin-binding sites and established location of reactive lysine, SH1 groups, and SH2 groups. The 37,000-M_r fragment is subunit of shorter S2. The 22,000-M_r fragment is putative hinge region lost in formation of short S2.

Actin Interaction Site

Isolating the S1 able to bind to actin (119) established that the actin-binding site is in the myosin head. Recent work has produced more detailed information on the location of this functionally important site. Yamamoto and Sekine (186) and Mornet et al. (114, 116) have shown that actin inhibits the proteolytic cleavage in the myosin head at the junction of the 50,000- and 22,000-M_r fragments. Conversely, after the split at the junction of the 50,000- and 22,000-M_r fragment, actin cannot activate the ATPase of S1, although cleavage at the junction of the NH_2- terminal end of the 25,000- and 50,000-M_r fragment leaves the activation essentially intact. Mornet et al. have also shown that it is not the cleavage at the junction of the 50,000 and 22,000-M_r peptide but the further degradation at the COOH-terminal end of the 22,000-M_r fragment that forms a slightly smaller 20,000-M_r fragment that leads to the loss of activation by actin.

Cross-linking of S1 and actin (115) with a soluble carbodiimide cross-linker that produces direct cross-linking between amino and carboxyl groups (0-length cross-linker) shows that both the 50,000-M_r region and the 20,000-M_r region of S1 are in contact with actin, which throws new light on the way myosin may bind to actin. Subfragment 1 binds to two actin monomers; when the actin and S1 are mixed in a ratio of 1:1, each actin monomer would be in contact with two S1s (Fig. 3). Cross-linking experiments show that the two S1s binding to the same pair of actins differ in their ability to be cross-linked by the soluble carbodiimide on activation of the actin carboxylates. The first S1 to bind to a given actin pair was readily cross-linked; the second, although bound, was a poor candidate for cross-linking. This weaker cross-linkability has been interpreted as resulting from a change in the actin monomers induced by S1 binding.

MYOSIN INTERACTION WITH ATP AND ITS ANALOGUES

Conformational Changes

Efforts have been made to define the changes in myosin structure that result from interaction with ATP. Because ATP or its analogues do not change the hydrodynamic properties of myosin or produce an appreciable change in the optical rotation or circular dichroism, whatever conformational changes take place are restricted to relatively small local regions of the molecule and do not significantly affect the polypeptide backbone of the molecule (46, 86). Recently ATP and analogues such as adenosine 5′-diphosphate (ADP) and inorganic pyrophosphate (PP_i) have been shown to produce differential changes in the rate of various steps at which limited enzymatic proteolysis takes place, resulting in the fragments discussed in PROTEOLYTIC FRAGMENTS, p. 258 (1, 108, 120, 159). This suggests that, although small, the conformational changes produced by these ligands may occur in regions at some distance from each other in the primary and possibly in the tertiary structure.

Ultraviolet Spectral Changes

The demonstration by Morita and Yagi (112, 113) of an ultraviolet difference spectrum on addition of ATP to HMM that decayed to the spectrum produced by ADP when ATP hydrolysis was complete not only indicated a localized conformational change induced by the ATP but furnished evidence for a structural change in myosin closely coupled with the enzymatic reaction. Morita and Yagi attributed changes in the ultraviolet absorption spectrum of HMM or S1 to changes in the absorption of tyrosine and tryptophan residues of the protein. Because the rate of decay of the ATP-induced spectral change agreed well with that expected from the rate of ATP hydrolysis, they interpreted the difference spectrum in terms of the formation of an enzyme-ATP complex, believed to be the predominant species during the steady state of ATP hydrolysis.

Electron Paramagnetic Resonance Spectra

Spectral changes correlated with the steady state of ATP hydrolysis were also revealed by EPR spectros-

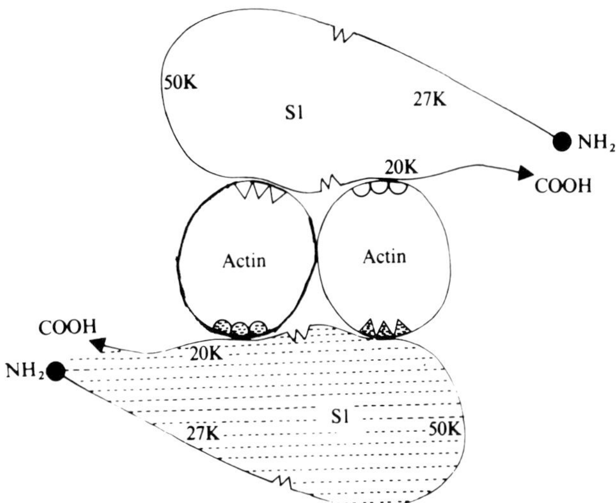

FIG. 3. Attachment of myosin head to 2 monomers in actin filaments. [From Mornet et al. (115). Reprinted by permission from *Nature*, copyright 1981 Macmillan Journals Limited.]

copy of myosin, HMM, or S1, spin labeled at the SH1 sulfhydryl group with a nitroxide free-radical–containing thiol reagent [see *Cysteine Residue Modification*, p. 261; (141, 142)] and by changes in the intrinsic tryptophan fluorescence of HMM (185). Both the changes in the EPR spectra and in fluorescence appear to reflect the same conformational change in the molecule; minor differences in the dependence on pH or ionic strength appear to be attributable to the introduction of the covalently bound spin label necessary for EPR measurements (140). The nature of the chemical state of myosin producing the altered EPR spectrum and fluorescence was interpretable in the light of kinetic studies on myosin-catalyzed hydrolysis of ATP. These studies showed that the hydrolysis of the terminal phosphate of ATP bound to the enzyme occurred much more rapidly (the so-called P_i burst; see the chapter by Webb and Trentham in this *Handbook*) than the dissociation of the resulting products; thus the predominant chemical species of myosin present during steady-state hydrolysis was recognized as a complex of the hydrolytic products ADP and P_i with myosin (92). The EPR spectrum and the enhanced fluorescence observed during the steady state differed from the corresponding spectral properties of the complex formed with added ADP and P_i, which led to the conclusion that the steady-state complex differed in conformation from the substrate enzyme or the final product complex.

Relation to ATPase Mechanism

Analysis of the kinetics of spectral changes accompanying ATP hydrolysis and comparison with spectral changes induced by nonhydrolyzable analogues of ATP and by analogues whose hydrolysis is characterized by the predominance of a substrate complex during the steady-state hydrolysis suggest that ATP itself induces a conformational change. This change takes place in two stages. The nonhydrolyzable analogue 5′-adenylyl imidodiphosphate [AMPPNP; (190, 191)] produces a spectral change similar to that produced by ADP (185). Results with adenosine 5′-*O*-(3-thiotriphosphate) (ATPγS) (45), which does not give rise to an initial burst of P_i liberation and does not produce maximal changes in fluorescence (7, 8) or EPR (143), suggest that the myosin substrate complex produces a smaller spectral change than does the product complex formed by hydrolysis and that the remaining spectral and conformational changes accompany the hydrolytic step. Direct kinetic studies showing that the increase in tryptophan fluorescence can be biphasic support this suggestion. The binding of ATP to myosin, which takes place in two steps, is accompanied by only part of the increase in fluorescence intensity. A final increase accompanies the hydrolytic step (71, 162).

The presence of an NH_2 group at position 6 of the nucleotide is essential for the full change in fluorescence. Nucleotides lacking this group produce small changes in fluorescence, ultraviolet absorption, or EPR, but the initial P_i burst is the same as with ATP (140). Inosine 5′-triphosphate (ITP) produces less tension in glycerinated fibers (49) than ATP, suggesting that the conformational change reflected in the fluorescence change may play a role in the force-generating process.

The conformation induced during steady-state hydrolysis requires the presence of a divalent metal ion, Mg^{2+} or Ca^{2+}, probably bound as a complex with the products ADP and P_i (93) to the enzymatic site as distinct from the divalent metal-binding site on the Nbs_2 light chain (9). The possibility that metal binding to the latter may be involved in the regulation of actin-myosin interaction has been raised. However, EPR studies on Mn^{2+} binding indicate that the dissociation of Ca^{2+} or Mg^{2+} from LC_2 is too slow to account for the rapid activation of muscle and tends to exclude LC_2 involvement in regulation (10).

The following abbreviated scheme, based on spectroscopic and kinetic studies of the interaction of ATP and its analogues with myosin, HMM, and S1, illustrates the conformational changes associated with ATP hydrolysis

$$\mathrm{M} + \mathrm{ATP} \rightleftharpoons \mathrm{M}^{*}\cdot\mathrm{ATP} \rightleftharpoons \mathrm{M}^{**}\cdot\mathrm{ADP}\cdot\mathrm{P_i} \rightleftharpoons \mathrm{M}^{*}\cdot\mathrm{ADP} \rightleftharpoons \mathrm{M} + \mathrm{ADP} + \mathrm{P_i}$$

The scheme includes three distinct forms of myosin (M, M*, and M**) having different spectral and conformational properties [see the chapter by Webb and Trentham in this *Handbook*; (162)]. It has been assumed that actin interacts with the M** complex, accelerating the release of products (162), but more recent evidence suggests that actin may interact with the ATP complex and the rate-limiting step may be the release of P_i (19).

Shriver and Sykes (146, 147) propose a classification of myosin states or conformations on the basis of ^{31}P NMR spectra of ADP and AMPPNP bound to S1. They suggest that two myosin states—reflected by the chemical shift (i.e., the spectral position) of the β-phosphorus resonance of the ligand—exist in a temperature-dependent equilibrium. These two states would not differ in fluorescence, but each of the states distinguishable by fluorescence could exist in two substates, each having a distinct NMR spectrum. Following the nomenclature for allosteric systems (108a), Shriver and Sykes propose a relaxed (R) and tense (T) state for myosin (cf. ref. 99); at a given temperature the relative population of the R and T states is different in different intermediate states of the ATPase cycle (see the chapter by Webb and Trentham in this *Handbook*). Shriver and Sykes suggest that R and T states may correspond to the conformation of the cross bridge when it is attached with a 90° or 45° attitude, respectively, to the actin filament. If this is true, a conformational state would exist in an isolated myosin head that would produce an optimal fit in one or the other attitude on attachment to actin; this suggestion need not imply that detached myosin cross bridges assume a preferred orientation. The unchanged rotational motion of myosin heads on nucleotide binding (100) is evidence against this preferred orientation. The views of Morales and Botts (110), who suggest that geometrically distinguishable attitudes of attached cross bridges correspond to different chemical states, appear to differ from those of Shriver and Sykes. More experimental and theoretical work is needed in this area.

Rod Conformational Changes

Recently researchers have shown that large conformational changes in the rod portion of smooth muscle myosin are deducible from various physicochemical measurements (153, 171) and directly demonstrable by electron micrographs of rotary-shadowed preparations (125, 171). The change occurs readily when the ionic strength in the presence of ATP is varied. At ionic strengths up to 0.2 M a form sedimenting at 10*S* dominates; at higher ionic strength a 6*S* peak is found. The 10*S* form was earlier thought to be caused by a dimer (154); it is now clear that it represents the folded form of the myosin molecule recognizable in electron micrographs. Folding of the tail of the smooth muscle myosin molecule occurs at two points, roughly dividing the rod into three equal portions. The hinge closest to the head-rod junction roughly corresponds to the skeletal myosin site at which bending may occur (53, 54). The ATP effect, which produces the 6*S*–10*S* transition, is most clear at an ionic strength of 0.2 M, where no aggregation occurs even in ATP absence (153). At lower ionic strength the effect is less clear because, in the absence of ATP, myosin aggregates and no 6*S* form is visible. With addition of ATP, aggregates disappear and the 10*S* species is formed. With arterial myosin (171) the 10*S* form is observed at 0.15 M KCl, even in the absence of ATP. Phosphorylation of both smooth muscle (154) and nonmuscle myosin (139) promotes filament formation and increases the resistance of filaments to ATP dissociation, suggesting that the control of filament formation by phosphorylation may play a role in the control of contraction (79). Electron-microscopic studies, however, show that in relaxed smooth muscle, myosin filaments, although dephosphorylated, do exist (149). This indicates that—at least in smooth muscle—dephosphorylation does not result in filament disaggregation, and relaxation does not depend on the disaggregation of filaments. Several researchers are investigating the role of phosphorylation in changing the myosin conformation in smooth muscle and nonmuscle systems. One unresolved question is whether phosphorylation promotes filament formation from the folded 10*S* form by first changing the conformation or whether the conformational change occurs after phosphorylation-promoted aggregation. Large conformational changes in the smooth muscle myosin rod portion raise the question whether similar changes may occur in the skeletal system. The preferential enzymatic proteolysis that leads to the formation of well-defined fragments in striated muscle rod is interesting in this context (12, 90), suggesting that proteolytic sites may be potential folding sites.

CHEMICAL MODIFICATION

In addition to serving as attachment sites for molecular probes, sulfhydryl groups of myosin or other amino acid residues can serve as conformational probes in reactions with modifiers (137, 144). The modification rate of cysteine or lysine residues of myosin has been used to detect changes induced by ATP and substrate analogues.

Cysteine Residue Modification

Myosin contains two well-characterized classes of reactive thiols, SH1 and SH2, each heavy chain containing one of each group. The most reactive —SH in skeletal muscle myosin is the so-called SH1 group, whose blocking leads to an increase in Ca^{2+}-ATPase and a loss of K^+-ATPase activity in the presence of ethylenediaminetetraacetic acid (EDTA). The reactivity of the SH1 group is reduced when myosin is in the state corresponding to the dominant species during ATP hydrolysis (137). The reactivity of the so-called SH2 sulfhydryl groups of myosin with alkylating agents and other sulfhydryl modifiers is rather low in the absence of nucleotides but greatly enhanced by MgATP or MgADP (144). This increased reactivity again indicates a change in myosin conformation, but here, because ADP is more effective, a conformational state different from that dominant during the steady state of ATP hydrolysis is involved. Actin also influences the reactivity of myosin SH groups (72). In myofibrils or muscle fibers under relaxing conditions, i.e., with MgATP and ethylene glycol-bis(β-aminoethylether)-*N*,*N*′-tetraacetic acid (EGTA) present, the interaction of sulfhydryl modifiers with the SH1 groups of myosin is favored; in rigor the labeling of the actin cysteine 373 is found. In this respect PP_i is as effective as ATP. Kamayama et al. (73) also reported enhancement by F actin of the MgATP-induced reactivity of the SH2 group accompanied by conformational changes. The effect depends on the formation of the hydrolysis products of ATP, because AMPPNP is ineffective (72).

Nine residues in the primary structure (35), which are located in a region of the myosin molecule close to the S1–S2 junction, separate SH1 and SH2 (13). The two sulfhydryls, SH1 and SH2, as shown by cross-linking with bifunctional thiol reagents, are in close proximity in the three-dimensional structure of the molecule (17). Molecular models of cross-linkers suggest that the two thiols when cross-linked are 12–14 Å apart in the absence of nucleotides. However, in the presence of a nucleotide, shorter bifunctional reagents can also form cross-links, indicating the distance is reduced to 5–7 Å. Reaction with Nbs_2, which results in a disulfide bond between the two thiols, suggests that their distance can change to as little as 2 Å with Mg^{2+}ADP binding (184).

SUBSTRATE TRAPPING. Yount and his colleagues found that cross-linking of these two thiol groups also traps nucleotides at the active site, which may account for the altered circular dichroism (17) of the SH1-SH2 cross-linked protein, which is similar to that induced by ATP or ADP addition to the native protein. The trapped nucleotides are released slowly with a half-life of ~5 days; however, on denaturation of the protein they are immediately released, indicating that the binding is not covalent (183). The nucleotide is bound at the active site as evidenced by the lack of binding of AMPPNP, a competitive inhibitor of myosin ATPase activity, to the cross-linked S1. When [γ-^{32}P]ATP is trapped, the radioactivity is released into the medium, but the ADP becomes trapped. Substrate trapping can also be obtained with cobalt-phenanthroline complexes in which cobalt is believed to form a bridge between the two sulfhydryls. Chelation of the sulfhydryl groups by cobalt suggests that the two thiols can approach to within 3–5 Å of each other in the cross-linked product (181). Loss of enzymatic activity parallels the extent of cross-linking, and preblocking of SH1 with *N*-ethylmaleimide or the bifunctional *p*-*N,N′*-phenylenedimaleimide (*p*PDM) prevents cobalt incorporation and subsequent trapping of ATP, verifying the involvement of both SH1 and SH2 groups in the cross-linking.

The stoichiometric trapping of Mg^{2+} and ADP as a 1:1 complex is consistent with the Mg^{2+}-nucleotide being the true substrate of myosin (180), as suggested by kinetic studies of ATP hydrolysis (93). Other nucleoside diphosphates, including cytidine 5′-diphosphate (CDP), guanosine 5′-diphosphate (GDP), and P_i, can also be trapped in stoichiometric amounts (180).

Nucleotide trapping was originally ascribed to a conformational change involving movement of groups located near the nucleotide-binding site. Accumulating evidence favors the active site being within the 25,000-M_r NH_2- terminal stretch of the myosin heavy chain [56, 125a, 158]; any conformational change detected in the distance between the two —SH groups is thus likely to be coupled with other changes in the active-site region that may be located some distance away.

Lysine Modification

Myosin modification with 2,4,6-trinitrobenzenesulfonate (TNBS), producing trinitrophenylated lysine derivatives, led to new insights into myosin structure. Trinitrophenylation decreases both Ca^{2+}- (82) and K-EDTA–ATPase activity of myosin and abolishes the rapid P_i burst, indicating that one or more lysine groups modified by TNBS are either involved in the ATPase center or their modification leads to structural changes affecting ATPase activity. These results have been interpreted in terms of there being one specific, more reactive, lysine per heavy chain, with other lysine groups reacting at a slower rate. The counterpart of the modification of the ATPase activity by trinitrophenylation is the decrease in the reactivity of the lysine group(s) in the presence of ADP or PP_i, suggesting a conformational change brought about by nucleotide binding that changes the lysine reactivity (106).

A variety of pieces of evidence indicating structural differences between various myosin types, viz., skeletal, cardiac, smooth muscle, ventricular, and atrial myosin, are further supported by recently found differences in reactivity toward TNBS (121, 150). Thus the phosphate burst of smooth muscle myosin was unaffected by trinitrophenylation; the phosphate burst of cardiac and skeletal myosin was first decreased and eventually lost. Cardiac and smooth muscle myosins differ from skeletal myosin in that spectra of trinitrophenyl residues bound to cardiac or smooth muscle myosins do not change on addition of pyrophosphate in contrast to skeletal myosin behavior.

The rapidly reacting lysine group has recently been located in the NH_2-terminal fragment (M_r 27,000) of the heavy chain (56, 106, 117), a fragment that has been shown to react with a photoaffinity analogue of ATP (158). Yount and his co-workers showed that the same region is involved in the trapping of nucleotides (R. G. Yount, unpublished observations). Hozumi and Muhlrad (56) detected two peptides differing by ~M_r 2,000 in their proteolytic digests and suggest, on the basis of the effect of pyrophosphate on the incorporation of trinitrophenyl residues into the two fragments, that they come from the two kinds of heads postulated by Tonomura's group.

Hiratsuka (55) recently reported a lysine residue reactive with an anilinonaphthalenesulfonyl derivative in a 6,000-M_r stretch between S1 and S2 of cardiac myosin. The fluorescence of the label changes on binding of myosin to actin, suggesting an actin-induced conformational change in the hinge region that would be some 200 residues from the putative actin-binding site (see *Actin Interaction Site*, p. 259).

TWO-HEADED NATURE OF MYOSIN

Are the Two Myosin Heads Identical?

Tonomura and his colleagues concluded from various observations that the two heads in each myosin molecule are not identical and that the difference resides in the heavy chains and not in the alkali light chains (106). Myosin heads differing by the criteria of

Tonomura et al. (for a comprehensive review reflecting the views of the Tonomura school see ref. 68) contain both A1 and A2 light chains. They reported that 1 mol of lysine per mol of myosin head is rapidly modified in the absence of pyrophosphate, although only 0.5 mol of lysine is rapidly modified in its presence. By column chromatography they separated two kinds of myosin heads in the form of S1; one head contains the lysine whose reactivity is decreased by pyrophosphate, suggesting that pyrophosphate produces a conformation change leading to a "buried state" of the lysine in one head.

Inoue et al. (67) and Miyanishi et al. (106) found an initial burst of 1 mol P_i/mol of myosin in contrast to the initial burst found in most other laboratories, being close to 2 mol/mol (see the chapter by Webb and Trentham in this *Handbook*). They found that of the two types of heads, separated by chromatography, the one that contains the PP_i-sensitive lysine does not give rise to a P_i burst; the other head is characterized by a burst approaching 1 mol P_i/S_1 (67, 69). No other workers have reported the separation of burst and nonburst myosin heads. Also, most laboratories report a burst approaching 2 mol/mol of myosin. The proposed explanations (38) of this discrepancy require further investigation.

Interactions of the Two Myosin Heads

The question of the functional significance of the two heads of myosin has prompted much theoretical and experimental effort, which so far has not produced a satisfactory answer.

VERTEBRATE STRIATED MUSCLE. Tonomura and his colleagues have extensively discussed the implications of their evidence for the nonidentity of the heads (3, 67, 68). They suggest that the burst head (see *Are the Two Myosin Heads Identical?*, p. 262) is responsible for tension development and that the other head controls interaction. However, chemical inactivation (133, 169) or proteolytic removal of one head (25, 94, 95) failed to produce differences between molecules with one or two active heads. Single-headed myosins hydrolyzed ATP at the same rate as did native myosin; actomyosin threads developed the same tension whether they contained single- or double-headed myosin. All this does not prove that head-head interactions do not take place or, if they do, that they are not important but only that such interactions are not essential for ATP hydrolysis or the development of contractile force. Schaub and Watterson (135) have reviewed evidence, based primarily on differences in the affinities of the two heads for nucleotides or divalent metals that suggests head-head interactions in vertebrate skeletal or cardiac myosin (136, 138, 176). The differences have been interpreted in terms of a model in which the two heads function alternately; while one is bound and develops tension the other is free and hydrolyzes ATP (cf. ref. 68).

MOLLUSCAN MUSCLE. Perhaps the strongest evidence for interactions between the two heads of myosin comes from work on myosin of the scallop *Aequipecten irradians* or *Placopecten magellanicus* (83). The actin-activated ATPase of this myosin is dependent on Ca^{2+} binding to myosin in which a regulatory light chain plays a central role. Removal by EDTA of one light chain per myosin molecule from either of the two myosin heads results in complete loss of regulation by Ca^{2+}, viz., actin-activated ATPase activity is unaffected but is insensitive to Ca^{2+}. Removal of the regulatory light chain from glycerinated fibers also renders tension development insensitive to Ca^{2+} (148). Recombination of the regulatory light chain with the unregulated myosin can restore regulation (80, 157). There is no apparent preference for removing the regulatory light chain bound to one or the other heavy chain. This is shown by experiments with myosin from which the regulatory light chain is removed after recombination with a radioactively labeled light chain; a second EDTA treatment removed only 50% of the radioactivity (78). Regulatory light chains from other molluscan myosins or the phosphorylatable light chains of myosins from other species, including vertebrates, whose actin-activated ATPase activity does not depend on Ca^{2+} binding to myosin, can reactivate the desensitized myosin from which one light chain has been removed.

If EDTA treatment is carried out at higher temperatures (30°C) both regulatory light chains can be removed (21). In this case regulation can be restored only if one of the recombined light chains has been obtained from myosin whose actin-activated ATPase is regulated by Ca^{2+} (145). The fact that the ATPase activity of S1 is unregulated whether or not it contains a regulatory light chain indicates that the regulation in the molluscan system may involve the junction between S1 and S2 regions of the myosin molecule (21), whereas the activity of single-headed myosin is fully regulated by Ca^{2+} provided the regulatory light chain is present. Recent electron-microscopic studies on actin decorated with molluscan S1, with or without the regulatory light chain, also indicate that the latter effects the myosin neck region (27, 175). The requirement that Ca^{2+} must bind to both myosin heads before actin can activate the activity of either also manifests the interaction between the two heads (20).

SMOOTH MUSCLE. Interaction between the two heads of smooth muscle (gizzard) myosin is suggested by the fact that activation of myosin ATPase activity by actin requires enzymatic phosphorylation of both of its 20,000-M_r light chains (131) located in each of the two heads; viz., neither head is active until both are phosphorylated. The fact that phosphorylation is an ordered process, i.e., occurring in two steps with the addition of the first phosphate being more rapid, could be interpreted in terms of phosphorylation of the first head inhibiting that of the other. On the other hand, the two stages of phosphorylation might reflect an effect of the packing symmetry of the two heads in the myosin molecule or a difference in the two heavy chains. Attempts to show an effect on the ATPase activity of striated muscle actomyosin have been inconclusive since Perrie et al. (129) discovered phosphorylation of striated muscle myosin LC_2 (104, 111, 128). Recent reports that myosin phosphorylation may affect cross-bridge turnover in an organized system (26, 28) will undoubtedly stimulate work on this point.

MOLECULAR MECHANISM OF CROSS-BRIDGE CYCLE

Beginning with the model proposed by A. F. Huxley (57)—involving a "sidepiece" attached to some elastic structure in a portion of myosin—the idea that intramolecular motion in myosin is essential for the sliding of the filaments, and hence for muscle shortening or tension development, has become firmly established. H. E. Huxley (62) formulated this motion more realistically in 1969, taking into account the by then established features of the myosin molecule and of the thick filament structure. He postulated two flexible regions, one between S1 and S2 and the other between the LMM and S2 of the myosin molecule (Fig. 4). The first region would allow rotation of the bound head both with respect to the S2 connection and the thin filament point of attachment, where the force generation is postulated; the second would allow lateral

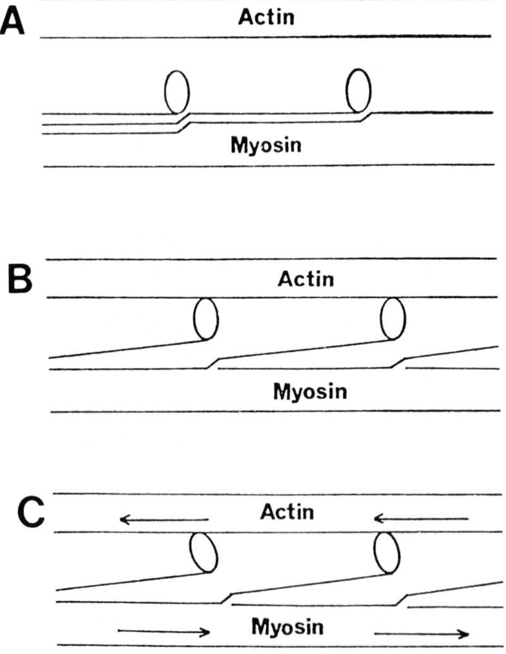

FIG. 4. Mechanism proposed for producing relative sliding movement of filaments. *A*: relaxed muscle. Cross bridges do not project far toward actin filament. *B*: during contraction or rigor, cross bridges attach to actin filament by bending at 2 flexible junctions. *C*: tilting of myosin head gives rise to movement of filaments past each other. [From H. E. Huxley (62). Copyright 1969 by the American Association for the Advancement of Science.]

movement of the cross bridge under conditions of shortening sarcomeres when the transverse distance between the thick and the thin filaments increases. Although it is customary to think of myosin heads attached to the thin filaments as carrying out rotational motion within certain angular limits relative to the filament axis, the actual situation may be more complicated. Several pieces of evidence raise questions about simple "rocking" models. Some of this evidence, such as the two-point attachment of the myosin heads to actin—which Amos et al. [Fig. 5; (2)] recently showed is compatible with three-dimensional reconstruction derived from electron micrographs—has already been alluded to (see *Actin Interaction Site*, p. 259). Other evidence on the behavior of probes under stretch is discussed in ORGANIZED SYSTEMS, p. 266. A. F. Huxley (58) also pointed out that other modes of molecular changes involving bending or stretching within myosin cannot be excluded.

Segmental Flexibility of Myosin

To understand muscle contraction at the molecular level requires information on segmental and global motions in myosin and on spatial and angular restrictions imposed on these motions by the geometry and molecular dynamics of the system. Regardless of the eventual model to be adopted, research on flexibility within the myosin molecules, either in their monomeric state or in their aggregated form, analogous to the thick filaments in vivo, has provided valuable insights. Lowey et al. (88) convincingly established the two-headed character of myosin in electron micrographs that clearly show the heads may assume different positions relative to the rod; this is also evident from recent electron micrographs of smooth muscle myosin (125, 171). Measurements of electric birefringence (53) producing an apparent length inconsistent with a rigid structure also support the existence of a flexible region in the rod corresponding to the second hinge. More recent work on the longer form of S2 (see PROTEOLYTIC FRAGMENTS, p. 258) localizes the flexible region within that part of the rod that spans ~40 nm from the S1-S2 hinge. Researchers have frequently noted that regions of higher proteolytic susceptibility in the myosin structure indicate a less rigid structure. It is therefore interesting that the myosin rod does contain a flexible region, as Burke et al. (16) deduced from comparing the temperature dependence of the optical rotation of the rod with that of LMM and de la Torre and Bloomfield (29) deduced from modeling the hydrodynamic properties of myosin. Subsequent studies have shown that the flexible region is in the longer but not in the shorter S2 (53, 172). Because the distance between the two forms of S2 has been found at the COOH-terminal end (89), the putative hinge can be located in that region ~40 nm from the first hinge. Recent work combining depolarized light scattering and proton magnetic resonance measurements

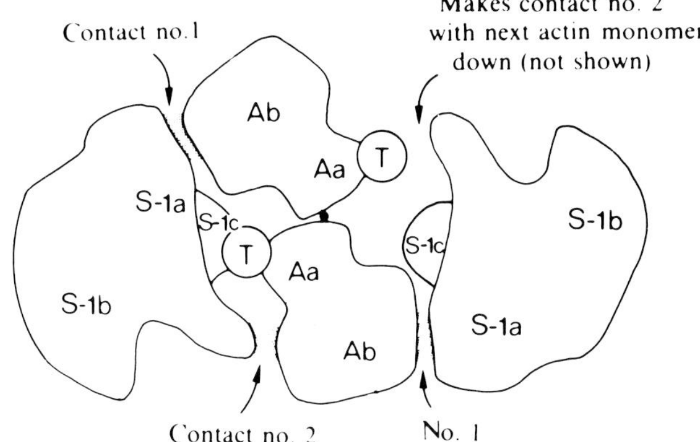

FIG. 5. Thin-filament structure permitting attachment of each myosin head to 2 actin monomers. [From Amos et al. (2). Reprinted by permission from *Nature*, copyright 1982 Macmillan Journals Limited.]

suggests that the flexible region is not made up of a random-coil structure (54). As discussed in *Rod Conformational Changes*, p. 261, according to electron-microscopic evidence the smooth muscle myosin rod contains two hinges. Electron micrographs reveal only one region in the striated muscle myosin rod that is consistent with a flexible hinge (34, 160).

Measurement of Correlation Time

MYOSIN AND ITS FRAGMENTS. Mendelson et al. (102) provided evidence for actual flexibility at the base of the myosin head by measuring the fluorescence-polarization decay of a probe bound to the head region of myosin or HMM. Although the molecular weights of myosin and S1 differ by a factor ≈5, the rotational correlation times of the bound probes differed by a factor ≤2. Measurements of correlation times by saturation transfer (ST) EPR, a modification of the EPR method sensitive to correlation times from 10^{-7} to 10^{-3} s (164) using rigidly bound spin label, gave the same relative values for the correlation times of myosin, HMM, and S1 (166, 168), confirming the results obtained by fluorescence (102). This indicates that the rotation of the principal magnetic axis of the spin label or the emission dipole of the fluorescent probe occurs about the short axis of an ellipsoidal S1. When assembled into filaments, spin-labeled or fluorescence-labeled myosin shows a 10- to 20-fold increase in the correlation time. Addition of ATP or Ca^{2+} does not change the correlation time of heads in myosin filaments monitored either by fluorescence-polarization decay (100) or ST EPR using a maleimide spin label (MSL) (168). Fortunately the MSLs that have been used in myosin studies do not respond to the local conformational changes produced by ATP (165) as does the iodoacetamide spin label (IASL) (141). Thus the MSL remains rigidly bound in the presence of ATP and its hydrolytic products and follows the motions of the protein or those of its segments. The effect on the correlation time of the assembly of myosin molecules into filaments may be related to the interactions proposed by Harrington and co-workers (see PROTEOLYSIS AS A CROSS-BRIDGE PROBE, p. 268) between myosin heads and rods of adjacent molecules making up the filament core.

INTERACTION WITH ACTIN. Saturation transfer EPR spectra of spin-labeled S1 bound to actin filaments have not shown rotational motion having correlation times <400 μs, the same correlation time being obtained when the spin probe is bound to actin complexed with unlabeled S1. The same results were obtained for acto-HMM, viz., the correlation time is the same whether the spin label was bound to HMM or to F actin. The observed correlation time is too fast to represent overall rotation of the complete actin filament and the attached myosin heads (167), which raises the possibility that reorientation of the myosin head in a contracting muscle fiber may be accompanied by reorientation of at least part of the actin monomer to which it is attached (cf. refs. 126, 127).

Local Fluctuations in Myosin Structure

Rigidity on the time scale of EPR experiments is consistent with limited local fluctuations in the head, which are most clearly demonstrated by the proton NMR spectra of S1 that exhibit a number of sharp peaks—representing highly mobile amino acid side chains—that disappear when S1 binds to actin (51, 52). Such rotations are characteristic of a number of proteins, suggesting a model for proteins, and are consistent with a model depicting a protein molecule as dense fluid composed of particles connected by flexible links (74–76). This type of local motion occurs on a nanosecond time scale, 10^{-8}–10^{-9} s. The fluctuations must involve relatively small linear displacement if S1 is to remain rigid on the microsecond to millisecond time scale. Kassab et al. (77), assuming that high susceptibility to proteolysis indicates a flexible structure, suggest that the residues responsible for the sharp peaks in the proton NMR spectrum of S1 attributable to their high mobility are localized in the 50,000/20,000-M_r joint region. The reported suppression of the rapid motions by actin would, according to them, fit the picture of actin interacting with that region. The fact, however, that titration with the paramagnetic ion Mn^{2+} or a negatively charged paramagnetic nitroxide compound failed to broaden to a significant extent the sharp peaks of S1 argues against the residues responsible for these peaks being on the surface (50, 52) and hence being accessible to proteolytic enzymes. Prince et al. (132) suggest that the most mobile residues are contributed by the A1 light chain and the difference between the spectra of S1 (A1) and S1 (A2) disappears with actin interaction. In this view the residues whose state is reflected in the NMR spectrum would not be at the proteolytic cleavage site.

ORGANIZED SYSTEMS

Motion of Myosin Heads

Selective and rigid spin labeling of the head of the myosin molecule in glycerinated myofibrils (70, 165) and glycerinated muscle fibers (163) has recently been achieved by methods used to attach fluorescent probes (31) to myosin or its fragments. For spin-labeled myofibrils in rigor the rotational correlation time of the heads is of the order of 1 ms, slightly longer than that for S1 bound to F actin. The long correlation time indicates either that at least 90% of the myosin heads in rigor are attached rigidly to the thin filaments or only 50% of the heads, one on each myosin molecule, are attached and they in turn immobilize the others. When ATP is added to labeled myofibrils the correlation time is reduced to that of myosin filaments. This short correlation time persists during the steady state when all the ATP has been hydrolyzed. During or after hydrolysis, Ca^{2+} does not affect the correlation time but simply shortens the time needed to return to the rigor state. In the presence of ATP the effect of Ca^{2+} reflects simply the acceleration of the actomyosin ATPase rate by Ca^{2+}. The same correlation time for rotation of the heads in the presence or absence of Ca^{2+}, within a 10% experimental error, suggests either that at least 90% of the myosin heads are detached or that the heads attached during the steady state of hydrolysis rotate faster than those in rigor.

Experiments have also been carried out under conditions yielding intermediate values for the correlation time, e.g., with nonhydrolyzable ligands such as pyrophosphate and AMPPNP. When the concentration of KCl, Ca^{2+}, and ATP analogues was varied and the temperature changed, the motional parameter changed in a manner suggesting that the rotation of heads is determined primarily by whether or not they are bound to the thin filaments, as shown with spin-labeled S1 by comparison of EPR data with the fraction of heads bound determined directly by sedimentation (70). These results may indicate that the bound heads rotate at a slower rate, which is determined by a motion within the thin filament, whereas the free heads rotate at the rapid rate characteristic of myosin filaments (167). Binding of pyrophosphate or AMPPNP to a head bound to actin does not alter its rotational motion while the head remains bound nor influence the rotation of a free head while it remains free but affects the rotation only indirectly, by changing the fraction of heads attached to the thin filaments. Whether ATP acts in the same manner as its analogues in influencing the rotation of the myosin head has not been determined.

Orientation of Myosin Heads

A considerable body of evidence is the basis of the swinging-cross-bridge–rotating-head theory. Early information on the rotational motion of cross bridges came from X-ray–diffraction and electron-microscopic studies (see the chapter by Haselgrove in this *Handbook*). Spectroscopic studies (109) began with the observation of Aronson and Morales (5) that the polarization of tryptophan fluorescence recorded from a muscle changed depending on whether the muscle was at rest, in rigor, or contracting. Dos Remedios et al. (30) showed that the perpendicular polarization ($P_{\perp}$) of fluorescence was greatest in relaxed muscle, decreased in contracting muscle, and further decreased in rigor when they obtained the same results with glycerinated rabbit psoas, glycerinated flight muscle of *Lethocerus americanus*, and living semitendinosus of *Rana pipiens*. With glycerinated psoas, $P_{\perp}$ increased with increasing sarcomere lengths when measurements were made on fibers in rigor but was not influenced by sarcomere length in resting muscle, i.e., in the presence of MgATP but absence of Ca^{2+}. Based on the distribution of tryptophan residues in myosin it was concluded that the changes in $P_{\perp}$ could be attributed to the S1 region and presumably represented changes in the S1 orientation.

Nihei et al. (124) obtained essentially similar results with a fluorescent dansyl label covalently bound to the S1 region, demonstrating that the differences in $P_{\perp}$ among rest, rigor, and contracting muscles depended on the presence of overlap between the thick and thin filaments. They concluded that the orientation of the cross bridge (i.e., S1) was dependent on the myosin-actin interaction. In the analysis of these data it was assumed that each value of $P_{\perp}$ represents a distinct orientation of the myosin head. However, as discussed in *Motion of Myosin Heads*, p. 266, EPR studies on myofibrils under resting conditions in the presence of MgATP and EGTA indicate that the S1 region is undergoing rapid rotational diffusion with rotational correlation times on the order of 1 μs (165) and cannot be considered to have a unique orientation. Therefore, $P_{\perp}$ must represent a time average of all the orientations in the S1 population. Some angular restriction for this rotational motion may exist, but the extent of such a restriction has yet to be established (101, 103, 163).

A recent approach used to study cross-bridge orientation involves measurement of linear dichroism of iodoacetyl tetramethyl rhodamine, which is either attached to myosin S1 diffused into glycerinated myofibrils or used for labeling in situ (14). In rigor, clear evidence for the orientation of the probe dipoles was found (80° relative to the myofibrillar axis). Relaxation or contraction abolished dichroism, suggesting cross-bridge disorder. A cross-bridge distribution intermediate between rigor and relaxation was imposed by MgAMPPNP and $MgPP_i$. Experiments with MgADP show a dichroic effect attributable to local conformational changes and point out possible problems with probes arising from the potential confusion of global changes in orientation or motion with local conformational changes resulting in changed probe motion—as already mentioned in MYOSIN AND ITS FRAGMENTS, p. 265.

X-ray–diffraction and electron-microscopic studies on glycerinated insect fibers in the presence of AMPPNP suggest that cross bridges remain attached but their orientation differs from that in rigor (91, 98); only the relaxed pattern is seen with ATP. Studies using EPR on glycerinated psoas fibers (163) and on glycerinated myofibrils (70) led to different results in that a fraction of the myosin heads appear dissociated, whereas those attached behave like rigor heads both with respect to motional (70) and orientational characteristics (163).

In glycerinated muscle fibers in rigor whose myosin heads had been selectively spin labeled with either IASL or MSL, Thomas and Cooke (163) obtained values of 68° and 82°, respectively, with conventional EPR spectroscopy, for the average angle between the fiber axis and the principal axis of the nitroxide spin label (NSL), with a narrow angular distribution within ~15° (163). The spectra support the conclusion that all heads in rigor are attached (165). Stretching the relaxed fibers or adding AMPPNP or PP_i resulted in an EPR spectrum reflecting increased disorientation of heads and suggesting that heads detach and undergo rotational motion on the submillisecond time scale (163). These results agree with measurements of the rotational motion of myosin heads by ST EPR (165) and suggest that AMPPNP and PP_i act by dissociating a fraction of the myosin heads. This view disagrees with the conclusion drawn from X-ray diffraction of glycerinated insect fibers (91, 98) that the effects of AMPPNP are attributable to changes in cross-bridge orientation and not to dissociation of a fraction of the cross bridges. Thomas and Cooke (163) argue that the rapid rotation of detached heads does not necessarily conflict with the appearance of well-defined reflections in the X-ray–diffraction pattern of muscles under relaxing conditions (63). They have estimated that angular fluctuations through an average angle of 45° relative to the fiber axis would not destroy the observed myosin layer lines. Moreover, a recent analysis, taking into account the relative orientation of the cross bridge and the principal axis of the probe, suggests that even with apparent disorder of the probe there may be considerable order in the cross-bridge arrangement. Thus the results of the EPR studies can be reconciled with the well-defined position of cross bridges in relaxed muscle indicated by the layer-line intensities in the X-ray pattern (cf. ref. 103).

The possibility that heads that remain bound to actin during ATP hydrolysis may rotate rapidly (165) cannot be ruled out but seems less likely in view of the finding that fluorescent (189) and EPR probes (24) on myosin heads that remain attached in contracting glycerinated psoas fibers assume the same well-defined angle with respect to the fiber axis as do those in rigor. Arata and Shimizu (4) also estimated the fraction of cross bridges attached to thin filaments in IASL fibers using conventional EPR, although this label does not remain rigidly immobilized in the presence of nucleotides (141–143) and thus may not provide information on orientation of heads or their rotational correlation time.

Without precise information on the relation of the probe's principal axis to the geometry of the macromolecule, e.g., S1, it is difficult to draw conclusions about the orientation of the macromolecule. Modeling studies allowing various angular distributions and motions of proteins and probes are useful in determining the limits of the predictive power of such measurements (103, 170). Torsional freedom about the S1 axis may produce considerable disorder of probe orientation even in the presence of significant order in the cross bridges themselves.

The apparent hydrodynamic rigidity of the head deduced from fluorescence (102) and EPR data (166, 168) is not inconsistent with experiments showing that when muscle fibers are stretched in rigor there is no change in the polarization of tryptophan fluorescence (30) or in the EPR spectrum of a spin label bound to the myosin head of stretched fibers (23). If a rigid S1 attached to actin is moving in a steep free-energy well (32), as Cooke (23) has pointed out, S2 may be stretched without changing the S1 pattern, a view consistent with the lack of change in the equatorial reflections in a stretched rigor muscle (122). On the other hand, if the attached S1 is in a shallow energy well the results could be interpreted in terms of a bending (hinge) region within S1 and the existence of a rigid S2. Such a hinge in S1 may, however, be stiff enough not to reveal any motion without an applied force. The part of S1 rigidly attached to actin would then have to contain the label. Possible differences between rigor and active cross bridges should be considered when applying these results to contracting muscle.

In a kinetic analysis of a previously described decrease in fluorescence on adding MgATP (96) of a fluorescein label attached to an SH group of LC_1, Marsh et al. (97) have shown that the decrease in fluorescence temporally coincides with the increase in tryptophan fluorescence accompanying ATP cleavage. Because the distance between the nucleotide-binding site and the LC_1 SH group is 5.5 nm (118), Marsh et al. (97) conclude that there must be some flexibility in the S1 if the nucleotide at the active site can produce an effect at such a large distance. The distance between the —SH landmark on the heavy chain and the —SH on the light chain (~4.5 nm) is not changed by MgATP (96). In the eventual mapping of the S1 region the distance of 2.6 nm, recently established by energy transfer, between the reactive lysine and the SH1 thiol (161) supplies another important datum. (See ref. 109 for a review of current myosin head topography.) The question arises whether the kind of flexibility that may be required to transmit an effect in a protein over some 5.0 nm would be detectable in experiments aimed at detecting motion.

FORCE GENERATION AND ELASTICITY

Rotating-Head Models

A. F. Huxley and Simmons (60, 61) were first to resolve on a millisecond time scale the time course of tension transients that arise when a stimulated single fiber exerting isometric tension is rapidly released by ~10 nm/half-sarcomere. In their original model (60, 61), the series elasticity shown to be associated with the cross bridges was thought to be localized in the S2 portion of the myosin molecule (Fig. 6). The head (S1) portion was thought to be able to assume different states characterized by the angle made with the thin filament, and the equilibrium between these states was considered a function of the cross-bridge tension. A. F. Huxley (58) emphasized, however, that the proposed interpretation of transients required only that the elasticity should reside somewhere in the cross bridge and did not depend on its being localized in the S2 portion. Thus equivalent models could be considered in which the S2 is rigid and the elasticity resides in the S1-actin junction or in S1 itself. Eisenberg et al. (33) developed a detailed model of this type. In this model there is no independent elastic element, and both force and elasticity result from the interaction of actin and the cross-bridge head. Broad free-energy wells allow a continuous change in free energy as a function of a geometric parameter, in this case an angle. Without the independent elastic element, transition to the tension-generating state does not require the stretching of a structure (32, 33). Both in the Huxley-Simmons and in the Eisenberg-Hill-Chen models, cross-bridge heads rotate, although the assumptions about an independent elastic element differ.

Helix-Coil Melting Model

Harrington (48) and Tsong et al. (172) have proposed another model that shares some features of the preceding two but differs significantly in that the heads would not rotate. The elasticity would be in the S2 portion, specifically in the hinge region between S2 and LMM that constitutes the difference between the shorter and longer forms of S2 (89). Tsong et al. (172) found a temperature-induced helix-coil transition in which 15%–25% of S2 assumes a random-coil structure at 37° and proposed that the random coil would behave in an elastic manner.

PROTEOLYSIS AS A CROSS-BRIDGE PROBE. Harrington and his colleagues stressed the importance of the interaction between the S2 moiety and the backbone of the thick filaments in stabilizing the helical form. With a combination of cross-linking and enzymatic proteolysis they were able to monitor the state of S2. Application of chymotryptic digestion has shown that myosin heads (22) and the S2 segment (174) are cross-linkable to the backbone of the myosin filament at neutral pH but not at pH ≥ 8, suggesting that the heads are held close to the backbone of the myosin filaments but are released at pH ≥ 8. This is consistent with EPR studies (168) that show a decrease in rotational correlation times of cross bridges or synthetic myosin filaments on increasing the pH. The region absent in the short S2, corresponding to a coiled coil having a length of ~220 Å and located at the LMM-HMM junction of the intact molecule (89), has been identified with the so-called sticky segment, viz., the backbone region to which the head attaches noncovalently (152). The release of S2 is highly cooperative and appears to be accompanied by an α-helix–random-coil conformational change in the S2-LMM hinge region as shown by an increased susceptibility to chy-

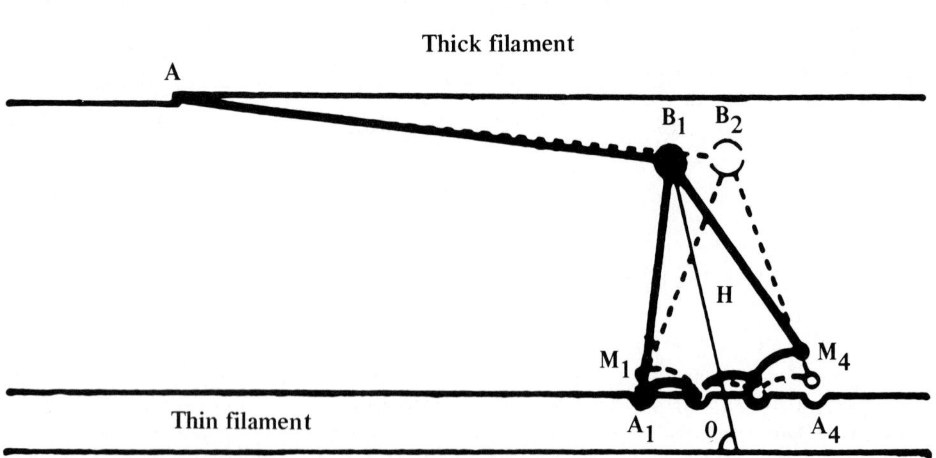

FIG. 6. Cross-bridge model. Different orientation of myosin heads corresponds to different stable states resulting, in this simple model, from pairs of M_iA_i, $M_{i+1}A_{i+1}$ contacts. As originally proposed, link AB contains instantaneous elasticity. *AB*, S2; *B*, S1-S2 hinge. [From A. F. Huxley and Simmons (60).]

motryptic proteolysis (22, 174). With this type of binding of S2 to the filament backbone only the S1 portion of the myosin molecule would be free to move; it would undergo rotational diffusion but would have no translational (radial) motion in a resting muscle. Such a restriction on motion of the cross bridge might account for changes in layer lines on activation (63) and for the observed restriction of rotational motion of the head on formation of myosin filaments.

Recently Ueno and Harrington (173) extended their cross-linking proteolysis studies to myofibrils and glycerinated fibers to include conditions corresponding to activation in living muscle. They showed that the proteolysis rates in the S2-LMM hinge region are enhanced in activating solutions, viz., those containing MgATP and Ca^{2+}, compared with both rigor and relaxing conditions (Fig. 7). Ueno and Harrington interpreted these experiments in terms of a release of the S2 and head portion of myosin from the core of the rod, not because of binding to actin or of interaction with ATP before binding to actin can take place but after heads hydrolyzing ATP bind to actin. This work forms the basis of the helix-coil contraction theory. According to the Harrington model the region close to the S2-LMM hinge would be both the site of elasticity and the source of the contractile force, in the sense that force develops because of the thermodynamic drive to form a coil (48) rather than by stretching of the coil because of a motion in the head portion. The mechanism by which binding to actin of the head bearing the products of ATP hydrolysis induces the release of S2 from the core, resulting in a state favoring the random coil over the α-helix, is not known. Harrington (47) suggested a mechanism involving the effect of proton release from ATP, hydrolyzed by a myosin head in one molecule, on the structure of an S2 segment spatially adjacent but belonging to another myosin molecule in the filament, which may play a role in this helix-coil transition.

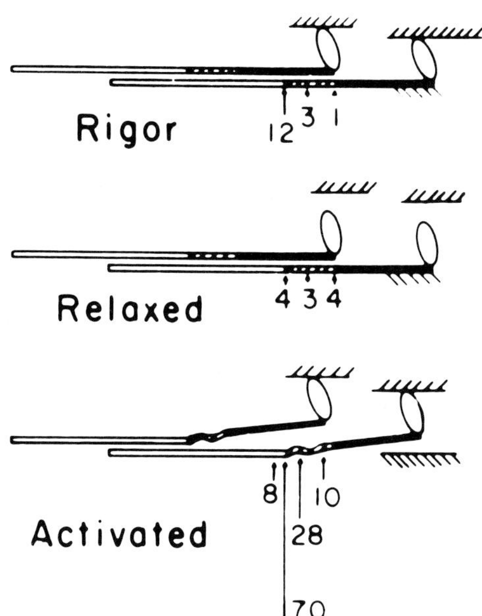

FIG. 7. Placing of force generator in hinge region between S2 and LMM with helix-coil transition as molecular basis of force development. Model does not require myosin head tilt. Numbers attached by arrows, magnitude of first-order rate constants of fragment formation under α-chymotryptic cleavage. Highest rate in hinge region under activating conditions. [From Ueno and Harrington (173).]

Actin Motions

The rigidity of the actin-myosin bond (167) and the internal modes of rotation or flexibility raise the possibility that elasticity might be related to the internal rotation observed in F actin (37, 126, 127, 167). The F-actin motions observed by quasielastic light scattering would be too slow (correlation times 10–100 ms) but those observed by ST EPR (correlation times 100–400 μs) could account for the fastest mechanical response.

X-Ray Studies

X-ray studies, discussed in detail in the chapter by Haselgrove in this *Handbook*, clearly indicate movement of masses associated with the myosin filament toward the actin filaments coupled with the transition from the relaxed to the activated state of muscle. Although the conventional view attributes these changes to radial movements of cross-bridge heads toward actin, the role of azimuthal changes of free cross bridges or of changes in the angular attitude of cross bridges attached to actin is also being considered. Biochemical evidence suggesting that activation of the actin-myosin system by Ca^{2+} may not involve a change in the fraction of attached cross bridges (18, 19) may affect the interpretation of X-ray data in terms of binding of heads to, or their dissociation from, actin filaments.

Recent time-resolved studies (64) using sophisticated electronic techniques and synchrotron-radiation studies show that the changes occurring on a millisecond time scale in the myosin layer-line pattern are closely correlated with the time course of tension development, strongly supporting the view that the activation process is closely linked with cross-bridge disordering. Studies combining mechanical and X-ray transients, again utilizing synchrotron-radiation and position-sensitive detectors, are equally promising for obtaining a better understanding of the changes occurring in cross bridges during the active muscle state (66). These studies have so far shown that although no significant changes occur in the myosin layer-line pattern and in the equatorial reflections of a muscle subjected to quick release or stretch, the changes in the 143-Å meridional reflection are consistent with a longitudinal change in the attached cross bridges. This provides rather direct evidence for rotation of cross bridges attached to actin in a contracting muscle.

Correlation Functions

Resolving whether cross-bridge movement in the attached state as distinct from the cyclic movement implicit in the attachment-detachment process itself is involved would be an important step toward understanding the molecular basis of muscle contraction and establishing a link between molecular changes demonstrated in the actin-myosin system in vitro and the organized systems in the isolated state and in vivo. A promising new approach involves an analysis of fluctuations of mechanical or optical parameters (109). Recent studies with labels presumably attached to myosin utilizing the analysis of correlation function suggest the existence of cyclic processes and frequencies (1–5 Hz) of the same order of magnitude as those involved in the ATPase reaction coupled to the contraction process (14). It is not yet sufficiently clear whether the frequency applies to the attachment-detachment cycle of the cross bridge or whether cyclic processes in the attached state are detected. Experiments measuring correlation between tension and an optical signal and between two optical signals reporting different processes are likely to bring new insights on the chemical basis of cross-bridge function (109).

Preparation of this manuscript and research by the authors described in it were supported by grants from the National Institutes of Health (HL-5949, HL-23249, HL-15391), the National Science Foundation, and the Muscular Dystrophy Association.

REFERENCES

1. AJTAI, K., L. SZILAGYI, AND E. N. A. BIRO. Study of the structure of HMM: vanadate complex. *FEBS Lett.* 141: 74–77, 1982.
2. AMOS, L. A., H. E. HUXLEY, K. C. HOLMES, R. S. GOODY, AND K. A. TAYLOR. Structural evidence that myosin heads may interact with two sites on F-actin. *Nature London* 299: 467–469, 1982.
3. ARATA, T., Y. MUKOHATA, AND Y. TONOMURA. Structure and function of the two heads of the myosin molecule. VI. ATP hydrolysis, shortening and tension development of myofibrils. *J. Biochem. Tokyo* 82: 801–812, 1977.
4. ARATA, T., AND H. SHIMIZU. Spin-label study of actin-myosin-nucleotide interactions in contracting glycerinated muscle fibers. *J. Mol. Biol.* 151: 411–437, 1981.
5. ARONSON, J. F., AND M. F. MORALES. Polarization of tryptophan fluorescence in muscle. *Biochemistry* 8: 4517–4522, 1969.
6. ASTBURY, W. T. Croonian lecture on the structure of biological fibres and the problem of muscle. *Proc. R. Soc. London Ser. B* 134: 303–328, 1947.
7. BAGSHAW, C. R., J. F. ECCLESTON, F. ECKSTEIN, R. S. GOODY, H. GUTFREUND, AND D. R. TRENTHAM. The magnesium ion-dependent adenosine triphosphatase of myosin. Two-step processes of adenosine triphosphate association and adenosine diphosphate dissociation. *Biochem. J.* 141: 351–364, 1974.
8. BAGSHAW, C. R., J. F. ECCLESTON, D. R. TRENTHAM, B. W. YATES, AND R. S. GOODY. Transient kinetic studies of the Mg^{2+} dependent ATPase of myosin and its proteolytic subfragments. *Cold Spring Harbor Symp. Quant. Biol.* 37: 127–135, 1972.
9. BAGSHAW, C. R., AND J. KENDRICK-JONES. Characterization of homologous divalent metal ion binding sites of vertebrate and molluscan myosins using electron paramagnetic resonance spectroscopy. *J. Mol. Biol.* 130: 317–336, 1979.
10. BAGSHAW, C. R., AND G. H. REED. The significance of the slow dissociation of divalent metal ions from myosin regulatory light chains. *FEBS Lett.* 81: 386–390, 1977.
11. BALINT, M., F. A. SRETER, I. WOLF, B. NAGY, AND J. GERGELY. The substructure of heavy meromyosin. The effect of Ca^{2+} and Mg^{2+} on the tryptic fragmentation of heavy meromyosin. *J. Biol. Chem.* 250: 6168–6177, 1975.
12. BÁLINT, M., L. SZILÁGYI, G. FEKETE, M. BLAZSÓ, AND N. A. BIRÓ. Studies on proteins and protein complexes of muscle by means of proteolysis. V. Fragmentation of light meromyosin by trypsin. *J. Mol. Biol.* 37: 317–330, 1968.
13. BALINT, M., I. WOLF, A. TARCSAFALVI, J. GERGELY, AND F. A. SRETER. Location of SH-1 and SH-2 in the heavy chain segment of heavy meromyosin. *Arch. Biochem. Biophys.* 190: 793–799, 1978.
14. BOREJDO, J., O. ASSULIN, T. ANDO, AND S. PUTNAM. Cross-bridge orientation in skeletal muscle measured by linear dichroism of an extrinsic chromophore. *J. Mol. Biol.* 158: 391–414, 1982.
15. BOREJDO, J., S. PUTNAM, AND M. F. MORALES. Fluctuations in polarized fluorescence: evidence that muscle cross bridges rotate repetitively during contraction. *Proc. Natl. Acad. Sci. USA* 76: 6346–6350, 1979.
16. BURKE, M., S. HIMMELFARB, AND W. F. HARRINGTON. Studies on the "hinge" region of myosin. *Biochemistry* 12: 701–710, 1973.
17. BURKE, M., E. REISLER, AND W. F. HARRINGTON. Effect of bridging the two essential thiols of myosin on its spatial and actin-binding properties. *Biochemistry* 15: 1923–1927, 1976.
18. CHALOVICH, J. M., P. B. CHOCK, AND E. EISENBERG. Mechanism of action of troponin-tropomyosin. Inhibition of actomyosin ATPase activity without inhibition of myosin binding to actin. *J. Biol. Chem.* 256: 575–579, 1981.
19. CHALOVICH, J. M., AND E. EISENBERG. Inhibition of actomyosin ATPase activity by troponin-tropomyosin without blocking the binding of myosin to actin. *J. Biol. Chem.* 257: 2432–2437, 1982.
20. CHANTLER, P. D., J. R. SELLERS, AND A. G. SZENT-GYÖRGYI. Cooperativity in scallop myosin. *Biochemistry* 20: 210–216, 1981.
21. CHANTLER, P. D., AND A. G. SZENT-GYÖRGYI, Regulatory light chains and scallop myosin. Full dissociation, reversibility and cooperative effects. *J. Mol. Biol.* 138: 473–492, 1980.
22. CHIAO, Y.-C. C., AND W. F. HARRINGTON. Cross-bridge movement in glycerinated rabbit psoas muscle fibers. *Biochemistry* 18: 959–963, 1979.
23. COOKE, R. Stress does not alter the conformation of a domain of the myosin cross-bridge in rigor muscle fibres. *Nature London* 294: 570–571, 1981.
24. COOKE, R., V. A. BARNETT, AND D. D. THOMAS. Measuring crossbridge angles with paramagnetic probes in rigor, relaxed and contracting muscle fibers (Abstract). *Biophys. J.* 37: 117a, 1982.
25. COOKE, R., AND K. E. FRANKS. Generation of force by single-headed myosin. *J. Mol. Biol.* 120: 361–373, 1978.
26. COOKE, R., K. FRANKS, AND J. T. STULL. Myosin phosphorylation regulates the ATPase activity of permeable skeletal muscle fibers. *FEBS Lett.* 144: 33–37, 1982.
27. CRAIG, R., A. G. SZENT-GYÖRGYI, L. BEESE, P. FLICKER, P. VIBERT, AND C. COHEN. Electron microscopy of thin filaments decorated with a Ca^{2+}-regulated myosin. *J. Mol. Biol.* 140: 35–55, 1980.
28. CROW, M. T., AND M. KUSHMERICK. Phosphorylation of myosin light chains in mouse fast-twitch muscle associated with reduced actomyosin turnover rate. *Science* 217: 835–837, 1982.
29. DE LA TORRE, J. G., AND V. A. BLOOMFIELD. Conformation of myosin as estimated from hydrodynamic properties. *Biochemistry* 19: 5118–5123, 1980.
30. DOS REMEDIOS, C. G., R. G. YOUNT, AND M. F. MORALES.

Individual states in the cycle of muscle contraction. *Proc. Natl. Acad. Sci. USA* 69: 2542–2546, 1972.

31. DUKE, J., R. TAKASHI, K. UE, AND M. F. MORALES. Reciprocal reactivities of specific thiols when actin binds to myosin. *Proc. Natl. Acad. Sci. USA* 73: 302–306, 1976.
32. EISENBERG, E., AND T. L. HILL. A cross-bridge model of muscle contraction. *Prog. Biophys. Mol. Biol.* 33: 55–82, 1978.
33. EISENBERG, E., T. L. HILL, AND Y. CHEN. Cross-bridge model of muscle contraction. Quantitative analysis. *Biophys. J.* 29: 195–227, 1980.
34. ELLIOTT, A., AND G. OFFER. Shape and flexibility of the myosin molecule. *J. Mol. Biol.* 123: 505–509, 1978.
35. ELZINGA, M., AND J. COLLINS. Amino acid sequence of a myosin fragment that contains SH-1, SH-2 and *N*-methylhistidine. *Proc. Natl. Acad. Sci. USA* 74: 4281–4284, 1977.
36. ENGELHARDT, V. A., AND M. N. LYUBIMOVA. Myosine and adenosinetriphosphatase. *Nature London* 144: 668–669, 1939.
37. FUJIME, S., AND S. ISHIWATA. Dynamic study of F-actin by quasielastic scattering of laser light. *J. Mol. Biol.* 62: 251–265, 1971.
38. FURUKAWA, K. I., A. INOUE, AND Y. TONOMURA. Extra burst of P_i liberation and formation of the myosin-phosphate-ADP complex at various concentrations of Mg^{2+} ions. *J. Biochem. Tokyo* 89: 1283–1292, 1981.
39. GAZITH, J., S. HIMMELFARB, AND W. F. HARRINGTON. Studies on the subunit structure of myosin. *J. Biol. Chem.* 245: 15–22, 1970.
40. GERGELY, J. Relation of ATPase and myosin (Abstract). *Federation Proc.* 9: 176, 1950.
41. GERGELY, J. Studies on myosin adenosine triphosphatase. *J. Biol. Chem.* 200: 543–550, 1953.
42. GERGELY, J. The interaction between actomyosin and adenosine triphosphate. Light scattering studies. *J. Biol. Chem.* 220: 917–926, 1956.
43. GERGELY, J., M. A. GOUVEA, AND D. KARIBIAN. Fragmentation of myosin by chymotrypsin. *J. Biol. Chem.* 212: 165–177, 1955.
44. GERSHMAN, L. C., A. STRACHER, AND P. DREIZEN. Subunit structure of myosin. III. A proposed model for rabbit skeletal myosin. *J. Biol. Chem.* 244: 2726–2736, 1969.
45. GOODY, R. S., F. ECKSTEIN, AND R. H. SCHIRMER. The enzymatic synthesis of thiophosphate analogs of nucleotide anhydrides. *Biochim. Biophys. Acta* 276: 155–161, 1972.
46. GRATZER, W. B., AND S. LOWEY. Effect of substrate on the conformation of myosin. *J. Biol. Chem.* 244: 22–25, 1969.
47. HARRINGTON, W. F. A mechanochemical mechanism for muscle contraction. *Proc. Natl. Acad. Sci. USA* 68: 685–689, 1971.
48. HARRINGTON, W. F. Origin of the contractile force in skeletal muscle. *Proc. Natl. Acad. Sci. USA* 76: 5066–5070, 1979.
49. HASSELBACH, W. Die Wechselwirkung verschiedener Nukleosidtriphosphate mit Aktomyosin in Gelzustand. *Biochim. Biophys. Acta* 20: 355–368, 1956.
50. HIGHSMITH, S. The dynamics of myosin and actin in solution are compatible with the mechanical features of the cross-bridge hypothesis. *Biochim. Biophys. Acta* 639: 31–39, 1981.
51. HIGHSMITH, S., K. AKASAKA, M. KONRAD, R. GOODY, K. HOLMES, N. WADE-JARDETZKY, AND O. JARDETZKY. Internal motions in myosin. *Biochemistry* 18: 4238–4243, 1979.
52. HIGHSMITH, S., AND O. JARDETZKY. Internal motions in myosin. *Biochemistry* 20: 780–783, 1981.
53. HIGHSMITH, S., K. M. KRETZSCHMAR, C. T. O'KONSKI, AND M. F. MORALES. Flexibility of myosin rod, light meromyosin and myosin subfragment 2 in solution. *Proc. Natl. Acad. Sci. USA* 74: 4986–4990, 1977.
54. HIGHSMITH, S., C.-C. WANG, K. ZERO, R. PECORA, AND O. JARDETZKY. Bending motions and internal motions in myosin rod. *Biochemistry* 21: 1192–1196, 1982.
55. HIRATSUKA, T. Actin-induced conformational changes around the reactive fluorescence-labeled lysyl residues located in the subfragment-1/subfragment-2 link region of cardiac myosin. *J. Biol. Chem.* 256: 10645–10650, 1981.
56. HOZUMI, T., AND A. MUHLRAD. Reactive lysyl of myosin subfragment 1: location on the 27k fragment and labeling properties. *Biochemistry* 20: 2945–2949, 1981.
57. HUXLEY, A. F. Muscle structure and theories of contraction. *Prog. Biophys. Chem.* 7: 255–318, 1957.
58. HUXLEY, A. F. Review lecture: muscular contraction. *J. Physiol. London* 243: 1–43, 1974.
59. HUXLEY, A. F., AND R. NIEDERGERKE. Structural changes in muscle during contraction. Interference microscopy of living muscle fibres. *Nature London* 173: 971–973, 1954.
60. HUXLEY, A. F., AND R. M. SIMMONS. Proposed mechanism of force generation in striated muscle. *Nature London* 233: 533–538, 1971.
61. HUXLEY, A. F., AND R. M. SIMMONS. Mechanical transients and the origin of muscular force. *Cold Spring Harbor Symp. Quant. Biol.* 37: 669–680, 1972.
62. HUXLEY, H. E. The mechanism of muscular contraction. *Science* 164: 1356–1366, 1969.
63. HUXLEY, H. E., AND W. BROWN. X-ray diffraction of vertebrate striated muscle during contraction and in rigor. *J. Mol. Biol.* 30: 383–434, 1967.
64. HUXLEY, H. E., A. R. FARUQI, M. KRESS, J. BORDAS, AND M. H. KOCH. Time resolved X-ray diffraction studies of the myosin layer line reflected during muscle contraction. *J. Mol. Biol.* 158: 637–684, 1982.
65. HUXLEY, H. E., AND J. HANSON. Changes in the cross-striations of muscle during contraction and stretch and their structural interpretation. *Nature London* 173: 973–976, 1954.
66. HUXLEY, H. E., R. M. SIMMONS, A. R. FARUQI, M. KRESS, J. BORDAS, AND M. H. KOCH. Millisecond time resolved changes in X-ray reflections from contracting muscle during rapid mechanical transients recorded using synchroton radiation. *Proc. Natl. Acad. Sci. USA* 78: 2297–2301, 1981.
67. INOUE, A., K. KIKUCHI, AND Y. TONOMURA. Structure and function of the two heads of the myosin molecule. V. Enzymatic properties of heads B and A. *J. Biochem. Tokyo* 82: 783–800, 1977.
68. INOUE, A., H. TAKENAKA, T. ARATA, AND Y. TONOMURA. Functional implications of the two-headed structure of myosin. *Adv. Biophys.* 13: 1–194, 1979.
69 INOUE, A., AND Y. TONOMURA. Separation of subfragment-1 of heavy meromyosin into two equimolar fractions with and without formation of the reactive enzyme-phosphate-ADP complex. *J. Biochem. Tokyo* 79: 419–434, 1976.
70. ISHIWATA, S., J. SEIDEL, AND J. GERGELY. Regulation by calcium ions of crossbridge attachment in myofibrils studied by saturation transfer EPR spectroscopy (Abstract). *Biophys. J.* 25: 1900a, 1979.
71. JOHNSON, K. A., AND E. W. TAYLOR. Intermediate states of subfragment 1 and acto-subfragment 1 ATPase: reevaluation of the mechanism. *Biochemistry* 17: 3432–3442, 1978.
72. KAMAYAMA, T. Actin induced local conformational change in the myosin molecule. III. Reactivity of S2 thiol and DTNB reactive thiols of porcine cardiac myosin. *J. Biochem. Tokyo* 87: 581–586, 1980.
73. KAMAYAMA, T., T. KATORI, AND T. SEKINE. Actin induced local conformational change in the myosin molecule. I. Effect of metal ions and nucleotides on the conformational change around a specific thiol group (S2) of heavy meromyosin. *J. Biochem. Tokyo* 81: 709–714, 1977.
74. KARPLUS, M., B. R. GELIN, AND J. A. MCCAMMON. Internal dynamics of proteins: short time and long time motions of aromatic sidechains in PTI. *Biophys. J.* 32: 603–618, 1980.
75. KARPLUS, M., AND J. A. MCCAMMON. Dynamics of folded proteins. *Nature London* 267: 585–590, 1977.
76. KARPLUS, M., AND J. A. MCCAMMON. The internal dynamics of globular proteins. *Crit. Rev. Biochem.* 9: 293–349, 1981.
77. KASSAB, R., D. MORNET, P. PANTEL, R. BERTRAND, AND E. AUDEMARD. Structural aspects of actomyosin interaction. *Biochimie* 63: 273–289, 1981.
78. KENDRICK-JONES, J. Role of myosin light chains in calcium regulation. *Nature London* 249: 631–634, 1974.
79. KENDRICK-JONES, J., AND J. M. SCHOLEY. Myosin-linked regulatory systems. *J. Muscle Res. Cell Motility* 2: 347–372, 1981.
80. KENDRICK-JONES, J., E. M. SZENTKIRALYI, AND A. G. SZENT-

GYÖRGYI. Regulatory light chains in myosin. *J. Mol. Biol.* 104: 747–775, 1976.
81. KOMINZ, D. R., E. R. MITCHELL, T. NIHEI, AND C. M. KAY. The papain digestion of skeletal myosin. *Biochemistry* 4: 2373–2382, 1965.
82. KUBO, S., S. TOKURA, AND Y. TONOMURA. On the active site of myosin A-adenosine triphosphatase. I. Reaction of the enzyme with trinitrobenzenesulfonate. *J. Biol. Chem.* 235: 2835–2839, 1960.
83. LEHMAN, W., AND A. G. SZENT-GYÖRGYI. Regulation of muscular contraction: distribution of actin control and myosin control in the animal kingdom. *J. Gen. Physiol.* 66: 1–30, 1975.
84. LOWEY, S. Myosin substructure: isolation of a helical subunit from heavy meromyosin. *Science* 145: 597–599, 1964.
85. LOWEY, S., AND C. COHEN. Studies on the structure of myosin. *J. Mol. Biol.* 4: 293–308, 1962.
86. LOWEY, S., AND S. M. LUCK. Equilibrium binding of adenosine diphosphate to myosin. *Biochemistry* 8: 3195–3199, 1969.
87. LOWEY, S., AND D. RISBY. Light chains from fast and slow muscle myosin. *Nature London* 234: 81–85, 1971.
88. LOWEY, S., H. S. SLAYTER, A. G. WEEDS, AND H. BAKER. Substructure of the myosin molecule. I. Subfragments of myosin by enzymatic degradation. *J. Mol. Biol.* 42: 1–29, 1969.
89. LU, R. C. Identification of a region susceptible to proteolysis in myosin subfragment 2. *Proc. Natl. Acad. Sci. USA* 77: 2010–2013, 1980.
90. LU, R. C., L. NYITRAY, M. BALINT, AND J. GERGELY. Localization of a region responsible for the low ionic strength insolubility of myosin (Abstract). *Biophys. J.* 41: 228a, 1983.
91. LYMN, R. W. Low-angle x-ray diagrams from skeletal muscle: the effect of AMP-PNP, a non hydrolyzed analogue of ATP. *J. Mol. Biol.* 99: 567–582, 1975.
92. LYMN, R. W., AND E. W. TAYLOR. Transient state phosphate production in the hydrolysis of nucleoside triphosphates by myosin. *Biochemistry* 9: 2975–2983, 1970.
93. MANDELKOW, E. M., AND E. MANDELKOW. Fluorometric studies on the influence of metal ions and chelators on the interaction between myosin and ATP. *FEBS Lett.* 33: 161–166, 1973.
94. MARGOSSIAN, S. S., AND S. LOWEY. Substructure of the myosin molecule. III. Preparation of single headed derivatives of myosin. *J. Mol. Biol.* 74: 301–311, 1973.
95. MARGOSSIAN, S. S., AND S. LOWEY. Substructure of the myosin molecule. IV. Interactions of myosin and its subfragments with adenosine triphosphate and F-actin. *J. Mol. Biol.* 74: 313–330, 1973.
96. MARSH, D. J., AND S. LOWEY. Fluorescence energy transfer in myosin subfragment-1. *Biochemistry* 19: 774–784, 1980.
97. MARSH, D. J., L. A. STEIN, E. EISENBERG, AND S. LOWEY. Fluorescently labelled myosin subfragment 1. Identification of the kinetic step associated with the adenosine 5′-triphosphate induced fluorescence decrease. *Biochemistry* 21: 1925–1928, 1982.
98. MARSTON, S. B., C. D. RODGER, AND R. T. TREGEAR. Changes in muscle crossbridges when β, γ-imido-ATP binds to myosin. *J. Mol. Biol.* 104: 263–276, 1976.
99. MARSTON, S. B., R. T. TREGEAR, C. D. RODGER, AND M. L. CLARKE. Coupling between the enzymatic site of myosin and the mechanical output of muscle. *J. Mol. Biol.* 128: 111–126, 1979.
100. MENDELSON, R. A., AND P. CHEUNG. Myosin crossbridges: absence of direct effect of calcium on movement away from the thick filaments. *Science* 194: 190–192, 1976.
101. MENDELSON, R. A., AND P. CHEUNG. Intrinsic segmental flexibility of the S-1 moiety of myosin using single-headed myosin. *Biochemistry* 17: 2139–2148, 1978.
102. MENDELSON, R. A., M. F. MORALES, AND J. BOTTS. Segmental flexibility of the S-1 moiety of myosin. *Biochemistry* 12: 2250–2255, 1973.
103. MENDELSON, R. A., AND M. G. A. WILSON. Three dimensional disorders of dipolar probes in a helical array. Application to muscle crossbridges. *Biophys. J.* 39: 221–228, 1982.
104. MICHNICKA, M., K. KASMAN, AND I. KAKOL. The binding of actin to phosphorylated and dephosphorylated myosin. *Biochim. Biophys. Acta* 704: 470–475, 1982.
105. MIHALYI, E., AND A. G. SZENT-GYÖRGYI. Trypsin digestion of muscle proteins. III. Adenosine triphosphatase activity and actin-binding capacity of the digested myosin. *J. Biol. Chem.* 201: 211–219, 1953.
106. MIYANISHI, T., A. INOUE, AND Y. TONOMURA. Differential modification of specific lysine residues in the two kinds of subfragment-1 of myosin with 2,4,6-trinitrobenzenesulfonate. *J. Biochem. Tokyo* 85: 747–753, 1979.
107. MIYANISHI, T., AND Y. TONOMURA. Location of the nonidentical two reactive lysine residues in the myosin molecule. *J. Biochem. Tokyo* 89: 831–839, 1981.
108. MÓCZ, G., R. C. LU, AND J. GERGELY. Nucleotide and metal effects on the structure of myosin subfragment 1 (Abstract). *Biophys. J.* 37: 38a, 1982.
108a. MONAD, J., J. WYMAN, AND J. P. CHANGEUX. On the nature of allosteric transitions: a plausible model. *J. Mol. Biol.* 12: 88–118, 1965.
109. MORALES, M. F., J. BOREJDO, J. BOTTS, R. COOKE, R. A. MENDELSON, AND R. TAKASHI. Some physical studies of the contractile mechanism in muscle. *Ann. Rev. Phys. Chem.* 33: 319–351, 1982.
110. MORALES, M. F., AND J. BOTTS. Molecular basis for chemomechanical energy transduction in muscle. *Proc. Natl. Acad. Sci. USA* 76: 3857–3859, 1979.
111. MORGAN, M., S. V. PERRY, AND J. OTTAWAY. Myosin light-chain phosphatase. *Biochem. J.* 157: 687–697, 1976.
112. MORITA, F. Interaction of HMM with Substrate. I. Difference in ultraviolet absorption spectrum between HMM and its Michaelis-Menten complex. *J. Biol. Chem.* 242: 4501–4506, 1967.
113. MORITA, F., AND K. J. YAGI. Spectral shift in heavy meromyosin induced by substrate. *Biochem. Biophys. Res. Commun.* 22: 297–301, 1966.
114. MORNET, D., R. BERTRAND, P. PANTEL, E. AUDEMARD, AND R. KASSAB. Proteolytic approach to structure and function of actin recognition sites in myosin heads. *Biochemistry* 20: 2110–2120, 1981.
115. MORNET, D., R. BERTRAND, P. PANTEL, E. AUDEMARD, AND R. KASSAB. Structure of the actin-myosin interface. *Nature London* 292: 301–306, 1981.
116. MORNET, D., P. PANTEL, E. AUDEMARD, AND R. KASSAB. The limited tryptic cleavage of chymotryptic S-1; an approach to the characterization of the actin site in myosin heads. *Biochem. Biophys. Res. Commun.* 89: 925–932, 1979.
117. MORNET, D., P. PANTEL, R. BERTRAND, E. AUDEMARD, AND R. KASSAB. Localization of the reactive trinitrophenylated lysyl residue of myosin ATPase site in the NH_2-terminal (27k domain) of the S1 heavy chain. *FEBS Lett.* 117: 183–188, 1980.
118. MOSS, D. J., AND D. R. TRENTHAM. Interaction of chromophoric nucleotide and nucleoside analogues and distance measurements in myosin subfragment 1 (Abstract). *Federation Proc.* 39: 1935, 1980.
119. MUELLER, H., AND S. V. PERRY. The degradation of heavy meromyosin by trypsin. *Biochem. J.* 85: 431–439, 1962.
120. MUHLRAD, A., AND T. HOZUMI. Tryptic digestion as a probe of myosin S-1 conformation. *Proc. Natl. Acad. Sci USA* 79: 958–962, 1982.
121. MUHLRAD, A., S. SRIVASTAVA, G. HOLLOSI, AND J. WIKMAN-COFFELT. Studies on the amino groups of myosin ATPase. Trinitrophenylation of reactive lysyl residues in ventricular and atrial myosins. *Arch. Biochem. Biophys.* 209: 304–313, 1981.
122. NAYLOR, G. R. S., AND R. J. PODOLSKY. X-ray diffraction of strained muscle fibers in rigor. *Proc. Natl. Acad. Sci. USA* 78: 5559–5563, 1981.
123. NEEDHAM, J., S. CHEN, D. M. NEEDHAM, AND A. S. G. LAWRENCE. Myosin birefringence and adenylpyrophosphate. *Nature London* 147: 766–768, 1941.

124. NIHEI, T., R. A. MENDELSON, AND J. BOTTS. The site of force generation in muscle contraction as deduced from fluorescence polarization studies. *Proc. Natl. Acad. Sci. USA* 71: 274–277, 1974.

125. OHNISHI, H., AND T. WAKABAYASHI. Electron microscopic studies of myosin molecules from chicken gizzard muscle: the formation of the intramolecular loop in the myosin tail. *J. Biochem.* 92: 871–879, 1982.

125a. OKAMOTO, Y., AND R. G. YOUNT. Identification of the active site peptide of myosin after photoaffinity labeling (Abstract). *Biophys. J.* 41: 298a, 1983.

126. OOSAWA, F. Dynamics of actin filament. In: *Muscle Contraction. Its Regulatory Mechanisms*, edited by S. Ebashi, K. Maruyama, and M. Endo. Berlin: Springer-Verlag, 1980, 165–172.

127. OOSAWA, F., S. FUJIME, S. ISHIWATA, AND K. MIHASHI. Dynamic property of F-actin and thin filament. *Cold Spring Harbor Symp. Quant. Biol.* 37: 277–285, 1972.

128. PEMRICK, S. The phosphorylated L_2 light chain of skeletal myosin is a modifier of the actomyosin ATPase. *J. Biol. Chem.* 255: 8836–8841, 1980.

129. PERRIE, W. T., L. B. SMILLIE, AND S. V. PERRY. A phosphorylated light-chain component of myosin from skeletal muscle. *Biochem. J.* 135: 151–164, 1973.

130. PERRY, S. V. The adenosinetriphosphatase activity of myofibrils isolated from skeletal muscle. *Biochem. J.* 48: 257–263, 1951.

131. PERSECHINI, A., AND D. J. HARTSHORNE. Phosphorylation of smooth muscle myosin: evidence for cooperativity between the myosin heads. *Science* 213: 1383–1385, 1981.

132. PRINCE, H. P., H. E. TRAYER, G. D. HENRY, I. P. TRAYER, D. C. DALGARNO, B. A. LEVINE, P. D. CARY, AND C. TURNER. Proton nuclear magnetic resonance spectroscopy of myosin subfragment 1 isozymes. *Eur. J. Biochem.* 121: 213–219, 1981.

133. REISLER, E. On the question of cooperative interaction of myosin heads with F-actin in the presence of ATP. *J. Mol. Biol.* 138: 93–108, 1980.

134. SARKAR, S., F. A. SRETER, AND J. GERGELY. Light chains of myosin from white, red, and cardiac muscles. *Proc. Natl. Acad. Sci. USA* 68: 946–950, 1971.

135. SCHAUB, M. C., AND J. G. WATTERSON. Symmetry and asymmetry in the contractile protein myosin. *Biochimie* 63: 291–299, 1981.

136. SCHAUB, M. C., J. G. WATTERSON, K. LOTH, AND P. G. WASER. Conformational relationships between distinct regions in the myosin molecule. *Biochimie* 61: 791–802, 1979.

137. SCHAUB, M. C., J. G. WATTERSON, AND P. G. WASER. Conformational differences in myosin. IV. Radioactive labelling of specific thiol groups as influenced by ligand binding. *Hoppe-Seyler's Z. Physiol. Chem.* 356: 325–339, 1975.

138. SCHAUB, M. C., J. G. WATTERSON, AND P. G. WASER. Evidence for head-head interactions for myosin and cardiac skeletal muscle. *Basic Res. Cardiol.* 72: 124–132, 1977.

139. SCHOLEY, J. M., K. A. TAYLOR, AND J. KENDRICK-JONES. Regulation of non-muscle myosin assembled by calmodulin-dependent light chain kinase. *Nature London* 287: 233–235, 1980.

140. SEIDEL, J. C. The effects of ionic conditions, temperature and chemical modification on the fluorescence of myosin during the steady state of ATP hydrolysis. *J. Biol. Chem.* 250: 5681–5687, 1975.

141. SEIDEL, J. C., AND J. GERGELY. The conformation of myosin during the steady state of ATP hydrolysis: studies with myosin spin labeled at the S1 thiol groups. *Biochem. Biophys. Res. Commun.* 44: 826–830, 1971.

142. SEIDEL, J. C., AND J. GERGELY. Investigation of conformational changes in spin-labeled myosin: implications for the molecular mechanism of muscle contraction. *Cold Spring Harbor Symp. Quant. Biol.* 37: 187–213, 1972.

143. SEIDEL, J. C., AND J. GERGELY. Electron spin resonance of myosin spin labeled at the S_1 thiol groups during hydrolysis of adenosine triphosphate. *Arch. Biochem. Biophys.* 158: 853–863, 1973.

144. SEKINE, T., AND M. YAMAGUCHI. Effect of ATP on the binding of *N*-ethylmaleimide to SH groups in the active site of myosin. *J. Biochem. Tokyo* 54: 196–198, 1963.

145. SELLERS, J. R., P. O. CHANTLER, AND A. G. SZENT-GYÖRGYI. Hybrid formation between scallop myofibrils and foreign regulatory light chains. *J. Mol. Biol.* 144: 223–245, 1980.

146. SHRIVER, J. W., AND B. D. SYKES. Phosphorus-31 nuclear magnetic resonance evidence for two conformations of myosin subfragment-1 · nucleotide complexes. *Biochemistry* 20: 2004–2012, 1981.

147. SHRIVER, J. W., AND B. D. SYKES. Energetics and kinetics of interconversion of two myosin subfragment-1 · adenosine 5'-diphosphate complexes as viewed by phosphorus-31 nuclear magnetic resonance. *Biochemistry* 20: 6357–6362, 1981.

148. SIMMONS, R. M., AND A. G. SZENT-GYÖRGYI. Reversible loss of calcium control of tension in scallop striated muscle associated with the removal of regulatory light chains. *Nature London* 273: 62–63, 1978.

149. SOMLYO, A. V., T. M. BUTLER, M. BOND, AND A. P. SOMLYO. Myosin filaments have non-phosphorylated light chains in relaxed smooth muscle. *Nature London* 294: 567–569.

150. SRIVASTAVA, S. K., Y. TONOMURA, AND A. INOUE. Modification of cardiac and smooth muscle myosins with 2,4,6-trinitrobenzenesulfonate. *J. Biochem. Tokyo* 86: 725–731, 1979.

151. STRAUB, F. B. Actin. In: *Studies from the Institute of Medical Chemistry, University of Szeged*, edited by A. Szent-Györgyi. Basel: Karger, 1942, vol. 2, p. 3–16.

152. SUTOH, K., K. SUTOH, T. KARR, AND W. F. HARRINGTON. Isolation and physico-chemical properties of a high molecular weight subfragment-2 of myosin. *J. Mol. Biol.* 126: 1–22, 1978.

153. SUZUKI, H., T. KAMATA, H. OHNISHI, AND S. WATANABE. Adenosine-triphosphate-induced reversible change on the conformation of chicken gizzard myosin and heavy meromyosin. *J. Biochem. Tokyo* 91: 1699–1706, 1982.

154. SUZUKI, H., H. ONISHI, K. TAKAHASHI, AND S. WATANABE. Structure and function of chicken gizzard myosin. *J. Biochem. Tokyo* 84: 1529–1542, 1978.

155. SZENT-GYÖRGYI, A. Studies on muscle. *Acta Physiol. Scand. Suppl.* 25: 1–128, 1945.

156. SZENT-GYÖRGYI, A. G. Meromyosins, the subunits of myosin. *Arch. Biochem. Biophys.* 42: 305–320, 1953.

157. SZENT-GYÖRGYI, A. G., E. M. SZENTKIRALYI, AND J. KENDRICK-JONES. The light chains of scallop myosin as regulatory subunits. *J. Mol. Biol.* 74: 179–203, 1973.

158. SZILÁGYI, L., M. BÁLINT, F. A. SRÉTER, AND J. GERGELY. Photoaffinity labelling with an ATP analog of the N-terminal peptide of myosin. *Biochem. Biophys. Res. Commun.* 87: 936–945, 1979.

159. SZILÁGYI, L., I. KURENNOY, M. BÁLINT, AND E. N. A. BIRO. Influence of ions and of ATP on the conformation of HMM studied by proteolysis. In: *Proteins of Contractile Systems*, edited by E. N. A. Biro. Budapest: Akad. Kiado, 1975, vol. 31, p. 47–59. (Proc. IX FEBS Meet.)

160. TAKAHASHI, K. Topography of the myosin molecule as visualized by an improved negative staining method. *J. Biochem. Tokyo* 83: 905–908, 1978.

161. TAKASHI, R., A. MUHLRAD, AND J. BOTTS. Spatial relationship between a fast-reacting thiol and a reactive lysine residue of myosin subfragment 1. *Biochemistry* 21: 5661–5668, 1982.

162. TAYLOR, E. W. Mechanism of actomyosin ATPase and the problem of muscle contraction. *Crit. Rev. Biochem.* 6: 103–164, 1979.

163. THOMAS, D. D., AND R. COOKE. Orientation of spin-labeled myosin heads in glycerinated muscle fibers. *Biophys. J.* 32: 891–906, 1980.

164. THOMAS, D. D., L. R. DALTON, AND J. S. HYDE. Rotational diffusion studied by passage saturation transfer EPR. *J. Chem. Phys.* 65: 3006–3024, 1976.

165. THOMAS, D. D., S. ISHIWATA, J. C. SEIDEL, AND J. GERGELY.

Submillisecond rotational dynamics of spin-labeled myosin heads in myofibrils. *Biophys. J.* 32: 873–889, 1980.

166. THOMAS, D. D., J. C. SEIDEL, AND J. GERGELY. The quantitative measurement of rotational motion of the subfragment-1 region of myosin by saturation transfer EPR spectroscopy. *J. Supramol. Struct.* 3: 376–390, 1975.
167. THOMAS, D. D., J. C. SEIDEL, AND J. GERGELY. Rotational dynamics of spin-labeled F-actin in the sub-millisecond time range. *J. Mol. Biol.* 132: 257–273, 1979.
168. THOMAS, D. D., J. C. SEIDEL, J. S. HYDE, AND J. GERGELY. Motion of subfragment-1 in myosin and its supramolecular complex: saturation transfer electron paramagnetic resonance. *Proc. Natl. Acad. Sci. USA* 72: 1729–1733, 1975.
169. TOKIWA, T., AND M. F. MORALES. Independent and comparative reactions of myosin heads with F-actin in the presence of adenosine triphosphate. *Biochemistry* 10: 1722–1727, 1971.
170. TREGEAR, R., AND R. A. MENDELSON. Polarization from a helix of fluorophores and its relation to that obtained from muscle. *Biophys. J.* 15: 455–467, 1975.
171. TRYBUS, K. M., T. W. HUIATT, AND S. LOWEY. A bent monomeric conformation of myosin from smooth muscle. *Proc. Natl. Acad. Sci. USA* 79: 6151–6155, 1982.
172. TSONG, T. Y., T. KARR, AND W. F. HARRINGTON. Rapid helix-coil transitions in the S-2 region of myosin. *Proc. Natl. Acad. Sci. USA* 76: 1109–1113, 1979.
173. UEÑO, H., AND W. F. HARRINGTON. Conformational transition in the myosin hinge upon activation of muscle. *Proc. Natl. Acad. Sci. USA* 78: 6101–6105, 1981.
174. UENO, H., AND W. F. HARRINGTON. Cross-bridge movement and the conformational state of the myosin hinge in skeletal muscle. *J. Mol. Biol.* 149: 619–640, 1981.
175. VIBERT, P., AND R. CRAIG. Three-dimensional reconstruction of thin filaments decorated with a Ca^{2+}-regulated myosin. *J. Mol. Biol.* 157: 299–320, 1982.
176. WATTERSON, J. G., L. KOHLER, AND M. C. SCHAUB. Evidence for two distinct affinities in the binding of divalent metal ions to myosin. *J. Biol. Chem.* 254: 6470–6477, 1979.
177. WEBER, A. The ultracentrifugal separation of L-meromyosin and actin in an actomyosin sol under the influence of ATP. *Biochim. Biophys. Acta* 19: 345–351, 1956.
177a. WEEDS, A. G., AND G. FRANK. Structural studies on light chains of myosin. *Cold Spring Harbor Symp. Quant. Biol.* 37: 9–17, 1982.
178. WEEDS, A. G., AND S. LOWEY. Substructure of the myosin molecule. II. The light chains of myosin. *J. Mol. Biol.* 61: 701–725, 1971.
179. WEEDS, A. G., AND B. POPE. Studies on the chymotryptic digestion of myosin. Effects of divalent cations on proteolytic susceptibility. *J. Mol. Biol.* 111: 129–151, 1977.
180. WELLS, J. A., M. SHELDON, AND R. G. YOUNT. Magnesium nucleotide is stoichiometrically trapped at the active site of myosin and its proteolytic fragments by thiol crosslinking reagents. *J. Biol. Chem.* 255: 1598–1602, 1980.
181. WELLS, J. A., M. M. WERBER, AND R. G. YOUNT. Inactivation of myosin subfragment 1 by cobalt (II)/cobalt (III) phenanthroline complexes. 2. Cobalt chelation of two critical SH groups. *Biochemistry* 18: 4800–4805, 1979.
182. WELLS, J. A., M. M. WERBER, AND R. G. YOUNT. Mechanism of inactivation of myosin subfragment 1 by cobalt (III) phenATP. A reinvestigation. *J. Biol. Chem.* 255: 7552–7555, 1980.
183. WELLS, J. A., AND R. G. YOUNT. Active site trapping of nucleotide crosslinking to sulfhydryl groups in myosin subfragment 1. *Proc. Natl. Acad. Sci. USA* 76: 4966–4970, 1979.
184. WELLS, J. A., AND R. G. YOUNT. Reaction of 5,5′-dithiobis(2-nitrobenzoic acid) with myosin subfragment 1: evidence for formation of a single protein disulfide with trapping of metal nucleotide at the active site. *Biochemistry* 19: 1711–1717, 1980.
185. WERBER, M. W., A. G. SZENT-GYÖRGYI, AND G. D. FASMAN. Fluorescence studies on heavy meromyosin substrate interaction. *Biochemistry* 11: 2872–2883, 1972.
186. YAMAMOTO, K., AND T. SEKINE. Interaction of myosin subfragment-1 with actin. I. Effect of actin binding on the susceptibility of subfragment-1 to trypsin. *J. Biochem. Tokyo* 86: 1855–1862, 1979.
187. YAMAMOTO, K., AND T. SEKINE. Interaction of myosin subfragment-1 with actin. II. Location of the actin binding site in a fragment of subfragment-1 heavy chain. *J. Biochem. Tokyo* 86: 1863–1868, 1979.
188. YAMAMOTO, K., AND T. SEKINE. Interaction of myosin subfragment-1 with actin. III. Effect of cleavage of the subfragment-1 heavy chain on its interaction with actin. *J. Biochem. Tokyo* 86: 1869–1881, 1979.
189. YANAGIDA, T. Angles of nucleotides bound to crossbridges in glycerinated muscle fibers at various concentrations of ϵ-ATP, ϵ-ADP and ϵ-AMPPNP detected by polarized fluorescence. *J. Mol. Biol.* 146: 539–560, 1981.
190. YOUNT, R. G., D. BABCOCK, W. BALLANTYNE, AND D. OJALA. Adenyl imidodiphosphate, an adenosine triphosphate analog containing a P-N-P linkage. *Biochemistry* 10: 2484–2489, 1971.
191. YOUNT, R. G., D. OJALA, AND D. BABCOCK. Interaction of P-N-P and P-C-P analogs of adenosine triphosphate with heavy meromyosin, myosin, and actomyosin. *Biochemistry* 10: 2490–2496, 1971.

CHAPTER 10

Electrical properties of striated muscle

RICHARD H. ADRIAN | *Physiological Laboratory, Cambridge, England*

CHAPTER CONTENTS

THE LAST 35 YEARS have seen an increase in our understanding of the mechanisms that produce electrical excitability. This electrophysiological knowledge has been successfully applied to axons, neurons, smooth muscle, cardiac muscle, and striated muscle. This chapter covers striated muscle and particularly amphibian twitch fibers. There is good reason to believe that most of the electrophysiological complexity of amphibian twitch fibers applies with only minor modification to mammalian fast- and slow-twitch fibers. The peculiarities of amphibian slow striated muscle, which are not described, are relevant to, at most, a few mammalian fibers with special functions, although they have considerable comparative importance (see, for instance, refs. 54–56).

Striated muscle fibers are large cylindrical cells and ideally must start to generate tension simultaneously in their entire cross section. The surface action potential therefore has to initiate a process that will affect the proteins in the middle of the fiber as rapidly as those near the surface, and they may be as much as 50 μm from the surface. The muscle fiber therefore must propagate a signal rapidly from the surface radially as well as along the fiber from end to end. Radial propagation in the network of the transverse tubular system (T system) is now reasonably well understood even if that understanding depends to an uncomfortable extent on indirect evidence about the ionic conductances of the tubular membrane. How the tubular signal reaches the sarcoplasmic reticulum and causes calcium ions to be released remains mysterious.

This chapter concentrates on the electrical properties of the surface and tubular membranes, at the expense of speculation about the interaction between the tubular membrane potential and the release of calcium from the sarcoplasmic reticulum. For a discussion of the latter question the reader is referred to L. L. Costantin's chapter on the "Activation of Striated Muscle" in the first volume of this *Handbook* section on the nervous system (37a). There is very active work in progress on the release and movement of intracellular calcium ion (33, 34, 85). I emphasize here the basic electrophysiological principles as they apply to striated muscle, in the belief that progress in the field depends on a sound grasp of this basic theory. I have gathered some otherwise rather scattered materials on cable theory, voltage clamping, and capacitance measurement in the hope that its presentation in one place will help students recognize its relevance. Readers interested only in the characteristics of the ionic currents in striated muscle need not involve themselves deeply in the first two sections on cable theory and voltage-clamp methods.

CABLE THEORY FOR STRIATED MUSCLE

The cable equation, known also as the telephone equation, was stated and solved by Lord Kelvin in 1855 (114). Kelvin wanted to know whether transatlantic communication by coaxial cable was a practical possibility given the imperfect insulators of that time. If the resistance of the core is r_i (in Ω/m) and the resistance and capacitance between the inside and outside of 1 m of cable is r_m (in $\Omega \cdot$m) and c_m (in μF/m), Kelvin showed that

$$\frac{1}{r_i}\frac{\delta^2 V}{\delta x^2} = \frac{V}{r_m} + c_m \frac{\delta V}{\delta t} \quad (1)$$

where $V(x, t)$ is the potential in the core of the cable.

Before Kelvin's work on submarine cables there had been a close relation between studies of electricity and excitability, so it was soon realized that Kelvin's equation could describe current flow in nerve and muscle. Kelvin's equation is a second-order linear differential equation in one dimension—the long axis of the cable or cell—and it adequately describes the distribution of potential along, for instance, a nonmyelinated nerve fiber. Striated muscle is morphologically complex, however, with transversely orientated membranes in the T system. It is important, therefore, to understand when the assumptions of one-dimensional cable theory are or are not valid.

Cable theory, in its physiological context, is a body of quantitative statements about current and potential that involve the geometry of the cell: it allows one to deduce the linear (and sometimes nonlinear) electrical properties (resistance, r_m; and capacitance, c_m) of the cell membrane from experimentally measured currents and potentials. The correctness of the deduced properties depends on knowing the shape of the cell and on adequately approximating the three-dimensional flow of current within the cell, in its membrane, and in its surroundings. See reference 79 for a comprehensive account of this material.

Full understanding of the flow of electric current within and without a striated muscle fiber, as much as in any other cell, depends therefore on the appropriate application of some form of Laplace's equation (46, 47, 111).

One can write for any isotropic conducting medium that the potential (V) due to current at any point not itself a source of current obeys the equation

$$\frac{\delta^2 V}{\delta x^2} + \frac{\delta^2 V}{\delta y^2} + \frac{\delta^2 V}{\delta z^2} = 0 \qquad (2)$$

where x, y, and z are any orthogonal coordinate system. A more relevant version of the same statement is in cylindrical coordinates r, θ, and x

$$\frac{1}{r}\frac{\delta}{\delta r}\left(r\frac{\delta V}{\delta r}\right) + \frac{1}{r^2}\frac{\delta^2 V}{\delta \theta^2} + \frac{\delta^2 V}{\delta x^2} = 0 \qquad (3)$$

This allows the properties of the membrane to be introduced into the boundary conditions on the region representing a cylindrical muscle fiber; the long axis of the fiber coincides with the x-axis, and the membrane is the cylindrical surface for which $r = a$. At any point on this surface the radially directed current (in A/cm^2) just within the membrane must equal the current passing across the membrane at this point (I_m)

$$-\frac{1}{R_i}\frac{\delta V}{\delta r}\bigg|_{r=a} = I_m \qquad (4)$$

where R_i is the resistivity of the inside of the fiber ($\Omega\cdot$cm). For a potential change (V_m) across the membrane that is everywhere small enough to ensure that the membrane resistance (R_m, $\Omega\cdot cm^2$) is ohmic and that the membrane capacitance (C_m, $\mu F/cm^2$) is linear

$$I_m = \frac{V_m}{R_m} + C_m\frac{\delta V_m}{\delta t} \qquad (5)$$

In Equation 5 the potential V_m is defined with respect to an isopotential external volume ($V_m = V_{r=a}$). In the steady state when $\delta V_m/\delta t = 0$

$$\frac{\delta V}{\delta r}\bigg|_{r=a} + \frac{R_i}{R_m}V_m = 0 \qquad (6)$$

It may be more useful to express this boundary condition in terms of the membrane resistance of unit length of fiber (r_m, $\Omega\cdot$cm) and the internal longitudinal resistance (r_i, Ω/cm), in which case Equation 6 becomes

$$\frac{\delta V}{\delta r}\bigg|_{r=a} + \frac{aV_m}{2\lambda^2} = 0 \qquad (7)$$

where λ is the length constant of the fiber and

$$\lambda^2 = \frac{r_m}{r_i} = \frac{aR_m}{2R_i} \qquad (8)$$

This boundary condition for Laplace's equation is referred to as a "mixed boundary condition" because it is a linear combination of the potential and its derivative normal to the boundary: a mixture of the Neuman boundary condition, which specifies only the derivative, and the Dirichelet condition, which specifies only the potential. Mixed boundary conditions arise in many physical problems: in heat conduction it is known as the radiation boundary condition (32). For a discussion of these questions see Peskoff (98).

If current is delivered by a micropipette impaling the striated muscle fiber, one can consider the source of the current to be a point. Mathematically the distribution of potential in the steady state will be given by a Green's function, which is a solution of Equation 3 inside a cylindrical boundary on which the potential is specified by Equation 6 (11, 46, 100). The more complex problem of a step function of current from a point source within a fiber in a medium of finite conductivity has been solved by Peskoff and Eisenberg (99).

Figure 1 shows the main features of the potential distribution in the steady state across the membrane of a fiber with a microelectrode current source located 5 μm below the membrane. The figure is taken from Adrian, Costantin, and Peachey (11), who computed the value of the membrane potential V_m (otherwise the value of the boundary potential $V_{r=a}$) for a source of current (I_0) at $r' < a$, $\theta' = 0^0$, and $x' = 0$. In this case

$$V_{r=a} = \frac{I_0 R_i}{2\pi a}\sum_{-\infty}^{+\infty}\cos n\theta \cdot \sum_{\beta}\frac{\beta\exp(-\beta x/a)\,J_n(\beta r'/a)}{[\beta^2 - n^2 + \frac{1}{4}(a/\lambda)^4]J_n(\beta)} \qquad (9)$$

where $J_n(\ )$ are Bessel functions of the first kind of order n, and the summation in β is over the positive roots of the equation

$$\frac{\beta J_{n-1}(\beta)}{J_n(\beta)} = n - \frac{a^2}{2\lambda^2} \qquad (10)$$

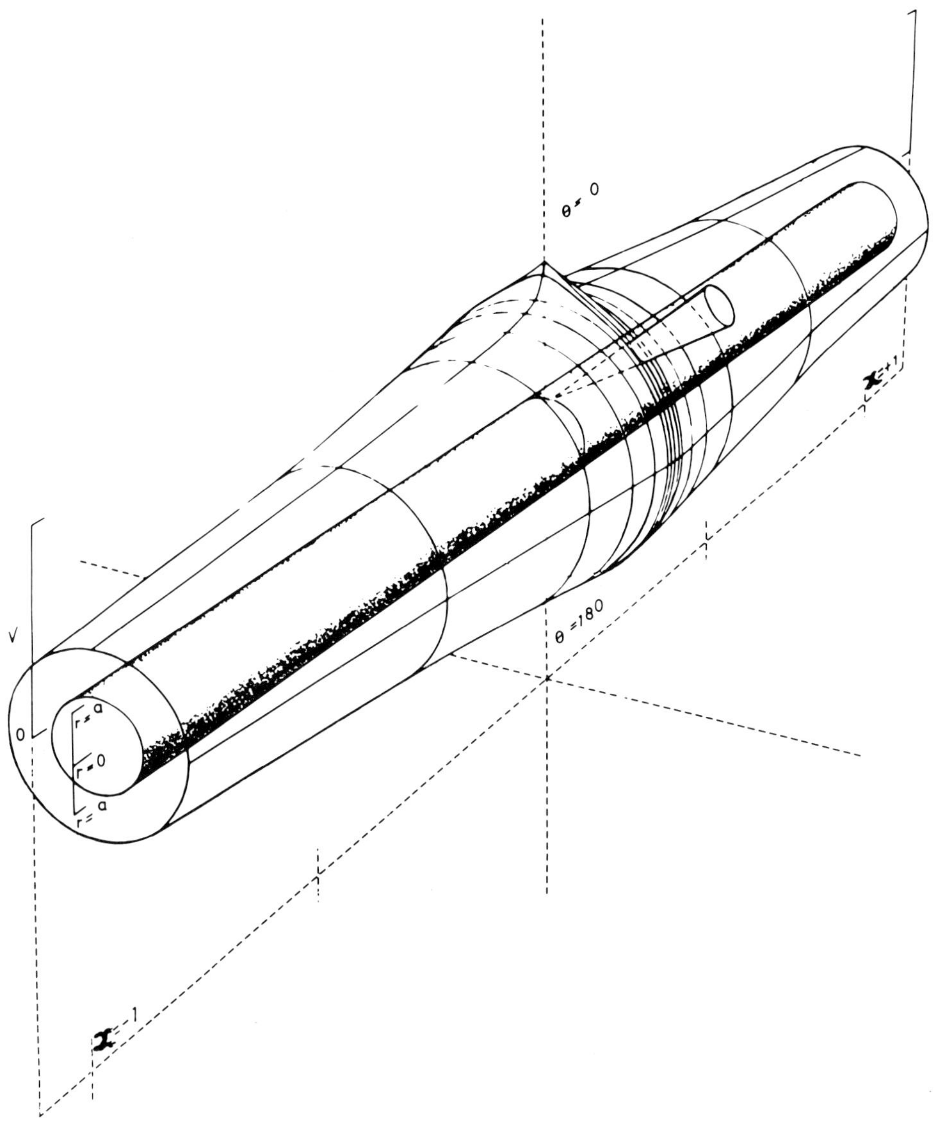

FIG. 1. Three-dimensional representation of potential ($V_{r=a}$; Eq. 9) across membrane at surface of a cylinder of specific resistivity R_i (200 Ω·cm) and membrane resistance R_m (1,000 Ω·cm²). Current is delivered from a point source represented as the tip of a microelectrode impaling the fiber. Microelectrode tip is at coordinates $x' = 0$, $\theta' = 0°$, $r' = 0.9a$ where a is the fiber radius (50 μm). Potential across membrane at any point on surface of cylinder is represented as radial distance between surface of cylinder and surface surrounding cylinder. Marks on x-axis are at ± 250 μm and ± 500 μm. [From Adrian, Costantin, and Peachey (11).]

Similar solutions are given in Falk and Fatt (47) and Eisenberg and Johnson (46). The latter authors give solutions that are substantially more convenient to compute than Equation 8, and they discuss in some detail the derivation of solutions to problems of three-dimensional current flow. Carslaw and Jaeger's book *Conduction of Heat in Solids* (32) is an important source of solutions (especially, in this context, chapter 14, section 13) because the equations governing the flow of heat and of current are very similar.

Despite the limitation that Figure 1 is for a unique set of conditions, the figure shows the main conclusion to be drawn from the analysis of the three-dimensional spread of current from a microelectrode in a muscle fiber. It is this: within 50 μm of the current-passing electrode the membrane potential is neither uniform in the circumference of the fiber nor is its longitudinal spread governed by the familiar steady-state solution of the cable equation

$$V = V_0 \exp(-x/\lambda) \qquad (11)$$

Figure 1 shows that there is a local change of potential (V) in the region of the current source, and it would be unsafe to use Equation 11 to extrapolate from or into the region around the current electrode, even though beyond that region Equation 11 would be appropriate in the steady state. As a practical consequence of this local state of affairs one should avoid a too close positioning of a current and voltage electrode in, for instance, a voltage-clamp arrangement. Moreover the dangers introduced by the local potential changes are greater at high frequencies of imposed potential or current, because the spatial distribution of the potential near the current source is much less affected by frequency than the potential distant from it. This point has been rightly emphasized by Valdiosera, Clausen, and Eisenberg (115).

An implicit assumption is involved in the application to cells of the equation developed by Kelvin to describe underwater cables (Eq. 1), that the flow of current (i) can be considered as occurring only in the direction of the longitudinal axis of the cell (along the x-axis) and that

$$\frac{\delta i}{\delta x} + i_m = 0 \tag{12}$$

where i_m is the current across the membrane in amperes per centimeter. It follows that the membrane current I_m (in A/cm^2) is

$$I_m = \frac{a}{2R_i}\frac{\delta^2 V}{\delta x^2} \tag{13}$$

but again this statement begs the question of how current reaches the membrane without flowing radially. One may, however, assume that just inside the membrane at $r = a$

$$\left.\frac{\delta V}{\delta r}\right|_{r=a} = -\frac{a}{2}\cdot\frac{\delta^2 V}{\delta x^2} \tag{14}$$

and that elsewhere the radial gradient of potential is ignorably small. Substituting from Equation 14 into Equation 7, which is the boundary condition for the three-dimensional problem considered earlier, one obtains the familiar cable equation for the steady state

$$\lambda^2\frac{d^2V}{dx^2} - V = 0 \tag{15}$$

or substituting into Equation 4 the more general Equation 13. Therefore it is hardly surprising that the complex solution of the three-dimensional problem (Eq. 9) should be equivalent to Equation 11 when $|x|$ is large. Note that this simplification arises generally because in excitable cells R_m is much greater than R_i, and therefore radial potential gradients in the cytoplasm of the cell are usually small enough to be ignored. For high-frequency currents this may not be the case because the membrane impedance may not be large compared to R_i.

The general solution of Equation 15 is

$$V = A\exp(x/\lambda) + B\exp(-x/\lambda) \tag{16}$$

where A and B are to be determined by the boundary conditions of the particular problem. This solution is for the steady state where the potential has reached an unchanging value everywhere. It can give information only about the membrane resistance (r_m) and the internal resistance (r_i). The transient solution, which describes how the potential varies from a distribution appropriate for one set of conditions (e.g., zero applied current) to another (e.g., constant applied current), includes information about the membrane capacitance (c_m,μF/cm) because the charge on that capacitance will alter.

In nerve and especially in nonmyelinated nerve, it is reasonable to consider that the membrane is a right circular cylinder and that there are no special regions of the surface. This is certainly not the case in striated muscle, and the assumption of a single time constant $\tau_m(r_m c_m)$ though widely made has given rise to difficulty. Nevertheless for the moment we shall assume (as did Kelvin) that the membrane current (i_m, A/cm) is given by

$$i_m = \frac{V_m}{r_m} + c_m\frac{\delta V_m}{\delta t} \tag{17}$$

Because

$$i_m = \frac{1}{r_i}\frac{\delta^2 V_m}{\delta x^2} \tag{18a}$$

$$\lambda^2\frac{\delta^2 V_m}{\delta x^2} - V_m = \tau_m\frac{\delta V_m}{\delta t} \tag{18b}$$

Setting $X = x/\lambda$ and $T = t/\tau_m$

$$\frac{\delta^2 V}{\delta X^2} - V = \frac{\delta V}{\delta T} \tag{19}$$

Substitution of $U = V\exp(T)$ gives

$$\frac{\delta^2 U}{\delta X^2} = \frac{\delta U}{\delta T} \tag{20}$$

which is an equation for which very many solutions are known for a wide variety of particular conditions (32, 38). In principle, therefore, it is possible to solve Equation 19 by finding the appropriately equivalent solution to Equation 20 and substituting $V = U\exp(-T)$. In practice this is not always a very useful way of finding solutions that involve delivering a constant current to a cell because the diffusional or heat flow equivalent of this boundary condition (integrated flux a constant) is not physically probable. It is more useful when the problem involves imposing a constant potential at some point in a cell (a point voltage clamp).

Among electrophysiologists the most widely known solution of Equation 18b is that given by Hodgkin and Rushton (70) for the case of a constant current delivered to the middle of a doubly infinite cable; that is, for a current I_0 (in A) at $x = 0$ for $t \geq 0$ with the cell extending from $x = \pm\infty$ where $V = 0$. Then

$$V(X, T) = \frac{I_0}{4}\sqrt{r_m r_i}[F_1(X, T) - F_2(X, T)] \quad (21)$$

where the functions of F_1 and F_2 include the complementary error function erfc

$$F_1(X, T) = \exp(-X)\operatorname{erfc}\left(\frac{X}{2\sqrt{T}} - \sqrt{T}\right) \quad (21a)$$

$$F_2(X, T) = \exp(X)\operatorname{erfc}\left(\frac{X}{2\sqrt{T}} + \sqrt{T}\right) \quad (21b)$$

and

$$\operatorname{erfc}(z) = 1 - \frac{2}{\sqrt{\pi}}\int_0^z e^{-\omega^2}\,d\omega \quad (21c)$$

This solution has been tabulated by Hodgkin and Rushton (70) and has been widely used.

For the case of a potential V_0 imposed at $x = 0$ for $t \geq 0$

$$V(X, T) = 1/2\,V_0[F_1(X, T) + F_2(X, T)] \quad (22)$$

see Carslaw and Jaeger (ref. 32, section 4.2).

We cannot always assume that the fiber is well represented by an infinite cable. This is uncomfortably true in striated muscle in which it may not be possible to locate the current-passing electrode sufficiently far ($\sim 5\lambda$) from both ends of the fiber. Hodgkin and Nakajima (69) give a solution useful for a short fiber. Based on the method of images, the solution is in the form of an infinite series, each term of which is the potential due to one of infinitely many equal current sources spaced in an infinite cable at $x = 2nl_3$ and at $x = 2nl_3 - 2l_1$ where $n = -\infty, \ldots -2, -1, 0, +1, +2, \ldots, +\infty$, and l_3 is the length of the short cable that has in it a current source at $x = 0$ and ends at $+l_2$ and $-l_1$. (Note that Hodgkin and Nakajima define the end of the fiber at $x = 0$.)

The series solution given by Hodgkin and Nakajima is very rapidly convergent, and in practice it may be sufficient to consider the potential as the sum of that due to three sources, at $x = 0$ and at the two image sources beyond the ends of the fiber at $x = 2l_2$ and $x = -2l_1$. In this restricted form for a constant current I_0 for $t \geq 0$ at $x = 0$ in a short fiber with ends at $-l_1$ and $+l_2$

$$\begin{aligned} V(X, T) \simeq \frac{I_0}{4}\sqrt{r_m r_i}[&F_1(X, T) + F_1(X + 2L_1, T) \\ &+ F_1(-X + 2L_2, T) - F_2(X, T) \\ &- F_2(X + 2L_1, T) - F_2(-X + 2L_2, T)] \end{aligned} \quad (23)$$

where, as before, $X = x/\lambda$, $L_1 = l_1/\lambda$, $L_2 = l_2/\lambda$, $T = t/\tau_m$ and $F_1(\ )$ and $F_2(\ )$ are given by Equations 21a and 21b. For a voltage V_0 imposed at $x = 0$ for $t \geq 0$

$$\begin{aligned} V(X, T) \simeq 1/2\,V_0[&F_1(X, T) + F_1(X + 2L_1, T) \\ &+ F_1(-X + 2L_2, T) + F_2(X, T) \\ &+ F_2(X + 2L_1, T) + F_2(-X + 2L_2, T)] \end{aligned} \quad (24)$$

Neither of these solutions is difficult to compute.

Alternative series representations of the potential in short cells can be obtained with Fourier expansions to solve the cable equation (Eq. 18). This was the method used by Kelvin, whose "short" cable stretched from London to New York. Some examples are given here because this method has very general applicability and forms the basis of the transient solution of the potential in the T system (8).

Consider this solution of Equation 20

$$U = A_n\cos(\alpha_n X)\exp(-\alpha_n^2 T) \quad (25)$$

Therefore

$$V = \sum_{n=1}^{\infty} A_n\cos(\alpha_n X)\exp[-(1 + \alpha_n^2)T] \quad (26)$$

will be a solution of Equation 19, the cable equation. The values given to A_n and α_n depend on the initial and boundary conditions of the problem.

Consider an imposed step change of potential V_0 at $x = 0$ in a short cable with ends at $\pm l$

$$V(X, T) = V_0\left\{\frac{\cosh|X| - L}{\cosh L} - \sum A_n\cos(\alpha_n X)\exp[-(1 + \alpha_n^2)T]\right\} \quad (27)$$

This solution is the steady-state distribution of potential (i.e., V at $T = \infty$) minus a term that is to be made identical initially (at $T = 0$) to the first term except at $X = \pm L$ where it is to be made equal to 0 by defining the values for α_n in terms of the roots of $\cos(\alpha_n L) = 0$ for $n = 1, 2, 3, \ldots, \infty$. Therefore $\alpha_n L = n\pi$ and $\alpha_n = n\pi/L$. At $X = 0$ the potential for $T > 0$ is V_0 and at all other points it grows toward its steady-state value because the second term in Equation 27 vanishes as $T \to \infty$.

At $T = 0$ therefore

$$\sum_1^{\infty} A_n\cos(\alpha_n X) = \frac{\cosh|X| - L}{\cosh L} = V(X, \infty) \quad (28)$$

Recalling that when $\cos(\alpha_n L) = 0$

$$A_n = \frac{2}{L}\int_0^L V(X, \infty)\cos(\alpha_n X)\,dX \quad (29)$$

$$V(X, T) = V_0\left\{\frac{\cosh(|X| - L)}{\cosh(L)} - \frac{2}{L\cosh(L)} \cdot \sum_{n=1}^{\infty}\frac{[\sinh(-L) + \alpha_n\sin(\alpha_n L)]\cos(\alpha_n X)}{1 + \alpha_n^2} \cdot \exp[-(1 + \alpha_n^2)T]\right\} \quad (30)$$

where $\alpha_n L$ are the positive roots of $\cos(\alpha_n L) = 0$; as before $\alpha_n = n\pi/L$ for $n = 1, 2, 3, \ldots$. By the same kinds of argument the potential in a short cable whose ends at $X = \pm L$ are clamped at V_L for $T > 0$ is

$$V(X, T) = V_L\left\{\frac{\cosh|X|}{\cosh(L)} - \frac{2}{L} \cdot \sum_{1}^{\infty} \frac{\alpha_n \cos(\alpha_n X)}{(1 + \alpha_n^2)\sin(\alpha_n L)} \exp[-(1 + \alpha_n^2)T]\right\} \quad (31)$$

where the values for α_n are defined by the positive roots of $\cos(\alpha_n L) = 0$. For a constant current I_0 delivered in the middle ($X = 0$) of a short cable with ends at $X = \pm L$

$$V(X, T) = \frac{I_0}{2}\sqrt{r_m r_i}\left\{\frac{\cosh(|X| - L)}{\sinh(L)} - \frac{\exp(-T)}{\sinh(L)} + \frac{2}{L} \cdot \sum_{1}^{\infty} \frac{[\cos(\alpha_n L) - \cos(\alpha_n X)\exp(-\alpha_n^2 T)]\exp(-T)}{1 + \alpha_n^2}\right\} \quad (32)$$

where $\sin(\alpha_n L) = 0$ (positive roots > 0). In this case the auxiliary equation is derived from the fact that at $X = \pm L$, $\delta V/\delta X = 0$.

Equations 32 and 31 are alternative solutions for Equations 23 and 24 with the condition that $L_1 = L_2$, i.e., that the current-passing electrode is at the middle of the fiber. Equation 30 applies for a one-dimensional analogy of the equation that has been used to describe the potential distribution in the T system (8).

The T system is a dense network of tubules extending across the entire cross section of the fiber, and it is reasonable to approximate it by a disk made up of two circular surfaces separated by a small space of thickness a and specific resistance R_i (in $\Omega \cdot$cm). Current flows across the surfaces (I_m, A/cm^2) and radially (I_r) in the intervening space. The sarcoplasm above and below the disk is treated as isopotential. Figure 2 shows the assumed geometry; radial symmetry is assumed. In order to show the parallel between one-dimensional and radially symmetrical cases, a solution will be given for the boundary conditions that are analogous with those that give rise to Equation 31, which is an imposed potential V_L at $r = l$, the edge of the disk.

The membrane current I_m at any value of the radius equals the change in radial current I_r at that radius

$$-\frac{\delta I_r}{\delta r} = 4\pi r I_m \quad (33)$$

But

$$\frac{\delta V_r}{\delta r} = \frac{-R_i I_r}{2\pi r a} \quad (34)$$

$$\therefore \frac{1}{r}\frac{\delta}{\delta r}\left(r\frac{\delta V_r}{\delta r}\right) = \frac{2R_i I_m}{a} \quad (35)$$

If

$$I_m = \frac{V}{R_m} + C_m\frac{\delta V_r}{\delta r} \quad (36)$$

which assumes as before that the current crosses the tubular membrane as a parallel combination of a linear resistance and capacitance, then

$$\frac{1}{r}\frac{\delta}{\delta r}\left(r\frac{\delta V_r}{\delta r}\right) = \frac{2R_i}{aR_m}\left(V + \tau_m\frac{\delta V_r}{\delta t}\right) \quad (37)$$

where $\tau_m = R_m C_m$. Change to the dimensionless variables $R = r/\lambda$ and $T = t/\tau_m$ and set $\lambda^2 = aR_m/2R_i$, then

$$\frac{1}{R}\frac{\delta}{\delta R}\left(R\frac{\delta V}{\delta R}\right) - V = \frac{\delta V}{\delta T} \quad (38)$$

[In the derivation and solution in Adrian, Chandler, and Hodgkin (8) the membrane capacitance and conductance and the lumen conductance are defined differently to take into account the morphological features of the T system and to relate them to fiber volume. Here they are defined in terms of the disk of Figure 2 in order to make the analogy with one-dimensional cases more clearly.]

Substitution of $U = V\exp[T]$ gives

$$\frac{1}{R}\frac{\delta}{\delta R}\left(R\frac{\delta U}{\delta R}\right) = \frac{\delta U}{\delta T} \quad (39)$$

Equation 39 is solved by

$$U(R,T) = A_n J_0(\alpha_n R)\exp(-\alpha_n^2 T) \quad (40)$$

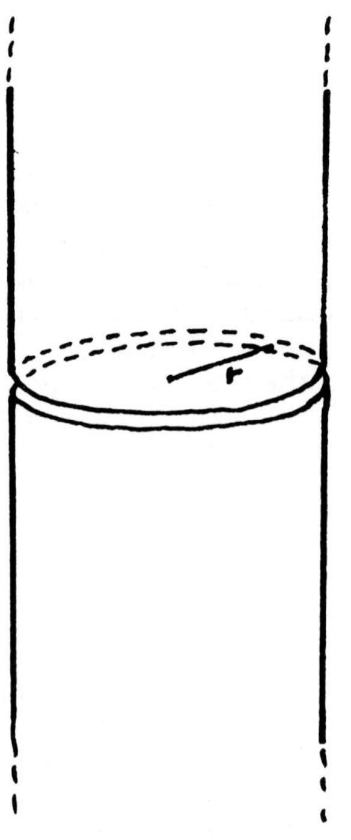

FIG. 2. Disk model of the transverse-tubular system.

where $J_0(\ )$ is a Bessel function of the first kind and zero order. So that

$$V(R,T) = \sum_{1}^{\infty} A_n J_0(\alpha_n R)\exp[-(1 + \alpha_n^2)T] \quad (41)$$

is a solution of Equation 38. As before we have to find values for A_n and α_n that satisfy the boundary and initial conditions (see ref. 32, section 7.4). In this case we make use of the relation that

$$A_n = \frac{2}{L^2 J_1^2(\alpha_n L)} \int_0^L R J_0(\alpha_n R)\, V(R,\infty) dR \quad (42)$$

when $J_0(\alpha_n R) = 0$. $J_0(\ )$ and $J_1(\ )$ are Bessel functions of zero and first order and $V(R,\infty)$ is the steady-state distribution of potential.

A particular experimental case that arises in striated muscle is the potential change that occurs in the T system when the potential across the surface membrane of the muscle fiber is abruptly changed. In terms of the disk model of Figure 2 the conditions are that for $T > 0$, $V(L,T) = V_L$; in other words, at the circumference of the disk the potential across the surfaces of the disk changes abruptly from 0 to V_L for $T > 0$. In this case

$$V(R,T) = V_L \left\{ \frac{I_0(R)}{I_0(L)} - \frac{2}{L} \cdot \sum_{1}^{\infty} \frac{\alpha_n J_0(\alpha_n R)}{(1 + \alpha_n^2) J_1(\alpha_n L)} \exp[-(1 + \alpha_n^2)T] \right\} \quad (43)$$

where the values for α_n are defined by the positive roots of $J_0(\alpha_n L) = 0$. Compare Equations 43 and 31. Both are made up of the steady-state potential from which is subtracted a series that is zero when $T \rightarrow \infty$ and at $T = 0$ is equal to the steady-state values except at the boundary ($X = \pm L$ or $R = L$) where it is zero. The forms of Equations 31 and 43 are identical after interchanging $I_0(x)$ and $\cosh(x)$, $J_0(x)$ and $\cos(x)$, and $J_1(x)$ and $\sin(x)$.

Solutions that involve the summation of infinite series are straightforward to compute for particular cases, even though care must be taken to check convergence. The ease with which they can be obtained has to be set against the difficulty of seeing the characteristics of the solution from the shape of the equation.

VOLTAGE-CLAMP METHODS FOR STRIATED MUSCLE

Although it is important to be able to describe expected changes in potential and current when membrane behavior is linear, the physiologically interesting behavior of the membrane of striated muscle, as of all excitable membranes, depends on its nonlinear conductances. This has been well recognized since the work of Cole and Hodgkin; but it has only recently been realized that the dielectric behavior of excitable cell membranes is also nonlinear. In this section I discuss some of the methods used to examine the nonlinear and sometimes time-dependent behavior of both the ionic conductances and the capacitance of the membrane.

Because the ionic conductances depend on the membrane potential, it is essential to be able to control that potential experimentally. An important feature of any reliable voltage-clamp method is whether it can achieve spatial uniformity and temporal invariance of membrane potential. Clamping squid giant axons usually involves long internal electrodes to measure potential and to pass current. The presence of these internal electrodes short-circuits the internal longitudinal resistance and goes a long way to ensure spatial uniformity. Even so the presence of a resistance in series with the membrane may give rise to a membrane potential that is neither spatially nor temporally uniform (112). The situation in striated muscle is much worse than in giant squid axons because it is not at all easy to insert internal longitudinal electrodes (but see ref. 41). Longitudinal spatial uniformity of voltage is almost impossible to achieve in striated muscle fibers. Without some knowledge of the degree of nonuniformity, the recorded current can be misleading, and it may be impossible to deduce the membrane current from it. It is not in general difficult to impose a particular shape (e.g., a step change) on the recorded potential, but it is difficult to be sure that the *recorded* potential accurately represents the membrane potential at every, or indeed at any, point on the membrane.

Information about ionic currents in striated muscle has been obtained by several kinds of clamping, perhaps better called quasi-clamping, techniques. There is certainly general agreement about the behavior of the currents, although there are detailed differences that may well depend on the particular uncertainties of particular methods. The methods themselves fall into two broad groups: those with internal microelectrodes and those with external electrodes with sucrose or Vaseline gaps to isolate a small patch of membrane. Each method has its characteristic compromises and dangers that must be understood if useful results are to be obtained. None of these methods provides any special means to control the potential of the T system. The degree of control in the T system is open to serious doubt, and if control has been achieved, it is certainly fortuitous.

Gap Methods

Essentially two variants of the gap method have been used on striated muscle. On isolated and intact muscle fibers Ildefonse and Rougier (77) employed a method developed by Rougier, Vassort, and Stämpfli (102) for atrial trabeculae. The fiber lies across three pools of solution that are electrically isolated by barriers of flowing sucrose solution. The narrow central pool contains an artificial "node" of membrane and is further demarcated by Vaseline seals. Current is applied between one outer pool and the central pool. Potential is measured between the central pool and the other outer pool containing isotonic KCl. The measured potential controls the current. Modifications of this method have been made by Léoty and Alix (87) and Poindessault, Duval, and Léoty (101). A more refined method based on the Dodge and Frankenhaeuser (42) method for myelinated nerve fibers has been developed by Hille and Campbell (30, 31, 64). The potential is measured by the method of Frankenhaeuser (49, 50). This method for clamping requires a third seal and two feedback amplifiers: one involved in measuring the potential and one to control it. The gap clamp of Hille and Campbell relies on Vaseline seals rather than sucrose gaps; however, it requires cut fiber ends in each end pool to reduce the resistance beween the pool and the inside of the fiber. There is some suggestion that using fiber segments may cause fiber damage.

There are several difficulties in gap methods that have been variously recognized and overcome. The most obvious is longitudinal nonuniformity of potential in the artificial node of the central compartment. The length of this compartment is usually 100–200 μm, which is certainly short in comparison with the DC length constant (λ, ca. 1.7 mm). But this is not the most relevant comparison. In a fiber with all its sodium channels open the length constant might be no more than 100–150 μm, which would allow substantial nonuniformity in a node of 100–200 μm. Indeed Hille and Campbell have recorded with a microelectrode the potential of the inside of the fiber just at the edge of the node next to the gap across which the current is delivered (ref. 64, Fig. 5). At the height of the sodium current this potential deviates from ground by 5 mV, which means there is a 5-mV variation of potential along the length of the artificial node. It is difficult to know how much this distorts the time course of the sodium current, but it certainly represents a departure from an ideal clamp. For mechanical reasons it is difficult to reduce the length of the central pool below 100 μm even though 100 μm may be dangerously long. Reduction of temperature and of external sodium ion concentration reduces the magnitude of the activated sodium current and thus of the potential nonuniformity.

A resistance in the central pool between the external membrane surface and the recording electrode will, when membrane currents are large, add a potential in series with the membrane potential. The sum of the membrane potential and this series potential is controlled by the feedback amplifier. Suitable compensation can be achieved by adding to the command signal, a compensatory signal of appropriate sign derived from the recorded membrane current. This certainly goes some way to eliminate the uncertainty and to impose a step change on the membrane potential, but there can be errors in the record of the membrane current, which arise because it is recorded as the potential developed across an impedance that is not a simple linear resistor. In their system Hille and Campbell (64) provide some correction for the behavior of this impedance; nevertheless the total result of both compensations is not ideal, and they remark that "our inability to find a routine practical way to determine the correct setting of the compensating dial [for series resistance] is unfortunate . . . since the time course of the sodium current varies significantly with the setting." Despite these reservations the Hille-Campbell method is the more reliable of the two gap methods, because considerable effort has been taken to find and mitigate the inherent problems.

Recently Kovács and Schneider (86) produced a simple and elegant variant of the gap method that has the advantage that tension and optical changes can be easily recorded under voltage control. The end of a cut fiber is made to protrude through a narrow channel in a partition and the tendon is attached to a tension recorder. Current is applied to the membrane by a potential across the partition, and the membrane potential is derived by combining this potential and a correction derived from the total current across the partition. The clamping amplifier compares this derived membrane potential with an appropriate command signal. The correct combination of the two signals that forms the recorded membrane potential is found with a recording microelectrode in the fiber; the derived potential is made to superimpose on the microelectrode record. In use the microelectrode is withdrawn so that movement can take place. The method depends on the resistances in the channel across the partition remaining fixed. It has been used to record the delayed potassium current (86) and, simultaneously, intramembrane charge movement and a Ca^{2+}-indicator dye signal (85).

Microelectrode-Clamping Methods

With two capillary microelectrodes, one to record membrane potential and one nearby to pass current, it is a simple matter to impose a step change of recorded membrane potential with a feedback amplifier. But the step change will only be in the region of the recording microelectrode (see, for instance, Eqs. 22 and 24). Some semblance of spatial uniformity can be achieved if the current-passing electrode is reasonably close to the end of a fiber. When this is the case the current delivered by the electrode consists largely of current flowing to the long part of the fiber, and a means of estimating the current passing across the membrane of the short end segment of the fiber is required.

In the clamping method of Adrian, Chandler, and Hodgkin (9), usually called the three-electrode method, three electrodes are spaced at $x = l$, $2l$, and $2l + l'$ from the end of a muscle fiber ($x = 0$). In general l is short compared with the steady-state space constant λ. In the steady state with a linear membrane conductance (g_m) the voltage distribution is therefore

$$V(x) = V_0 \cosh \frac{x}{\lambda} \tag{44}$$

where $\lambda = (r_i g_m)^{-1/2}$.

The potentials measured at $x = l$ and $x = 2l$ are V_1 and V_2. Usually V_1 is the controlled voltage, and we are interested in the membrane current i_m(in A/cm) at that potential. Consider the measurable quantity

$$\Delta V = V_2 - V_1 = V_0[\cosh(2l/\lambda) - \cosh(l/\lambda)] \tag{45}$$

Now

$$V_0 = i_m/[g_m \cosh(l/\lambda)] \tag{46}$$

where i_m and g_m are, respectively, the membrane current at V_1 and membrane conductance of unit length of fiber

$$\Delta V = \frac{i_m}{g_m} \cdot \frac{\cosh(2l/\lambda) - \cosh(l/\lambda)}{\cosh(l/\lambda)} \tag{47}$$

expanding the hyperbolic cosines as series

$$\Delta V = \frac{i_m}{g_m} \cdot \frac{\frac{3}{2!}\left(\frac{l}{\lambda}\right)^2 + \frac{15}{4!}\left(\frac{l}{\lambda}\right)^4 \cdots}{1 + \frac{1}{2!}\left(\frac{l}{\lambda}\right)^2 \cdots} \tag{48}$$

and if l/λ is sufficiently small

$$\Delta V \simeq \frac{3 i_m l^2}{2 g_m \lambda^2} \tag{49}$$

$$i_m \simeq \frac{2\Delta V}{3 r_i l^2} \tag{50}$$

This simple relation between the membrane current and the recorded potential ($V_2 - V_1$) is approximate. From Equations 45 and 46 we know that

$$i_m = \frac{\Delta V g_m \cosh(l/\lambda)}{\cosh(2l/\lambda) - \cosh(l/\lambda)} \tag{51}$$

therefore if p is a correction factor such that

$$\frac{2\text{p}\Delta V}{3 r_i l^2} = \frac{\Delta V g_m \cosh(l/\lambda)}{\cosh(2l/\lambda) - \cosh(l/\lambda)} \tag{52}$$

$$\text{p} = \frac{3}{2} l^2 \frac{\cosh L}{\cosh 2L - \cosh L} \tag{53}$$

where $L = l/\lambda$. Therefore p is a function of the length constant and the electrical spacing and gives, for the steady state and provided the membrane conductance is linear, the error that is involved in assuming that ΔV is proportional to the membrane current (Eq. 50). Equation 51 is strictly valid if g_m is not a function of voltage, but this is less of a disadvantage than it seems at first sight as p is close to 1 for $L < 2$. This suggests that R_m could fall to, say, 50 $\Omega \cdot \text{cm}^2$ for spacing $l = 250$ μm. It is worth considering two other conditions: where the membrane conductance is negative and where there is a significant current in the membrane capacitance. If the membrane conductance is negative, then in the steady state the potential near the end of the fiber is

$$V = V_0 \cos(x/\lambda) \tag{54}$$

where $\lambda = (r_i |g_m|)^{-1/2}$ and by the same argument as before

$$i_m \simeq \frac{2\Delta V \text{p}'}{3 r_i l^2} \tag{54a}$$

where

$$\text{p}' = -\frac{3}{2} L^2 \frac{\cos L}{\cos 2L - \cos L} \tag{55}$$

where as before $L = l/(r_i |g_m|)^{-1/2}$. Insofar as there are few steady-state situations with a uniformly negative membrane conductance, p′ is less useful than p. The behavior of p′ as a function of L, however, serves to emphasize the dangers of regenerative currents: p′ is 0.95 for $L = 0.65$ and drops to 0 for $L = 1.57$ ($\pi/2$). During the peak inward sodium current, $|g_m|$ may be 1.3 mmho/cm and λ is ~100 μm. With an electrode spacing of 250 μm, L is 2.5 and is well beyond the safe limit for reliable estimation of membrane current from ΔV. Kass, Siegelbaum, and Tsien (81) recently applied a similar analysis to a three-electrode clamp of short Purkinje fibers.

To apply the three-electrode method to the measurement of membrane capacitance, first consider the nature of muscle membranes. Previous methods for measuring capacitance have depended on choosing a particular equivalent circuit to represent the linear electrical properties of the cell surface, and measured "capacitance" only has meaning in terms of that equivalent circuit. In striated muscle, however, the structure of the fiber surface is complex, and it is far from clear how this should be reflected in an equivalent circuit. Clearly the impedance of the striated membrane cannot be represented by a single resistance and single capacitor in parallel. This basic analogue serves well for very many excitable cells, but for striated muscle it is necessary to add at least one alternative pathway for current consisting of a resistance and capacitor in series (47).

This minimum necessary modification certainly represents the current pathway across the membrane of the T system. Because this is itself a radially directed "cable," it is plainly an oversimplification to represent it by a single time constant in an equivalent circuit. A good deal of effort has been put into refining the electrical representation of the T system without the emergence of any clearly preferred representation (47,

90, 104, 115). An alternative approach has been to employ some operational definition of capacitance that is independent of any assumed equivalent circuit.

Essentially we seek a measurement of effective capacitance defined as the ratio between the voltage imposed at a particular point in a cell and the charge required to impose that potential; the charge is taken as the time integral of the transient current, that is, the current that does not flow through purely resistive membrane pathways. Hodgkin and Rushton (70) point out that Equation 21 for $V(X,T)$ in an infinite cable has the property that the total charge on the cable rises and falls exponentially on the make and break of a constant current. For an internal electrode delivering current at $x = 0$ (cable ends at $\pm\infty$) and a constant current (I_0) made at $t = 0$

$$c_m \int_{-\infty}^{+\infty} V(x,t)\mathrm{d}x = \tau_m I_0[1 - \exp(-t/\tau_m)] \quad (56)$$

The total charge placed on the cable at $t = \infty$ will be

$$c_m \int_0^{\infty}\int_{-\infty}^{+\infty} V(x,t)\mathrm{d}x\mathrm{d}t = \tau_m I_0 \quad (57)$$

and this will be true whether a constant current has been delivered at $x = 0$ or a step of potential has been forced at $x = 0$. Now if we consider Equation 22, which applies to a clamp step to V_0 at $x = 0$

$$V(X,T) = \tfrac{1}{2}V_0\left[\exp(-X)\mathrm{erfc}\left(\frac{X}{2\sqrt{T}} - \sqrt{T}\right) + \exp(X)\mathrm{erfc}\left(\frac{X}{2\sqrt{T}} + \sqrt{T}\right)\right] \quad (58)$$

the current delivered by the electrode is (with error function erf)

$$I_0(T) = \frac{-2}{r_i\lambda}\left(\frac{\mathrm{d}V}{\delta X}\right)_{X=0} = \frac{2V_0}{\sqrt{r_m r_i}}\left[\mathrm{erf}(\sqrt{T}) + \frac{\exp(-T)}{\sqrt{\pi T}}\right] \quad (59)$$

At $T = \infty$, $I(\infty) = 2V_0/\sqrt{r_m r_i}$; therefore the transient part of the current is

$$I(T) - I(\infty) = \frac{2V_0}{\sqrt{r_m r_i}}\left[\mathrm{erf}\sqrt{T} + \frac{\exp(-T)}{\sqrt{\pi T}} - 1\right] \quad (60)$$

so that the total transient current is

$$\int_0^{\infty}[I(T) - I(\infty)]\mathrm{d}t = \frac{\tau_m V_0}{\sqrt{r_m r_i}} = c_m\lambda V_0 \quad (61)$$

Since $I(\infty) = 2V_0/\sqrt{r_m r_i}$

$$\int_0^{\infty}[I(T) - I(\infty)] = \frac{\tau_m I(\infty)}{2} \quad (62)$$

Therefore the integral of the transient part of the electrode current is exactly one-half the total charge on the cable. (This proof is from A. L. Hodgkin.) Equation 61 allows one to measure c_m in an infinite cable if λ is known. The membrane capacitance is the ratio of the integral of the transient current in a point voltage clamp to the product of λ_∞ and the magnitude of the step

$$c_m = \frac{1}{V_0\lambda}\int_0^{\infty}[I(T) - I(\infty)]\mathrm{d}t \quad (63)$$

This relation is a particular case of a much more general proposition that allows us to define an effective membrane capacitance (c_m) in terms of the integral of the transient current. What follows is a summary of the arguments developed by Schneider and Chandler (105) and by Adrian and Almers (5, 6).

Consider the admittance $y(p)$ between the terminals of a network

$$y(p) = i(p)/v(p) \quad (64)$$

where $i(p)$ and $v(p)$ are the Laplace transforms of the current and voltage and p here is the dummy transform variable (to be distinguished from p in Eq. 53). The DC conductance of the network is given by

$$g = \lim_{p\to 0} y(p) \quad (65)$$

Let a voltage displacement $v(t)$ be applied at $t = 0$ such that

$$\lim_{t\to\infty} v(t) = v(\infty) \quad (66)$$

and if $i(t)$ is the current that flows into the network as a result of $v(t)$, one can define the transient part of the current as

$$i_{tr}(t) = i(t) - v(t)g \quad (67)$$

Laplace transformation and rearrangement give

$$\int_0^{\infty} e^{-pt}i_{tr}(t)\mathrm{d}t = pv(p)\frac{y(p) - y(0)}{p} \quad (68)$$

$$\therefore \int_0^{\infty} i_{tr}(t)\mathrm{d}t = \lim_{p\to 0} pv(p)\frac{y(p) - y(0)}{p} \quad (69)$$

From the final value theorem and the definition of the derivative

$$\frac{1}{v(\infty)}\int_0^{\infty}[i(t) - v(t)g]\mathrm{d}t = \left.\frac{\mathrm{d}y(p)}{\mathrm{d}p}\right|_{p=0} = C_{eff} \quad (70)$$

and this provides a definition of effective capacitance (C_{eff}) for any network whose admittance function at $p = 0$ has at least one derivative with respect to p and for any voltage waveform, oscillatory or otherwise, provided it reaches a steady value (5).

Consider a cable made up of elements each with an admittance $y(p)$ and joined by resistances $r_i\mathrm{d}x$ where r_i is the longitudinal resistance of unit length of fiber.

Let the ends of the fiber be at $x = \pm l$, and the middle of the fiber be at $x = 0$ where the current (I_0) and voltage (V_0) are measured. Assuming further that the network contains only linear elements, the complex admittance of the cable is

$$Y_0(p) = \frac{I_0(p)}{V_0(p)} \tag{71}$$

As before $I_0(p)$ and $V_0(p)$ are the Laplace transforms of I_0 and V_0. By cable theory

$$Y_0(p) = 2\tanh[l/\lambda(p)]\,[y(p)/r_i]^{1/2} \tag{72}$$

where

$$\lambda(p) = [y(p)r_i]^{-1/2} \tag{73}$$

Differentiating Equation 72 and setting $p = 0$

$$\left.\frac{dY(p)}{dp}\right|_{p=0} = \lambda\tanh(l/\lambda) \cdot \left[\frac{l/\lambda}{\cosh(l/\lambda)\sinh(l/\lambda)} + 1\right]\left.\frac{dy(p)}{dp}\right|_{p=0} \tag{74}$$

As before

$$\left.\frac{dY(p)}{dp}\right|_{p=0} = \frac{1}{V_0(\infty)}\int_0^\infty\left[I_0(t) - \frac{2}{\sqrt{r_m r_i}}V_0(t)\right]dt \tag{75}$$

and if

$$\left.\frac{dy(p)}{dp}\right|_{p=0} = c_{eff} \tag{76}$$

then it follows that

$$c_{eff} = \frac{\int_0^\infty\left[I_0(t) - \frac{2}{\sqrt{r_m r_i}}V_0(t)\right]dt}{V_0(\infty)\lambda\tanh(L)\left[\frac{L}{\cosh(L)\sinh(L)} + 1\right]} \tag{77}$$

where $L = l/\lambda$ and c_{eff} is the effective capacitance of the element making up the cable.

The expression $\lambda\tanh(L)\{L\cdot[\cosh(L)\sinh(L)]^{-1} + 1\}$ takes values between $2l$ and λ for $0 \le L < +\infty$. For $L \to \infty$, which is an infinite cable

$$c_{eff} = \frac{1}{V_0(\infty)\lambda}\int_0^\infty\left[I_0(t) - \frac{2}{\sqrt{r_m r_i}}V_0(t)\right]dt \tag{78}$$

For $L \to 0$, which is for electrodes at the middle of a very short fiber

$$c_{eff} = \frac{1}{2lV_0(\infty)}\int_0^\infty\left[I_0(t) - \frac{2}{\sqrt{r_m r_i}}V_0(t)\right]dt \tag{79}$$

and this holds to 1% for $L \le 0.1$.

For an imposed voltage $V_0(\infty)$ at $x = 0$ from $t = 0$ (point clamp), the integral in Equations 78 and 79 is

$$\int_0^\infty\left[I_0(t) - \frac{2}{\sqrt{r_m r_i}}V_0(t)\right]dt = \int_0^\infty[I_0(t) - I_0(\infty)]dt \tag{80}$$

and for a constant current $I_0(\infty)$ from $t = 0$

$$\int_0^\infty\left[I_0(t) - \frac{2}{\sqrt{r_m r_i}}V_0(t)\right]dt = I_0(\infty)\int_0^\infty\left[1 - \frac{V_0(t)}{V_0(\infty)}\right]dt \tag{81}$$

It is thus equally easy to determine c_{eff} with a constant current or an imposed step of voltage. It is perhaps worth illustrating the meaning of the effective capacitance (C_{eff}) with respect to two simple equivalent circuits. In Figure 3*A*

$$y(p) = G_m + pC_s + \frac{pC_T}{pR_sC_T + 1} \tag{82}$$

$$\left.\frac{dy(p)}{dp}\right|_{p=0} = C_s + C_T = C_{eff} \tag{83}$$

In Figure 3*B*

$$y(p) = G_m + pC_S + \frac{pC_TR_T + 1}{pC_TR_TR_s + R_s + R_T} \tag{84}$$

$$\left.\frac{dy(p)}{dp}\right|_{p=0} = C_S + C_T\left(\frac{R_T}{R_s + R_T}\right) \tag{85}$$

Both these circuits can be made electrically equivalent in the steady state by appropriate choice of elements, but in Figure 3*B* the effective capacitance is less than the sum of the capacitors.

Returning to the three-electrode–clamp measurement of membrane capacitance we have defined the effective capacitance as

$$C_{eff} = \frac{1}{v(\infty)}\int_0^\infty[i_m(t) - g_m v(t)]\,dt \tag{86}$$

In terms of three electrodes at the end of the fiber, $v(\infty)$ and $v(t)$ in Equation 86 are, respectively, $V_1(\infty)$ and $V_1(t)$

$$i_m(t) \simeq \frac{2[V_2(t) - V_1(t)]}{3r_i l^2} \tag{87}$$

$$g_m(t) \simeq \frac{2[V_2(\infty) - V_1(\infty)]}{3V_1(\infty)r_i l^2} \tag{88}$$

Inserting these expressions into Equation 86 gives

$$r_i c_{eff} \simeq \frac{2}{3V_1(\infty)l^2}\int_0^\infty\left[V_2(t) - \frac{V_2(\infty)}{V_1(\infty)}V_1(t)\right]dt \tag{89}$$

As Schneider and Chandler (105) have pointed out, this measurement of capacitance is independent of

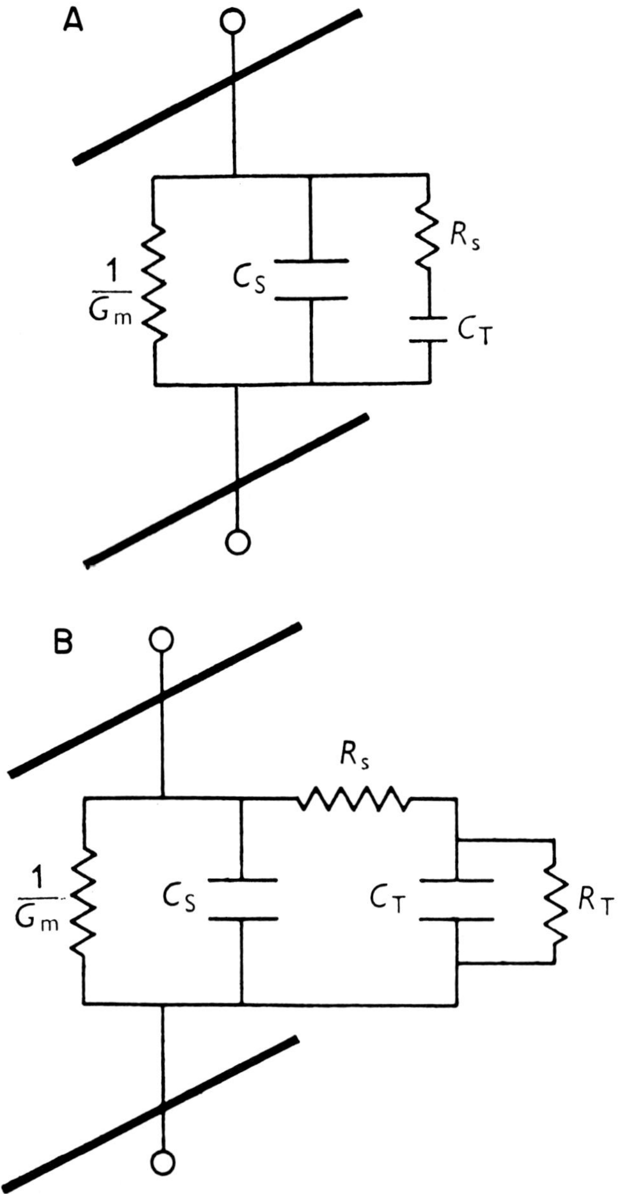

FIG. 3. Circuits referred to in text to illustrate the definition of effective capacitance by means of Equation 70. [From Adrian and Almers (5).]

any knowledge of λ (cf. Eq. 78, which can be used to define c_{eff} in terms of the electrode current delivered to the center of an infinite cable). This relation can be made precise by deriving a correction factor h analogous to p (Eq. 53) such that

$$c_{\text{eff}} = \frac{2\text{h}}{3V_1(\infty)r_i l^2} \int_0^\infty \left[V_2(t) - \frac{V_2(\infty)}{V_1(\infty)} V_1(t)\right] dt \quad (90)$$

$$\text{h} = \frac{3L}{(3 - \tanh^2(L)) \sinh(L)} \quad (91)$$

As with p (Eq. 53), the correction factor h is a function of L ($= l/\lambda$), and provided L is small, h is close to 1. As might be expected, h deviates from 1 more rapidly than p. Both Schneider and Chandler (105) and Adrian and Almers (6) have considered the effects of current leak at the electrodes. They conclude that whereas electrode leaks can seriously affect measurements of conductance, their effect on capacitance measurements is small.

Although it is possible to obtain the necessary measurements from photographic records of I_0, V_1, and ΔV, it would be cumbersome and time consuming. Moreover the necessary integrations and manipulations are easily done on a minicomputer that can store appropriate records in the form of digitized arrays. In general this has been done; outline descriptions of the procedures are given in, for instance, Chandler, Rakowski, and Schneider (33), Adrian and Almers (6), Adrian and Marshall (14), and Adrian and Rakowski (17).

A variant of the three-electrode method has been used to examine the membrane currents of mammalian fibers. These have also been examined by gap methods (43–45, 97). Adrian and Marshall (14) inserted three electrodes at specified distances from each other in the middle of a fiber, rather than at its end. For the spacings in Figure 4 the membrane current is given by

$$i_m(t) \simeq \frac{1}{l}\left\{\frac{I_0(t)}{2} - \frac{\Delta V(t)}{r_i l}\right\} \quad (92)$$

where

$$\Delta V(t) = V_1(t) - V_2(t) \quad (93)$$

$$g_m \simeq \frac{1}{V_1(\infty)l}\left\{\frac{I_0(\infty)}{2} - \frac{\Delta V(\infty)}{r_i l}\right\} \quad (94)$$

$$c_{\text{eff}} \simeq \frac{1}{2lV_1(\infty)} \int_0^\infty \left[I_0(t) - \frac{V_1(t)}{V_1(\infty)} I_0(\infty)\right] dt - \frac{1}{r_i l^2 V_1(\infty)} \int_0^\infty \left[\Delta V(t) - \frac{V_1(t)}{V_1(\infty)} \Delta V(\infty)\right] dt \quad (95)$$

It is possible by similar arguments to define factors analogous to p and h that make these equations exact for a membrane with linear properties.

The above analysis of three-electrode methods is only correct for fibers with uniform cylindrical geometry and linear properties. It takes no account of three-dimensional current flow (e.g., see CABLE THEORY FOR STRIATED MUSCLE, p. 275) and is in varying degrees inadequate if the membrane conductance or capacitance is nonlinear with voltage or changes with time. Time-independent nonlinearity of conductance (not involving negative-slope conductances) does not give rise to serious error provided l is kept small with respect to the λ that would hold at the maximum value of the conductance. Negative-slope conductances and rates of change of conductance that impose sufficiently rapid changes of potential on the mem-

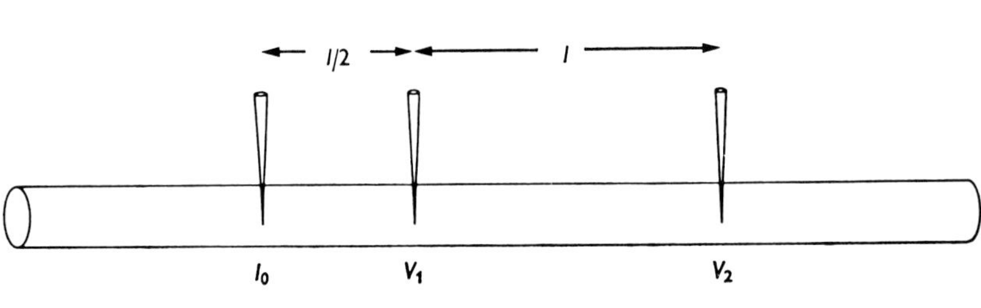

FIG. 4. Arrangement of microelectrodes in three-electrode method adapted to the center of a long cylindrical fiber. Fiber ends are to be understood to be several (more than, say, 5λ) length constants away from $x = 0$. [From Adrian and Marshall (14).]

brane removed from V_1 can be expected to give rise to substantial errors. It is perhaps surprising that these three-electrode methods give any valid information about the sodium and potassium currents of the action potential (84). Low temperature and reduction of external sodium-ion concentration, which respectively slow and reduce the sodium current, improve the reliability (14, 81).

Gap-clamp methods (31, 77) have much the same inherent cable limitations; however, because the clamping current is delivered through a relatively low impedance they can be made fast. Indeed the center-fiber three-electrode method (14) is more or less the equivalent of a gap clamp with a "gap" of width l centered on the V_1 electrode, and it is unlikely that a gap clamp will be anymore spatially uniform than is that system. Adrian and Marshall (14) found it necessary to work at low temperature and at about a tenth of the normal sodium concentration to avoid spatial instability. Their gap width was 250 μm. Sodium concentrations that gave an outward electrode current caused the potential between $x = 0$ and $x = l/2$ (see Fig. 3) to repolarize as inward membrane current developed. The result was sodium current that activated and was then inactivated ($m \rightarrow 0$) in the left-hand part of the gap and sodium current that activated and inactivated ($h \rightarrow 0$) in the middle of the gap. With gaps of 100 μm Campbell and Hille (31) worked at 5°C and Ildefonse and Rougier (77) at room temperature; both groups used a normal sodium concentration. During the peak inward sodium current, Campbell and Hille measured a swing in the negative direction of internal potential as large as 5 mV at one end of their gap (but not at the other), and this could itself cause a substantial deactivation of sodium conductance at that end. The question has to be asked whether any of the investigations of sodium current in striated muscle can be said to be strictly reliable.

When considering the results of voltage-clamp studies on muscle, contraction and its possible consequences cannot be ignored. In microelectrode clamping it is usual to use hypertonic solutions at low temperature to prevent movement. Fibers in hypertonic solutions at room temperature rapidly deteriorate, but even though survival is apparently good at low temperature, the raised tonicity will alter the ionic strength of the sarcoplasm and the volume of the fiber. It may also interfere with the morphological relationships of the T tubules and the sarcoplasmic reticulum. In gap methods, on the other hand, if movement occurs the geometry of the gap may alter. Heavy water, dantrolene sodium, formaldehyde, and tetracaine have all been used to interfere with contraction, but these may themselves have actions on the ionic currents. No wholly satisfactory way of avoiding these uncertainties has been found.

ACTION POTENTIAL IN STRIATED MUSCLE

The detailed reconstruction of the action potential in striated muscle has depended heavily on the principles developed by Hodgkin and Huxley (67) to describe the sodium and potassium currents in the squid axon. The special features in striated muscle involve its morphological complexity and how this is to be expressed in the mathematical reconstruction. Before dealing with that question the currents of the action potential are briefly described.

Sodium Current

The rapid inward current in striated muscle is abolished by tetrodotoxin (TTX) and is absent in sodium-free solutions. Its reversal potential is substantially positive to 0 mV and appears to alter appropriately with alterations of either external or internal [Na]. The kinetic behavior of this sodium current is adequately described by the scheme proposed by Hodgkin and Huxley for the sodium current in squid axons, but the reliability of the experimental measurements would hardly allow much weight to be put on the similarity of experimental and calculated current.

Sodium current is a function of the membrane potential (E) and time (t)

$$I_{Na}(E, t) = m^3h\, \bar{I}_{Na}(E) \qquad (96)$$

where m and h are parameters with values between 0 and 1. They are functions of membrane potential and time. The current-voltage relation of the membrane if m and h equal 1 is $\bar{I}_{Na}$.

Hodgkin and Huxley showed that in squid axon

$$\bar{I}_{Na} = \bar{g}_{Na}(E - E_{Na}) \tag{97}$$

stating that the instantaneous conductance is linear. Adrian, Chandler, and Hodgkin (9) assumed this relation for the sodium current in striated muscle although they did not show experimentally that it was so. Ildefonse and Rougier (77) and Campbell and Hille (31) examined the instantaneous current-voltage relation for the inward current and used a constant-field equation (57, 68) to describe $\bar{I}_{Na}$

$$\bar{I}_{Na} = \bar{P}_{Na}[Na]_o \frac{F^2E}{RT} \cdot \frac{\exp[(E - E_{Na})F/RT] - 1}{\exp(EF/RT) - 1} \tag{98}$$

(Campbell and Hille introduce a further small empirical modification into the equation for $\bar{I}_{Na}$.)

Changes of m and h are defined by first-order transitions

$$\frac{dm}{dt} = \alpha_m(1 - m) - \beta_m m \tag{99}$$

$$\frac{dh}{dt} = \alpha_h(1 - h) - \beta_h h \tag{100}$$

from which

$$m = m_\infty - (m_\infty - m_0)\exp(-t/\tau_m) \tag{101}$$

$$h = h_\infty - (h_\infty - h_0)\exp(-t/\tau_h) \tag{102}$$

with

$$m_\infty = \alpha_m/(\alpha_m + \beta_m)\tau_m = (\alpha_m + \beta_m)^{-1} \tag{103}$$

$$h_\infty = \alpha_h\ (\alpha_h + \beta_h)\tau_h \quad = (\alpha_h + \beta_h)^{-1} \tag{104}$$

The voltage dependence of the rate constants is empirically represented by equations of the following form, unaltered except for numerical values, from the equations for squid axon

$$\alpha_m = \bar{\alpha}_m(E - \bar{E}_m)/(1 - \exp[(\bar{E}_m - E)/V_{\alpha m}]) \tag{105}$$

$$\beta_m = \bar{\beta}_m \exp[(\bar{E}_m - E)/V_{\beta m}] \tag{106}$$

$$\alpha_h = \bar{\alpha}_h \exp[(\bar{E}_h - E)/V_{\alpha h}] \tag{107}$$

$$\beta_h = \bar{\beta}_h/(1 + \exp[(\bar{E}_h - E)/V_{\beta h}]) \tag{108}$$

Table 1 shows the values for various parameters derived in the four principal studies of sodium current in frog skeletal muscle. In view of the differences and uncertainties of technique, it is perhaps surprising that the agreement is so good!

Potassium Current

The delayed potassium currents in striated muscle have not been fully characterized although a number of interesting features have been established.

Moore (93) first commented on the difficulty of recording large delayed outward currents in striated muscle fibers. The records of Ildefonse and Rougier (77) show little or no delayed outward current, and Campbell and Hille (31) comment on its absence in their cut fiber preparations. Adrian, Chandler, and Hodgkin (9) show clear records of delayed outward current and analyze its kinetic behavior in terms of a Hodgkin and Huxley model

$$I_K(E, t) = n^4\bar{I}_K(E) \tag{109}$$

where

$$\bar{I}_K(E) = \bar{g}_K(E - E_K) \tag{110}$$

which in this case was shown to hold reasonably well for $-100\ mV < E < 0\ mV$. The rate of change of n was controlled by the usual first-order equation with voltage-dependent rate constants

$$\alpha_n = \bar{\alpha}_n(E - \bar{E}_n)/(1 - \exp[(\bar{E}_n - E)/V_{\alpha n}] \\ \beta_n = \bar{\beta}_n \exp[(\bar{E}_n - E)/V_{\beta n}] \tag{111}$$

with

$$\bar{\alpha}_n \cong 0.003/ms \tag{112}$$

$$\bar{\beta}_n \cong 0.013/ms^{-1} \text{ at } 2°C \tag{113}$$

$$-45\ mV < \bar{E}_n < -40\ mV \tag{114}$$

$$V_{\alpha n} = 7\ mV \tag{115}$$

$$V_{\beta n} = 40\ mV \tag{116}$$

They showed that the delayed outward potassium current was subject to an inactivation process similar to the inactivation of the sodium current, but apart from noting that the time constant of the inactivation was voltage and temperature dependent (with a value of ~0.5 s at −20 mV and 20°C), they did not attempt to incorporate an inactivation variable into the formal description of the potassium current. Inactivation of the delayed potassium current was not unexpected since Nakajima, Iwasaki, and Obata (94) had already shown that depolarization in high-potassium solutions inactivates the delayed potassium current. Inactivation rates for the potassium system are relatively slow, and it is probably reasonable to ignore potassium inactivation in calculating single action potentials. It is possible, however, that in the course of a train of action potentials the potassium system could be considerably inactivated. Indeed repolarization is markedly slowed in later action potentials of trains even at quite low frequencies [10/s; (60)].

Clearly this potassium current in striated muscle can be completely eliminated by prolonged depolarization, and to this extent it appears to be a more labile system than that in the squid giant axon. In the experiments of Ildefonse and Rougier (77) and Campbell and Hille (31), however, it is not clear how much the apparent absence of delayed outward currents can be accounted for by some form of this inactivation or whether their absence is due to some damage involved in isolation.

An unexpected finding (10) was that the outward delayed current was made up of two components, one

TABLE 1. *Parameters of Kinetic Models for the Sodium Current in Frog and Mammalian Skeletal Muscle*

	Ildefonse and Roy (78) *Rana esculenta*, 20°–23°C	Adrian et al. (9) *Rana temporaria*, 1°–3°C	Campbell and Hille (31) *Rana pipiens*, 5°C	Pappone (97) Rat, 12°C
$\bar{\alpha}_m$, ms^{-1}	0.35	0.04	0.04	0.115
$\bar{\beta}_m$, ms^{-1}	5.0	0.41	0.46	0.55
$\bar{E}_m$, mV	−57	−42	−42	−63.5
$V_{\alpha m}$, mV	5.0	10.0	10.0	6.8
$V_{\beta m}$, mV	13.7	18.0	18.0	37
$\bar{\alpha}_h$, ms^{-1}	0.001	0.003	0.00012	0.00323
$\bar{\beta}_h$, ms^{-1}	7.4	0.65	0.9	1.75
$\bar{E}_h$, mV	−25	−41	−25	−46
$V_{\alpha h}$, mV	11.0	14.7	11.0	25
$V_{\beta h}$, mV	13.6	7.6	13.6	10

fast and one slow. Both components showed inactivation, but the analysis of the rates of activation and inactivation was complicated because inactivation of the fast component took place at approximately the same time as activation of the slow. In a voltage-clamp depolarization at 2°C–3°C (10)

> the slow system contributes relatively little at first and can be ignored during the first 50 msec. It reaches a maximum when the fast component has fallen to about one-third and is then about one-half the fast component in amplitude. Both fast and slow components are inactivated, the former nearly completely and the latter to perhaps one-third.

The equilibrium potentials for the fast and slow channels appeared to differ by about 10 mV, the slow being the more negative. It is not, however, clear that the measured zero-current potentials were free from uncertainty due to local ion accumulation or tubular capacitative current (15).

Stanfield (108) has shown that both potassium channels are affected by tetraethylammonium (TEA) ion, although the affinity of the slow channels for TEA is substantially less than that of the fast channels. Apparently TEA slowed the activation rate of the fast channel. At a time when the slow channel was not yet activated, 58 mM TEA reduced $\bar{g}_K$ by about 90% and slowed the rate constant controlling the activation to about 20% of its normal value. Some part of the slowing may have been due to the activation of the slow component, which is substantially less affected by TEA.

Lynch (89) has confirmed and extended the description of the two delayed current channels in striated muscle. With short fibers (lumbricalis longissimus digiti IV) and a two-electrode voltage clamp at 5°C, he has shown that most fibers have a variable mixture of two delayed outward currents; one with n^4 kinetics (τ = 7.8 ms at 0 mV) and a second with n^2 kinetics (τ = 90 ms at 0 mV). Some fibers have only one of these currents. Tetraethylammonium (115 mM) and 4-aminopyridine (1 mM) block >95% of the fast current and ~50% of the slow current. The slow current is eliminated by 1 mM diethylpyrocarbonate. Reducing the pH increases the activation rate of the slow component.

The functional significance of the slow component is obscure, but it is possible that it is related to the potassium conductance seen in many cells, which is activated when intracellular calcium concentration rises (91).

The voltage thresholds for the activation of contraction and of delayed outward current are sufficiently close to raise the question whether they are close because contraction relies in some way on the development of outward current. Agents such as Ca^{2+} and foreign anions shift these thresholds in similar directions (36, 80, 88). Heistracher and Hunt (62) concluded that there is a difference in the shifts produced by foreign anions even if the difference is not large, and that delayed potassium current is not responsible for contractile activation. Adrian, Chandler, and Hodgkin (8) showed that the strength-duration relations of delayed current and contraction were different; the conductance change at the onset of contraction was not constant. It now appears that although both contraction and delayed potassium current are activated at comparable membrane potentials and although both are inactivated and both can be reactivated (reprimed) by repolarization, the two processes are independent. Where they have been studied in detail the kinetics of activation, inactivation, and repriming in each system are not identical, even if they are similar. The similarity is perhaps not very surprising because both contraction and delayed outward current are processes that have to be activated by the depolarization of the action potential. Several studies have been made of the repriming of the delayed potassium current. Unfortunately none of them distinguished the fast from the slow delayed current, so that it is difficult to assess the apparently complex kinetics of the repriming process. Heistracher and Hunt (63) showed that after depolarization, repolarization restores along a sigmoid time course the ability to respond to a further depolarization by contraction and potassium current. Hodgkin and Horowicz (65) had already demonstrated that the steady-state repriming of contraction depends on membrane potential; Heistracher and Hunt (63) showed that the rate of the sigmoid contraction repriming is likewise dependent on membrane potential. Argibay and Hutter (22) showed that the rate of repriming at any particular potential could be made to depend on the duration of the preceding inactivating depolarization. Repriming was more rapid when the inactivating period was short. Adrian and Rakowski (17), in a recent study with fibers depolarized in hypertonic Ringer's solutions with a high rubidium sulphate concentration (40 mM) at 10°C, did not see early nonexponential repriming. They concluded that repriming was taking place in two stages. Little can be said to summarize these rather scattered findings except that repriming is not a first-order process.

Calcium Current

The existence of activable calcium current in striated muscle was first suggested by the slow spike activity reported by Beaty and Stefani (26) in the absence of chloride and with delayed potassium current suppressed by TEA. These slow spikes were absent in a Ca^{2+}-free solution and abolished by Mn^{2+}, Co^{2+}, and D 600. Similar slow responses have been reported by Bernard, Cardinaux, and Potreau (27) in frog skeletal fibers in the presence of high Ba^{2+} concentrations. Subsequently several authors have shown the presence of an inward Ca^{2+} current in voltage-clamp studies (26, 103, 109). Because it is very slow this Ca^{2+} current has been studied at temperatures between 20°C and 26°C. Sanchez and Stefani (103) remark that its "time to peak is several seconds at 2–6°C." Even at 20°C the time to peak is several hundred milliseconds. It activates at about −40 mV and reverses in the potential range +20 to +40 mV. The maximum inward Ca current is about 0.1 mA/cm^2 (cf. maximum inward Na current of 2.4 mA/cm^2). The inward Ca current is inactivated by depolarization. Half-inactivation is produced by 2.4 s at −40 mV.

The role of a very slow inward Ca^{2+} current is uncertain. It is unlikely to be activated in the course of a single twitch and thus cannot play a role in the action potential or in the immediate activation of contraction. Moreover twitches continue normally for many minutes when the external [Ca] is reduced to very low levels (24). It could be activated in the course of maintained activity and would account for the increased Ca fluxes during activity (39, 40).

Action-Potential Calculations

Armed with formal descriptions of the sodium and potassium currents in striated muscle, it is reasonable to ask how many of the characteristic features of the muscle action potential are reproducible by calculation and to answer that a good many of them are reproducible provided a large number of rather arbitrary assumptions is accepted. These assumptions principally concern the electrical consequences of the structure of the T system and the distribution of the active conductances between the fiber surface and the tubular membrane.

Given the behavior of the sodium and potassium currents for times short enough to exclude any appreciable inactivation of the latter or activation of slow potassium or calcium currents, there is no reason to suppose that an action-potential spike will not be generated when appropriate conductances are inserted into the equation for a uniformly propagating potential wave in a uniform longitudinal cable (67)

$$\frac{d^2V}{dt^2} = \frac{2\theta^2 R_i}{a}\left\{I_L(E) + I_{Na}(E, t) + I_K(E, t) + C_m\frac{dV}{dt}\right\} \tag{117}$$

$V = E - V_R$, where V_R is the resting potential and θ is the propagation velocity. There are, however, two important reasons for thinking that such a calculation would be misleadingly simplified. First, the capacitance of striated muscle does not behave as if it were a single linear element; second, the active sodium and potassium currents are not necessarily confined to the geometric fiber surface but could also be present in the membrane of the T system. [The calculations referred to here and subsequently in this section are computer-executed solutions of simultaneous nonlinear differential equations. In general they have been based on a modified fourth-order Runge-Kutta procedure as described by Fitzhugh (48).]

It has been pointed out that the membrane impedance of striated muscle is not accurately represented by a resistance and capacitance in parallel (47). The simplest equivalent circuit that could reproduce the measured AC impedance is shown in Figure 3*A*. The series combination R_sC_T here represents the resistance of the tubular lumen and the capacitance of the tubular wall. With this equivalent circuit as a representation of the relation of tubular to surface capacitance and making the assumption that the sodium and potassium channels are only in the fiber surface membrane, the equations for the propagated action potential become

$$\frac{d^2V}{dt^2} = \frac{2\theta^2 R_i}{a}\left\{I_L(E) + I_{Na}(E,t) + I_K(E,t) + C_m\frac{dV}{dt} + \frac{V - V_T}{R_s}\right\} \tag{118}$$

$$\frac{dV_T}{dt} = \frac{V - V_T}{R_sC_T} \tag{119}$$

where V_T is the potential across the capacitance C_T. The leak current I_L is assumed to be a linear function of $(E - E_L)$. This approach was adopted by Adrian, Chandler, and Hodgkin (9), and Figure 5 shows a comparison between recorded and calculated action potentials. They noted the following discrepancies (9):

(1) the conduction velocity and rate of rise of the action potential was smaller than that observed experimentally;

(2) the experimental action potential of 2°C has a flatter maximum than the theoretical one; (3) the falling phase of the theoretical action potential merges rather smoothly into the negative after-potential and does not give the dip which is often seen in records from muscle.

It is clear in Figure 5 that V_T, the potential that represents the potential across the tubular wall, lags considerably behind the potential change in the surface of the fiber (V).

In these calculations the T system is represented by a single lumped combination of resistance and capacitance ($R_s C_T$). Taken literally this means that there is a resistance at the mouths of the tubules that is very large in comparison to the luminal resistance. This hypothetical resistance, which might result from an effective scarcity of tubular mouths (76) or from a narrowing or tortuosity of the peripheral tubule, has been called an access resistance (15). In the limit if the access resistance is larger than the tubular lumen resistance, the tubular capacitance will appear to be lumped; if the tubular lumen resistance is larger than the access resistance, the tubular capacitance will appear to be distributed in the cross section of the fiber. The fact that the magnitude of the membrane capacitance is proportional to the fiber diameter strongly suggests that a large part of the membrane capacitance of striated muscle is physically located in the tubular system (69).

Important studies of the AC impedance of striated muscle have attempted to define the degree to which the tubular capacitance is lumped or distributed (47, 90, 104, 115). Measurement of impedance especially at high frequency is beset with considerable technical difficulty and all these studies agree that neither extreme of wholly lumped or wholly distributed is as satisfactory as something in between; neither access resistance nor lumen resistance can be ignored. However, this middle ground is fairly wide, and there is no precise agreement about the magnitude of access and luminal resistances. Nevertheless impedance measurements suggest that any access resistance is a relatively small fraction of total radial resistance (see the chapter by R. S. Eisenberg in this *Handbook*).

Treating the tubular capacitance as if it were distributed in the cross section of the fiber introduces a further degree of complexity in calculating action potentials (15). One may assume uniform propagation along the fiber and use this assumption to convert the cable equation from a partial differential to an ordinary differential equation, but uniform propagation will not occur in a radially symmetrical network like the T system. One has therefore to resort to a rather less elegant procedure and decompose the tubular system into a number of segments, writing equations for the membrane currents in each segment and equations for the current between adjacent segments [see, for instance, Crank (ref. 38, chapter 10)]. The circular shape of the tubular system has to be represented by systematic change in the magnitude of the circuit elements in each segment, so that each segment represents an annulus of the tubular system.

Details of this procedure are given by Adrian and Peachey (15); Figures 6 and 7 show the main conclusions from their calculations. What follows is taken

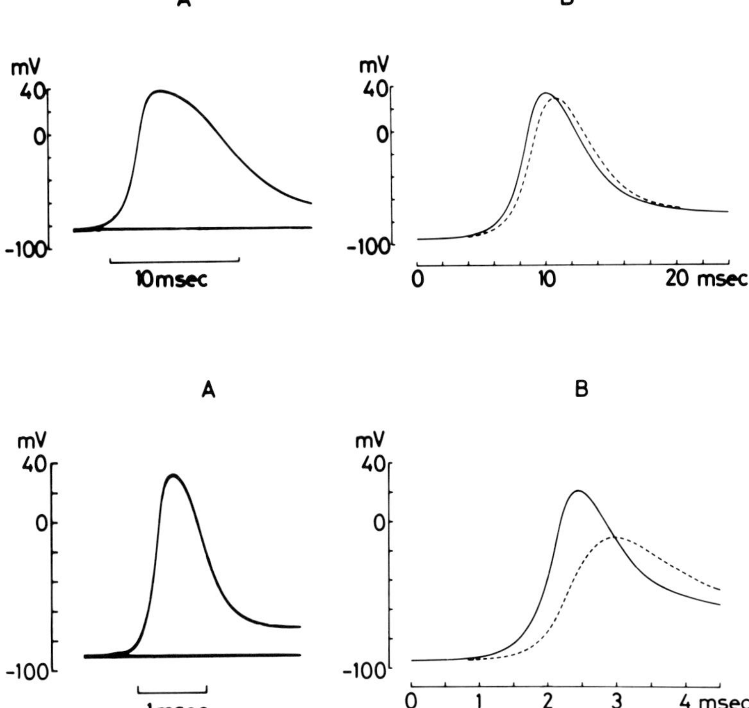

FIG. 5. Recorded (by S. Nakajima) and calculated action potentials for frog striated muscle. *A*: recorded action potential at 3.3°C (*above*) and 21.8°C (*below*). *B*: action potentials calculated at 2°C (*above*) and 20°C (*below*) by Eqs. 118 and 119. *Dotted lines* are V_T, the potential across the capacitance representing the tubular wall (C_T) in the membrane equivalent circuit shown in Fig. 3*A* (but shown there without any elements to represent potential-dependent ionic currents). [From Adrian, Chandler, and Hodgkin (9).]

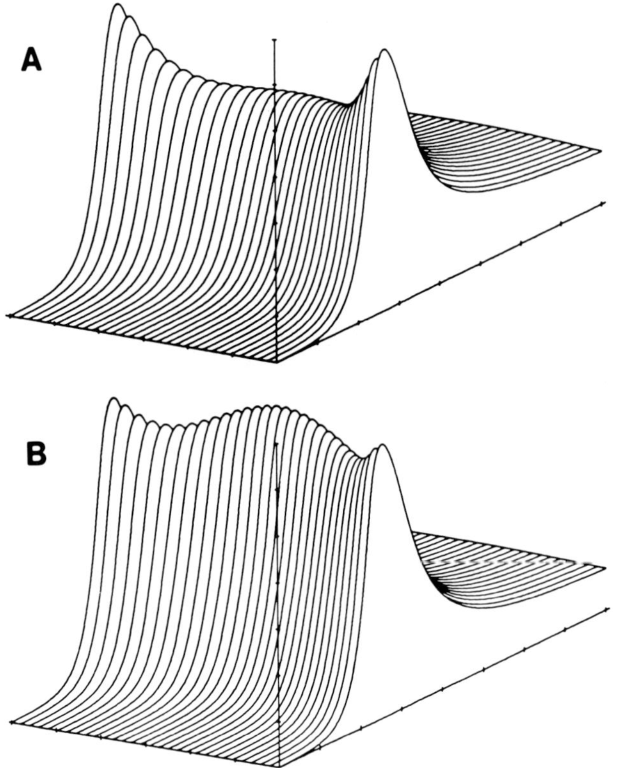

FIG. 6. Calculated action potentials across surface of a fiber and across wall of T system at various radial distances. Coordinates: *vertical*, potential in 20-mV divisions; *horizontal to the left*, the fiber diameter divided into 6 equal divisions; *horizontal to the right*, time in 1-ms divisions. In both calculations no additional resistance is assumed at entrances of the tubular system (access resistance = 0 $\Omega \cdot cm^2$). *A*: no activable sodium or potassium current in tubular system. *B*: activable sodium and potassium currents in tubular system are assumed. [From Adrian and Peachey (15).]

more or less directly from their paper. Four calculations are plotted with a three-dimensional surface whose coordinates are potential, time, and position on the diameter of the fiber. The lines on these surfaces represent the time course of the potential change, that is the action potential, which occurs across the surface membrane and across the tubular membrane at various radial distances: the individual curves are what would be recorded between an electrode in the sarcoplasm and an electrode in the tubule. Each set of action potentials is what would be recorded if one could insert an electrode into a T tubule and advance it in steps from one side of a fiber along a diameter to the other side. In all four figures the fiber diameter is 100 μm; the total capacitance (surface plus tubular) is 7.65 $\mu F/cm^2$; the conductivity of the tubular lumen is 10 mS/cm (conductivity of Ringer's solution = 12 mS/cm). The structure of the tubular network is described by three parameters (8): the volume fraction of the muscle occupied by the tubular system ($\rho = 0.003$); the volume-surface ratio of the tubules ($\zeta = 10^{-6}$ cm); a factor to express the tortuosity of the radial current pathway ($\sigma = 0.5$). (See the chapter by R. S. Eisenberg in this *Handbook* for a discussion of morphological parameters.) The saturating sodium and potassium conductances of the fiber surface were, respectively, 180 mS/cm^2 and 41.5 mS/cm^2. The temperature is taken as 20°C.

Figure 6*A* shows the calculation for a tubular system without activable sodium and potassium currents and with no additional resistance (access resistance) at the entrances of the tubular system. In this reconstruction the surface action potential rises and falls slowly and propagates at 109 cm/s. Neither of these failings is improved by adding sodium and potassium currents to the tubular membrane (Fig. 6*B*: tubular sodium conductance 67.5 mS/cm^2 *fiber* surface, tubular potassium conductance 9.5 mS/cm^2 *fiber* surface). These calculations suggest that the low propagation velocity is due to the large total capacitance; a substantial reduction would certainly increase the propagation velocity. However, the measurements of Hodgkin and Nakajima (69) suggest that 7.65 $\mu F/cm^2$ is an appropriate value for a diameter of 100 μm. Alternatively, a substantial increase in the limiting sodium conductance of surface would increase the rate of rise of the action potential and the propagation velocity. The measurement of $\bar{g}_{Na}$ by Campbell and Hille (31) suggests that 180 mS/cm^2 may be low by about 50%, but this does not improve matters very much as the conduction velocity varies as approximately the fifth root of the limiting sodium conductance [see, for instance, calculations on squid axon, Adrian (3)].

The effect of the tubular capacitance in slowing propagation can be overcome by decoupling the surface and tubular systems to some extent by introducing a resistance at the entrance of the tubular system so that it lies between the bulk of the extracellular fluid and the fluid of the tubular lumen. Figure 7*A* shows the calculation for a tubular system without activable currents and with an access resistance of 150 $\Omega \cdot cm^2$. An access resistance of this magnitude makes little difference to the measured membrane resistance and low-frequency capacitance, but the rates of rise and fall of the action potential are now reasonably rapid, and the propagation velocity is nearly doubled at 200 cm/s (measured velocity about 250 cm/s). In the presence of such an access resistance activable sodium and potassium currents become necessary if a reasonably large potential change is to occur across the tubular lumen at the middle of the fiber. They do not much alter the longitudinal propagation velocity. The four action potentials in Figures 6 and 7 differ only in two features: the presence and absence of the access resistance and the presence and absence of activable sodium and potassium current in the tubular wall. Of these calculated action potentials Figure 7*B* is a better approximation to experimentally recorded action potentials than the other three. The calculations of Figures 6 and 7 are based on a model with a specified geometry and a good many numerical parameters, not all of which can be given experimentally determined values. It is certainly possible that other geometries and other numerical values might do as well or better than this model. Because the required calculation requires considerable computer time, exploration of alternative models has not been extensive. In particular it is possible that the disk model used to represent the tubular system may cease to be appropriate for the high frequencies that correspond to the rising phase of the action potential. The paucity of tubular openings and an effective length constant for those frequencies comparable to the diameter of a myofibril could reduce the tubular capacitance to be charged during the initial stages of the surface action potential (see the chapter by R. S. Eisenberg in this *Handbook*).

It seems reasonable to conclude that the action potential of a striated muscle fiber has no features that cannot be explained in terms of the structure of the fiber and of the activable sodium and potassium currents present both in the fiber surface and in the tubular wall (25, 37, 83).

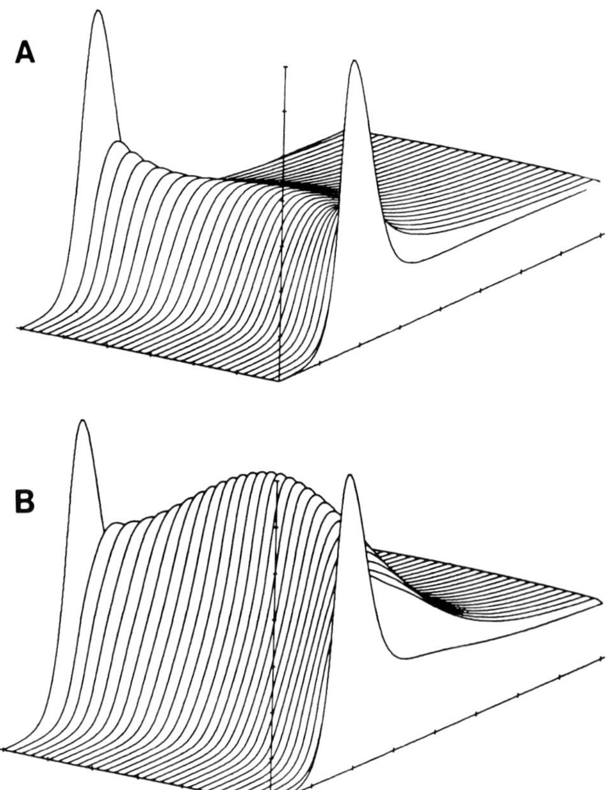

FIG. 7. Calculated action potentials across surface of a fiber and across wall of T system at various radial distances. Coordinates as in Fig. 6, and all parameters of calculation in *A* and *B* are same as in Fig. 6*A* and *B*, respectively, with the exception of access resistance of 150 $\Omega \cdot cm^2$. [From Adrian and Peachey (15).]

CURRENTS IN THE INACTIVE MEMBRANE

At the resting potential, net ionic current across the membrane is zero; for small (<5-mV) deviations of potential the membrane current in striated muscle is carried largely by potassium and chloride ions. In frog fibers the chloride transport number is about 0.7, and in mammalian fibers it may be even larger (71, 72). In frog twitch fibers the resting membrane conductance is about 0.3 mS/cm^2; in round figures therefore at the resting potential the potassium conductance is 0.1 mS/cm^2 and the chloride conductance is 0.2 mS/cm^2. These conductances are expressed for unit area of fiber surface even though the ionic currents may be across both surface and tubular membranes. Gage and Eisenberg (51, 52) conclude, on the basis of experiments in which the tubular system is disrupted by osmotic shock, that the chloride conductance is mainly in the surface membrane. Almers (19) concludes that more than 80% of the potassium conductance is in the tubular membrane. Although this evidence is indirect, one might suppose that the density of the channels that carry potassium ions in the resting state is the same in the surface and tubular membranes, but that the chloride channels occur only in the surface membrane. Although this is probably true for frog, other distributions may hold for other species.

Potassium Conductance

The channels that carry potassium ions through the resting membrane must be distinguished at once from those responsible for the activable potassium currents of the action potential. The latter, often called the "delayed rectifier" channels, have an instantaneous current-voltage relation that is essentially linear; the former allow large potassium currents into the fiber but only very small potassium currents in an outward direction and indeed may close very nearly completely when the driving force on the potassium ion is large and outwardly directed. This characteristic nonlinear current-voltage relation has earned this channel the name of "inward rectifier." The behavior of the two potassium channels toward the rubidium ion is completely different. Rubidium not only fails to cross the inwardly rectifying channel but blocks it to the passage of potassium ions. The delayed rectifier channel allows the passage of both rubidium and potassium ions essentially without discriminating between them (2).

The inability to pass large outward potassium currents in isotonic potassium sulfate solutions was first described by Katz (82). Ten years later, by investigating changes in the resting potential produced by changes in the external concentrations of both potassium and chloride, Hodgkin and Horowicz (65) showed that the permeability of potassium was strikingly variable, whereas that of chloride was relatively constant. Also the permeability of potassium was reduced whenever the circumstances demanded a movement of potassium ions out of the fiber. They found that the potassium permeability can depend on the external potassium concentration even when the membrane potential remained unaltered; this makes the behavior of the inwardly rectifying channel very different from the delayed rectifying channel. The former acts as a true valve for potassium movement, closing when the driving force is outward and opening when the driving force is inward; the latter opens over a particular range of membrane potential (ca. −50 mV) and allows potassium ions to pass regardless of the direction in which they are moving.

Figure 8 shows the relation between the inwardly rectifying potassium current and the membrane potential. Potential steps are imposed on the membrane of a fiber by a three-electrode clamp (10). For hyperpolarizing steps of potential the large inward currents are not maintained but decline to a steady-state value in a second or so. Adrian and Freygang (12) attributed the slow fall in conductance to depletion of potassium ions in the T tubules by the inward current. Such depletion occurs if the current removes potassium ions across the tubular membrane at a rate that is faster than potassium can diffuse into the tubular system by way of its surface openings. Hodgkin and Horowicz (66) described differences in the rate at which the potential changes in response to rapid changes of external ion concentration. Such changes in chloride ion concentration affect the membrane potential rapidly; changes in potassium ion concentration affect the potential after a delay. These findings were also explained in terms of diffusion delays in the tubular system. The findings were consistent with the chloride permeability being in the fiber surface and the inwardly rectifying potassium channels being largely in the tubular wall.

Nevertheless the explanation is complicated by knowing that tubular depletion cannot account for all the time-dependent changes in the inward current. Depletion cannot account for a negative slope frequently seen in the steady-state current-voltage relation at large hyperpolarizations. Almers (19, 20) suggested that the inwardly rectifying channel was gated, because it was necessary to suppose that there was a slow permeability change at large hyperpolarizations. He showed that the temperature coefficients of the rates at which the conductance diminished were different at different hyperpolarized potentials. For small hyperpolarizations the temperature coefficient was small; for larger hyperpolarizations it was large. In an elegant analysis he suggested that potassium ion depletion occurs, but that there is also a time-dependent permeability change in the tubular membrane. Inwardly rectifying channels appear to close slowly at potentials more negative than −130 mV. Standen and Stanfield (107) have shown that this closing or blocking depends on the presence of sodium ions in the external solution. It does not take place if sodium is replaced by 2-amino-2-hydroxymethyl-1,3-propanediol (Tris), TEA ions, or lithium.

The blocking action of rubidium ions on the inward rectifier has been mentioned. In fact the alkali cations (other than potassium itself and lithium) and the

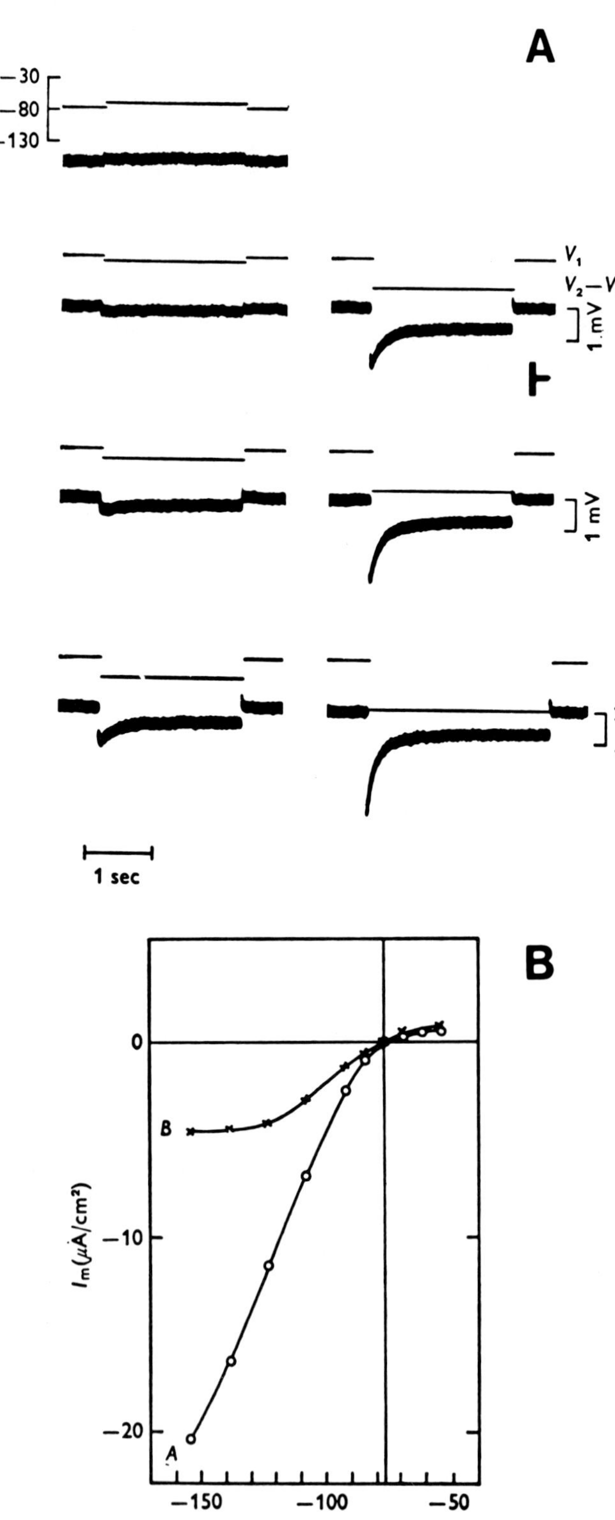

FIG. 8. *A*: records of currents required to impose voltage steps of long duration on a muscle fiber. Three-electrode method with fiber in an isotonic sulfate Ringer's solution with 5 mM K at 1.5°C. Current for hyperpolarization is initially large but decays with time constant 0.5–1 s. *B*: initial (*open circles*) and final (*crosses*) current plotted against membrane potential during imposed potential step. Outward current is positive. [From Adrian, Chandler, and Hodgkin (10).]

alkaline earth cations seem to interfere with the passage of potassium, and the degree of interference depends on the potential at which the current is measured. Absence of sodium, as mentioned above, prevents the slow reduction of current at large depolarizations, and in the presence of varying concentrations of sodium the slow reduction occurs at different potentials, appearing at more positive potentials as the sodium concentration is increased. Cesium causes a voltage-dependent block of inward potassium current (53) as do barium and strontium (106). Similar findings have been reported in the eggs of starfish (58, 59) and tunicates (96). These complex interactions suggest that potassium ions and the blocking ions may be competing for intramembrane (or perhaps intrachannel) sites and that the occupancy by a blocking ion depends on the affinity of the ion for the site and on the local ion concentration at the site, which will be dependent on the potential there. The blocking action of external cations then depends on their moving into the channels from the outside (110). The inwardly rectifying behavior of the potassium current may depend on an internal cation (not identified) moving from the inside of the fibers when the current is outward and rapidly occupying a blocking site in the channel (106). Several models have been proposed to account for inwardly rectifying behavior, which does not only occur in striated muscle (23, 35).

It is hard to give a convincing reason for these complexities in the potassium channel that is open at the resting potential. Its behavior is altogether different from the leak current in squid nerve, which, at least at the resting potential, is linear and must be carried largely by potassium ions. On the other hand it resembles the inwardly rectifying potassium channel in cardiac muscle [I_{K2}; Noble and Tsien (95)], even though the voltage dependence of its opening and closing is such that it is always open at all physiologically likely membrane potentials. Therefore, unlike I_{K2}, the potassium current through the inward rectifier in striated muscle cannot generate repetitive activity. By allowing only very small outward potassium movement the channel may sometimes prevent a dangerous escape of intracellular potassium, such as might occur in traumatic damage to a muscle mass. Alternatively the low resistance to inward potassium movement would prevent large hyperpolarizations that would otherwise occur when an electrogenic sodium pump was turned on fully (18). Neither of these reasons provides a very convincing teleology for the presence of the inward rectifier in striated muscle, but its presence in other tissues may mean that it fulfills some fairly general role in the membrane function of cells.

Chloride Conductance

The resting potassium conductance of striated muscle is insensitive to pH. The opposite is true for the resting chloride conductance. The chloride conductance varies by nearly an order of magnitude between pH 5.0 and 9.8. The relation of chloride conductance to pH is sigmoid; the midpoint of the relation is at about pH 7 and the conductance is high in alkaline solutions (28, 73, 74). The direction of this striking variation is the reverse of what would be expected if the chloride channel were lined with weakly ionized groups. For such a channel an increase in permeability would be expected when the pH falls and the membrane takes on positive charge (92).

Copper, zinc, and uranyl ions in low concentration (10^{-4} M) substantially reduce the chloride permeability when it is high; other divalent ions, in particular calcium, have little or no effect (74). Iodide, bromide, and nitrate also decrease the chloride permeability (1, 61, 74). Hutter and Warner (74) propose that the chloride permeability depends on the affinity of a membrane protein for chloride and that the affinity is affected by pH and some cations. They suggest that the controlling factor may be the charge on an imidazole grouping.

In two additional papers Hutter and Warner (75) and Warner (116) explore the effects of pH on the current-voltage relations and the time dependence of the chloride current. Substituting rubidium for potassium they show first that the rubidium current is small and linear. At pH 7.4 the chloride current behaved in accordance with the expectation of the constant-field equation (57, 68) with a constant permeability, but inward currents were not maintained and declined with a time constant of about 100 ms. At pH 9.8 inward current reached a saturating value even early in a voltage step; in the course of a long pulse it declined with a time constant of about 200 ms. At pH 5 the conductance for inward current was low for small steps of potential and larger for large steps of potential; the conductance rose slowly in the course of a long-lasting step.

Though of interest for the mechanism of chloride permeation, these complexities of behavior have no obvious physiological significance. Because the chloride current is always small, it plays a relatively minor part in the currents of the action potential. It certainly plays a part in the stable working of a muscle fiber, however, and it is important for two reasons. The behavior of the resting potassium permeability is such that any small depolarizations will reduce the potassium permeability; this in turn could depolarize further. A relatively large resting chloride permeability reduces the likelihood of such a regenerative depolarization. A second effect of the chloride conductance is protection of the surface membrane of a muscle fiber from depolarization as a result of potassium accumulating in the T system. A single action potential may increase the potassium concentration in the tubular lumen by about 0.5 mM (15), and the released potassium diffuses from the tubular system in about a second. A brief tetanus may therefore produce a large excess of potassium in the tubular system depolarizing it. The extent to which this will depolarize the surface membrane will depend critically on the conductance

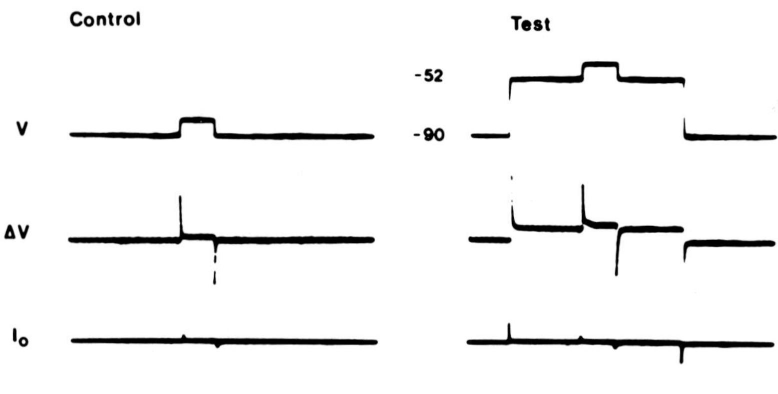

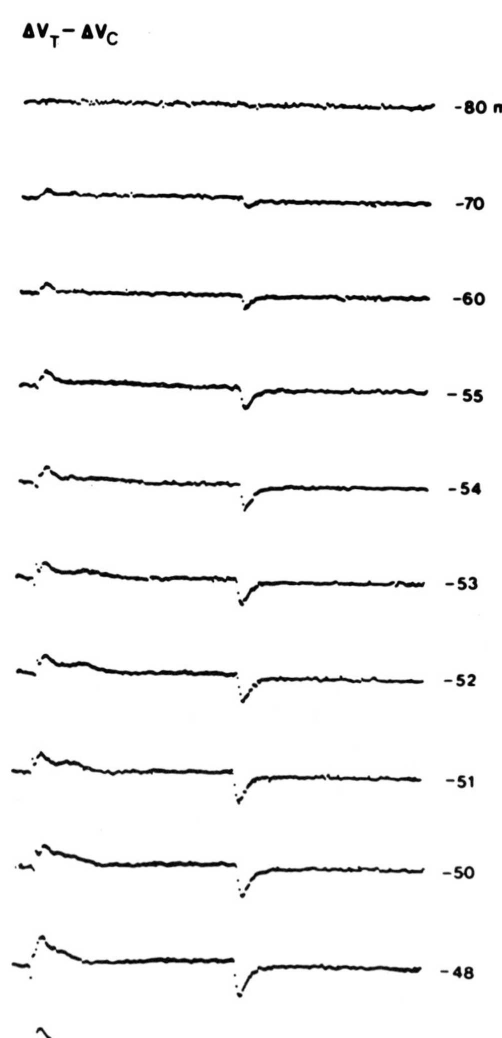

FIG. 9. *Above*: records of membrane potential (V), membrane current (ΔV), and electrode current (I_0) for control and test 10-mV steps of V at 2.5°C. Control step is from −90 mV; test step from −52 mV. Membrane capacity at control and test potential (C_C, C_T) is determined from integral of transient part of membrane current at "on" and "off" of 10-mV step. *Below*: point-by-point differences in membrane currents ($\Delta V_T - \Delta V_C$) for test and control steps. These records show, for various starting potentials, current that is not present in the control step from −90 mV. Note that the kinetics of this additional polarization current can be complex. In both sets of records the 10-mV step lasts for 128 ms. Three-electrode clamp; fiber in a hypertonic solution designed to minimize ionic currents. [From Adrian and Peres (16).]

of the surface and tubular membranes; the greater the surface conductance the less the surface depolarization. Clinically the results of a low chloride conductance are seen in the condition myotonia congenita (29, 113). This hereditary muscular condition occurs in humans and in goats. In both the primary fault is a very low chloride conductance in striated muscle. As a result of this abnormality, intense muscular activity

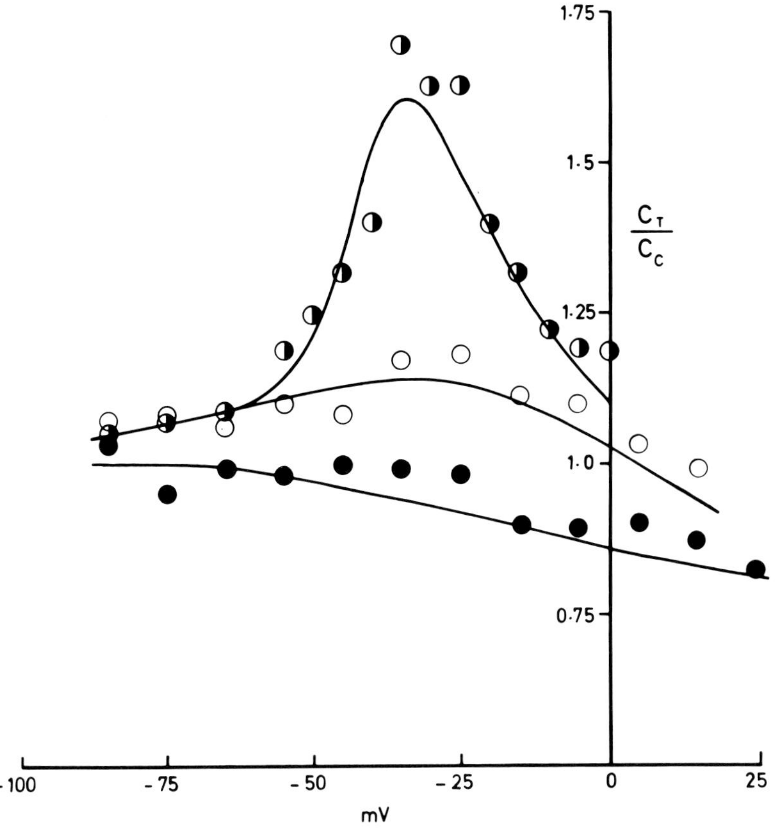

FIG. 10. Voltage dependence of nonlinear membrane capacity (C_T:C_C). For all curves, C_C measured at −90 mV; C_T at membrane potential indicated on abscissa. Membrane potential was held at −90 mV (*half-filled circles*), −40 mV (*open circles*), and −20 mV (*filled circles*) except during the measurements of capacity (as in Fig. 9). Note that the behavior of the nonlinear capacity depends on the holding potential. [From Adrian (4). Reproduced, with permission, from *Annu. Rev. Biophys. Bioeng.*, vol. 7, ©1978 by Annual Reviews, Inc.]

results in an uncontrollable tetanus that may last several seconds. It appears that tubular potassium accumulation resulting from the initial voluntary activity depolarizes the surface membrane and generates repetitive and self-maintained firing there (7, 13). Once this has happened cessation of impulses in the motor nerve does not bring the contraction to an end.

Voltage-Dependent Membrane Capacitance

In recent years it has become apparent that the behavior of the membrane dielectric in striated muscle is nonideal. Its polarization is not a linear function of voltage nor is it instantaneous. The membrane dielectric shows both saturation and loss (21). Interest in these dielectric properties arises in connection with the gating of voltage-dependent processes, for instance, ionic conductances and contraction, and it follows a long period during which an ideal membrane capacitance of 1 $\mu F/cm^2$ had assumed the status of a biological constant. In almost all calculations of action potentials (including those in Figs. 5, 6, and 7) in very many different excitable cells, an ideal membrane dielectric has been assumed. We can now say that the magnitude of nonlinearities is unlikely to impose easily detectable changes in the shape of action potentials, even though they may have quite large (ca. 25%) effects on the conduction velocity (3).

Variation in the measured capacitance of striated muscle was first clearly shown by Schneider and Chandler (105). They used a method of measuring capacitance that depended on the integral of the charging current (e.g., see VOLTAGE-CLAMP METHODS FOR STRIATED MUSCLE, p. 281). They showed that for a small or large potential step the integrals of the transient current at the beginning and end of the step were equal, which must be the case if the currents arise by polarization of the dielectric, but that these integrals were not a linear function of the size of the potential step. Their results have been confirmed and extended (6, 16). The most direct way of investigating the voltage dependence of capacitance is to measure the integral of the transient currents at the beginning and end of a 10-mV potential step imposed by a voltage clamp from a variable initial potential. In this way one can compare the required polarization charge for a 10-mV step from a control potential at −90 mV and from a test potential at any other part of the accessible potential range. Figure 9 shows the test and control potential steps with the recorded "membrane currents." The records are from a sartorius muscle fiber and a three-microelectrode clamp at its pelvic end. The fiber is in a solution that is hypertonic to prevent movement and in which ionic current is as far as possible minimized by suppression (TTX and TEA) or by replacement of permeable species (SO_4^{2-} for Cl^- and Rb^+ for K^+). The ratio of the transient current integrals will give the ratio (C_T:C_C) of the membrane capacitance at test and control potential. The point-by-point differences [i_m (test) − i_m (control)] give the time course of the polarization currents that are present in the 10-mV step from the test potential and that do not occur in the control 10-mV step.

Figure 10 shows $C_T{:}C_C$ from the same fiber under three conditions. For all curves C_C was measured at −90 mV, but when not measuring C_C or C_T the membrane potential was held at −90 mV (half-filled circles), −40 mV (open circles), and −20 mV (filled circles). Clearly the capacitance is not independent of voltage under any of these circumstances, although the form of the dependence depends on the holding potential. The maximum value of C_T is not far short of twice C_C. The results in Figure 10 are consistent with the earlier finding of Chandler, Rakowski, and Schneider (34) that intramembrane charge is immobilized by prolonged depolarization. In no part of a wide potential range (−200 mV to +100 mV) are the polarization currents wholly linear. However, it seems probable that several nonlinear components may contribute differently at various potentials. Separation of the complex polarization currents into components is still uncertain (4). Although the magnitude of the potential-dependent capacitance may seem surprising, the multitude of components is probably not when one remembers the number of voltage-regulated processes already described for striated muscle: Na conductance, two K conductances, calcium current, and contraction (all of which both activate and inactivate), and inward rectification (which activates for $V < -140$ mV) (20).

The author expresses his indebtedness and thanks to numerous colleagues, especially to those with whom he has worked in the laboratory.

REFERENCES

1. Adrian, R. H. Internal chloride concentration and chloride efflux of frog muscle. *J. Physiol. London* 156: 623–632, 1961.
2. Adrian, R. H. The rubidium and potassium permeability of frog muscle membrane. *J. Physiol. London* 175: 134–159, 1964.
3. Adrian, R. H. Conduction velocity and gating current in the squid giant axon. *Proc. R. Soc. London Ser. B* 189: 81–86, 1975.
4. Adrian, R. H. Charge movement in the membrane of striated muscle. *Annu. Rev. Biophys. Bioeng.* 7: 85–112, 1978.
5. Adrian, R. H., and W. Almers. Membrane capacity measurements on frog skeletal muscle in media of low ion content. *J. Physiol. London* 237: 573–605, 1974.
6. Adrian, R. H., and W. Almers. Charge movement in the membrane of striated muscle. *J. Physiol. London* 254: 339–360, 1976.
7. Adrian, R. H., and S. H. Bryant. On the repetitive discharge in myotonic muscle fibres. *J. Physiol. London* 240: 505–515, 1974.
8. Adrian, R. H., W. K. Chandler, and A. L. Hodgkin. Kinetics of mechanical activation in frog muscle. *J. Physiol. London* 204: 207–230, 1969.
9. Adrian, R. H., W. K. Chandler, and A. L. Hodgkin. Voltage clamp experiments in striated muscle fibres. *J. Physiol. London* 208: 607–644, 1970.
10. Adrian, R. H., W. K. Chandler, and A. L. Hodgkin. Slow changes in potassium permeability in skeletal muscle. *J. Physiol. London* 208: 645–668, 1970.
11. Adrian, R. H., L. L. Costantin, and L. D. Peachey. Radial spread of contraction in frog muscle fibres. *J. Physiol. London* 204: 231–257, 1969.
12. Adrian, R. H., and W. H. Freygang. The potassium and chloride conductance of frog muscle membrane. *J. Physiol. London* 163: 61–103, 1962.
13. Adrian, R. H., and M. W. Marshall. Action potentials reconstructed in normal and myotonic muscle fibres. *J. Physiol. London* 258: 125–143, 1976.
14. Adrian, R. H., and M. W. Marshall. Sodium currents in mammalian muscle. *J. Physiol. London* 268: 223–250, 1977.
15. Adrian, R. H., and L. D. Peachey. Reconstruction of the action potential in frog sartorius muscle. *J. Physiol. London* 235: 103–131, 1973.
16. Adrian, R. H., and A. Peres. Charge movement and membrane capacity in frog muscle. *J. Physiol. London* 289: 83–97, 1979.
17. Adrian, R. H., and R. F. Rakowski. Reactivation of membrane charge movement and delayed potassium conductance in skeletal muscle fibres. *J. Physiol. London* 278: 533–557, 1978.
18. Adrian, R. H., and C. L. Slayman. Membrane potential and conductance during transport of sodium, potassium and rubidium in frog muscle. *J. Physiol. London* 184: 970–1014, 1966.
19. Almers, W. Potassium conductance changes in skeletal muscle and the potassium concentration in the transverse tubules. *J. Physiol. London* 225: 33–56, 1972.
20. Almers, W. The decline of potassium permeability during extreme hyperpolarization in frog skeletal muscle. *J. Physiol. London* 225: 57–83, 1972.
21. Almers, W., R. H. Adrian, and S. R. Levinson. Some dielectric properties of muscle membrane and their possible importance for excitation-contraction coupling. *Ann. NY Acad. Sci.* 264: 278–292, 1975.
22. Argibay, J. A., and O. F. Hutter. Voltage clamp experiments on the inactivation of the delayed potassium current in skeletal muscle fibres. *J. Physiol. London* 232: 41P–43P, 1973.
23. Armstrong, C. M. Interaction of tetraethylammonium ion derivatives with the potassium channels of giant axons. *J. Gen. Physiol.* 58: 413–437, 1971.
24. Armstrong, C. M., F. M. Bezanilla, and P. Horowicz. Twitches in the presence of ethylene glycol bis(β-aminoethyl-ether)-*N,N'*-tetraacetic acid. *Biochim. Biophys. Acta* 267: 605–608, 1972.
25. Bastian, J., and S. Nakajima. Action potential in the transverse tubules and its role in the activation of skeletal muscle. *J. Gen. Physiol.* 63: 257–278, 1974.
26. Beaty, G. N., and E. Stefani. Calcium dependent electrical activity in twitch muscle fibres of the frog. *Proc. R. Soc. London Ser. B* 194: 141–150, 1976.
27. Bernard, C., J. C. Cardinaux, and D. Potreau. Long duration responses and slow inward current obtained from isolated skeletal muscle fibres with barium ions. *J. Physiol. London* 256: 18P–19P, 1976.
28. Brooks, A. E., and O. F. Hutter. The influence of pH on the chloride conductance of skeletal muscle. *J. Physiol. London* 163: 9P–10P, 1962.
29. Bryant, S. H. The electrophysiology of myotonia, with a review of congenital myotonia of goats. In: *New Developments in Electromyography and Clinical Neurophysiology*, edited by J.E. Desmedt. Basel: Karger, 1972.
30. Campbell, D. T. Ionic selectivity of the sodium channel of frog skeletal muscle. *J. Gen. Physiol.* 67: 295–307, 1976.
31. Campbell, D. T., and B. Hille. Kinetic and pharmacological properties of the sodium channel of frog skeletal muscle. *J. Gen. Physiol.* 67: 309–323, 1976.
32. Carslaw, H. S., and J. C. Jaeger. *Conduction of Heat in Solids* (2nd ed.). Oxford: Oxford Univ. Press, 1959.
33. Chandler, W. K., R. F. Rakowski, and M. F. Schneider. A non-linear voltage dependent charge movement in frog skeletal muscle. *J. Physiol. London* 254: 245–283, 1976.
34. Chandler, W. K., R. F. Rakowski, and M. F. Schneider.

Effects of glycerol treatment and maintained depolarization on charge movement in skeletal muscle. *J. Physiol. London* 254: 285–316, 1976.

35. CLEEMANN, L., AND M. MORAD. Potassium currents in frog ventricular muscle: evidence from voltage clamp currents and extracellular K accumulation. *J. Physiol. London* 286: 113–143, 1979.
36. COSTANTIN, L. L. The effect of calcium on contraction and conductance thresholds in frog skeletal muscle. *J. Physiol. London* 195: 119–132, 1968.
37. COSTANTIN, L. L. The role of sodium current in the radial spread of contraction in frog muscle fibers. *J. Gen. Physiol.* 55: 703–715, 1970.

37a. COSTANTIN, L. L. Activation in striated muscle. In: *Handbook of Physiology. The Nervous System*, edited by J.M. Brookhart and V.B. Mountcastle. Bethesda, MD: Am. Physiol. Soc., 1977, sect. 1, vol. I, pt. 1, chapt. 7, p. 215–259.

38. CRANK, J. *The Mathematics of Diffusion*. Oxford: Oxford Univ. Press, 1956.
39. CURTIS, B. A. Ca fluxes in single twitch muscle fibers. *J. Gen. Physiol.* 50: 255–267, 1966.
40. CURTIS, B. A. Calcium efflux from frog twitch muscle fibers. *J. Gen. Physiol.* 55: 243–253, 1970.
41. DAVIES, P. W. Voltage clamp measurements on skeletal muscle fibers with low resistance internal electrodes (Abstract). *Federation Proc.* 33: 401, 1974.
42. DODGE, F. A., AND B. FRANKENHAEUSER. Membrane currents in isolated frog nerve fibre under voltage clamp conditions. *J. Physiol. London* 143: 76–90, 1958.
43. DUVAL, A., AND C. LÉOTY. Ionic currents in mammalian fast skeletal muscle. *J. Physiol. London* 278: 403–423, 1978.
44. DUVAL, A., AND C. LÉOTY. Ionic currents in slow twitch skeletal muscle in the rat. *J. Physiol. London* 307: 23–41, 1980.
45. DUVAL, A., AND C. LÉOTY. Comparison between the delayed outward current in slow and fast twitch skeletal muscle in the rat. *J. Physiol. London* 307: 43–57, 1980.
46. EISENBERG, R. S., AND E. A. JOHNSON. Three-dimensional electrical field problems in physiology. *Prog. Biophys. Mol. Biol.* 20: 1–65, 1970.
47. FALK, G., AND P. FATT. Linear electrical properties of striated muscle fibres observed with intracellular electrodes. *Proc. R. Soc. London Ser. B* 160: 69–123, 1964.
48. FITZHUGH, R. Theoretical effect of temperature on threshold in the Hodgkin-Huxley nerve model. *J. Gen. Physiol.* 49: 989–1005, 1966.
49. FRANKENHAEUSER, B. A method for recording resting and action potentials in the isolated myelinated nerve fibre of the frog. *J. Physiol. London* 135: 550–559, 1957.
50. FRANKENHAEUSER, B., B. D. LINDLEY, AND R. S. SMITH. Potentiometric measurement of membrane action potentials in frog muscle fibres. *J. Physiol. London* 183: 152–166, 1966.
51. GAGE, P. W., AND R. S. EISENBERG. Capacitance of the surface and transverse tubular membrane of frog sartorius muscle fibers. *J. Gen. Physiol.* 53: 265–278, 1969.
52. GAGE, P. W., AND R. S. EISENBERG. Action potentials, afterpotentials, and excitation-contraction coupling in frog sartorius fibers without transverse tubules. *J. Gen. Physiol.* 53: 298–310, 1969.
53. GAY, L. A., AND P. R. STANFIELD. Cs^+ causes a voltage-dependent block of inward K currents in resting skeletal muscle fibres. *Nature London* 267: 169–170, 1977.
54. GILLY, W. F., AND C. S. HUI. Mechanical activation in slow and twitch skeletal muscle fibres of the frog. *J. Physiol. London* 301: 137–156, 1980.
55. GILLY, W. F., AND C. S. HUI. Membrane electrical properties of frog slow muscle fibres. *J. Physiol. London* 301: 157–173, 1980.
56. GILLY, W. F., AND C. S. HUI. Voltage-dependent charge movement in frog slow muscle fibres. *J. Physiol. London* 301: 175–190, 1980.
57. GOLDMAN, D. E. Potential, impedance, and rectification in membranes. *J. Gen. Physiol.* 27: 37–60, 1943.
58. HAGIWARA, S., S. MIYAZAKI, W. MOODY, AND J. PATLAK. Blocking effects of barium and hydrogen ions on the potassium current during anomalous rectification in the starfish egg. *J. Physiol. London* 279: 167–185, 1978.
59. HAGIWARA, S., S. MIYAZAKI, AND N. P. ROSENTHAL. Potassium current and the effect of cesium on this current during anomalous rectification of the egg cell membrane of a starfish. *J. Gen. Physiol.* 67: 621–638, 1976.
60. HANSON, J., AND A. PERSSON. Changes in the action potential and contraction of isolated frog muscle after repetitive stimulation. *Acta Physiol. Scand.* 81: 340–348, 1971.
61. HARRIS, E. J. Anion interaction in frog muscle. *J. Physiol. London* 141: 351–365, 1958.
62. HEISTRACHER, P., AND C. C. HUNT. The relation of membrane changes to contraction in twitch muscle fibres. *J. Physiol. London* 201: 589–611, 1969.
63. HEISTRACHER, P., AND C. C. HUNT. Contractile repriming in snake twitch muscle fibres. *J. Physiol. London* 201: 613–626, 1969.
64. HILLE, B., AND D. T. CAMPBELL. An improved vaseline gap voltage clamp for skeletal muscle fibers. *J. Gen. Physiol.* 67: 265–293, 1976.
65. HODGKIN, A. L., AND P. HOROWICZ. The influence of potassium and chloride ions on the membrane potential of single muscle fibres. *J. Physiol. London* 148: 127–160, 1959.
66. HODGKIN, A. L., AND P. HOROWICZ. The effect of sudden changes in ionic concentrations on the membrane potential of single muscle fibres. *J. Physiol. London* 153: 370–385, 1960.
67. HODGKIN, A. L., AND A. F. HUXLEY. A quantitative description of membrane current and its application to conduction and excitation in nerve. *J. Physiol. London* 117: 500–544, 1952.
68. HODGKIN, A. L., AND B. KATZ. The effect of sodium ions on the electrical activity of the giant axon of the squid. *J. Physiol. London* 108: 37–77, 1949.
69. HODGKIN, A. L., AND S. NAKAJIMA. The effect of diameter on the electrical constants of frog skeletal muscle fibres. *J. Physiol. London* 221: 105–120, 1972.
70. HODGKIN, A. L., AND W. A. H. RUSHTON. The electrical constants of a crustacean nerve fibre. *Proc. R. Soc. London Ser. B* 133: 444–479, 1946.
71. HUTTER, O. F., AND D. NOBLE. The chloride conductance of frog skeletal muscle. *J. Physiol. London* 151: 89–102, 1960.
72. HUTTER, O. F., AND S. M. PADSHA. Effect of nitrate and other anions on the membrane resistance of frog skeletal muscle. *J. Physiol. London* 146: 117–132, 1959.
73. HUTTER, O. F., AND A. E. WARNER. The pH sensitivity of the chloride conductance of frog skeletal muscle. *J. Physiol. London* 189: 403–425, 1967.
74. HUTTER, O. F., AND A. E. WARNER. The effect of pH on the ^{36}Cl efflux from frog skeletal muscle. *J. Physiol. London* 189: 427–460, 1967.
75. HUTTER, O. F., AND A. E. WARNER. The voltage dependence of the chloride conductance of frog muscle. *J. Physiol. London* 227: 275–290, 1972.
76. HUXLEY, A. F., AND R. E. TAYLOR. Local activation of striated muscle fibres. *J. Physiol. London* 144: 426–441, 1958.
77. ILDEFONSE, M., AND O. ROUGIER. Voltage-clamp analysis of the early current in frog skeletal muscle fibre using the double sucrose-gap method. *J. Physiol. London* 222: 373–395, 1972.
78. ILDEFONSE, M., AND G. ROY. Kinetic properties of the sodium current in striated muscle fibres on the basis of the Hodgkin-Huxley theory. *J. Physiol. London* 227: 419–431, 1972.
79. JACK, J. J. B., D. NOBLE, AND R. W. TSIEN. *Electrical Current Flow in Excitable Cell.* London: Oxford Univ. Press, 1975.
80. KAO, C. Y., AND P. R. STANFIELD. Action of some anions on the electrical properties and mechanical threshold of frog twitch muscle. *J. Physiol. London* 198: 291–309, 1968.
81. KASS, R. S., S. A. SIEGELBAUM, AND R. W. TSIEN. Three micro-electrode voltage clamp experiments in calf cardiac Purkinje fibres: is slow inward current adequately measured? *J. Physiol. London* 290: 201–225, 1979.

82. KATZ, B. Les constantes électriques de la membrane du muscle. *Arch. Sci. Physiol.* 3: 285–300, 1949.
83. KIRSCH, G. E., R. A. NICHOLS, AND S. NAKAJIMA. Delayed rectification in the transverse tubules. Origin of late afterpotential in frog skeletal muscle. *J. Gen. Physiol.* 70: 1–21, 1977.
84. KOOTSEY, J. M. Voltage clamp simulation. *Federation Proc.* 34: 1343–1349, 1975.
85. KOVÁCS, L., E. RÍOS, AND M. F. SCHNEIDER. Calcium transients and intramembrane charge movement in skeletal muscle fibres. *Nature London* 279: 391–396, 1979.
86. KOVÁCS, L., AND M. F. SCHNEIDER. Contractile activation by voltage clamp depolarization of cut skeletal muscle fibres. *J. Physiol. London* 277: 483–506, 1978.
87. LÉOTY, C., AND J. ALIX. Some technical improvements for the voltage clamp with the double sucrose gap. *Pfluegers Arch.* 365: 95–97, 1976.
88. LORCOVIC, H., AND C. EDWARDS. Threshold for contraction and delayed rectification in muscle. *Life Sci.* 7: 367–370, 1968.
89. LYNCH, C. Kinetic and biochemical separation of delayed rectifier currents in frog striated muscle. *Biophys. J.* 21: 55a, 1978.
90. MATHIAS, R. T., R. S. EISENBERG, AND R. VALDIOSERA. Electrical properties of frog skeletal muscle fibers interpreted with a mesh model of the tubular system. *Biophys. J.* 17: 57–93, 1977.
91. MEECH, R. W., AND N. B. STANDEN. Potassium activation in *Helix aspersa* neurones under voltage clamp: a component mediated by calcium influx. *J. Physiol. London* 249: 211–239, 1975.
92. MEYER, K. H., AND J. F. SIEVERS. La perméabilité des membranes. I. Théorie de la perméabilité ionique. *Helv. Chim. Acta* 19: 649–664, 1936.
93. MOORE, L. E. Voltage clamp experiments on single muscle fibers of *Rana pipiens*. *J. Gen. Physiol.* 60: 1–19, 1972.
94. NAKAJIMA, S., S. IWASAKI, AND K. OBATA. Delayed rectification and anomalous rectification in frog's skeletal muscle membrane. *J. Gen. Physiol.* 46: 97–115, 1962.
95. NOBLE, D., AND R. W. TSIEN. Outward membrane currents activated in the plateau range of potentials in cardiac Purkinje fibres. *J. Physiol. London* 200: 205–231, 1969.
96. OHMORI, H. Inactivation kinetics and steady-state current noise in the anomalous rectifier of tunicate egg cell membranes. *J. Physiol. London* 281: 77–99, 1978.
97. PAPPONE, P. A. Voltage clamp experiments in normal and denervated mammalian skeletal muscle fibres. *J. Physiol. London* 307: 377–410, 1980.
98. PESKOFF, A. Green's function for Laplace's equation in an infinite cylindrical cell. *J. Math. Phys.* 15: 2112–2120, 1974.
99. PESKOFF, A., AND R. S. EISENBERG. A point source in a cylindrical cell: potential for a step-function of current inside an infinite cylindrical cell in a medium of finite conductivity. Los Angeles, CA: UCLA, 1974. (Tech. Rep. UCLA-ENG-7421.)
100. PESKOFF, A., R. S. EISENBERG, AND J. P. COLE. Potential induced by a point source of current inside an infinite cylindrical cell. Los Angeles, CA: UCLA, 1973. (Tech. Rep. UCLA-ENG-7303.)
101. POINDESSAULT, P. J., A. DUVAL, AND C. LÉOTY. Voltage clamp with double sucrose gap technique. External series resistance compensation. *Biophys. J.* 16: 105–120, 1976.
102. ROUGIER, O., G. VASSORT, AND R. STÄMPFLI. Voltage clamp experiments on frog atrial heart muscle fibres with the sucrose gap technique. *Pfluegers Arch.* 301: 91–108, 1968.
103. SANCHEZ, J. A., AND E. STEFANI. Inward calcium current in twitch muscle fibres of the frog. *J. Physiol. London* 283: 197–209, 1978.
104. SCHNEIDER, M. F. Linear electrical properties of the transverse tubules and surface membrane of skeletal muscle fibers. *J. Gen. Physiol.* 56: 640–671, 1970.
105. SCHNEIDER, M. F., AND W. K. CHANDLER. Effects of membrane potential on the capacitance of skeletal muscle fibers. *J. Gen. Physiol.* 67: 125–163, 1976.
106. STANDEN, N. B., AND P. R. STANFIELD. A potential- and time-dependent blockade of inward rectification in frog skeletal muscle fibres by barium and strontium ions. *J. Physiol. London* 280: 169–191, 1978.
107. STANDEN, N. B., AND P. R. STANFIELD. Potassium depletion and sodium block of potassium currents under hyperpolarization in frog sartorius muscle. *J. Physiol. London* 294: 497–520, 1979.
108. STANFIELD, P. R. The effect of tetraethylammonium ion on the delayed currents of frog skeletal muscle. *J. Physiol. London* 209: 209–229, 1970.
109. STANFIELD, P. R. A calcium dependent inward current in frog skeletal muscle fibres. *Pfluegers Arch.* 368: 267–270, 1977.
110. STANFIELD, P. R., F. M. ASHCROFT, AND T. D. PLANT. Gating of a muscle K^+ channel and its dependence on the permeating ion species. *Nature London* 289: 509–511, 1981.
111. TAYLOR, R. E. Cable theory. In: *Physical Techniques in Biological Research. Electrophysiological Methods*, edited by W. L. Nastuk. New York: Academic, 1963, vol. 6, pt. B.
112. TAYLOR, R. E., J. W. MOORE, AND K. S. COLE. Analysis of certain errors in squid axon voltage clamp measurements. *Biophys. J.* 1: 161–202, 1960.
113. THOMSEN, J. Tonische Krämpfe in willkürlich beweglichen Muskeln in Folge von erebter psychischer Disposition (Ataxis muscularis?). *Arch . Psychiatr. Nervenkr.* 6: 702–718, 1876.
114. THOMSON, W. (LORD KELVIN). On the theory of the electric telegraph. *Proc. R. Soc. London* 7: 382–399, 1855.
115. VALDIOSERA, R., C. CLAUSEN, AND R. S. EISENBERG. Impedance of frog skeletal muscle fibers in various solutions. *J. Gen. Physiol.* 63: 460–491, 1974.
116. WARNER, A. E. Kinetic properties of the chloride conductance of frog muscle. *J. Physiol. London* 227: 291–312, 1972.

CHAPTER 11

Impedance measurement of the electrical structure of skeletal muscle

ROBERT S. EISENBERG | *Department of Physiology, Rush Medical College, Chicago, Illinois*

CHAPTER CONTENTS

MUSCLES ARE COMPLEX STRUCTURES that use chemical energy to perform mechanical work. The mechanisms that control the transduction of chemical energy into mechanical work are associated with the membrane systems of muscle fibers and so are easily studied by electrophysiological techniques designed to measure the properties of membranes.

The membrane systems of skeletal muscle are quite complex and have obviously been specialized by evolution to help perform the control mechanisms required. I briefly discuss the evolutionary specialization of muscle structure in the light of molecular and developmental biology before dealing with our main subject. After all, it is much easier to figure out how a machine works if you have some idea of how and why it was designed! Structural complexity extends beyond muscle; the basic structural patterns of membranes are repeated in many tissues (26). Therefore impedance techniques, the main subject of this chapter, are potentially useful in many other areas of biology, wherever structural specialization helps a tissue to function.

The structural specialization of muscle is only one example of the mechanisms of gene expression and cellular differentiation that allow a genome, common to all cells in the body, to produce cells highly specialized for particular functions. Evidently, it is much easier for evolution to modify an existing gene or gene product than it is to create a new one. The fundamental organelles and macromolecules of all cells are quite similar. Tissues are specialized more often by elaboration of common organelles and macromolecules than by synthesis of new ones. Many of the enzymes, structural proteins, and organelles of muscle fibers are not very different from those of other cells, but their structural organization is strikingly specialized.

Conservation of genetic information may be an important evolutionary principle; put another way, creation of new genetic information is evolutionarily difficult. That is probably why lower eucaryotes have a segmented structure (basically a periodic repeat of the expression of a single set of genes) and why even higher vertebrates have so much symmetry in their anatomy. Surprisingly large changes in final structure (and function) can be produced by simple changes in the rate of growth of a particular substructure. For example, Hampé [as described by Gould (50)] showed that "minor quantitative changes in the timing of development [could lead to] a change in arrangement of the entire ankle area." Similarly many structural complexities of muscle fibers may be the result of minor changes in the rate or pattern of expression of genes. Thus much structural specialization could be produced from a rather limited genome. The similar specialization of membranes in many tissues—the similar use of invaginations and infoldings with different distribution of ionic conductances and active transport systems—argues for a related genetic and developmental origin. Techniques for analysis of structural complication [see Eisenberg and Mathias (35)], including impedance measurements, are thus of general biological interest because structural complexity is a common evolutionary strategy for specialization and adaptation.

Skeletal muscle fibers illustrate the uses of structural complexity. They have a variety of membrane systems, most with specific and well-known functions directly related to contraction. The three main membrane systems are the outer membrane, the T system, and the sarcoplasmic reticulum (SR). The electrical properties of the surface and T-system membrane, and of the solution within the T system, are important determinants of the shape, conduction velocity, and radial spread of the action potential and so are of direct physiological interest. Many of these properties can be determined by impedance measurements.

Even the outer membrane of skeletal muscle fibers is structurally complex. It is not a smooth cylinder; it has irregular shallow folds that allow the fiber to stretch and infolded pockets called caveolae (27, 105) of unknown function.

The T system of skeletal muscle is formed by tubular infoldings of the outer membrane; these tubules branch predominantly in the transverse plane (hence the name T system) to surround the myofibrils and to be in close contact with the SR. Some of the caveolae seem independent of the T system, but a substantial fraction of the caveolae are part of the T system and connect the tubular system and the extracellular space. Indeed tubules probably open into caveolae and are not otherwise connected to the surface membrane.

The sarcoplasmic reticulum is a separate compartment within the muscle; its membrane is not continuous with that of the T system. A substantial gap separates the T membrane and the adjacent SR membrane, a gap accessible to solutes in the sarcoplasmic solution [Eisenberg, Mathias, and Gilai (30); Franzini-Armstrong (41)]. The gap between T system and SR is spanned by well-delineated structures called *pillars* [Eisenberg and Gilai (29); Eisenberg, Mathias, and Gilai (30); Somlyo (96); Eisenberg and Eisenberg (28a)] and amorphous material called *feet* [reviewed in Franzini-Armstrong (42)]. The lumen of the SR is inaccessible to large molecules in the bathing solution that diffuse easily into the lumen of the T system. The possibility that small ions can flow and carry electrical current from T system to SR has recently been discussed at length by Mathias, Levis, and Eisenberg (68). Whatever the validity of their speculations, clearly the SR must be considered a separate compartment from the T system, electrically linked to the T system, if at all, by a specialized system with a specialized molecular structure and function.

The function of each membrane system of muscle is important for contraction. The surface membrane conducts the action potential longitudinally down the fiber, allowing nearly simultaneous contraction of longitudinally distant sarcomeres. The T system conducts the action potential radially into the depths of the fiber, allowing nearly simultaneous contraction of radially distant myofibrils. The T system profoundly alters the shape and longitudinal conduction velocity of the action potential (4, 47). The SR releases calcium in response to an action potential, thus initiating contraction; subsequently it reaccumulates calcium for another twitch.

Each of the membrane systems thus has a distinct functional role; each membrane must therefore be expected to have distinct electrical properties resulting from the differences in molecular structure and in the currents that cross the membranes. The different membrane systems have distinct lipid and protein composition. The density and even type of macromolecular conductors (e.g., sodium channels) must be expected to differ in various membranes.

One must then measure the electrical properties of each membrane. Someday electrical measurements will be made on preparations isolated by biochemical techniques. Eventually the individual membranes and membrane macromolecules will be recovered and purified from homogenized muscle, just as enzymes are recovered and purified today. In the meantime, and even then, there are some advantages to measuring the properties of the membranes of muscles in their natural state within a living muscle fiber.

The electrical properties of muscle fibers can be divided into two categories, linear and nonlinear. The distinction is made because of different analytical techniques. Linear properties (which are independent of the size of the signal used to measure them, like the capacitance of lipid bilayers) can be analyzed with the general theory of linear systems, which is a highly developed and powerful branch of electrical engineering and applied mathematics [see Cooper and McGillem (22) for an introductory text]. Most of the important derivations and results of linear-system theory are in the frequency domain, with the idea of impedance used to relate the sinusoidal output to the sinusoidal input of the linear system. Unknown linear systems are usually best characterized by impedance functions because of the central role of impedance functions in linear-system theory.

Nonlinear properties (which vary with the size of the applied signal, like the ionic conductances of nerve fibers) are much harder to analyze because no general theory describes their complex behavior. Indeed nonlinear systems have such a variety of behavior that a general theory may not be possible. [For example, the general theory of nonlinear systems called Wiener kernel analysis (63, 93, 93a) has been shown to have serious intrinsic limitations (80, 81).] Nonlinear systems are not usually measured in the frequency domain or characterized by impedance functions because such functions do not easily describe complex nonlinear behavior. (See refs. 45, 63, and 104 for exceptions to this statement.) Rather, the behavior of nonlinear systems is usually measured in the time domain, where it is more easily described.

Why should one be interested in the linear electrical properties of biological systems, when their natural activity is usually nonlinear? Linear properties are interesting for several reasons. They describe the biophysical properties of resting membranes; they describe all the electrical properties of some cellular components, like the lumen of the T system; and they are the resting basis for natural activity. Linear properties can also be analyzed in much more detail than nonlinear properties because a general theory of linear properties is known. Thus the contribution of each membrane system to the linear properties of a muscle fiber can be determined, but it has not yet been possible to perform such a structural analysis of nonlinear properties.

A structural analysis has several steps (35): the structure must be described and measured, assumptions must be made concerning the qualitative properties of each membrane, the expected properties of a cell with that structure and those membranes must be predicted theoretically, the electrical properties of the cell must be measured, and the measurements must be compared with theoretical predictions. If the confrontation of structure, theory, and measurements is satisfactorily resolved, the measurements can then yield reliable estimates of the resistance and capacitance of the various components, membrane systems, and extracellular spaces of the cell. Several of the steps are far more difficult for nonlinear systems than linear systems. In particular the qualitative assumptions concerning membrane properties, the theoretical prediction of electrical properties, and the measurement of electrical parameters with high resolution are very difficult with a nonlinear system. Analysis of linear systems is much easier; they have much less diverse behavior than nonlinear systems. The powerful techniques of linear-system theory are also a great help. Therefore structural analysis so far has been confined to linear systems.

The linear electrical properties of biological preparations can be measured in a number of ways. Sometimes the properties can be deduced from the natural electrical activity of the preparation. For example, the shape and conduction velocity of the action potential can itself be used to estimate some of the linear properties of a muscle fiber [reviewed in Jack, Noble, and Tsien (58)]. Usually, however, the system must be artificially perturbed to measure the electrical properties. For impedance measurements with microelectrodes, current is usually applied and the resulting voltage is recorded. Voltage can also be applied, with a voltage-clamp system, and the resulting current recorded [Fishman, Poussart, and Moore (40) is a recent reference to this technique applied to axons]. The voltage-clamp technique has recently been used for microelectrode recording of impedance (J. L. Rae, R. T. Mathias, and R. S. Eisenberg, unpublished observations) and has advantages.

Whether the perturbation applied to the system is a sinusoidal current or voltage, the result is an impedance measurement: as originally defined, impedance (or its reciprocal admittance) measures the response to experimentally applied sinusoidal currents or voltages, or at least that was the original definition. The definition now must be generalized to include the response to perturbations that are the sums of sinusoids, for example, the response to white noise. The essential characteristic of impedance measurements is that they are made in the frequency domain, whether the perturbing signal is a simple sinusoid or a more complex waveform. Impedance analysis does not analyze directly the time course of the applied signal and its response; rather, the applied signal and response are decomposed into their sinusoidal components by Fourier analysis, and the frequency dependence of the amplitude and phase delay of those components is studied.

Analysis in the frequency domain is justified, despite its apparent complexity (in algebra, if not logic), by the resulting sensitivity and resolution of the measurements. Measurements in the frequency domain typically provide more resolution, by at least an order of magnitude, than direct analysis of time-varying signals.

Impedance measurements are thus made by recording the sinusoids resulting from sinusoids applied to the preparation. Sinusoids are characterized by three parameters: size (i.e., amplitude), phase, and frequency. The amplitude of the sinusoid is its peak value [or equivalently, its root-mean-square value]; the phase angle is the normalized delay between applied current and recorded voltage. In a linear system, the frequency of the sinusoidal response measured is the same as the frequency of the sinusoidal perturbation applied to the system. The frequency of the applied signal is known and thus does not need to be measured. Impedance measurements then involve two quantities: the ratio of the amplitude of recorded voltage to applied current and the normalized delay (phase angle) between the same two signals.

The amplitude of the impedance and its phase angle depend on the frequency of applied current, because the properties of the components of a muscle depend on frequency. The capacitive properties of membranes ensure that both the amplitude and delay (i.e., phase angle) of currents are different at different frequencies. Impedance must therefore be measured at a variety of frequencies if the electrical properties are to be completely specified. The phase angle and magnitude of the impedance (i.e., the amplitude) are functions of frequency. To specify the electrical properties of the muscle fiber one must measure those functions over a band of frequencies wide enough to determine the biologically significant behavior of the muscle. Typically this band of frequencies has been from 0.1 Hz to 10 kHz, although information over a wider bandwidth might be of interest.

The experimental impedance data may be treated in a variety of ways. Measurements of phase angle and magnitude can be converted into other forms, with various algebraic formulas. Such conversions are quite natural and proceed without effort because of a convenient property of impedance functions: they can be described by complex numbers. The phase angle between sinusoidal current and voltage can be written as the phase angle of a complex number, and the relative amplitude of the sinusoids can be written as the magnitude of the same complex number. The impedance of a preparation is simply a complex function of frequency. At any one frequency the phase angle of that complex function is the normalized delay between sinusoidal current and sinusoidal voltage of that frequency; the magnitude is the relative magnitude of the same two signals. The use of complex numbers and complex algebra to describe impedance functions is well described in textbooks of electrical engineering [e.g., Desoer and Kuh (25)]. Although the algebra has the name "complex," and that name is often thought appropriate by biologists, the rules of complex arithmetic and algebra are the same as, and thus as simple as, those of real arithmetic and algebra. Indeed, complex numbers were discovered (or should we say invented?) because without them one sometimes cannot solve equations involving only real quantities. For example, the solutions of quadratic equations usually involve the square root of minus one.

The reader unfamiliar with complex arithmetic will find that the few days of work necessary to learn to manipulate complex numbers and penetrate the psychological energy barrier will make many disciplines accessible. Indeed, without the knowledge of complex arithmetic little biological use can be made of many results of physics, engineering, or applied mathematics. Practical exercises and the needed theory of complex arithmetic are presented in many texts of college algebra.

Some confusion has been produced by the different descriptions of complex numbers and thus impedance functions. Early workers preferred to describe the rectangular components of complex numbers and impedances, whereas later workers prefer to use the amplitude and phase angle. The relation of these two representations is straightforward. Just as any point can be described by its rectangular coordinates x and y or its polar coordinates ρ and θ, so can any impedance or complex number be described by its real and imaginary component or its amplitude and phase. (The real component is neither more nor less tangible than the imaginary component. The name *real* is simply an unfortunate historical synonym for x coordinate; the name *imaginary* is a synonym for y coordinate.) Later workers and electrical engineers prefer to describe impedance functions by their amplitude and phase for a number of practical reasons, particularly because phase plots are such a sensitive measure of the properties of many systems. Conversion of impedance data from one representation to another is no more complicated than conversion from polar to rectangular coordinates.

In fact the question of the proper representation of impedance functions is somewhat academic now. Measurement, computation, and theory are done largely by computers that directly perform complex arithmetic without explicit reference to the components of the complex number. Only the output programs, meant for human evaluation, convert these complex numbers into phase angles and magnitudes or real and imaginary parts.

Figure 1 illustrates the sensitivity of impedance measurements compared with transient measurements and the sensitivity of phase plots compared with other impedance plots. I calculate the response of a simple resistance-capacitance (RC) circuit that contains the essential features of many biological preparations. The circuit contains a series resistance (R_s), a "membrane" resistance of 2,000 Ω, and a "membrane" capacitance of 6 μF. Plots are given in Figure 1 for two different values of R_s, 0 and 100 Ω. The responses shown are either to sinusoids or to a step function of current. The response to sinusoids is plotted in three ways: *1*) as the phase angle of the impedance versus log frequency, *2*) as the magnitude versus log frequency, and *3*) as the real part of the impedance versus the imaginary part of the impedance (often called a Cole-Cole or Nyquist plot). The response to a 1-μA step function of current is also shown.

Consider first the response to a step function. The effect of R_s is rather small and can be seen most clearly only at very short times. Indeed the shape of the transient response is independent of the value of R_s. The constancy of shape causes serious difficulties in the real world. If there is instrumental confusion at short times (as is usually the case) or if the system is somewhat distributed (either spatially or statistically), the initial jump in the waveform is obscured. Then the value of R_s cannot be determined with any accuracy.

Figure 2 shows the responses of a more relevant circuit, one that is a lumped approximation to the electrical properties of 1 cm^2 of the outer membrane of a frog muscle fiber together with its associated T system. The two curves shown are for two different values of R_s, 200 and 300 Ω.

Figures 1 and 2 clearly show that the phase plot is much more sensitive than the other plots. The size and more importantly the shape of the phase plot vary substantially as parameters change value. This is not a special property of the circuits illustrated but is a rather general finding. In fact as circuit complexity increases, the advantages of the phase plot increase, and the advantages of impedance measurements in general also increase. This point is discussed at some length in Eisenberg and Mathias (35), where reference is made to some of the applied mathematics literature comparing analysis of frequency domain and time domain. We also consider integrals of transients and show that such integrals may be more helpful than the transients themselves in characterizing linear systems. In fact integrals of transients may sometimes be more helpful than impedance measurements.

Impedance measurements are important in muscle physiology. They allow specification of the linear prop-

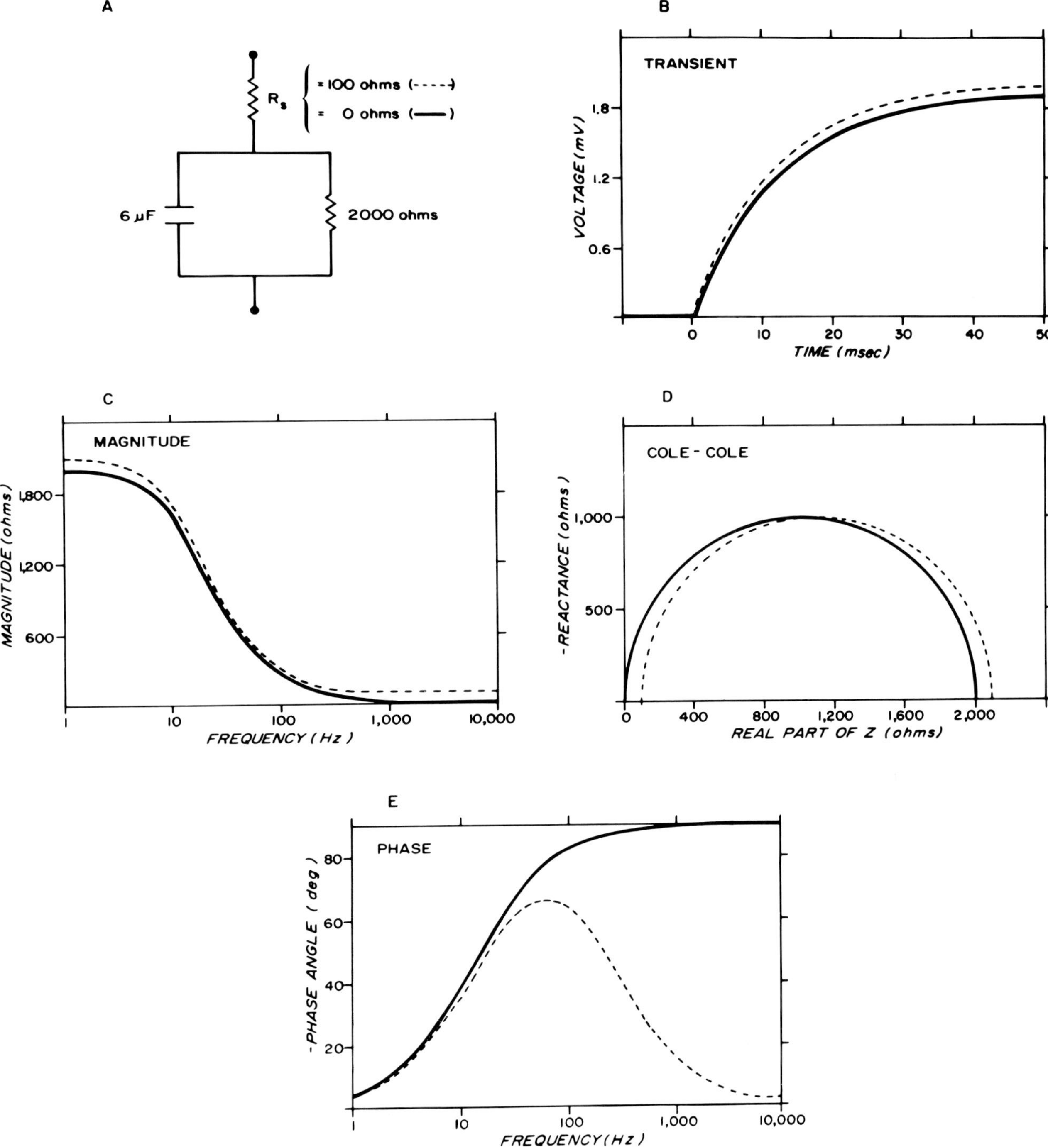

FIG. 1. *A*: simple circuit with 2 different values of series resistance. Other panels show response of the circuit plotted in different ways. *B*: transient response to a step function of current (1 μA) applied at time 0. *Dashed line*, response with 100-Ω series resistance, is a vertical displacement of response with no series resistance (*solid line*). Therefore these responses are hard to tell apart and are hard to use to measure the series resistance. *C*: magnitude of impedance of circuit measured with sinusoidal currents of the frequency shown on the abscissa. The effect of a series resistance is upward displacement of the curve without change in shape. *D*: plot of imaginary part of the impedance vs. real part of the impedance. Although frequency is not an explicit variable, variation of frequency and the subsequent variation in the real and imaginary parts of the impedance produce the curve. Again the effect of a series resistance is a simple translation of the curve without change in shape. *E*: phase angle between sinusoidally applied current and voltage. Effects of series resistance are substantial, making it easy to measure series resistance.

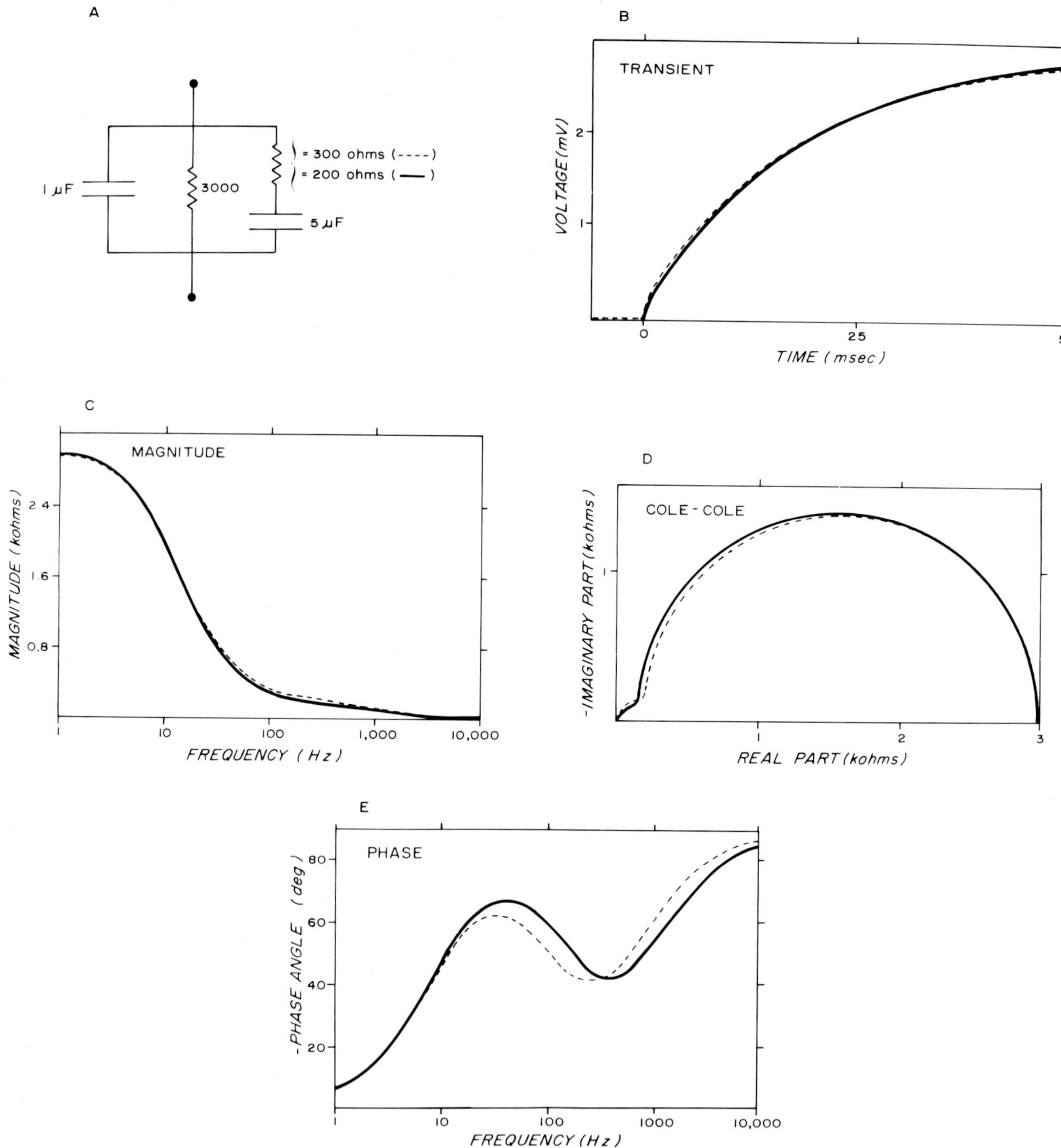

FIG. 2. *A*: lumped approximation to properties of 1 cm^2 of surface membrane and associated T system of frog skeletal muscle with 2 different values of series resistance indicated. *B*: transient response of lumped circuit to a step function of applied current. Tiny difference between the 2 curves makes measurement of series resistance difficult from transient responses. *C*: magnitude of the response to sinusoidal currents of different frequencies. Effect of series resistance is small, making measurement difficult. *D*: a plot of imaginary vs. real part of the impedance. Effects of series resistance and of the 1-μF capacitor are hard to see in this plot. *E*: phase angle between sinusoidally applied current and voltage. Effects of series resistance are substantial, making it easy to measure series resistance.

erties of the muscle fiber with a high degree of resolution. Combined with the appropriate morphological measurements and theory, impedance measurements can determine the resting electrical properties of several components of a muscle fiber—the surface membrane and T system, at least. Knowledge of the resting properties is important in itself and also gives insight into many of the active properties.

METHODS AND TECHNIQUES

The main advantage of impedance measurements is their accuracy and resolution. This advantage, however, can also be a disadvantage. Impedance measurements are just as sensitive to the properties of the recording system as they are to the properties of a muscle fiber. Artifact is more apparent in the frequency domain than in the time domain. Techniques and recording systems developed for transient measurements are usually unsatisfactory for impedance measurements.

It has taken a number of years and the work of many laboratories to develop reliable methods of measuring impedance from single cells with microelectrodes. Other methods are undoubtedly possible but have not yet been tested on previously studied preparations. I therefore pay most attention to microelectrode methods that have been extensively used and tested by several laboratories.

Microelectrode Techniques

The basic plan of measurement was introduced by Falk and Fatt (38). They inserted one microelectrode into a muscle fiber to pass sinusoidal current from the fiber interior to an external electrode in the bath. They recorded the induced potential with another microelectrode inserted into the fiber. The phase angle and relative delay of the two signals determined the input impedance $Z(j\omega)$; Z (in Ω) is a complex number, a function of $j\omega$ (in rad/s). The angular frequency ω equals $2\pi f$, where f is the frequency (in Hz), and $j = (-1)^{1/2}$. The input impedance is a property of the whole length of the muscle fiber, the sarcoplasm, the outer membrane, and the inner (i.e., tubular and perhaps SR) membranes as well. Moreover Z is simply related to r_i (in Ω/cm), to the resistance of the sarcoplasm in a unit length of fiber, and to the shunt admittance y in a unit length of fiber (in S/cm)

$$Z(j\omega) = \tfrac{1}{2}\,(r_i/y)^{1/2} \tag{1}$$

the resistance r_i is related to the resistivity R_i (in $\Omega \cdot$cm) by $r_i = R_i/\pi a^2$, where a is the radius (in cm).

Falk and Fatt (38) interpreted the shunt admittance y as the result of all current flows from sarcoplasm to the extracellular space. They allowed it to have two components, the admittance y_s of the surface membrane (in S/cm) and the admittance y_e of the inner membranes (also in S/cm)

$$y = y_s + y_e \tag{2}$$

where $y_s = G_s + j\omega C_s$; that is, the admittance of the surface membrane consists of the conductance of the surface membrane G_s (in S/cm) and the capacitance C_s of the surface membrane (in F/cm). The linear properties of the T system are given by y_e, which is properly described later.

The formula of Falk and Fatt (38) requires some justification. First, it must be understood that their equation is assumed and not derived. A derivation must proceed from the fundamental laws of the electric field and statements of the structure of a muscle fiber; such a derivation for a tubular system is only recently available [R. T. Mathias, personal communication; see Peskoff (86) for a related derivation for a system of clefts]. Second, Falk and Fatt (38) assumed that the only significant electrical property of the sarcoplasm was its resistance—they did not allow the sarcoplasm or SR to have an impedance. This assumption has been shown to be correct experimentally by Schneider (94) and Mobley, Leung, and Eisenberg (72, 73).

Falk and Fatt (38) assumed, for the most part, that the membrane capacitance behaved ideally, with a phase angle of 90°. This assumption has been questioned on the basis of early impedance measurements on suspensions of cells [reviewed in Cole (20)], which were interpreted as evidence for a membrane capacitance with a reduced phase angle of about 70°. Hanai and co-workers (6, 51) have shown, however, that the theory used by early workers to interpret the impedance of suspensions was incorrect: it did not properly describe conductors with thin membranes, and it did not properly describe cells of nonspherical shape. When a revised theory is used, the impedance data do not require a membrane capacitance with a reduced phase angle. Membrane capacitors of 90° phase angle produce essentially perfect fits to impedance data from suspensions of cells.

Early impedance measurements on axons were also taken as evidence for a reduced phase angle of the membrane capacitance. The recent results of Fishman, Poussart, and Moore, and other references cited therein (40), together with the work of Takashima and Schwan (99), show that the linear properties of squid axons are highly sensitive to corrections for series resistance, to the length of the axon from which measurements are made, and to reactive current that flows through the sodium (i.e., tetrodotoxin-sensitive) and potassium (i.e., tetraethylammonium-sensitive) channels. (A reactive current is one that is delayed or advanced in time from its driving voltage: it has a phase shift. Currents through capacitors and inductors are reactive, whereas currents through resistors are not. Currents through time-dependent ionic conductances are generally shifted in phase. If the perturbing signal is sufficiently small to make the time-dependent ionic conductance quasi-linear, the current through an ionic channel can be described as an ionic reactance.)

The deviations from a phase angle of 90° reported by Cole and colleagues can probably be explained by the effects just listed, without invoking an imperfect membrane capacitance.

There are certain important technical difficulties in the measurements of Falk and Fatt (38). The first is the difficulty of interpreting results in which the source of current is very small, almost a point. The resulting three-dimensional effects are not trivial and can be made negligible only by the special precautions taken by Mathias, Eisenberg, and Valdiosera (67). Little more is said here about such effects since they have been extensively analyzed and reviewed (3, 32, 34, 87).

The other type of problem arises from the stray capacitances around the microelectrode and in the devices attached to the microelectrode. Since microelectrodes have impedances of the order of tens of megohms, and measurements are needed to frequencies of many kilohertz, stray capacitances of tenths of picofarads are serious problems. Indeed one capacitance—the capacitance between the top of the current microelectrode and the top of the voltage-recording electrode—needs to be smaller than 10^{-15} F to be negligible! Falk and Fatt (38) and subsequently Eisenberg (31) (their graduate student) faced these difficulties without operational amplifiers. They refined the standard microelectrode recording apparatus [Fatt and Katz (39); Nastuk and Hodgkin (77)] and made corrections (determined by measurement to a large extent) for the capacitive artifact. Despite the care with which the corrections were made (both experimentally and analytically), the size of the correction at frequencies above 1 kHz was disquieting and must bring into question the accuracy of their measurements. Freygang et al. (46) used a new recording circuit [suggested by A. Bak (46)] that, at least in principle, was much less sensitive to capacitive artifact. They did not extend their measurements beyond 1 kHz, however, because of difficulties in implementation. Without measurements in the frequency range 1–10 kHz, it is difficult to be sure of the amount of artifact in the lower frequency ranges. Artifact is often obvious in the higher frequency range because it introduces spurious maxima/minima into impedance plots or produces "unallowed" (i.e., unanticipated) behavior. In the lower frequency range the artifact does not produce such dramatic behavior and thus is not so obvious. Qualitatively invisible artifacts can be quantitatively quite significant, and one cannot be sure of the quantitative reliability of data taken with a limited frequency range. Although these are fairly serious criticisms, Gilai (48), Nicolaysen (78), and Schneider (94), all of whom used versions of the circuit of Freygang et al. (46), seem not to have substantial error in results from the frequency range below 800 Hz.

Circuits have also been made that try to compensate for some or all of the stray capacitances. Such circuits have not been very successful, because of *1*) difficulties in implementing an accurate negative capacitance, *2*) difficulties in adjusting the value of the negative capacitance to precisely compensate the actual stray capacitance, and *3*) the instability of the stray capacitances in and around microelectrodes. Even when implemented with modern electronics [e.g., Suzuki, Rohlicek, and Fromter (98)], the reliability of circuits with negative capacitance must be demonstrated by measurements in the frequency domain, preferably of phase angle.

Valdiosera, Clausen, and Eisenberg (100) modified the recording circuit of A. Bak (46) and made measurements with small and measured artifact up to 10 kHz. They showed that all the artifacts identified by Falk and Fatt (38) could be made negligible but that a significant artifact remained. The significant artifact was caused by capacitive coupling between the interior of the microelectrodes and the bathing solution. This artifact had not been previously recognized because its frequency dependence is similar to that of the interelectrode artifact. The current through the capacitances between the microelectrode interior and bath flows through the resistance of the bathing solution, produces a substantial extracellular potential, and thus distorts the recorded potential. Coupling into the bath could be limited but not removed by painting the microelectrodes with a conducting silver paint. The painting technique, introduced (I believe) by Valdiosera, Clausen, and Eisenberg (100), also reduces the interelectrode capacitance to negligible amounts.

The circuitry used by Valdiosera, Clausen, and Eisenberg (100) was accurate but inconvenient. It requires the repeated measurement of the resistance of the voltage microelectrode, since the gain of the circuit depends on the microelectrode resistance. In their circuit the microelectrode resistance also appears as a resistive load on the muscle fiber, typically drawing some 10 nA of DC from the fiber. The DC can be removed in a more complex version of the circuit, independently developed by R. T. Mathias (personal communication) and Sachs and Specht (91). Those workers applied feedback to the noninverting input of the voltage-recording amplifier [marked $\mathbf{A}(j\omega)$ in Fig. 2 of ref. 100]. The feedback was derived from the DC component of the output of that amplifier. By sensing and feeding back only the DC component (with, for example, a low-pass filter circuit with bandwidth from DC to 0.01 Hz), Mathias and Sachs removed the resistive load on the muscle fiber.

The circuit of Valdiosera, Clausen, and Eisenberg (100), either in its original or modified form, gives the widest reported bandwidth with microelectrodes because it is the only circuit that permits the bath to be at ground potential while the top of the voltage-recording microelectrode is also held close to ground potential. This arrangement minimizes current through the stray capacitance from the inside of the microelectrode to the bath and ground. One early implementation had a bandwidth (−3-dB point) of some 300 kHz with microelectrode attached, and this bandwidth undoubtedly could be extended with newer amplifiers if necessary.

Despite the spectacular bandwidth of the Valdiosera circuit, it remains inconvenient. If the top of the microelectrode is at virtual ground while the bath is also close to ground, there must be current flow through the microelectrode (driven by the membrane potential of the muscle fiber). In fact the Valdiosera circuit actually measures that current flow and not the membrane potential! Thus determination of the size of the membrane potential with this circuit requires the microelectrode resistance to be known, a serious inconvenience. Mathias, Rae, and Eisenberg (69, 70) therefore developed another wide-band circuit, which keeps the top of the voltage-recording microelectrode close to ground potential. Their circuit avoids the practical difficulties of the Valdiosera circuit because it does not require current to flow through the microelectrode, but the new circuit has some limitation in bandwidth.

Mathias, Rae, and Eisenberg modified the feedback-follower circuit of Eisenberg and Gage (33) first by shielding the microelectrode with conductive paint (69) and then by adding circuitry to allow direct recording of the current flowing through the preparation (70). The article by Mathias, Rae, and Eisenberg (70) contains extensive discussion and detailed diagrams of a practical circuit that allows measurement to some 10 kHz with little or no capacitive artifact. With this circuit it is possible to measure impedance reliably, conveniently, and over a sufficiently wide bandwidth.

Of course microelectrodes are not the only way to record potential within a muscle fiber. Hille and Campbell (53), for example, have recorded intracellular potential with a modification of the Vaseline-gap apparatus previously used on vertebrate nerve. One might expect that such a system could give an even wider bandwidth than the circuits previously discussed because high-impedance microelectrodes are not involved, and such is probably the case. The history of recording with microelectrodes suggests that a certain degree of caution is appropriate, however: between the principle and the reality lurks the hidden artifact! Until the artifacts of the Hille-Campbell arrangement are measured and analyzed in the frequency domain, it will not be safe to assume they are negligible.

Analysis of Sinusoidal Data

The earliest records of impedance with microelectrodes (31, 38, 94) were measured with oscilloscopes using Lissajous patterns photographed and analyzed by hand. This procedure was not speedy, typically requiring 2 days of film reading and computation with tables of trigonometric functions to acquire 24 data points. Further, although the variance of the estimates appeared quite small, even with signal-to-noise ratios of 2–4, the possibility of systematic errors was always present. Thus it seemed wise to use instrumentation rather than eye and brain to measure phase angle and amplitude.

A variety of instruments can be used for this purpose, ranging from the phase meter of Freygang et al. (46), to the phase-sensitive detectors of Valdiosera, Clausen, and Eisenberg (100), to the computer programs of Nicolaysen (78). I do not discuss these implementations, since they undoubtedly will be supplanted by the time this chapter is published. The instrumentation to measure impedance (phase and amplitude or real and imaginary parts) clearly should be accurate, insensitive to contaminating noise, and quick and easy to operate. Automation in data acquisition is desirable since the results must be entered into a computer for subsequent analysis. Of course the cheaper and less complex the instrumentation, the better. Although many of these characteristics are obtainable from the instrumentation that measures sinusoids, others are not. It is particularly difficult to measure rapidly with sinusoids, because all measurements must be made one frequency at a time with each measurement delayed until a steady state is reached and noise is averaged out. Averaging the response at one frequency takes a substantial amount of time, depending on the signal-to-noise ratio. Even if the signal far exceeds the noise, one must average for something like $10/f$ seconds, where f is the frequency of the sinusoid being measured. Thus the total duration of the measuring period is mostly determined by the low-frequency points, and measurements at many frequencies must take a long time [see Bendat and Piersol (ref. 10, chapt. 8) and Magrab and Blomquist (ref. 62, p. 81) for a quantitative analysis of the duration of analog measurement].

The requirement for a long duration of measurement is an example of a law familiar to experimenters called "the conservation of troubles." The price paid for the improved sensitivity and resolution of sinusoidal methods is the longer duration of the measurements. Sinusoidal measurements provide much more accurate information about a system but are much slower than transient measurements.

The problems associated with measurements of long duration are serious in biology, particularly when microelectrodes are used. Most biological preparations have random drift in their properties on a slow time scale; most physiological preparations also drift systematically, toward death. Because penetration by microelectrodes accentuates both random and systematic drifts, the measurements of biological impedance need to be done as quickly as possible. The faster the measurements are made, the more successful experiments can be done, and the greater are the range of experimental conditions that can be investigated, including conditions that eventually damage the fiber.

The speed of measurement of sinusoids can be improved considerably by swept-frequency methods (48) and by automating those measurements with a digital computer (78). These changes, however, do not provide a qualitative improvement in the measurement of sinusoids. The most important limitation on the speed of measurement of sinusoids is inherent in the method, as already pointed out: measurement at a given frequency requires many periods of the sinusoid at that frequency. Thus the total duration of the experiment is set largely by the lowest frequency points measured. These in turn are set by the longest functionally important time constants of the system and the resolution (i.e., number of frequency points) required to determine the experimental properties of the system, as well as the signal-to-noise ratio at each frequency. In practice, measurement of 24 data points at frequencies between 1 Hz and 10 kHz takes many minutes.

Impedance Analysis With Fourier Techniques

One way to decrease the duration of the experiment is to apply all sinusoids at once. If the perturbation applied to the system were the sum of sinusoids of many frequencies, it would be possible, at least in principle, to measure the response to that single perturbation. Then one could determine the response to all the frequencies represented in the perturbing signal. In other words, if a broad-band signal is applied to a muscle fiber and the resulting output is analyzed into its component frequencies, one should be able to measure the response (of a noise-free system) over the entire frequency range from a single measurement. The duration of that measurement would be the duration necessary to determine the response to the lowest frequency component. For example, to measure the response of a muscle fiber from 1 Hz to 10 kHz (or to any higher frequency for that matter), it would be necessary to take data just long enough to determine the response at 1 Hz.

The preceding paragraph describes the principles of Fourier analysis with white-noise input. If the perturbing signal is noise, it contains energy at all frequencies. If the response to that applied signal is decomposed by Fourier analysis into its frequency components, then sufficient data are available to determine the broad-band response, even from a short-duration record. One must acquire enough data to determine the lowest frequency point, but the higher frequency points are free, as it were.

Of course the higher frequency points are only free in principle. The implementation of this Fourier analysis is not trivial, and the number of frequency points computed is an important determinant of the cost of the Fourier analysis.

The Fourier analysis of signals is well described in the engineering literature, although perhaps it is not so well known to physiologists. Therefore a fairly extensive listing of references may be useful. Cooper and McGillem (22) provided a textbook that assumes little background and provides a clear and elementary introduction to the analysis of linear systems, including a few chapters on Fourier analysis. The other references concentrate on Fourier analysis. The book by Koopmans (60) is moderately difficult but very useful and should be accessible to most readers comfortable with calculus. The books by Papoulis (82, 83) are advanced with a rather personal approach, but contain a wealth of useful information. The book by Oppenheim and Schafer (79) is advanced, elegant, but rather abstract. Brillinger (15) and Hannan (52) provide statistical analysis and proofs of the relevant theorems; despite their rigor the results of the analysis can be read by the nonstatistician, although the proofs of the theorems are more difficult. A number of books are excellent on specialized subjects. For example, Brigham (14) includes an outstanding discussion of the digital (i.e., discrete) Fourier transform and presents ingenious and useful graphs to explain the relation of the discrete and continuous Fourier transforms; For a long time, Bendat and Piersol (10, 11) provided the only references with a reasonably complete and practical discussion of impedance measurements with Fourier techniques. Carter (15a) and Kay and Marple (58a) have recently added significantly to this literature.

This is not the place, and I am certainly not the author, to attempt a brief synthesis of this literature. There are several critical results, however, that seem important enough to present here, even though they are not original. A practically oriented tutorial treatment of impedance measurements with Fourier techniques would be helpful to both physiologists and engineers. Perhaps when the technology of Fourier measurements reaches maturity, such a review will appear in the engineering literature and supplant the next few paragraphs.

The first step in a Fourier analysis is the conversion of the analog signal into numbers. The conversion process involves many pitfalls, most of which have been removed from presently available instrumentation. One problem for digital measurements remains in much equipment designed for transient measurements. Impedance measurements require simultaneous measurement of the input and output to determine phase (i.e., time delay), whereas transient measurements often do not. It is not sufficient to measure one signal, then the other (as is often sufficient for transient measurements). Rather, the jitter and delay between the measurements must be small compared to the period of the signal with the highest frequency of interest. That is the only way to avoid artifactual phase errors. Analog-to-digital (A/D) converters are available with the feature of "simultaneous sample and hold" and the jitter and delay in such converters are negligible in the frequency range of interest here.

The central difficulty in digital Fourier analysis is the discrete nature of the numbers used to represent a continuous signal. The numbers are measured and computed with a finite number of digits, and the numbers represent samples at a finite number of times. In contrast, the analog signals from the muscle fiber are continuous in both amplitude and time. The quantization of the amplitude of digital signals need not be a problem now, although early A/D converters (still found on some instruments) often were not sufficiently linear for phase measurements. The linearity of present 12-bit A/D converters and the word length of minicomputers are sufficient (if properly used) to make this source of error negligible. The programmer should be aware, however, that computations of the power in a waveform usually require the temporary use of double precision, and power computations are needed for estimates of impedance.

Quantization in the time domain is more serious,

however. Here the physiological investigator reaches limits set by the speed of A/D converters, the size and cost of memory, and the speed of Fourier analysis of blocks of many time points. These factors set the practical limits of resolution and bandwidth for impedance measurements.

The fundamental difficulty caused by sampling (i.e., quantization) in time is aliasing, the inability to distinguish different waveforms ("aliases") if insufficient samples or too low a sampling rate is used. In fact one might expect that no finite amount of sampling could allow waveforms to be distinguished, since no finite number of (x, y) coordinates can specify a function! Luckily, however, the physical origin of our analog waveforms avoids this problem. If a waveform of physical origin (waveforms that are a tiny subset of all possible functions) contains no energy above the so-called folding frequency F_f (which equals half the sampling rate S), then it can be reconstructed uniquely from its samples, according to the sampling theorem (see engineering references 10, 11, 14, 15, 22, 52, 60, 79, 82, 83 already cited). Ambiguity arises only if there is energy in the analog waveform above the folding frequency. If there is energy above the folding frequency, however, the ambiguity produced by aliasing is a necessary consequence of sampling *and cannot be removed once the digital samples are taken* without a priori knowledge of the signal sampled.

Figure 3 illustrates the problem. If digital samples are taken at a rate of $S = 8/s$ (samples shown as filled circles in Fig. 3), a sinusoid with a frequency of 4 Hz cannot be distinguished from a sinusoid of 0 Hz (horizontal line shown). Similarly, sampling at 5/s (open circles) cannot distinguish a sinusoid of 1-Hz frequency from a sinusoid of 4-Hz frequency. A sinusoid of frequency greater than half the sampling rate cannot be distinguished from a sinusoid of frequency less than half the sampling rate. Similarly a waveform with energy at frequencies above half the sampling rate will not be distinguishable from a waveform with all its energy below half the sampling rate. In fact the energy density $E(f_0)$ at a frequency f_0 (in Hz, with $f_0 \leqslant S/2$) cannot be distinguished from energy at the frequencies $S \pm f_0$, $2S \pm f_0$, ..., $nS \pm f_0$, and so on, where n is any integer. The total energy $\hat{E}(f_0)$ is the sum of the energies $E(f_n)$ at all the frequencies $f_n = nS \pm f_0$ (summation over n) and not the energy density $E(f_0)$ at the single frequency f_0 that one would wish to measure.

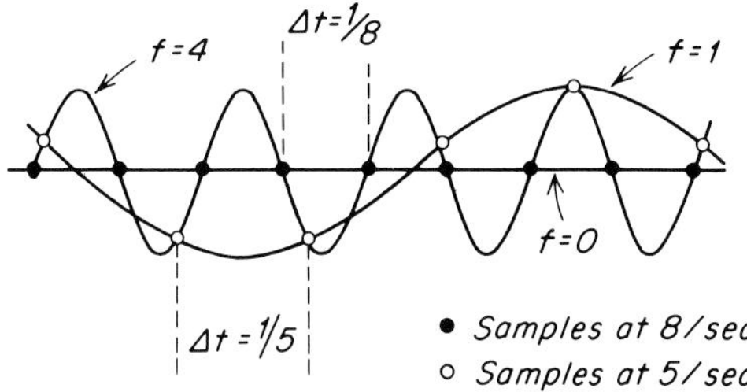

FIG. 3. Three sinusoids show effects of digital sampling. Samples taken at 8/s (*filled circles*) from a sinusoid of 4-Hz frequency are the same as samples taken from a sinusoid of 0 Hz (i.e., DC). Thus samples taken at this rate cannot distinguish between the 2 sinusoids—the sinusoids are said to be aliases of one another. Similarly samples taken at 5/s (*open circles*) from a sinusoid of 1-Hz frequency cannot be distinguished from samples from a sinusoid of 8 Hz; they also are aliases. Aliasing is a direct consequence of sampling. Once digital samples are taken, aliases cannot be distinguished. Precautions can be taken before sampling to minimize problems of aliasing.

Sampling at an infinite rate would clearly remove the problem of aliasing. This is not possible, however, nor can it be approached with present-day technology. There are serious technological limitations on the speed of high-resolution A/D converters, although these will disappear with the growth of technology. There is also a limit on the number of data points that can be handled in subsequent digital Fourier analysis, however, and this limitation is unlikely to disappear in the next few decades. If a waveform is sampled at high speed, a large amount of data is acquired, perhaps more than is actually needed and more than can be easily stored or rapidly computed. Thus samples should be taken as frequently as necessary but as seldom as possible.

One method of sampling has been suggested that might avoid aliasing of a waveform containing energy at all frequencies. If samples are taken at random time intervals [see Masry and Lui (65)], aliasing does not occur. Masry's scheme requires sampling at arbitrarily short intervals (i.e., at arbitrarily high rates) and eventually produces an infinite number of samples in a given frequency range. The theoretical advantages of random sampling may not survive the practical restrictions of a limited sampling rate and a finite number of samples in a given frequency range. In any case, simulations including these and other practical limitations are needed before Masry's scheme could be safely applied to unknown systems.

Although manipulation of periodic sampling cannot avoid aliasing, manipulation of the analog waveform can. If the analog signals that will be digitized contain no significant energy above the so-called folding frequency F_f, they can be uniquely specified by their samples. There will then be no aliasing. Filtering of the input signals (in steep low-pass, so-called antialiasing filters) circumvents aliasing, because after the filtering, there is no energy present to alias. The use of such filters has an added benefit, which applies to transient measurements as well. The steep low-pass filters decrease the amount of noise energy at irrelevant frequencies. Thus the filtering used to remove aliasing also significantly improves signal-to-noise ratios.

Some of the details of filtering, which are critical to the implementation of impedance measurements, are not well discussed in the literature, at least to my knowledge. I present analysis only of analog low-pass filtering. Instruments recently made by Hewlett-Packard (e.g., model 5420A) use a combination of analog and digital low-pass filters with great success (as determined by direct measurement), but the techniques involved are largely proprietary and so I am not able to discuss them in a critical manner. [See Patkay, Chu, and Wiggers (84) for an outline presentation of the digital technique.]

An idealized low-pass filter is shown in Figure 4 in a conventional logarithmic plot. The steep filters actually used in most antialiasing schemes have more complex characteristics, but the idealized filter characteristic shows the important points. The ordinate of the plot represents the gain of the filter (on a logarithmic scale), and the abscissa represents the log frequency. The bandwidth of the filter is called B_w and the cutoff frequency is called $F_A = kB_w$, where k is a constant determined by the steepness of the filter. Where M is the average slope of the filter characteristic between B_w and F_A in decibels per octave, $k = 2 \times 10^{A/M}$. The cutoff frequency is the frequency F_A at which a signal is attenuated by A, a value large enough to ensure no significant effects of aliasing compared with other errors. If $-A$ is 70–100 dB (i.e., 0.03%–0.001%), most workers assume that there will be no significant effect of aliasing from frequencies above F_f. Aliasing is caused by the total energy of the incoming signal at frequencies above F_f; therefore the low-pass filter must attenuate the total energy above F_f sufficiently to eliminate significant aliasing at any one frequency below F_f. This is not a stringent requirement in typical physiological situations but can be limiting in some applications where there is a tremendous concentration of energy in a small frequency band somewhere above F_f.

Figure 5 shows the optimal relationship between the filter characteristics and the sampling rate, with linear scales. A linear scale is used because the distribution of aliases (described previously) occurs on a linear frequency scale, not a logarithmic one. The optimal relationship between sampling and filter characteristics is determined by two conditions: *1*) that signals in the usable band, extending to B_w, be free of aliasing and *2*) that the sampling frequency S be as close to B_w as possible. These conditions are met by setting the folding frequency as shown, with F_f lying between B_w and F_A. The relationship illustrated of $F_f = \frac{1}{2}(F_A + B_w)$ satisfies both conditions optimally.

The sampling rate $S = 2F_f = F_A + B_w$ must be much larger than twice the usable frequency B_w because the low-pass filter is not infinitely steep. Consequently many of the samples taken and many of the computations subsequently made on those samples are wasted. The wasted samples must be taken and the computations made to perform Fourier analysis on the frequencies below B_w. The wasted samples are not useful, however, because they give results in the frequency range between B_w and F_A, a range in which there is significant aliasing. Indeed the fraction of usable frequency points (those uncontaminated by aliasing) is simply $2/(1 + k)$. If the filter were infinitely steep, k would equal 1 and no samples would be wasted. If the low-pass filter were a typical Butterworth filter with a slope of 24 dB/octave ($k = 7.5$), only about 20% of the computed frequency points

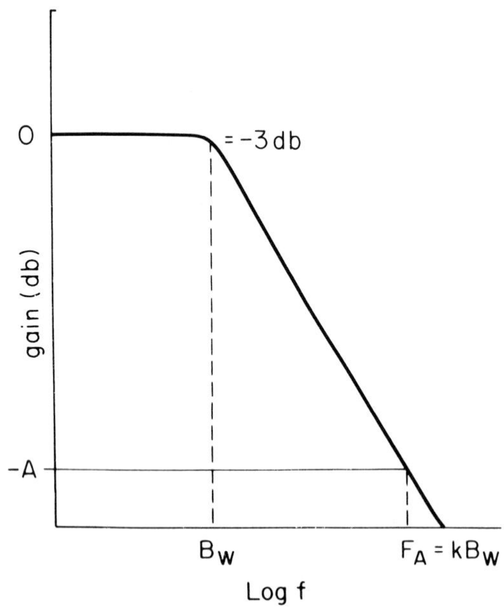

FIG. 4. Idealized filter response shown in a log-log plot. Ordinate is the gain in dB. Frequency at which the gain is −3 dB is shown as B_w; frequency at which the gain is down $-A$ dB is shown as $F_A = kB_w$. Filters recommended for use in impedance measurements have more complicated responses, with ripple in the pass band (DC to B_w), nonlinear dependence on frequency, and a finite amount of gain in any range of frequencies. All these features of practical filters are introduced to allow a very steep dependence of gain on frequency, i.e., as small a value of k as possible.

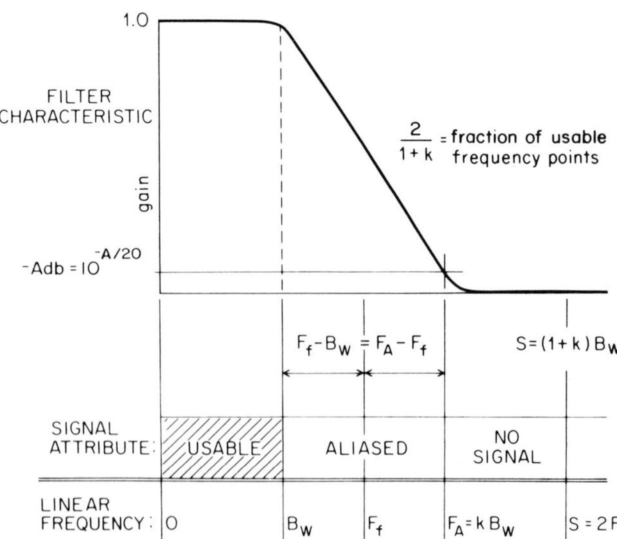

FIG. 5. Optimal relation between sampling rate, bandwidth, and folding frequency. All signals above B_w contain aliased energy. Adjustment of the folding frequency to halfway between B_w and F_A allows closest approach of F_A to B_w without introduction of aliased energy below B_w. This adjustment maximizes bandwidth and fraction of usable frequency points. Linear plot is used for convenience. Filter is shown with a limiting gain at high frequencies to be more realistic.

would be useful for $A = -70$ dB. Even if the filter slope were 48 dB/octave ($k = 2.7$), which is the steepest Butterworth filter available commercially (to my knowledge), only some 50% of the points would be useful. To minimize unnecessary computation and thus minimize cost while maximizing bandwidth and resolution, it is important to have the steepest filter possible. These are called Cauer elliptic filters (61) and are currently available with slopes of 110 dB/octave ($k = 1.6$), allowing about 75% of the computed points to be used.

Instrumentation Noise

With the procedures just discussed, it is possible to measure impedance with wide-band signals analyzed by Fourier methods. The only quantities directly used to estimate impedance are the power and cross-power spectra. These have been computed in two different ways. In the early engineering literature, before the discovery of the fast Fourier transform algorithm, power spectra were computed from correlation functions. That is, correlation and cross-correlation functions (defined in engineering texts previously cited) were computed from the input- and output-voltage waveforms. Then a Fourier transform of these correlation functions was taken to determine the power and cross-power spectra.

After the discovery of the fast Fourier transform, it was much faster to measure the power spectra directly from the discrete Fourier transforms of the input and output signals. Thus almost all measurements of power spectra with Fourier transforms use the following formulas

$$\begin{aligned} G_{xx} &= X(f) \cdot X^* (f) \\ G_{yy} &= Y(f) \cdot Y^* (f) \\ G_{xy} &= X^* (f) \cdot Y(f) \end{aligned} \tag{3}$$

where f is the frequency; a superscript * indicates the complex conjugate of the Fourier transforms $X(f)$ and $Y(f)$ of the analog waveforms $x(t)$ and $y(t)$; G_{xx}, G_{yy}, and G_{xy} indicate the power spectra of the input, the output, and the cross power between input and output, respectively.

The power spectra defined in Equation 3 are computed for a single series of time points, usually between 128 and 2,048 points, called a block of data. To measure impedance in the presence of contaminating noise, it is necessary to average several such blocks of data; we use the notation $G_{xx}{}^k$ to indicate the kth block of data. Certain other difficulties arise if the signals are contaminated by instrumentation noise; these are worth mentioning, since they have not been well reviewed in the literature, at least to my knowledge.

Figure 6 shows a typical physiological situation in which an input signal $x(t)$ is applied to a muscle fiber. The Fourier transform of the input signal is called $X(f)$, and the muscle fiber is described by its transfer function $H(f)$, i.e., its impedance. The input is supposed to be measured without the addition of contaminating noise, but the output is contaminated with noise. The idealized output, free of noise, is called $y(t)$, and the Fourier transform of that output is called $Y(f)$. The recording amplifier and associated electronic devices introduce a noise $n(t)$, giving the output $\hat{y}(t)$ actually available for measurement; $\hat{y}(t)$ is the best estimate available of the true output $y(t)$. Figure 6 distinguishes between the effects of uncorrelated contaminating noise arising in the instrumentation, called $n(t)$ or "noisy noise," and the input signal $x(t)$, which may or may not be stochastic (i.e., noise), depending on the choice of the investigator. The input signal $x(t)$ must be wide band, with energy at many frequencies, but whether it is stochastic or periodic, with energy at many frequencies (i.e., pseudorandom), is not significant here.

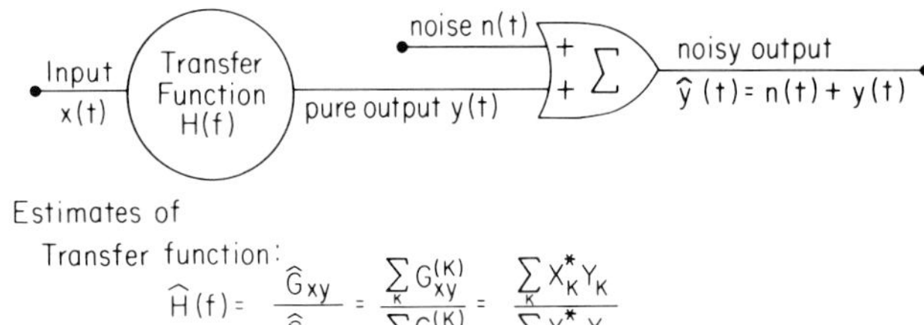

Estimates of Transfer function: $\hat{H}(f) = \dfrac{\hat{G}_{xy}}{\hat{G}_{xx}} = \dfrac{\sum_K G_{xy}^{(K)}}{\sum_K G_{xx}^{(K)}} = \dfrac{\sum_K X_K^* Y_K}{\sum_K X_K^* X_K}$

FIG. 6. Instrumentation noise in the output signal. Transfer function $H(f)$ might be impedance of a muscle fiber. Input $x(t)$ is applied current. Noise-free measurements of $x(t)$ are assumed to be available. Pure output $y(t)$ is voltage that would be measured in the absence of instrumentation noise. Noise $n(t)$ is noise introduced by voltage-recording amplifier and associated electronic devices. Noisy output $\hat{y}(t)$ is the sum of pure output and noise; $\hat{y}(t)$ is the best available estimate of membrane voltage. Transfer function should be estimated from estimates $\hat{G}_{xy}(f)$ and $\hat{G}_{xx}(f)$ of cross-power and power spectra, respectively. Those estimates should be the mean of cross power and power recorded from k blocks of data, as indicated. Cross power and power of each block of data are determined from the Fourier transforms $X(f)$ and $Y(f)$ of signals $x(t)$ and $y(t)$, respectively. *Complex conjugate. Other estimates of the transfer function (e.g., made by dividing the power spectra and then averaging) lead to incorrect results, as discussed by Bendat and Piersol (10).

The proper method of estimating impedance functions in the presence of noise is given by Bendat and Piersol (10, 11). They have shown that the only correct estimate of the transfer function, i.e., the impedance (in the statistical sense that it is unbiased and of reasonable variance), is the one shown with a circumflex in Figure 6. In this estimate of impedance the power spectra G_{xx} and G_{xy} of each block of data must be computed; the estimates of the power spectra of each block are then averaged to form the estimate of the power spectra. The only correct estimate of impedance is the ratio of the averaged power spectra shown in Figure 6. One must not average the Fourier transforms and then compute the transfer function, nor can one compute transfer functions from each block of data and then average those estimates.

Bendat and Piersol (10, 11) also analyze systems where the measurement of the input signal $x(t)$ is corrupted by noisy noise, a noise that is not an input to the system being studied (see Eq. 6.122 in ref. 10). Some setups used to measure the impedance of muscle fall into this category, where the current flowing through the muscle fiber is measured with circuits that introduce noise. In those setups, estimates of the amplitude of an impedance can be biased by the noisy noise, but estimates of phase are not. Bendat and Piersol show that a signal-to-noise ratio of 10 (in power terms) can produce about a 10% underestimate of the amplitude of the impedance.

The discussion just presented assumes, of course, that both the current applied and the voltage recorded from the muscle fiber are measured and that both are used to compute the power spectrum and cross-power spectrum. When the input signal is known in advance and thus need not be measured each time it is applied to the preparation, impedance can be measured without simultaneous measurement of both input and output and without computation of input, output, and cross-power spectra [see, e.g., the work of Poussart and colleagues (89) and Clausen and Fernandez (18)]. When microelectrodes are used, however, it is not possible to know the input signal beforehand. The microelectrode resistance fluctuates substantially during the experiment, and these effects cannot be removed with sufficient accuracy at high frequencies by a constant-current circuit (70). Thus microelectrode measurements of impedance require measurement of the current applied to the muscle fiber. The classic methods described here therefore seem advisable and the simpler methods seem likely to give difficulty.

Manipulation of Impedance Data

A number of manufacturers make instruments that measure impedance by the Fourier techniques just described. These instruments allow measurements at between 100 and 800 frequency points (corresponding to between 256 and 2,048 time points in each block of data) and at frequencies up to ~50 kHz. The major difficulty with such machines is the embarrassment of riches. They provide more data than can be dealt with easily. The techniques for reducing the amount of data and putting the data into conventional formats are important and have been described elsewhere (69, 70).

Theory and Curve Fitting

The next steps in impedance analysis are the fitting of theory and the determination of circuit parameters. Both require a theoretical description of the electrical structure of the preparation. For skeletal muscle there is wide agreement concerning the appropriate theory. The longitudinal spread of current away from the current microelectrode is accurately described by traditional one-dimensional cable theory [reviewed by Jack, Noble, and Tsien (ref. 58, chapt. 3)]. The frequency dependence of the impedance data and the presumptive radial spread of potential in the T system require more analysis (see ref. 58, chapt. 6).

The radial spread of current within the T system of muscle is governed by cable equations similar to those governing longitudinal spread down unmyelinated nerve. The potential change across the T-system membrane is not uniform, just as the potential across a nerve fiber is not uniform and for a similar reason: significant potential drops occur in long narrow volumes of saline and across membranes. In nerve fibers the potential drops occur longitudinally within the saline solution that fills the axon. In the T system the potential drops occur radially within the saline solution that fills the extracellular lumen of the T system. The radial variation of potential in the T system is produced by current flow in the high resistance of an extracellular space; the radial variation of potential within the sarcoplasm is negligible. Thus the longitudinal potential drops in nerve fibers occur intracellularly, whereas the radial potential drops in the T system occur extracellularly. This difference between axonal and T-system cable theory is important conceptually but trivial analytically. It does not change the form of the cable equations.

A more important difference is produced by the shape of the T system. The T system is embedded in a roughly cylindrical muscle fiber, which gives the system a roughly circular outer boundary. This geometry implies that the radial spread of potential will be described by cylinder functions instead of exponentials; the cylinder functions are in fact the modified Bessel functions I_n and K_n of integral order, usually with order $n = 0$ or 1.

Cable theory for the T system and cable theory for an unmyelinated fiber are conceptually different. The nerve fiber is usually considered infinitely long, at least in the mind's eye, whereas the diameter of a muscle fiber, and thus of the outer boundary of the T system, is finite. The T system is analogous to a nerve fiber, but a nerve fiber of finite length. The length of the axon analogous to the T system (measured in units of axonal length constants) is equal to the radius of a muscle fiber, measured in units of T-system length constants. The finite size of the axon and T system constrains the flow of current and makes the spread of potential quite different from that in axons of infinite length. In an axon of finite length, or a T system, current cannot flow away to infinity. Rather it is reflected off the end (or center) of the system. These reflections add to the potential that would be present in an infinitely long axon. Thus there is much less decrement of potential in an axon of finite length or a T system than there would be in an axon of infinite length.

Of course the T system is not an axon of finite length. It has radial symmetry and so the spread of potential in the T system is described by Bessel functions, whereas an axon of finite length is described by exponentials. This radial symmetry forces a convergence of current flow near the center of the fiber, which is not present in the axon of finite length.

Nonetheless the electrical properties of finite lengths of terminated axon are surprisingly close to those of radially symmetric T systems if the comparison is made between properly normalized systems, systems normalized to have the same total amount of membrane (R. A. Levis, R. T. Mathias, and R. S. Eisenberg, unpublished observations). In fact these systems are sufficiently similar that they may be difficult to distinguish with measurements at experimentally accessible frequencies.

Electrical Models of the T System

The fundamental cable equations describing current flow in the T system are used to compute the admittance y_e in Equation 2. These equations were first given by Falk and Fatt (38) in their "distributed" model of the T system. Falk and Fatt described the T system as if it were a disk, the faces of the disk being the tubular membrane and the space between the faces being filled with a saline solution. The circumference of the disk coincided with the circumference of the muscle fiber. Adrian, Chandler, and Hodgkin (2) and Schneider (94) described the T system more realistically as a branching network of tubules. Such a network can be described as a disk (if the amount of membrane area and luminal volume is properly written), but only crudely, since current flow in a network clearly cannot be the same as current flow in a disk. The branching of the tubules obviously will have important effects on the radial flow of current. For example, *1)* a branched network will have a larger radial resistance than the disk; and *2)* when the frequency is high enough, or the length constant short enough, the discrete nature of a network of branching tubules will dominate, and a tubular network cannot be described as a disk even approximately. Adrian et al. (2) dealt with the first effect by introducing a tortuosity factor to describe the extra radial resistance to current flow. They computed this tortuosity factor for several regular models of the T system and used it to analyze the resistivity of the solution in the lumen of the tubules.

The tortuosity factor of Adrian et al. (2) is certainly needed to reconcile the properties of a network with the disk equations, but their factor is incomplete. The radial resistance of the T system must depend on the amount of twisting of the tubules in the T network. The path length for radial current flow will clearly be much longer in a network of convoluted tubules than in a network of straight tubules; thus the radial resistance must be higher in the convoluted network. Since the length of the tubules did not enter into their equations or definition of tortuosity, a factor is obviously missing.

A simple derivation of the missing factor can be found in Eisenberg, Mathias, and Rae (36). We related the effective radial resistance (and by inference the tortuosity factor) to the morphometric parameters of the T-system network, including the length of the tubules. Our simple derivation is justified mathematically by the rigorous work of Mathias, Eisenberg, and Valdiosera (67), who considered the distribution of potential in a random network made of branching tubules.

Mathias, Eisenberg, and Valdiosera (67) treated the T system as a random branching mesh that could be divided (by an explicit geometrical construction) into concentric shells. If the potential within each shell was averaged over the circumferential location, the potential within the T system (and thus its impedance) could be calculated accurately, with no other assumptions. In this case the T-system admittance (the reciprocal of impedance) is described by a first-order nonlinear difference equation (ref. 67, Eq. 36), which can be dealt with rapidly and trivially by computers, since a difference equation is a computer program.

Mathias, Eisenberg, and Valdiosera (67) compared their mesh model of the T system with earlier models by constructing accurate analytical approximations to the solution of their difference equation. They showed that the mesh model was a simple generalization of the disk model of Falk and Fatt (38) and later workers (2, 94). The mesh model included the effects of the branching and wiggling of the tubules that might be expected. When the length constant of the T system was large compared with the mesh size, the mesh expression had precisely the same form as the disk expression, but there was no explicit tortuosity factor requiring separate analysis, as in the work of Adrian et al. (2). Rather, the morphometric properties of the T system appeared directly in the solution of the mesh equations. If one then adopts the definition of a tortuosity factor introduced by Adrian et al. (2), one can compute the tortuosity factor of any network from its morphometric parameters. The resulting expression for the tortuosity factor (ref. 67, Eq. 29) includes the dependence on the length of tubule and the number of branches per node that one might intuitively expect.

When the length constant of the T system is sufficiently short, the analysis of the mesh clearly must differ from that of the disk either in the form presented by Falk and Fatt (38) or in the form presented by Adrian et al. (2) and Schneider (94). The mesh expression must approach the admittance of a number of unbranched tubules in parallel, whereas disk expressions—even those including a tortuosity factor—cannot have this property. In fact the expression derived by Mathias, Eisenberg, and Valdiosera (ref. 67, Eq. 43) has just the required behavior under conditions of short length constant or high frequency.

Despite the involved mathematics of the derivation of the mesh model (67), the result is pleasingly simple. At low frequencies, when the length constant is long, the mesh model has the same form as the disk model, with a generalization of the definition of the tortuosity factor. At high frequencies, when the length constant is short, the mesh model behaves like a set of tubules in parallel. In fact the complexity of the mathematics of the mesh model is misleading, since its main result can be derived (36) just as simply as the disk model itself.

There is practical significance to the behavior of the T system and mesh model at high frequencies or short length constants. During an action potential, both conditions occur and the spread of current within the T system might be expected to be better described by a mesh than by a disk model. Indeed preliminary calculations of propagating action potentials (R. A. Levis, R. T. Mathias, and R. S. Eisenberg, unpublished observations) have shown sensitivity to the properties of the mesh and give results different from calculations with a disk model.

Other models of the T system have been suggested. Falk and Fatt (38) used a lumped model in which all the membranes of the T system were supposed to be in series with the same resistance. They assumed that the radial drop of potential in the resistance of the lumen of the tubules was negligible compared with the drop of potential in a resistor elsewhere, presumably at the mouth of the tubules. The lumped model was certainly a useful (if crude) approximation and is still useful [see, e.g., ref. 67, which shows how the lumped model is an analytical approximation to the mesh or disk model]. The existence of significant decrement of potential within the T system under many physiological conditions has always been apparent, however, both from qualitative experimental results [e.g., Huxley and Taylor (57); Endo (37); Gonzalez-Serratos (49); Adrian, Costantin, and Peachey (3)] and from consideration of the shape and size of the tubules. The shape and size of the lumen of the T tubule guarantee significant potential decrement in the radial direction under many physiological conditions.

Peachey and Adrian (4, 85) generalized the lumped model by placing a single large resistance at the mouth of the tubules. This access resistance was supposed to be of the same order as the total radial resistance of the rest of the T system. Thus approximately half the radial drop in potential would occur across the access resistance and approximately half would occur across the radial dimension of the fiber. Mathias, Eisenberg, and Valdiosera (ref. 67, Eqs. 47–49) give general expressions for the effect of an access impedance on the impedance of any model of the distributed T system. In *Impedance Measurements of Normal Frog Fibers*, p. 317, I discuss the experimental evidence concerning the access resistance and show that if the access resistance exists at all, it must have a value much smaller than the effective radial resistance of the tubular meshwork.

A generalization of the analysis of the T system considers it a branching network of extracellular space that penetrates the muscle fiber. As such it can be described in much the same way as the extracellular space within a syncytial tissue. (A syncytial tissue is made of many cells electrically coupled together with a narrow extracellular space between the cells.) Eisenberg, Barcilon, and Mathias (32) derived the partial differential equations and boundary conditions that describe syncytial tissues, and these have been solved by Peskoff (86) for cylindrical syncytia with clefts between cells. R. T. Mathias (personal communication) has solved the syncytial equations for cylindrical tissues containing tubular networks and has shown that the disk or mesh model appears in the solution naturally, without further assumptions. Mathias finds that the potential close to the current microelectrode is quite complex, much more so than assumed by Valdiosera et al. [(101); but see the caption of their Fig. 2]. The solution for the radial variation of potential away from the current electrode (and thus impedance) assumes the form used by Falk and Fatt (38) and later workers (2, 94) in the field, namely, the form given in Equations 1 and 2.

The mesh theory of the T system thus seems an adequate description of the known structural complexities. All the parameters of the theory can be determined experimentally by a combination of electrical and morphometric measurements. Measurements of the frequency dependence of the muscle impedance can then be used to determine the parameters of the theory and thereby check its validity.

Necessity for Morphometry

The electrical properties of muscle fibers depend on the structure and organization of their membrane systems as much as on the properties of the individual membranes themselves. This fact, which applies to the electrical properties of all cells and tissues (35), implies the importance of structural analysis, both description of the qualitative structure and measurement of the amounts of the various structures.

For example, the electrical properties of muscle fibers depend in a critical way on the amount of T membrane and of surface membrane. In a muscle fiber of small diameter, there is much less T membrane in relation to outer membrane than in a fiber of large diameter. Thus the T system influences the electrical properties of small fibers less than large fibers. Some of the electrical properties can be measured independent of impedance measurements [Hodgkin and Nakajima (55, 56)].

The importance of the total amount of membrane in determining electrical properties is obvious, but the theoretical implications are sometimes forgotten. When one compares different models of the same tissue, it is essential that the different models contain the same amount of membrane area. If the disk model is compared with a mesh model, if a model with branching tubules is compared with one without branching, or if a model containing clefts is compared with one containing tubules, care must be taken to ensure that the amount of membrane is the same in all cases. The easiest way to ensure morphological comparability is to write the models in terms of morphological parameters. Morphometric parameters and electrical parameters are of equal importance in determining the measured properties, and suppression of morphometric parameters by combination into "effective" parameters is more likely to hide errors than to reveal truth.

The morphometric parameters of interest in a particular preparation and their measurement are an important subject beyond the scope of this chapter. This subject is discussed, with reference to the appropriate stereological literature, in the chapter by B. R. Eisenberg in this *Handbook* and by Eisenberg and Mathias (35).

RESULTS OF IMPEDANCE MEASUREMENTS

Impedance Measurements of Normal Frog Fibers

Many of the results of early impedance measurements are reviewed by Cole (20) and by Schanne and Ruiz-P.-Ceretti (92). Falk and Fatt (38) first showed that the impedance of muscle fibers could not be explained without reference to the T system. The dependence of impedance on frequency was far more complex than that of an axon and showed the general kind of behavior expected from a T system connected in parallel with a surface membrane. This result is now taken for granted but was quite important at the time it was made, since the patency of the T system was still then in question.

Comparison of impedance results from several laboratories is complicated by the evolution of techniques, theories, and interpretations through the years. Nonetheless the measurements by Falk and Fatt (38) and Freygang et al. (46) of the properties of fibers in normal solutions have been largely supplanted by the results of Schneider (94), Valdiosera, Eisenberg, Mathias, and Clausen (67, 100–102) because the earlier measurements had a significant possibility of artifact, did not extend over a sufficient frequency range, and were done at an unknown sarcomere length. Indeed the results of Valdiosera, Clausen, and Eisenberg (100–102) are also subject to serious criticism because the microelectrodes were placed close together. This placement of microelectrodes is not appropriate for the theory they used.

The discussion in this chapter is based on the results of Mathias, Eisenberg, and Valdiosera (67) without meaning to slight the significance of earlier work. They measured the impedance of single muscle fibers with microelectrodes placed to minimize three-dimensional effects. They interpreted their results with the mesh model of the tubular system and made measurements from 1 Hz to 10 kHz with small and measured artifact. Their main findings, which in most cases confirmed the qualitative results of earlier papers, were the following:

1. The electrical properties depended steeply on sarcomere length. The biological variance in measurements was too large to allow detailed interpretation of this dependence on sarcomere length. Furthermore morphometric data were not (and are not) available at different sarcomere lengths.
2. The capacitance of the surface membrane measured 1.1 $\mu F/cm^2$, where the area implicit in the measurement is that of a smooth unfolded outer membrane. Although this value seems large, it is easy to explain if a substantial fraction of the caveolae appear as part of the surface membrane.
3. The specific capacitance of the wall of the tubules is 1.4 $\mu F/cm^2$ of tubular membrane area. This is substantially larger than expected, implying either that the T membrane has unusual thinness or dielectric constant, or that the area measurements used were incorrect, or that some current is flowing across membranes other than the T system, for example, through the membranes of the SR.
4. The conductance of the tubular membrane could not be determined because potential decrements within the T system are small at DC. Under those conditions any distributed model of the T system—disk, mesh, or whatever—approaches the lumped model and shares the property that parallel conductances (i.e., the conductance of the surface membrane and the conductance of the tubular membrane) cannot be separated. This is an inconvenient property of resting muscle that can be modified by changing conditions. When the DC tubular length constant is shortened, usually by increasing the resistance of the lumen of the tubules, radial decrement can be large enough to allow measurement of the tubular conductance (1).
5. The resistivity of the tubular lumen was ~140 $\Omega \cdot cm$ compared with the resistivity of ~90 $\Omega \cdot cm$ for the extracellular bathing solution. The difference is certainly significant and requires discussion. Errors in the electrical measurements are unlikely to produce this difference, since estimates of the resistivity are determined by the low- to middle-frequency data and so are quite reliable. Furthermore a similar discrepancy appears in a wide variety of measurements of the T system [see Nakajima and Bastian (74) for references and discussion]. Errors in the morphological measurements used to compute the resistivity are possible and may explain the discrepancy in estimates. It seems more likely, however, that some structural property of the muscle fiber was not properly included in the theory used to interpret the data. One possibility is that some of the apparent radial resistance comes from current flow into the SR (68). Another possible source of error in the estimate of radial resistance comes from structural complexities in the T system itself. S. Page and L. D. Peachey (personal communication) found that the T system has a small circular cross section in regions where it is not associated with the terminal cisternae of the SR. Such regions might have more radial resistance than predicted by the

mesh model, which assumes all tubules have the same cross section. In fact the mesh model assumes all tubular parameters are radially uniform. Even if the volume fraction and surface-to-volume ratio of these circular tubules are measured correctly by the procedures of Mobley and Eisenberg (71), use of their average parameters in the mesh model may not properly describe the radial resistance of a nonuniform T system.

The impedance measurements of Valdiosera, Eisenberg, Mathias, and Clausen (67, 100–102) bear directly on the value of the access resistance to the T system postulated by Peachey and Adrian (4, 85). Valdiosera, Clausen, and Eisenberg (102) showed that the impedance data were incompatible with a substantial value of the access resistance; only a small amount (1/7) of the total radial resistance was lumped into an access resistance at the mouth of the tubules. Mathias, Eisenberg, and Valdiosera (67) then showed that even this small amount of access resistance produced a significant misfit to experimental data taken with precautions to minimize three-dimensional effects. Thus there is clearly no experimental reason to postulate the existence of an access resistance.

Other Preparations of Skeletal Muscle

Impedance measurements have now been performed on crab skeletal muscle (31), scorpion muscle (48), and hagfish muscle (78). The work on crab muscle is difficult to interpret because of the dearth of structural information and the plethora of potential artifact. The work on scorpion and hagfish muscle is notable because in these preparations the T system consists of short unbranched tubules. The finding that the resistivity of the tubular lumen in the scorpion is close to that of Ringer solution is striking and if confirmed would suggest that the different result in frog muscle is caused by structural complication. Whether the relevant structural complexity of frog muscle is the branching, the density of T-SR junctions, or the variation of diameter of the tubules is not clear and deserves further investigation.

Impedance Measurements of Muscle Fibers in Various Conditions

Freygang et al. (46) were the first to study the impedance of muscle fibers under various experimental conditions. They were particularly interested in the effects of hypertonic solutions, presumably because hypertonic solutions paralyze muscle fibers. Rather surprisingly Freygang et al. (46) found that the capacitance of the T system increased markedly in hypertonic solutions [confirmed by Valdiosera, Clausen, and Eisenberg (102)]. Indeed, Almers [(5) and personal communication] has confirmed the result by measuring integrals of transients from the same fiber in both normal and hypertonic Ringer's solutions.

There may be some artifact or error in the measurements in hypertonic solutions, perhaps associated with the general state or low resting potential of such fibers. Most likely, however, the increased capacitance in hypertonic solutions reflects an increase in the area of membrane across which current can flow. Morphological measurements are needed to see if the increase in area is in the T system. If not, one might suspect that current was flowing into the SR under these hypertonic conditions. A combination of impedance measurements under voltage-clamped conditions (to control possible effects of depolarization in hypertonic fibers) and morphometric measurements might resolve these questions. The qualitative morphological findings of Franzini-Armstrong et al. (43) and the microprobe measurements of Somlyo et al. (97) do not rule out this possibility, in my opinion. Other interpretations of their (43) images seem possible, and microprobe measurements (97) are probably not sensitive enough to detect concentration changes produced by leakage through the small ionic conductance that has recently been postulated (68) to link the T system and SR.

Impedance has also been measured in solutions of various conductivities (67, 78, 102). These measurements show that the conductivity of the lumen of the tubules varies linearly with the extracellular conductivity and so provide additional evidence, if such were needed, that the lumen is filled with extracellular solution. The absolute value of the luminal conductivity in these solutions is not explained entirely; the luminal conductivity is less by almost a factor of 2 than that of the bathing solution. The possible explanations for this discrepancy have already been discussed.

Finally, impedance has been measured in glycerol-treated fibers in which the T system has been substantially disrupted (102). Eisenberg and Eisenberg (28) [confirmed by Franzini-Armstrong, Venosa, and Horowicz (44)] have shown that only a small fraction of the T system is accessible to extracellular marker under these conditions. The possibility had been raised [Nakajima, Nakajima, and Peachey (76)] that glycerol treatment drastically increases the radial resistance to current flow without actually disrupting the tubular system. The increase in radial resistance would be enough to prevent the diffusion of extracellular marker but might not represent an actual disconnection of the T system from the extracellular space. That is, current (carried by small ions) might penetrate where markers did not.

Surprisingly, impedance measurements differentiate between a muscle fiber containing a T system with a very high radial resistance and a muscle fiber containing a disrupted T system [Valdiosera, Clausen, and Eisenberg (ref. 102, Fig. 10)]. The best fit to impedance data from glycerol-treated fibers gave a striking result: the tubular capacitance (per unit area of outer membrane) is only 0.4 $\mu F/cm^2$, suggesting that some 90% of the T system is unavailable for current flow, in reasonable agreement with the morphological results of Eisenberg and Eisenberg (28) and in close agreement with those of Franzini-Armstrong et al. (44). Furthermore Valdiosera, Clausen, and Eisenberg (102) showed that the impedance data could not be fitted with a model including the capacitance of a resting fiber and a series resistance, no matter how large the value of that series resistance.

The impedance measurements of Valdiosera, Clausen, and Eisenberg (102) give estimates of the radial resistance in glycerol-treated fibers that allow direct evaluation of the suggestion of Nakajima et al. (76) that the radial resistance is very high in glycerol-treated fibers. Valdiosera, Clausen, and Eisenberg (102) found that the effective radial resistance, computed using a lumped model of the T system in glycerol-treated fibers, was some 70 times larger than that in normal fibers. Of course the effective radial resistance depends linearly on the volume fraction of tubules. Thus the effective radial resistance would be expected to be some 10 times higher in glycerol-treated fibers than in normal fibers, because only 10% of the T system is left in such fibers. Thus the radial resistivity (as opposed to effective radial resistance) apparently is increased by a factor of 7 in glycerol-treated fibers. This increase is probably the result of collapse of the tubular lumen and could explain the slow diffusional phenomena observed by Nakajima et al. (76).

The capability of impedance measurements to distinguish between similar but distinct explanations of the properties of glycerol-treated fibers is a striking example of the utility of the method, at least under these circumstances.

Comparison With Other Results

Different kinds of measurements of the linear electrical properties of skeletal muscle agree quite well [see Nakajima and Bastian (74) and Chandler and Schneider (17) for some numerical comparisons]. Measurements with transient techniques (1, 17, 55, 56), measurements with estimates of diffusion constants (7, 37, 59, 75), and impedance measurements (67, 102) are in good agreement, well within the range expected because of different experimental conditions, different morphometric assumptions, and possible experimental errors.

Thus measurements of the properties of the T system derived from the properties of the whole muscle fiber seem to have reached a certain state of maturity. The maturity of the measurements of T-system properties does not imply a similar development in their interpretation, however.

DISCUSSION

Electrical properties of skeletal muscle have been studied intensely for perhaps two logical reasons, as well as the psychological reason that such study was a natural and seductive sequel to earlier work on nerve fibers. The logical reasons are *1*) to determine the parameters of the various membrane systems and compartments of a muscle fiber and *2*) to study the mechanism by which excitation of the surface membrane produces contraction of the myofibrils deep within a fiber, a process called excitation-contraction (EC) coupling.

The first step in EC coupling is the radial spread of potential within the T system. The measurement and the analysis of this spread of potential have a long history, reviewed in Costantin (23, 24) and Nakajima and Bastian (74). The measurement of impedance has contributed importantly to the study of the spread of potential in the T system. The linear properties of a muscle fiber put severe constraints on theories of the radial spread of potential, even though the distribution and properties of nonlinear conductances within the T system must be known to calculate the radial spread of the action potential [Adrian and Peachey (4)].

The radial spread of the action potential probably is not a critical step in determining the physiological aspects of EC coupling, although of course radial spread is an essential step. The system more likely to be a critical determinant of EC coupling is the junction between T system and SR.

Impedance measurements have had a small part in the analysis of the T-SR junction, but may well have an important function in the future. For example, if the mechanism of coupling between T system and SR is simply the flow of ionic current across the T-SR junction (68), one way to measure that current is with impedance measurements. Alternatively, if the mechanism of coupling is by remote control, that is, by a mechanism with the essential features of the rigid-rod model suggested by Chandler, Rakowski, and Schneider (16), impedance measurements still have a role to play. In that model, a component of capacitive current, called nonlinear charge movement, is supposed to arise from the movement of a voltage-sensing macromolecule within the T membrane. The sensor molecule remotely controls calcium release from the distant membrane of the SR and at the same time contributes to the capacitive current flowing across the T membrane. Impedance techniques might measure the capacitive current associated with the movement of the sensor more accurately than transient methods.

Impedance Measurements of Nonlinearities

Of course it is difficult to make impedance measurements of charge movement in muscle. Charge movement in skeletal muscle is nonlinear and my discussions so far have concerned linear systems.

The measurement and interpretation of linear measurements from nonlinear biological systems are difficult problems that have been worked on for a number of years [see the references in Fishman et al. (40)]. Although the results are inconclusive, some of the problems and principles of a linear analysis of a nonlinear system can be mentioned. These problems apply to two cases of physiological interest: the analysis of nonlinear charge movement by impedance techniques and the analysis of the distribution of nonlinear ionic conductances (e.g., K conductance) by impedance techniques.

Is an impedance analysis of a nonlinear process worth doing? If the measurement of a transient response and the interpretation of that response by traditional methods are able to explain the biological properties of interest, there seems little to be gained by an impedance analysis. On the other hand, if there is a biological need (e.g., in the analysis of nonlinear charge movement in skeletal muscle), then perhaps the extra resolution of impedance measurements will be worth the novelties and difficulties inherent in a linear analysis of a nonlinear system.

An impedance analysis of a nonlinear preparation can be performed if the system is time invariant, if the system can be linearized by the voltage clamp, and if all the membranes in the preparation have the same potential across them. That is, *1)* if the potential in the T system is uniform, *2)* if the perturbing signal is the sum of a step function (to turn on or, as physiologists say, "activate" the nonlinearity) and a sufficiently small wide-band signal, and *3)* if the nonlinear conductances of the membranes reach a steady state after activation, the system is no longer nonlinear under the conditions of a single voltage-clamp measurement and an impedance analysis is possible. These conditions may be hard to achieve in important situations (since a sufficiently small signal is very small indeed in the potential range where ionic conductances vary steeply with potential, near threshold). One still cannot interpret the results of such experiments. If these conditions are met, however, the measurement is meaningful.

These conditions are not met for the most interesting of the biological conductances, the sodium channel, even when that channel is embedded in a nondistributed system like a squid axon containing an axial wire. The conductance there is transient even under voltage-clamp conditions; that is, the conductance turns on (activates), turns off, and inactivates. Such conductances cannot be measured by simply taking the Fourier transform of the transient current because the transform as usually defined does not apply to time-varying systems. (The Fourier transform of a time-varying system confuses the transient properties of the system and the impedance of the system, when impedance is defined as some time-average property of the time-varying system.) The definition of a Fourier transform can be generalized for use in a time-varying system [(64); ref. 82, p. 440–447; ref. 83, p. 304]; other methods are used to process signals derived from human speech (88, 90) and nonstationary current fluctuations (21, 95). The utility of these generalizations for impedance measurements and their advantages over other methods of analysis are not yet known, however. At present an impedance analysis of a time-varying system cannot be made.

Linear measurements from stationary (i.e., time-invariant) nonlinear systems (such as the steady state of the K-conductance system of the squid) can be interpreted, however, if the system is linearized with the voltage clamp and satisfies the conditions previously discussed. The interpretation must proceed in several steps and deal with formidable problems.

The impedance of each membrane must first be separated into its components before the contributions of a particular conductance system can be identified. These components include the linear capacitance, presumably a property of the lipid of the membrane; the ionic conductance through each conductance system; and the "ionic reactance" (as I like to call it) of each conductance system. The ionic reactance is the result of the time delay and consequent phase shift of each ionic conductance. The phase shift ensures that, in the neighborhood of a given potential, each ionic conductance will behave like a combination of capacitors, inductors, and resistors. The ionic reactance is produced by a combination of the nonlinear and active (i.e., energy-requiring) properties of ionic channels. Thus ionic reactances have properties distinct from those of capacitors and inductors or from the properties of lipid bilayers. For example, ionic reactances depend on the concentration of ions moving through the ionic channel (since the concentrations set the chemical potential energy available to drive this active process), and they disappear in the presence of drugs that specifically block ionic movement through those channels. These special properties of ionic reactances make it possible to distinguish them from the linear properties of the rest of the membrane.

The construction of an explicit linearized model of a membrane is straightforward once one has models of the individual ionic reactances. The models of the ionic reactances may not be quite as simple as often assumed, however. Although the simple linearization of the nonlinear properties of an ionic conductance is straightforward [first reported by Hodgkin and Huxley (54)], this linearization is not sufficient to determine an ionic reactance. One must demonstrate, and not assume, that higher-order terms in the expansion of the ionic conductance are uniformly small, that is, are small under all the experimental conditions of interest. This point is not pedantic but practical, since there are many conditions (e.g., near threshold) where one must expect the contribution of higher-order terms to be substantial. Theoretical analysis of the linearization process is clearly needed, but simulations are more convincing. The best check of the linearization process is a mock experiment in which the Hodgkin-Huxley equations are programmed, a sinusoidal (or wide-band) input is applied, and the resulting output is computed. A correct linearization procedure will give precisely the same results as the simulation.

If full advantage is taken of the variety of selective drugs presently available, an impedance analysis of a time-invariant, nondistributed nonlinearity seems possible. Such an analysis has been started by Fishman,

Poussart, and Moore (40) on squid axon and by Mathias, Ebihara, Lieberman, and Johnson (66) on tissue-cultured aggregates of heart muscle.

The extension to a muscle fiber will not be easy, however. First, a method is needed to separate the properties of the measured impedance into the properties of the T membrane and surface membrane. Such a method requires knowledge of the resting capacitance and conductance of the surface and tubular membranes and the conductivity of the tubular lumen. That is, it requires prior structural analysis of the nonionic reactances. Furthermore one must consider the effects of variation in DC potential within the T system. In the nonlinear case the DC potential in the T system is a function of the properties and distribution of the ionic reactances and of the linear properties of the T system. Thus the analysis of ionic reactances of a distributed system like the T system may well require an explicit distributed model of the nonlinearities, a shell model of the sort constructed numerically by Adrian and Peachey (4). Such numerical models are possible, but they present formidable computational problems and have not yet been used to interpret impedance measurements, to my knowledge.

Other Methods

Many of the difficulties of existing impedance measurements on muscle arise from their essentially composite nature and their paucity of spatial information. Impedance measurements have been confined to only a few spatial locations [see, however, Schneider (94) and Mathias, Eisenberg, and Valdiosera (67)] and so have not measured the spatial distribution of potential with much accuracy. Furthermore the impedance measured is always the combination (see Eq. 2) of the properties of the surface and inner membranes. It would be much better if one could measure the T-system potential directly: the measurement would be independent of the properties of the surface membrane and so would no longer be a composite; the spatial resolution would far exceed that available with microelectrodes.

Optical measurements of membrane potential, for example, with potentiometric dyes [see Cohen and Salzburg (19) for a review], hold great promise. They should allow direct measurement of the distribution of potential, although arrangements such as that used by Blinks (13) may be necessary to avoid confusion in the optical path. Optical measurements certainly should allow measurement of T-system properties independent of the surface membrane. Of course the relative amplitude and phase angle between applied current and light signals from different locations are also quite susceptible to impedance analysis as described in this paper.

For these reasons I expect optical measurements of potential in the T system and SR to answer important questions in muscle physiology, and a great deal of work is in progress right now with these techniques to make transient measurements of natural activity (8, 9, 12, 103). These methods will have their ambiguities, mostly arising from the unknown interaction of dye with membranes of different compositions, but optical measurements of impedance may also be successful in teaching us more about how a muscle contracts.

It is a pleasure to thank Rick Mathias, Rick Levis, Jim Rae, and Brenda Eisenberg, who have been comrades in making and interpreting impedance measurements through many years. Their criticisms and comments on this manuscript provided considerable help and some comfort.

The original work described here has been supported by a series of grants from the American Heart Association, the Muscular Dystrophy Association, and the National Institutes of Health.

REFERENCES

1. Adrian, R. H., and W. Almers. Membrane capacity measurements on frog skeletal muscle in media of low ion content. *J. Physiol. London* 237: 573–604, 1974.
2. Adrian, R. H., W. K. Chandler, and A. L. Hodgkin. The kinetics of mechanical activation in frog muscle. *J. Physiol. London* 204: 207–230, 1969.
3. Adrian, R. H., L. L. Costantin, and L. D. Peachey. Radial spread of contraction in frog muscle fibres. *J. Physiol. London* 204: 231–257, 1969.
4. Adrian, R. H., and L. D. Peachey. Reconstruction of the action potential of frog sartorius muscle. *J. Physiol. London* 235: 103–131, 1973.
5. Almers, W. Gating currents and charge movements in excitable membranes. *Rev. Physiol. Biochem. Pharmacol.* 82: 95–190, 1978.
6. Asami, K., T. Hanai, and N. Koizumi. Dielectric approach to suspensions of ellipsoidal particles covered with a shell in particular reference to biological cells. *Jpn. J. Appl. Physiol.* 19: 359–365, 1980.
7. Barry, P. H., and R. H. Adrian. Slow conductance changes due to potassium depletion in the transverse tubules of frog muscle fibers during hyperpolarizing pulses. *J. Membr. Biol.* 14: 243–292, 1973.
8. Baylor, S. M., and W. K. Chandler. Optical indications of excitation-contraction coupling in striated muscle. In: *Biophysical Aspects of Cardiac Muscle*, edited by M. Morad and M. Tabatabai. New York: Academic, 1978, p. 207–228. (Proc. Cardiac Muscle Symp., May 1977, Shiraz, Iran.)
9. Baylor, S. M., W. K. Chandler, and M. W. Marshall. Studies in skeletal muscle using optical probes of membrane potential. In: *Regulation of Muscle Contraction Coupling*, edited by A. D. Grinnell and M. A. B. Brazier. New York: Academic, 1981, p. 97–127.
10. Bendat, J. S., and A. G. Piersol. *Random Data: Analysis and Measurement Procedures*. New York: Wiley-Interscience, 1971.
11. Bendat, J. S., and A. G. Piersol. *Engineering Applications of Correlation and Spectral Analysis*. New York: Wiley-Interscience, 1980.
12. Bezanilla, F., and P. Horowicz. Fluorescence intensity changes associated with contractile activation in frog muscle stained with Nile Blue-A. *J. Physiol. London* 246: 709–735, 1975.
13. Blinks, J. R. Influence of osmotic strength on cross-section and volume of isolated single muscle fibres. *J. Physiol. London* 177: 42–57, 1965.

14. BRIGHAM, E. O. *The Fast Fourier Transform.* Englewood Cliffs, NJ: Prentice-Hall, 1974.
15. BRILLINGER, D. R. *Time Series: Data Analysis and Theory.* New York: Holt, Rinehart & Winston, 1975.
15a. CARTER, G. C. *Coherence Estimation.* New London, CT: Naval Underwater Systems Center, 1981.
16. CHANDLER, W. K., R. F. RAKOWSKI, AND M. F. SCHNEIDER. Effects of glycerol treatment and maintained depolarization on charge movement in skeletal muscle. *J. Physiol. London* 254: 285–316, 1976.
17. CHANDLER, W. K., AND M. F. SCHNEIDER. Time-course of potential spread along a skeletal muscle fiber under voltage clamp. *J. Gen. Physiol.* 67: 165–184, 1976.
18. CLAUSEN, C., AND J. FERNANDEZ. A low-cost method for rapid transfer function measurements with direct application to biological impedance analysis. *Pfleugers Arch.* 390: 290–295, 1981.
19. COHEN, L. B., AND B. M. SALZBERG. Optical measurement of membrane potential. *Rev. Physiol. Biochem. Pharmacol.* 83: 36–88, 1978.
20. COLE, K. S. *Membranes, Ions and Impulses: A Chapter of Classical Biophysics.* Los Angeles: Univ. of California Press, 1968.
21. CONTI, F., B. NEUMCKE, W. NOUNER, AND R. STAMPFLI. Conductance fluctuations from the inactivation process of sodium channels in myelinated nerve fibres. *J. Physiol. London* 308: 217–239, 1980.
22. COOPER, G. R., AND C. D. MCGILLEM. *Methods of Signal and System Analysis.* New York: Holt, Rinehart & Winston, 1967.
23. COSTANTIN, L. L. Contractile activation in skeletal muscle. *Prog. Biophys. Mol. Biol.* 29: 197–224, 1975.
24. COSTANTIN, L. L. Activation in striated muscle. In: *Handbook of Physiology. The Nervous System*, edited by J. M. Brookhart and V. B. Mountcastle. Bethesda, MD: Am. Physiol. Soc., 1977, sect. 1, vol. I, pt. I, chapt. 7, p. 215-259.
25. DESOER, C. A., AND E. S. KUH. *Basic Circuit Theory.* New York: McGraw-Hill, 1969.
26. DORMER, K. J. *Fundamental Tissue Geometry for Biologists.* New York: Cambridge Univ. Press, 1980.
27. DULHUNTY, A. F., AND C. FRANZINI-ARMSTRONG. The relative contribution of the folds and caveolae to the surface membrane of frog skeletal muscle fibres at different sarcomere lengths. *J. Physiol. London* 250: 513–539, 1975.
28. EISENBERG, B. R., AND R. S. EISENBERG. Selective disruption of the sarcotubular system in frog sartorius muscle. *J. Cell Biol.* 39: 451–467, 1968.
28a. EISENBERG, B. R., AND R. S. EISENBERG. The T-SR junction in contracting single skeletal muscle fibers. *J. Gen. Physiol.* 79: 1–19, 1982.
29. EISENBERG, B. R., AND A. GILAI. Structural changes in single muscle fibers after stimulation at a low frequency. *J. Gen. Physiol.* 74: 1–16, 1979.
30. EISENBERG, B. R., R. T. MATHIAS, AND A. GILAI. Intracellular localization of markers within injected or cut frog muscle fibers. *Am. J. Physiol.* 237 (*Cell Physiol.* 6): C50–C55, 1979.
31. EISENBERG, R. S. The equivalent circuit of single crab muscle fibers as determined by impedance measurements with intracellular electrodes. *J. Gen. Physiol.* 50: 1785–1806, 1967.
32. EISENBERG, R. S., V. BARCILON, AND R. T. MATHIAS. Electrical properties of spherical syncytia. *Biophys. J.* 25: 151–180, 1979.
33. EISENBERG, R. S., AND P. W. GAGE. Ionic conductances of the surface and transverse tubular membranes of frog sartorius fibers. *J. Gen. Physiol.* 53: 279–297, 1969.
34. EISENBERG, R. S., AND E. A. JOHNSON. Three dimensional electrical field problems in physiology. *Prog. Biophys. Mol. Biol.* 20: 1–65, 1970.
35. EISENBERG, R. S., AND R. T. MATHIAS. Structural analysis of electrical properties. *Crit. Rev. Bioeng.* 4: 203–232, 1980.
36. EISENBERG, R. S., R. T. MATHIAS, AND J. L. RAE. Measurement, modelling and analysis of the linear electrical properties of cells. *Ann. NY Acad. Sci.* 303: 342–354, 1977.
37. ENDO, M. Entry of fluorescent dyes into the sarcotubular system of the frog muscle. *J. Physiol. London* 185: 224–238, 1966.
38. FALK, G., AND P. FATT. Linear electrical properties of striated muscle fibres observed with intracellular electrodes, *Proc. R. Soc. London Ser. B* 160: 69–123, 1964.
39. FATT, P., AND B. KATZ. An analysis of the end-plate potential recorded with an intracellular electrode. *J. Physiol. London* 115: 320–370, 1951.
40. FISHMAN, H. M., D. POUSSART, AND L. E. MOORE. Complex admittance of Na^+ conduction in squid axon. *J. Membr. Biol.* 50: 43–63, 1979.
41. FRANZINI-ARMSTRONG, C. Studies of the triad. II. Penetration of tracers into the junctional gap. *J. Cell Biol.* 49: 196–203, 1971.
42. FRANZINI-ARMSTRONG, C. Structure of sarcoplasmic reticulum. *Federation Proc.* 39: 2403–2409, 1980.
43. FRANZINI-ARMSTRONG, C., J. E. HEUSER, T. S. REESE, A. P. SOMLYO, AND A. V. SOMLYO. T-tubule swelling in hypertonic solutions. A freeze substitution study. *J. Physiol. London* 283: 133–140, 1978.
44. FRANZINI-ARMSTRONG, C., R. A. VENOSA, AND P. HOROWICZ. Morphology and accessibility of the "transverse" tubular system in frog sartorius muscle after glycerol treatment. *J. Membr. Biol.* 14: 197–212, 1973.
45. FRENCH, A. S., AND E. G. BUTZ. Measuring the Wiener kernels of a nonlinear system using the fast Fourier transform algorithm. *Int. J. Control* 17: 529–539, 1973.
46. FREYGANG, W. H., JR., S. I. RAPOPORT, AND L. D. PEACHEY. Some relations between changes in the linear electrical properties of striated muscle fibers and changes in ultrastructure. *J. Gen. Physiol.* 50: 2437–2458, 1967.
47. GAGE, P. W., AND R. S. EISENBERG. Action potentials, after potentials, and excitation-contraction coupling in frog sartorius fibers without transverse tubules. *J. Gen. Physiol.* 53: 298–310, 1969.
48. GILAI, A. Electromechanical coupling in tubular muscle fibers. II. Resistance and capacitance of one transverse tubule. *J. Gen. Physiol.* 67: 343–367, 1976.
49. GONZALEZ-SERRATOS, H. Inward spread of activation in vertebrate muscle fibres. *J. Physiol. London* 212: 777–799, 1971.
50. GOULD, S. J. Hen's teeth and horse's toes. *Nat. Hist.* 89: 24–28, 1980.
51. HANAI, T., K. ASAMI, AND N. KOIZUMI. Dielectric theory of concentrated suspensions of shell spheres in particular reference to the analysis of biological cell suspensions. *Bull. Inst. Chem. Res. Kyoto Univ.* 57: 297–305, 1979.
52. HANNAN, E. J. *Multiple Time Series.* New York: Wiley, 1970.
53. HILLE, B., AND D. T. CAMPBELL. An improved Vaseline gap voltage clamp for skeletal muscle fibers. *J. Gen. Physiol.* 67: 265–293, 1976.
54. HODGKIN, A. L., AND A. F. HUXLEY. A quantitative description of membrane current and its application to conduction and excitation in nerve. *J. Physiol. London* 117: 500–544, 1952.
55. HODGKIN, A. L., AND S. NAKAJIMA. The effect of diameter on the electrical constants of frog skeletal muscle fibres. *J. Physiol. London* 221: 105–120, 1972.
56. HODGKIN, A. L., AND S. NAKAJIMA. Analysis of the membrane in frog muscle. *J. Physiol. London* 221: 121–136, 1972.
57. HUXLEY, A. F., AND R. E. TAYLOR. Local activation of striated muscle fibres. *J. Physiol. London* 144: 426–441, 1958.
58. JACK, J. J. B., D. NOBLE, AND R. W. TSIEN. *Electric Current Flow in Excitable Cells.* Oxford, UK: Oxford Univ. Press, 1975.
58a. KAY, S. M., AND S. L. MARPLE. Spectrum analysis: a modern perspective. *Proc. IEEE* 69: 1380–1418, 1981.
59. KIRSCH, G. E., R. A. NICHOLS, AND S. NAKAJIMA. Delayed rectification in the transverse tubules. *J. Gen. Physiol.* 70: 1–21, 1977.
60. KOOPMANS, L. H. *The Spectral Analysis of Time Series.* New York: Academic, 1974.
61. LAM, H. Y. *Analog and Digital Filters: Design and Realization.* Englewood Cliffs, NJ: Prentice-Hall, 1979.

62. MAGRAB, E. B., AND D. S. BLOMQUIST. *The Measurement of Time-Varying Phenomena.* New York: Wiley 1971.
63. MARMARELIS, P. Z., AND V. Z. MARMARELIS. *Analysis of Physiological Systems: The White-Noise Approach.* New York: Plenum, 1978.
64. MARMARELIS, V. Z. A single-record estimator for correlation functions of nonstationary random processes. *Proc. IEEE* 69: 841-842, 1981.
65. MASRY, E., AND M. C. LUI. A consistent estimate of the spectrum by random sampling of the time series. *SIAM J. Appl. Math.* 28: 793–810, 1975.
66. MATHIAS, R. T., L. EBIHARA, M. LIEBERMAN, AND E. A. JOHNSON. Linear electrical properties of passive and active currents in spherical heart cell clusters. *Biophys. J.* 36: 221–242, 1981.
67. MATHIAS, R. T., R. S. EISENBERG, AND R. VALDIOSERA. Electrical properties of frog skeletal muscle fibers interpreted with a mesh model of the tubular system. *Biophys. J.* 17: 57–93, 1977.
68. MATHIAS, R. T., R. A. LEVIS, AND R. S. EISENBERG. Electrical models of excitation contraction coupling and charge movement in skeletal muscle. *J. Gen. Physiol.* 76: 1–31, 1980.
69. MATHIAS, R. T., J. L. RAE, AND R. S. EISENBERG. Electrical properties of structural components of the crystalline lens. *Biophys. J.* 25: 181–201, 1979.
70. MATHIAS, R. T., J. L. RAE, AND R. S. EISENBERG. The lens as a non-uniform syncytium. *Biophys. J.* 34: 61–83, 1981.
71. MOBLEY, B. A., AND B. R. EISENBERG. Sizes of components in frog skeletal muscle measured by methods of stereology. *J. Gen. Physiol.* 66: 31–45, 1975.
72. MOBLEY, B. A., J. LEUNG, AND R. S. EISENBERG. Longitudinal impedance of skinned frog muscle fibers. *J. Gen. Physiol.* 63: 625–637, 1974.
73. MOBLEY, B. A., J. LEUNG, AND R. S. EISENBERG. Longitudinal impedance of single frog muscle fibers. *J. Gen. Physiol.* 65: 97–113, 1975.
74. NAKAJIMA, S., AND J. BASTIAN. Membrane properties of the transverse tubular system of amphibian skeletal muscle. In: *Electrobiology of Nerve, Synapse, and Muscle,* edited by J. P. Reuben, D. P. Purpura, M. V. L. Bennett, and E. R. Kandel. New York: Raven, 1976, p. 243–268.
75. NAKAJIMA, S., Y. NAKAJIMA, AND J. BASTIAN. Effects of sudden changes in external sodium concentration on twitch tension in isolated muscle fibers. *J. Gen. Physiol.* 65: 459–482, 1975.
76. NAKAJIMA, S., Y. NAKAJIMA, AND L. D. PEACHEY. Speed of repolarization in glycerol treated frog muscle fibres. *J. Physiol. London* 234: 465–480, 1973.
77. NASTUK, W. L., AND A. L. HODGKIN. The electrical activity of single muscle fibers. *J. Cell. Comp. Physiol.* 35: 39–73, 1950.
78. NICOLAYSEN, K. The spread of the action potential through the t-system in hagfish twitch muscle fibers. *Acta Physiol. Scand.* 96: 29–49, 1976.
79. OPPENHEIM, A. V., AND R. W. SCHAFER. *Digital Signal Processing.* Englewood Cliffs, NJ: Prentice-Hall, 1975.
80. PALM, G., AND T. POGGIO. The Volterra representation and the Wiener expansion: validity and pitfalls. *SIAM J. Appl. Math.* 33: 195–216, 1977.
81. PALM, G., AND T. POGGIO. Wiener-like system identification in physiology. *J. Math Biol.* 4: 375–381, 1977.
82. PAPOULIS, A. *Probability, Random Variables and Stochastic Processes.* New York: McGraw-Hill, 1965.
83. PAPOULIS, A. *Signal Analysis.* New York: McGraw-Hill, 1977.
84. PATKAY, J. D., F. CHU, AND H. A. WIGGERS. Front-end design for digital signal analysis. *Hewlett-Packard J.* 29: 9–13, 1977.
85. PEACHEY, L. D., AND R. H. ADRIAN. Electrical properties of the transverse tubular system. In: *Structure and Function of Muscle* (2nd ed.), edited by G. Bourne. New York: Academic, 1972, vol. I, p. 1–30.
86. PESKOFF, A. Electrical potential in cylindrical syncytia and muscle fibers. *Bull. Math. Biophys.* 41: 183–193, 1979.
87. PESKOFF, A., AND R. S. EISENBERG. Interpretation of some microelectrode measurements of electrical properties of cells. *Annu. Rev. Biophys. Bioeng.* 2: 65–79, 1973.
88. PORTNOFF, M. Time-frequency representation of digital signals and systems based on short-time Fourier analysis. *IEEE Trans. Acoust. Speech Signal Process.* 28: 55–69, 1980.
89. POUSSART, D., L. E. MOORE, AND H. M. FISHMAN. Ion movements and kinetics in squid axon. I. Complex admittance. *Ann. NY Acad. Sci.* 303: 355–379, 1977.
90. RABINER, L. R., AND R. W. SCHAFER. *Digital Processing of Speech Signals.* Englewood Cliffs, NJ: Prentice-Hall, 1978.
91. SACHS, F., AND P. SPECHT. Fast microelectrode headstage for voltage clamp. *Med. Biol. Eng. Comput.* 19: 316–320, 1981.
92. SCHANNE, O. F., AND E. RUIZ-P.-CERETTI. *Impedance Measurements in Biological Cells.* New York: Wiley-Interscience, 1978.
93. SCHETZEN, M. *The Volterra and Wiener Theories of Nonlinear Systems.* New York: Wiley-Interscience, 1980.
93a. SCHETZEN, M. Nonlinear system modeling based on the Wiener theory. *Proc. IEEE* 69: 1557-1573, 1981.
94. SCHNEIDER, M. F. Linear electrical properties of the transverse tubules and surface membrane of skeletal muscle fibers. *J. Gen. Physiol.* 56: 640–671, 1970.
95. SIGWORTH, F. J. Covariance of nonstationary sodium current fluctuations at the node of Ranvier. *Biophys. J.* 34: 111–133, 1981.
96. SOMLYO, A. V. Bridging structures spanning the gap at the triad of skeletal muscle. *J. Cell Biol.* 80: 743–750, 1979.
97. SOMLYO, A. V., H. SHUMAN, AND A. P. SOMLYO. Elemental distributions in striated muscle and the effects of hypertonicity. *J. Cell Biol.* 74: 828–857, 1977.
98. SUZUKI, K., V. ROHLICEK, AND E. FROMTER. A quasi-totally shielded, low capacitance glass microelectrode with suitable amplifiers for high frequency intracellular potential and impedance measurements. *Pfluegers Arch.* 378: 141–148, 1978.
99. TAKASHIMA, S., AND H. P. SCHWAN. Passive electrical properties of squid axon membrane. *J. Membr. Biol.* 17: 51–68, 1974.
100. VALDIOSERA, R., C. CLAUSEN, AND R. S. EISENBERG. Measurement of the impedance of frog skeletal muscle fibers. *Biophys. J.* 14: 295–315, 1974.
101. VALDIOSERA, R., C. CLAUSEN, AND R. S. EISENBERG. Circuit models of the passive electrical properties of frog skeletal muscle fibers. *J. Gen. Physiol.* 63: 432–459, 1974.
102. VALDIOSERA, R., C. CLAUSEN, AND R. S. EISENBERG. Impedance of frog skeletal muscle fibers in various solutions. *J. Gen. Physiol.* 63: 460–491, 1974.
103. VERGARA, J., F. BEZANILLA, AND B. M. SALZBERG. Nile blue fluorescence signals from cut single muscle fibers under voltage or current clamp conditions. *J. Gen. Physiol.* 72: 775–800, 1978.
104. WEINER, D. D., AND J. F. SPINA. *Sinusoidal Analysis and Modeling of Weakly Nonlinear Circuits: With Application to Nonlinear Interference Effects.* New York: Van Nostrand Reinhold, 1980.
105. ZAMPIGHI, G., J. VERGARA, AND F. RAMÓN. On the connection between the transverse tubules and the plasma membrane in frog semitendinosus skeletal muscle. Are caveolae the mouths of the transverse tubule system? *J. Cell Biol.* 64: 734–740, 1975.

CHAPTER 12

Inward spread of activation in twitch skeletal muscle fibers

HUGO GONZALEZ-SERRATOS | *Department of Biophysics, University of Maryland School of Medicine, Baltimore, Maryland*

CHAPTER CONTENTS

THERE IS A FINITE TIME between the action potential and the initiation of the mechanical activation of twitch skeletal muscle cells. This delay (shown in Fig. 1) represents the time required for development of the links necessary to couple the action potential to contractile activation. The possibility that this delay might include one or more steps was probably first recognized in 1873 by Engelmann (28) and in 1881 by Retzius (89). They were aware of the need for a link between excitation and contraction but not of the delay.

In 1895 Biedermann (13) identified the first step in the sequence as a change in the membrane potential. He concluded that whenever there was a muscle contraction, there was a preceding change in membrane potential, the action potential. Another early finding showed that when a whole skeletal muscle was stimulated by increased current steps, the contractile force was proportional to the current applied. Because the action potential that initiated the contraction was known to follow the all-or-none law, a question arose about whether the contractile activation of whole muscles followed the all-or-none mechanism or if the initiation of contraction was dissociated from the action potential. In 1922 Adrian (1) answered this question in a very ingenious manner. He demonstrated that the relation between stimulus and response, recorded as an electric activity of the muscle cells, was discontinuous and the response rose in a series of steps (Fig. 2). The steps coincided with the excitation of a new fiber or groups of fibers, as verified by direct microscopic observations. Between each step the electric response remained constant although the stimulus was increased. He concluded that individual skeletal muscle fibers obeyed the all-or-none law and the graded activation seen in whole muscle was due to recruitment of individual muscle cells. The existence of the action potential is, however, not the only condition necessary to initiate the contraction. As Gelfan (38) showed in 1933, a graded mechanical response can be produced by graded depolarization of single muscle fibers. We now recognize that the contraction of normal twitch-type striated muscle fibers is always followed by either an action potential or a depolarization of the sarcolemma (Fig. 1*C*, *D*). Deplorization is not necessarily followed by mechanical activation, however, as illustrated in Figure 1*A*, *B*. Later it became clear that there was a sequence of physiological reactions triggered by the initial excitatory event in the sarcolemma linking it to the final mechanical response. Sandow (92) called this chain of events the "excitation-contraction" (EC) coupling system.

INWARD SPREAD OF THE EXCITATORY PROCESS

Assuming that the sarcolemmal action potential is linked to the contraction, how does a change in potential at the surface membrane influence myofibrils that may be as much as 90 μm away? The reduction and/or inversion of the sarcolemmal potential taking place across a membrane approximately 70–100 nm could not be expected to directly affect any structure located more than a very few nanometers from the membrane. Therefore some physical process or link must occur by which myofibrils several tens of thousands of nanometers away from the surface will be activated to contract. The spread of surface depolarization across the muscle cell is the subject of this chapter.

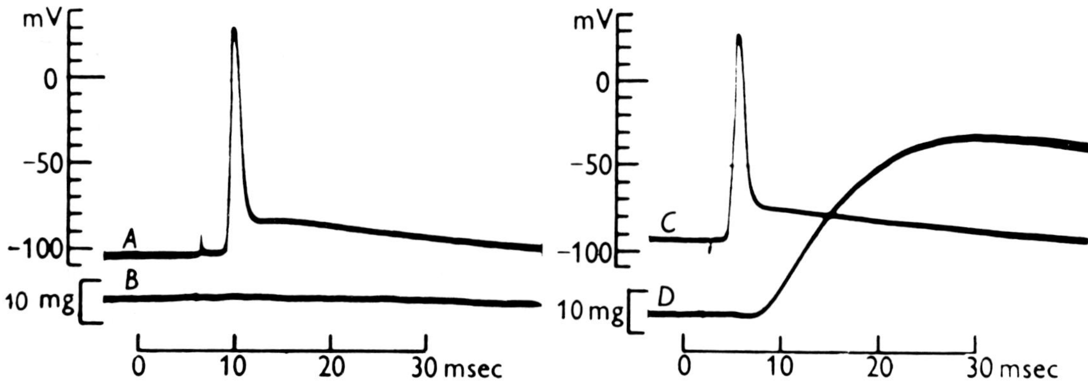

FIG. 1. Electrical (A, C) and mechanical (B, D) responses of a single muscle fiber recorded with an internal electrode and a transducer in hypertonic solution (*left*) and in normal Ringer's fluid (*right*). Temperature, 20°C; fiber diameter, 140 μm. [From Hodgkin and Horowicz (49).]

Development of the Problem

In 1947 Heilbrunn and Wiercinski (45) suggested that the simplest possibility for coupling excitation to contraction would be to liberate a substance from the sarcolemma during depolarization. This substance would diffuse inward to trigger the mechanical activation of the myofibrils. When cut skeletal twitch muscles placed in a Ca-free solution were exposed to various ions, mechanical activation was induced at different levels. Sodium and potassium ions produced only weak contractions, whereas calcium produced by far the most powerful contractions. Although the experiment obviously had many drawbacks, they correctly concluded that Ca^{2+} was the most important ion for producing muscle contraction. They proposed that Ca^{2+} enters the myoplasm through the surface membrane during depolarization and diffuse along the cross section of the muscle cell, sending a wave of myofibrillar mechanical activation from the surface to the center of the fiber.

In 1948 Hill (46) proposed that if diffusion of Ca^{2+} or another substance was the trigger for contraction, the rapidity of the contraction phase and the time available for diffusion of the hypothetical activating substance to reach the myofibrils in the center of the fiber should agree. He compared the time needed for a substance to diffuse into the center of a fiber with the time available to do it. To calculate the diffusion time he stated the corresponding equation assuming that a substance x is liberated at time $t = 0$ on the entire surface of a cylinder of radius a. He further assumed that substance x diffuses into the cylinder

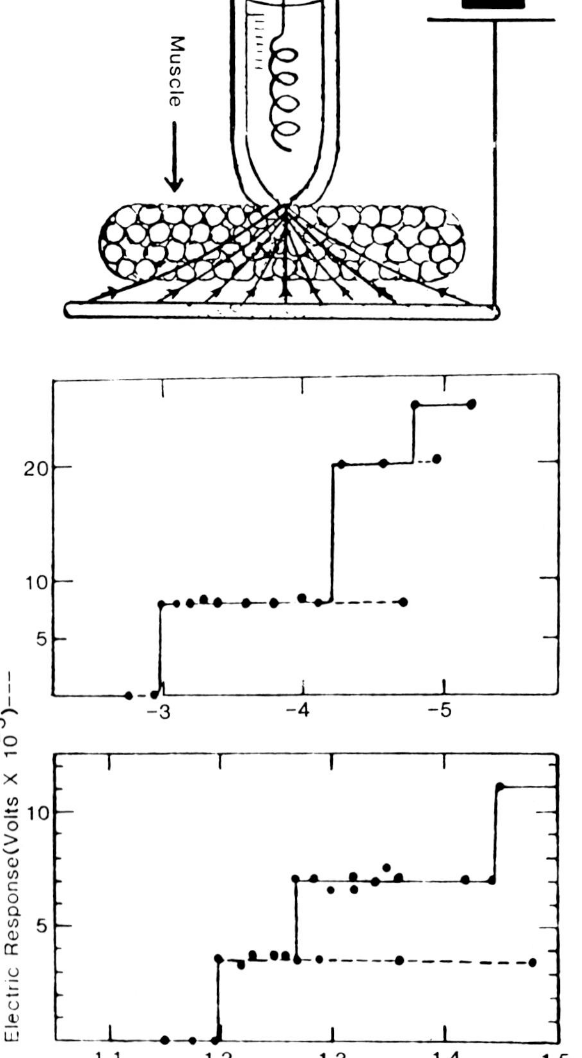

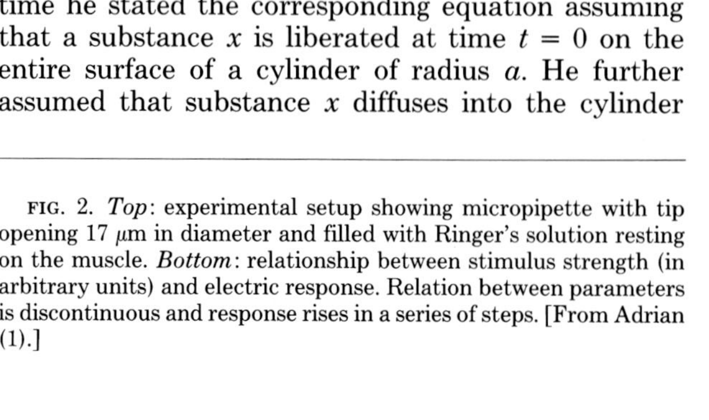

FIG. 2. *Top*: experimental setup showing micropipette with tip opening 17 μm in diameter and filled with Ringer's solution resting on the muscle. *Bottom*: relationship between stimulus strength (in arbitrary units) and electric response. Relation between parameters is discontinuous and response rises in a series of steps. [From Adrian (1).]

but not toward the outside, that it is not consumed but will react with the myofibrils, and that it will have a diffusion constant k. Assuming y is the concentration at time t at a point r from the center of the fiber and y_∞ is the final concentration after diffusion is completed, Hill devised the corresponding differential equation with the following solution

$$\frac{y}{y_\infty} = 1 + \sum_{\alpha_1, \alpha_2, \cdots} \frac{J_0(\alpha r/a)}{J_0(\alpha)} e^{-a2kt/a^2} \tag{1}$$

where α_1, α_2, $\cdots$ are the positive roots of $J_1(\alpha)$ and J_1 is the Bessel function of order 1. The solution relating y/y_∞ to kt/a^2 in Hill's paper is plotted in Figure 3 for a different r. To use this plot we need to solve first kt/a^2. Assuming a muscle fiber with a diameter of $2a$ = 100 μm that gives $a = 0.005$ cm and a diffusion constant k of 5×10^{-6} cm^2/s, therefore

$$\frac{kt}{a^2} = \frac{5 \times 10^{-6} t}{(0.005)^2 \text{ cm}^2}$$

and $kt/a^2 = 0.2t$. The question then is whether in this fiber the hypothetical substance can diffuse fast enough to affect all the cross-sectional area during the time given by the tension development of the twitch. At 0°C the contraction phase of a twitch is of the order of 0.3–0.5 s (frog). For example, taking 0.2 s as the necessary time for diffusion, $t = 0.2$ s and $kt/a^2 = 0.2\ t = 0.04$ s. In Figure 3 for $kt/a^2 = 0.04$, the corresponding $y/y_\infty = 0.02$ for $r = 0$ for the substance x to diffuse to the center of the fiber. Since the substance increased only 0.02 times, diffusion was not fast enough to arrive in time. Hill further proved that the mismatch was larger if temperature was increased. The remaining possibility was that during a single twitch not all of the cross-sectional area was activated, only an outer ring of myofibrils. If this was true, diffusion of a substance might explain the inward spread of activation. In 1949 he concluded from indirect experiments that the entire cross-sectional area might be activated (47). Gonzalez-Serratos (39, 42) later showed directly that all the myofibrils in the cross-sectional area of a muscle fiber are activated during a twitch. Nevertheless it is possible that minute amounts of Ca^{2+} are needed to trigger the contraction ($y/y_\infty = 0.02$). In 1955 Niedergerke (82) demonstrated in a very elegant experiment that when calcium is injected into a muscle fiber in a concentration large enough to produce contraction, this contraction remains well localized at the injection site and does not initiate a wave of contraction toward the center of the fiber (Fig. 4). Thus it was clearly shown (despite later

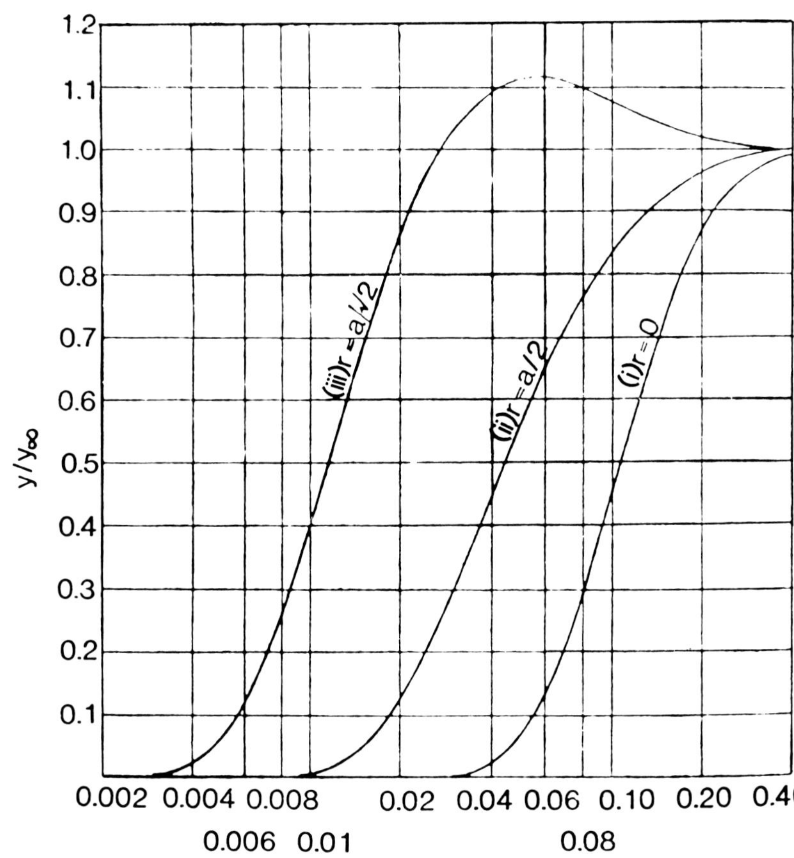

FIG. 3. Calculated relation (Eq. 2) between $y/y\infty$ and kt/a^2, with kt/a^2 given on logarithmic scale. *Curves i, ii,* and *iii* are for points on axis and points $0.5a$ and $0.707a$ distant from the axis, respectively. [From Hill (46).]

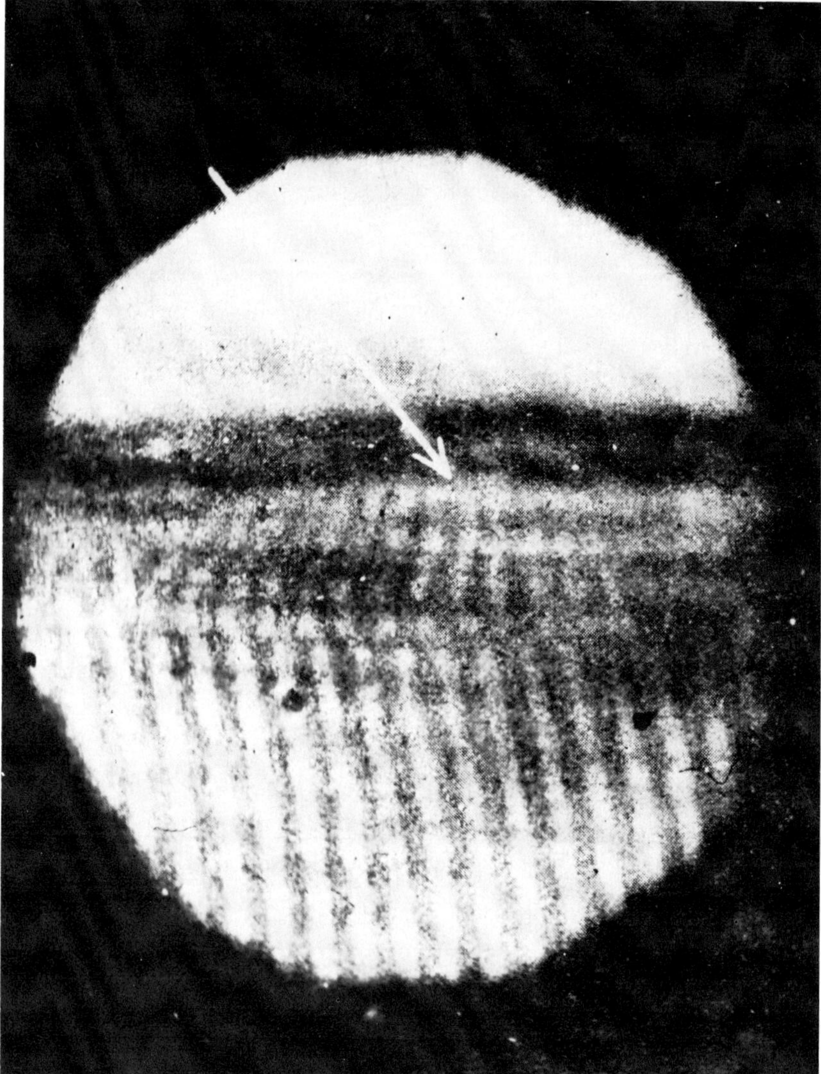

FIG. 4. Part of muscle fiber photographed a few seconds after intracellular application of Ca at place indicated by *arrow*. Fiber was stretched to ~120% of its resting length. I bands are clear; edge of fiber is out of focus. [From Niedergerke (82).]

claims that Ca^{2+} flow from the outside is the mechanism triggering contraction) that diffusion of Ca^{2+} into the fiber was not the mechanism of inward spread of activation. Since diffusion was ruled out, it became necessary to postulate the existence of another specific mechanism of inward spread of the excitatory process.

Role of the Action Potential

Two facts were clearly established: *1*) there is an action potential on the surface membrane and *2*) it is followed, after a few milliseconds, by contraction of all myofibrils. The next challenge was to discover how the triggering mechanism, set by the surface action potential, spread from the surface to the center of the fiber. The action potential is a short-lasting change of the potential difference that exists across the resting surface membrane and may be responsible for the initiation of contraction either by the currents it produces or the depolarization itself.

The proposition that the step between the action potential and the initiation of the contraction might be the internal current generated by the sarcolemmal action potential seemed simple and attractive. If the action potential's current was sufficient to flow throughout the whole muscle cell nothing else would be needed. This would provide the necessary intermediary mechanism that would affect all the myofibrils. Could an action potential produce a significant current in the myoplasmic contents of the muscle cell? The current flow (i) can be calculated by

$$i = \frac{E}{r_i} \tag{2}$$

where E is the voltage change produced by the action potential per distance covered by it ($\partial V/\partial x$) and r_i is the myoplasm resistance. Substituting $\partial V/\partial x$ for E in Equation 2 gives

$$i_{long} = \frac{1}{r_i}\frac{\partial V}{\partial x} \quad (3)$$

x can be found from the conduction velocity θ of the action potential, $\theta = \partial x/\partial t$, and thus $\partial x = \theta \partial t$. Substituting ∂x for $\theta \partial t$ in Equation 3

$$i_{long} = \frac{1}{r_i \theta}\frac{\partial V}{\partial t} \quad (4)$$

r_i can be calculated from the specific resistance (R_i) of the myoplasm (200 $\Omega\cdot$cm) $r_i = R_i/A$ where A is the cross-sectional area; therefore for a fiber of radius a = 50 μm, then $A = 2 \times 3.14 \times (5 \times 10^{-3})^2$ cm^2 = 75 $\times$ 10^{-6} cm^2, and thus

$$r_i = \frac{200\ \Omega\cdot\text{cm}}{75 \times 10^{-6}\text{cm}^2} = 2.65 \times 10^6\ \Omega\cdot\text{cm}^{-1} \quad (5)$$

With θ = 100 cm/s, we can calculate $\partial V/\partial x$. If the change in membrane potential is 100 mV during 0.25 ms then the distance covered during those 25 ms $x = \theta t$ = 100 $\times$ 2.5 $\times$ 10^{-4} cm$\cdot$s$^{-1}\cdot$ = 250 $\times$ 10^{-4} cm; therefore

$$\frac{\partial V}{\partial x} = \frac{100 \times 10^{-3}\ \text{V}}{25 \times 10^{-3}\ \text{cm}} = 4\ \text{V/cm} \quad (6)$$

If we take R_i for any fiber, from Equation 3

$$i_{long} = \frac{1}{R_i}\frac{\partial V}{\partial x} = \frac{1}{200} \times 4\ \Omega^{-1}\cdot\text{cm}^{-1}\cdot\text{V}\cdot\text{cm}^{-1}$$

$$= 0.02\frac{V}{\Omega} \times \frac{1}{\text{cm}^2} = 2 \times 10^{-2}\ \text{A}\cdot\text{cm}^{-2}$$

and for a particular fiber with a = 50 μm the current flow is

$$i_{long} = \frac{1}{r_i} = \frac{\partial V}{\partial x}$$

$$= \frac{1}{2.65 \times 10^6} \times 4\ \Omega^{-1}\cdot\text{cm}^{-1}\cdot\text{V}\cdot\text{cm}^{-1}$$

$$= 1.2 \times 10^{-6}\ \text{A}$$

This is sufficient current considering the amount found to flow in other excitable tissues during activation [see, e.g., Fatt and Katz (33)].

The change in membrane potential as estimated above during an action potential produces a gradient of about 4 V/cm during the depolarization phase of the action potential. This gradient can initiate other excitatory processes, but it would require a link between the sarcolemma and all the myofibrils to reach the center of the fiber. When these ideas were developed such a link was unknown, making the current-flow proposition the most attractive.

In 1953 Bay, Goodall, and Szent-Györgyi (9) described the so-called window-field theory, which states that in a series of resistances placed across an electric field there is a point in the center of the field between the cathode and the anode electrodes that is neither positive nor negative, as illustrated in Figure 5, but through which current must flow despite the lack of difference in potential at this point. Based on this theory, Csapo and Suzuki (22) reasoned that if they placed a sartorius muscle, which is composed of parallel fibers, with its long axis perpendicular to the electrode plates, when they created an electric field there should be a small region midpoint between the tendons where no difference in membrane potential exists. Current would flow through the interior of the fibers in this area, however. If contraction occurred at a midpoint between tendons, it would be interpreted as clear proof that current flow was the contraction trigger. There would be no need for an excitatory process traveling across the muscle cell. Their results, illustrated in Figure 5, showed that if the potential was measured along the muscle, there was indeed an area (although not well defined) with no difference in

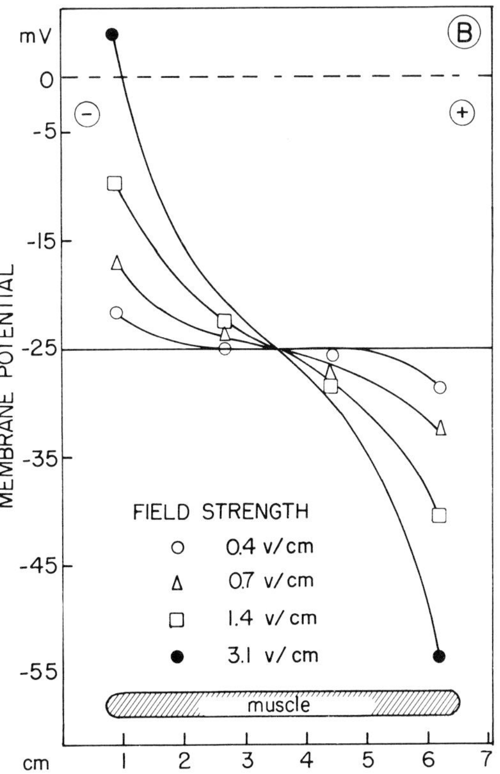

FIG. 5. Changes in membrane potential of turtle retractor penis along length of K-depolarized (nonpropagating) muscle during application of DC field. Stimulus, longitudinal DC of different strengths. 20°C, $[K]_o$ = 24 mM. Cathodal half always depolarized, whereas anodal half always polarized during stimulation, leaving membrane potential unchanged in center portion. Extent of change in membrane potential is a function of field strength. [From Sakai and Csapo (91).]

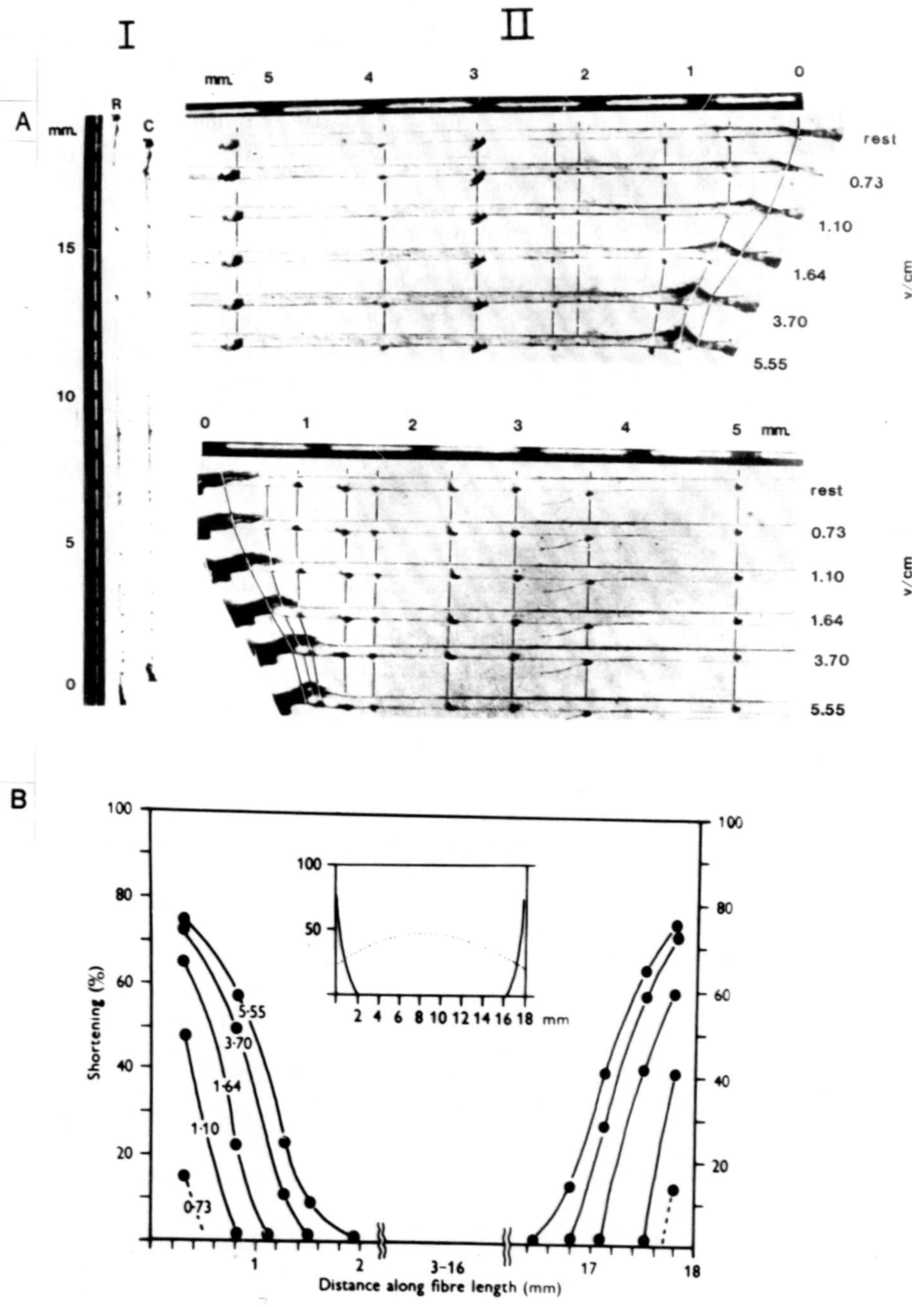

FIG. 6. Isotonic shortening of isolated single muscle fiber from frog semitendinosus. *A*: photographs of reversible isotonic AC contractures in a nonpropagating fiber. *I*: photographs of whole length of fiber marked with graphite particles. R, resting fiber; C, longitudinal AC field at 5 V/cm (100 cycles/s). *II*: enlargements of end portions of fiber with all frames aligned with one mark placed at distance of ~5 mm from the ends. *Upper row* of each set shows resting fiber; those below show effect of AC field, with numbers indicating each field strength. *Black lines*, displacement of the graphite granules. *B*: extent and degree of shortening along fiber during longitudinal AC stimulation (100 cycles/s); field strength (V/cm, rms) indicated by numbers on curves. Ordinate, relative shortening of each length element; abscissa, distance along length of fiber, with the midregion strongly compressed. *Inset*, distribution of shortening along whole fiber (*solid line*); *dotted line*, example of results (V/cm, 60 cycles/s) from Csapo and Suzuki (ref. 22; Fig. 3). [From Sten-Knudsen (96).]

potential. They measured the movement of different portions along the muscle and found that the whole muscle shortened but that shortening was much more powerful in the region without a potential difference (see Fig. 6*B*, dotted line of *inset*). They concluded that current flow was the important link to trigger contraction and that depolarization was not necessary to initiate it.

Other experiments that seemed to support this hypothesis were described by Natori and Isojima (81); some were done in skinned fibers in 1954 by Natori (80). They applied current between two electrodes placed 1.5 mm apart in the myoplasm and observed a contraction with 1.5 V (or more). Since there was no sarcolemma, they concluded that current was the triggering factor.

In their studies of local responses, Brown and Sichel (15) demonstrated that when a transverse current was applied to a muscle with plate electrodes placed parallel to its long axis, a larger shortening was observed on the cathodic side, where the membrane potential depolarized more than on the anodic portion. Apparently current was not the triggering factor for contraction. As early as 1946 Kuffler (70) described experimental results regarding current and depolarization. He reasoned that if depolarization was the triggering mechanism, only the depolarized portion of the muscle cell would contract. He depolarized a muscle cell with K^+ or acetylcholine placed on a small area of the muscle cell and with a microscope observed a clear, sustained contraction. Furthermore passing an anodic current with a microelectrode in the same area inhibited the K contracture, despite the fact that current was flowing. This supported the hypothesis that depolarization of the sarcolemma was the triggering mechanism for contraction.

In 1954 Sten-Knudsen (95), with the window-field theory as a basis, attempted to solve the problem using small bundles of muscle fibers. He soon realized that geometrical uncertainties dictated the use of isolated single muscle cells, which he used in 1960 to repeat the experiment (96). The results shown in Figure 6*A* for an AC field are plotted in Figure 6*B*. They clearly indicate that there is no shortening in the midpoint between the tendons after applying either an AC or DC field. The contraction occurred on the cathodic side of the field. The magnitude of shortening increased either toward the cathode or with the strength of the field applied. It is difficult to compare these results with those of Csapo and Suzuki (22) for whole muscle. Hagiwara and Watanabe (44) did an experiment similar to those of Natori and Isojima (81) in muscle cells but in some cases treated the sarcolemma with procaine to make it inexcitable. They inserted two microelectrodes and passed longitudinal current between them. Without treatment there was no mechanical response up to 2×10^{-6} A; with procaine treatment they could increase the current without causing contraction. From the experiments of Natori and Isojima (81) it can be estimated that with a threshold of 1.5 V and the electrodes 1 mm apart, given $r_i = 2 \times 10^6\ \Omega \cdot cm^{-1}$, the current passed between the electrodes was on the order of 8×10^{-6} A, which is approximately 4 times the one used by Hagiwara and Watanabe. It undoubtedly produced a contraction, but this may not indicate whether current is the link between the sarcolemmal action potential and the triggering of the contraction. In 1960 Hodgkin and Horowicz (51) showed that when isolated muscle fibers were quickly superfused with solutions containing different potassium concentrations (solution covering all the muscle cell was changed in 0.5 s), there was a positive relationship between the force produced and the potassium concentration, as shown in Figure 7. Mechanical activation was not due to the presence of potassium per se, but to the degree of depolarization. Furthermore there was a clear threshold for mechanical activation set by a given membrane potential level

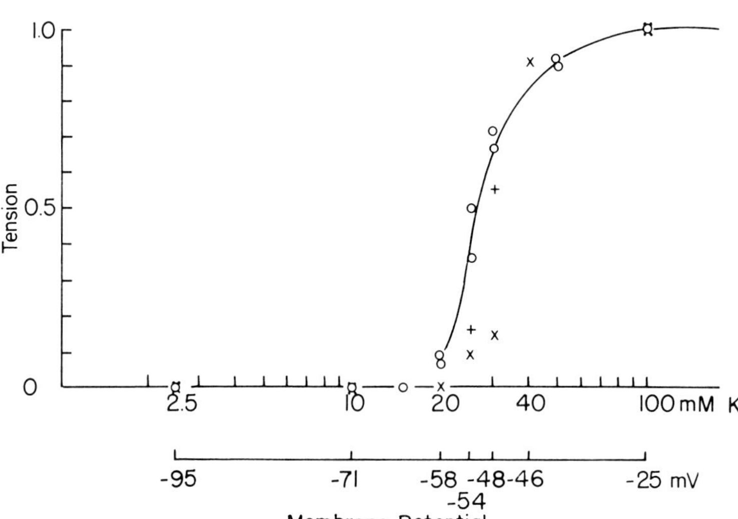

FIG. 7. Relation between peak tension and K concentration or membrane potential (○ and +, only tension was measured; +, tension; ×, tension and membrane potential were measured). Numbers on *lower scale* are internal potentials measured at same time as tension. Scale for K concentration is logarithmic and for potential is approximately linear; difference in scale corresponds to 45 mV for a 10-fold change. Choline Ringer's solution was used, with K replacing choline. Temperature, 18°C. [From Hodgkin and Horowicz (51).]

(−55 mV in the absence of Na_o). It is difficult to see how a current can occur between different portions of the sarcolemma once a steady depolarization is reached all along the muscle cell, and yet the muscle cells contract for several seconds. The overall conclusion from the results of the experiments have given strong evidence that depolarization is the important initial factor in the chain of events that trigger contraction.

New Facts and Theories

Evidence showed that depolarization was the mechanism linking the sarcolemmal action potential to the contraction, but the problem of the mechanism by which this change of sarcolemmal potential spread into the muscle fiber remained unsolved. In an attempt to solve this problem, Huxley and his colleagues (56, 58, 63–66) published a series of papers that became a milestone in muscle physiology and experimental design. Since diffusion and current were ruled out, they reasoned that there must be a specialized pathway to transmit the excitatory signal into the muscle cell. The type of excitatory signal spreading into the muscle remained unidentified, but they decided first the pathway should be understood. They reasoned that if they could produce a depolarization beyond mechanical threshold only across a very small area (e.g., a circular spot 1–1.5 μm diam) of the sarcolemma without changing the membrane potential elsewhere, then they would observe with a high-power microscope only the area of depolarization. They expected the change in membrane potential to cause a contraction only if the area of sarcolemma depolarized covered the surface attachment of one of the hypothetical structures along which inward activation would occur. Three experimental conditions were needed: *1)* a very localized depolarization produced by passing current through a micropipette with an opening around 1.5 μm in diameter, *2)* the means to distinguish optically between anisotropic and isotropic bands through a high-power polarizing or phase microscope suitable for thick specimens (this type of microscope was not commercially available), and *3)* a micromanipulator to produce such small movements of the micropipette that it could be placed smoothly against the sarcolemma without penetrating it and also to permit side movements of less than 1 μm (also not available). Huxley (55, 57) designed and built both the microscope and the micromanipulator.

The next question was whether the current across the area covered by the mouth of the stimulating pipette during a test depolarization would be small enough so as not to trigger an action potential. The surface covered by the pipette was 3×10^{-8} cm^2; therefore if during depolarization with a 100-mV pulse the resistance across that area drops to around 30 Ω/cm^2, the current flowing through the area should be about 1×10^{-10} A. During an action potential the current density is of the order of 2 nA/cm^2 (79); the current flowing through the area covered by the pipette should be approximately 6×10^{-11} A. The current flow during an action potential is approximately 10^{-7} A. Therefore, as long as the seal between the mouth of the micropipette and the surrounding medium is large, the current passing with a 100-mV depolarization remains in the neighboring sarcolemma (Fig. 8). Results obtained in frog twitch fibers are illustrated in Figure 9. During depolarization with the pipette placed in the middle of the A band and in the A-I region, there was no contraction. With the pipette in the middle of the I band the sarcomere under the pipette contracted and the two half I bands in front of the pipette decreased in size when the A bands moved toward the center of the I band, revealing mechanical activation. When the sarcomere under the pipette mouth contracted, the two adjacent sarcomere bands 2 μm away did not contract. Increasing the stimulating current in the I band produced a further penetration of inward spread of contraction, graded and of no more than 10 μm, whereas there was no lateral spread of activation. There was no suggestion of an all-or-none behavior, because with a further increase in the current, the fiber went into a full contraction and became damaged.

When the first experiments were reported, the Z line was the obvious possible explanation for the inward spread of activation (64). During a meeting, however, after Huxley presented his paper, J. D. Robertson (90) showed an electron micrograph he had taken from lizard striated muscle. He indicated a special transversely oriented tubular structure localized not at the level of the Z line but two per sarcomere (Fig. 10) at the level of the A-I junction. He raised the possibility that this structure might be involved in the inward spread of activation. [For a review on the sequence of events see Huxley's 1967 Croonian Lecture (60).]

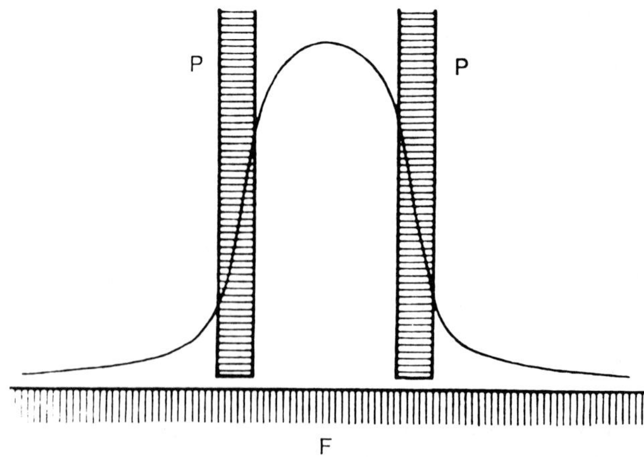

FIG. 8. Distribution of potential on surface of muscle fiber when pulse is applied to pipette, as determined in model experiments. Walls of pipette (P) and gap between tip of pipette and surface of fiber (F) are drawn to scale. [From Huxley and Taylor (66).]

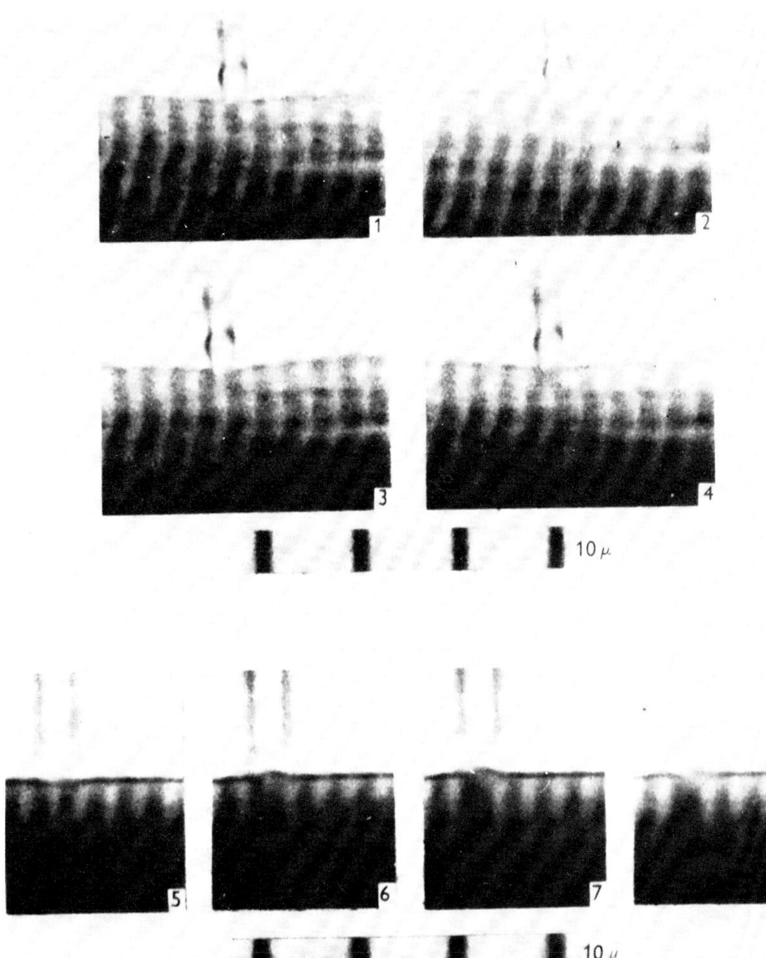

FIG. 9. *Frames 1–4:* edge of isolated frog muscle fiber with pipette in contact. Polarized light was compensated so that A bands appear dark. Pipette was applied in *1* and *2* to an A band and in *3* and *4* to an I band. *Left* picture is taken just before and *right* picture during a negative pulse applied to the pipette; a contraction is produced only if pipette is opposite an I band (*frame 4*). *Frames 5–8:* successive frames from a cinefilm (16 frames/s) showing shortening induced by local depolarization of frog fiber. Polarized light was compensated so that A bands appear dark. Onset of a negative pulse applied to pipette occurs between *frames 5* and *6*. [From Huxley and Taylor (66).]

When Huxley and Taylor (65, 66) repeated the local stimulation experiments in crab and lizard muscle cells that have larger sarcomere spacings, they found a different pattern. Depolarization produced contraction in these muscles only when the micropipette was placed at the border of the A-I bands, ruling out the Z disk as a possible transmitter of inward excitatory signals.

Morphological Evidence

In 1953 Bennett and Porter (11) rediscovered a series of internal membranes in the skeletal muscle. The original description made in 1902 by Veratti (100) was completely ignored until after this rediscovery. In 1957 Porter and Palade (88) reconstructed the sarcoplasmic reticulum (SR) from electron micrographs. They also described a distinct structure composed of a central element and two lateral sacs. Because it was formed by three units it was named the triad. It was shown that in amphibians the triad is localized at the level of the Z line (see Fig. 11 and 12). Robertson (90) showed that the same structure in lizards is localized in the boundaries of the I-A band. Huxley and Taylor (66) used this as a basis to propose that activation spreads inward through the triads. Porter and Palade (88) showed that in mammalian and crustacean muscles the localization is approximately 0.5 μm from the Z line, but in crustacean muscles the structure is composed of two elements rather than three, forming a dyad. Another consequence of the localization in mammals, reptiles, and crustaceans is that there are two triads or dyads per sarcomere, whereas amphibians have only one triad per sarcomere.

Hypothesis

In 1958 Huxley and Taylor (66) proposed the following hypothesis. *1)* The inward spread of activation occurs through the triads. *2)* Within the limits of depolarization used, the spread is not an all-or-none process. *3)* The inward spread of excitation is graded like an electrotonic spread along a cable whose intensity decays with distance. *4)* Since in the frog the spots where inward activation was found were spread 5 μm apart along the perimeter of the fiber, in a 100-μm-diameter fiber during an action potential traveling at 100 cm/s there are an estimated 2,000 spots under the

5-ms duration of the action potential above mechanical threshold. This high density of active spots would probably permit an inward activation all along the cross-sectional area of the fiber. *5*) They defined the functional contractile unit as each half sarcomere on both sides of a Z line, because local activation could not spread sideways further than that.

Morphological Corroboration

Huxley and his collaborators clearly based their hypothesis on experimental findings. Nevertheless some aspects needed further corroboration. For example, if inward spread of activation takes place through the triads, one of its elements should be a continuous structure that passes from one myofibril to the other and from the surface to the center of the fiber, and it should be open or have a continuity with the sarcolemma.

In 1959 Huxley (58) published for the first time an electron micrograph showing that the central element of the triad was continuous from myofibril to myofibril (Fig. 11). At nearly the same time Andersson-Cedergren (7) published the same finding and called this element the transverse or T system. In 1964 Franzini-Armstrong and Porter (35), and Peachey in 1965 (85), using better fixation and different muscle preparations, clearly confirmed the continuity of the T system (Fig. 12).

Both Franzini-Armstrong and Porter in fishes and Peachey in frogs showed that the central element,

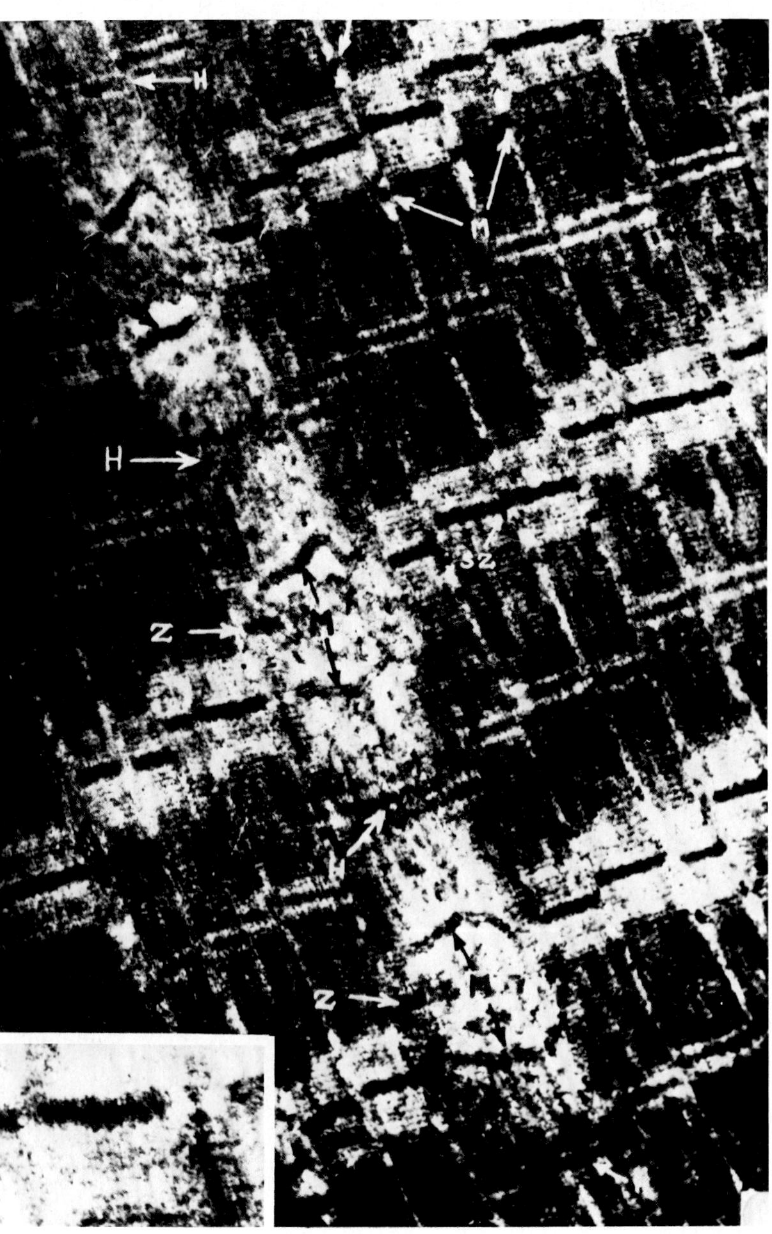

FIG. 10. Longitudinal section of a lizard leg muscle fiber. Note pairs of double membranes (*arrows M*) or tubules lying in sarcoplasm immediately adjacent to this grazed myofibril associated roughly with edges of A bands. In a favorable spot in which Z bands of 2 adjacent myofibrils are in register, some dense material can be seen in sarcoplasm between Z bands (*arrows Z*). × 33,000. *Inset*, × 69,000. [From Robertson (90).]

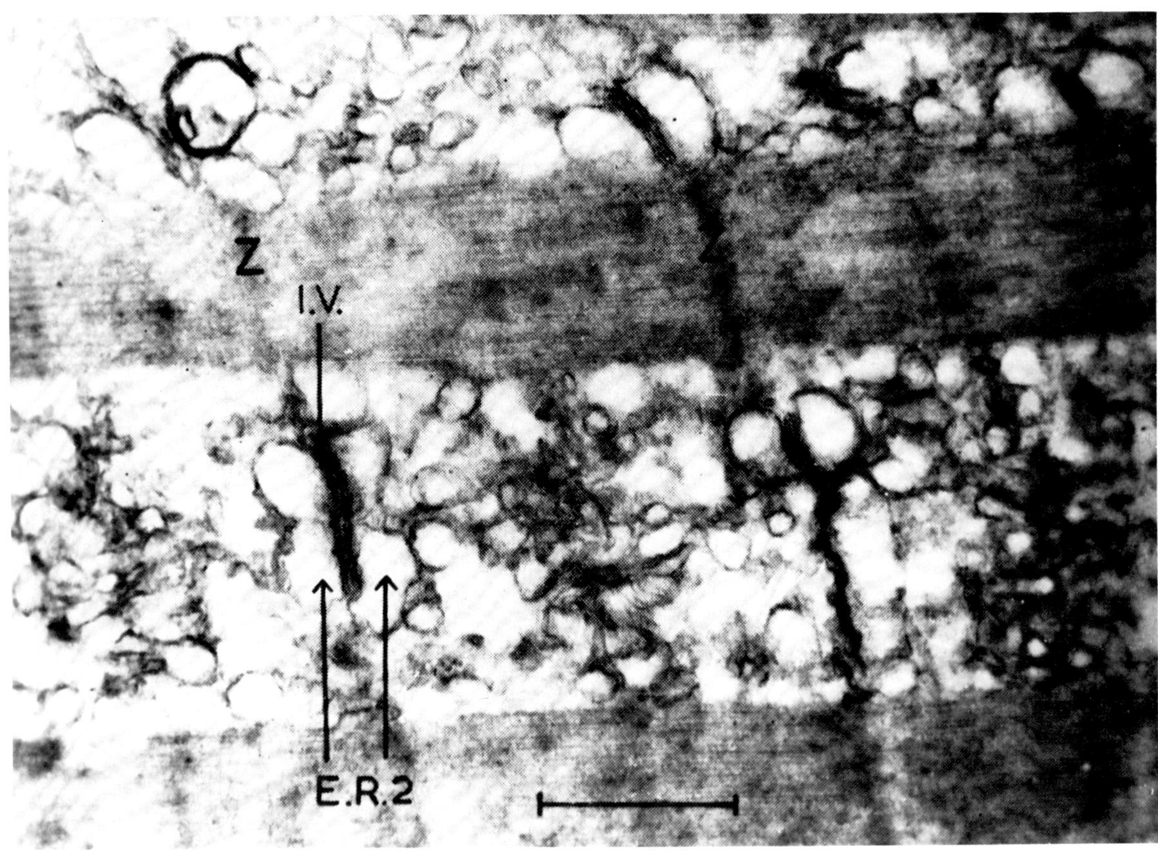

FIG. 11. Frog muscle SR. Triads consisting of I-band vesicles (*E.R.2*) and intermediary vesicles (*I.V.*) at level of each Z line [Porter and Palade's nomenclature (88)]. Middle element of each triad appears to be a continuous structure rather than a row of small vesicles. Fixed in buffered 1% OsO_4; no further staining. Scale bar, 0.5 μm. [From Huxley (58).]

which could be regarded as a tubule, is an independent structure and separated from the lateral elements. The last are called the terminal cisternae (TC) and are part of the SR (Fig. 12).

In 1961 Smith (94) showed that in insect muscles one of the elements of the triad had continuity with the sarcolemma and opened to the extracellular space. The same was true for crab muscles (87, 93) and fishtail muscle (35). Most of the physiological experiments have been done in frog muscles, where concrete experimental design and interpretation of results were based on the assumption that the T tubules were open to the extracellular space and had continuity with the sarcolemma [Hodgkin and Horowicz (50) and Adrian and Freygang (5)], but neither condition could be demonstrated when those experiments were published. Therefore they took a different approach to demonstrate continuity with the extracellular space. If T tubules were open to the extracellular space, it seemed reasonable that large molecules unable to move through the sarcolemma might diffuse into the T-tubule space. The next step was to find an appropriate marker molecule and the means to detect it. In 1964 Endo (26), in an isolated live muscle cell that had been incubated with a fluorescent dye, observed under a fluorescence microscope that *1)* during washout the dye was localized along the middle portion of the I band (where the T tubules should be) and *2)* the washout times corresponded to the diffusion times of a substance previously accumulated in a volume similar to that of the T system (25, 27). At approximately the same time Huxley (67) and Page (84) clearly showed with electron microscopy that in a frog muscle incubated in ferritin prior to fixation, the ferritin filled only the T-system space (Fig. 13) and not the SR or the myoplasm.

After these studies it was clear that the T system is a continuous network of tubules opened to extracellular space and separated from the TC (see Fig. 12). Openings were found in frog muscles (Fig. 14), showing that the T-tubule membranes were invaginations of the sarcolemma. Recently Peachey showed clearly and impressively, using 5-μm-thick sections in tridimensional electron micrographs, that all the features of the tubule network are very similar to what was reconstructed from two-dimensional high-resolution electron micrographs. New details from this work are discussed in the chapter by Peachey in this *Handbook*.

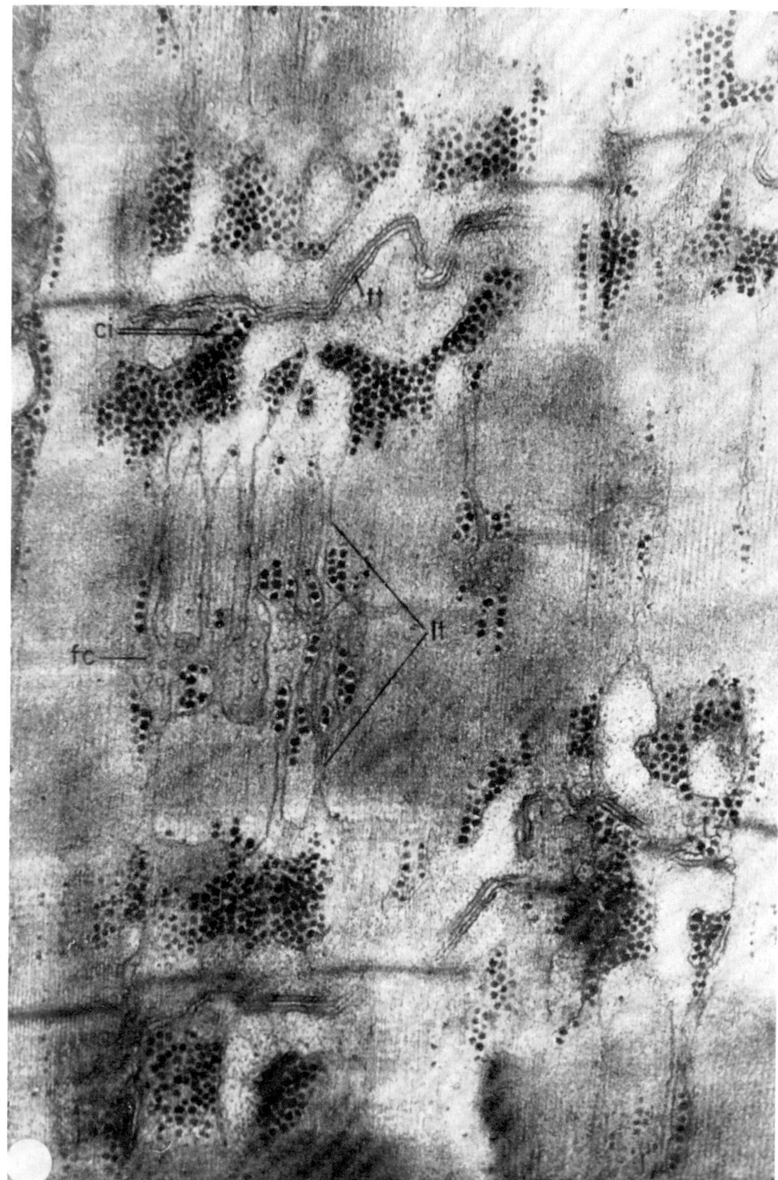

FIG. 12. Longitudinal section showing extensive face view of SR. Near *top*, transverse tubule (*tt*) can be followed for almost 2 μm as a continuous structure. Discontinuity in terminal cisterna (*ci*) is indicated. *lt*, Longitudinal tubules; *fc*, fenestrated collar. × 44,000. [From Peachey (85).]

MECHANISM OF INWARD SPREAD OF ACTIVATION

Some Physiological Properties of the T-Tubule System

One early question was whether the T-tubule membrane, like the sarcolemma, is selectively permeable to ions. Some of the experiments published as part of a series of now-classic papers by Hodgkin and Horowicz (50, 51) dealt with this problem. They reasoned that one way to estimate the accessibility of selective sites for ion permeability was to produce a sudden change in the composition of the fluid surrounding an isolated muscle fiber and to observe the changes in membrane potential measured with a microelectrode. If a sudden change in external concentration of a particular ion affected the outside membrane, it would produce an almost immediate change in membrane potential. If the tubule membrane had no permeable sites for that ion, during the sudden return to the original external concentration of the ion, the membrane potential should rapidly return to the original resting membrane potential. Since the concentration of an ion in the T-tubule space requires time to equilibrate with the external solution after a sudden change to a different concentration, there should be a slower change in membrane potential during the washout period providing the tubule membrane is permeable to the ion. Figure 15 summarizes the experimental results obtained when this idea was tested. When $[Cl^-]_o$ was suddenly decreased, depolarization responses to both the decrease and increase of $[Cl^-]_o$ had very similar time courses, indicating that the T-tubule membrane has a very low Cl permeability. A similar result was found when $[K^+]_o$ was rapidly increased. During the fast washout period the repolarization was very slow compared with the membrane potential change in response to high K concentration and Cl washout. This indicates that the T-tubule membrane is permeable to K ions. Furthermore the larger the $[K^+]_o$, the slower the response to a sudden return to low K concentration; also if fibers of different diameters are exposed to the experimental solution, the larger the diameter, the slower the time course of the repolarization response (Fig. 15). The depolarization was essentially the same for all fibers. When the volume occupied by K ions was estimated from the repolarization responses, it corresponded to 0.2%–0.5% of the fiber volume. Peachey (85) calculated from electron micrographs that the T-tubule volume is approximately 0.3% of the fiber volume. Nakajima, Nakajima, and Peachey (78) confirmed this conclusion. Using the glycerol treatment described by Howell and Jenden (54), they showed that the OFF response disappeared after the T system was disconnected from the sarcolemma. Adrian and Freygang (5) and Freygang et al. (36) expanded this type of experimental research based on the reasoning of Hodgkin and Horowicz. Their results supported the idea that the T-tubule membrane is permeable to K ions and not permeable to Cl ions, whereas the sarcolemma is permeable to both.

Some Electrophysiological Properties of the T-Tubule System

The first measurements of linear electrical properties of the frog striated skeletal muscle (sartorius) were reported in 1935 by Bozler and Cole (14) and in 1936 by Cole and Curtis (19). They obtained a capacitance of 1–2 $\mu F/cm^2$ between the inside and outside of the muscle cell. Twelve years later Katz (68) and Fatt and Katz (33) estimated a transmembrane capacitance of 6 $\mu F/cm^2$. Furthermore, in a study of the linear properties of crustacean leg muscle fibers, Fatt and Katz (34) found in some instances a capacity of approximately 40 $\mu F/cm^2$, and in the crayfish Fatt and Ginsborg (32) calculated a capacity of approximately 20 $\mu F/cm^2$. These measurements were too high for a biological dielectric membrane. Other biological membranes were known to have 1 $\mu F/cm^2$ capacitance value [for a review see Cole (18)]. The large capacitance suggested an extra membrane attached to the sarcolemma, but this membrane could not be found.

This discrepancy led Falk and Fatt (30) to propose in 1964 that the different values might be due to the

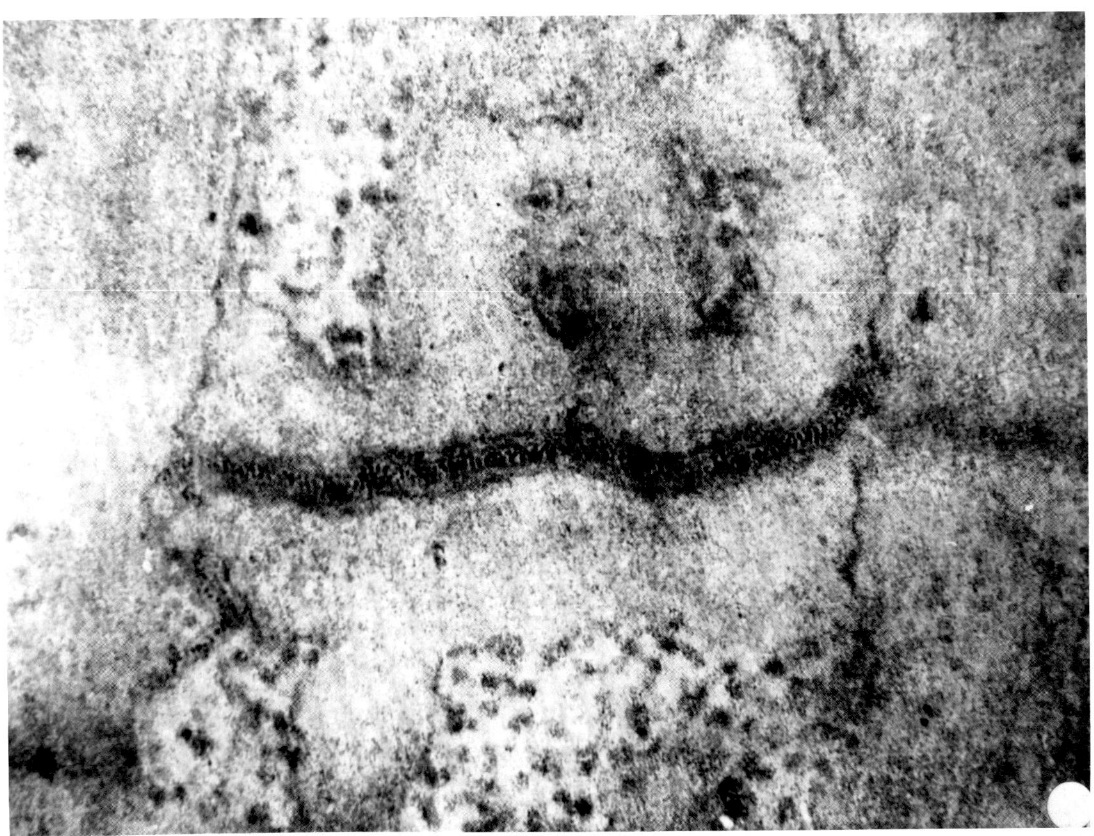

FIG. 13. Triad from muscle soaked in Ringer's solution containing 15% ferritin. Ferritin particles fill central element of triad. × 85,000. [From Page (84).]

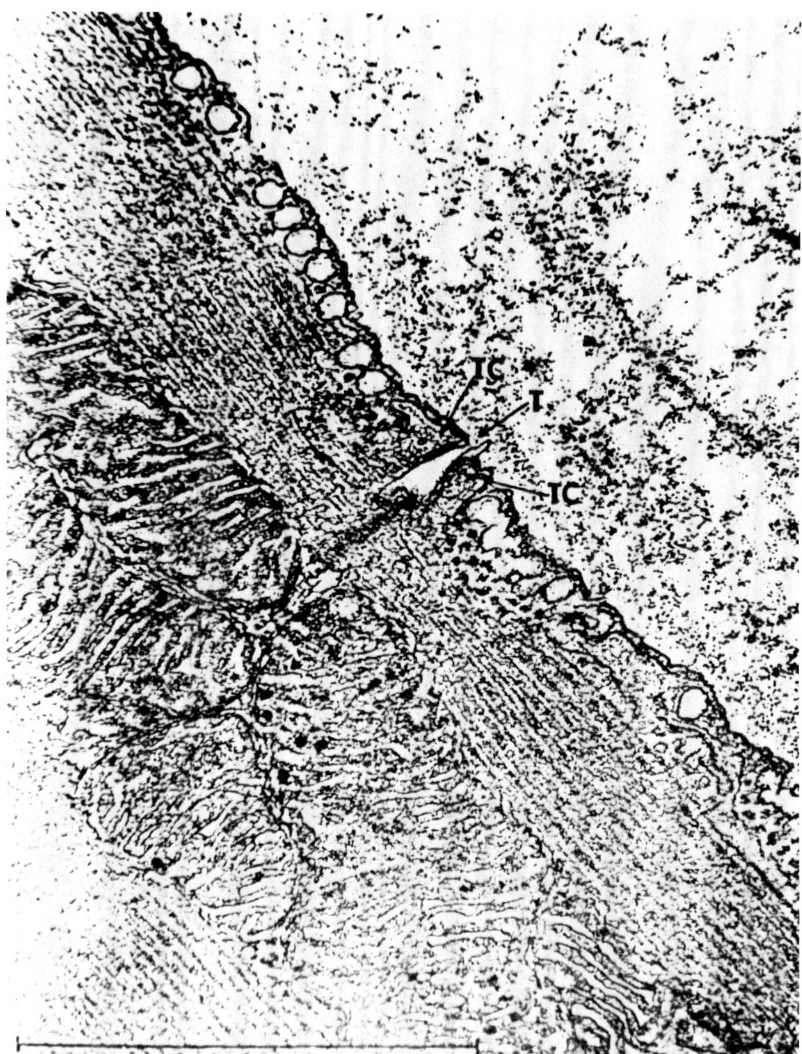

FIG. 14. Electron micrograph of longitudinal section of muscle fiber from semitendinosus muscle of a frog (*Rana temporaria*). Triad is formed by 2 terminal cisternae (*TC*) of SR adjacent to a transverse tubule (*T*). Constricted mouth of this transverse tubule suggests a possible source of access resistance. [From Peachey and Adrian (86).]

difference in technique used by the two groups as well as differences in species. The major difference in technique was that Bozler and Cole (14) and Cole and Curtis (19) calculated the capacitance from impedance measurements at frequencies between 1 kHz and 1 MHz, whereas the measurements of Katz (68) and Fatt and Katz (33) corresponded to frequencies of approximately 10 Hz.

Before pursuing the question of why different frequencies would yield such different capacitance values, the effects of AC current on resistance-capacitance (*RC*) currents are reviewed briefly. Capacitance is not measured directly; it is calculated from electric impedance measurements. In a capacitor the term capacitive reactance (X_c) takes the place of resistance to the current flow. In a series circuit composed of a capacitor and a resistor (Fig. 16*A*), the total opposition to the current flow is called impedance (*Z*) and is the sum of the resistance (*R*) due to the resistor and the reactance (X_c). When the switch (S) of the circuit is closed at time $t = 0$, there is an immediate change in voltage (V) that appears between V and V_g. With the step in voltage, there is also an immediate surge of current (*i*) that begins flowing charge onto or off the plates of the capacitor. Charge cannot cross the dielectric material, so it builds up and a voltage (V_c) appears across the plates of the capacitor. The voltage opposes the flow of charge with the same polarity, which reduces current flow in the circuit. The net result, illustrated in Figure 16*A*, *B*, is a large immediate flow in current followed by a slow exponential decline to zero. In contrast, V_c at $t = 0$ would be zero followed by an exponential growth due to the charge built up until $V_c = V$, when the current would decline to zero. When S is opened the same process is repeated but in the opposite direction, current flow reverses, and V_c declines to zero. Thus for any time *t* the current is not in phase and current will lead the voltage. Once the transient flow of current has disappeared, when there is no change in voltage, current will not flow

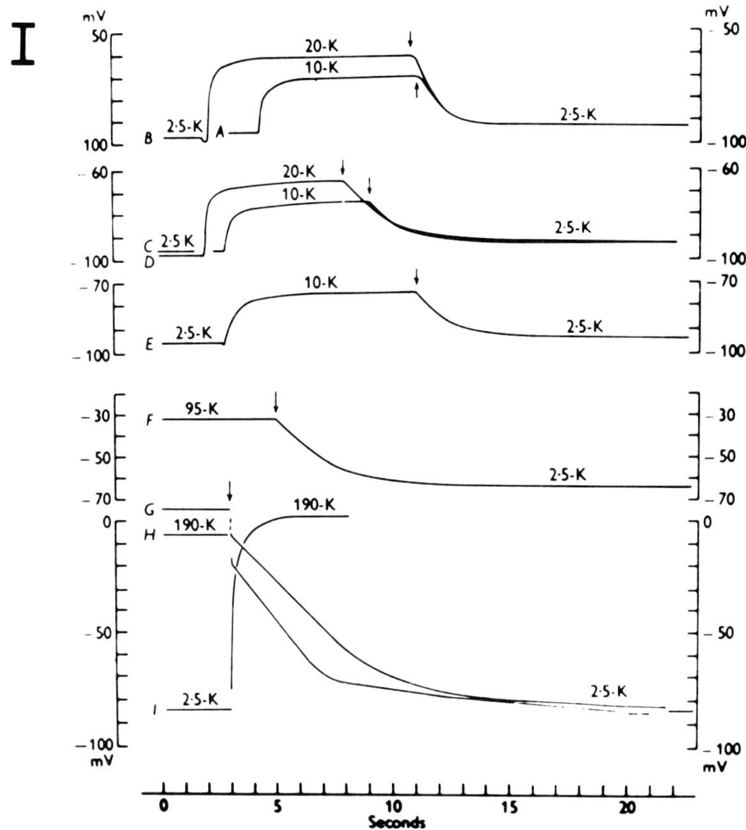

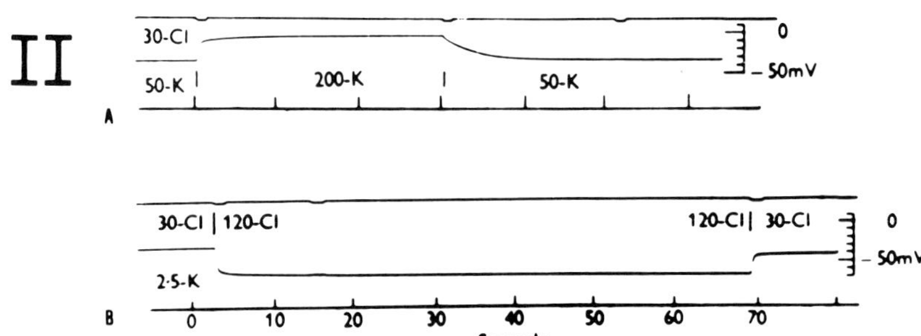

FIG. 15. Effect of changing $[K]_o$ and $[Cl]_o$ on membrane potential. *I*: repolarization in 2.5 mM K, 120 mM Cl (or 214 mM Cl) after depolarization with elevated K. Potassium concentration in mM shown on records; temperature, 18°–21°C. Corresponding fiber diameters were: A and B, 74.5 μm; C and D, 138 μm; E, 119 μm; F, 132 μm; G, 83 μm; H and I, 62 μm. B and D were shifted downward 3 and 6 mV, respectively, to superimpose end of records. In F the fiber was in high K for 1.7 min, in G for 11 min, and in H for 3 min. E and F were recorded with a microelectrode filled with 3 M KCl in the external circuit; the others were recorded with an agar-Ringer electrode externally. H and I were rescaled; the others are tracings. Fiber did not contract in any case except I, where it developed maximum tension for 1.5 s and then relaxed with a time constant of ~1 s. *II*: comparison of effect of changing $[K]_o$ at constant $[Cl]_o$ (record A) with effect of changing $[Cl]_o$ at constant $[K]_o$ (record B, 2.5 mM K). Chloride was replaced with SO_4 and K with Na. *Lower line*, internal potential; *upper line*, transducer output. Fiber diameter, 134 μm; temperature, 22°C. [From Hodgkin and Horowicz (50).]

even if V or V_c has certain constant (DC) values. Therefore from Ohm's law, the resistance for a DC applied voltage is ∞. The more rapidly the switch is connected and disconnected, the more charge will move per second and X_c will decrease. One important characteristic of X_c is its frequency dependence, which is expressed as $X_c = 1/\omega C$, where $\omega = 2\pi f$, f is the frequency at which the current is alternating, and C is the capacitance. If a sinusoidal current is applied the same equation holds, and the current leads the voltage

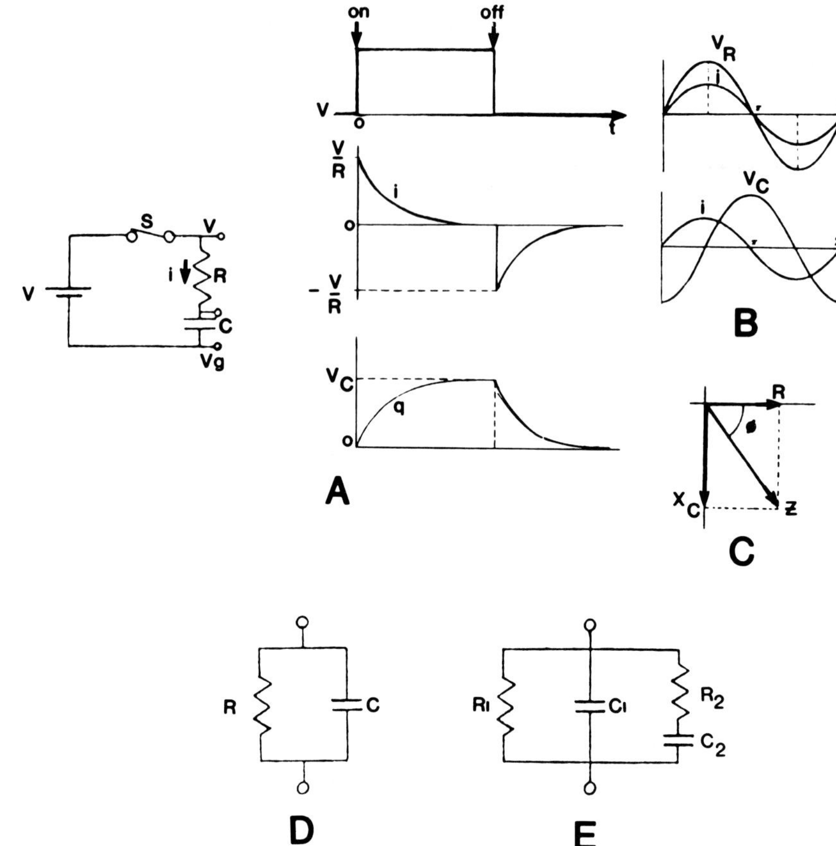

FIG. 16. Resistance (R) and capacitance (C) circuits. *Top left*, a series RC circuit with a battery (V), a switch (S), a resistor (R), and a capacitor (C). V and Vg, terminals from which measurements can be made. Direction of current flowing (i) when switch is closed is indicated. *A*: current V/R (*middle trace*) and voltage V_C (*bottom trace*) transient changes measured across the capacitor when a square voltage pulse (V on *top trace*) is applied by turning on and off S. q, Charge built up on capacitor; o, time at which S is closed; t, time. *B*: sinusoidal voltage is applied instead of a square voltage pulse as in *A*. Abscissas represent angle (=180°) between voltage recorded across resistance (V_R, *top trace*) or capacitor (V_C, *bottom trace*) and current (i). C: vectorial components of impedance (Z) resulting from resistance (R) and reactance (X_C) separated by a phase angle ϕ. *D* and *E*: 2 parallel RC circuits. *D* is a simple 2-branch parallel circuit with R and C in parallel, whereas *E* is a 3-branch circuit with R and C in parallel to each other and to the 3rd, a branch where R and C are in series with each other.

by 90° (Fig. 16*B*) and leads in the series *RC* circuit (Fig. 16*A*). The impedance is the sum of the resistance plus the reactance X_c, each having its own value. Since they differ in angle, $\boldsymbol{Z}$ can be considered the sum of two vectors (Fig. 16*C*). The current sinusoidal wave leads the voltage sinusoidal wave by an angle between 0° and 90°, depending on the ratio of resistance and capacitance. Whereas current and voltage are in phase in a purely resistive circuit, a circuit composed of both resistance and capacitance will have a phase angle that depends on the ratio of reactance to resistance. An angle with impedance vector $\boldsymbol{Z}$ will be the resultant vectorial addition of the two vectors $|\boldsymbol{X_c}|$ and $|\boldsymbol{R}|$ (Fig. 16*C*).

It follows that the phase angle (ϕ) can be calculated by $\tan \phi = |\boldsymbol{X_c}|/|\boldsymbol{R}|$. The value of ϕ will depend on the ratio of X_c to R so that when the resistance is near zero, the phase angle is nearly 90° and the impedance is almost entirely due to the reactance; however, when $R \gg X_c$, ϕ approaches zero and impedance is almost entirely due to R. There are several ways to express this dependence, but unfortunately the equations are complicated. For the purpose of this chapter, it is sufficient to realize that the absolute value of Z can be calculated with this geometric concept. In a series *RC* circuit, $Z = \sqrt{R^2 + X_c^2}$, but since $X_c^2 = (\frac{1}{2}\pi fC)^2$, then $Z = \sqrt{R^2 + 1/(2\pi fC)^2}$. Since $Z^2 = R^2 + \frac{1}{4}\pi^2 f^2 C^2$, the Z must be inversely related to the frequency of current applied to the circuit. At very high frequencies, X_c approaches zero and the circuit behaves as if composed of a resistance.

In a parallel *RC* circuit (Fig. 16*D*) the absolute impedance value can be expressed

$$|\boldsymbol{Z}| = \frac{1}{\sqrt{\frac{1}{R^2} + (2\pi fC)^2}} \tag{7}$$

There is also a phase angle between X_c and R whose value depends on the ratio of R to X_c. Since $X_c = \frac{1}{2\pi fC}$, it appears ϕ is a function of the frequency applied.

The capacitance is not measured directly but is calculated from equations similar to Equation 7 [for a more detailed discussion of the method see Falk and Fatt (30) and Cole (18)]. There are two ways to calculate the linear electrical properties. One is by plotting X_c versus R for the impedance measurement at different frequencies and then the corresponding theoretical locus impedance plots to see which best fits the experimental observation. Another way is to plot ϕ at different frequencies and measure the impedance. Provided the errors introduced are corrected (30), this method is easier to use and has better resolution [see, e.g., Freygang et al. (37) and Valdiosera et al. (99)].

If both the series and parallel circuits are combined (Fig. 16*E*), the branch that would be better seen in an impedance plot will depend on the particular frequency at which the measurement is done, the ratio of C_2/C_1, and the ratio of R_2/R_1. The analytical solution has been published by several authors (18, 24, 30, 37, 99). Falk and Fatt (30) reasoned that the discrepancies between the capacitance measurements Katz made at 10 Hz and those Cole made at 10^4 Hz could be a strong indication of an extra capacitance located in parallel with the surface membrane capacitance and lying along separate channels. They also proposed that a resistance in series, connected to one of these capacitances and not to the other, joined the two branches. The existence of an extra capacitance in the circuit was also suggested by the discovery of a capacitance of 20 μF/cm^2 in crayfish (32) and of 40 μF/cm^2 in crab muscles (34). There seemed to be a correlation between capacitance per unit area of muscle fiber surface and fiber diameter, suggesting the excess capacity could arise from channels running from the surface to the center of the fiber. They reasoned that the presence of an *RC* circuit with two time constants could be detected by measuring impedance over a frequency range of 1-10^3 Hz. This measurement was made by passing current through a microelectrode and recording the voltage with another microelectrode somewhere in the center of the fiber, very carefully shielding the microelectrodes, the gap between them, and the cables to eliminate the stray capacitance that might appear in the system. The quantitative analysis of the experimental data considered the correction of remaining stray capacitance. Falk and Fatt (30) presented their results as an *X-R* plot of impedance measurements (Fig. 17). They chose the *X-R* plot instead of a plot of the magnitude of *Z* against phase angle ϕ because it let them weigh all the points equally. The experimental error introduced is constant for all points in the *X-R* plot, whereas in a *Z*-ϕ plot (ref. 30, Fig. 9) the error varies with frequency. Figure 17 shows the characteristic impedance of a muscle fiber between a point in the fiber and the outside for the frog sartorius in a complex-plane plot. Two theoretical impedance loci are shown in Figure 17*A*, one for an *RC* parallel circuit with one time constant and the other for a two-branch circuit with two time constants (one *RC* in series connected to an *RC* in parallel). Although at high frequencies (above 10 kHz) and at very low frequencies (below 5 Hz) the two loci are similar, they clearly differ at all intermediate frequencies. The difference is more obvious at around 100 Hz. In Figure 17*B* the experimental measurements, corrected for stray capacitances, are shown as dots superimposed on the theoretical curve for the model with two time constants, drawn as a continuous line. They concluded that the twitch muscle cells are composed of two branches, one representing the surface membrane R_m and C_m and the other corresponding to the inner channels with R_e and C_e in series. The R_e and C_e are in parallel with R_m and C_m.

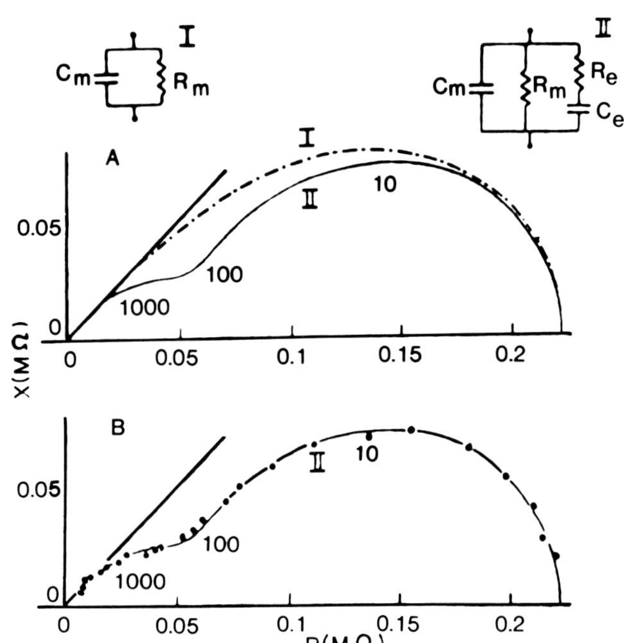

FIG. 17. Impedance-locus plots. *A*: theoretical impedance locus. *Dot-dashed line*, impedance locus for model of inside-outside admittance shown at *upper left* (*I*), fitted to limiting value of R obtained at low frequencies. *Solid line*, locus for more complicated model with 2 time constants of inside-outside admittance shown at *upper right* (*II*), with additional parameters R_e/R_m and C_e/C_m adjusted to give best fit of observations. *B*: impedance-locus plots obtained with intracellular microelectrodes from frog sartorius muscle fiber. Current-applying and voltage-recording electrodes were placed close together distant from the fiber ends. *Filled circles*, after correction for stray capacitances around microelectrodes. Measurements made at frequencies (6/decade) from 1 cycle/s to 10 kilocycles/s; frequencies (cycles/s) are labeled on a few points. Theoretical impedance locus for model with 2 time constants is superimposed (*solid line*). [Adapted from Falk and Fatt (30).]

Mechanism of Inward Spread of the Excitatory Process

Falk and Fatt (30) questioned the location of R_e and C_e in the inner channels and proposed that C_e and R_e

arose from two adjacent membranes presumably in the triad. The C_e would come from the membrane forming the wall of the middle element of the triad, and the R_e would arise from the membrane belonging to the lateral element of the triads. The model represented the path between the adjacent walls of the T tubules to the TC (C_e), into the TC, and from the SR to the myoplasm (R_e).

Several questions then arise, particularly since the resistance R_x of the inner path of the tubules (inner part of the T tubules is connected to the external solution) is considered very low. Given this type of circuit, what would be the delay of activation between the surface membrane action potential and a potential across the C_e-R_e branch (29, 30)? What would be the mechanism of the inward spread of activation of the excitatory process along the tubule system? Since diffusion of a substance was ruled out as a mechanism of inward spread of activation, two possible mechanisms exist to carry the mechanical triggering information from the surface to the center of the fiber. Either the action potential is confined to the sarcolemma and the inward spread occurs by passive electronic conduction through the tubules or the sarcolemmal action potential propagates along the T system and produces an electrical regenerative tubule action potential traveling toward the center of the fiber. If the length constant of the T-tubule system (λ_T) in the muscle cell is as large or several times larger than the radius (a) of a fiber, a tubule action potential is not essential to spread from the surface to the axis and activate the whole cross section of a muscle fiber. If $\lambda_T < a$, however, for the whole cross section to be activated a regenerative depolarization must travel along the T tubules.

For a contraction to occur, the relevant surface membrane potential must reach mechanical threshold, which in this case is approximately −55 mV (51). Thus, in order for the whole cross-sectional area of a muscle cell to be mechanically activated, the tubular membrane potential in the axis of the fiber must be at or below −55 mV. For a steady passive depolarization there is a drop in the tubular membrane potential between the surface and the axis of the fiber produced by the leak of current across the tubular membrane. How much more the surface potential must be depolarized for the axis tubular membrane to be at −55 mV depends on the value of λ_T.

Consider a very simple situation, the space constant for the tubule $\lambda_T^2 = \bar{G}_L/\bar{G}_w$, where $\bar{G}_w$ is the conductance of the tubule walls per unit volume and $\bar{G}_L$ is the conductance of the tubule lumen per unit length (2). According to the model proposed by Falk and Fatt (30), later called model 1 by Falk (29), if $\bar{G}_L$ is very large and $\bar{G}_w$ is relatively small then λ_T would be very large, several times larger than a. Sandow (92) estimated the fractional value of a sarcolemmal potential would be 0.82 at the axis of a fiber with a radius of 50 μm. Since electronic propagation of current was enough to reach the axis, if the surface membrane potential had been depolarized from, for example, −90 mV to approximately +20 mV, the tubules in the axis of the fiber should have had a membrane potential of +3.5 mV, well beyond mechanical threshold. A regenerative signal traveling down the tubule system to reach the center of the fiber was not needed for full mechanical activation. That alone, however, was not a necessary or sufficient condition to rule out the tubule action potential.

According to the model for two time constants, the delay between the activation of surface myofibrils and of central myofibrils (those in the axis of the fiber) should be negligible [see Valdiosera et al. (99)]. This means the excitatory signal must travel along the T-system membranes at a very high velocity and all the myofibrils in the cross section are activated instantaneously during a twitch. The equivalent network proposed in 1964 by Falk and Fatt (30) represented a lumped circuit. To include possible delays of activation between surface and axial myofibrils as reported by Gonzalez-Serratos (40) in 1966, Falk (29) represented the same network in a distributed fashion in model 1. The delay discussed for either type of network was between the T tubules and the TC and provided no interval between the activation of superficial and axial myofibrils.

If an experimental technique allowing a direct measurement of the activation of individual myofibrils could be found, the existence of a delay in activation of superficial and central myofibrils could be verified. Measurement of the speed of the inward spread of activation during a twitch might also be possible. Unfortunately the most straightforward feature of the microscopic appearance of an isolated skeletal muscle fiber, the striations, cannot be used to indicate the onset of activation. At or above the slack length of a fiber, Huxley and Niedergerke (62) showed that the relative changes in width of A and I bands depend only on the length of the fiber and are the same during active shortening or during passive stretch and release. Therefore above 2.0–2.1 μm per sarcomere space [Brown, Gonzalez-Serratos, and Huxley (16)], if a few superficial myofibrils shorten actively, they affect the striation spacings of the more radial myofibrils due to mechanical coupling and shorten them passively [see also Huxley and Gordon (61)]. Hence changes in striation spacings per se are not reliable indicators of activity.

In 1966 and 1971 Gonzalez-Serratos (40, 42) approached the solution of this problem by expanding observations during DC stimulation (61) and during potassium contractures (39), showing that some myofibrils close to the surface appeared straight, whereas others near the axis of the fiber were wavy. The straight myofibrils apparently were undergoing an active contraction, whereas the wavy ones were being passively shortened. An isolated muscle fiber was placed in gelatin, and the block of gelatin was compressed along the fiber axis until all the myofibrils were wavy. The fiber was stimulated electrically to produce a twitch. Under stimulation the active myofibrils would straighten and the others would remain wavy. The entire process was recorded with high-speed cinemicrophotography. The cinemicrographs showed a clear delay in activation between the superficial and central myofibrils (see Fig. 18). The time course of the decrease in wave height from superficial and central myofibrils was measured as shown in Figure 19*A*. The velocity of the inward spread of the tubular excitatory process was calculated from the delay of activation between a given superficial myofibril and a central one and from the distance that separated them. Figure 19*A* also shows the delay for the same myofibrils decreased as the temperature increases. In other words, the propagation velocity of the tubule excitatory process increases with increased temperature. In this particular case the calculated velocities were 2.4, 3.1, and 6.9 cm/s at 6°, 12°, and 19°C, respectively, and the corresponding measured delays were 3.13, 2.2, and 1.3 ms. The average velocity of inward propagation along the T system obtained from the experimental results was 7 cm/s at 20°C. Figure 19*B* shows the relationship between the velocity of inward spread of activation and the temperature.

From these data a Q_{10} of 2.13 can be calculated. It was also shown (ref. 41, Fig. 40; ref. 42, plate 4) that when the propagation of the twitch along the longitudinal axis of the fiber failed (indicating failure of the sarcolemmal action potential propagation), it was accompanied by a failure of radial propagation. This was in clear contrast to the whole cross-sectional activation seen during normal twitches.

If the tubule membrane is assumed to have the same properties as the surface membrane, then the velocity (θ_T) at which an action potential should travel along the T system can be calculated. If the specific electric membrane properties, the current density through the membrane during the action potential, and its time course remain the same for fibers of different diameters, then the velocity of the surface action potential (θ_s) can be written as $\theta_s^2 = k\text{D}$ where D is the diameter of the fiber and k is a constant (48, 69). This constant can be calculated from the results of Katz (68), with θ_s^2 and D measured in frog muscle fibers, and it is of the order of 43×10^4 m/s^2. Since it was assumed that the tubules have the same properties as the surface membrane, with the calculated k and a diameter of 0.05 μm for the tubules (85), θ_T should be about 5 cm/s, which is of the same order of magnitude as the velocity of inward activation ob-

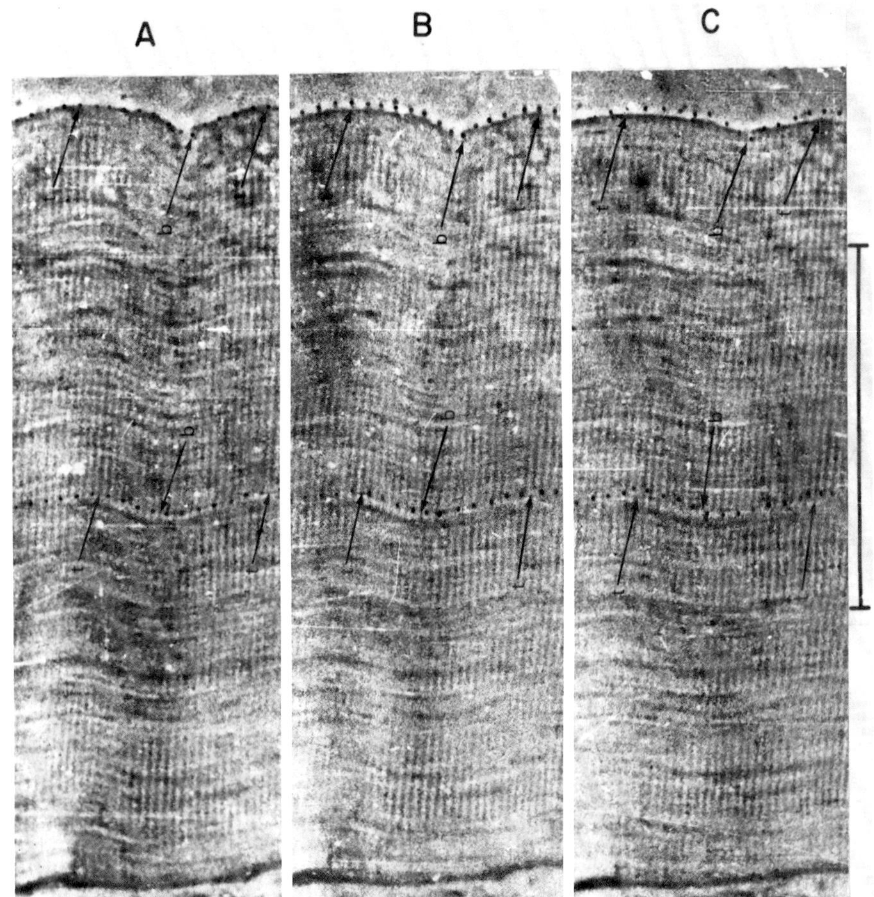

FIG. 18. Delay of activation between superficial and central myofibrils. *A*: wavy myofibrils before stimulation; *dots* have been drawn over a myofibril on edge and near center. *Arrows t* and *b* indicate top and bottom of waves, respectively, in *A–C*. *B* and *C*: wavy myofibrils, with *dots* drawn in exactly the same positions as in *A*. In *B*, edge myofibril has started to contract, whereas myofibril near center has same height as before. In *C*, height of central myofibril has decreased compared with *dots*, showing it has begun to flatten. Time interval between *B* and *C*, 2.5 ms; calibration bar, 100 μm. [From Gonzalez-Serratos (42).]

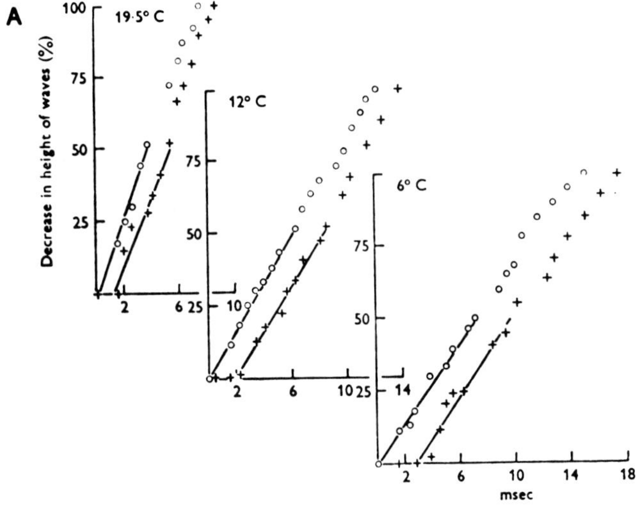

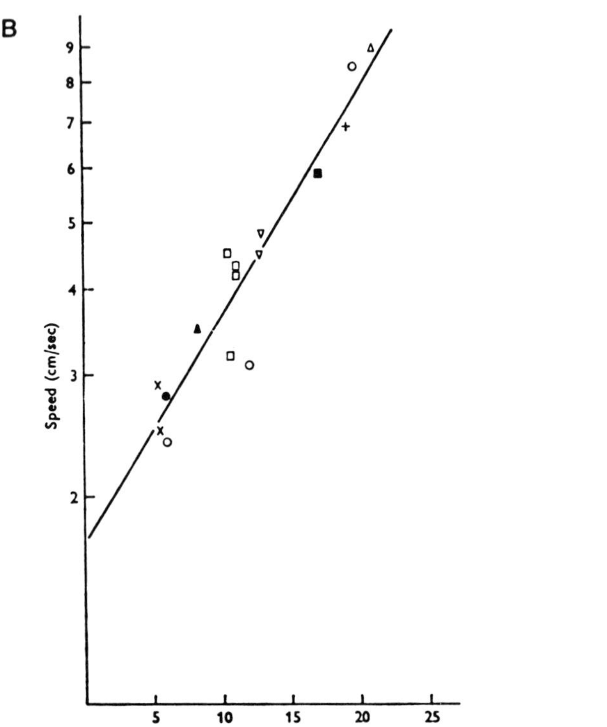

FIG. 19. Velocity of inward spread of activation and effect of temperature. *A*: time course of straightening of myofibrils of same fiber but at different temperatures. ○, Myofibrils near surface; ×, myofibrils near center. *B*: relationship between velocity of inward spread of activation and temperature. Velocity is on logarithmic scale. Each symbol indicates a different experiment. [From Gonzalez-Serratos (42).]

tained experimentally. All this indicated for the first time that the propagation of the excitatory process along the tubules was probably a regenerative process like an action potential rather than a passive one.

Another indication of a regenerative action potential traveling along the T system came from the experiments published in 1967 by Sugi and Ochi (98). They showed that when several sarcomeres were covered by a macropipette for passing current, similar to the one used by Huxley and collaborators, stimulation caused a contraction to spread around the perimeter of the fiber at a velocity of 0.8–6 cm/s at room temperature. Strickholm (97) found that a local contraction could also spread across the center of the fiber.

In 1980 Nakajima and Gilai (72) used an entirely different approach to measure the radial conduction velocity of the wave of depolarization through the T system. They studied what they called the "optical action potential" of isolated muscle cells from *Xenopus*. They measured absorption signals from the muscle fibers stained with potential-sensitive dyes rhodanine and merocyanine oxazolone, as described in their earlier paper (74). Since these dyes do not penetrate the cell membrane, clearly the optical signals that appear during stimulation come from combined sarcolemmal and T-system membranes and not from the SR. Stimulation caused several optical changes, but the first wave seemed to represent the action potential. When the optical and intracellular action potentials were recorded simultaneously, the optical wave was slower than the action potential. The peak of the electrical recorded action potential appeared 0.55 ms earlier than the peak of the optical wave. They interpreted the slowness of the optical wave as being due to the contribution of the action potential spread radially along the T system. When the velocity (θ) of inward spread of the tubule action potential was calculated by obtaining the best fit between the optical signal and the delay along the T tubules of the electrical signal due to a given θ, they found that at 24°C the best fit was obtained with a tubule conduction velocity of 6.4 cm/s when an access delay of 133 μs was introduced. This radial conduction velocity agrees with the value Gonzalez-Serratos (42) had obtained earlier. A simple explanation of the results of Nakajima and Gilai was that the assumptions on which Gonzalez-Serratos' conclusion and their analysis were based are probably correct.

If inward propagation is determined by an electrotonic current flow, a different equivalent electric circuit of the T system must be devised to accommodate the delays described above. Falk (29) calculated the responses of three electrical models based on the circuits proposed earlier by Falk and Fatt (30) and discussed the results in relation to data Gonzalez-Serratos (40, 41) had presented in 1966 and 1967. The delay in the first model was between the T tubules and the TC. This model therefore provides no interval between activation of superficial and central myofibrils and is excluded by the results just described and those of Adrian, Costantin, and Peachey (4), Costantin (21), and Hodgkin and Nakajima (52, 53). The other models introduced a finite lag in the inward conduction by assuming a finite resistance along the T tubules, appearing in series with the capacity of the tubule membrane. In the second model, when the entire series resistance was placed in the tubules, the calculated delays were too great. In model 3 much of the series resistance was placed outside the tubule and therefore did not contribute to the lag in inward conduction; with the actual values taken from the paper, the calculated delays are too small. It appeared that a case intermediate between models 2 and 3 might be selected to match the experimental delays, but it is not obvious whether it would satisfactorily fit all aspects of impedance measurements.

At around the same time Adrian, Chandler, Costantin, Hodgkin, and Peachey were interested in the same types of problems. Their approach was to control the voltage across the sarcolemma using a two-microelectrode voltage-clamp system, as described previously by Costantin (20), and to study the electrophysiological responses of the T-tubule system to step depolarizations of the surface membrane. Although Adrian, Chandler, and Hodgkin (2) were primarily interested in the kinetics of mechanical activation studied by changing several parameters of the depolarization pulses, they questioned how quickly and completely a sudden change in the sarcolemma potential would spread along the tubule system. They expanded the theoretical treatment used earlier by Falk. Assuming that the chloride conductance was uniformly spread throughout the membrane system, the calculated tubule space constant for a fiber with a radius of 40 μm would be 100 μm. Conversely, if most of the chloride conductance was localized in the surface membrane as proposed by Eisenberg and Gage (23), the estimated λ_T would be about 170 μm. In theory there was no need for a tubule action potential to activate all myofibrils in the cross-sectional area of a fiber. At the same time, Adrian, Costantin, and Peachey (4) designed an experimental method to estimate λ_T. By knowing the solution of the steady-state equation of tubule transmembrane potential as a function of the degree of radial penetration and sarcolemmal depolarization, the first step was to find the sarcolemmal membrane potential that produced the first signs of mechanical threshold in most superficial myofibrils. Once this value was determined, the membrane potential was decreased further to find the necessary superficial displacement required for the radial myofibrils to reach mechanical threshold. To control the membrane potential, the fiber was bathed with Ringer's solution containing tetrodotoxin (TTX), and the membrane potential was displaced to the desired values with the two-microelectrode voltage-clamp system (2, 20). Since the longitudinal space constant is much larger than the fiber circumference, the depolarization would be nearly uniform around the circumference of the fiber sarcolemma even though it would not be uniform along the longitudinal axis. They chose the changes of sarcomere spaces as a signal of mechanical activation; presumably sarcomere shortening would indicate mechanical activation. Once these two values were obtained and the radius of the fiber was measured, they could be applied to a particular solution of the steady-state equation for displacement of the tubule transmembrane potential, given previously by Adrian et al. (2). From this equation and experimental measurements, the value of λ_T could be estimated.

The partial differential equation of displacement of transmembrane potential along the tubule walls of the T system was given by Adrian et al. (2). The equation describes the change in tubule transmembrane potential (u) from its value at rest at any radial distance r from the fiber longitudinal axis in the center as follows

$$\kappa \frac{\partial^2 u}{\partial r^2} + \frac{\kappa}{r}\frac{\partial u}{\partial r} = \frac{u}{\tau_w} + \frac{\partial u}{\partial t} \tag{8}$$

where κ is the ratio of effective radial conductivity of tubule lumen per unit of fiber length ($\bar{G}_L$) to the capacitance of tubular membrane per unit of fiber volume ($\bar{C}_w$). Since the dimensions of $\bar{G}_L$ are in siemens per centimeter and those of $\bar{C}_w$ are in farads per cubic centimeter, $\kappa = \bar{G}_L/\bar{C}_w$ in square centimeters per second and is called the propagation constant. The time constant of the tubule walls τ_w is therefore defined as $\bar{C}_w/\bar{G}_w$; $\bar{G}_w$ is the conductance of the tubule membrane per unit of fiber volume (S/cm^3).

A steady-state solution of Equation 8 was given first by Falk (29) and then by Adrian et al. (2). The simplified solution given by Adrian et al. (4) expressed the ratio of change of tubule transmembrane potential (u_r) anywhere in a radial direction along the T tubules, to the degree of change of steady-state depolarization u_a at the surface of a fiber of radius a ($r = a$) as follows

$$\frac{u_r}{u_a} = \frac{I_0(r/\lambda_T)}{I_0(a/\lambda_T)} \tag{9}$$

where I_0 is the zero-order hyperbolic Bessel function. If λ_T is known, the change u_r can be predicted for a given u_a and radius a. The question, however, was which λ_T to choose. In the same paper λ_T was calculated for $a = 40$ μm from

$$R_T = \frac{\lambda_T I_0(a/\lambda_T)}{\bar{G}_L I_1(a/\lambda_T)} \tag{10}$$

where R_T is the resistance of the tubule system referred to the unit area of fiber surface in ohms per square centimeter and I_1 is the first-order hyperbolic Bessel function. With this equation, λ_T was 100 μm when the electric characteristics of the surface and tubule membranes were assumed to be identical. When the resting conductance was divided between the fiber surface and the T system in proportion to their areas, λ_T was reduced to 81 μm; when all the potassium conductance and 25% of the chloride conductance were assigned to the T system, λ_T was increased to 105 μm. They calculated the steady-state potential change across the tubule walls in a 50-μm-radius fiber for λ_T between the limits of 120 and 60 μm. The corresponding profiles of steady-state potential change for $\mu_a = 35$ mV, a depolarization from −90 to −55 mV on the surface membrane ($r = a$), are shown in Figure 20*A*. If the tubule space constant was 60 μm it would be necessary to depolarize the tubule walls at the center of the fiber ($r = 0$) another 5–6 mV to reach a tubule membrane potential value similar to mechanical threshold (U_t). Therefore if the myofibrils were activated at all points where the T-tubule membrane potential reached mechanical threshold (U_t), then the surface depolarization V_c (at $r = a$) required for mechanical threshold to be reached in the center of the fiber (at $r = 0$) would be expressed by

$$U_t/V_c = \frac{1}{I_0(a/\lambda_T)} \tag{11}$$

Adrian, Costantin, and Peachey (4) further reasoned that if mechanical threshold was the same all along the T system, U_t would be equal to the surface depolarization necessary to activate the most superficial myofibrils (V_s). They concluded that by measuring the depolarization needed to just reach mechanical activation for the most superficial myofibrils (V_s) and how much more the sarcolemma should be depolarized (V_c) to see the first signs of myofibril contraction in the axis of the fiber (i.e., the surface depolarization needed to just activate the entire cross section), λ_T could be estimated from these experimental measurements applied to the last equation.

After obtaining the necessary experimental observations, they concluded that λ_T was larger than the radius of the fiber and varied with it (Fig. 20*B*). For example, for a fiber having a radius of 50 μm, λ_T would be 79 μm [Fig. 6 and Table 2 of Adrian et al. (4)]. They reported that by injecting artificial action potentials through the microelectrode for passing current in the presence of TTX, the magnitude of the action potentials was just enough to activate the entire cross-sectional area. Therefore this short-lasting depolarization would have a very small safety factor. Although this did not rule out the existence of a tubule action potential, it did suggest the inward spread of a regenerative process along the T system was not necessary to excite the entire cross section.

Gonzalez-Serratos (39, 41) had found earlier that during isotonic potassium contractures some centrally located myofibrils apparently were not activated. Based on this observation, he later proposed (43) this might indicate that during steady depolarizations beyond mechanical threshold λ_T was less than a. If so, the amount of depolarization needed to reach mechanical threshold would be independent of fiber diameter,

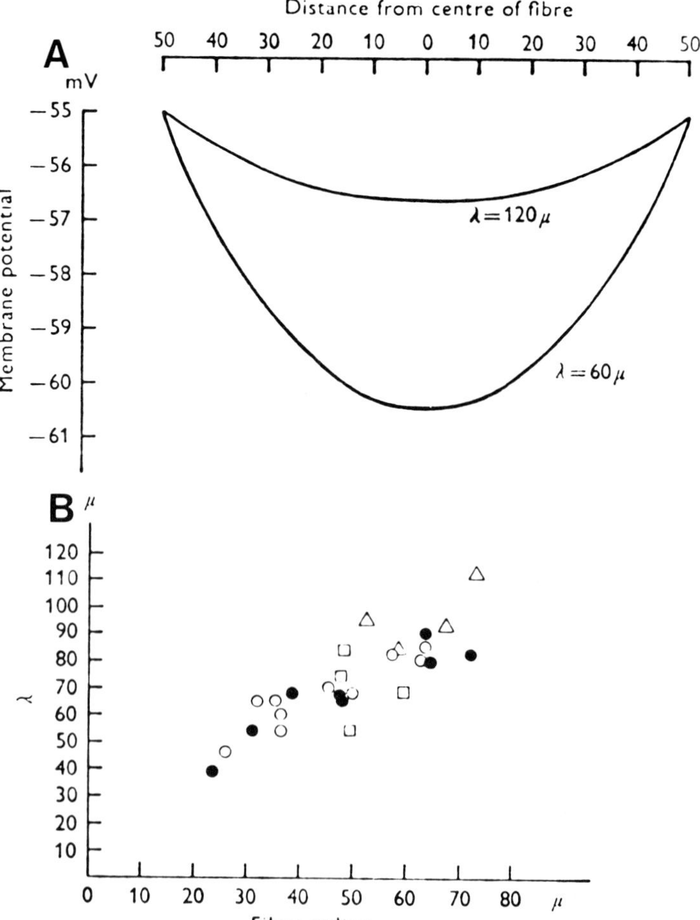

FIG. 20. Tubular space constant. *A*: steady-state potential across wall of tubule system [Eq. 2 of Adrian et al. (4)] when potential difference across surface membrane of fiber is altered from −90 to −55 mV (u_a = 35 mV; see Eq. 11). Potential distribution is shown for 2 tubule length constants (λ_T, 120 and 60 μm). Diameter of fiber is 100 μm. *B*: calculated values of λ_T [based on experimental results applied to Eq. 3 of Adrian et al. (4)] plotted against fiber radius. *Open circles*, fibers in Ringer's solution; *filled circles*, fibers in hypotonic Ringer's solution; *open triangles*, fibers in tetraethylammonium Ringer's solution; *open squares*, fibers in sucrose Ringer's solution. [From Adrian et al. (4).]

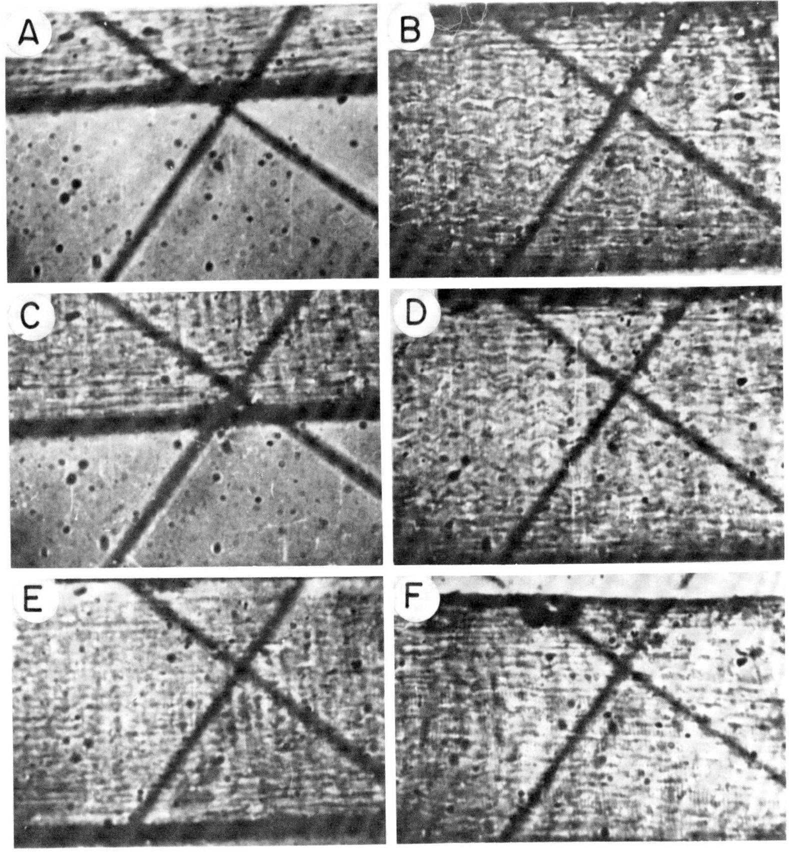

FIG. 21. Sample photomicrographs from a cinerecording selected at different times during isotonic contracture in 60 mM K. Sample pictures selected at following times after contracture started: *A*, 0.43 s; *C*, 0.65 s; *E*, 0.78 s; *B*, 2.2 s; *D*, 2.3 s; and *F*, 3.7 s. Contracture reached plateau between *D* and *F*. Elongation due to relaxation started in *F*. Shortening of fiber can be followed as a movement to *right* of any piece of connective tissue. During tetanic stimulation with 50 shocks/s fiber shortened same amount but myofibrils remained straight without forming waves. Calibration bar, 100 μm; temperature, 5°C. [From Gonzalez-Serratos (43).]

but the depolarization needed to produce maximal tension would vary with fiber diameter. This hypothesis was tested in isolated muscle fibers by producing uniform steady depolarizations with different concentrations of external potassium; the force or the shortening produced by the contractures was recorded with cinemicrophotography or with an isometric transducer. The isotonic contractures developed axial wavy myofibrils when the sarcomere spacings decreased below 2 μm (Fig. 21), indicating that the central core of myofibrils was less than fully activated or not activated at all. The measurement of sarcomere spaces in the wavy myofibrils suggested that they were not activated. The isometric contractures showed the membrane potential V_t at which mechanical threshold was reached averaged -48.85 ± 2.65 mV in 14 fibers whose diameters varied from 30.4 to 82.4 μm. In contrast the membrane potential V_m at which maximum tension was reached varied from -12.5 mV for the larger fibers to -30 mV for the smaller ones. Therefore the span between V_t and V_m decreased as the fiber radius became shorter. The relationship $V_m - V_t$ against a gave a slope of 6.1 mV/10 μm: i.e., for each 10-μm increment in fiber radius for a, it would be necessary to depolarize the surface membrane by another 6.1 mV to obtain maximal tension. Assuming that part of the increment $V_m - V_t$ was required for going from mechanical threshold to maximum tension by a given group of myofibrils at any position within the fiber and that λ_T is independent of a, λ_T was roughly estimated with the same type of equation (Eq. 11) proposed by Adrian et al. (4)

$$V_c = V_{sm} I_0(a/\lambda_T) \qquad (12)$$

where V_c is the resting membrane potential minus V_m and V_{sm} represents the depolarization required for maximal activation of myofibrils at any point in the fiber. Here V_{sm} was estimated as the value V_c for $a = 0$ by extrapolating the regression line calculated from the experimental results of V_c against a to $a = 0$, as shown in Figure 22. When different values of λ_T were computed with Equation 12, it was found that taking λ_T as 26 μm, the regression line of V_c against a could be roughly fit with $I_0(a/\lambda_T)$.

There are difficulties in the experimental measurement of λ_T attempted with steady depolarizations. The work of Adrian et al. (4) indicated mechanical coupling between the superficial and central myofibrils during the contraction. In their study and in that of Gonzalez-Serratos (43) the membrane potential was depolarized beyond the value where membrane conductance increases appreciably (delayed rectification) as de-

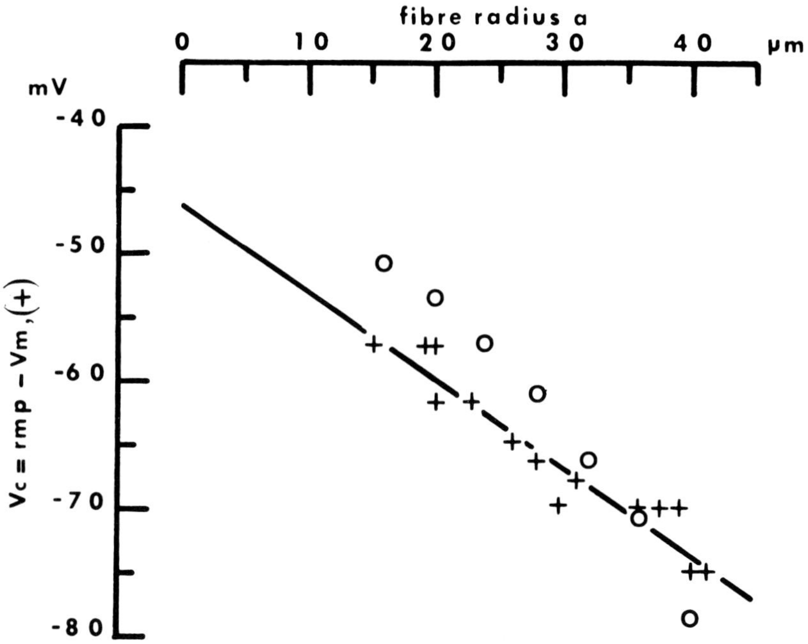

FIG. 22. Relationship between V_c and fiber radius a. *Crosses*, experimental results. *Continuous line*, regression line of V_c against a. *Circles* correspond to $V_c = V_s J_0(a/\lambda_T)$ when $V_s = V_{sm}$ at $a = 0$, which is 46.2 mV and $\lambda_T = 26\mu m$. Values of a chosen were similar to ones found experimentally.

scribed by Nakajima, Iwasaki, and Obata (76) and Costantin (20). This might change $\bar{G}_w$ and therefore λ_T, making the inward spread less effective than predicted by the theory (2, 4). In Gonzalez-Serratos' study another problem was the diffusion of K^+ up the tubules. Although this process is slow, it could influence the results. In general it is doubtful whether the transmembrane potential across the T tubules in the core around the axis of the fiber is clamped. Adrian and Peachey (6) calculated that the potential across the tubule membrane in the axis region would not be controlled by voltage-clamping steps imposed on the surface membrane.

The normal triggering mechanism for contractions is not a prolonged sarcolemmal depolarization but a brief depolarization and repolarization, the action potential. The cable theory, as demonstrated by Hodgkin and Nakajima (52, 53, 75) predicts that a brief exponential depolarization like the foot of the action potential would spread less effectively than a prolonged depolarization. They calculated the space constant during the foot of the action potential (λ_{Tf}), would be approximately 6–8 μm; therefore only a small outer ring of the tubular network would be effectively depolarized at high frequencies.

In 1970 Costantin (21) pointed out that although the measurements of λ_T done by Adrian, Costantin, and Peachey (4) indicated $\lambda_T > a$, delayed rectification might be present in the T tubules and the findings of Gonzalez-Serratos (40–42) were possibly more compatible with a regenerative process traveling along the tubules. Since the experiments of Adrian et al. (4) were done in the presence of TTX, the existence of a sodium-regenerative process in the T tubules in normal muscle fibers could not be ruled out. Costantin (21) therefore repeated the experiments done by Adrian et al. (4) with fibers bathed by Ringer's solution containing different sodium concentrations and no TTX. The pattern of mechanical activation differed from that found previously in the presence of TTX. With prolonged depolarizations (200 ms) in Ringer's solution, with 50% sodium once the depolarization needed to just activate the superficial myofibrils was reached, either the entire cross section of the fiber became activated or 1–2 mV of further depolarization were required. With brief depolarizations (2–5 ms) the same results were obtained in some fibers, but in others the more centrally located myofibrils were activated before the superficial ones (Fig. 23). The radial spread of contraction could be reduced by either lowering the external sodium concentration or by adding TTX to the bathing solution. These results clearly indicated that a sodium current in the T-tubule membrane contributed to the tubule spread of the excitatory process, as in an action potential. They strongly supported the existence of a sodium-regenerative process in T tubules.

The results of Adrian et al. (4) led Bezanilla, Caputo, Gonzalez-Serratos, and Venosa (12) to reason that if the spread of an excitatory process along the tubules is purely passive and the safety factor for a short depolarization like the action potential is very small, then decreasing the amplitude of the action potential by lowering the external Na^+ concentration should lead to incomplete activation of the fiber. This should diminish twitch tension or cause the appearance of nonactivated myofibrils. On the other hand, if there was an action potential in the tubules, twitch tension should be unchanged when external sodium concentration was lowered, provided there was sufficient Na^+ for generating an action potential. Because of the large area of tubule membrane and its geometric disposition, described in 1965 by Peachey (85), fast repetitive stimulation at low external sodium concentration should deplete the tubules of Na^+ below the concentration necessary to produce the tubule action potential. Bezanilla et al. (12) could distinguish between these possibilities by recording force development of a single fiber during a twitch and at high-frequency tetanic stimulation and by cinemicrophotographic recording during isotonic twitches and tetanic stimulations. Both types of experiments were done with normal and low external sodium concentrations. In low-sodium solutions, twitch tension was not modified very much. Tetanic tension was also initially similar to that in a normal-sodium Ringer's solution but then fell smoothly to a new, much lower level during the rest of the stimulation. During the isotonic contractions in low external sodium concentrations, wavy myofibrils appeared in the center of the fiber and spread toward the periphery (Fig. 24). Initially the central wavy myofibrils actively contracted but later became inactive. Wavy myofibrils never appear in normal Ringer's solution under the conditions used in these experiments. Action potentials recorded during the tetanic stimulation in normal Ringer's solution decreased in size as stimulation continued. Their magnitude could be the same or smaller than those recorded during tetanic stimulation in low-sodium Ringer's solution when mechanical inactivation had already appeared, indicating that the presence of inactive myofibrils was not due to changes in the size of the action potential in low sodium. The results were explained on the basis of Na^+ depletion in the more central region of the tubule network that would decrease the sodium concentration in this area below the concentration necessary to produce action potentials. The results further supported the proposition that the tubule membrane undergoes an increase in Na^+ permeability during activation, and the increase in permeability can be regenerative.

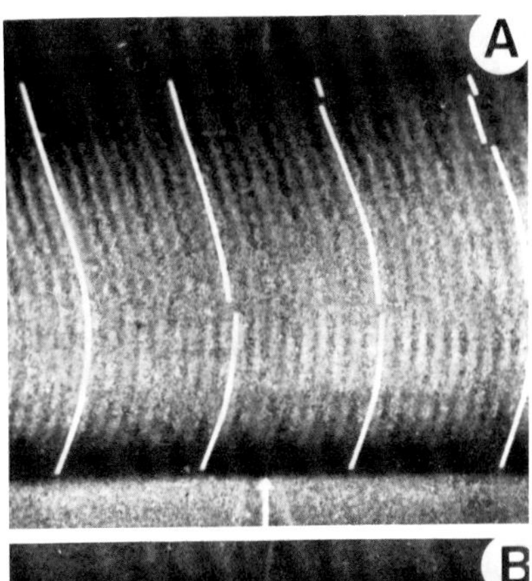

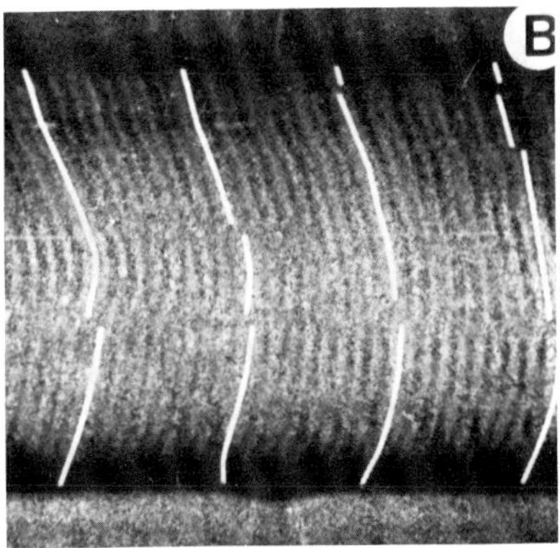

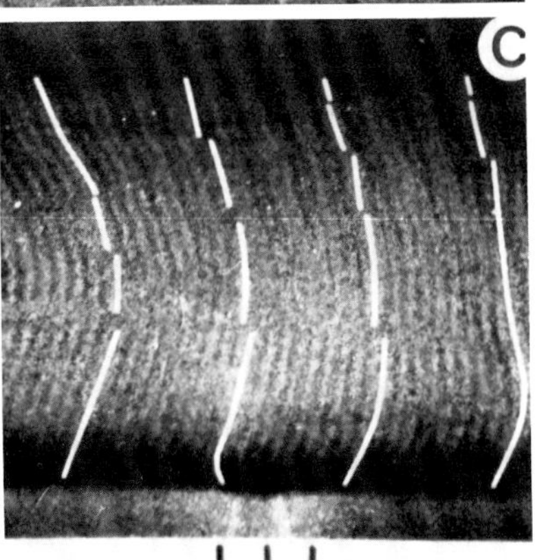

FIG. 23. Frames from cinefilm of relaxed muscle fiber (*A*) and of maximum contraction elicited by train of 3-ms depolarizing pulses (*B* and *C*). *A*: holding potential, −90 mV; sarcomere length, 3.57 μm. *Arrow* indicates site of insertion of current-passing electrode. Voltage-recording electrode can be seen on opposite side of fiber. *B*: 43-mV depolarizing pulses; axial sarcomeres have shortened to 3.34 μm. *C*: 44-mV depolarizing pulses; axial sarcomere length, 3.12 μm; superficial sarcomere length, 3.40 μm. Small localized contraction can be seen in region of current electrode in *B* and *C*. Bathing solution, 54 mM sodium Ringer's. Grid spacing, 10 μm. White lines in each frame mark every 9th sarcomere. Sarcomere length determined as mean of 20 sarcomeres. [From Costantin (21).]

By 1973 it was clear that the signal process traveling along the T-tubule network from the surface to the axis of a muscle fiber was probably an action potential. Qualitatively the tubule action potential would be generated by changes in the sodium conductance (and probably in K conductance also), like the sarcolemmal action potential. The tubule action potential had not been recorded, and therefore any analysis of the electrophysiologic characteristics that might generate the tubule action potential could not be judged directly. Nevertheless, due to the morphological characteristics of the T system, a change in tubule membrane potential would be reflected on the surface membrane potential [Hodgkin and Horowicz (50), Eisenberg and Gage (23), and Nakajima et al. (78)]. If the surface-recorded action potential could be accurately constructed by giving the proper qualitative and quantitative electrophysiological characteristics to changes in membrane potential in the tubule and sarcolemma during excitation beyond the action potential's threshold, the nature, conduction velocity, and shape of the tubule action potential could be predicted. In 1970 Adrian, Chandler, and Hodgkin (3) attempted to reconstruct the surface-recorded action potential from frog striated muscles. They based the reconstruction on the equivalent circuit where the T system was

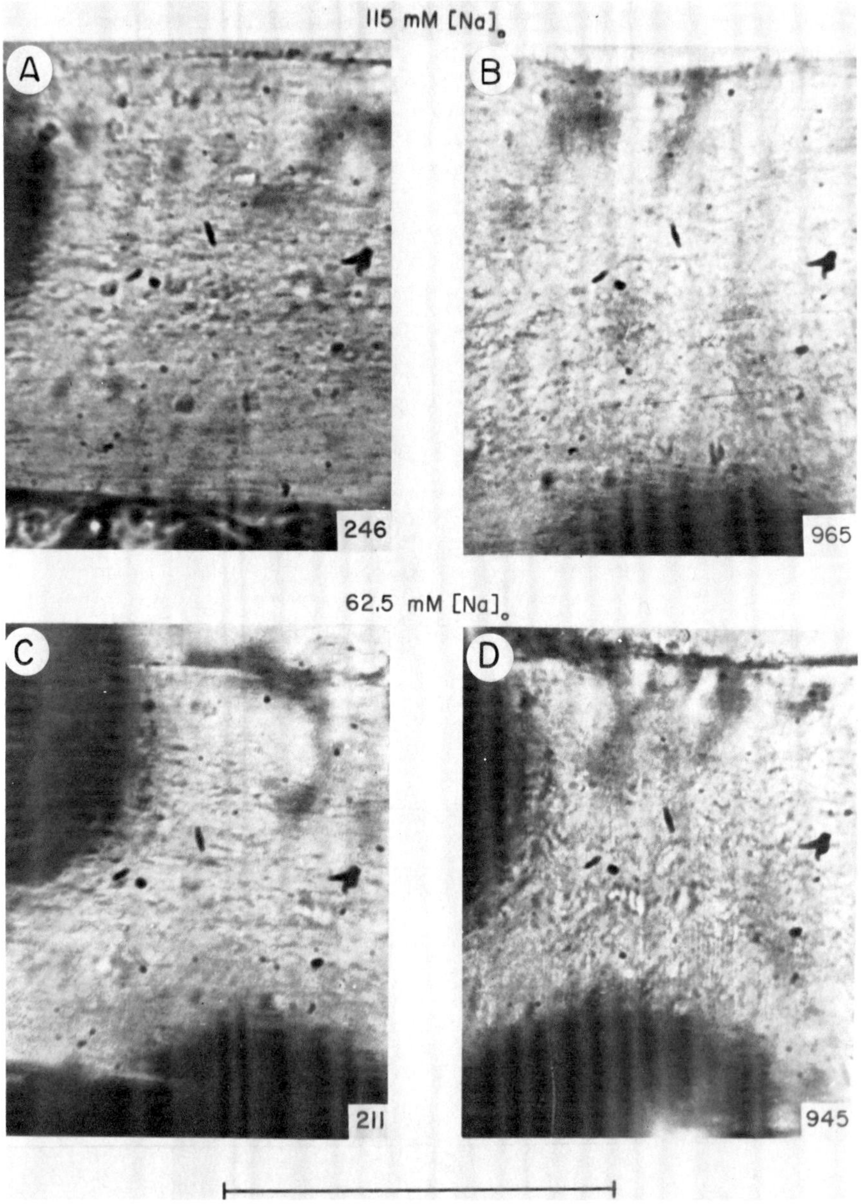

115 mM [Na]$_o$

A 246 B 965

62.5 mM [Na]$_o$

C 211 D 945

FIG. 24. Sample pictures from a cinerecording (100 frames/s) of isotonic contraction of isolated muscle fiber during tetanic stimulation (70 shocks/s). In *A* and *B* the fiber was in normal Ringer's solution; in *C* and *D* it was in 62.5 mM [Na^+]. Times at which pictures were taken after beginning of tetanus were as follows: *A*, 246 ms; *B*, 965 ms; *C*, 211 ms; and *D*, 945 ms. Calibration bar, 100 μm. Water-immersion objective, × 40; numerical aperture, 0.75. [From Bezanilla et al. (12).]

represented by linear electrical properties and did not undergo changes in sodium conductance during the inward spread of the excitatory wave. They pointed out that this might be the reason for the deficiencies in the reconstructed action potential. In 1973 Adrian and Peachey (6, 86) did the experiments again, but this time they reconstructed the action potential with a distributed-parameter equivalent circuit that represented the tubule system as a 16-element-system radial cable. Therefore the model had 17 time constants. They also took into account the tubule ionic currents carried by sodium and potassium. [For a description of the mathematical derivations and solutions, see the original papers (6, 86).] Once the proper equations were solved, they did several reconstructions, modifying various parameters: *1*) the access tubule resistance was assumed to be zero and the ionic currents in the tubule walls linear; *2*) the access tubule resistance was zero, but there were activable sodium and potassium currents in the tubule wall; *3*) the access tubule resistance was 150 Ω/cm^2, and again the ionic current in the tubule walls was linear; and *4*) the access tubule resistance was 150 Ω/cm^2, and there were activable sodium and potassium currents. The time course of the superficial action potential, shape of the afterpotential, and the conduction velocity could best be described by the model where the parameters mentioned in *4* were taken into account. The action potentials reconstructed from the calculations with parameters *3* and *4* are shown in Figure 7, in the chapter by Adrian in this *Handbook*.

Further support for the existence of a regenerative

tubule process involving active changes of sodium permeability came from experimental results reported by Caputo and DiPolo (17). They added Dextran 15 to the bathing solution and found that ion diffusion into and out of the T system was delayed. They then examined the influence of Dextran 15 on the ability of a fiber to recover its twitch when the external solution was rapidly changed from no sodium to 45 mM sodium. On a fiber previously exposed to Dextran 15, recovery of the twitch was much slower. This observation was explained by proposing that the presence of the Dextran 15 slowed the entry of sodium ions into the T system and therefore delayed the return of the regenerative tubule excitatory process. Bastian and Nakajima (8) showed that injecting previously recorded action potentials in the node of isolated single muscle cells clamped with a double sucrose-gap technique produced smaller outputs of twitch tension in fibers bathed with TTX or a sodium-free solution than in fibers with normal Ringer's solution and without TTX. Nakajima et al. (77) arrived at the same conclusion by measuring and calculating diffusion times due to sudden changes of sodium or potassium ions in the bathing solution.

Consideration of all the experiments, results, and propositions described in this chapter shows how, after the clear statement of the problem on the inward spread of activation by Hill, the experiments of Huxley and his colleagues opened one of the most extensive and changing fields of muscle research: EC coupling. Several important facts were discovered between 1948 and the present, but so far we have not been able to clearly and unmistakably record the tubule action potential. An intense effort has been made in this area of research by Landowne (71), Vergara and Bezanilla (101), Oetliker, Baylor, and Chandler (83), Nakajima Gilai, and Dingeman (74), and Baylor and Chandler (10). It is hoped that the tubule action potential soon will finally be "seen." The experimental approach used in 1922 by Adrian has recently been adapted with great success by several laboratories. Adrian used a pipette with a 17-μm tip, but Huxley, Taylor, and Straub used a 1.5-μm pipette and later others used micropipettes with tips of around 0.5 μm for recording and controlling transmembrane potentials. Although often neglected, the use of microscope observations related to cell function has added important observations and conclusions.

Like the progress from the study of whole muscle to the study of single fibers, and from single fibers to myofibrils, Adrian's conceptual approach (2) combining the use of microscope observations with physiological results may find further expression in the future study of components of a single sarcomere, as predicted in Huxley's 1967 Croonian Lecture (60).

I am grateful to Dr. L. D. Peachey and Dr. G. McClellan for help in the preparation of the manuscript.

The preparation of the manuscript was supported by a grant from the National Institutes of Health (5R01-NS-17048-01) and the Muscular Dystrophy Association of America, Inc.

REFERENCES

1. Adrian, E. D. The relation between the stimulus and the electric response in a single muscle fibre. *Arch. Neerl. Physiol.* 7: 330–332, 1922.
2. Adrian, R. H., W. K. Chandler, and A. L. Hodgkin. The kinetics of mechanical activation in frog muscle. *J. Physiol. London* 204: 207–230, 1969.
3. Adrian, R. H., W. K. Chandler, and A. L. Hodgkin. Voltage clamp experiments in striated muscle fibres. *J. Physiol. London* 208: 607–644, 1970.
4. Adrian, R. H., L. L. Costantin, and L. D. Peachey. Radial spread of contraction in frog muscle fibres. *J. Physiol. London* 204: 231–257, 1969.
5. Adrian, R. H., and W. H. Freygang. Potassium conductance of frog muscle membrane under controlled voltage. *J. Physiol. London* 163: 104–114, 1962.
6. Adrian, R. H., and L. D. Peachey. Reconstruction of the action potential of frog sartorius muscle. *J. Physiol. London* 235: 103–131, 1973.
7. Andersson-Cedergren, E. Ultrastructure of motor end plate and sarcoplasmic components of mouse skeletal muscle fiber as revealed by three-dimensional reconstructions from serial sections. *J. Ultrastruct. Res. Suppl.* 1: 5–191, 1959.
8. Bastian, J., and S. Nakajima. Action potential in the transverse tubules and its role in the activation of skeletal muscle. *J. Gen. Physiol.* 63: 257–278, 1974.
9. Bay, Z., M. C. Goodall, and A. Szent-Györgyi. The transmission of excitation from the membrane to actomyosin. *Bull. Math. Biophys.* 15: 1–13, 1953.
10. Baylor, S. M., and W. K. Chandler. Optical indications of excitation-contraction coupling in striated muscle. In: *Biophysical Aspects of Cardiac Muscle*, edited by M. Morad and S. Smith. New York: Academic, 1978, p. 207–228.
11. Bennett, H. S., and K. R. Porter. An electron microscope study of sectioned breast muscle of the domestic fowl. *Am. J. Anat.* 93: 61–105, 1953.
12. Bezanilla, F., C. Caputo, H. Gonzalez-Serratos, and R. A. Venosa. Sodium dependence of the inward spread of activation in isolated twitch muscle fibres of the frog. *J. Physiol. London* 223: 507–523, 1972.
13. Biedermann, W. *Elektrophysiologie.* Jena: Fischer, 1895, p. 149–272.
14. Bozler, E., and K. S. Cole. Electric impedance and phase angle of muscle in rigor. *J. Cell. Comp. Physiol.* 6: 229–241, 1935.
15. Brown, D. E. S., and F. J. M. Sichel. The isometric contraction of isolated muscle fibers. *J. Cell. Comp. Physiol.* 8: 315–328, 1936.
16. Brown, L. M., H. Gonzalez-Serratos, and A. F. Huxley. Electron microscopy of frog muscle fibres in extreme passive shortening. *J. Physiol. London* 208: 86P–88P, 1970.
17. Caputo, C., and R. DiPolo. Ionic diffusion delays in the transverse tubules of frog twitch muscle fibres. *J. Physiol. London* 229: 547–557, 1973.
18. Cole, K. S. *Membranes, Ions and Impulses: A Chapter of Classical Biophysics.* Berkeley: Univ. of California Press, 1968.
19. Cole, K. S., and H. J. Curtis. Electric impedance of nerve and muscle. *Cold Spring Harbor Symp. Quant. Biol.* 4: 73–89, 1936.
20. Costantin, L. L. The effect of calcium on contraction and conductance thresholds in frog skeletal muscle. *J. Physiol. London* 195: 119–132, 1968.
21. Costantin, L. L. The role of sodium currents in the radial spread of contraction in frog muscle fibers. *J. Gen. Physiol.* 55: 703–715, 1970.

22. Csapo, A., and T. Suzuki. The effectiveness of the longitudinal field, coupled with depolarization in activating frog twitch muscles. *J. Gen. Physiol.* 41: 1083–1098, 1958.
23. Eisenberg, R. S., and P. W. Gage. Ionic conductances of the surface and transverse tubular membranes of frog sartorius fibers. *J. Gen. Physiol.* 53: 279–297, 1969.
24. Eisenberg, R. S., and E. A. Johnson. Three-dimensional electrical field problems in physiology. *Prog. Biophys. Mol. Biol.* 20: 1–65, 1970.
25. Endo, M. Entry of a dye into the sarcotubular system of muscle. *Nature London* 202: 1115–1116, 1964.
26. Endo, M. Staining of a single muscle fibre with fluorescent dyes. *J. Physiol. London* 172: 11P, 1964.
27. Endo, M. Entry of fluorescent dyes into the sarcotubular system of the frog muscle. *J. Physiol. London* 185: 224–238, 1966.
28. Engelmann, T. W. Mikroskopische Untersuchungen Fiber die quergestreifte Muskelsubstanz. Zweiter Articol. Die thatige Muskelsubstanz. *Pfluegers Arch. Gesamte Physiol. Menschen Tiere* 7: 155–188, 1873.
29. Falk, G. Predicted delays in the activation of the contractile system. *Biophys. J.* 8: 608–625, 1968.
30. Falk, G., and P. Fatt. Linear electrical properties of striated muscle fibres observed with intracellular electrodes. *Proc. R. Soc. London Ser. B* 160: 69–123, 1964.
31. Fatt, P. An analysis of the transverse electrical impedance of striated muscle. *Proc. R. Soc. London Ser. B* 159: 606–651, 1964.
32. Fatt, P., and B. L. Ginsborg. The ionic requirements for the production of action potentials in crustacean muscle fibres. *J. Physiol. London* 142: 516–543, 1958.
33. Fatt, P., and B. Katz. An analysis of the end-plate potential recorded with an intracellular electrode. *J. Physiol. London* 115: 320–370, 1951.
34. Fatt, P., and B. Katz. The electrical properties of crustacean muscle fibres. *J. Physiol. London* 120: 171–204, 1953.
35. Franzini-Armstrong, C., and K. R. Porter. Sarcolemmal invaginations constituting the T system in fish muscle fibers. *J. Cell Biol.* 22: 675–696, 1964.
36. Freygang, W. H., S. I. Rapoport, and L. D. Peachey. Some relations between changes in the linear electrical properties of striated muscle fibers and changes in ultrastructure. *J. Gen. Physiol.* 50: 2437–2458, 1967.
37. Freygang, W. H., Jr., D. A. Goldstein, D. C. Hellam, and L. D. Peachey. The relation between the late afterpotential and the size of the transverse tubular system of frog muscle. *J. Gen. Physiol.* 48: 235–263, 1964.
38. Gelfan, S. The submaximal responses of the single muscle fibre. *J. Physiol. London* 80: 285–295, 1933.
39. Gonzalez-Serratos, H. Differential shortening of myofibrils during contractures of single muscle fibres. *J. Physiol. London* 179: 12P–14P, 1965.
40. Gonzalez-Serratos, H. Inward spread of contraction during a twitch. *J. Physiol. London* 185: 20P–21P, 1966.
41. Gonzalez-Serratos, H. Studies on the Inward Spread of Activation in Isolated Muscle Fibres. London: London University, 1967. PhD dissertation.
42. Gonzalez-Serratos, H. Inward spread of activation in vertebrate muscle fibres. *J. Physiol. London* 212: 777–799, 1971.
43. Gonzalez-Serratos, H. Graded activation of myofibrils and the effect of diameter on tension development during contractures in isolated skeletal muscle fibres. *J. Physiol. London* 253: 321–339, 1975.
44. Hagiwara, S., and A. Watanabe. The effect of tetraethylammonium chloride on the muscle membrane examined with an intracellular microelectrode. *J. Physiol. London* 129: 513–527, 1955.
45. Heilbrunn, L. V., and F. J. Wiercinski. The action of various cations on muscle protoplasm. *J. Cell. Comp. Physiol.* 29: 15–32, 1947.
46. Hill, A. V. On the time required for diffusion and its relation to processes in muscle. *Proc. R. Soc. London Ser. B*: 135: 446–453, 1948.
47. Hill, A. V. The abrupt transition from rest to activity in muscle. *Proc. R. Soc. London Ser. B*: 136: 399–420, 1949.
48. Hodgkin, A. L. A note on conduction velocity. *J. Physiol. London* 125: 221–224, 1954.
49. Hodgkin, A. L., and P. Horowicz. The differential action of hypertonic solutions on the twitch and action potential of a muscle fibre. *J. Physiol. London* 136: 17P, 1957.
50. Hodgkin, A. L., and P. Horowicz. The effect of sudden changes in ionic concentrations on the membrane potential of single muscle fibres. *J. Physiol. London* 153: 370–385, 1960.
51. Hodgkin, A. L., and P. Horowicz. Potassium contractures in single muscle fibres. *J. Physiol. London* 153: 386–403, 1960.
52. Hodgkin, A. L., and S. Nakajima. The effect of diameter on the electrical constants of frog skeletal muscle fibres. *J. Physiol. London* 221: 105–120, 1972.
53. Hodgkin, A. L., and S. Nakajima. Analysis of the membrane capacity in frog muscle. *J. Physiol. London* 221: 121–136, 1972.
54. Howell, J. N., and D. J. Jenden. T-tubules of skeletal muscle: morphological alterations which interrupt excitation-contraction coupling (Abstract). *Federation Proc.* 26: 553, 1967.
55. Huxley, A. F. A high-power interference microscope. *J. Physiol. London* 125: 11P–13P, 1954.
56. Huxley, A. F. Local activation of striated muscle from the frog and the crab. *J. Physiol. London* 135: 17P–18P, 1956.
57. Huxley, A. F. Das Interferenz-Mikroskop und seine Anwendung in der biologischung. *Naturwissenschaften* 7: 189–196, 1957.
58. Huxley, A. F. Local activation in muscle. *Ann. NY Acad. Sci.* 81: 446–452, 1959.
59. Huxley, A. F. The links between excitation and contraction. *Proc. R. Soc. London Ser. B* 160: 486–488, 1964.
60. Huxley, A. F. The Croonian Lecture, 1967. The activation of striated muscle and its mechanical response. *Proc. R. Soc. London Ser. B*: 178: 1–27, 1971.
61. Huxley, A. F., and A. M. Gordon. Striation patterns in active and passive shortening of muscle. *Nature London* 193: 280–281, 1962.
62. Huxley, A. F., and R. Niedergerke. Measurement of the striation of isolated muscle fibres with the interference microscope. *J. Physiol. London* 144: 403–425, 1958.
63. Huxley, A. F., and R. W. Straub. Local activation and interfibrillar structures in striated muscle. *J. Physiol. London* 143: 40P–41P, 1958.
64. Huxley, A. F., and R. E. Taylor. Function of Krause's membrane. *Nature London* 176: 1068, 1955.
65. Huxley, A. F., and R. E. Taylor. Local activation of striated muscles from the frog and the crab. *J. Physiol. London* 135: 17P–18P, 1956.
66. Huxley, A. F., and R. E. Taylor. Local activation of striated muscle fibres. *J. Physiol. London* 144: 426–441, 1958.
67. Huxley, H. E. Evidence for continuity between the central elements of the triads and extracellular space in frog sartorius muscle. *Nature London* 202: 1067–1071, 1964.
68. Katz, B. The electrical properties of the muscle fibre membrane. *Proc. R. Soc. London Ser. B* 135: 506–534, 1948.
69. Katz, B. *Nerve, Muscle and Synapse.* New York: McGraw-Hill, 1966.
70. Kuffler, S. W. The relation of electric potential changes to contracture in skeletal muscle. *J. Neurophysiol.* 9: 367–377, 1946.
71. Landowne, D. Changes in fluorescence of skeletal muscle stained with merocyanine associated with excitation-contraction coupling. *J. Gen. Physiol.* 64: 5a, 1974.
72. Nakajima, S., and A. Gilai. Action potentials of isolated single muscle fibers recorded by potential-sensitive dyes. *J. Gen. Physiol.* 76: 729–750, 1980.
73. Nakajima, S., and A. Gilai. Radial propagation of muscle action potential along the tubular system examined by poten-

tial-sensitive dyes. *J. Gen. Physiol.* 76: 751–762, 1980.
74. NAKAJIMA, S., A. GILAI, AND D. DINGEMAN. Dye absorption changes in single muscle fibers: an application of an automatic balancing circuit. *Pfluegers Arch.* 362: 285–287, 1976.
75. NAKAJIMA, S., AND A. L. HODGKIN. Effect of diameter on the electrical constants of frog skeletal muscle fibers. *Nature London* 227: 1053–1055, 1970.
76. NAKAJIMA, S., S. IWASAKI, AND K. OBATA. Delayed rectification and anomalous rectification in frog's skeletal muscle membrane. *J. Gen. Physiol.* 46: 97–115, 1962.
77. NAKAJIMA, S., Y. NAKAJIMA, AND J. BASTIAN. Effects of sudden changes in external sodium concentration on twitch tension in isolated muscle fibers. *J. Gen. Physiol.* 65: 459–482, 1975.
78. NAKAJIMA, S., Y. NAKAJIMA, AND L. D. PEACHEY. Speed of repolarization and morphology of glycerol-treated frog muscle fibres. *J. Physiol. London* 234: 465–480, 1973.
79. NASTUK, W. L., AND A. L. HODGKIN. The electrical activity of single muscle fibers. *J. Cell. Comp. Physiol.* 35: 39–73, 1950.
80. NATORI, R. The property and contraction process of isolated myofibrils. *Jikeikai Med. J.* 1: 119–126, 1954.
81. NATORI, R., AND C. ISOJIMA. Excitability of isolated myofibrils. *Jikeikai Med. J.* 9: 1–8, 1962.
82. NIEDERGERKE, R. Local muscular shortening by intracellularly applied calcium. *J. Physiol. London* 128: 12P, 1955.
83. OETLIKER, H., S. M. BAYLOR, AND W. K. CHANDLER. Simultaneous changes in fluorescence and optimal retardation in single muscle fibers during activity. *Nature London* 257: 693–696, 1975.
84. PAGE, S. The organization of the sarcoplasmic reticulum in frog muscle. *J. Physiol. London* 175: 10P–11P, 1964.
85. PEACHEY, L. D. The sarcoplasmic reticulum and transverse tubules of the frog's sartorius. *J. Cell Biol.* 25, Suppl. 3: 209–231, 1965.
86. PEACHEY, L. D., AND R. H. ADRIAN. Electrical properties of the transverse tubular system. In: The *Structure and Function of Muscle. Physiology and Biochemistry* (2nd ed.), edited by G. H. Bourne. New York: Academic, 1973, vol. 3.
87. PEACHEY, L. D., AND S. F. HUXLEY. Transverse tubules in crab muscle. *J. Cell Biol.* 23: 70A–71A, 1964.
88. PORTER, K. R., AND G. E. PALADE. Studies on the endoplasmic reticulum. III. Its form and distribution in striated muscle cells. *J. Biophys. Biochem. Cytol.* 3: 269–300, 1957.
89. RETZIUS, G. Zur Kenntnis der quergentreiften Muskelfaser. *Biol. Untersuch.* 1: 1–26, 1881.
90. ROBERTSON, J. D. Some features of the ultrastructure of a reptilian skeletal muscle. *J. Biophys. Biochem. Cytol.* 2: 369–380, 1956.
91. SAKAI, T., AND A. CSAPO. Contraction without membrane potential change. In: *The Structure and Function of Muscle* (1st ed.), edited by G. H. Bourne. New York: Academic, 1960, p. 228.
92. SANDOW, A. Excitation-contraction coupling in skeletal muscle. *Pharmacol. Rev.* 17: 265–320, 1965.
93. SELVERSTON, A. Structure and function of the transverse tubular system in crustacean muscle fibers. *Am. Zool.* 7: 515–525, 1967.
94. SMITH, D. S. The structure of insect fibrillar fly muscle. Study made with special reference to the membrane system of the fibre. *J. Biophys. Biochem. Cytol.* 10, Suppl. 4: 123–159, 1961.
95. STEN-KNUDSEN, O. The ineffectiveness of the "window field" in the initiation of muscle contraction. *J. Physiol. London* 125: 396–404, 1954.
96. STEN-KNUDSEN, O. Is muscle contraction initiated by internal current flow? *J. Physiol. London* 151: 363–384, 1960.
97. STRICKHOLM, A. Local sarcomere contraction in fast muscle fibres. *Nature London* 212: 835–836, 1966.
98. SUGI, H., AND R. OCHI. The mode of transverse spread of contraction initiated by local activation in single frog muscle fibers. *J. Gen. Physiol.* 50: 2167–2176, 1967.
99. VALDIOSERA, R., C. CLAUSEN, AND R. S. EISENBERG. Circuit models of the passive electrical properties of frog skeletal muscle fibers. *J. Gen. Physiol.* 63: 432–459, 1974.
100. VERATTI, E. Ricerche Zulla fine struttura della fibra muscolare striata Memorie 1st lomb. *Sci. Lett.* (*Ll. Sci. Math. Nat.*) 19, 97–133, 1902.
101. VERGARA, J., AND F. BEZANILLA. Fluorescence changes during electrical activity in frog muscle stained with merocyanine. *Nature London* 259: 684–686, 1976.

Optical studies of excitation-contraction coupling using voltage-sensitive and calcium-sensitive probes

STEPHEN M. BAYLOR | *Department of Physiology, University of Pennsylvania, Philadelphia, Pennsylvania*

CHAPTER CONTENTS

THE ACTIVITY of a wide variety of cells is controlled by changes in membrane potential and/or changes in cytoplasmic calcium (Ca^{2+}) levels. A vertebrate skeletal muscle cell, such as a frog twitch fiber, is one example. In this cell, on a time scale of milliseconds, an action potential on the surface membrane is followed by a transient rise in myoplasmic calcium and soon thereafter by a rapid increase in force.

The mechanism whereby depolarization of the surface membrane results in an increase in myoplasmic calcium is called the excitation-contraction (EC) coupling process and is known to involve activity in a twitch fiber's internal membrane systems: the transverse-tubular system (T system) and the sarcoplasmic reticulum (SR). The T system is the structure responsible for the rapid spread of an activation signal throughout the fiber cross section whereas the SR membranes contain the release and reuptake sites for Ca^{2+}. T-system activity undoubtedly depends on the electrical spread of a voltage signal from the surface membrane, as these systems are in direct electrical and chemical continuity (e.g., refs. 40, 48, 56). How a voltage change across the walls of the T system leads to Ca^{2+} release from the SR membranes, however, is a more complicated problem. An anatomical basis for some type of signal transfer has been visualized at the triadic junction (42) where these membrane systems are in close physical proximity, but direct electrochemical continuity, at least at rest, appears unlikely (see, e.g., the chapter by R.S. Eisenberg in this *Handbook* and ref. 90).

One promising experimental line toward elucidating the voltage dependence of this process involves the measurement of charge-movement currents, a phenomenon first detected by Schneider and Chandler (86) and subsequently investigated in detail by a number of laboratories (1, 4, 6, 30, 51, 52, 53, 77, 85, 87). The original hypothesis proposed to explain this current was that it reflected movement of charged groups in the T-system membranes from resting to activating positions and once in the activating position enabled Ca^{2+} release to proceed from adjacent SR membranes (86).

A second experimental approach toward learning more about the events of EC coupling has involved measurement of optical signals that precede or accompany Ca^{2+} release. Since muscle fibers transmit light readily and have many structurally interpretable optical properties (for a review, see ref. 55) the use of optical techniques is attractive. However, because muscle fibers move soon after stimulation the problem created by movement artifacts in the optical records might also be anticipated to set important limitations on the use of such techniques. Early experimental efforts were successful in measuring changes in the intrinsic optical properties of frog muscle after stimulation but before fiber movement. The signals monitored, however, such as changes in scattering (27, 44, 84), diffraction (45), or birefringence (39), did not at that time lend themselves readily to interpretation in terms of specific events underlying EC coupling.

Beginning with the work of Jöbsis and O'Connor (57) an important new step was taken in optical studies of EC coupling in muscle cells. These investigators attempted to expose the cell interior to an extrinsic optical probe—the calcium-sensitive indicator dye murexide (71)—that they hoped would give rise to a signal having a specific interpretation, namely, it might directly reflect the rise and fall of myoplasmic free calcium. Dye exposure involved an indirect technique, via intraperitoneal injection into the living animal, with permeation through muscle membranes possibly assisted in some experiments by dimethylsulfoxide. Three types of information were obtained as evidence that the optical signal from an isolated muscle after dye injection did, at least in some cases, likely reflect changes in myoplasmic calcium: *1*) a component of the signal was detected that depended on exposure to dye, *2*) a temporal comparison of this component with other known physiological signals verified that it had an appropriate time course, and *3*) the spectral features of the signal showed a wavelength dependence consistent with that expected for calcium.

In Figure 1*A* the signal attributed to the presence of murexide (lower trace, a differential recording involving three wavelengths of light) began after stimulation but before the tension response (upper trace), reached a peak in the rising phase of the tension response, and returned approximately to the base line at the peak of the tension response. Furthermore its time course was quite different from the overall light-scattering change in the muscle (middle trace), a change not expected to be specific for calcium. Figure 1*B* shows that the optical response had spectral properties appropriate for calcium. Differential wavelength combinations on either side of the null (isosbestic) wavelength for the calcium-murexide reaction were chosen and measurements were made from two different muscles. As expected for a calcium-dye signal, the waveforms had similar time courses but opposite polarity.

An important limitation in this method for tracking calcium was the variable success seen in achieving dye penetration into muscle cells following the intraperitoneal injection, as it was difficult to adjust conditions so that significant dye uptake into a viable muscle was achieved (F. F. Jöbsis, personal communication). Nevertheless this work was an important first step in the use of indicator dyes to monitor calcium transients in muscle, a technique that was not reproducibly and reliably carried out until more than a decade later (see *Arsenazo III Signals in Intact Fibers*, p. 372).

Success in measuring a second type of optical signal reflecting a specific physiological event was first reported in studies with neuronal cells (35, 93). For example, in experiments on squid giant axon a variety of optical signals have now been detected that rapidly track changes in membrane electrical activity (for reviews, see refs. 37, 100). The first signals detected, such as changes in intrinsic scattering and intrinsic

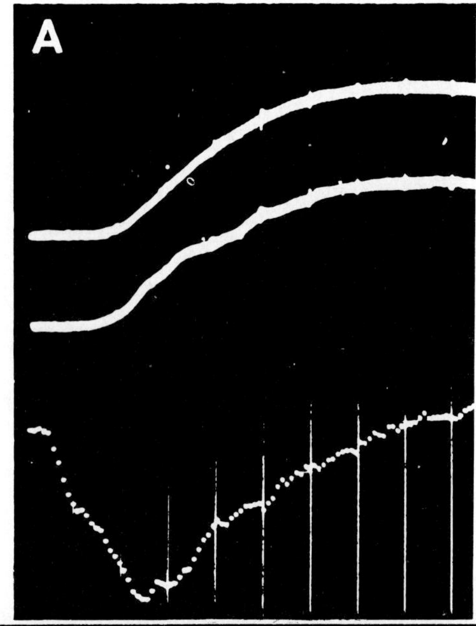

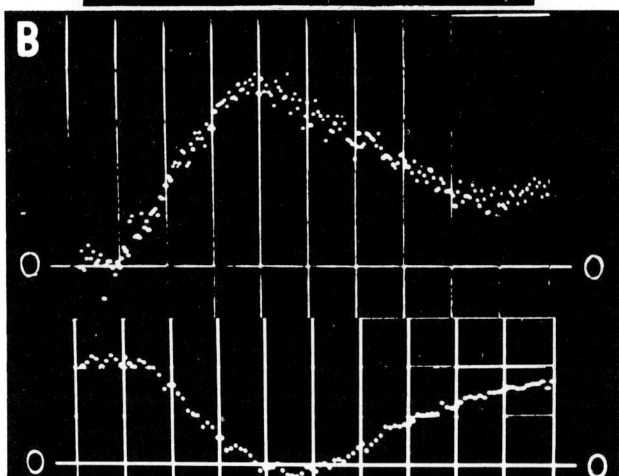

FIG. 1. Kinetics of Ca^{2+}-murexide complex in toad muscle after action potential stimulation. An increase in transmission is in the upward direction. *Vertical lines* provide a time scale at every 25 ms. Effects of 4 series of 10 contractions. *A*: time relations between tension development (*upper trace*), light scattering (*middle trace*), and formation of Ca^{2+}-murexide complex (*lower trace*). Formation was approximated by subtracting transmission changes at 440 and 505 nm, wavelengths relatively insensitive to Ca, from transmission change at 470 nm, a wavelength corresponding to a peak in Ca^{2+}-murexide difference spectrum. The subtraction procedure was designed to minimize interference from nonspecific effects. Stimulus delayed 12 ms after start of sweep; 12°C. *B*: time relation of optical response at 2 wavelengths on opposite sides of isosbestic point for Ca^{2+}-murexide reaction. *Upper trace,* 540 nm (relative to 505 and 580 nm); *lower trace*, 470 nm (relative to 440 and 505 nm). Stimulus delayed 25 ms from start of sweep. Results on 2 preparations from different toads; 9°C–10°C. [From Jöbsis and O'Connor (57).]

birefringence, were small and required extensive signal averaging (e.g., intrinsic birefringence signal, Fig. 2*A*). However, signals subsequently detected that depend on staining the axonal membrane with extrinsic probes give changes many times larger and are easily resolved in a single sweep (e.g., the absorbance change from the dye WW375, Fig. 2*B*). For many such signals voltage-clamp experiments (33, 38, 78) have verified that the optical changes primarily reflect changes in membrane potential and not changes in membrane current or permeability.

As the techniques for making potential-related optical measurements in neurons progressed, interest developed in making similar measurements in muscle cells, where, by analogy, signals might also be expected to reflect changes in membrane potential. Such signals could be particularly useful in studies of EC coupling because they might provide a means for tracking potential changes across a fiber's internal membranes, which are not directly accessible to study with conventional electrical techniques. Signals in muscle, however, might not monitor only membrane electrical activity by identical mechanisms giving rise to the signals from neuronal membranes. As one way for checking on this possibility, the optical properties of the neuronal signals have been used as a standard against which the muscle signals can be compared.

This review summarizes recently reported experi-

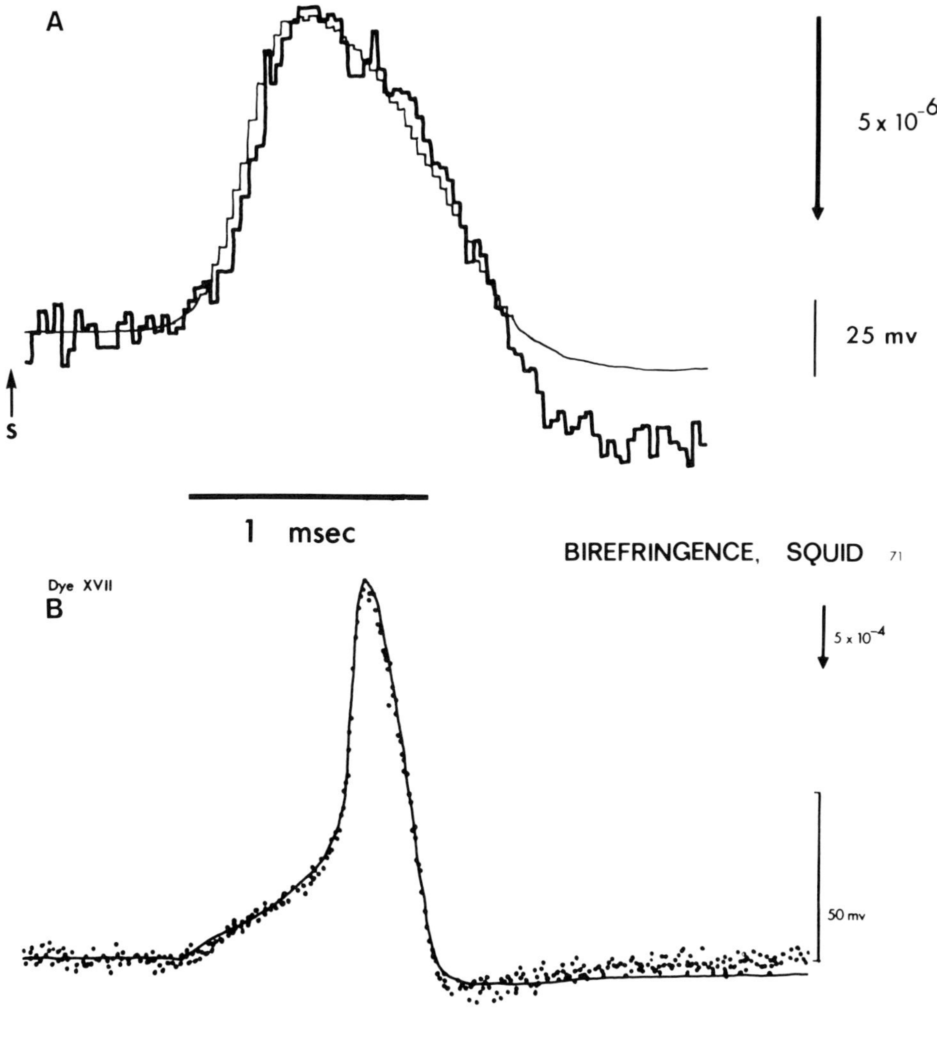

FIG. 2. Simultaneous recordings of action potential (*less-noisy trace*) and optical change from squid giant axon. *Arrow* calibrates fractional change in light intensity, ΔI/I. *A*: intrinsic birefringence change, i.e., signal detected with axon positioned between crossed polarizers oriented at ±45° to fiber axis. Time constant for optical recording, 24 μs; number of sweeps averaged, 2,030; 14°C. *B*: extrinsic absorbance change after staining with WW375, a merocyanine-rhodanine dye. Time constant for optical recording, 5 μs; number of sweeps averaged, 32; room temperature (21°C–23°C); dye exposure, 10 min with a concentration of 0.2 mg/ml. [*A* from Cohen et al. (32); *B* from Ross et al. (78).]

ments from a number of laboratories where optical signals from amphibian twitch fibers have been measured in hopes of tracking rapid changes in both membrane potential and myoplasmic calcium levels. In addition to focusing on new results of physiological interest, the chapter attempts to point out where unexpected experimental results have been encountered and where possible complications in the interpretations might exist.

OPTICAL SIGNALS SENSITIVE TO CHANGES IN SURFACE POTENTIAL AND T-SYSTEM POTENTIAL

The first study designed to look specifically for potential-related optical signals in skeletal muscle, analogous to the signals first detected in axons, was reported by Carnay and Barry (28). In these experiments, bundles of approximately 50 fibers were stretched out in normal Ringer's solution and stimu-

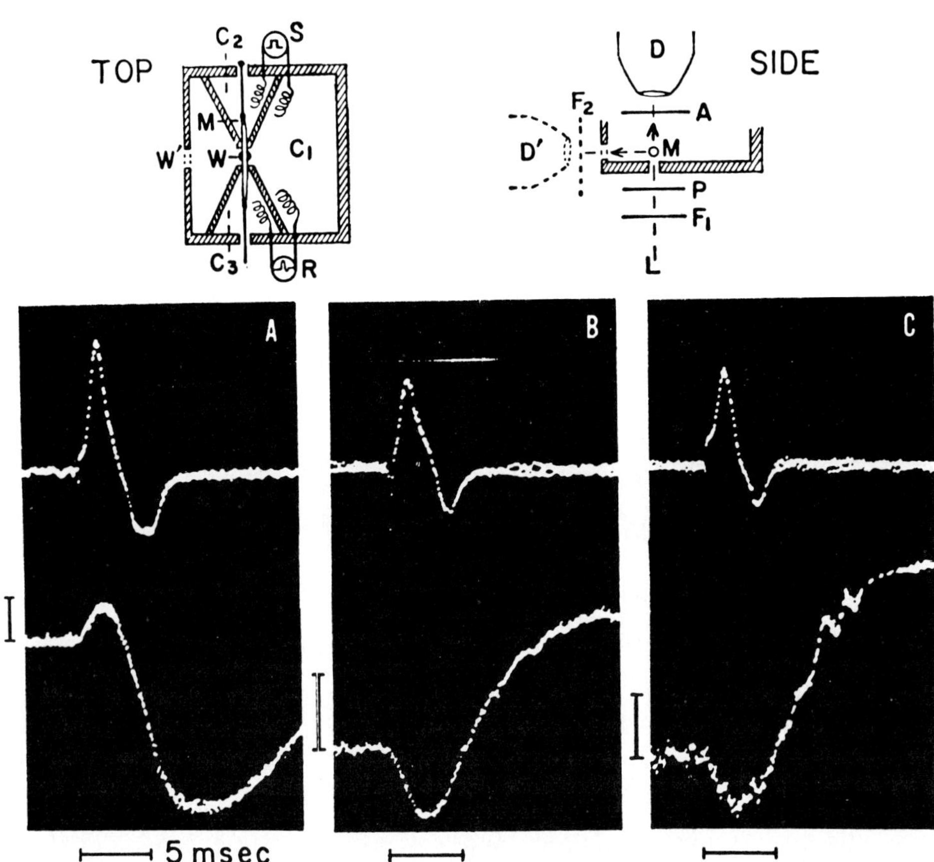

FIG. 3. *Top*: schematic diagram (top and side views) of recording chamber and optical arrangement used for detection of changes in scattering, birefringence, and fluorescence of skeletal muscle fibers of *Rana pipiens* after electric stimulation. M, muscle fibers; S, stimulating electrodes; R, recording electrodes; W and W′, windows for illumination and detection; L, light source; F_1, interference filter; F_2, sharp-cut filter; P and A, polarizer and analyzer, respectively; and D (or D′), photomultiplier at 0° (or 90°). *Bottom*: records of changes in light intensity (*lower traces*) coincident with externally recorded action potentials (*upper traces*). Optical signals represent changes in light scattering (*A*) recorded with photodetector in position D′, changes in birefringence (*B*) recorded with photodetector in position D and with polarizer and analyzer in place and oriented at ±45° with respect to the fiber axis, and changes in fluorescence of muscle fibers stained with pyronine B (*C*) recorded with photodetector in position D′ and with F_1 and F_2 in place (F_1 selects dye excitation wavelengths near 550 nm, and F_2 selects emission wavelengths beyond 610 nm). Different muscle preparations were used in each record. Upward deflection of *lower trace* represents an increase in light intensity. CAT computer was used to record both the action potentials and the optical signals. *Vertical bars* represent an increase of 2×10^{-4} (*A* and *B*) and 10^{-4} (*C*) times the resting level of illumination. Dye staining with pyronine B involved a 10-min exposure using a concentration of 0.05 mg/ml. Normal Ringer's solution; 22°C; signal-averaging was used. [From Carnay and Barry (28). Copyright 1969 by the American Association for the Advancement of Science.]

lated to give propagated action potentials. External action currents (Fig. 3*A*–*C*, upper traces) were recorded along with three types of optical signals (Fig. 3*A*–*C*, lower traces): intrinsic scattering (*A*), intrinsic birefringence (*B*), and extrinsic fluorescence due to staining with pyronine B (*C*). In each case light-intensity changes were detected having generally similar time courses, with the earliest deflection occurring approximately coincident with the passage of the action potentials. Because of this temporal coincidence and the general similarity to results from axons, these earliest optical changes were presumed to reflect electrical activity across membranes, although a separation into possible contributions from surface, T-system, and SR membranes did not appear warranted at that time (see also ref. 10). It was suggested that the later deflection in the optical records, in each case of opposite polarity to the early deflection, might reflect structural changes accompanying latency relaxation.

Intrinsic Birefringence Signal: First Component

Because of the likelihood that an optical signal from a bundle of fibers would reflect a temporal dispersion of single cell events, Baylor and Oetliker (16) undertook the study of the intrinsic birefringence signal using the intact single-fiber preparation. Fiber movement was reduced by increasing the tonicity of the Ringer's solution (47), and the action potential was recorded with an internal microelectrode. By this procedure the early decrease in intrinsic birefringence was resolved into two components not attributable to fiber movement. The small first component, with a fractional change in light intensity on the order of 10^{-5}, appeared to be relatively independent of tonicity (Fig. 4*A*) and, in three-times-hypertonic (3T) Ringer's solution, had a time course closely similar to the transmembrane action potential measured within the site of optical recording (Fig. 4*B*). As for axons a change in optical retardation was shown to be the most likely optical mechanism underlying this signal. Unfortunately, because of the small size of the first component and the limited number of action potentials that can be elicited from a muscle fiber in strongly hypertonic solution, it was not determined whether the wavelength dependence and spatial distribution of the signal were also identical to the axonal signal. However, because of its general similarity to the signal in Figure 2*A*, the first component was attributed primarily to the action potential on the surface membrane.

On the other hand the amplitude of the larger and more slowly developing second component (Fig. 4*B*, second peak; also see *Intrinsic Birefringence Signal: Second Component*, p. 364) was shown to depend strongly on tonicity. For example, in normal Ringer's solution the peak of the second component was approximately 100 times larger than that of the first component and its rapid rate of rise prevented resolution of the first component (Fig. 4*A*). Furthermore two-microelectrode, current-clamp experiments in the presence of tetrodotoxin (TTX), which blocks sodium conductance and regenerative voltage changes in the T system, indicated that the second component could not be attributed directly to potential spread into the T system. Rather, it was only observed when surface and T-system membranes were depolarized about 30

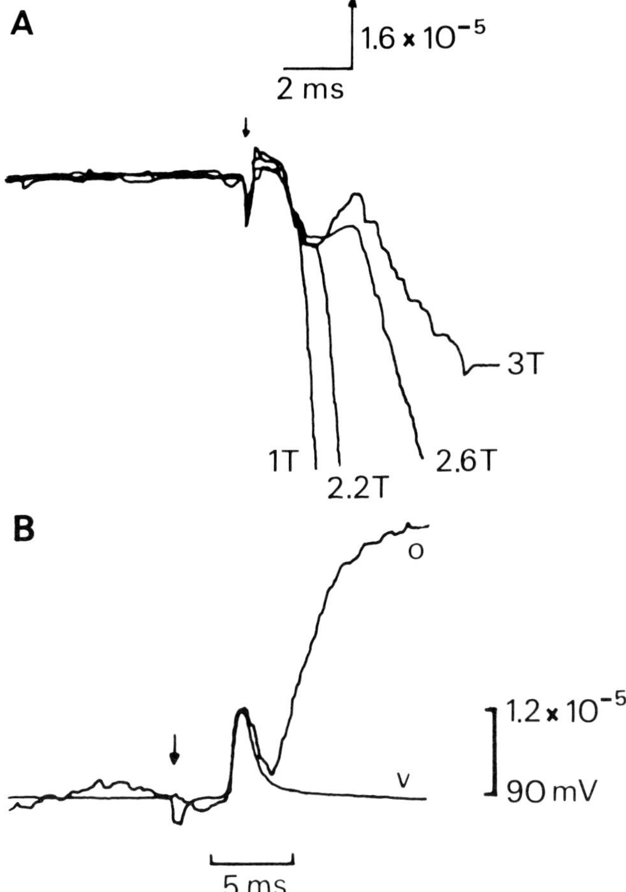

FIG. 4. Intrinsic birefringence signal from intact single fibers of *Rana temporaria*. Room temperature (19°C–23°C). *A*: separation of 1st and 2nd components. Optical recordings of fractional intensity changes from the same fiber in Ringer's solutions of various tonicities superimposed by lining up the stimulus artifact (*arrow*): normal tonicity (1T), 120 mM NaCl; 2.2T, 270 mM NaCl; 2.6T, 320 mM NaCl; 3T, 370 mM NaCl Ringer's solution. In 1T Ringer's solution the 2 components cannot be distinguished temporally; in 3T Ringer's solution the 1st component, with a time to peak of about 2 ms after stimulation, is kinetically distinct from the second component, which is still rising at end of record. Each trace is the average of 64 sweeps. Optical recording was a 500-μm field, 1.5 mm from stimulus cathode. *B*: optical (o) and intracellular voltage (v) recordings taken simultaneously in 3T Ringer's solution (370 mM NaCl). Optical trace is inverted to facilitate comparison with action potential. Upper vertical calibration refers to the optical trace, and the lower to the potential trace, each of which is an average of 300 sweeps. Optical recording was 7 mm from stimulus cathode. [From Baylor and Oetliker (16).]

mV or more from the resting level, i.e., into the range of potentials where calcium release from the SR was likely to become significant (2, 49). Under the assumption that the second component reflected a membrane potential change, the authors considered the SR membranes to be the only possible candidates (16). However, these experiments did not rule out the possibility that the second component might reflect events unrelated to membrane potential, e.g., early changes in the myofilaments subsequent to calcium binding (19, 92).

Not convincingly resolved in these experiments was an optical signal likely to reflect changes in T-system potential. However, some current-clamp experiments at potentials below the threshold for contractile activation, where effects from the second component were negligible, produced rapid birefringence changes in response to membrane potential but of opposite polarity to that expected from either the surface membrane alone or the second component (19). It was proposed that contributions from the T-system membranes might, on balance, outweigh the contributions of the surface membranes to these signals. A possible explanation suggested for the finding that these current-clamp experiments did not always produce a signal of consistent polarity was that the amplitude and polarity of the T-system contribution should depend on both the total amount and net orientation of T-system membranes with respect to the light path. The total amount varies with fiber diameter (75), whereas the net orientation might depend on fiber diameter, sarcomere length, and possibly other variables.

Signals From Impermeant Potentiometric Dyes

In general, the large number of dyes that have been used successfully in neurons to monitor changes in membrane potential (38, 78) can be divided into two classes: *1*) membrane permeant ones (e.g., pyronine B, Fig. 3*C*), which tend to give two-component and sometimes multicomponent responses to potential changes and *2*) membrane impermeant ones (e.g., WW375, Fig. 2*B*), which tend to give rapid, single-component responses. However, with either class of dye the problem of multicomponent signals is usually greater at higher dye concentrations (78).

Each class of dye might have a particular use in muscle cell studies. For example, permeant probes added to the bath should stain surface, T system, and SR membranes (see *Signals From Membrane-Permeant Dyes*, *Simultaneous Comparisons of Signals from Birefringence and Membrane-Permeant Dyes*, and *Vesicular Preparations*, p. 364–366 for further discussion of signals from these dyes). On the other hand impermeant probes, unless introduced into the myoplasm, should stain only surface and T-system membranes. Since the quantity of T-system membranes exceeds that of the surface membrane severalfold (64, 75, 76), one might expect to see predominantly T-system signals from impermeant dyes, assuming signal amplitude is proportional to membrane area. However, the latter assumption might be in error if, for example, staining of membranes was not homogeneous, the orientation of the membrane with respect to light path was an important determinant of signal amplitude, or if there were substantial radial variations in the amplitude and time course of the T-system action potential. Therefore the exact basis for explaining any given dye signal is a question requiring experimental investigation.

The first reported signal from an impermeant dye in skeletal muscle was that seen with merocyanine 540, a dye that is quite toxic to axonal membranes in the presence of light and oxygen. This dye also gave a relatively large signal in muscle (61, 68, 70, 96) with a time course appropriate to some combination of surface and T-system action potentials. The relatively severe toxicity of this dye to skeletal muscle membranes, however, made detailed quantitative studies difficult to carry out and interpret [cf. results from studies of cardiac muscle with this dye where large signals have been recorded in the apparent absence of toxicity (65)].

As impermeant potentiometric dyes without measurable toxicity became available from axonal studies, they were also tested in skeletal muscle. For example, a small concentration of WW375 (Fig. 2*B*) appeared nontoxic to single fibers; also following stimulation it gave an absorbance change with a large signal-to-noise ratio and a time course appropriate to some combination of surface and T-system action potentials (11). In addition the wavelength dependence of this signal was shown to be similar, although not identical in all cases, to that found in axon membranes (78). To the extent that the spectral features agree with those in axons, this result supports the idea of a common underlying mechanism (i.e., a rapid, single-component response to a change in membrane potential) as the source of the signal. To the extent they disagree, however, the result raises questions of whether the dye behavior in muscle membranes might reflect other mechanisms not seen in axons. Alternatively the authors suggested that the unanticipated features observed in muscle might be explained solely in terms of geometric effects arising from the differing orientations of surface and T-system membranes (11).

Figure 5*A* shows results from an experiment by Nakajima and Gilai (67) on a single twitch fiber from *Xenopus laevis* in which the absorbance change after staining with WW375 (upper trace) was recorded simultaneously with the surface action potential measured by an internal microelectrode (lower trace). The time courses of the two events were significantly different, with the peak of the optical signal systematically lagging behind the peak of the action potential by about 0.5 ms. This result stands in contrast to that seen in axons (Fig. 2*B*) but is in the direction to be expected if the dye signal in muscle substantially

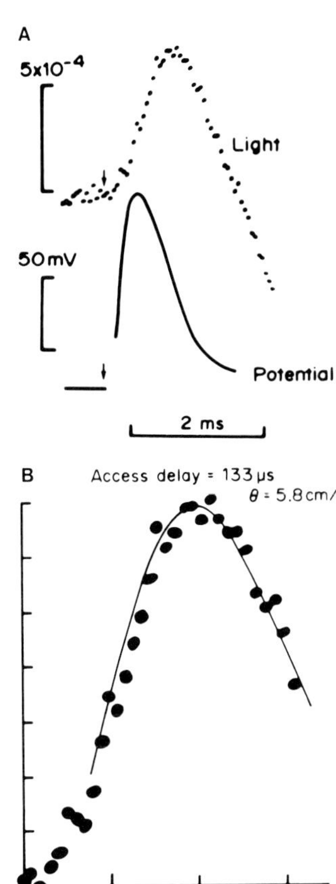

FIG. 5. *A*: simultaneous recordings of optical signals (*upper trace*) and intracellularly recorded action potentials (*lower trace*) in a single muscle fiber of *Xenopus laevis* stained with WW375 (100 μg/ml) for 15 min. Optical signal was signal-averaged by an averager, and action potential represents the average of the photographs of the 4 spikes. Optical calibrations refer to ΔI/I; the wavelength was 702 nm; slit size = fiber diameter × 500 μm. *Arrows* indicate start of massive stimulation. Fiber diameter, 108 μm; sarcomere length, 2.6 μm; room temperature (25°C). Response time constant of optical system was 25 μs and that of the electrical system was 30 μs. *B*: estimation of radial conduction velocity of tubular action potential by analysis of simultaneously recorded optical and electrical signals. *Continuous curve* is the best-fit optical signal calculated from the experimentally determined electrical signal (action potential) obtained by adjusting values of access delay and radial conduction velocity. *Filled circles,* recorded optical signal. Normalizing factors were introduced to the *continuous curve* to make height approximately the same as optical signal. Data are from experiment illustrated in *A*. [From Nakajima and Gilai (67).]

reflects changes in T-system potential. For example previous computations for frog muscle had indicated that the peak of the T-system action potential might lag behind that of the surface action potential with delays at this temperature varying between 0.1 and 1.5 ms (3).

As modeled by Nakajima and Gilai (67) the time course of the optical signal observed in Figure 5*A* could be satisfactorily explained (Fig. 5*B*) under the assumptions that *1*) the optical signal responds only to membrane potential and without kinetic delay (cf. Fig. 2*B*); *2*) it arises from changes in surface and T-system potential only, with amplitude contributions in proportion to anatomical membrane area; and *3*) the T-system action potential has the same shape as the surface action potential but starts at the outer perimeter of the muscle cell after a small access delay (on the order of 0.1 ms in Fig. 5*B*) and then propagates toward the fiber center with a constant conduction velocity. The best-fit value obtained from this analysis for the radial conduction velocity was of physiological interest because it averaged about 6 cm/s at 25°C (5.8 cm/s in Fig. 5*B*) and therefore agreed closely with the radial conduction velocity for an activation signal estimated with a high-speed cinematographic method by Gonzalez-Serratos [7–8 cm/s at 20°C in frog muscle (43)]. Thus the dye signal appeared to represent a spatial and temporal integration of changes in surface and T-system potential and to confirm that the radial conduction velocity for activation is 6–8 cm/s at 20°C–25°C.

Additional information concerning the behavior of the WW375 absorbance signal in muscle membranes was obtained in intact single-fiber experiments from frog (*Rana temporaria*) carried out in 3T D_2O Ringer's solution, in which movement artifacts and non-dye-related transmission effects in the optical traces were likely to be negligible (15). By means of more extensive signal averaging a careful comparison could be made of the amplitude and time course of the optical signal at three different wavelengths, each with two forms of polarized light (Fig. 6*A*). If all of the signals monitored only surface and T-system action potentials, without delay and in constant proportion, their time courses would be expected to be identical although their relative amplitudes might vary. However, the results comparing time courses (Fig. 6*B*) indicated the presence of at least two underlying temporal processes, since four of the six waveforms (570 nm, 0°; 690 nm, 0°; 750 nm, 0°; 750 nm, 90°) had identical time courses, whereas the other two waveforms (570 nm, 90°; 690 nm, 90°) were somewhat slower. The authors suggested two possible explanations not distinguished by the experiments for this temporal discrepancy: *1*) two underlying physiological events, e.g., surface and T-system action potentials, that are signaled in different proportions in the 570-nm, 90° and 690-nm, 90° traces than in the other traces or *2*) the presence of a second component to the absorbance change, e.g., one that tracks membrane potential with a somewhat different delay than the first component.

A second difference between these results in hypertonic D_2O Ringer's solution on frog muscle (14) and those reported by Nakajima and Gilai (67) in isotonic H_2O Ringer's solution on toad muscle concerns the spectral and polarization dependence of the amplitude of the absorbance signal. In the experiment of Figure 6 the spectral and polarization features are closely similar to those reported in axons [although this is not always the case in frog muscle (11, 14)], whereas in the toad experiments they are consistently different

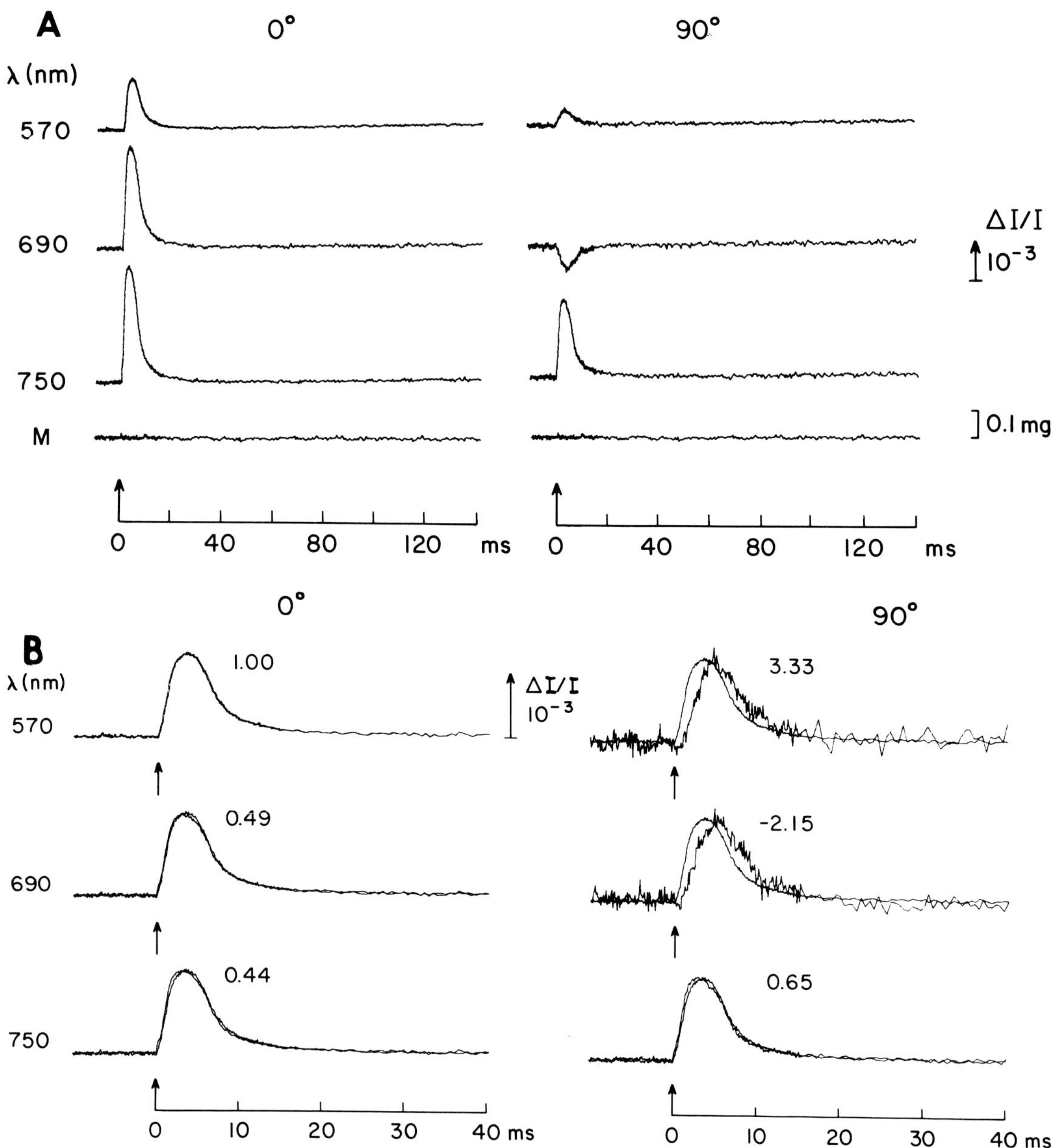

FIG. 6. Wavelength and polarization dependence of the WW375 transmission change from a single fiber of *Rana temporaria* after action potential stimulation in 3T D_2O Ringer's solution. *A*: original records of fractional changes in light intensity. 0° indicates that light polarized at 0° to fiber's axis was used, and 90° indicates that light polarized at 90° to fiber's axis was used. Wavelength is indicated alongside the 0° traces. M is tension response. Optical traces obtained with a 27 × 300-μm slit and traces signal-averaged as follows: 570 nm, 0°, 64 times; 690 nm, 0°, 32 times; 750 nm, 0°, 8 times; 570 nm, 90°, 32 times; 690 nm, 90°, 16 times; 750 nm, 90°, 4 times. *B*: results of fitting 570-nm, 0° waveform by scaling the other optical traces shown in *A*. The least-squares fitting constants are shown alongside each optical trace. The 570-nm, 90° trace and the 690-nm, 90° trace are noisy traces. The 570-nm, 0° trace is not well fitted by their scaled versions, indicating more than a single temporal process. [From Baylor et al. (15).]

from axonal results. At present the exact basis for these differences does not appear to be well understood (see Discussion in ref. 66).

Another preparation where signals from impermeant potentiometric dyes have been examined is the cut single-fiber preparation (46). Using *Rana catesbeiana* fibers at 10°C, Vergara and Bezanilla (97, 98) compared electrical and optical signals using two different impermeant dyes: the absorbance dye WW375 (as in Figs. 2*B*, 5, and 6) and the fluorescence dye WW781 (34). With WW375 (Fig. 7*A*) the action potential recorded electrically only slightly preceded the optical change (a result not obviously inconsistent with that in Fig. 5, however, considering the difference in temperature), whereas WW781 gave a signal dramatically slower than the action potential (Fig. 7*B*). Although the dye concentrations used for the experiments of Figure 7 were higher (0.5–1 mg/ml) than concentrations giving detectable signals with these dyes from intact single fibers [0.01–0.1 mg/ml (11, 15, 66, 67)], the difference between *A* and *B* strongly suggests that not all impermeant potentiometric dyes behave identically in the same muscle preparation in all situations.

This discrepancy was investigated further in voltage-clamp experiments in a half-sodium Ringer's solution without TTX (98). In the case of a step depolarization of the surface membrane from −100 mV to −40 mV, the WW375 signal revealed one principal component that followed surface membrane potential with a delay of a small fraction of a millisecond. Under similar conditions the WW781 signal showed a first component having a greater delay, on the order of several milliseconds, and in addition showed a large and obvious second component that was temporally correlated with notches in the current record. This second component was attributed to a membrane event, namely, a lack of voltage control in the T system. Because the second component was not seen with WW375, Vergara and Bezanilla (98) concluded that in cut fibers WW375 gives a single component that monitors primarily changes in surface potential and not T-system potential, whereas WW781 was presumed to give a predominantly T-system signal. The discrepancy between this conclusion for cut fibers stained with WW375 and that for intact single fibers (see discussion of Figs. 5 and 6, p. 360–362) has no obvious explanation, although differences in preparation, dye concentration, and wavelength and polarization characteristics of the light are obvious candidates for future investigation.

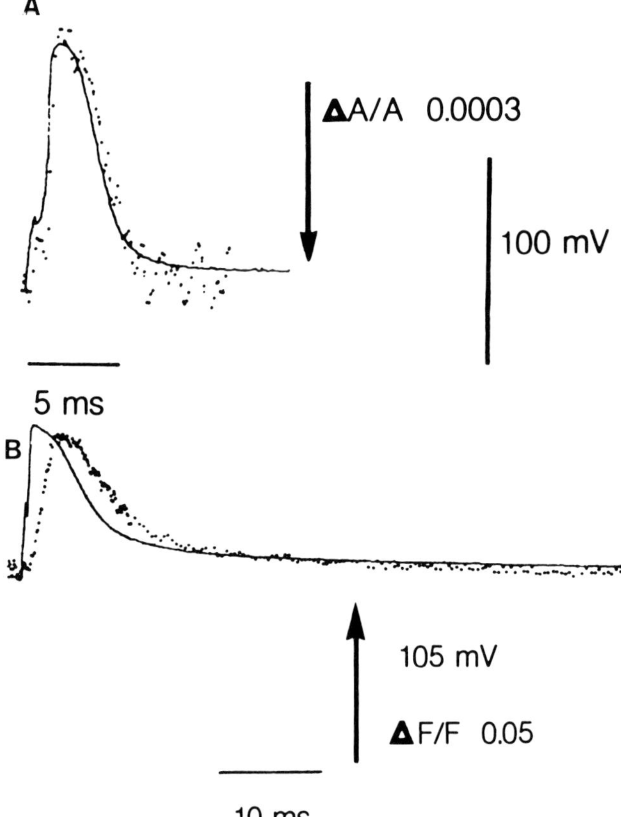

FIG. 7. Simultaneous recordings of optical signals and action potentials after staining of cut single fibers of *Rana catesbeiana* with impermeant potentiometric dyes. In both parts of the figure the noisier records are optical traces. *A*: absorbance change from WW375 (1 mg/ml) obtained with 750-nm light at 10°C. *B*: fluorescence change from WW781 (approx. 0.5 mg/ml). Average of 4 sweeps. Excitation was with 625-nm light; fluorescence was measured with a 665-nm, cut-on filter at 10°C. [From Vergara and Bezanilla (98).]

In summary, signals from muscle fibers stained with impermeant dyes have amplitudes, time courses, and spectral and polarization characteristics that are in general agreement with what might be expected on the basis of axonal studies, under the assumption that membrane potential change is the principal underlying event signaled. However, a comparison of the signals seen when using the same dye on different preparations and different dyes on the same preparation has revealed several unexpected features, suggesting that new physiological conclusions concerning muscle membranes should be drawn with caution. In particular it is possible that these dyes do not always stain surface and T-system membranes uniformly and it appears likely that they do not always give a single component response tracking potential change across these membranes in a constant proportion independent of the wavelength and polarization of the light. Nevertheless the possibility of obtaining rather direct information concerning potential spread into the T system with this technique would appear to make carefully controlled studies with this class of dyes an important endeavor.

OPTICAL SIGNALS POSSIBLY SENSITIVE TO CHANGES IN SR POTENTIAL

If the voltage of the SR membrane changes substantially during a twitch, it might be possible to see relatively large optical signals reflecting this event, since the area of SR membrane in a frog twitch fiber typically exceeds that of the surface membrane by a factor close to 100-fold and the area of surface plus T system by a factor close to 10-fold (64, 75, 76). In particular an SR signal might be the predominant signal seen in measuring an intrinsic change (e.g., changes in birefringence), a change dependent on permeant probes added to the bath, or a change dependent on impermeant probes introduced into the myoplasm. Whether any given signal does monitor SR potential, however, is a somewhat speculative conclusion, as direct electrical recording across SR membranes with microelectrode techniques appears to be ruled out by considerations of size. Also recent evidence from electron-probe analysis is consistent with there being little or no resting potential across the SR (89, 90). Furthermore no independent evidence indicates that a significant SR potential change accompanying Ca^{2+} release has to take place, although such a voltage change might be either a direct trigger for or direct result of Ca^{2+} release. Rather, evidence favoring an SR voltage interpretation of an optical signal must be indirect but might rely on *1*) temporal comparisons with known physiological events to establish a reasonable time course; *2*) a comparison of the optical features of the signal, such as wavelength and polarization dependence, with those of analogous signals that arise from potential changes in other membrane systems; and *3*) temporal comparisons among the class of optical signals that appear to be reasonable candidates on the basis of criteria like *1* and *2*, to check for internal consistency in the interpretation.

Intrinsic Birefringence Signal: Second Component

The relatively large second component of the intrinsic birefringence signal (Fig. 4*B*) begins soon after depolarization of the surface membrane. Furthermore its overall time course from a highly stretched fiber where movement artifacts were minimized was seen to peak early in the rising phase of the residual tension response (17), appropriate for a possible SR signal (for examples in a normal Ringer's solution, see Fig. 9). Also, its optical properties (18) were closely similar to features in axons that are characteristic of a membrane potential mechanism. These observations led to the proposal that this signal might reflect an SR potential change (16, 19).

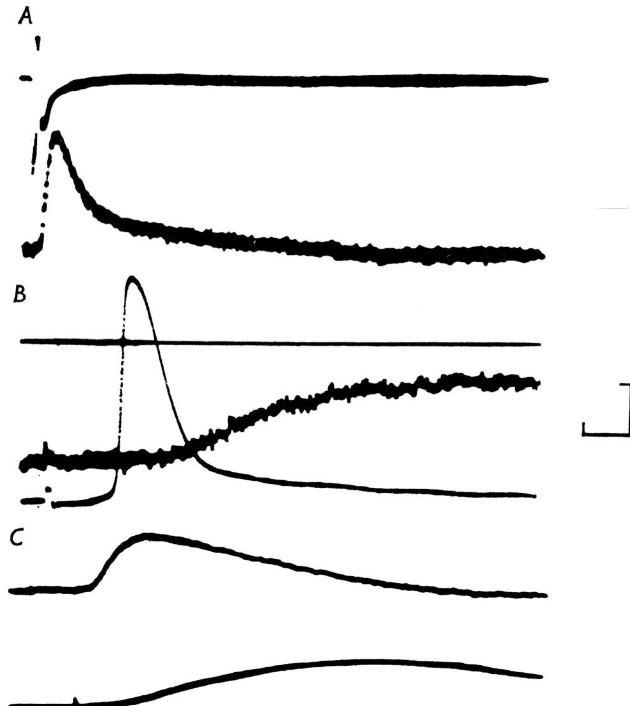

FIG. 8. Nile blue fluorescence change from whole muscle of *Rana pipiens* after action potential stimulation. *A*: external action currents (*upper trace*) and fluorescence signal (*lower trace*) in response to one supramaximal stimulus. Time calibration bar is 50 ms; fluorescence calibration bar is 2 mV. Resting fluorescence, 0.78 V. Temperature, 17.9°C. *B*: relation of intracellular action potential to fluorescence signal. *Upper trace*, external 0-potential reference; *middle trace*, fluorescence signal; *lower trace*, internal potential. Time calibration bar is 2 ms. Calibration for internal potential is 25 mV and for fluorescence is 2 mV. Resting fluorescence, 0.9 V; 25°C. *C*: time relation of fluorescence to mechanical response. *Upper trace*, fluorescence signal in response to single stimulus; *lower trace*, tension response. Time calibration bar is 10 ms for both traces; tension calibration bar is 28 mg; fluorescence calibration bar is 10 mV; 23.5°C. [From Bezanilla and Horowicz (22).]

Signals From Membrane-Permeant Dyes

A second, independent line of experiments that followed the work of Carnay and Barry (28) was begun by Bezanilla and Horowicz (22), who stained whole frog muscle with Nile blue A added to the bath, in the expectation of detecting signals related to membrane potential. In axons, Nile blue gave a relatively large and fairly rapid response to membrane potential (31) and had properties consistent with it being membrane permeant (99). In muscle, after external stimulation, a large increase in Nile blue fluorescence was detected, which followed the action potential but preceded the residual tension response (Fig. 8*A–C*). Moreover in current-passing experiments in the presence of TTX, the signal appeared only at depolarizations near or above the contractile threshold, ruling out the possibility that the principal component of the signal reflected change in surface and/or T-system potential. In addition the signal amplitude increased when chloride was replaced with nitrate and decreased when H_2O Ringer's solution was replaced with D_2O Ringer's solution, agents known respectively to potentiate and depress the twitch response. The pattern of evidence was therefore consistent with the possibility that the signal arose from some step in EC coupling. A potential change across the SR membranes near the time of calcium release was proposed (22).

Simultaneous Comparisons of Signals From Birefringence and Membrane-Permeant Dyes

From the experiments described above, the time course and other physiological features of the Nile blue fluorescence signal and intrinsic birefringence signal (second component) appeared similar, supporting the idea that they reflected the same underlying physiological event. An obvious check on this interpretation would be to measure both signals simultaneously on the same preparation to see if their time courses were identical.

This experiment was attempted on the intact single-fiber preparation in hypertonic Ringer's solution but was made technically difficult due to a toxic effect of Nile blue on single fibers (70). At a reduced dye concentration (0.1 μg/ml rather than 10 μg/ml) where pharmacological effects could not be detected, the birefringence and Nile blue signals were noted to start approximately at the same time. However, the small signal-to-noise ratio of the fluorescence change obtained at this dye concentration did not permit a completely satisfactory temporal comparison.

A more accurate comparison (15) was made in subsequent experiments on single fibers, carried out in normal Ringer's solution at a somewhat higher dye concentration (0.5 μg/ml). In these experiments the time course of the birefringence signal recorded before and after staining with Nile blue was identical, indicating that Nile blue at this concentration did not significantly change the birefringence signal. However, the time course of the Nile blue signal was substantially slower than that of birefringence (Fig. 9*A*): birefringence had a time to peak of 8.5 ms, and the Nile blue signal had a time to peak of 24.5 ms (16°C). Thus the conclusion was reached that the two optical signals could not both be rapid monitors of the same underlying physiological event. Not ruled out by the experiments, however, was the possibility that both signals could be tracking the same event but with substantially different delays.

In these experiments a similar comparison was made between the intrinsic birefringence signal and the fluoresence decrease from an indodicarbocyanine dye. This dye had also been selected as a membrane-permeant dye that gave a large potential-related signal in axons (dye 122 in ref. 38). As first noted in hypertonic Ringer's solution (70), the signal from this dye in normal Ringer's solution showed a time course through time to peak that was closely similar to that of the birefringence signal; however, the falling phases of the signals differed somewhat (Fig. 9*B*). The time to peak for birefringence was 9 ms and for cyanine fluorescence was 11 ms (16°C), supporting the conclusion that these signals could be tracking the same underlying event with similar delays. However, the presence of other components in the fluorescence change from this dye, particularly easily seen at low dye concentrations (15), made it difficult to draw a more specific interpretation.

One general conclusion from the experiments comparing the signals from birefringence and the membrane-permeant dyes in the same preparation, there-

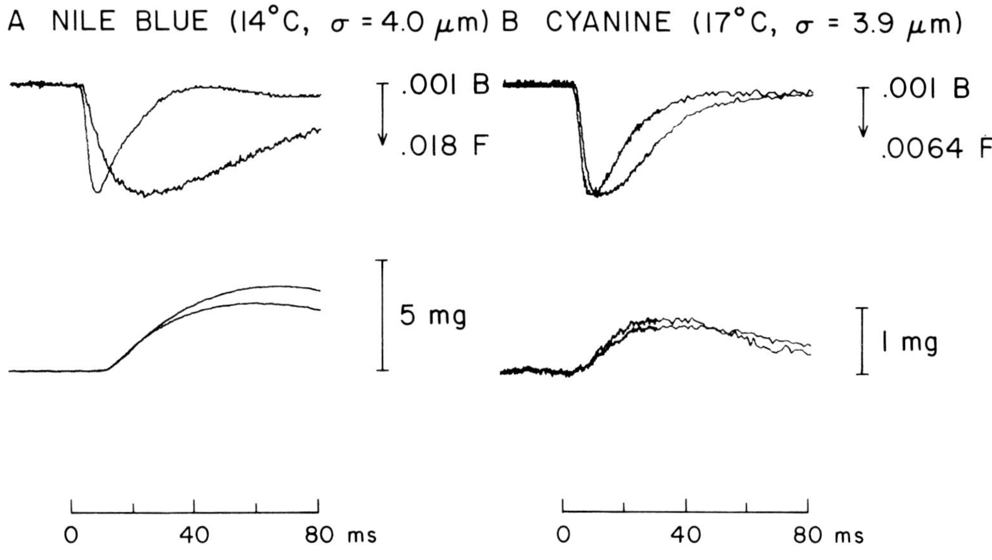

FIG. 9. Temporal comparison of intrinsic birefringence signal and fluorescence signals from single muscle fibers of *Rana temporaria* stained with membrane-permeant dyes. In both experiments action potentials were elicited by an external shock occurring at 0 ms on the horizontal time calibration. In both parts of figure, $\Delta I/I$ calibration applies to birefringence and $\Delta F/F$ calibration applies to fluorescence trace. *A*: *upper traces* show birefringence and Nile blue signals. Birefringence signal peaks earlier than Nile blue signal. Birefringence recorded in Ringer's solution before dye; fluorescence recorded after exposing fiber to Ringer's solution containing 0.5 μg/ml Nile blue. Birefringence was obtained with white light and signal-averaged twice. Nile blue was a single sweep, obtained with a 570-nm primary filter, 90° polarized light, and a 645-nm secondary filter. *Lower traces* show tension records; larger response was recorded after dye and shows that Nile blue caused a small potentiation of the twitch. *B*: *upper traces* show birefringence and downward cyanine signals; *lower traces* show tension. Birefringence signal decays more rapidly than cyanine signal. Birefringence recorded in Ringer's solution before and fluorescence recorded after adding 1 μg/ml of cyanine dye. Birefringence trace was signal-averaged twice and obtained with a 570-nm filter. Cyanine signal, a single sweep, was obtained with a 570-nm primary filter, unpolarized light, and 695-nm secondary filter. [From Baylor et al. (15).]

fore, was that unexpected complexity had been encountered that did not have a clear-cut interpretation. While it could be that all signals tracked SR potential but with variable delays, a second possibility, that some or possibly all such signals might reflect other underlying events, was raised (15).

Vesicular Preparations

Another experimental approach that has raised questions about the interpretation of signals in muscle from permeant potentiometric dyes comes from their use on SR vesicle preparations. Oetliker (69) reported that isolated SR vesicles exposed to the indodicarbocyanine dye produced a sigmoid fluorescence decrease as a function of changes in pCa from eight to five. A similar change was also detected in vesicles made calcium permeable by the ionophore X537A, vesicles digested by phospholipase A, and also with the purified SR adenosine triphosphatase (ATPase) alone. Therefore the signal from this dye in the intact fiber might reflect changes in calcium binding to the SR ATPase in response to changes in myoplasmic calcium.

Russell et al. (80) reported that vesicles exposed to oxacarbocyanine dyes, which are chemically similar to the indodicarbocyanine dyes, give at least two fluorescence changes that probably do not simply track diffusion potentials across the SR. One signal appears to be driven by changes in Ca^{2+} and adenosine triphosphate (ATP) binding to high-affinity sites on the membrane, whereas a second may be driven by changes in Ca^{2+}, Mg^{2+}, or K^{+} binding to low-affinity sites. The authors suggested that these signals could reflect changes in membrane surface potential caused by ion binding. Whatever the exact mechanism, these findings also raise questions about using membrane permeant dyes to track changes in SR membrane potential in a simple fashion.

Use of Impermeant Dyes to Possibly Stain SR Membranes

The complexity of signals from the permeant dyes is perhaps not entirely surprising as the presence of multicomponent signals was a prominent feature when these dyes were used in axons. On the other hand the impermeant dyes, as a class, tend to have more desirable characteristics. Used in low concentrations, they often give a single-component response to membrane voltage that is rapid (time constant: a small fraction of a ms) and linear (37). Therefore the use of impermeant dyes to stain SR membranes could represent a technical improvement because a more consistent pattern might be obtained if a voltage change across the SR was the underlying event signaled. The main technical difficulty would be finding a way to expose the SR membranes to the impermeant dyes.

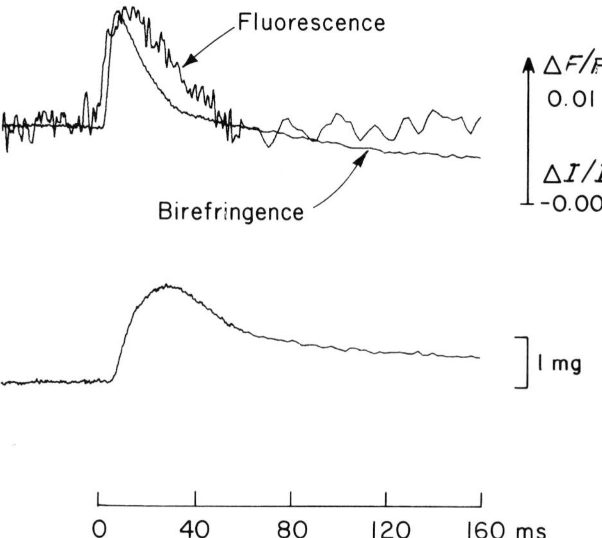

FIG. 10. *Upper traces*, temporal comparison of intrinsic birefringence signal and fluorescence signal due to the injection of impermeant dye WW781 (intact single fiber from *Rana temporaria*). Birefringence obtained after WW781 had been iontophoresed into myoplasm. Birefringence trace (single sweep) was obtained with white light and is plotted upside down; fluorescence trace (signal-averaged 31 times) obtained with 630-nm primary filter, unpolarized light, and 695-nm secondary filter. *Lower trace*, tension. Field of optical recording, 300 μm; fiber diameter, 80 μm; sarcomere spacing, 4.5 μm; normal Ringer's solution; 19°C. [From Baylor et al. (15).]

INJECTION OF IMPERMEANT DYES INTO INTACT FIBERS. One obvious solution to this problem might be to inject the impermeant dyes into the myoplasm, for example, by pressure or iontophoresis. Some success in carrying out this type of experiment on intact single fibers was reported by Baylor et al. (15). After iontophoresis of WW781 (the fluorescent dye used in Fig. 7*B*) a signal was detected that had a time course distinctly slower than the signal related to the action potential seen after external staining but was generally similar to the second component of the birefringence signal measured just prior to injection (Fig. 10). However, because of technical difficulties associated with dye injections of this sort, a comparison of the optical properties of this signal with those attributed to surface and/or T-system signals from this dye (15, 97, 98) has not yet been done. The detection of this signal must therefore be regarded as a preliminary, although encouraging, finding.

IMPERMEANT DYES ON SKINNED FIBERS. A second way of exposing SR membranes to the impermeant dyes is to use the skinned-fiber preparation and simply add the dye to the bath. Experiments of this type were first reported by Fabiato and Fabiato (41) and subsequently by Best et al. (20, 21), in which optical changes were detected when Ca^{2+} release from the SR was induced by either substituting chloride for an impermeant anion or by reducing external potassium. Although the mechanism for inducing calcium release in this way may or may not be relevant to the normal EC coupling process, the preparation allows for important control experiments. The signal reported by Best et al., which preceded the time course of the tension response, depended on staining the preparation with NK2367—a dye (chemically similar to WW375) that was first used to monitor membrane potential changes in neurons (78) and also gave an absorbance change in muscle that timed closely with the action potential (66). Furthermore the detection of the NK2367 signal in skinned fibers required prior loading of the SR with calcium and its amplitude was correlated with the amount of calcium released during stimulation, as inferred from the magnitude of the tension response. Importantly the signal was not detected when tension production was induced by increasing calcium in the bath surrounding a stained but unloaded fiber. Thus the signal had the properties expected if it depended on the movement of Ca^{2+} across the SR membranes.

To further test whether this dye could give signals in response to SR potential changes, potassium-substitution experiments were carried out in the presence of valinomycin, when the dominant SR membrane permeability was expected to be to potassium. An optical change was detected that approximated a linear function of the log of the external K^+ concentration (Fig. 11), in support of the idea that a membrane diffusion potential could be the underlying event signaled. Under the assumption that the signal seen in the presence of valinomycin could be used as a calibration for the stimulated-release signal, the sign and magnitude of the latter signal would be explained if the outside of the SR became approximately 0.1 V positive relative to the inside. Thus Ca^{2+} might be the ion responsible for generating the presumed potential change seen during the stimulated release (21).

An important further question concerning the characteristics of the signal driven by potassium substitution in the presence of valinomycin is the extent to which its spectral and polarization dependence might resemble that of the stimulated-release signal and the signal reported by Nakajima and Gilai (66) that comes from the surface and T-system membranes. (These features might be generally similar if a membrane potential change is the underlying mechanism in all cases.) However, because of the technical difficulty of reproducibly imposing changes in the skinned-fiber preparation by ion substitution, Best et al. (21) were able to determine the spectral shape at only a few points, which were not sufficient to permit a completely satisfactory comparison with the data of Nakajima and Gilai.

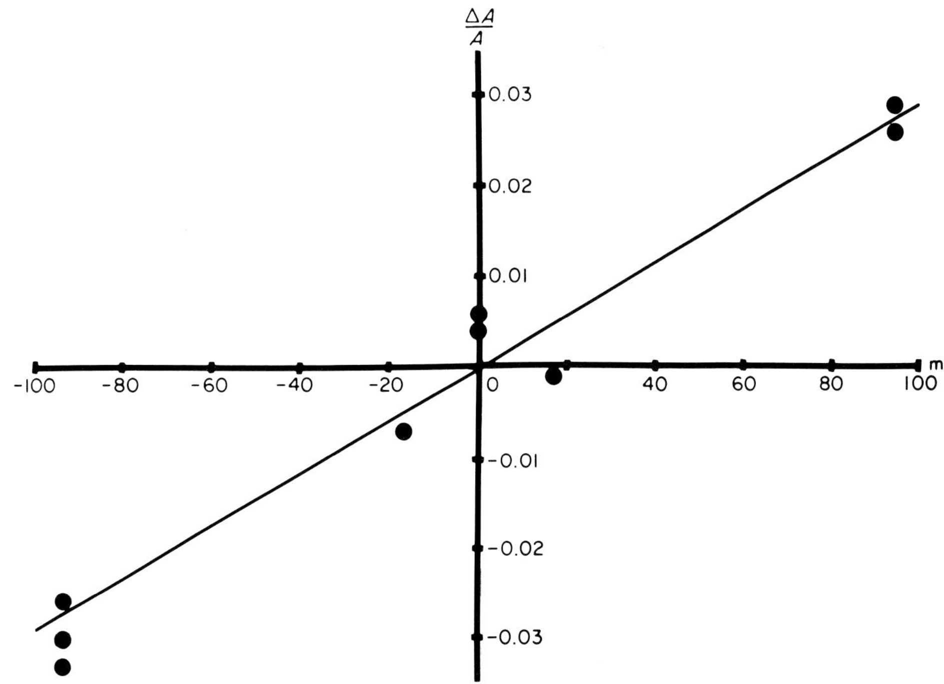

FIG. 11. Absorbance change from a skinned fiber of *Xenopus laevis* stained with impermeant dye NK2367 (0.2 mg/ml) as a function of changes in bath K^+ concentration after exposure of fiber to valinomycin. Scale on abscissa has been converted to mV by Nernst relationship, under the assumption that the SR membrane potential behaves as a potassium electrode. A straight-line relationship has been fit to the data by method of least squares. [From Best et al. (21).]

Voltage-Clamp Studies

Although the exact relationship of these possible SR signals to either the release of Ca^{2+} from the SR or the rise in myoplasmic calcium remains undetermined, they all seemed to reflect some step or steps in the EC coupling process subsequent to transverse-tubular depolarization. It was therefore of interest to observe their kinetic and steady-state properties in voltage-clamp experiments in hopes of learning more about the mechanisms underlying the signals and the mechanisms underlying the EC coupling process.

CHANGES IN INTRINSIC TRANSMISSION. The first study of an optical signal in voltage-clamped single fibers was reported by Kovacs and Schneider (60), who used the cut-fiber preparation to investigate changes in intrinsic transmission during activation. Such changes in frog muscle following soon after the action potential had been investigated previously on whole muscle (44, 45), bundles of fibers (10, 28), and intact single fibers (17, 18). The earliest changes seen in highly stretched fibers in which intensity changes had been detected in the direction of the light path (0°) were a decrease followed by an increase in transmitted light (17, 18, 28). Thus when interference from myofilament activity was minimized, the earliest change in both optical retardation and 0° transmission was a decrease, as might be expected by analogy with the earliest changes in axons thought to monitor membrane electrical activity (36).

Figure 12*A* shows examples of 0° transmission changes in response to different levels of membrane potential during a 60-ms pulse for a cut fiber at 4°C exposed to TTX and tetraethylammonium (TEA). For hyperpolarization or small depolarizations from the holding potential (traces *a* and *b*), little or no optical signal was seen. For larger depolarizations, however, increases in transmitted light began after a substantial delay, reached a plateau or peak during the pulse, and decayed approximately monoexponentially following the end of the pulse (decay time constant: 35–85 ms). The polarity of this change was therefore opposite to the earliest signal that followed an action potential in highly stretched fibers. Because no comparable signal was seen in traces *a* and *b*, the signal elicited by larger depolarizations was unlikely to reflect simply changes

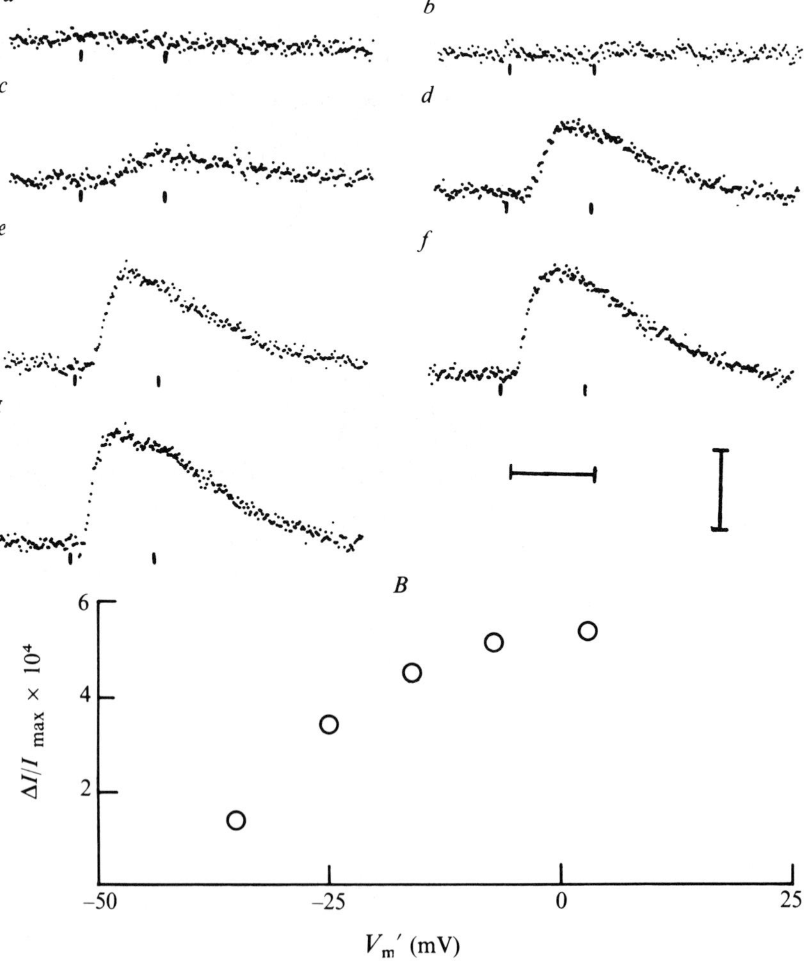

FIG. 12. Changes in intrinsic transmission from a cut fiber of *Rana pipiens* as a function of pulse amplitude under voltage-clamp conditions. Fiber was exposed to tetrodotoxin (TTX) and tetraethylammonium (TEA) at 3.9°C. *A*: ΔI/I records for 60-ms pulses to the following values of membrane potential (mV): *a*, −165; *b*, −44; *c*, −35; *d*, −25; *e*, −16; *f*, −7; *g*, +3. Each record is a single sweep. Horizontal calibration bar represents 60 ms; vertical calibration bar represents 4×10^{-4}. *B*: maximum ΔI/I as a function of membrane potential during pulse for records in *A*. [From Kovacs and Schneider (60).]

in surface or tubular potential. Rather the steady-state voltage dependence of the signal amplitude (Fig. 12*B*) was generally similar to that previously described for the charge-movement phenomenon (86), as would be expected if the movement of a single charged group controlled a single Ca^{2+}-release site and thereby controlled the optical signal. However, the delays in the rising phase of the optical signals were greater than those directly attributable to the kinetics of charge movement measured on the intact fiber. It was suggested that if charge movement controlled the transmission changes, the delays might be explained if either *1*) the optical signal reflected some change one or more steps removed from charge movement or *2*) more than one charged group was required to move before generating the change giving rise to the optical signal.

CHANGES IN NILE BLUE FLUORESCENCE. Studies of the Nile blue fluorescence signal were also made under voltage-clamp conditions by Vergara et al. (99) using the cut-fiber preparation (Fig. 13*A*). Little or no signal was detected for hyperpolarizations or small depolarizations, whereas for depolarizations near the contractile threshold, the signal started with a delay, then reached a plateau or peak late in the 50-ms pulse (15°C), and decayed approximately monoexponentially following the end of the pulse. For larger potential steps the signal had a faster rate of rise and an earlier and larger peak or plateau amplitude, although the decay time constant was, to a first approximation, independent of the voltage during the pulse. The general kinetic features of the intrinsic transmission change (Fig. 12*A*) and of the extrinsic fluorescence change (Fig. 13*A*) thus appear to be quite similar. However, in view of the temperature difference for the two experiments, this might be considered surprising since the decay rate constant of the Nile blue signal in intact fibers has a large Q_{10} [~7 for temperatures between 10°C and 16°C (22)].

The amplitude of the Nile blue signal plotted against membrane potential also showed a sigmoid activation curve (Fig. 13*B*), similar to the voltage dependence of the transparency change (Fig. 12*B*) and of charge movement. However, in carrying out a quantitative model Vegara et al. (99) noted that the dependence of signal amplitude on membrane potential might be explained equally well by independent participation of two charged groups (continuous curve), each with a voltage dependence slightly less steep than that calculated for a single-group fit (dashed line).

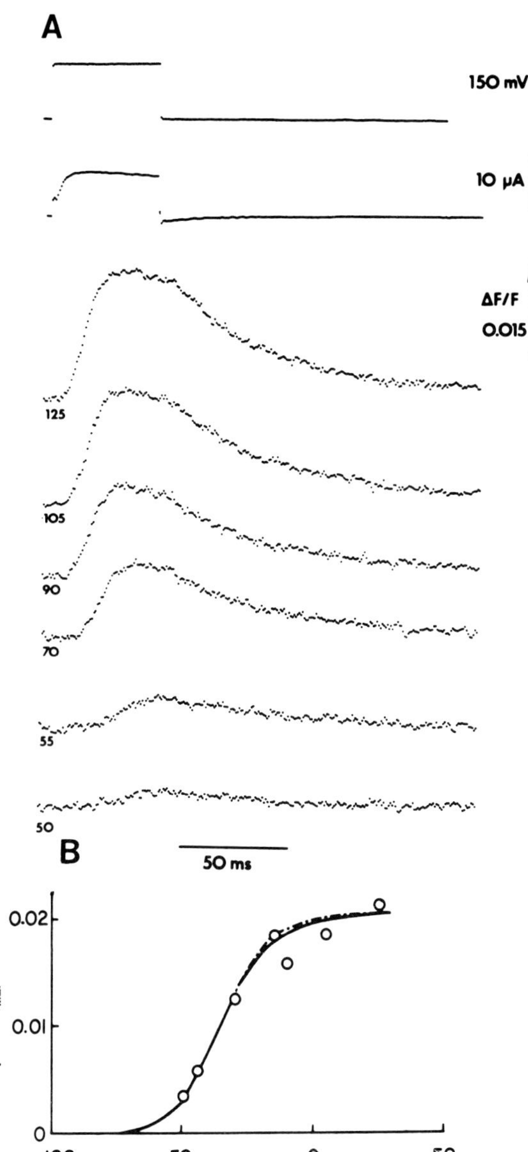

FIG. 13. Fluorescence signals from a cut fiber of *Rana catesbeiana* stained with Nile blue (0.5–2 µg/ml) as a function of pulse amplitude under voltage-clamp conditions. *A*: *1st trace,* sample voltage pulse of 125 mV; *2nd trace,* sample current for 125-mV pulse, *3rd–8th traces,* fluorescence signals associated with depolarizing voltage steps of the magnitudes indicated from a holding potential of −100 mV. Fiber was exposed to a Na-free, 115 mM tetramethylammonium solution; 15°C. *B*: peak amplitude of fluorescence change in *A* as a function of membrane potential during pulse. *Circles* are experimental peak values of ΔF/F plotted as a function of absolute membrane potential; *dashed line* corresponds to $\Delta F/F = 0.0205/[1 + \exp([V + 35]/9)]$; *continuous curve* corresponds to $\Delta F/F = 0.0462/[1 + 1.2(1 + \exp[-(V + 40)/12])^2]$, where V = absolute membrane potential (mV). [From Vergara et al. (99).]

CHANGES IN BIREFRINGENCE AND CYANINE FLUORESCENCE. Voltage-clamp experiments on intact single fibers exposed to TTX and TEA were carried out by Baylor and Chandler (11), who investigated the second component of the intrinsic birefringence signal and fluorescence changes from the indodicarbocyanine dye. In addition to observing the general saturating sigmoid voltage dependence over a wide range of potentials, these authors examined in more detail the features of the optical signals near the threshold for contraction (e.g., the birefringence signal, Fig. 14*A*). The signals were first observed at membrane potentials 5–10 mV below the threshold for detectable movement (measured either visually or by a sensitive tension transducer) as might be expected for an underlying event in the sequence of steps leading to contractile activation. Furthermore both the amplitude and maximum rate of change of the signals were remarkably steep with voltage, increasing *e*-fold for a 2.5- to 4.5-mV change in potential (see Fig. 14*B* for the analysis of the maximum rate of change of the birefringence signal). Although the precise way in which the optical signals might be related to calcium had not been determined, the experiments suggested that calcium release from the SR was likely to be more strongly dependent on the voltage change across surface and T-system membranes than previously supposed. In particular the data argued against the proposal that the originally described component of charge movement, detected in strongly hypertonic solution and seen to increase *e*-fold in amplitude for 8–13 mV (1, 30, 86), controls the Ca^{2+}-release sites in the SR in a simple one-to-one fashion (86). Rather the steep voltage dependence of the optical signal might be more readily explained if three or four such charged groups independently gated a single calcium-release site (cf. ref. 50) or if several components of charge, each with a similar voltage steepness, participated in a series of voltage-dependent steps (cf. ref. 8). Alternatively the optical signals and calcium release at threshold might be more immediately related to another component of charge movement, which is seen in less strongly hypertonic solution (1, 4, 53, 54) and may have a steeper voltage dependence than the originally described component.

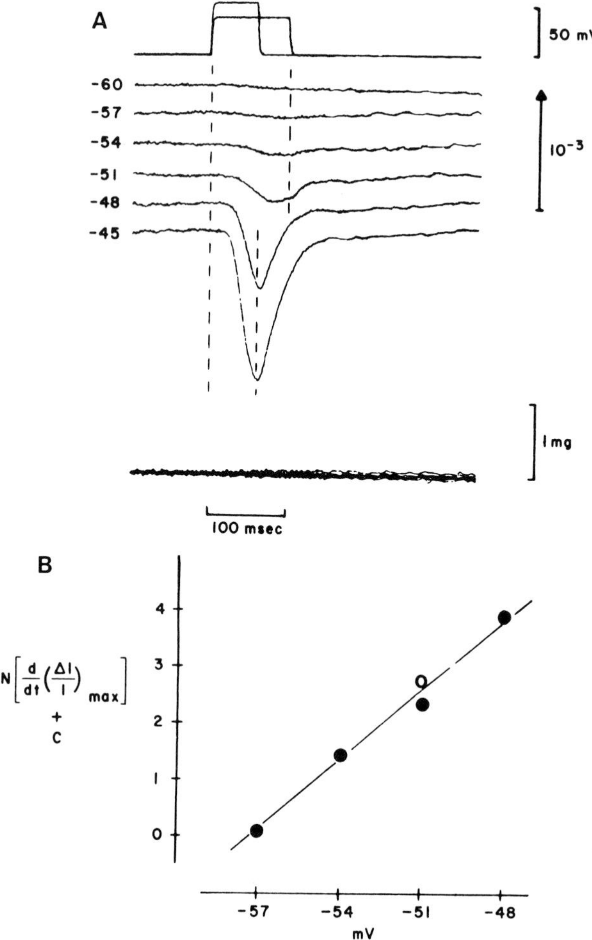

FIG. 14. *A*: birefringence signals near contractile threshold in a voltage-clamp experiment on a highly stretched single fiber of *Rana temporaria* exposed to TTX and TEA. *Upper traces* show 2 voltage pulses—100 ms and 60 ms in duration; *middle traces* show birefringence records; *lower traces* show superimposed tension records. All traces are single sweeps. *Dashed vertical lines* mark beginning and end of the pulses. Sarcomere spacing was 3.9 μm at site of optical recording in the middle of the fiber. Illumination was with a narrow transverse slit (about 60 μm wide) of white light positioned about 50 μm from voltage-sensing microelectrode. Resting potential of fiber was −90 mV; holding potential was −100 mV. Numbers to the *left* of optical traces indicate membrane potential (mV) during pulse; 10°C. *B*: logarithmic plot of maximum rate of change of birefringence signal vs. membrane potential during pulse. *Solid circles*, from records in *A*; *open circles*, from a bracketing record during run. *Straight line* was drawn by eye; its slope corresponds to an *e*-fold change per 2.5 mV. Scale for ordinate has been arbitrarily shifted. [From Baylor and Chandler (11).]

To summarize, these various studies demonstrated that a variety of optical signals can be detected having an appropriate time course and voltage dependence that might be indicative of a significant underlying change in SR potential occurring near the time of Ca^{2+} release. However, no strong evidence had been produced to support this interpretation for any of the signals. Rather, further study of the signals had revealed unexpected temporal relationships as well as the presence of multiple components. Nevertheless the hypothesis that the optical signals reflect a step (or steps) closely related to calcium appeared to be generally supported.

OPTICAL SIGNALS SENSITIVE TO CHANGES IN MYOPLASMIC CALCIUM

Luminescence Response From Aequorin

The first completely reproducible method for tracking calcium transients in skeletal muscle involved the use of aequorin, a photoluminescent protein that in combination with calcium can emit light (88). Its first successful intracellular use was tracking calcium transients in cannulated barnacle muscle fibers (9). In frog twitch fibers, however, it was more practical to introduce aequorin into the myoplasm by pressure injection through a microelectrode (79).

Figure 15*A* shows an aequorin response and the tension response reported by Blinks et al. (25) from an injected single twitch fiber in response to one action potential, and Figure 15*B* shows the averaged response to seven action potentials. The increased light emission, reflecting elevated calcium levels in the myoplasmic space occupied by aequorin, started slightly before the change in tension, reached a peak approximately halfway through the rising phase of tension, and declined to less than 50% of its peak value at the

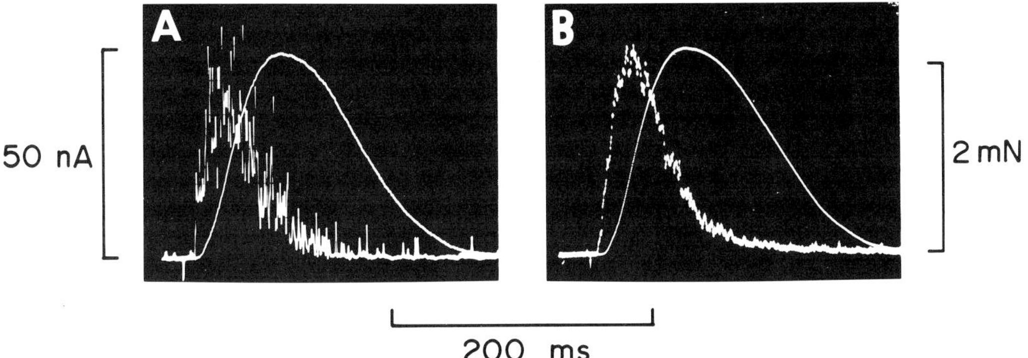

FIG. 15. Luminescent and mechanical responses in isometric twitches from a single fiber of *Rana temporaria* injected with aequorin. Striation spacing, 2.3 μm; temperature, 10°C. *A*: records of light (*noisy trace*) and force from a single rested-state contraction. *B*: 7 such twitches have been averaged to reduce photomultiplier shot noise. Time of stimulus is indicated by the vertical mark below the base line. (Note: recent improvements in techniques of light collection now allow a single-sweep signal-to-noise ratio for aequorin response comparable to that seen for averaged response in *B*—see, e.g., ref. 24a.) [From Blinks et al. (25).]

time tension reached its maximum value. Thus the light signal appeared capable of tracking calcium transients in the myoplasm occurring on the time scale of a twitch. However, because in a stopped-flow measurement in cuvette the change in light emission from aequorin in response to a step change in calcium has a time constant in the range of 10–15 ms at 10°C (24), it is likely that the signal in Figure 15 does not track the free-calcium transient effectively instantaneously. In addition the aequorin response in the fiber is probably not a linear monitor of changes in free calcium because cuvette calibrations indicate that for micromolar levels of calcium the response varies approximately as $[Ca^{2+}]^{2.5}$ (5). On the other hand an advantageous feature of the aequorin signal is the small fraction of released calcium (perhaps a few percent) that must bind to the indicator to give the signal in Figure 15. In addition there appears to be an absence of movement artifacts in the light trace, even for a fiber at a normal sarcomere spacing generating a substantial tension response. These and other advantages and disadvantages of the aequorin technique for tracking calcium in amphibian twitch fibers have been discussed (24, 25).

With the availability of the higher-affinity calcium-indicator dyes like arsenazo III (26, 95), dichlorophosphonazo III (also called chlorophosphonazo III) (76, 101), and antipyrylazo III (82) for use in biological preparations, it was natural that these dyes might be applied to skeletal muscle cells as another method for gaining information concerning calcium and the EC coupling process. One possibly troublesome feature of these dyes is that they are not entirely specific indicators for calcium; they also give large absorbance changes in cuvette in response to changes in H^+ and Mg^{2+}. Thus their use inside cells could be complicated if substantial changes in H^+ or Mg^{2+} occurred simultaneously with changes in Ca^{2+}.

A second disadvantage is that the stoichiometry of the dye reaction with calcium is not well understood in all cases. The first reports on stoichiometry implied that the dyes reacted in a one-to-one fashion with calcium, with an effective dissociation constant at neutral pH in the range of hundreds of micromoles per liter for antipyrylazo III (82), tens of micromoles per liter for arsenazo III (58, 83), and a few micromoles per liter for dichlorophosphonazo III (101). However, some subsequent studies have reported a more complicated stoichiometry in the case of both arsenazo III [(73, 94); R.Y. Tsien, unpublished observations] and antipyrylazo III (73), with one calcium–two dye complexes and two calcium–two dye complexes reported in addition to one calcium–one dye complexes. One implication of these results, if correct, is that the apparent dye sensitivity for calcium depends on total dye concentration. Therefore attempts to convert absorbance signals inside cells to levels of cytosolic free calcium on the basis of cuvette measurements may be considerably influenced by which calcium and dye concentrations are used for the calibrations and which assumptions are made concerning stoichiometry.

A third problem concerns the speed of the complexation reaction. One possible advantage of the indicator dyes over aequorin is the faster rates observed for the calcium-dye reactions in cuvette [with reported time constants: a small fraction of a ms for antipyrylazo III (83), less than 2 ms for dichlorophosphonazo III (101), and 2–3 ms for arsenazo III (83)]. If these numbers are applicable to myoplasmic conditions, the speed of the antipyrylazo response should probably be sufficiently fast for tracking calcium transients in amphibian skeletal muscle without introducing kinetic delays. However, in the case of dichlorophosphonazo III and arsenazo III it is not entirely clear that the dye reactions are effectively instantaneous for tracking calcium under all conditions—e.g., the calcium transient at warm temperatures in response to an action potential or a strongly positive voltage-clamp pulse.

Arsenazo III Signals in Intact Fibers

Miledi et al. (63) reported the first successful intracellular use of arsenazo III in twitch fibers, to measure Ca^{2+} transients in frog costocutaneous muscle. Interference from movement artifacts in the optical records was reduced by stretching the fibers to a sarcomere spacing of about 3.6 μm, and dye was injected into individual fibers by iontophoresis, usually to a concentration in myoplasm not exceeding 0.3 mM. Absorbance changes during activity could then be recorded under both action potential and voltage-clamp conditions.

In Figure 16*A* the lower trace shows the intracellularly recorded action potential and the upper trace shows light-intensity changes recorded at a single wavelength of light (532 nm) after dye injection. The biphasic optical response was presumed to reflect an early decrease in absorbance caused by the calcium-dye reaction and a delayed increase in absorbance caused by a small remaining movement artifact. On the other hand the middle trace was recorded differentially using a pair of wavelengths (532 nm and 602 nm) for which movement-related signals, expected to have the same polarity as a function of wavelength, would tend to cancel, whereas a calcium-dye signal, which should have opposite polarity at these two wavelengths, would summate. Under the assumptions that the absorbance change measured in this differential recording mode reflects only a change in the amount of calcium-dye complex and that cuvette calibrations for calcium and dye are applicable to intracellular conditions, it was inferred that the peak myoplasmic free-calcium level during a twitch at 7°C averages about 5 μm and is reached 15–20 ms after the action potential. Therefore, although extensive checks were not carried out to control for possible interference from other effects (e.g., simultaneous absorbance changes due to H^+ or Mg^{2+}), the differential-wavelength method appeared to give reasonable estimates for calcium.

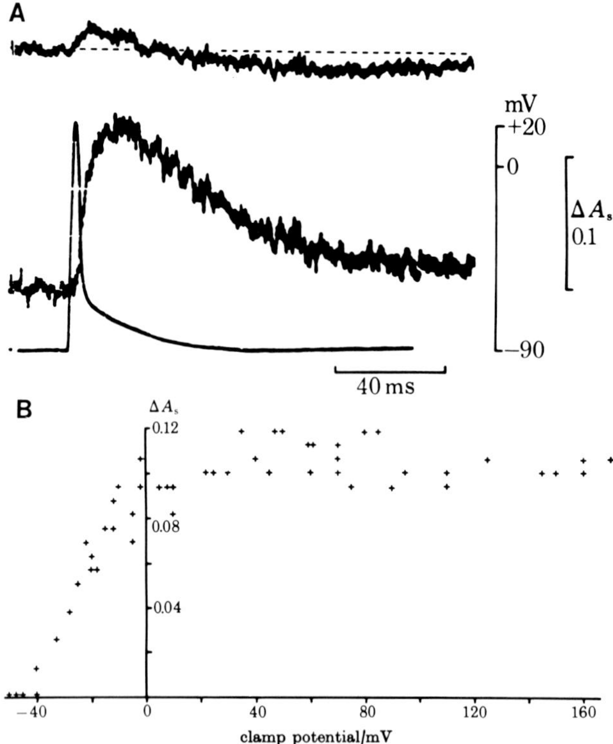

FIG. 16. Absorbance changes from a costocutaneous muscle fiber of *Rana temporaria* injected with arsenazo III. *A*: action potential conditions; 7.5°C. *Upper trace* is (minus) the absorbance record at 532 nm. *Middle trace* is the absorbance change at 602 nm minus the change at 532 nm, with the difference normalized by the resting absorbance at 532 nm. Subtraction procedure is designed so nonspecific changes tend to cancel, whereas changes on opposite sides of the isosbestic wavelength (approx. 570 nm) will summate. *Lower trace,* intracellularly recorded action potential. *B*: analysis of voltage-clamp records; 7°C. Relation between membrane potential and amplitude of the differentially recorded (602 nm relative to 532 nm) and normalized optical signal for a depolarizing pulse of 10-ms duration to the level indicated. Holding potential, −75 mV. [From Miledi et al. (63).]

The effects of surface and T-system depolarization on the absorbance signals were investigated further in voltage-clamp experiments with TTX and TEA. One type of experiment determined the amplitude of the optical transient in response to a 10-ms potential step to a variety of membrane voltages (Fig. 16*B*). The threshold for a just-detectable signal occurred at about −40 mV and thereafter the signal followed a saturating sigmoid shape. Furthermore even at strongly positive potentials (up to +170 mV) no falloff from the maximal amplitude of the absorbance change was evident. Because the electrochemical driving force on calcium would be greatly reduced, if not reversed, at these positive potentials, it was concluded that calcium entry across the surface or T-system membranes is not required for the response. This conclusion was further supported in voltage-clamp experiments in which free calcium in the bath was reduced below 10^{-7} M by chelation with EGTA [ethylene glycol-bis(β-aminoethylether)-*N,N'*-tetraacetic acid], with little or no change in the relation between membrane potential and the optical response [cf. a similar conclusion reached by Armstrong et al. (7) on the basis of action potential experiments].

Subsequently Baylor et al. [(12, 13); see also ref. 29] carried out similar experiments on intact single fibers injected with either arsenazo III, phenol red, or arsenazo I. Phenol red was used to check the magnitude of possible simultaneously occurring H^+ changes and arsenazo I checked for H^+ and Mg^{2+} changes. The signals detected by these two dyes during a twitch were small and indicated that myoplasmic pH probably changes by no more than 0.01 units and free Mg^{2+} by no more than 0.1 mM. Therefore any contribution to the arsenazo III absorbance signals due to these ions was likely to be small in comparison with that of a calcium signal (e.g., the 650-nm trace in Fig. 17*A*). However, after injection of arsenazo III, absorbance measurements made with two forms of polarized light (parallel and perpendicular to the fiber axis) showed unexpectedly large differences at some wavelengths, indicating the presence of an anisotropic (dichroic) component to the dye signal. This type of signal is not expected for changes in dye interactions with other molecules in solution as the absorbance change produced by this mechanism should give equal amplitude signals using the two forms of polarized light. In addition an isotropic component was detected that was prominent under some recording conditions. The time course of the dichroic component could be determined by taking the difference between absorbance records detected at any one wavelength using the two forms of polarized light, since by definition the isotropic component would cancel by taking differences. By this means the isotropic and dichroic components were seen to overlap in time course and precede the residual tension response. Furthermore the relative amplitudes of the two components varied with both dye concentration and wavelength. At lower dye concentrations (0.2–0.3 mM) both components were present in approximately equal amounts, whereas at higher dye concentrations (greater than 0.5 mM) the isotropic component predominated. Moreover the amplitude of the dichroic signal showed no isosbestic point, but rather it varied with wavelength approximately as did the resting absorbance of the dye. The mechanism proposed to explain the dichroic component was that some subpopulation of dye molecules must undergo a change in orientation during activity.

An example of the isotropic component of the arsenazo III signal is given in Figure 17*A*. Absorbance measurements after an action potential are shown at six wavelengths with one form of polarized light in a fiber injected with a relatively high concentration of dye, approximately 0.6–0.8 mM. (In this experiment, other records taken with both forms of polarized light indicated that interference from the dichroic component was negligible.) The 750-nm trace, taken at a wavelength that is beyond the absorption band of the dye, was flat, as would be expected if intrinsic changes were small and the high stretch (sarcomere spacing: approx. 4.0 μm) had successfully eliminated movement artifacts. This conclusion was also confirmed by the 570-nm trace, a wavelength that is close to an isosbestic point for the arsenazo III reactions with Ca^{2+}, Mg^{2+}, or H^{+}. At the other four wavelengths, however, substantial absorbance changes were seen, having differing amplitudes but essentially identical temporal waveforms. The pattern of the records was therefore consistent with the idea that only one underlying process was signaled. Furthermore the relative amplitude of the signal versus wavelength approximately agreed with cuvette calibrations previously reported for an arsenazo III–calcium difference spectrum (58). It was concluded that this isotropic signal, readily detected at higher dye concentrations, primarily reflected changes in myoplasmic calcium, with negligible interference from other processes if recordings were made with light at 650–660 nm. This result stands in contrast to that reported by Miledi et al. [(63); see also ref. 74], who monitored the difference between absorbance changes using 602-nm and 532-nm light and concluded that a relatively low concentration of arsenazo (not exceeding 0.3 mM) was best suited for monitoring the calcium transient.

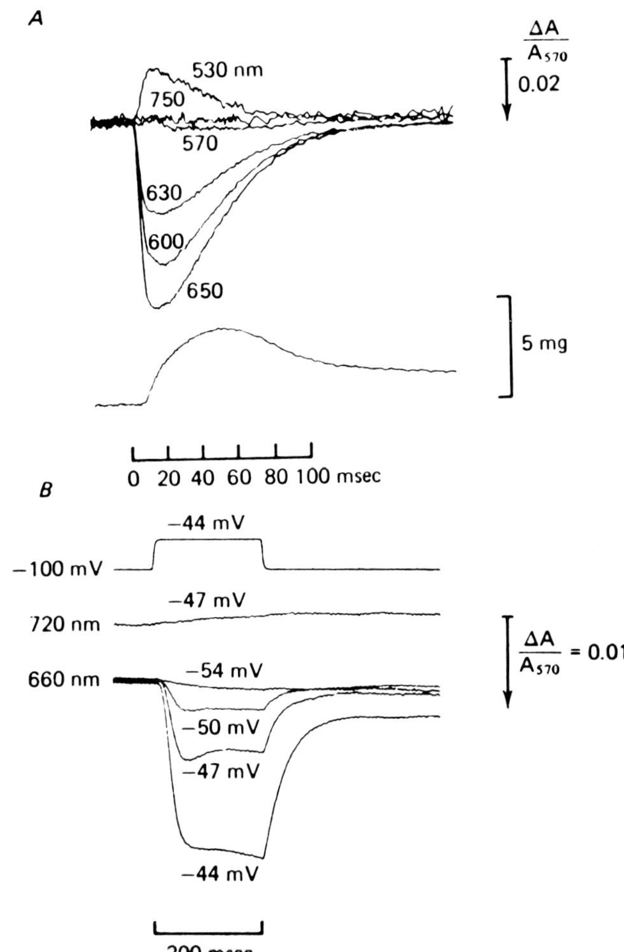

FIG. 17. Changes in transmission recorded from highly stretched intact single fibers of *Rana temporaria* injected with relatively high concentrations of arsenazo III. *A*: action potential conditions. *Upper traces* show superimposed optical records taken at wavelengths indicated with light polarized transversely (90°) to the fiber axis. *Lower trace* is the residual tension response. External shock occurred at 0 ms on the horizontal time axis. Sarcomere spacing, 4.0 μm; 16°C; normal Ringer's solution; 0.6–0.8 mM arsenazo III. *B*: voltage-clamp conditions. *Upper trace* shows a sample 200-ms voltage pulse. *Middle trace* is the transmission change at 720 nm, which is representative of non-dye-related effects. *Lower traces* are superimposed transmission changes at 660 nm for steps of potential to the levels indicated. Holding potential, −100 mV; sarcomere spacing, 3.9 μm; 16°C; D_2O Ringer's solution; 0.8 mM arsenazo III; 90° polarized light. [From Baylor et al. (13).]

Figure 17*B* shows results from a voltage-clamp experiment in the presence of TTX and TEA, designed to look at the voltage-dependence of calcium release near threshold. This experiment, at a relatively high arsenazo concentration (0.8 mM), was carried out in D_2O Ringer's solution to reduce movement artifacts, although essentially the same results were seen with H_2O Ringer's solution. The 660-nm trace, where the calcium signal was largest in the action potential experiments, was assumed to primarily reflect changes in myoplasmic free Ca^{2+} during and after the 200-ms voltage step to the membrane potentials indicated. This signal was seen to begin at a threshold level near −54 mV and to be strongly voltage dependent, changing *e*-fold in amplitude for approximately each change in potential of 3–4 mV. Therefore the tentative conclusion first reached in studies of the possible SR signals concerning the steep voltage dependence of calcium release (see, e.g., Fig. 14) was confirmed by direct measurements of myoplasmic calcium with arsenazo III.

Charge-Movement Currents and Antipyrylazo III Signals in Cut Fibers

Kovacs et al. (59) were the first to report experiments on the cut-fiber preparation designed to measure calcium transients using indicator dyes. These experiments extended previous studies by Horowicz and Schneider (51, 52) correlating the properties of charge-movement currents with mechanical activation, in which a just-visible movement had been used to qualitatively ascertain the presence of elevated myoplasmic calcium levels (51, 52, 87). The dye chosen for the measurements was antipyrylazo III, since it easily diffused from the cut ends of the fiber into the region of the optical and electrical recording. Optical changes were measured at 790 nm, a wavelength beyond the absorption band of the dye, as a check on intrinsic and movement-related signals, and at 720 nm and 550 nm, two wavelengths where large Ca^{2+} signals would be expected but would have opposite polarity since these wavelengths lie on opposite sides of the isosbestic point for the antipyrylazo-calcium reaction (82). At the latter two wavelengths, relatively large signals of opposite polarity were seen, having similar but not identical time courses. However, if correction was made for a small component having the same time course as the 790-nm signal, the remaining signals at 550 and 720 nm had identical time courses, as would be expected if one underlying process was signaled. The contribution from the non-dye-related signal to the 720-nm change appeared to be negligible in most circumstances, and absorbance changes at this wavelength, which are also relatively insensitive to H^+ and Mg^{2+} changes (82), were assumed to give a linear monitor of myoplasmic free Ca^{2+}. It was then possible in this preparation to simultaneously record both calcium-related signals and charge-movement currents under voltage-clamp conditions (Fig. 18).

After a 100-ms step of potential (Fig 18*A*, lowest trace) to various levels, the kinetic and steady-state properties of the calcium-related signals (Fig. 18*A*, upper traces) and charge-movement currents (Fig. 18*B*) could be compared. The threshold potential for detection of the calcium signal (between −50 and −40 mV) was more positive than that for detection of charge movement, suggesting that some finite amount of charge must move before significant calcium release takes place. Moreover, as the voltage level during the step was made more positive, increasing amounts of charge movement were seen, along with increasing magnitudes of the calcium signal, as expected if the amount of calcium that was released was related to the amount of charge that had moved.

An analysis of the relative time courses of the electrical and optical events was also consistent with the possibility that charge movement is causally related

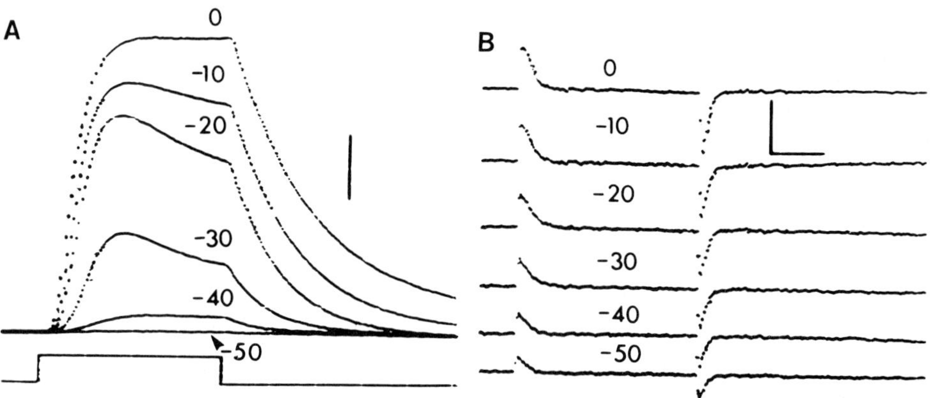

FIG. 18. Voltage dependence of Ca transients and intramembrane charge movement for a cut fiber of *Rana pipiens* exposed to TTX and TEA. *A*: superimposed ΔA signals at 720 nm for 100-ms depolarizing pulses to indicated values of membrane potential (mV). Each record is average of 6 determinations with no correction for fiber movement. Calibration bar corresponds to $\Delta A_{720}/A_{550}$ of 1.4×10^{-2}. Pulse is diagrammed below records. *B*: records of intramembrane charge-movement currents for same pulses as in *A*. Vertical calibration denotes 3.2 μA/μF, and the horizontal calibration denotes 30 ms; holding potential, −100 mV; sarcomere spacing, 3.5 μm; 3°C. Concentration of antipyrylazo III was 1 mM. [From Kovacs et al. (59).]

to calcium release. Qualitatively, it can be seen in Figure 18 that the time course of the currents appears to precede that of the calcium signal. This observation was made more quantitative by first describing the time course of the absorbance change after the ON of the voltage step as the sum of two exponential functions plus a constant. The ON transition time was by definition the time interval after the step change in potential during which the optical trace failed to satisfy the two-exponential description. This time interval decreased as the voltage step increased and was closely correlated with the time required for completion of the charge movement. Typically the ON transition time corresponded closely to the time required to achieve approximately 95%–98% of the total ON charge movement. Therefore the kinetic description supported the hypothesis that charge movement is a necessary preliminary step that controls calcium release. The subsequent two-exponential time course of the calcium transient was interpreted to indicate that calcium is redistributed between three effective compartments, with voltage-dependent but time-independent rate coefficients. The most likely explanation for the three calcium-containing compartments was considered to be the myoplasmic pool (accessible to the dye) plus the release and reuptake pools of the SR.

On the other hand the time course of the absorbance record after the return of the voltage to the holding potential involved a single-exponential description, again if one allowed for an OFF transition time taken as the interval during which the exponential description was not satisfactory. In this case, however, only 16%–86% of the charge movement had returned from the activating position during the OFF transition time. The explanation proposed for this observation was that several charged groups might participate in the gating of a single Ca^{2+}-release site or that charge movement might return to the resting position in several sequential steps. A final point concerned the voltage dependence of the single-exponential rate constant describing the decay of the optical signal. This parameter decreased with increasing voltages during the step, and it was suggested that the effect of voltage to increase myoplasmic calcium may involve not only an increased rate of release from the SR but a decreased rate of uptake [cf. a similar conclusion reached by Stephenson and Podolsky from studies on calcium movements in skinned fibers (91)].

Comparison of Signals From Calcium-Indicator Dyes on the Same Preparation

The above experiments suggest that under the proper recording conditions it is possible to monitor changes in myoplasmic calcium levels with negligible interference from other processes, in intact fibers with arsenazo III or in cut fibers with antipyrylazo III. As a check on the consistency of these interpretations, it would be desirable to compare the calcium signals obtained with both dyes on the same preparation. Unfortunately, because of factors such as the overlapping absorption spectra of the two indicators, it would appear technically difficult to carry out a satisfactory simultaneous comparison on the same region of the same fiber.

Using different fibers, however, Palade and Vergara (72, 73) have compared the characteristics of both arsenazo III and antipyrylazo III signals in the cut-fiber preparation. Figure 19*A* shows an example from a fiber injected with arsenazo III where absorbance was recorded at three wavelengths after action-potential stimulation. The relative amplitudes of these signals versus wavelengths show a pattern similar to that seen in the intact fiber (Fig. 17*A*), suggesting that the signals reflect a calcium component. However, their time courses are not identical, as a later time to peak is observed at shorter wavelengths. Therefore, in contrast to the results seen in the intact fiber at a high dye concentration, more than one underlying process must make substantial contributions to these signals. The source of the additional process(es) was not determined in these experiments, but changes in H^+ or Mg^{2+} were considered unlikely, as was possible interference from a dichroic signal. After exposure of myoplasm to antipyrylazo III, qualitatively similar absorbance signals (not shown) were also observed in response to action-potential stimulation. A comparison of results from the different fibers, however, suggested possible systematic differences in the signals from the two dyes. Whereas the rising phase and time to peak of the antipyrylazo III signal (recorded at 710 nm) and the arsenazo III signal (recorded at 660 nm) were judged to be closely similar, the antipyrylazo signal was reported to have a more rapid return to the base line than the arsenazo III signal.

Voltage-clamp experiments were also carried out by Palade and Vergara with both antipyrylazo III and arsenazo III (Fig. 19*B* and *C*). Rather surprisingly the absorbance changes elicited by large steps in potential (e.g., to +20 mV) were seen to have obviously different temporal waveforms after exposure to the two different dyes. Whereas the antipyrylazo III signal (Fig. 19*B*) always reached a peak and then decayed before the end of a large, long-lasting pulse [as reported by Kovacs, Rios, and Schneider (59) if corrections were made for movement artifacts], the arsenazo III signal (Fig. 19*C*) always continued to rise throughout a strongly positive pulse. Although this difference has not been satisfactorily explained, the result supports the possibility that either *1*) one or both of the dyes significantly change the calcium transient or *2*) more than one process largely contributes to one or both of the dye signals.

Some progress toward sorting out some of the complexity observed intracellularly may have been reached in comparing the characteristics of signals from three calcium-indicator dyes (arsenazo III, antipyrylazo III, and dichlorophosphonazo III) used on the intact single-fiber preparation (15). When the sig-

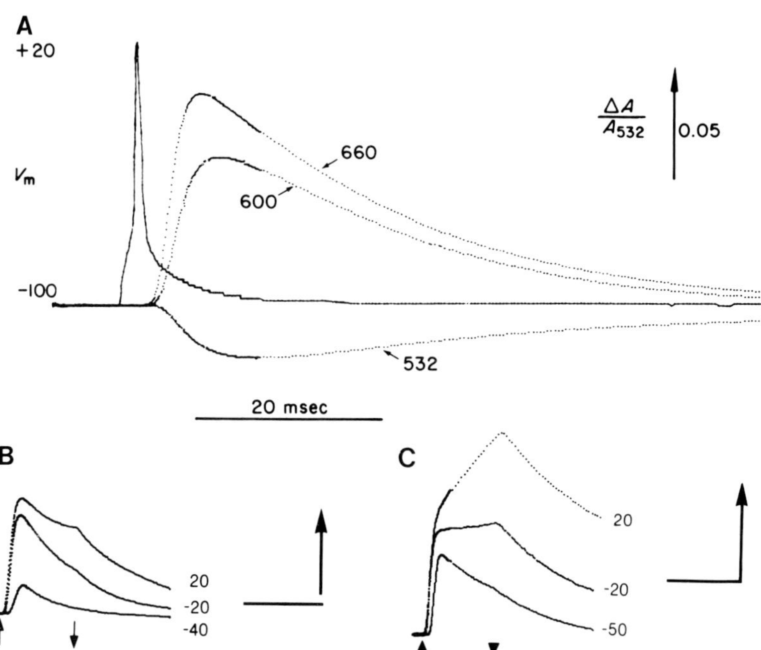

FIG. 19. Absorbance signals from cut fibers of *Rana temporaria* and *Rana catesbeiana* exposed to Ca-indicator dyes. *A*: action potential conditions with arsenazo III; 21°C. Superimposed traces show the electrically recorded action potential (earliest deflection, left calibration) and absorbance records at indicated wavelengths (later deflections, right calibration). *B*: voltage-clamp conditions with 1 mM antipyrylazo III; 10°C. Ringer's solution without TTX. Horizontal calibration is 50 ms; vertical calibration is 0.02 units of the absorbance change at 710 nm minus the fractional transmission change at 790 nm and normalized by the resting absorbance at 550 nm. *C*: voltage-clamp conditions with arsenazo III; 10°C. Ringer's solution without TTX. Horizontal calibration is 50 ms; vertical calibration is 0.2 units of the absorbance change at 660 nm minus the fractional transmission change at 740 nm and normalized by the resting absorbance at 532 nm. [From Palade and Vergara (73).]

nals observed from these dyes over a range of dye concentrations under single action potential conditions were analyzed as a function of wavelength and polarization, at least three qualitatively different components could be detected. The earliest component seen with all dyes was isotropic and had a spectrum closely similar to the calcium-dye difference spectrum measured in cuvette for small amounts of added calcium. Furthermore through time to peak the time course of the calcium signal was approximately the same for all dyes, as judged indirectly by comparison with the intrinsic birefringence signal used as a temporal bench mark [cf. Suarez-Kurtz and Parker (92), who reported a similar time of onset for the birefringence signal and the arsenazo III signal]. Thus the signal from all three dyes appeared to have at least one component that tracks myoplasmic calcium with a similar, although undetermined, delay. Starting soon after the calcium component, the dichroic component was observed, most easily seen with either arsenazo III or dichlorophosphonazo III. Finally, after return of the calcium and dichroic components to the base line (about 0.2 s after stimulation, 16°C–21°C), a second isotropic signal was evident, most easily seen with antipyrylazo III or dichlorophosphonazo III. The spectrum for the late change approximately agreed with cuvette calibrations for a small increase in either pH or Mg^{2+}, and it was suggested that this myoplasmic change might reflect the net hydrolysis of phosphocreatine after the twitch (cf. ref. 62). Thus the experiments indicated that the three dyes, at least under action potential conditions with movement artifacts eliminated, give qualitatively similar signals, reflecting the presence of at least three underlying physiological events. However, the relative proportions of the various components seen with any given dye or of any given component comparing different dyes depend on experimental circumstances, such as dye concentration and the wavelength and polarization of light used to make the measurement. The extent to which a similar analysis would be successful in decomposing the signals seen from the three dyes after tetanic stimulation or in voltage-clamp experiments remains a question for future investigation.

CONCLUSIONS

A number of studies have now been reported in which optical signals were measured from amphibian skeletal muscle fibers in the hope of tracking specific steps in the EC coupling process, including changes in surface and T-tubular potential, possible SR potential changes, and changes in myoplasmic free-calcium levels. The progress of this research has seen a general trend toward collecting signals from smaller numbers of muscle cells and smaller regions of single cells, as well as the introduction of techniques for making optical measurements with the cut-fiber preparation. At the same time the amount of optical information collected from a given type of experiment has increased, with more complete data being collected according to wavelength and polarization. Emphasis has also increased on comparing several types of optical signals that may monitor the same event and on comparing both optical and electrical data in the same fiber. To some extent these trends reflect the recognition of previously unanticipated problems in carrying out and interpreting optical experiments on muscle cells. For example, in the case of all three classes of signals, evidence has pointed to the existence of multiple components in signals that were originally considered to be single component. Although the presence of multiple components has introduced considerable complexity to the process of identifying the mechanism responsible for any single component, it is also possible that the total information eventually obtained may be usefully increased. Future experiments will therefore probably reflect more carefully controlled optical measurements, both in characterizing the signals in muscle cells and in simpler systems where the underlying optical mechanisms can be more easily studied (e.g., squid axon membranes, vesicular preparations, lipid bilayers, and cuvette solutions).

Nevertheless the muscle studies already completed have contributed new information about the EC coupling process. For example, in highly stretched fibers injected with arsenazo III or antipyrylazo III, signals can be recorded during a twitch that are likely to be more rapid and linear monitors of myoplasmic free calcium than the signal from aequorin. Such signals should therefore be able to contribute importantly to a more quantitative understanding of the rates of calcium release, binding, and reuptake under these conditions. In voltage-clamp experiments the signals from these dyes, as well as from the probes of possible SR potential change, have helped to characterize the time course and voltage dependence of calcium release in the absence (or near absence) of ionic currents, as well as the relationship between charge-movement currents and myoplasmic calcium. The availability of the optical signals is therefore generally useful for constraining possible models proposing how information in tubular depolarization may be coupled to changes in the SR membranes that result in calcium release. It is likely that the possibility of using optical methods to acquire information about EC coupling not readily available through other techniques will continue to be a sufficient impetus for future developments.

The author is grateful to his colleagues—in particular, Drs. W. K. Chandler and M. W. Marshall—for discussions.

The preparation of the manuscript was supported by the National Science Foundation (Grant PCM77-25163) and the American Heart Association (Grant 79-630).

S. M. Baylor is an Established Investigator of the American Heart Association.

REFERENCES

1. Adrian, R. H., and W. Almers. Charge movement in the membrane of striated muscle. *J. Physiol. London* 254: 339–360, 1976.
2. Adrian, R. H., W. K. Chandler, and A. L. Hodgkin. The kinetics of mechanical activation in frog muscle. *J. Physiol. London* 204: 207–230, 1969.
3. Adrian, R. H., and L. D. Peachey. Reconstruction of the action potential of frog sartorius muscle. *J. Physiol. London* 235: 103–131, 1973.
4. Adrian, R. H., and A. Peres. Charge movement and membrane capacity in frog muscle. *J. Physiol. London* 289: 83–97, 1979.
5. Allen, D. G., J. R. Blinks, and F. G. Prendergast. Aequorin luminescence: relation of light emission to calcium concentration—a calcium-independent component. *Science* 195: 996–998, 1977.
6. Almers, W., and P. M. Best. Effects of tetracaine on displacement currents and contraction of frog skeletal muscle. *J. Physiol. London* 262: 583–611, 1976.
7. Armstrong, C. M., F. M. Bezanilla, and P. Horowicz. Twitches in the presence of ethylene glycol-bis(β-aminoethylether)-*N*, *N'*-tetraacetic acid. *Biochim. Biophys. Acta* 267: 605–608, 1972.
8. Armstrong, C. M., and W. F. Gilly. Fast and slow steps in the activation of sodium channels. *J. Gen. Physiol.* 74: 691–712, 1979.
9. Ashley, C. C., and E. B. Ridgeway. On the relationships between membrane potential, calcium transient and tension in single barnacle muscle fibres. *J. Physiol. London* 209: 105–130, 1970.
10. Barry, W. H., and L. D. Carnay. Changes in light scattered by striated muscle during excitation-contraction coupling. *Am. J. Physiol.* 217: 1425–1430, 1969.
11. Baylor, S. M., and W. K. Chandler. Optical indications of excitation-contraction coupling in striated muscle. In: *Biophysical Aspects of Cardiac Muscle*, edited by M. Morad. New York: Academic, 1978, p. 207–228.
12. Baylor, S. M., W. K. Chandler, and M. W. Marshall. Arsenazo III signals in frog muscle (Abstract). *Biophys. J.* 25: 141A, 1979.
13. Baylor, S. M., W. K. Chandler, and M. W. Marshall. Arsenazo III signals in singly dissected frog twitch fibres (Abstract). *J. Physiol. London* 287: 23P–24P, 1979.
14. Baylor, S. M., W. K. Chandler, and M. W. Marshall. Comparison of optical signals in frog muscle obtained with three calcium indicator dyes (Abstract). *Biophys. J.* 33: 150A, 1981.
15. Baylor, S. M., W. K. Chandler, and M. W. Marshall. Studies in skeletal muscle using optical probes of membrane potential. In: *Regulation of Muscle Contraction: Excitation-Contraction Coupling*, edited by A. D. Grinnell and M. A. B. Brazier. New York: Academic, 1981, p. 97–130.
16. Baylor, S. M., and H. Oetliker. Birefringence experiments on isolated skeletal muscle fibres suggest a possible signal from the sarcoplasmic reticulum. *Nature London* 253: 97–101, 1975.
17. Baylor, S. M., and H. Oetliker. A large birefringence signal preceding contraction in single twitch fibres of the frog. *J. Physiol. London* 264: 141–162, 1977.
18. Baylor, S. M., and H. Oetliker. The optical properties of birefringence signals from single muscle fibres. *J. Physiol. London* 264: 163–198, 1977.
19. Baylor, S. M., and H. Oetliker. Birefringence signals from surface and T-system membranes of frog single muscle fibres. *J. Physiol. London* 264: 199–213, 1977.
20. Best, P. M., J. Asayama, and L. E. Ford. Optical absorption changes in skinned muscle fibers during calcium release (Abstract). *Biophys. J.* 25: 140A, 1979.
21. Best, P. M., J. Asayama, and L. E. Ford. Membrane voltage changes associated with calcium movement in skinned muscle fibers. In: *Regulation of Muscle Contraction: Excitation-Contraction Coupling*, edited by A. D. Grinnell and M. A. B. Brazier. New York: Academic, 1981, p. 161–173.
22. Bezanilla, F., and P. Horowicz. Fluorescence intensity changes associated with contractile activation in frog muscle stained with Nile Blue A. *J. Physiol. London* 246: 709–735, 1975.
23. Bezanilla, F., and J. Vergara. Fluorescence signals from skeletal muscle fibers. In: *Biophysical Aspects of Cardiac Muscle*, edited by M. Morad. New York: Academic, 1978, p. 229–254.

24. Blinks, J. R. Measurement of calcium ion concentrations with photoproteins. *Ann. NY Acad. Sci.* 307: 71–85, 1978.

24a. Blinks, J. R. Applications of aequorin. In: *Bioluminescence and Chemiluminescence: Basic Chemistry and Analytical Applications*, edited by M. A. DeLuca and W. D. McElroy. New York: Academic, 1981, p. 243–248.

25. Blinks, J. R., R. Rudel, and S. R. Taylor. Calcium transients in isolated amphibian skeletal muscle fibres: detection with aequorin. *J. Physiol. London* 277: 291–323, 1978.

26. Brown, J. E., L. B. Cohen, P. De Weer, L. H. Pinto, W. N. Ross, and B. M. Salzberg. Rapid changes of intracellular free calcium concentration: detection by metallochromic indicator dyes in squid giant axon. *Biophys. J.* 15: 1155–1160, 1975.

27. Buchthal, F., G. G. Knappeis, and T. Sjöstrand. Optisches Verhalten der quergestreiften Muskelfaser im natürlichen Licht. *Skand. Arch. Physiol.* 85: 225–257, 1939.

28. Carnay, L. D., and W. H. Barry. Turbidity, birefringence and fluorescence changes in skeletal muscle coincident with the action potential. *Science* 165: 608–609, 1969.

29. Chandler, W. K. Voltage dependence of calcium release in vertebrate skeletal muscle fibers. In: *Muscle Contraction*, edited by S. Ebashi, K. Maruyama, and M. Endo. New York: Springer-Verlag, 1980, p. 411–420.

30. Chandler, W. K., R. F. Rakowski, and M. F. Schneider. A non-linear voltage dependent charge movement in frog skeletal muscle. *J. Physiol. London* 254: 245–283, 1976.

31. Cohen, L. B. Changes in neuron structure during action potential propagation and synaptic transmission. *Physiol. Rev.* 53: 373–418, 1973.

32. Cohen, L. B., B. Hille, and R. D. Keynes. Changes in axon birefringence during the action potential. *J. Physiol. London* 211: 495–515, 1970.

33. Cohen, L. B., B. Hille, and R. D. Keynes. Analysis of the potential-dependent changes in optical retardation in the squid giant axon. *J. Physiol. London* 218: 205–237, 1971.

34. Cohen, L. B., K. Kamino, S. Lesher, C. H. Wang, A. S. Waggoner, and A. Grinvald. Possible improvements in optical methods for monitoring membrane potential (Abstract). *Biol. Bull. Woods Hole, Mass.* 153: 419, 1977.

35. Cohen, L. B., R. D. Keynes, and B. Hille. Light scattering and birefringence changes during nerve activity. *Nature London* 218: 438–441, 1968.

36. Cohen, L. B., R. D. Keynes, and D. Landowne. Changes in light scattering that accompany the action potential in squid giant axon: potential-dependent components. *J. Physiol. London* 224: 701–725, 1972.

37. Cohen, L. B., and B. M. Salzberg. Optical measurements of membrane potential. *Rev. Physiol. Biochem. Pharmacol.* 83: 35–88, 1978.

38. Cohen, L. B., B. M. Salzberg, H. V. Davila, W. N. Ross, D. Landowne, A. S. Waggoner, and C. H. Wang. Changes in axon fluorescence during activity: molecular probes of membrane potential. *J. Membr. Biol.* 19: 1–36, 1974.

39. Eberstein, A., and A. Rosenfalck. Birefringence of isolated muscle fibers in twitch and tetanus. *Acta Physiol. Scand.* 57: 144–166, 1963.

40. Endo, M. Entry of fluorescent dyes into the sarcotubular system of frog muscle. *J. Physiol. London* 185: 224–238, 1966.

41. Fabiato, A., and F. Fabiato. Variations of the membrane potential of the sarcoplasmic reticulum of skinned cells from cardiac and skeletal muscle detected with a potential-sensitive dye (Abstract). *J. Gen. Physiol.* 70: 6A, 1977.

42. Franzini-Armstrong, C. Studies of the triad. I. Structure of the junction in frog twitch fibers. *J. Cell Biol.* 47: 488–499, 1970.

43. Gonzalez-Serratos, H. Inward spread of activation in vertebrate muscle fibres. *J. Physiol. London* 212: 777–799, 1971.

44. Hill, D. K. Changes in transparency of muscle during a twitch. *J. Physiol. London* 108: 292–302, 1949.

45. Hill, D. K. The effect of stimulation on the diffraction of light by striated muscle. *J. Physiol. London* 119: 501–512, 1953.

46. Hille, B., and D. T. Campbell. An improved Vaseline gap voltage clamp for skeletal muscle fibers. *J. Gen. Physiol.* 67: 265–293, 1976.

47. Hodgkin, A. L., and P. Horowicz. The differential action of hypertonic solutions on the twitch and action potential of single muscle fibres (Abstract). *J. Physiol. London* 136: 17P, 1957.

48. Hodgkin, A. L., and P. Horowicz. The effect of sudden changes in ionic concentrations on the membrane potential of single muscle fibres. *J. Physiol. London* 153: 370–385, 1960.

49. Hodgkin, A. L., and P. Horowicz. Potassium contractures in single muscle fibres. *J. Physiol. London* 153: 386–403, 1960.

50. Hodgkin, A. L., and A. F. Huxley. A quantitative description of membrane current and its application to conduction and excitation in nerve. *J. Physiol. London* 117: 500–544, 1952.

51. Horowicz, P., and M. F. Schneider. Membrane charge movement in contracting and non-contracting skeletal muscle fibres. *J. Physiol. London* 314: 565–593, 1981.

52. Horowicz, P., and M. F. Schneider. Membrane charge movement at contraction thresholds in skeletal muscle fibres. *J. Physiol. London* 314: 595–633, 1981.

53. Huang, C. L.-H. Charge movement components in skeletal muscle (Abstract). *J. Physiol. London* 305: 31P, 1980.

54. Hui, C. S. Effect of dantrolene sodium on charge movement in frog twitch muscle fibers (Abstract). *Biophys. J.* 33: 152A, 1981.

55. Huxley, A. F. Muscle structure and theories of contraction. *Prog. Biophys. Biophys. Chem.* 7: 255–318, 1957.

56. Huxley, A. F., and R. E. Taylor. Local activation of striated muscle fibres. *J. Physiol. London* 144: 426–441, 1958.

57. Jöbsis, F. F., and M. J. O'Connor. Calcium release and reabsorption in the sartorius muscle of the toad. *Biochem. Biophys. Res. Commun.* 25: 246–252, 1966.

58. Kendrick, N. C., R. W. Ratzlaff, and M. Blaustein. Arsenazo III as an indicator for ionized calcium in physiological salt solutions: its use for determination of the CaATP dissociation constant. *Anal. Biochem.* 83: 433–450, 1977.

59. Kovacs, L., E. Rios, and M. F. Schneider. Calcium transients and intramembrane charge movement in skeletal muscle fibres. *Nature London* 279: 391–396, 1979.

60. Kovacs, L., and M. F. Schneider. Increased optical transparency associated with excitation-contraction coupling in voltage-clamped cut skeletal muscle fibres. *Nature London* 265: 556–560, 1977.

61. Landowne, D. Changes in fluorescence of skeletal muscle stained with merocyanine associated with excitation-contraction coupling (Abstract). *J. Gen. Physiol.* 64: 5A, 1974.

62. MacDonald, V. W., and F. F. Jöbsis. Spectrophotometric studies on the pH of frog skeletal muscle: pH change during and after contractile activity. *J. Gen. Physiol.* 68: 179–195, 1976.

63. Miledi, R., I. Parker, and G. Schalow. Measurement of calcium transients in frog muscle by the use of arsenazo III. *Proc. R. Soc. London Ser. B* 198: 201–210, 1977.

64. Mobley, B. A., and B. R. Eisenberg. Sizes of components in frog skeletal muscle measured by methods of stereology. *J. Gen. Physiol.* 66: 31–45, 1975.

65. Morad, M., and G. Salama. Optical probes of membrane potential in heart muscle. *J. Physiol. London* 292: 267–295, 1979.

66. Nakajima, S., and A. Gilai. Action potentials of isolated single muscle fibers recorded by potential-sensitive dyes. *J. Gen. Physiol.* 76: 729–750, 1980.

67. Nakajima, S., and A. Gilai. Radial propagation of muscle action potential along the tubular system examined by potential-sensitive dyes. *J. Gen. Physiol.* 76: 751–762, 1980.

68. Nakajima, S., A. Gilai, and D. Dingeman. Dye absorption changes in single muscle fibers: an application of an automatic balancing circuit. *Pfluegers Arch.* 362: 285–287, 1976.

69. Oetliker, H. Studies on the mechanism causing optical excitation-contraction coupling signals in skeletal muscle (Abstract). *J. Physiol. London* 305: 26P–27P, 1980.

70. Oetliker, H., S. M. Baylor, and W. K. Chandler. Simultaneous changes in fluorescence and optical retardation in

single muscle fibres during activity. *Nature London* 257: 693–696, 1975.

71. OHNISHI, T., AND S. EBASHI. Spectrophotometrical measurement of instantaneous calcium binding of the relaxing factor of muscle. *J. Biochem. Tokyo* 54: 506–511, 1963.
72. PALADE, P. Calcium transients in cut single muscle fibers (Abstract). *Biophys. J.* 25: 142A, 1979.
73. PALADE, P., AND J. VERGARA. Detection of Ca^{++} with optical methods. In: *Regulation of Muscle Contraction: Excitation-Contraction Coupling*, edited by A. D. Grinnell and M. A. B. Brazier. New York: Academic, 1981, p. 143–160.
74. PARKER, I. Use of Arsenazo III for recording calcium transients in frog skeletal muscle fibers. In: *Detection and Measurement of Free Ca^{++} in Cells*, edited by C. Ashley and A. K. Campbell. Amsterdam: North-Holland, 1979, p. 269–285.
75. PEACHEY, L. D. The sarcoplasmic reticulum and transverse tubules of frog's sartorius. *J. Cell Biol.* 25: 209–231, 1965.
76. PEACHEY, L. D., AND R. F. SCHILD. The distribution of the T-system along the sarcomeres of frog and toad sartorius muscles. *J. Physiol. London* 194: 249–258, 1968.
77. RAKOWSKI, R. F. Reprimed charge movement in skeletal muscle fibres. *J. Physiol. London* 281: 339–358, 1978.
78. ROSS, W. N., B. M. SALZBERG, L. B. COHEN, A. GRINVALD, H. V. DAVILA, A. S. WAGGONER, AND C. H. WANG. Changes in absorption, fluorescence, dichroism and birefringence in stained giant axons: optical measurement of membrane potential. *J. Membr. Biol.* 33: 141–183, 1977.
79. RUDEL, R., AND S. R. TAYLOR. Aequorin luminescence during contraction of amphibian skeletal muscle (Abstract). *J. Physiol. London* 233: 5P–6P, 1973.
80. RUSSELL, J. T., T. BEELER, AND A. MARTONOSI. Optical probe responses on sarcoplasmic reticulum—oxacarboncyanines. *J. Biol. Chem.* 254: 2040–2046, 1979.
81. SCARPA, A. Kinetics and energy-coupling of Ca^{++}-transport in mitochondria. In: *Calcium Transport in Contraction and Secretion*, edited by E. Carafoli, F. Clementi, W. Drabikowski, and A. Margreth. Amsterdam: North-Holland, 1975, p. 65–76.
82. SCARPA, A., F. J. BRINLEY, AND G. DUBYAK. Antipyrylazo III, a "middle range" Ca^{++} metallochromic indicator. *Biochemistry* 17: 1378–1386, 1978.
83. SCARPA, A., F. J. BRINLEY, T. TIFFORT, AND G. DUBYAK. Metallochromic indicators of ionized calcium. *Ann. NY Acad. Sci.* 307: 86–111, 1978.
84. SCHAEFER, H., AND H. GOPFERT. Aktionsstrom und optisches Verhalten des Frosch Muskels in ihrer zeitlichen Beziehung zur Zuckung. *Pfluegers Arch. Gesamte Physiol. Menschen Tiere* 238: 684–708, 1937.
85. SCHLEVIN, H. H. Effects of external calcium concentration and pH on charge movement in frog skeletal muscle. *J. Physiol. London* 288: 129–158, 1979.
86. SCHNEIDER, M. F., AND W. K. CHANDLER. Voltage dependent charge movement in skeletal muscle: a possible step in excitation-contraction coupling. *Nature London* 242: 244–246, 1973.
87. SCHNEIDER, M. F., AND P. HOROWICZ. Membrane charge movement at contraction thresholds (Abstract). *Biophys. J.* 25: 201A, 1979.
88. SHIMOMURA, O., F. H. JOHNSON, AND Y. SAIGA. Microdetermination of calcium by aequorin luminescence. *Science* 140: 1339–1340, 1963.
89. SOMLYO, A. V., H. SHUMAN, AND A. P. SOMLYO. Elemental distribution in striated muscle and effects of hypertonicity: electron probe analysis of cryo sections. *J. Cell Biol.* 74: 828–857, 1977.
90. SOMLYO, A. V., A. P. SOMLYO, H. GONZALEZ-SERRATOS, H. SHUMAN, AND G. MCCLELLAN. Sarcoplasmic reticulum, mitochondria and excitation-contraction coupling in smooth and striated muscle. In: *Regulation of Muscle Contraction: Excitation-Contraction Coupling*, edited by A. D. Grinnell and M. A. B. Brazier. New York: Academic, 1981, p. 199–223.
91. STEPHENSON, E. W., AND R. J. PODOLSKY. The regulation of calcium in skeletal muscle. *Ann. NY Acad. Sci.* 307: 462–476, 1978.
92. SUAREZ-KURTZ, G., AND I. PARKER. Birefringence signals and calcium transients in skeletal muscle. *Nature London* 270: 746–748, 1977.
93. TASAKI, I., A. WATANABE, R. SANDLIN, AND L. CARNAY. Changes in fluorescence, turbidity, and birefringence associated with nerve excitation. *Proc. Natl. Acad. Sci. USA* 61: 883–888, 1968.
94. THOMAS, M. V. Arsenazo III forms 2:1 complexes with Ca and 1:1 complexes with Mg under physiological conditions. *Biophys. J.* 25: 541–548, 1979.
95. VALLIERES, J., A. SCARPA, AND A. P. SOMLYO. Subcellular fractions of smooth muscle: isolation, substrate utilization and Ca^{++} transport by main pulmonary artery and mesenteric vein mitochondria. *Arch. Biochem. Biophys.* 170: 659–669, 1975.
96. VERGARA, J., AND F. BEZANILLA. Fluorescence changes during electrical activity in frog muscle stained with merocyanine. *Nature London* 259: 684–686, 1976.
97. VERGARA, J., AND F. BEZANILLA. Tubular membrane potentials monitored by a fluorescent dye in cut single muscle fibers (Abstract). *Biophys. J.* 25: 201A, 1979.
98. VERGARA, J., AND F. BEZANILLA. Optical studies of E-C coupling with potentiometric dyes. In: *Regulation of Muscle Contraction: Excitation-Contraction Coupling*, edited by A. D. Grinnell and M. A. B. Brazier. New York: Academic, 1981, p. 67–77.
99. VERGARA, J., F. BEZANILLA, AND B. M. SALZBERG. Nile Blue fluorescence signals from cut single muscle fibers under voltage or current clamp conditions. *J. Gen. Physiol.* 72: 775–800, 1978.
100. WAGGONER, A. Optical probes of membrane potential. *J. Membr. Biol.* 27: 335–346, 1976.
101. YOSHIKAMI, S., AND W. A. HAGINS. Calcium in excitation of vertebrate rods and cones: retinal efflux of calcium studied with dichlorophosphonazo III. *Ann. NY Acad. Sci.* 307: 545–561, 1978.

Pharmacological investigations of excitation-contraction coupling

CARLO CAPUTO | *Centro de Biofísica y Bioqúimica, Instituto Venezolano de Investigaciones Científicas, Caracas, Venezuela*

CHAPTER CONTENTS

EXCITATION-CONTRACTION COUPLING is a term that originally designated the series of events that, starting with the propagated action potential, activates contraction in muscle fibers (248). This term has become enormously popular, and its use has been extended to cover the events related to contractile activation in the absence of action potentials, by depolarizing the membrane other ways, and even in the absence of membrane depolarization [e.g., with caffeine (18)]. Although lax (250), this practice is followed in this chapter because of the widespread use of the term.

Muscle function has been pharmacologically investigated since the last century, and numerous drugs and experimental manipulations that affect excitation-contraction coupling (ECC) have been found. Unfortunately none of these substances, as pointed out recently (82), affects a definite step in ECC specifically, as do some drugs that are specific for other phenomena, such as tetrodotoxin for membrane excitability and curare for neuromuscular transmission. Nevertheless characterizing the effects of some of the substances that alter ECC has proved somewhat valuable because it has helped to establish criteria for the participation of certain phenomena in ECC and to establish the localization of these phenomena at levels of structure not readily accessible with conventional experimental techniques. Frog skeletal twitch fibers and more recently isolated single fibers have come into such general use that most of this chapter refers to work carried out with these preparations. However, other preparations are considered when necessary.

EXCITATION-CONTRACTION COUPLING PHENOMENA

The phenomena related to contractile activation have been clearly covered in Costantin's (67) chapter in the 1977 edition of the *Handbook* section on the nervous system.

Active State

In vertebrate fast-twitch skeletal muscle fibers the physiological event that under normal conditions leads to contractile activation is the action potential, which starts at the end-plate region and propagates longitudinally along the sarcolemma and radially along the membranes of the transverse tubules (T tubules).

The transient depolarization associated with the action potential is responsible for starting the chain of

ECC events and leads to massive release of Ca^{2+} from the terminal cisternae of the sarcoplasmic reticulum (SR) (67, 249). Ample evidence from different techniques (68, 69, 292–294) shows that most of the Ca^{2+} in muscle fibers is stored in the SR elements preferentially in the terminal cisternae. Calcium is sequestered and released by the SR by mechanisms that are described in detail in the chapter by Martonosi and Beeler in this *Handbook*. At its peak the action potential brings the fiber interior, in a fraction of a millisecond, to about 30 mV, inside positive, from a resting membrane potential of −95 mV. This condition is almost completely reversed in less than 4 ms. Yet the first signs of mechanical activity are detectable only 1 or 2 ms after the peak of the action potential (155), as shown in Figure 1. For an isometric-tension recording the maximum twitch tension is reached 20 or 30 ms after the peak of the action potential, when the electrical changes associated with it have completely disappeared. The relaxation phase of the twitch prolongs this response to more than 100 ms.

According to Hill (149), immediately after stimulation and before one can detect signs of contractile activity, muscle fibers reach a state of full activity, termed the *active state*, during which the fiber resistance to stretch increases. Hill suggested that the twitch lagged behind contraction during the active state because the contractile elements of the fiber have to stretch the series-elastic elements to develop tension. In a single twitch the active state does not last long enough for the series-elastic elements to stretch completely; therefore twitch tension does not reach its maximal possible value. Because of the damping effect of the series-elastic elements, tension development and relaxation during a twitch lag behind the rising and decaying phases of the active state. On the other hand, during a tetanus, repetitive stimulation prolongs the active state enough so the contractile elements have time to stretch the series-elastic elements and so the fiber can develop its maximal possible tension.

Recently several attempts have been made to explain the time course of the active state with some of the phenomena that participate in ECC. For instance Edman and Kiessling (87) proposed that the intensity of the active state may follow a time course that depends on the concentration of a Ca–contractile-protein complex whose kinetics are determined by the release of Ca^{2+} from and its reuptake by the SR. Calcium indicators such as the photoprotein aequorin (17, 41, 241) or the dyes arsenazo (22, 211) and antipyrylazo (188) have allowed the time course of the transient increase in Ca^{2+} concentration to be studied; the results support the idea of an early start of the active state.

Figure 2 schematically shows the time relationship between the active state, the aequorin Ca signal, and the isometric force during a single fiber twitch at 5°C. The decay of the light signal precedes the decay of active state and is almost complete by the time maximum force is attained. This agrees with the possibility that the active state parameter indicates protein-bound Ca^{2+} (87).

Regulation of Calcium Release

The mechanism that regulates Ca release from the SR during contractile activity has not yet been defined, in spite of a large body of experimental work. The inaccessibility of the SR to conventional electrophysiological measurements has impeded gathering direct information on the nature of the events that cause Ca release. Under physiological conditions the depolarization of the surface and T-tubule membranes is the electrical signal that triggers Ca release. There are, however, many uncertainties about the way this signal is transmitted to the SR membrane and about subsequent events at the level of this membrane.

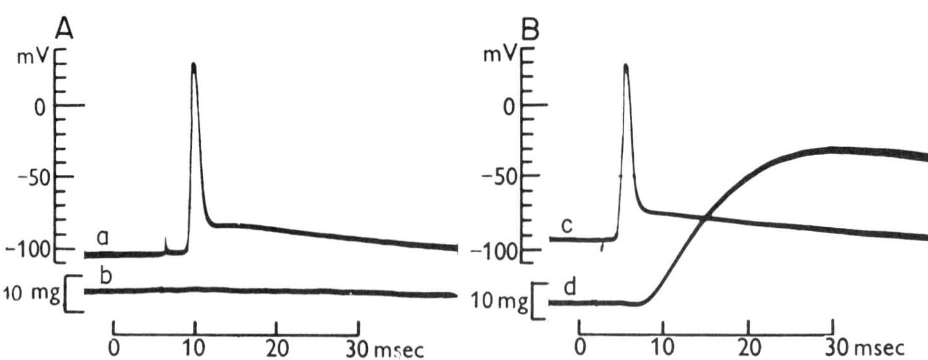

FIG. 1. Simultaneous recording of electrical and contractile responses of frog single muscle fiber in hypertonic (*A*) and normal (*B*) Ringer's solution. Action potentials (*a* and *c*) were recorded with an intracellular microelectrode; a transducer measured twitch tension (*b* and *d*). While immersed in hypertonic fluid of 270 mM NaCl (instead of 120 mM), fiber resting potential was slightly increased, action potential basically not modified, and twitch tension completely inhibited (*a* and *b*). This effect on twitch tension is rapidly reversed when fiber is exposed to normal Ringer's solution (*d*). Fiber diameter, 140 μm; 20°C. [From Hodgkin and Horowicz (155).]

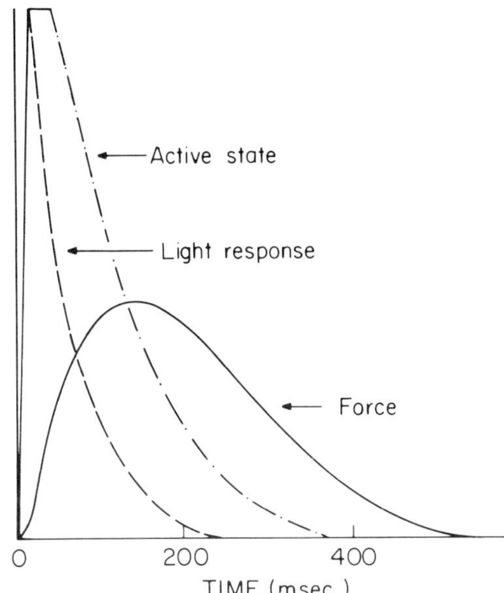

FIG. 2. Time courses of isometric tension, active state, and aequorin light signal during twitch of frog single muscle fiber at 5°C. Force trace records single muscle fiber from *Rana pipiens*; light-response trace redrawn from ref. 41 and scaled for twitch time course. Active-state trace combines ideas and results of Hill (149) and Edman and Kiessling (87).

Information between the T tubules and the SR membrane is probably transmitted at the junction between these membranes (123). At the triad the membranes of the T tubules and of the SR terminal cisternae are not in close apposition but are separated by a gap of about 110–130 Å (124). This gap appears partially bridged by electron-dense feet (124, 125) and pillars (261) that extend from the terminal cisterna membranes to the T-tubule membranes.

The interior of the feet appears to be electron opaque and occupied by dense material that may anchor the feet to the SR membrane (125). On the other hand the pillars, which are much less numerous, have an electron-lucent interior, and their number appears to increase after low-frequency stimulation (90) and potassium depolarization but not after caffeine contractures (89a), indicating that their formation might be a cause and not an effect of Ca release. The hypothesis that pillar formation might be a step in ECC is interesting, and pharmacological interventions may prove important in testing it. Information on the effect of pharmacological agents that modify ECC of these structures unfortunately is not yet available.

Much evidence supports the hypothesis that the nonlinear intramembrane charge movement, which occurs at the level of the tubule membranes, links membrane depolarization with Ca release (1, 256). The feet or pillars might be the structural basis for this coupling mechanism; the number of charged groups necessary to account for the charge movement and the number of electron-dense feet localized between the tubular and the SR membrane appear to be related (124a). Almers (9) and Adrian in his chapter of this *Handbook* have detailed descriptions of charge movement and its possible involvement in ECC. Charge movement, if involved in ECC, would provide the voltage sensitivity required for Ca release.

An alternate model recently proposed by Mathias et al. (207) is also based on pillars at the junction between the T-tubule SR, which might serve as transient conductive pathways. According to this theoretical model the electrical signal usually interpreted as representing nonlinear capacitative currents associated with intramembrane charge movement reflects ionic currents flowing through the interiors of the pillars, which could either be formed transiently during excitation or preexist and be transiently conductive. It has also been pointed out, however, that the formation of pillars during ECC might provide the structural basis for the remote control model (58) proposed to explain the nonlinear charge movement (89a).

Mechanically Effective Period

How membrane depolarization leads to Ca release from the SR is not well understood and is one area where research efforts are most concentrated. Contractile activation starts at the threshold of the membrane potential, measured by different techniques (2, 3, 66, 157) as about −50 mV. The action potential initiates Ca release by depolarizing the membrane beyond the contractile threshold. The possibility of potentiating the twitch with NO_3^- (151, 181) first suggested that tension development during a twitch could be modulated. The quantitative relationship between membrane potential and tension output could not be established by using the action potential to trigger contractions, however, since this signal, because of its all-or-none nature, could hardly be modulated in amplitude or duration.

Based on the results of Hodgkin and Horowicz (157) with K-depolarization contractures, Sandow, Taylor, and Preiser (255, 274), under a variety of experimental conditions, related the changes in the membrane potential during an action potential with the tension output of a twitch. In particular they explained the potentiating action of several compounds. Their explanation depended on the assumption that Ca release in response to an action potential is limited to the interval during which the membrane potential is more positive than the contractile threshold. This interval, termed the *mechanically effective period*, is the most useful parameter for determining contractile output during a twitch. In frog skeletal muscle it lasts about 1.5 ms at room temperature and about 5 ms at 4°C.

Figure 3 relates the mechanically effective period to the action potential time course. Effective extension of this period is achieved either by lowering the contractile threshold or by prolonging the action poten-

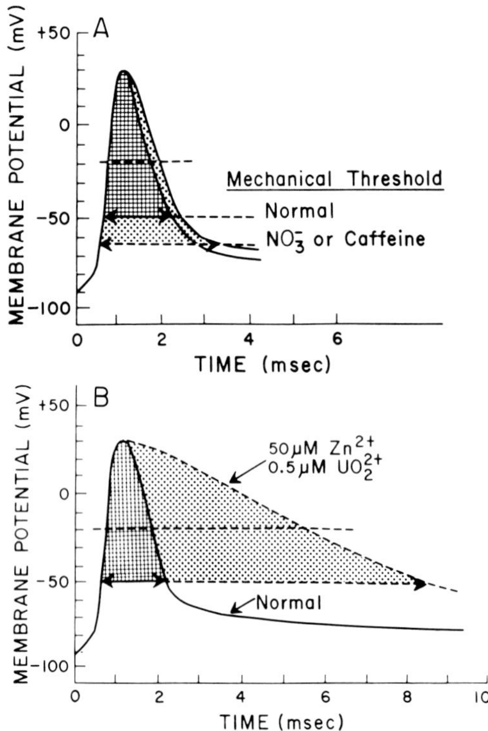

FIG. 3. Role of action potential in ECC with different contractile potentiators. Voltage and temporal features are typical for frog muscle fibers at 20°C. *A*: how contractile potentiators of type A (nitrate or caffeine) prolong the mechanically effective period (*arrowed bars*), by lowering contractile threshold from −50 mV to about −64 mV. *Dashed line* at about −20 mV represents the level of mechanical saturation. *B*: extent that type B potentiators (zinc and uranyl ions) prolong the action potential and thus the mechanically effective period. [From Sandow et al. (255).]

tial. In both cases the consequence is an increase in the amount of contractile activator released as later confirmed in experiments with aequorin (198). This interpretation is also supported by voltage-clamp studies in which contractile activation was graded (66) and tension output was increased either by increasing the amplitude or the duration of short depolarizing pulses (28, 29, 145).

Contractile Threshold

The three-electrode, voltage-clamp technique, originally developed by Adrian et al. (3), and the two-electrode version of it (2) have been increasingly used to study phenomena related to ECC, including intramembrane charge movement. When applied to preparations whose voltage cannot be controlled along the entire length, this technique has been most useful for obtaining information on contractile activation at membrane potentials near the contractile threshold (2). In fact, in the region of the muscle fiber near the electrodes, good clamping conditions can be achieved and direct or photographic observation of movement can be made through a microscope. Thus the contractile threshold could be precisely determined (65, 78, 184, 185), allowing study of the effects of several extraneous ions and different substances on contractile activation. Because the membrane potential threshold for contractile activation is very close to that for delayed rectification, much work has been carried out to determine whether a causal relationship could exist between these two phenomena.

The possibility of differentially affecting the two thresholds prompted the use of several agents that modify the contractile threshold. The lyotropic anions that potentiate muscle contraction by lowering the contractile threshold (158) lowered the threshold for the delayed rectifier as well (184). Experiments with sulfate and quaternary ammonium cations yielded the same results, pointing to a close parallelism between the two phenomena (186). A causal relationship between delayed rectifier and contractile activation could be discarded, however, because of experiments in which the kinetics of mechanical activation was compared to that of the delayed rectifier (2). Relatively long pulses of amplitude below the contractile threshold activated delayed rectification; short pulses of amplitude sufficient to activate contraction did not turn on the delayed rectifier. Thus the strength-duration curves of the two phenomena appear to be different, indicating that they are casually, not causally, related.

The similarity of action of different ions on the contractile and the K conductance thresholds suggests, however, that a similar mechanism underlies both phenomena. It was thought that Ca^{2+} adsorbed at the outer edge of the membrane caused a shift in the threshold for excitability in squid axons(121). The screening of fixed charges by Ca^{2+} could change the electric field within the membrane and cause the shift in threshold. A similar mechanism was suggested for the effect of the lyotropic anions on the contractile threshold (158). Large shifts in the contractile threshold are also produced by Ca^{2+}, Mg^{2+}, H^+, and La^{3+} (14, 61, 65, 78, 80a) and have been explained by binding and screening of negative fixed charges. Evidence favoring this view has been obtained with neuraminidase (80), which removes negative charges associated with sialic acids from the membrane, and ruthenium red (79), which is though to bind to and neutralize them. Both produced shifts of several millivolts in the contractile threshold.

Potassium Contracture

Because the action potential is an all-or-none phenomenon that can be modulated only over short ranges of amplitude and duration, studies of ECC have used other means to achieve fiber depolarization.

The membrane potential in muscle fiber is practically determined by the ratio of external and internal K concentrations (156); therefore changes in the $[K]_o$ can depolarize the membrane to the desired values. The study of K contractures in frog single muscle

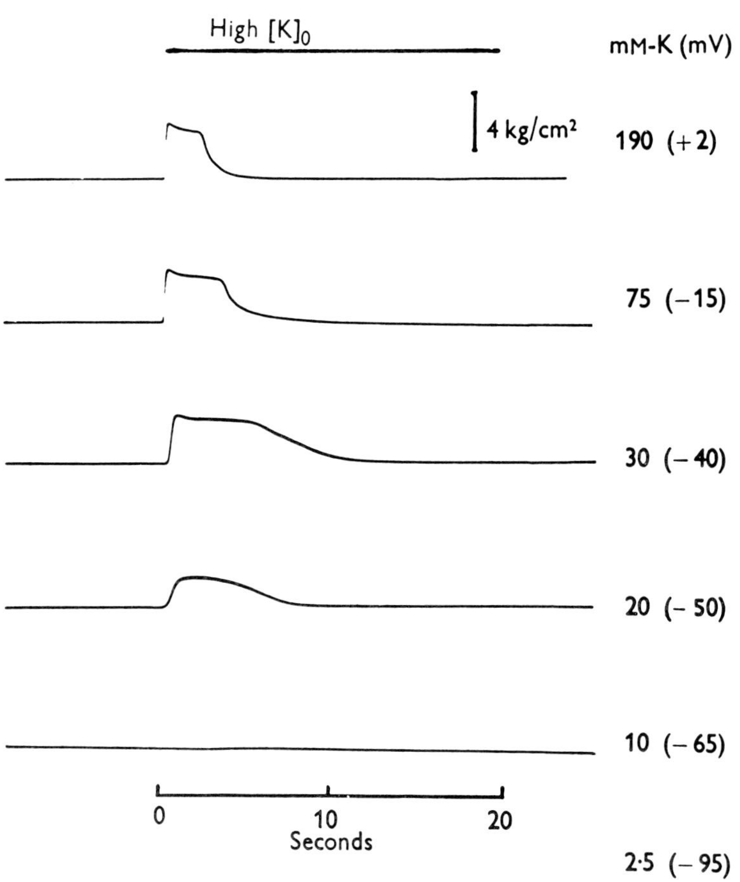

FIG. 4. Time course of K contractures of single muscle fiber tested with K concentrations (values with corresponding membrane potential). Before inducing contractures, fiber was exposed to a Na-free, choline solution to avoid twitching. [From Hodgkin and Horowicz (157).]

fibers started by Kuffler (192) led to the elegant work of Hodgkin and Horowicz (157), which has yielded much information on several phenomena involved in ECC. When K concentration in the external medium is raised, the fiber develops tension to a maximal value, which diminishes very slowly for several seconds and then falls rapidly to complete relaxation even though the fiber membrane remains depolarized. Examples of K contractures elicited by different K concentrations are shown in Figure 4. The time course of a K contracture is potential dependent because with lower K concentrations the duration of the plateau and of the fast relaxation phase are prolonged. These results have shown that tension output of single muscle fibers is related to the logarithm of the external K concentration and hence to the fiber membrane potential by a steep S-shaped curve with tension starting at about −55 mV and reaching saturation at about −40 mV. Voltage-clamped short muscle fibers of the frog have also given curves of the same type (53), as shown in Figure 5.

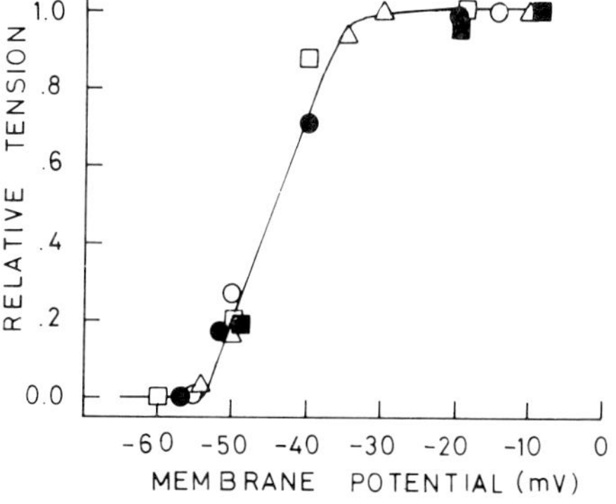

FIG. 5. Relationship between peak tension as a fraction of maximum tension and membrane potential of muscle fibers under voltage-clamp conditions. *Symbols*, results from 5 different fibers of m. lumbricalis IV digiti of frog that were approximately 1.5 mm long and voltage clamped with 2 microelectrodes inserted in their middles. Holding potential, −100 mV; depolarizing pulse, ≥1 s; 20°C–22°C. [From Caputo and de Bolaños (53).]

After a K contracture, for the fiber to develop tension again, its membrane must be repolarized to critical values of membrane potential for given periods of time—i.e., the fiber must be reprimed for a second response to depolarization (73, 157). Steady-state repriming depends on the membrane potential; for a second response equal to the first, the membrane must be repolarized above −50 mV. No repriming is achieved if the membrane potential remains below −30 mV. The relationship between repriming of contractility and membrane potential is a steep inverted S-shaped curve, which looks like a mirror image of the

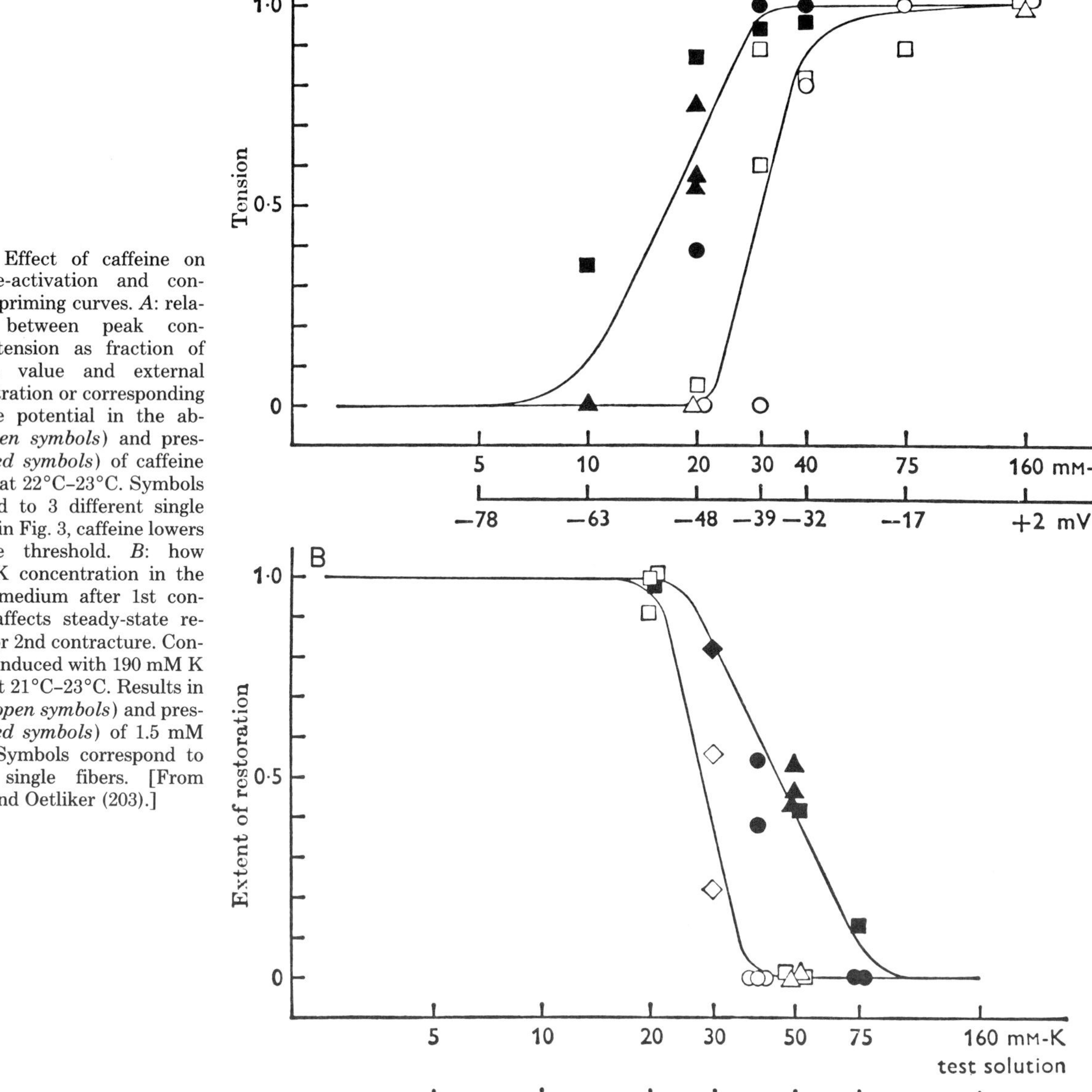

FIG. 6. Effect of caffeine on contractile-activation and contractile-repriming curves. *A*: relationship between peak contracture tension as fraction of maximum value and external K concentration or corresponding membrane potential in the absence (*open symbols*) and presence (*filled symbols*) of caffeine (1.5 mM) at 22°C–23°C. Symbols correspond to 3 different single fibers. As in Fig. 3, caffeine lowers contractile threshold. *B*: how external K concentration in the recovery medium after 1st contracture affects steady-state repriming for 2nd contracture. Contractures induced with 190 mM K medium at 21°C–23°C. Results in absence (*open symbols*) and presence (*filled symbols*) of 1.5 mM caffeine. Symbols correspond to different single fibers. [From Lüttgau and Oetliker (203).]

curve relating tension to membrane potential (see Fig. 6). This repriming process appears necessary only for contractions elicited by membrane depolarization, since a fiber can develop caffeine contractures even when depolarized (18, 203). Translocation of Ca^{2+} at the level of the SR structures might be one step involved in contractile repriming. In fact radioautographic techniques (292, 293, 294) have shown that during tetanic contractions Ca^{2+} originally released from the terminal cisternae reappears in the SR, first at the level of the longitudinal elements and then again in the terminal cisternae. These intracellular translocations of Ca^{2+}, which follow activity, are not, however, the voltage-dependent step for contractile repriming because they occur even when the fibers, after a K contracture, remain exposed to the high-K solution (294). The voltage sensitivity for contractile repriming, as well as for contractile activation, could reside in the intramembrane charge movement (see the chapter by Adrian in this *Handbook* and refs. 1 and 256). In fact contractile repriming does appear to be linked with the recovery of charge movement after membrane depolarization (4).

The decrease or inactivation of the peak tension of a test contracture caused by preceding conditioning depolarization is also related to the state of contractile refractoriness (122). The relationship between contractile activation, contractile repriming, inactivation, and membrane potential depends on the external Ca concentration (61, 73, 122, 201) and may be affected differently by drugs like caffeine and local anesthetics (52, 203). Figure 6 shows the effect of caffeine on both the activation and repriming curves.

The membrane potential also controls the time course of K contractures because the duration of the plateau is shorter and the rate of spontaneous relaxation is higher with high K concentrations (157). At low temperatures the time course of K contractures can be greatly prolonged and the repriming process delayed (50). Therefore these responses can be cut short by sudden repolarization of the membrane and resumed again after a second depolarization (51). The second tension reaches the same level that it had at the moment of the interruption, independently of when this occurred. This suggests that during a K contracture Ca^{2+} is released throughout the response and that a fixed amount is released under a given condition. The time course of K contractures can be altered in different ways. Figure 7 shows how it can be shortened in the presence of low Ca^{2+} concentrations or local anesthetics. High Ca^{2+} concentrations (122, 201) or drugs like caffeine (52), imipramine (12), and La (see *Lanthanum*, p. 400) can also prolong the responses, indicating that the exhaustion of a fixed store of activator does not determine the spontaneous relaxation during a K contracture, since the amount released can be modulated in different ways. Another explanation of the transient nature of these prolonged responses is that Ca release is activated when the fibers are depolarized and then is inactivated at a rate dependent on the membrane potential (51). Figure 8 shows such a mechanism for the control of Ca release. Some types of pharmacological agents that affect ECC could prolong or shorten the time course of the inactivation process shown in this figure.

Tension Development With Voltage Clamp

A two-microelectrode, voltage-clamp technique has been applied to short (2-mm) muscle fibers dissected from the scale muscles of the garter snake (145) and the lumbricalis muscle of the frog (28, 29, 53); with two

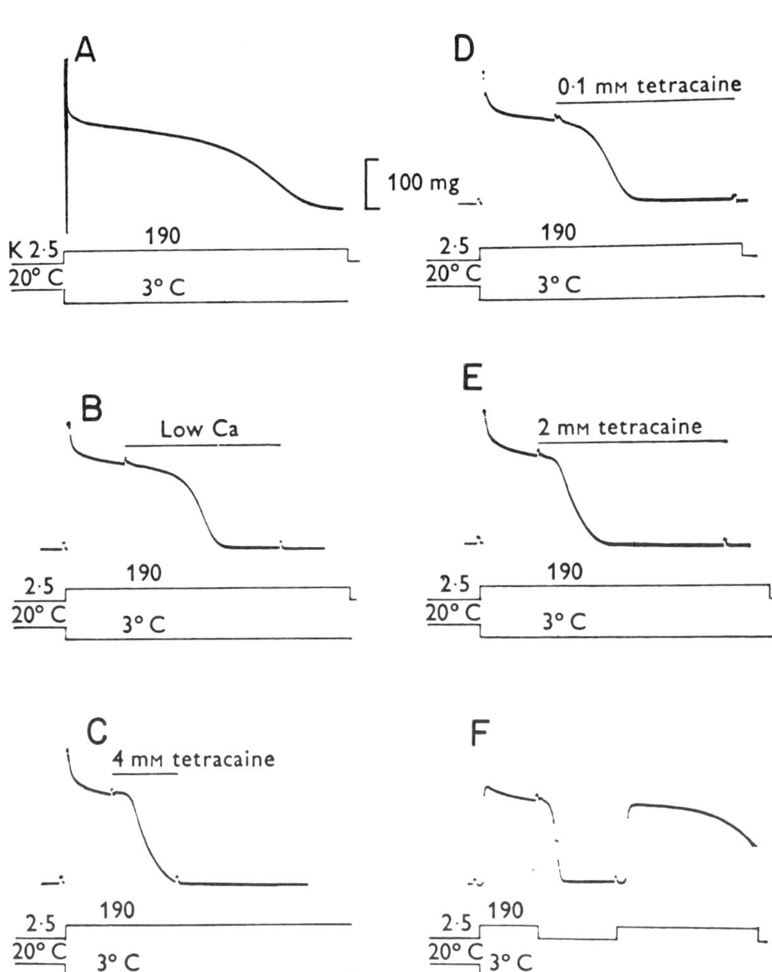

FIG. 7. Changes in the onset and time course of relaxation of K contractures of single muscle fibers produced by different concentrations of tetracaine and at a low Ca concentration (≃ 10 μM free Ca). Contractures at 3°C have a prolonged time course. Tetracaine speeds up onset of relaxation; sudden repolarization of fiber causes faster relaxation. Fiber diameter, 81 μm. [From Caputo (51).]

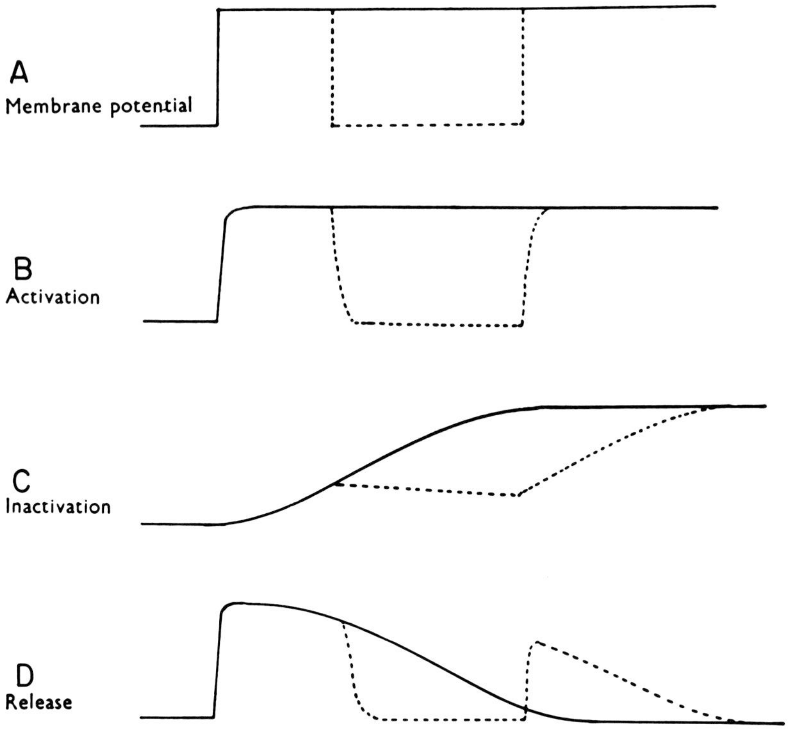

A
Membrane potential

B
Activation

C
Inactivation

D
Release

FIG. 8. Time course of Ca release during a K contracture. *A*: membrane potential. *B* and *C*: time courses of activation and inactivation processes of mechanism that controls Ca release. *D*: time course of Ca release. *Dashed lines*, result of sudden changes in membrane potential caused by K-concentration changes as in Fig. 7*F*. [From Caputo (51).]

microelectrodes inserted in the center of the fiber, the clamp system can effectively control most of the fiber length because the length constant of these fibers is only about 2 mm. With this technique maximal tension of the fibers in response to voltage-clamp depolarizing pulses under a variety of experimental conditions has been recorded. Most of the results from this preparation have confirmed those from K contractures. In general the contractile-activation curves from voltage-clamp conditions appear to be steeper than those from K^+ depolarizations. The reason for this behavior may be the diffusional delays that appear to limit K^+ depolarization (133). Even under voltage-clamp conditions, however, steepness of the curve and the contractile threshold may vary widely. These variations, which may depend on the state of each particular fiber, must be taken into account when comparing contractile-activation curves with other curves describing the membrane potential dependency of other phenomena such as charge movement (1, 256) and fluorescence signals (284).

With voltage-clamp techniques the kinetics of contractile repriming can be studied in snake muscle fibers at 20°C with better time resolutions. In fact these fibers are substantially reprimed when they are repolarized at −100 mV for less than 1 s (146). Besides depending on the fiber membrane potential, contractile repriming is greatly delayed by procaine at relatively low concentrations (147). This delay appears to be reversed, however, with repriming at more negative membrane potentials (−150 mV). Drugs like caffeine can also shift the potential dependency of contractile repriming in the opposite direction (203).

Calcium Indicators

The most direct evidence for an increase in the myoplasmic free-Ca^{2+} concentration during contractile activation has been derived from studies of the Ca-sensitive photoprotein aequorin (17, 41, 241, 276) and other Ca indicators (22, 188, 211). The first study of ECC events to apply aequorin successfully used the giant muscle fiber of the barnacle (17). Since then aequorin has been injected into frog single muscle fibers to study contraction (41, 241), thus obtaining the time relationships between light emission and force development under different experimental conditions. In Figure 2, after a single stimulus, light emission and force development start at about the same time, with light emission reaching its peak and declining before force. During a series of twitches at a frequency of 5 Hz, light emission increased during the first twitch and then declined, whereas force increased because of the staircase phenomenon (64). Calcium-release capacity, however, did not decline during repetitive activity, since during tetanic stimulation, and even when tetanic force had become saturated, light emission increased. During K contracture, however, the light-emission time course differs from the force time course for maximal contractures, as shown in Figure 9.

These records indicate that the aequorin response

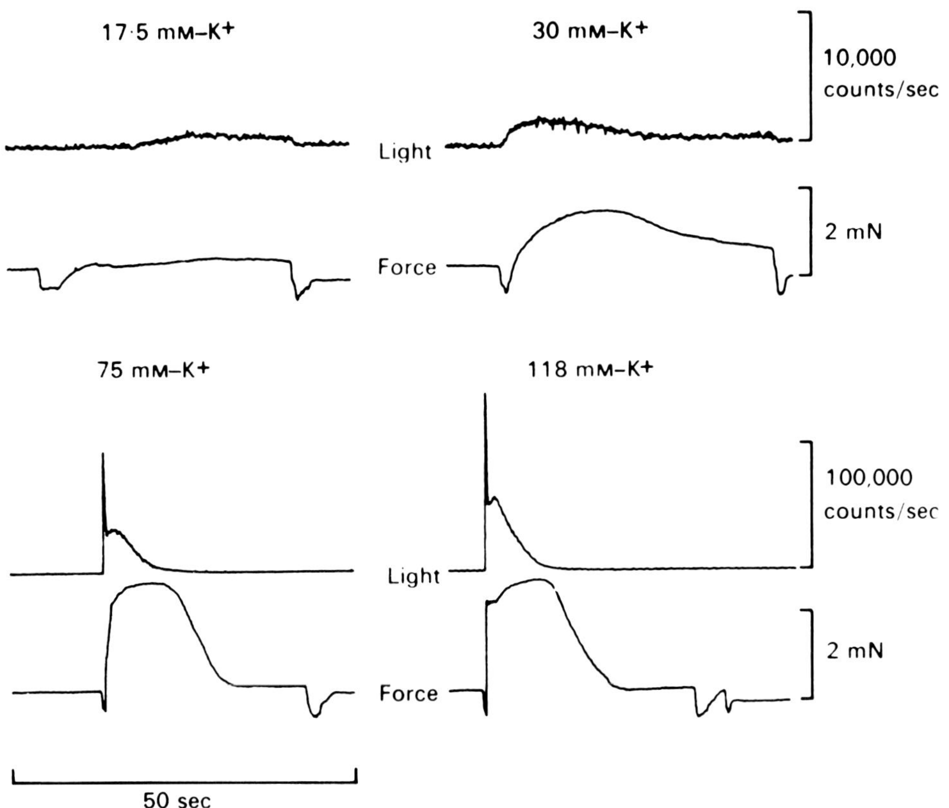

FIG. 9. Comparison between time courses of aequorin luminescence signals and mechanical responses during K contractures of single muscle fiber at 15°C with different K concentrations. Note different calibrations for light signals. [From Blinks et al. (41).]

might measure, not the Ca^{2+} released, but the Ca concentration in equilibrium with the contractile filaments and with other intracellular Ca-binding sites (45). Although the use of aequorin may be limited (40) it has proved useful in determining the effect of several experimental interventions on Ca release (198, 273).

Other Ca indicators, such as arsenazo III, have also been injected for studying Ca release (22, 211). The application of Vaseline-gap, voltage-clamp techniques to cut segments of skeletal muscle fibers has great potential (154, 188, 189, 284). Although they cannot measure force, the techniques allow the study of contractile activation in the membrane potential region near contractile thresholds, and more importantly they allow the fiber intracellular space to be exposed to different impermeable substances like Ca buffers, fluorescent dyes, and Ca indicators, which may diffuse into the fiber through its cut ends. Charge movement can also be measured with this technique (188). Thus more detailed information on the Nile-blue–fluorescence signal under voltage-clamp conditions could be obtained. The metallochromic dye antipyrylazo (AP) III has been used to monitor changes in the concentration of myoplasmic-free Ca^{2+} because it reacts rapidly with Ca and shows Ca-dependent absorbance changes at 720 and 550 nm (188). Antipyrylazo III Ca transients have been recorded simultaneously with intramembrane charge movement. The results indicate that charge movement precedes and therefore may control Ca release. Figure 10 shows simultaneous recordings of charge movement and AP III Ca transients at different membrane potentials (J. F. Vergara and C. Caputo, unpublished observations).

Calcium-Induced Calcium Release

Normally, with voltage-clamp experiments or with potentiators of contraction, Ca release from the SR can be modulated. Under particular conditions, however, a regenerative Ca release can be obtained (94, 97, 110).

This kind of release occurs in the skinned-fiber preparation, developed originally by Natori (221), which is obtained by mechanically peeling off the surface membrane of muscle fiber under oil. With Ca-buffering agents like ethylene glycol-bis(β-aminoethylether)-N,N^1-tetraacetic acid (EGTA) the skinned-fiber preparation allows different ions and other substances to be applied directly into the myofibrillar space and the Ca^{2+} concentration to be held at the desired levels (111, 112). Several investigators have used this preparation to study the properties of both

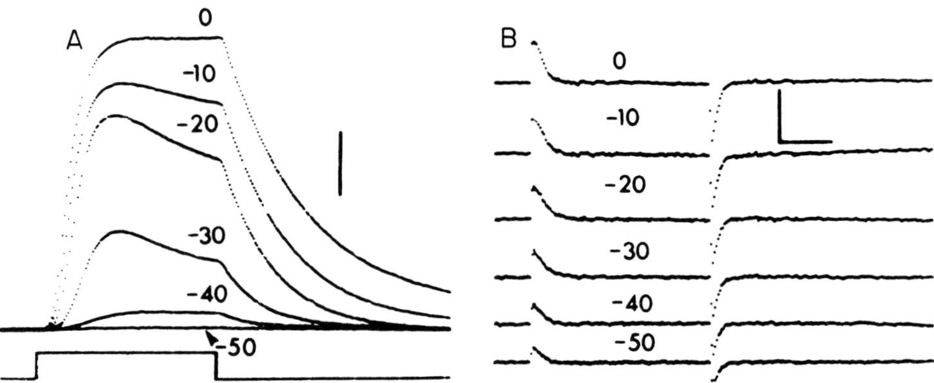

FIG. 10. Voltage dependence of Ca transients and intramembrane charge movement of a cut muscle fiber segment under voltage-clamp conditions at 3°C. *A*: average of 6 determinations of light absorbance changes of antipyrylazo III at 720 nm for 100-ms pulses of different amplitude. Fiber had holding potential of −100 and was depolarized to values shown near each record. Calibration, ratio of A_{720}/A_{550} of 1.4×10^{-2}. *B*: intramembrane charge-movement currents for same pulses. Vertical calibration for charge movement, 3.2 $\mu A\ \mu F^{-1}$; horizontal calibration, 30 ms. Fiber stretched 3.46 μm per sarcomere to diminish movement artifacts. [From Kovacs et al. (188). Reprinted by permission from *Nature*, copyright 1979, Macmillan Journals Ltd.]

contractile machinery and the SR. The ability of the SR to release or accumulate Ca^{2+} can be demonstrated in this preparation under a variety of experimental conditions. In skinned fibers the development of contraction, which demonstrates Ca release from the SR, can be obtained after electrical stimulation (70, 71, 221), alteration in the ionic composition of the bathing medium (71, 95, 214), or the use of drugs such as caffeine (96). Most interestingly, with this preparation Ca release has also been induced by an increase in the concentration of the medium free Ca^{2+}, giving origin to the concept of Ca-induced Ca release (94, 97, 110).

When skinned muscle fibers are exposed to solutions containing about 10^{-6} M Ca^{2+} the SR may accumulate this cation. After the SR has been preloaded with Ca, exposing the preparation to a relatively high Ca^{2+} concentration (10^{-4} M) induces a fast transient contractile response of maximal amplitude caused by a massive release of Ca from the SR. Several authors (97, 111, 112) think Ca-induced Ca release may be important in ECC of skeletal muscle fibers under physiological conditions. One great difficulty with this hypothesis is that Ca-induced Ca release appears to be an all-or-none phenomenon, while normal contractile responses in intact fibers appear to be graded. The high Ca concentration necessary to induce further Ca release does not support the physiological explanation for the role of Ca-induced Ca release. This is not a strong objection, however, because a high Ca concentration must be attained only in restricted regions, such as the junction between the T tubules and the SR, which may be readily accessible to extracellular Ca^{2+}. Furthermore much lower Ca concentrations are needed for further Ca release under certain experimental conditions—e.g., the presence of caffeine (96) or a low concentration of Mg (268). Although the Ca-induced–Ca-release mechanism for contractile activation of striated muscle may not be relevant to ECC (97), under normal conditions it appears to be important in cardiac muscle activation (102).

Depolarization-Induced Calcium Release

The possibility of contractile activation by electrical stimulation in skinned fibers was demonstrated originally by Natori (221) and confirmed by other authors (70, 71). Also this preparation, bathed in a medium containing an impermeant anion such as propionate and a high K concentration, contracts transiently when exposed to a medium that contains Cl^- or when the K concentration is reduced (71, 268, 269). These Cl^--induced or low K-induced releases of Ca have been generally referred to as *depolarization-induced Ca releases.* If the SR membrane were permeable to these ions, sudden elevation of Cl^- or reduction of K^+ in the extrareticular space would make the interior of the SR more negative than the exterior, as when the fiber membrane is depolarized. These membrane changes at the level of the SR of skinned fibers, because of alterations in the ionic composition, could cause the Ca release. However, resealing the T tubules and maintaining connections between the transverse-tubule system (T system) and the SR might also be important in depolarization-induced Ca release in skinned fibers (71). Possibly the connections beween the T tubules and the SR remain intact, thus providing the structural basis for the depolarization-sensitive coupling between these structures. If the tubule mouths spontaneously sealed, the lumena of these structures would make a closed compartment separated from the myofibrillar space by the tubular membrane, across which a potential could develop as a consequence of an asymmetric ion distribution between the sealed lumena of the T systems and the myofibrillar space. Because electrical activation in skeletal muscle is abolished after membrane depolarization, one might expect the membrane system of the skinned segment to be depolarized and hence inactivated.

The response of skinned fibers to electrical stimulation therefore implies that after the surface membrane is removed, excitability must be restored in some way, probably by repolarization of the membrane elements. This could occur if the tubules resealed after their disruption from the surface membrane and if the K content in the T tubule lumena decreased because of the activity of the Na pump. Reestablishing a K gradient across the internal membranes would then cause the generation of a resting potential across these membranes with the lumena of the internal membrane system more positive than the myofibrillar space that is in contact with the bathing solution. In the work of Costantin and Podolsky (71) the contractile response of the skinned-fiber preparation to electrical stimulation was abolished in the presence of cardiac glycosides. Strophanthin, by blocking the Na pump, would prevent the development of a membrane potential difference and the reestablishment of excitability. Once the conditions for excitability are reestablished, changes in the ionic composition of the medium that is bathing the myofibrillar space can cause contractile activation.

When skinned-fiber preparations are incubated in EGTA-buffered media with the concentration of free Ca^{2+} set above the concentration threshold, the rate of tension development is much slower than expected from diffusion consideration alone. This delay has been attributed to the Ca^{2+} uptake by the SR because agents that destroy the capacity of the SR to sequester Ca cause much faster tension development (148). In studying the effects of pharmacological interventions on the Cl^--induced Ca release it is important to consider that Ca uptake occurs at the same time, thus affecting the magnitude of the net Ca concentration increase. For instance, raising the Mg^{2+} concentration in the myofibrillar space from 1 to 3 mM inhibits the force developed by the skinned fiber exposed to high Cl^- (112, 279). Stimulation of the Ca uptake mechanism by the SR appears to cause this action, since Mg^{2+} can be antagonized by agents that inhibit Ca uptake, like Cd^{2+} and low temperature (269). Low temperature, however, may also lower the rate of Ca release in response to depolarization in intact fibers.

In the skinned-fiber preparation the Cl^--induced Ca release and Ca-induced Ca release appear to differ in Ca preloading requirements and the effects of local anesthetics, Mg^{2+}, and adenosine 5′-triphosphate (ATP) (278). Chloride-induced Ca release requires less preloading of Ca^{2+}, is slightly stimulated by procaine and not inhibited by tetracaine, and is not affected by Mg^{2+} or ATP. Calcium-induced Ca release on the other hand requires massive preloading of Ca^{2+}, is inhibited by local anesthetics and Mg^{2+}, and is stimulated by ATP. These differences show that the two mechanisms are completely independent; the differences may not be absolute, however, because recently it has been found that Mg^{2+} at a high concentration affects both mechanisms by stimulating Ca uptake by the SR. Furthermore the preloading requirements may differ only quantitatively because a certain degree of preloading is necessary for obtaining release, independent of the stimulus applied. These uncertainties suggest a possible common basis for these two mechanisms. For instance, an initially small amount of Ca^{2+}, released from the SR in response to membrane potential changes, might trigger further Ca release. Under this modality in an intact fiber extracellular Ca^{2+} would not be necessary to trigger Ca release.

Membrane Potential Changes at SR Level

The apparently homogeneous distribution of the intracellular ions (except Ca^{2+}) between the myoplasm and the SR interior (262, 263) makes the presence of a resting membrane potential between these two compartments highly improbable. Potential changes caused by conductance changes of the SR membrane to some specific ion or the massive outflow of Ca^{2+} from the SR, however, could cause membrane potential changes at the level of the SR membrane.

The inaccessibility of the SR to conventional electrical measurements makes it impossible to test directly for eventual membrane potential changes in the SR during contractile activation. Recently, however, it has become possible to measure optical signals associated with membrane potential changes (63). Because these signals can be detected far from the site where they are generated, they may be useful for monitoring potential changes at the membrane level of some structures (e.g., the SR), which are otherwise inaccessible. During contractile activity of isolated single muscle fibers the birefringence changes that might be associated with ECC can be measured. In fact, besides two small, early signals (23, 24, 25) that are thought to be associated with electrical events at the surface and T-tubule membranes (25), two large and distinct birefringence signals may be detected after stimulation (23, 24). The first begins shortly after the rising phase of the action potential and precedes contraction; the second follows the tension time course and is clearly associated with contraction.

Pharmacological interventions have proved useful for distinguishing these two signals because several procedures that affect tension development of muscle fibers appear to diminish them in different proportions. In fact treatment with hypertonic solutions, exposure to D_2O, or different degrees of stretch effectively reduce the tension time course more than the early large birefringence signal. With contractile output reduced by hypertonic treatment this early signal can be differentially increased by NO_3^-, which is a well-known contractile potentiator. Although this signal still might be related to mechanical activity during latency relaxation, or even to Ca binding to troponin, it more likely reflects a step in ECC prior to tension development (226) and more specifically a potential change in the SR membrane.

Extrinsic fluorescence signals in muscle fibers stained with Nile blue A have also been associated with electrical events during ECC (30, 284). They might be related to potential changes at the level of the SR membrane when the lipid solubility of Nile blue A is taken into account and the signals given by this substance and those given by other impermeant fluorescent dyes are compared. Although impermeant dyes bind only at the surface and T-system membranes, permeant dyes stain SR membranes as well. The flourescence signals generated by these compounds are expected to be proportional to the magnitude of the membrane potential change and the size of the stained membrane area. Because in frog skeletal muscle the approximate surface:T system:SR membrane ratio for a 100-μm fiber is 1:7:90, one would expect the signal from the SR membrane to predominate. Accordingly, although impermeant fluorescent dyes such as merocyanine 540 may monitor electrical potential changes at the level of the surface and T-system membranes (283) and closely follow the time course of the surface action potential, other permeable dyes such as Nile blue A and indocarbocyanine give signals that are not proportional to either the surface or the T-system membrane potential; they follow a much slower time course than the surface action potential and therefore have been associated with SR membrane potential changes.

The first experiments in which fluroescence signals were obtained with Nile blue A used whole sartorius muscles mounted in a chamber with triangular, liquid electrodes to achieve longitudinally uniform membrane depolarizations (30). This arrangement enables the muscle to be stimulated directly or a current to be passed through the triangular electrode, permitting longitudinally uniform depolarizations of the muscle fibers. When the muscles were electrically stimulated and the action potential of a single muscle fiber was recorded intracellularly with a microelectrode, the fluorescence signal started soon after the peak and early in the falling phase of the action potential. It was found that the magnitude of the fluorescence signal could be graded by increasing the strength of the depolarizing pulse above a certain threshold value. The signal in response to long depolarizing pulses was not greater than that in response to short pulses. The curve describing the relationship between the fluorescence signal and the current passing through the triangular electrode was a steep S shape like that of the tension-potential relationship; furthermore the threshold for the fluorescence signal was the same as the contractile threshold. However, it began before any detectable tension increase, peaked soon after the start of tension development, and ended before tension reached its maximum.

The fluorescence signal in response to a single stimulus was markedly potentiated when NO_3^- was substituted for Cl^- in the bathing medium and was depressed when the Ringer's solution was prepared with deuterated water. Furthermore the fluorescence signals were suppressed in the presence of the local anesthetics procaine and tetracaine, which also suppressed contractile output (55).

Extrinsic fluorescence measurements under voltage-clamp and current-clamp conditions with short segments of single muscle fiber confirmed the results obtained with whole muscle and provided information on the fluorescence signal and its nonlinear dependency on membrane potential (284). The curves relating peak amplitude and maximum rise rate of the fluorescence signals with the fiber membrane potential are S shaped and reminiscent of the contractile-activation curve although the relationship is less steep and covers a wider range of potentials. These results support the view that Nile blue A effectively monitors SR membrane potential changes. One point not yet resolved, however, is whether these changes of the SR membrane potential are the cause or a consequence of Ca release. Calcium release could be produced after potential-dependent changes in the SR membrane, e.g., a change in the potential-dependent Ca^{2+} conductance, or currents carried primarily by Ca^{2+} could cause the potential change across the SR membrane. In this case the controlling mechanism for Ca release could be a phenomenon at the level of the T-tubule membrane near the SR junction and linked to Ca gates in the SR (e.g., the charge movement). Accordingly intramembrane charge movement acting as a voltage sensor in T-tubule membrane could remotely control the Ca gates of the SR membrane. Another possibility is the mechanism of Ca-induced Ca release.

Although the birefringence and extrinsic fluoresence changes suggest changes of the SR membrane potential associated with Ca release, recent work with isolated SR vesicles shows that fluorescence changes with different potentiometric dyes normally thought to monitor membrane potential changes might be caused by binding Ca or ATP to SR membranes (225, 242, 243). Some of these dyes may respond to surface potential changes caused by the electrostatic effect of bound Ca (243); therefore fluorescence changes detected with these compounds may not be associated with changes in the SR membrane potential but only reflect changes in the intracellular Ca^{2+} concentration. These considerations point to the need for further work to establish the occurrence of membrane potential changes at the level of the SR and their relationship to Ca release.

PHARMACOLOGICAL AND EXPERIMENTAL MODIFICATIONS OF ECC

Effect of Extracellular Calcium

The role of extracellular Ca^{2+} in ECC has been the object of numerous studies and much controversy for a long time. In the early 1940s Heilbrunn and Wiercinski (144) demonstrated that Ca^{2+} was the only ion of those normally present in muscle that, when injected at very low concentrations, could cause rapid shortening of muscle fibers. Before these experiments were published Heilbrunn had proposed (143) that different types of stimulation could cause release of Ca^{2+} from the surface or outer regions of the muscle fibers and that this Ca^{2+}, entering the cell, could induce a contractile response. Based on theoretical calculations and on the experimentally determined length of the delay between stimulation and the onset of contraction, Hill (149, 150) showed, however, that diffusion of any substance from the surface to the interior of a muscle fiber would be much too slow to account for contractile activation. With remarkable insight Hill concluded that the inward propagation of the surface signal had to occur by a process rather than by diffusion of some substance. In 1952 in his famous review where the term "excitation-contraction coupling" first appeared, Sandow (248) expounded the Heilbrunn hypothesis once more, proposing a kind of exchange diffusion that, helped by electrostatic attractions between Ca^{2+} and myofibrils, might hasten transport to the center of the fiber of the Ca^{2+} liberated at the surface. Experimental evidence pointing to the involvement of extracellular Ca in ECC (36, 119, 259) soon strengthened this view.

Furthermore the demonstration by Huxley and Taylor (169) of local activation at the level of the Z line in frog fast-twitch muscle fibers indicated a structural specialization that permitted the inward spread of surface depolarization. This study, the rediscovery of the T system (233), and the clear demonstration that the T tubules open into the extracellular space (170) verified that the Ca^{2+} could enter the fiber or be released from the surface membrane at short diffusional distances from the contractile sites.

Bianchi and Shanes (36) provided evidence of extra influxes of Ca^{2+} during single twitches and K contractures. In whole sartorius muscles bathed in a solution containing 1 mM Ca^{2+}, they measured an extra influx of 0.2 pM/cm^2 per impulse. When NO_3^- replaced Cl^- as the main anion in the external medium, an increase in the influx per impulse amounting to 60% was observed; the resting influx was unaffected. Calcium influx in the presence of NO_3^- increased with the increase of the area under the potentiated twitch; both amounted to 60%. This exact agreement suggested a direct relationship between twitch height and Ca entry.

During K contractures Ca influx also substantially increased. More recently Ca-influx determinations with single muscle fibers gave values of 0.34, 0.73, and 1 pM/cm^2 per impulse in media containing 0.5, 1, and 1.8 mM Ca^{2+}, respectively (74). The hypothesis that Ca entry is the link between excitation and contraction was further strengthened when such a link was broken by removing Ca from the external medium (119, 120, 267). In a study with whole toe muscles Frank (119) showed that K contractures could be abolished after exposure to Ca-free solutions. Several divalent cations, however, some of which do not produce a contractile response when injected intracellularly (e.g., Ni^{2+} and Mg^{2+}), can substitute for Ca^{2+} to maintain ECC (52a, 120, 200). Furthermore caffeine contractures can be obtained in Ca-free solutions when K contractures have been abolished (120).

On the basis of these results it was proposed that Ca^{2+} was necessary for maintaining the coupling by an action at or near a membrane site. Foreign divalent cations or low concentrations of caffeine were thought to release Ca^{2+} from surface sites in or on the muscle and this Ca^{2+} was thought to replace the Ca^{2+} lost in the Ca-free solution by diffusion. The idea that Ca^{2+} is necessary for maintaining coupling at the level of the membrane was further justified through the work of several other authors (72, 86, 175, 177). Modified Ca concentrations affect the electrical properties of muscle fibers; in fact the maximal rising rate of the action potential decreases with increasing Ca concentrations, suggesting that the Na^+ current during activity decreases in proportion to the increase in Ca (175). Excess Ca^{2+} also causes marked increases in both the magnitude and time constants of the negative afterpotential, while reduced Ca^{2+} decreases them. More importantly, in Ca-free solution the resting membrane potential is reduced, leading to a loss of excitability (86, 177).

The failure of contractility induced by electrical stimulation in the absence of external Ca^{2+} was studied with whole sartorius muscle. Edman and Grieve (86) concluded that Ca^{2+} was essential for maintaining normal resting potentials and for producing the action potential and that in its absence loss of excitability was the main cause of complete mechanical failure. Progressive decline of the twitch that preceded complete failure could be accounted for by the diminishing action potential in Ca-free solutions. Jenden and Reger (177) showed that the fall in the resting potential contributed to the effect of Ca-free solution on the mechanical output, pointing out that in the absence of Ca^{2+} the fiber became mechanically refractory at a higher (more negative) membrane potential.

These authors concluded that Ca^{2+} was required in the extracellular fluid for the maintenance of some property that regulated the inward transmission of excitation. The importance of changes in the resting membrane potential caused by external Ca deprivation on the mechanical tension-development capacity of muscle fibers was stressed by Curtis (72), who obtained contractile responses to depolarizing pulses in fibers bathed in Ca-free Ringer's solution by passing a hyperpolarizing current through the fiber, which restored the normal resting potential before the onset of the depolarizing pulse. These results supplied additional evidence that a change in the coupling mechanism in Ca-free solution occurs. More recent work, in which Ca deprivation produced a shift in the contractile thresholds, confirms this view (16, 61, 78, 201).

The effect of extracellular Ca^{2+} on different elements of ECC has been most successfully studied with frog single muscle fibers. This preparation shows that reduction of extracellular Ca^{2+} causes a marked shortening of the plateau of K contractures (see Fig. 7) and a shift of the curve that describes the steady-state relation between membrane potential and the contractile system toward a more negative potential. These results confirm the earlier suggestion that a low Ca concentration causes a shift in the inactivation curve (51, 201).

With single muscle fibers diffusion delays are minimized and rapid equilibration with the external medium can be achieved. When single muscle fibers are exposed to a low or a very low external Ca concentration they maintain their ability to develop contraction for a long time (16, 54). After exposure to a Ca-free solution a potentiation of the twitch occurs, which is maintained for at least 150 twitches when the fiber is stimulated at 1 twitch/s. The eventual decline in tension output is probably caused by depolarization of the membrane, which develops slowly. In fact, fibers in Ca-free Ringer's solution with normal or slightly reduced resting potentials always developed tension when suddenly depolarized by increased K. Thus external Ca^{2+} does not appear to intervene directly in contractile activation. However, Ca^{2+} in partially protected compartments like the T tubules still might remain at a concentration high enough to allow this Ca^{2+} to trigger further Ca release. Although Ca entering the fiber during membrane depolarization might not be sufficient to activate all the contractile sites, it could trigger further Ca release from the SR. Armstrong et al. (16) objected to this hypothesis because they effectively lowered the free-Ca^{2+} concentration to about 10^{-9} mM with 1 mM EGTA. Even in the presence of EGTA, single muscle fibers maintained their twitching ability for a long time. Therefore these experiments, besides providing evidence that extracellular Ca^{2+} plays no role in the generation of action potentials in muscle fibers, indicated that Ca^{2+} in the T tubules could not be involved in triggering the release of Ca^{2+} from the SR because the calculated influx was about one calcium ion per sarcomere. However, the possibility that 1 mM EGTA might not remove all free Ca^{2+} from the T system has been explored with a higher EGTA concentration (80 mM) (20). With this concentration the fiber membrane depolarizes; therefore the fibers must be hyperpolarized to evoke action potentials. Then action potentials of nearly normal amplitude (80 mV) evoked no visible contraction. Similar results were obtained when citrate was substituted for EGTA. It was proposed therefore that Ca^{2+} in some protected extracellular compartment is the source of a Ca influx during depolarization, which enhances further release of Ca^{2+} from the terminal cisternae of the SR. More recently it has been shown, however, that, even in the presence of 80 mM EGTA, fibers can develop tension in response to electrical stimulation in the presence of Mg^{2+} (204). Therefore external Ca deprivation appears to affect the coupling efficiency.

Recent electrophysiological evidence (11a, 26, 247) points to substantial inward Ca currents during membrane depolarization in frog muscle fibers. These Ca currents are greatly diminished after glycerol treatment, indicating that Ca^{2+} enters through the T-tubule membranes (222). The kinetics of these currents is much too slow to be important in contractile activation. Their magnitude, however, suggests a substantial role in the normal functioning of these cells. In fact an entry of 1×10^{-10} mol/cm^2 external surface has been estimated (222). This entry should raise the intracellular Ca^{2+} level to about 10^{-4} M in a fiber of 60 μm diameter.

Because of this observation and the sizable inward Ca currents, it has been suggested that these currents might be used to sustain the time course of prolonged responses such as K contractures (247). In the absence of external Ca^{2+} the first important effect on K contractures is the disappearance of the plateau and shortening of the time course of these responses (54, 201).

Like many other divalent cations, Ni^{2+} appears to maintain ECC almost as well as Ca^{2+} without participating in contractile activation (109, 200). In fact these ions do not activate the MgATP-induced syneresis of isolated myofibrils (109). On the other hand Ca^{2+} currents are greatly diminished in the presence of Ni^{2+} (11a). It has been shown in whole toe muscle and more recently in single muscle fibers, however, that when Ni^{2+} substitutes for Ca^{2+}, K contractures can be obtained with a time course identical to that obtained in normal Ca-containing media (52a, 200).

Therefore the fate of the Ca^{2+} that enters the fiber in currents is questioned. In the absence of these currents and with the ECC mechanism protected by other divalent cations, the mechanical output of muscle fibers during different types of contractile responses are not appreciably changed. Possibly the Ca released from the SR far exceeds that entering the fiber; the contribution of the entering Ca^{2+} would then be negligible.

Also, the myoplasmic Ca-buffering systems (45), localized in the diffusional path between the entry and contractile sites, may efficiently dispose of the entering Ca^{2+}; they are less effective with the Ca released from the SR because the release sites are nearer to the contractile sites.

Effect of Hypertonic Solutions

Hypertonic solutions have been widely used to block or decrease contractility, thereby reducing movement artifacts during different types of electrical measurement in muscle fibers. Although tension output is markedly reduced in solutions made two- or three-times hypertonic by the addition of nonpenetrating solutes, electrical properties like the resting membrane potential and the action potential are not much affected [see Fig. 1; (155)]. Whole sartorius muscles exposed to hypertonic solutions are more resistant to passive stretch and have a greatly reduced intrinsic speed of shortening during isotonic contractions, and reduced rates of relaxation during isometric contractions. The duration of the active state and the intensity of activation heat, however, are not changed much in hypertonic (up to 3 times) solutions (161). These results indicate mainly that the effect of hypertonic solutions on muscle contractility is due to a direct action on the contractile apparatus rather than on the coupling mechanism although other effects on this process may also be detected.

Muscle fibers exposed to solutions of altered tonicity (hyper- or hypotonic) usually give predictable volume changes, assuming the fibers behave like quasi-perfect osmometers (39, 49, 81). X-ray measurements have confirmed that these changes are reflected at a level of the filament lattice where volume decreases in hypertonic solutions (239). The loss of fiber-solvent water in hypertonic solutions increases viscosity and ionic strength of the intracellular medium; these changes, and particularly the second one, may explain the reduced tension output if they affect the contractile-protein interactions (134). In isolated crayfish muscle fibers bathed in hypertonic media, tension induced by intracellular injection of Ca declines steeply with increasing external tonicity (15). Furthermore, in chemically skinned frog fiber preparations where the membranes are removed by detergent, the contractile-protein response to decreased medium pCa (EGTA controlled) decreases with increased ionic strength of the bathing medium (135). Hypertonic solutions, however, may also affect the ECC mechanism; caffeine contractures and depolarization-elicited contractions appear to be affected differently by them. In two-times-hypertonic solutions, contractures induced by low (3–5 mM) caffeine concentrations are not depressed but potentiated (47). In three-times-hypertonic solutions that abolish tetanic and K-contracture tension, 10% of maximal caffeine-contracture tension can be obtained (159). Furthermore some evidence suggests that signals associated with Ca release and Ca release itself may be diminished in hypertonic media (260). Because contractile tension induced by an exogenous supply of Ca^{2+} diminishes with increases in external tonicity or internal ionic strength of the medium, it is clear that these conditions impair contractile mechanisms and that the effects on the coupling mechanism are minor (134). Whole muscles (152) and single muscle fibers (196) immersed in hypertonic solutions develop a small (<10% tetanic tension), long-lasting, graded, and reversible resting tension that is not affected by tetracaine and is generated with the same time course as the fiber-volume changes (196).

With single muscle fibers a transient component of tension can be detected when the fibers are exposed to hypertonic media. These hypertonic contractures increase as tonicity increases, reaching a maximal value of about one-third of normal tetanic tension at 2.5 times normal tonicity. These contractures, which may last tens of seconds at room temperature, occur independently of the fiber membrane potential and are abolished by tetracaine (196). In these respects they resemble caffeine contractures and are probably caused by Ca released from the SR in response to morphological changes occurring when the fibers are immersed in hypertonic media (125).

Hypertonic solutions have a relevant effect on the intracellular membrane systems of muscle fibers. Early electron-microscope studies revealed that swollen vesicles, identified as altered elements of the triads, could be visualized at levels of the I band even though the fibers themselves appeared shrunken with clearly reduced interfibrillar spaces (37). This observation indicated that the swollen elements were continuous with the extracellular space; the possibility that they were the terminal cisternae of the SR was important for the hypothesis about the compartmentalization of the intracellular structures. In fact, swelling of SR elements would indicate that this compartment is extracellular or at least that it might open to the extracellular space under certain conditions. This could explain certain features of the osmotic behavior of muscle fibers and would add to the explanation that the Ca-release mechanism transmits information from the T-tubule membranes to the SR for contractile activation.

There has been much controversy on whether swelling occurs at the level of the T tubules or at the level of the terminal cisternae of the SR. Although there is some indirect physiological evidence that the T tubules swell when muscles are placed in hypertonic solutions with excess sucrose or in solutions of low ionic strength (236), most of the evidence for selective swelling of either compartment has been obtained with electron-microscope studies with different experimental procedures and different fixatives (38, 236). Transverse-tubule swelling is best seen when sucrose is used as the hypertonic agent and osmium is the fixative; SR swelling is observed when aldehydes or acrolein are the fixatives and NaCl raises the tonicity (38). Therefore the possibility of fixation artifacts has made it difficult to decide which one of the observations indicates real change. The swelling of the T tubules in hypertonic solutions did not appear to be artifactual, however, because it was reversible and independent of the sucrose concentration in the fixative solution (236).

Recently, using rapid freezing instead of chemical fixation for preparing samples for electron microscopy seems to have eliminated artifacts during fixation. In these studies only the T tubules appear swollen, not the elements of the SR (125).

An interesting effect of hypertonic solutions involves the ionic distribution in the fiber interior. Although under normal conditions no compartmentalization is observed, after treatment with hypertonic solutions, swollen vacuoles that could be filled with solutes from the extracellular space (e.g., NaCl and isethionate) were observed. Furthermore Ca^{2+} was translocated to the longitudinal tubules of the SR (262).

Transverse-Tubule Disrupture (Glycerol Treatment)

Treatment of muscle fibers with hypertonic solutions prepared with 400 mM glycerol followed by reexposure to normal Ringer's solution results in the uncoupling of contraction from excitation (129, 130, 162). This effect is accompanied by a decrease in the low-frequency membrane capacity and structural modification of the T system. At a low frequency under normal conditions the membrane capacity of muscle fibers, expressed per unit area of surface membrane, is about 7 $\mu F/cm^2$, considerably higher than that of other membranes—squid axon membrane, for example, is 1 $\mu F/cm^2$ (129). The presence of the T-tubule membrane network, which is electrically coupled to the surface membrane, accounts for this substantial difference. After glycerol treatment the low-frequency capacity of the muscle fiber membrane is reduced to about 2 $\mu F/cm^2$, suggesting that the tubular network has been mostly uncoupled from the surface membrane. Electron-microscope studies with an electron-dense extracellular marker have provided morphological evidence of the alterations caused by glycerol treatment in the morphology of the T system (89, 190). Depending on the marker, between 90% and 98% of the T tubules are disconnected from the surface-membrane openings to the external medium (126). Thus glycerol treatment appears to separate the properties of the surface membrane from those of the T system and topologically localizes different phenomena.

Contractile responses to electrical depolarization are abolished after glycerol treatment because the T tubules are the pathway for inward spread of depolarization from the surface membrane to the junction between the T tubules and the SR. A large fraction of the intramembrane charge movement is also removed after this treatment, evidence that it might be an important step in ECC (58). After glycerol treatment muscle fibers appear to be depolarized by 10–30 mV. This depolarization develops with time and is diminished and delayed by adding extra divalent cations (5 mM Ca^{2+} + 5 mM Mg^{2+}) (91). The ability to disrupt the T system after osmotic shock is not specific to glycerol; it also occurs with other penetrating solutes such as ethylene glycol (258), propylene glycol, urea, and acetamide (49). Of these substances glycerol and urea are less permeable but they certainly penetrate muscle fibers (49). With lower glycerol concentrations (110–220 mM) (191) or other permeable substances such as ethylene glycol, acetamide, etc. (49), twitch tension may be recovered after disappearing when the fibers are reimmersed in the normal Ringer's solution. With ethylene glycol at a high concentration (1,095 mM) depolarization of the fiber membrane is less conspicuous and action potentials with quasi-normal negative afterpotentials may be recorded (258). Recently a new method for uncoupling excitation contraction in frog muscle based on 1.5–2 M formamide containing Ringer's solution was described. One advantage of this method is that with short exposures (15–30 min) to the formamide solution, neuromuscular transmission is not impaired (75).

It has been reported that under some experimental conditions, muscle fibers exposed to hypertonic solutions may be protected from their effect. For instance when single muscle fibers and whole muscles were exposed to a solution made hypertonic by 430 mM glycerol, twitch tension declined transiently and then recovered its normal value (297). However, the volume decrease (measured by weighing the muscles) was sustained when tension was recovered. Thus fiber contractility was restored even though the fibers remained dehydrated. Similar results were obtained with urea but not with other solutes. On the other hand, when single muscle fibers are exposed to hypertonic solutions prepared with penetrating solutes, such as ethylene glycol, propylene glycol, and acetamide, fiber volume and twitch tension initially decline and then recover their original values in a parallel way (49). Glycerol and urea appear to be less permeable; therefore the recovery time of twitch tension and volume is longer. Therefore the muscle's failure to recover weight after the loss caused by exposure to hypertonic glycerol solutions may be attributed to a too short recovery time ($<$ 1 h for whole muscles). The partial recovery of the twitch of whole muscles can be explained if only the few outermost fibers recover their normal twitch and volume values. Recently Miyamoto and Hubbard (212) reinvestigated this matter and confirmed that, in hypertonic glycerol solutions, muscle weight is recovered after the initial decrease.

These authors also reinvestigated the report (128) that presoaking muscles in isotonic KCl protects them against the contractile failure normally expected in hypertonic solutions prepared with two-times hypertonic NaCl. When exposed to isotonic KCl, the muscles gained water, which entered the fiber after the K^+ and Cl^-. After this swelling, hypertonic NaCl solutions caused these muscles to dehydrate less than muscles not presoaked in isotonic KCl, thereby accounting for the protective effect of this treatment.

Effects of Anions

INORGANIC ANIONS. It has long been known that several anions potentiate muscular contractions elicited by different types of stimuli. Zoethout (298), in 1908, showed that I^- and to a lesser degree Br^- sensitized muscles to contract in response to normally subthreshold K^+ concentrations. Later the ability of different anions to potentiate contraction was tested. The relative effectiveness of these anions followed the lyotropic series $Cl^- < Br^- < NO_3^- < ClO_3^- < I^- < SCN^-$ (160, 205, 285). Kahn and Sandow (181), using supramaximal electrical stimuli transversely applied in the absence and presence of Br^-, NO_3^-, and I^- ensured a response from all the fibers in the muscle and confirmed that such anions markedly potentiated the twitch but not the tetanus. Because of the magnitude of stimulus they could conclude that the twitch potentiation of whole muscle was caused by intrinsic potentiation of the twitch of each fiber and not by recruitment of additional fibers. By an extracellular recording of action potentials they also showed that the potentiated twitches were associated with single action potentials, which were unchanged in amplitude and in duration. This was confirmed in later work, in which, with intracellular microelectrodes, only minor modifications of the action potential time course were induced by I^-, Br^-, or NO_3^- (101).

The potentiation of twitch tension in the presence of these foreign anions has been attributed to a prolongation of the active state (151, 238) caused by a process occurring at the surface membrane. Thus contractile activation, once started by membrane excitation, does not proceed independently of the triggering process but rather is controlled and determined by some process, "which does not occur inside but at the surface" of muscle fibers (151). The anions of the lyotropic series affect membrane properties of excitable cells, as well as the duration of the active state, without altering the duration of the action potential much. Replacing Cl^- with Br^-, NO_3^-, or I^- increases the membrane resistance more than twofold (166). These effects result because Cl^- contributes most of the membrane conductance (156); their replacement by less-permeant anions result in a decreased membrane conductance (165, 215). However, these conductance decreases per se are not immediately relevant to the problem of ECC because lowering the external pH may also reduce the Cl^- conductance (167) without causing effects like those the lyotropic anions produce on the contractile phenomena.

More recent studies by Hodgkin and Horowicz (158) show that NO_3^- and other foreign anions also change the contractile threshold for K contractures. These anions appear to affect the mechanism that enables the membrane potential to control the contractile process. Therefore an understanding of this effect and knowing its location could help clarify the ECC mechanism. Hodgkin and Horowicz, working with single muscle fibers to avoid diffusion delays, showed that NO_3^- potentiation is established with a short delay (2–3 s) after a solution change (Fig. 11). With their technique, Hodgkin and Horowicz could demonstrate that this delay was not caused by experimental limitations, since Na^+-free solutions instantaneously abolished excitation of the fibers. Therefore they concluded that NO_3^- must diffuse into a restricted region to produce its effect, suggesting that diffusion into the T tubules caused the delay. They also showed, using K contractures, that NO_3^-, as well as potentiating the twitch, shifted the relationship between peak tension developed during the contracture and the K concentration, which determines the fiber membrane potential. According to these effects NO_3^- and the other anions of the lyotropic series are type A potentiators because they prolong the mechanically effective period by lowering the contractile threshold [(255, 274); see Fig. 3]. Other agents that prolong the duration of the action potential are known as type B potentiators (255).

Subsequently the changes in contractile threshold produced by foreign anions were more precisely measured with voltage-clamp techniques and visual observations of movement (184). These studies were designed to test whether contractile activation was causally related to the onset of the delayed rectifier since under normal conditions the two phenomena appear to start at the same membrane potential value.

ORGANIC ANIONS. Some organic anions, depending on the group and size of the hydrocarbon chain, when substituted for Cl^- also can induce changes in ECC. Some induce marked changes in the shape of the action potential by increasing the negative afterpotential and causing repetitive firing in response to a single stimulus (113). This increased excitability of the muscle fiber membrane is reversed by raising the external Ca concentration. These organic anions then enhance twitch tension in this order: γ-hydroxybutyrate > propionate > formate > acetate > methanesulfonate > hexanesulfonate > propanesulfonate. Butyrate, on the other hand, was found to depress twitch tension.

These anions affect the relationship between contracture tension and the external K concentration differently. Most lower the mechanical threshold; hexanoate and butyrate, however, increase the mechanical threshold and decrease the maximal contracture tension.

Interestingly, although K contractures of whole toe muscle appear unaffected by pH changes between 5 and 9 (114, 199), in the presence of organic anions a great sensitivity develops so that a small pH reduction can reduce K contractures (117). Changes in membrane potential do not explain these effects. Penetration of the undissociated organic molecule in the interior of the fiber may be responsible for them in part or pH changes may favor the interactions of these organic substances with membrane groups leading to a modification of the potential-dependent step in ECC. More detailed work on single muscle fibers is necessary to clarify this process.

Effects of Cations

Divalent cations affect ECC in a variety of ways (88). They can substitute for Ca^{2+} in the maintenance

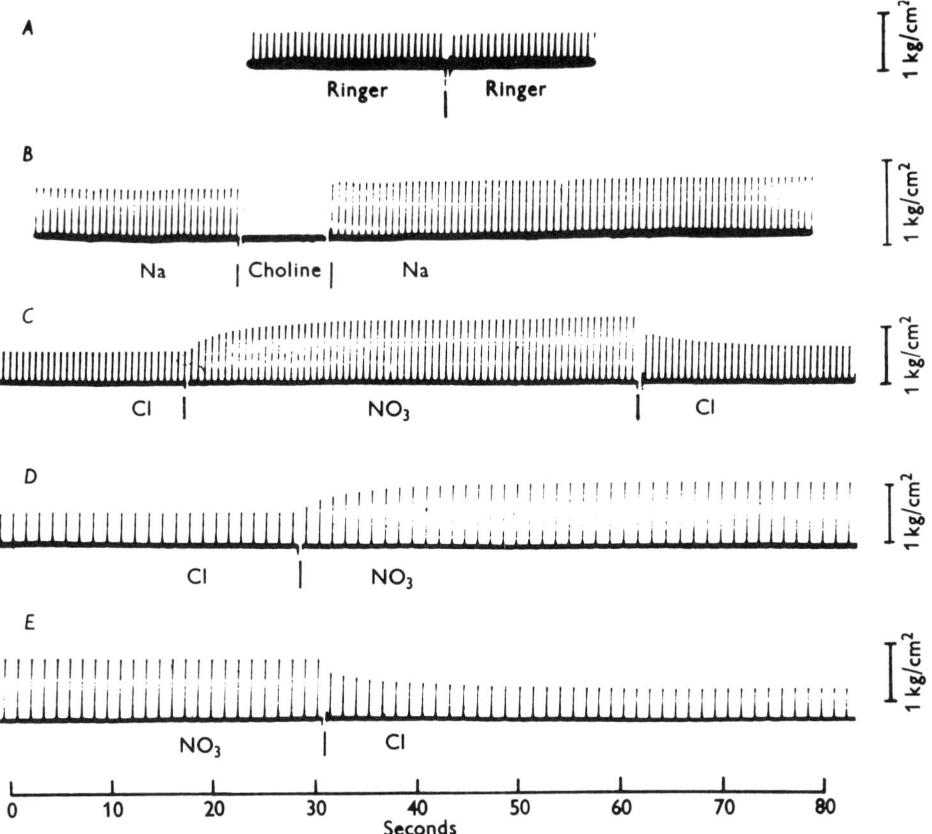

FIG. 11. Effect of NO_3^- on twitch tension in a single muscle fiber during rapid solution changes. *A*: small artifact caused by sudden flow of solution. *B*: effectiveness of solution change system in abolishing twitch tension when normal Ringer's solution is substituted with Na-free, choline solution. Abrupt loss of twitch indicates effectiveness of solution change. *C*, *D*, and *E*: time course of twitch potentiator and decay of potentiation when NO_3^- Ringer's solution is flushed into and out of chamber. In *C* fiber was stimulated at 1.56 Hz and in *D* and *E* at 0.78 Hz. Exponential time constant for ON effect, 3–4 s; for OFF effect, 2–3 s; fiber diameter, 122 μm; 19°C. [From Hodgkin and Horowicz (158).]

of normal contractile functions, act as contractile potentiators, or produce contractile uncoupling. Since the work of Frank (120), carried out with whole muscles (extensor digituorum longus IV), the failure of K contractures when this preparation is bathed in Ca-free media has been prevented with different degrees of effectiveness by adding Cd^{2+}, Be^{2+}, Ni^{2+}, Co^{2+}, Mg^{2+}, Sr^{2+}, Mn^{2+}, and Fe^{2+}; other cations are ineffective, such as Ba^{2+} and Pb^{2+}, or could even produce irreversible inhibition of contractile activity, such as Hg^{2+}.

Some of these cations, depending on their concentration, can produce a dual effect: thus a low concentration (1 mM) of Mn^{2+} sustains K contractures in Ca-free media and prevents progressive depolarization of muscle fiber membrane in the absence of Ca^{2+}; a high concentration (>10 mM) of Mn^{2+} inhibits contracture (62, 228).

POTENTIATION BY DIVALENT CATIONS. *Zinc.* The original report that Zn^{2+}, at very low concentrations, potentiates twitch (252) led to more detailed studies that clarified its mechanism, as well as that of other cations that appear to have a similar effect (173, 253). Zinc is normally present in muscle tissue at a relatively high concentration [about 1 mM (84)] and appears to enhance contractility of glycerol-extracted muscle fibers at a much lower concentration (1 μM) indicating that most of it is in a bound state in the fiber. Its effects as a contractile potentiator in intact fibers, however, appear to be exerted at the level of the fiber membrane. In the presence of Zn^{2+} (5–50 μM) the twitch, but not the tetanus, tension is potentiated. Both the rising and relaxation phases of the twitch are prolonged, indicating that the active state is prolonged but not intensified (173). Similar potentiations of twitch tension, also by prolonging the active state, are induced by Be^{2+}, Ba^{2+}, Cd^{2+}, Ni^{2+}, Cu^{2+}, Pb^{2+}, and UO_2^{2+} (253). These ions prolong the active state by a marked delay of the repolarization phase of the action potential [(206, 275); see also Fig. 3]. Thus these compounds may be classified as type B potentiators (255).

Interestingly Zn^{2+}, Cd^{2+}, and other anionic potentiators inhibit the active uptake and increase the passive binding of Ca at the level of the membrane of isolated SR (57). Although this could contribute to their potentiating action, it is not known whether these cations could penetrate the fiber and reach the SR membrane. The effect, however, might be related to the ability of these ions to bind more tightly than Ca^{2+} to the fiber membranes. The time course of potentiation by Zn^{2+}, although slower than that by NO_3^-, is rapid enough to indicate that Zn^{2+} acts at the fiber surface. In experiments on the same muscles NO_3^- potentiation occurred with a half time of 6–12 s and potentiation with 50 μM Zn^{2+} developed with a half time of 96 s, after an initial lag phase of about 12 s. Zinc potentiation reverses much more slowly when Zn^{2+} is washed out with normal Ringer's solution (253). Up to concentrations of 2.5 mM, Zn^{2+} does not affect the fiber resting potential; at concentrations between 0.05 (185) and 0.5 mM (206) it causes an appreciable increase in the fiber membrane resistance without affecting the thresholds for contraction or for the delayed rectifier (185). At very low concentrations (0.05 mM), however, Zn^{2+} prolongs the action potential (206, 255) by reducing the intensity of the outward K current through the delayed rectifier and also by affecting the development rate of this current (185). In this respect Zn^{2+} acts very much like tetraethylammonium (TEA), which also inhibits the delayed K conductance (265). One significant difference, however, is that Zn^{2+} does not affect the resting K conductance, while TEA does. The increase in the membrane electrical resistance in the presence of Zn^{2+} is caused by interference with the Cl^- conductance in the resting membrane (266).

Barium. Barium ions, which also are effective as contractile potentiators, behave very much like TEA, since besides affecting the delayed rectifier, they also greatly diminish the resting K conductance. In fact in normal Cl^- Ringer's solution, Ba^{2+} does not induce membrane depolarization whereas in sulfate solution (180) addition of Ba^{2+} at a low concentration decreases the K conductance and causes fiber depolarization (264). Barium ions produce long-lasting action potentials in crustacean and frog muscle fibers (237). Frog muscle fibers in the presence of this ion may show two types of response. In most cases the repolarization phase of the action potential is greatly slowed down. This is explained by the drastic reduction of K conductance by Ba^{2+} (264). In a few cases a second regenerative response with a long-lasting plateau follows the normal rapid depolarization phase of the action potential. This response has been explained by the development of a Ba^{2+} conductance, which causes a net inward Ba^{2+} current like the slow Ca inward current (237). Recent work with single muscle fibers under voltage-clamp conditions has provided interesting results on the effect of Ba^{2+} on contractile activity (234). Because voltage clamping was achieved by the double sucrose-gap technique, tension development could not be directly registered at the fiber end but could be estimated by placing the prolonged shaft of the transducer tangential to the fiber segment lying in the test-node portion of the double-sucrose gap. With this arrangement, in the presence of a high Ba^{2+} concentration (76 mM), two components of tension development, the first potential dependent and the second current dependent, could be visualized, inhibited by Mn^{2+}, and greatly affected by glycerol treatment. Because contractile proteins have a low affinity for Ba^{2+}, these ions entering the fiber most probably do not directly activate tension; an interesting possibility is that Ba^{2+} might release Ca from the SR by a mechanism analogous to the Ca-induced Ca release (234). However, a high Ba^{2+} concentration (76 mM) would then be a strict requirement, since equimolar substitution (1.8 mM) of Ba^{2+} for Ca^{2+} cannot reverse the changes induced by Ca-free solutions on the time course of contractile responses to prolonged depolarizations (53a).

UNCOUPLING BY DIVALENT CATIONS. Divalent cations, depending on their concentration, may or may not play a dual role; several divalent cations at relatively high concentraions increase the contractile threshold and act as contractile uncouplers. One of these, which has been extensively studied, is Mn^{2+}.

Manganese ions. Manganese ions at concentrations between 3 and 10 mM progressively inhibit both twitch and tetanus tension in massively stimulated whole muscles to complete although reversible block (228). In normal Ringer's solution 10 mM Mn^{2+} hyperpolarizes the fiber membrane about 10 mV without affecting the membrane resistance. The increase in membrane resistance in isotonic K_2SO_4 media indicates a decrease of the K conductance (62). The amplitude of the action potential is not affected although the threshold for its appearance is markedly increased, its duration appreciably prolonged, and the negative afterpotential increased (62, 228, 246). At concentrations between 10 and 20 mM, Mn^{2+} markedly shifts the contractile threshold for K contractures of single fibers from −48 to −33 mV, shifting the contractile-activation curve also, without diminishing the maximal tension much.

At these concentrations Mn^{2+} does not diminish the membrane depolarization induced by increased K concentrations. The decrease or abolition of K contractures obtained with submaximal K concentrations can thus be explained by the activation curve shift; in fact tension in response to 75 mM K is greatly reduced although contracture tension elicited by 190 mM K is not much affected and the duration of this response is prolonged (62). At low temperatures Mn^{2+} does not affect development of caffeine contracture nor diminish its increased sensitivity to this drug (246). The inhibitory effects of Mn^{2+} both on the twitch (62) and on low K contractures rapidly disappear, indicating a surface membrane action. These effects could in principle be explained by a reduction in their membrane permeability to Ca^{2+}. In fact Mn^{2+} does reduce inward Ca currents in barnacle muscle fibers and other excitable cells.

However, because neither peak tension nor contractile-response time courses depend solely on external Ca^{2+} and because Mn^{2+} affects the contractile threshold considerably, Mn^{2+}, like other divalent and trivalent cations at high concentrations, probably interferes with ECC at the triadic junction.

EFFECTS OF TRIVALENT CATIONS. *Lanthanum.* Lanthanum ions can have one of two effects on ECC phenomena, depending on their concentration. Between 0.05 and 0.3 mM, they produce reversible and increasing potentiation of the twitch, characterized by a prolonged latent period, an increase in the rate of tension development, and a prolonged relaxation phase (13). This potentiation is probably indirectly caused by a prolongation of the action potential, which increases the duration of the mechanically effective period although much less conspicuously than other type B potentiators. At 7°C the action potential, measured at −25 mV, increases from about 4 to 6 ms in the presence of 0.3 mM La^{3+} (13). Even at a low concentration (0.1 mM), La^{3+} increases the mechanical threshold for K contractures of single muscle fibers from −50 to −35 mV (13, 80a), thus qualitatively simulating the effect of large external Ca concentrations (201). Between 0.1 and 1 mM, La^{3+} does not change the membrane resting potential and prevents the depolarization caused by Ca-free solution.

Higher than 0.5 mM, La^{3+} diminishes the depolarization caused by increased K concentrations and impairs the generation of action potentials, thus causing contractile failure in response to electrical stimulation. Lanthanum also prolongs the time course of K contractures severalfold and causes only a small decrease in the peak tension (14). This prolongation is observed also in Ca-free media.

In whole sartorius muscle 1 mM La^{3+} markedly reduces K contractures (80 mM), perhaps by interfering with membrane depolarization. Nitrates reduce this effect. However, caffeine contractures were not diminished but potentiated (290). Lanthanum also inhibits Ca uptake by isolated fragments of the SR (21). This action may not be related to the prolongation of the relaxation phase of twitches or K contractures, however, because trivalent ions do not permeate the plasma membranes (56). More probably La^{3+} affects the mechanism of Ca release from the SR by prolonging its time course.

Other lanthanide ions. Other trivalent ions of the lanthanide series reduce twitch tension at low concentrations. Electron-microscope studies show that these ions are deposited on the external side of the surface membrane of intact fibers, leading to the conclusion that they do not penetrate the fibers. Lanthanide ions more effectively inhibit the twitch response of cardiac muscle than of skeletal muscle (56, 138). For cardiac muscle the uncoupling effect of divalent and trivalent cations is thought to be caused by their ability to displace surface-bound Ca^{2+} and their effectiveness is thought to depend on the size of the nonhydrated ionic radius (194). Contractile activation in skeletal muscle probably depends less on membrane-bound Ca^{2+} and more likely on the stabilizing role of Ca^{2+} at the junction of the SR and T tubules. The uncoupling action of La^{3+} as well as that of some divalent cations may be caused by displacement of Ca by these cations at these junctions, which could change the coupling efficiency.

Drugs That Activate or Potentiate Contraction

CAFFEINE. Normally, membrane depolarization is the first step for contractile activation of muscle fibers. Caffeine activates the contractile mechanism, however, without producing any appreciable change in the membrane potential (18, 59). Furthermore it can induce contractures even in muscles bathed in isotonic K solutions and thus depolarized and in a refractory state. Therefore caffeine seems to activate Ca release, bypassing those steps of ECC that depend on the fiber membrane potential. In addition to this capability, at lower concentrations caffeine also acts as contractile potentiator and causes important changes in several phenomena related to ECC (203). Examples of different actions of caffeine are illustrated in Figure 12. The potentiation of the twitch by caffeine is indirectly caused by lowering the contractile threshold without significantly changing the shape of the action potential (98). Therefore caffeine is a type A potentiator (255).

The speed with which caffeine potentiates twitch in frog single muscle fibers suggests a site of action near or at the junction between T-tubule membranes and the SR (208, 251, 279). Therefore in several ways the action of caffeine is similar to that of other potentiators, such as the anions of the lyotropic series. For these other compounds, however, changes in the mechanical threshold may involve membrane surface charges and reduction of surface potentials caused by the higher adsorbability of these anions to the fiber membrane (121), whereas caffeine is uncharged and therefore should act by some other mechanism.

Besides acting more slowly than NO_3^- (131, 208), the speed of twitch potentiation by caffeine seems to depend on the stimulation frequency (296). Thus although at 1–5 Hz maximal potentiation occurs in less than 5 s, at 0.1 Hz maximal potentiation takes over 20 s. This observation is puzzling because at higher concentrations, caffeine induces contracture with a very short delay. In the contractile actions of caffeine probably no extracellular Ca^{2+} is involved; the drug acts by directly releasing Ca^{2+} from the SR since undiminished contractures can be elicited repeatedly and for a long time in the virtual absence of external Ca^{2+} (47). Caffeine induces modification in Ca^{2+} movements in and out of the fibers (31, 44, 174), however, and for crayfish muscle fibers it induces Ca^{2+} electrogenesis by changing the normally graded responses into Ca spikes, which are insensitive to tetrodotoxin (TTX) (59).

Caffeine could inhibit the active, ATP-dependent, Ca^{2+} uptake by the SR (227, 286). This tentative

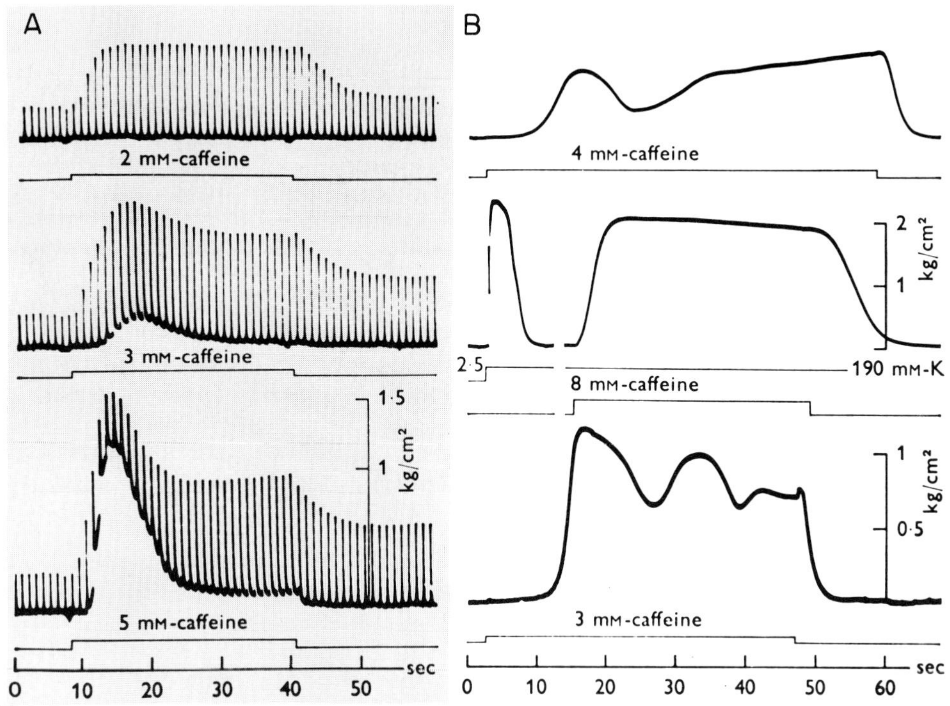

FIG. 12. Effect of caffeine at different concentrations on single muscle fibers at 21°C–23°C. *A*: effects of 2, 3, and 5 mM caffeine on twitch tension of fiber 109 μm in diameter. *B*: contractures obtained with 4, 8, and 3 mM caffeine and a fiber 145 μm in diameter, either polarized or depolarized. [From Lüttgau and Oetliker (203).]

interpretation is strengthened by the demonstration that low temperatures increase the effectiveness of caffeine so that normally subthreshold concentrations of the drug cause strong contractures (245). In the presence of ATP, 8 mM caffeine can release massive amounts of Ca^{2+} from loaded vesicles of fragmented SR of the frog (287). However, this release could be the result of reduction in the SR's ability to accumulate Ca^{2+} and of reduction in the rate of Ca^{2+} uptake. This interpretation was based on the demonstration that caffeine-induced Ca^{2+} release was diminished with low internal Ca^{2+} concentrations and that caffeine did not increase the rate of Ca outflow from the SR in a Ca-free medium (286). In the presence of ATP, Ca release is difficult to characterize since Ca uptake is occurring simultaneously. Firm evidence that caffeine as well as other drugs can induce Ca release from the SR has been obtained with SR vesicles loaded with Ca^{2+} and with a limited supply of ATP (103). After the pump activity has exhausted ATP, massive drug-induced Ca^{2+} release can be clearly demonstrated. Thus several compounds that potentiate contractility and prolong the time course of K contractures were found to be effective in promoting Ca^{2+} release.

Experiments with intact fibers also support the idea that the main effect of caffeine is in inducing Ca^{2+} release. In fact even with caffeine concentrations sufficient to induce contracture, the fibers maintain their ability to relax. This evidence is based on the demonstration that tetanuses and K contractures, with almost normal relaxation phases, may be superimposed on caffeine contractures (52, 203). Moreover prompt relaxation by exposure to tetracaine can suddenly terminate maximal caffeine contractures (203). This effect of tetracaine is caused by the block of Ca^{2+} release, induced either by caffeine or by membrane depolarization. Therefore the principal effect of caffeine is on the mechanism of Ca^{2+} release, although its inhibition of the Ca^{2+} uptake mechanism may also contribute. In fact there may be a normal Ca^{2+} leak from the SR into the myoplasm supported by a large concentration gradient and balanced by the ATP-driven Ca^{2+} pump. Caffeine at a concentration insufficient to cause Ca^{2+} release might reduce the pump activity, leading to an increase in the myoplasmic free Ca^{2+}. Reduced activity of the SR Ca^{2+} pump could explain the slow initial relaxation rate after a tetanus (229).

An increased but still subthreshold intracellular free-Ca^{2+} concentration achieved either by subthreshold Ca^{2+} release or by interference with the Ca^{2+} pump could explain how caffeine lowers the contractile threshold and potentiates twitch. This is supported by the observation that in the presence of low caffeine concentrations asynchronous sarcomere activation causes localized movement (232). This activity does not cause tension development because the contracting sarcomeres shorten at the expense of the nonactive ones. At low concentrations caffeine also greatly increases the basal oxygen consumption in both normal and K-depolarized muscles (213), in a way that is similar to the Solandt effect, produced by moderately high (10–20 mM) K concentrations (142). This effect is blocked by procaine (224) and is probably caused by increased Ca^{2+} concentration in the myoplasm (223).

Other than an increase in the myoplasmic free Ca^{2+} the lowering of the contractile threshold induced by caffeine could be caused by an increased sensitivity of the coupling system to membrane depolarization. This explanation is supported by recent work with Ca^{2+}-sensitive microelectrodes in which no change in the myoplasmic free-Ca^{2+} concentration was induced by 1 or 2 mM caffeine (J. R. Lopez et al., unpublished observations). Besides producing a shift of the contractile-activation curve toward more negative potentials, caffeine also causes the contractile-repriming curve to shift toward more positive potentials [Fig. 6; (203).] This indicates that in the presence of caffeine, contractile activation may occur over a broader range of membrane potentials than usual. In amphibian muscle fibers, caffeine may induce contractures even with the fibers depolarized. Some of these contractures, depending on the drug concentration, do not appear to relax spontaneously although in some cases tension may oscillate. In crustacean muscle fibers, caffeine contractures are not sustained and relax spontaneously (60); then a repriming process, like that necessary for K contractures, must occur before a second response to caffeine can be elicited.

Anions of the lyotropic series effectively increase the sensitivity of muscle fibers to caffeine (116, 209) for the development of contractures. Caffeine contractures on the other hand can be stopped by local anesthetics such as procaine and tetracaine, which also effectively block Ca^{2+} release in response to membrane depolarization (51, 203). Therefore the mechanisms responsible for Ca^{2+} release in both cases appear to have some similarities. Although both lyotropic anions and caffeine effectively change the contractile threshold, there are some differences in their mode of action. In fact although NO_3^- (substituted for Cl^-) causes a rapid contracture in muscles exposed to 20 mM K^+, caffeine produces this effect but with a slower time course (131).

The speed with which caffeine potentiates twitch in frog single muscle fibers suggests an action site at or near the junction of the T tubules and the SR. On the other hand caffeine is highly permeable (32) and its action site for inducing contractures could be intracellular. In frog fibers intracellular injection of caffeine with a micropipette could not induce contractions, although injection on the external side produces a localized response (18). In invertebrate muscle fibers, intracellular injection of caffeine by hydrostatic pressure or catelectronic current pulses appears to induce contractile responses (59); however, the complex geometry of the surface membrane, with deep invaginations, suggests that the drug might act at the level of the surface membrane facing the lumena of the clefts. Results conflict on whether caffeine contractures are abolished after glycerol treatment, which disrupts the T system. Although disruption of the T tubules does not impair the ability of frog toe muscles to develop caffeine contractures (162), later work with whole muscles indicated that in winter frog caffeine-contracture peak tension was reduced by about 40% after glycerol treatment and in spring frog was not affected (245). In more recent work it has been found that in glycerol-treated single muscle fibers, caffeine-contracture peak tension and the rate of tension development are markedly reduced but not completely abolished (217), indicating that because caffeine is readily permeable in muscle fibers, although the T tubules are disrupted, it may penetrate the fiber membrane and reach the SR to cause Ca release (216). Interestingly foreign anions such as SCN^- and NO_3^- stopped potentiating caffeine contracture after glycerol treatment (217), suggesting that caffeine may release Ca^{2+} directly from the SR membrane. The results confirm, however, that contractile potentiation caused by foreign anions is mediated at the junction between the T-tubules and the SR.

In frog muscle after NO_3^- induced potentiation of the twitch, addition of caffeine (1 mM) causes further potentiation. When the inverse order is followed, however, adding NO_3^- after caffeine, less NO_3^- potentiation is achieved, indicating that caffeine may partially inhibit the NO_3^- effect. Mammalian skeletal muscles are less sensitive to NO_3^- and caffeine, and in this preparation maximal potentiation of the twitch is obtained with either agent. Subsequent addition of the other does not produce further potentiation (46).

Interestingly, for dystrophic mouse muscles pretreatment with either of these potentiators does not prevent further potentiation by the other. Furthermore tetanic tension in these diseased muscles is also potentiated by NO_3^- or caffeine, indicating defects in the coupling mechanisms that can be overcome by contractile potentiators (46). Mammalian muscles normally do not respond with contractures in the presence of caffeine, even at high concentrations; after denervation, however, they can (137).

When sarcomeres are relatively short, tension development declines with a decrease in muscle-fiber activation, which the appearance of wavy myofibrils in the core of the shortening fiber shows (240). A graded decline of contractile force during active shortening in a tetanus can also demonstrate this deactivation (85). Although a decrease of Ca release in shortened fibers could explain this decrease, shortening may also reduce the degree of interaction between A and I filaments. With 1.3-μm sarcomeres the fibers develop no tension when stimulated tetanically. In the presence of caffeine (3 mM), however, 35% of maximal tetanic tension can be obtained (240).

At a lower concentration (0.5 mM) caffeine can also reduce the depressive effect of active shortening (85).

QUININE AND QUINIDINE. Since 1939 both quinine and its optical isomer quinidine have been known to markedly affect muscle contractility and neuromuscular transmission (140). Injection of quinine hydrochloride at low concentrations in the tibialis anterior muscle of the cat causes a great potentiation of twitch tension. In the frog a smaller potentiation may be observed only in isolated, curarized, directly stimulated muscles because quinine, like curare, blocks neuromuscular transmission and masks its potentiating action in indirectly stimulated muscles (140).

More recent work has shown definitively that quinine and quinidine prolong the active state in frog muscles (193); they also prolong the duration of the action potentials, thus increasing the mechanically effective period (98, 106). Furthermore quinidine lowers the contractile threshold for K contractures in frog single muscle fibers (12). Thus the active state is prolonged by two mechanisms, one affecting the duration of the action potential and the other affecting the contractile threshold. The second mechanism is probably related to the ability of these drugs to release Ca.

In fact, although they both may reduce the rate of Ca accumulation by the SR (43), quinidine promotes Ca release from both heavy and light fractions of the SR (103). At a concentration of 5×10^{-5} M it prolongs the time course of K contractures of single muscle fibers; at 3×10^{-3} M it effectively elicits quinidine contractures whose peak tension amounts to about one half of tetanic tension. The quinidine contractures occur whether the fibers are depolarized by high K concentrations or bathed in a Ca-free medium (12). Quinine at 1 mM induces twitch potentiation in whole frog muscle and causes a marked increase in Ca outflow and uptake (174). The increase in Ca efflux persists in muscles bathed in Ca-free ethylenediaminetetraacetic acid (EDTA) media. These effects are much larger at higher drug concentrations, which cause contracture. The site of quinine action for these effects on Ca mobilization is probably intracellular, since they are potentiated when pH is raised, causing an increase in the uncharged and more permeable variety of the quinine molecule (172).

Most of these quinine and quinidine actions point to a similarity with caffeine. Some differences, however, indicate that the action sites of these drugs may differ. In fact procaine, which inhibits caffeine contractures and caffeine-induced Ca release, does not impair the action of quinine and quinidine (172). Furthermore, after repeated caffeine contractures, when this drug can induce no further response, quinine can still elicit a contracture (27). After prolonged exposure or repeated stimulation the quinine-induced twitch potentiation is not sustained and tension decays to very low values. Failure of the action potential probably causes this, as supported by the finding that quinine and quinidine have effects similar to those of procaine on the electrical activity of muscle fibers (106).

In crab striated muscle fibers quinine does not affect the contractile threshold. Furthermore it causes transient twitch potentiation that soon declines because of a decrease in both the resting and action potentials of the fiber membrane. In depolarized crab fibers quinine cannot produce contractures (163).

RYANODINE. Ryanodine is a neutral alkaloid that produces irreversible contractures in vertebrate muscles at a relatively low (1 mM) concentration (176). In whole muscles that are not allowed to shorten, ryanodine may cause individual fibers to rupture during development of rigor (42). Development of ryanodine contractures is not accompanied by substantial changes in the resting membrane potential (42, 179) and may occur also in depolarized muscles. In this respect the action of ryanodine resembles that of caffeine. However, there are also marked differences between these two drugs. One is the temperature sensitivity of muscles to their action; contrary to what happens with caffeine (245), at low temperatures muscle fibers appear to be less sensitive to ryanodine and the onset of ryanodine contractures is much delayed (141). At a low concentration (0.2 mM) ryanodine greatly prolongs the relaxation phase of twitches (257). The delayed relaxation results in development of steady tension when muscles are stimulated to frequencies higher than 1 Hz (187). Ryanodine also progressively depresses twitch tension, which results in contractile failure after prolonged activity. This effect of ryanodine is partially reversed by caffeine or quinidine (187). In the presence of ryanodine, K-induced contractures lose their typical relaxation phase and become sustained (33).

Ryanodine-induced rigor is not caused by interference with myofibrillar contractility or by ATP depletion (42, 257). In isolated, fragmented SR, ryanodine reduces this system's capacity for active uptake of Ca^{2+} in terms of ATP split per Ca^{2+} transported (104). This drug is particularly effective in reducing the Ca^{2+}-uptake capacity of the heavier part of the SR (105). However, it also induces Ca^{2+} release from the SR (103).

Most of the ryanodine effect can be explained because it affects mainly the Ca^{2+}-uptake capacity of the SR. Contractile failure when muscles are repeatedly stimulated in the presence of this drug might indicate depletion of Ca^{2+} in the SR stores. Although ryanodine increases both the uptake and release of Ca^{2+} in whole muscles (6) it has a larger effect on efflux, thus causing a net Ca loss (33).

NICOTINE. Since the work of Langley (195) it has been known that nicotine can induce contractures in vertebrate muscles. In the sartorius muscle of the frog it caused a phasic response that, depending on the concentration of the drug, might later be followed by a sustained contracture. A nicotine-induced Ca^{2+} release from the SR similar to that induced by caffeine probably caused this sustained contracture. The initial rapid response is probably caused by the depolarizing action of nicotine at the end-plate zone and is abolished by a curare treatment of the muscle (195). Furthermore this depolarization is transitory and the normal resting potential is rapidly reestablished (277).

When single muscle fibers stimulated at 1 Hz are exposed for the first time to nicotine, depolarization of the end plate causes an increased response followed by a twitch failure, which lasts only for a few seconds, and then activity resumes with potentiated twitches. A second exposure to nicotine causes only twitch potentiation with a time course like that observed with caffeine. Nicotine can also prolong the K contractures by affecting the mechanism that determines the time course of Ca^{2+} release, as illustrated in Figure 13. Nicotine increases the uptake and release of Ca^{2+} in frog sartorius muscle (6). In depolarized muscles, both Ca^{2+} uptake and sustained contracture induced by nicotine are decreased (288). The effectiveness of nicotine increases at alkaline pH, indicating that the nonionized form of nicotine is the moiety that penetrates the cell to cause Ca^{2+} release (289).

VERATRUM ALKALOIDS. Pure ester alkaloids cevadine and veratridine as well as veratrine at very low concentrations prolong the late phase of the action potential (99, 106). Repetitive firing is followed by a stable depolarized state in fully veratrinized muscles. Thus the contractile response of veratrinized muscle fibers to a simple stimulus may be a tetanus followed by a contracture (192). These effects of veratrum alkaloids depend on external Na^+ (106, 282) and thus differ from the effects of other agents that prolong the action potential duration. Particularly from work in myelinated nerve fibers it is clear that these substances affect the mechanism of inactivation of the Na^+-conductance system (281).

Drugs That Depress Contraction

LOCAL ANESTHETICS. Local anesthetic amines such as procaine and tetracaine block impulse conduction in nerve and muscle fibers by interfering with both the Na- and K-conductance mechanisms (127, 272). This action on excitable cells is thought to take place at a level on the cytoplasmic side of the membrane.

For squid giant axons and frog myelinated nerves the anesthetic potency of tertiary and some quaternary amines, externally applied, depends on the pH of the medium (153, 218). Furthermore the quaternary forms of some of these molecules are only anesthetic when applied intracellularly (127). Therefore it has been proposed that local anesthetics, externally applied, penetrate the axon membrane in the uncharged form (127, 218, 153) and, once inside, dissociate into the cationic form, which according to Narahashi and Yamada (219) is the active one. The fact that benzocaine, which has no charge, is an effective anesthetic, however, indicates that the presence of a charged

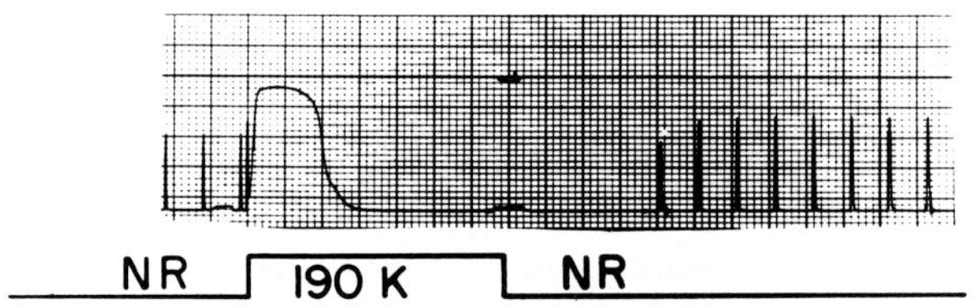

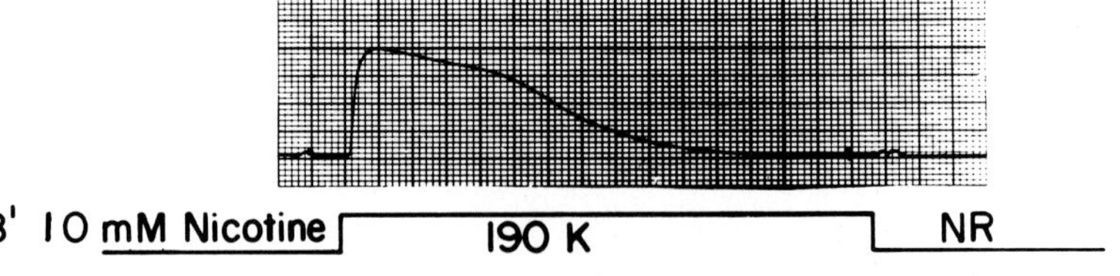

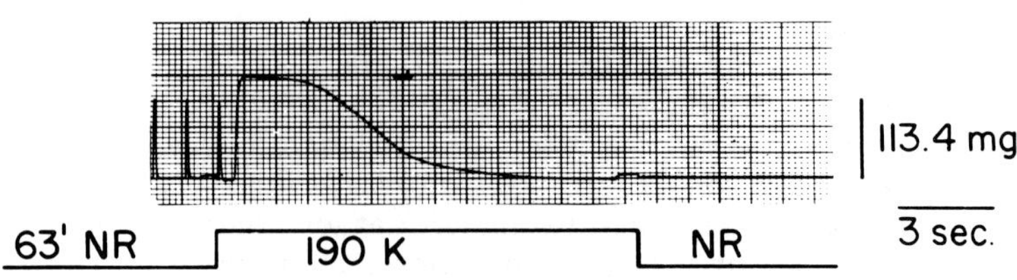

FIG. 13. Effect of nicotine (10 mM) on time course of K contracture of single muscle fiber. NR, normal Ringer's solution. At this concentration nicotine did not cause a contracture even after 8-min exposure. The time course of maximal K contractures, however, was markedly prolonged, consistent with an effect on inactivation mechanism for Ca release shown in Fig. 8. Nicotine effect appears partially reversible. (From C. Caputo, unpublished experiment.)

cationic group in the molecule is not an indispensable requisite for their action (153). Although there might be some argument against it, the view that these molecules penetrate more easily in the uncharged form appears well supported experimentally (153).

This information may be needed to understand the action of local anesthetics in muscle fibers. Besides anesthetizing the muscle fiber membrane, several local anesthetics affect ECC in a different way. Procaine, tetracaine, and others interfere with this process by diminishing or blocking Ca release from the SR (35); lidocaine facilitates it and even produces contractures (34).

In 1963 it was shown that procaine and tetracaine competitively inhibit caffeine by blocking the contractures induced by this drug and the associated increases in Ca fluxes in both polarized and depolarized muscles (107). The possibility that complexation of caffeine with these local anesthetics explained the effects was ruled out by a series of control experiments in the presence of an excess concentration of caffeine that showed that the inhibitory action of local anesthetics depended on the free concentration of these substances (107).

A direct effect of local anesthetics on the mechanism of Ca release from SR has also been demonstrated by inducing contraction by other means, e.g., with K contractures and Ca-induced Ca release (52, 278).

Procaine. At very low (10 μM–1 mM) concentrations (280) procaine appears to enhance Ca release during single twitches, as evidenced by increased peak tension (up to 1.6 times) and aequorin luminescence (up to 2.3 times). This stimulation is probably aided by prolongation of the action potential (100, 106, 171) and can occur if the K-conductance system is more sensitive than the Na one to low procaine concentrations. In 1980, however, Baker and Shapiro (19) showed that procaine (25 mM), tetracaine (2.5 mM), and other anesthetic agents such as urethane and chloroform appear to increase the affinity of aequorin for Ca^{2+}, producing more light emission at a constant level of Ca^{2+}. At higher concentrations procaine abolishes the action potential and can block caffeine contractures (107). At relatively high concentrations procaine markedly shortens the time course of contractile responses of short muscle fibers of the snake under voltage-clamp conditions (147) and can slow down the repriming process so that when the fibers are repeatedly depolarized each depolarization produces a smaller response than the previous one until complete contractile failure ensues (147). The curve describing the relationship between repriming and membrane potential is also shifted toward more negative membrane potential values. For frog muscle fibers, the effect of procaine on K contractures is debatable (52, 55, 278). At 2–5 mM, procaine clearly cuts short the time course of K contractures induced at low temperatures (51). At physiological pH, however, procaine cannot effectively reduce tension during K contractures in intact fibers (100) or depolarization-induced Ca release in skinned fibers, whereas it can effectively abolish Ca-induced Ca release (278), diminish tension in voltage-clamped short muscle fibers of the frog, and decrease the nonlinear Nile blue fluorescence signal normally observed when muscle fibers are depolarized (55). Preliminary experiments with frog single muscle fibers showed that procaine's ability to block K contracture is largely pH dependent; in fact although at pH 7.2 K contractures are only slightly affected, at pH 9 complete block is produced (M. E. Sanchez and C. Caputo, unpublished observations). Procaine can also abolish the increase in oxygen consumption that occurs when frog muscles are exposed to elevated K concentrations or to caffeine (224).

Therefore these different results probably can be explained by differences in the number of procaine molecules that in the uncharged form penetrate the interior of the muscle fibers either because of species differences or different pH conditions. Clarification of this point is necessary because the ability of procaine to block Ca-induced Ca release and its alleged inability to block K contractures is an argument against the idea that Ca-induced Ca release is significant to contractile activation in frog skeletal muscle fibers under physiological conditions (97).

The anesthetic action of procaine in abolishing the action potential without changing the membrane resting potential is potentiated by organic anions (115). The rapid action of these anions (which follow the series: hexanoate, butyrate, propionate, acetate, hydroxybutyrate, and formate) suggests that they act at a level of the external side of the membrane. Interestingly they potentiate the effect of procaine on K contractures of whole toe muscles. The action of benzocaine on the other hand, at an equally effective anesthetic concentration, is not affected by these anions.

Tetracaine. Although there may be some doubt about the effectiveness of procaine, tetracaine is recognized as very effective in blocking Ca release in response to a variety of stimuli. Thus 0.1 mM tetracaine can cut short both caffeine contractures (203) and prolonged K contractures obtained at a low temperature [(51); see Fig. 7]; at a higher concentration (1 mM) tetracaine abolishes both types of responses. Tetracaine, as well as procaine, effectively abolishes the nonlinear Nile blue fluorescence signal (55), which may indicate potential change at the level of the SR membrane.

Because of its large effect on both the delayed K conductance and contractile activation tetracaine has been used to test the relationship between these two phenomena and charge movement (8, 11). Delayed K conductance is reduced to about half its normal value in the presence of 2 mM tetracaine; the curve describing its voltage dependency shifts along the voltage axis about 25 mV toward more positive potential values. The kinetics of the delayed K channels also slows down in the presence of 2 mM tetracaine, but displacement currents are not greatly affected. Thus the curve describing the voltage dependency of charge movements shifts only 5 mV and the kinetics of charge movement are not affected. These results suggest that charge movement does not have a role in gating K channels (8).

The strength-duration curve for the threshold of contractile activation shifts toward longer duration. At 5°C the rheobasic potential of −35.6 mV for a 0.4-s pulse becomes −20 mV for a 1.95-s pulse. At the same temperature a pulse, no matter how strong, must last longer than 70 ms to effectively induce contraction in the presence of 2 mM tetracaine. At this concentration tetracaine does not affect the response of chemically skinned fibers to solutions with lowered pCa, indicating that reduced contractility in intact fibers is caused by an effect of tetracaine on the Ca-release mechanism and not by decreased sensitivity of the contractile proteins to Ca^{2+}. Therefore if charge movement represents the voltage-sensitive step in the chain of ECC events tetracaine affects Ca release at a later stage (11).

Even though tetracaine does not appear to change the most important characteristics of charge movement, it effectively abolishes a component of the charge-movement signal, as visualized under certain circumstances (162a, 162b; J. Vergara and C. Caputo, unpublished observations). It is usually referred to as a hump, or Q_Y, and appears as a slow nonexponentially decaying component (5).

Figure 14 illustrates the effect of 0.5 mM tetracaine on charge movement and Ca signals associated with voltage pulses to −20 mV in a voltage-clamped cut frog muscle fiber. At this concentration the drug abolishes both the Ca signal and the Q_Y component of charge movement, suggesting some relationship between them. Recall (see *Membrane Potential Changes at SR Level*, p. 391) that tetracaine also reduces the extrinsic fluorescence signal in muscle fibers stained with Nile blue A (55).

DANTROLENE. Dantrolene is a peripherally acting muscle relaxant that does not affect the electrical properties of muscle fibers nor the neuromuscular transmission (92, 93). At low concentrations (< 10 μM) it causes a marked reduction in twitch tension and a significant but small decrease in tetanic tension (235). With single muscle fibers, twitch tension declines to about 20% of the initial value in a few seconds indicating that dantrolene acts at the level of the fiber membrane, possibly at the triadic junction (C. Caputo, unpublished observations). In whole muscles the K-contracture peak tension and the area under the tension are greatly reduced (235). With single fibers, however, dantrolene mainly affects the time courses

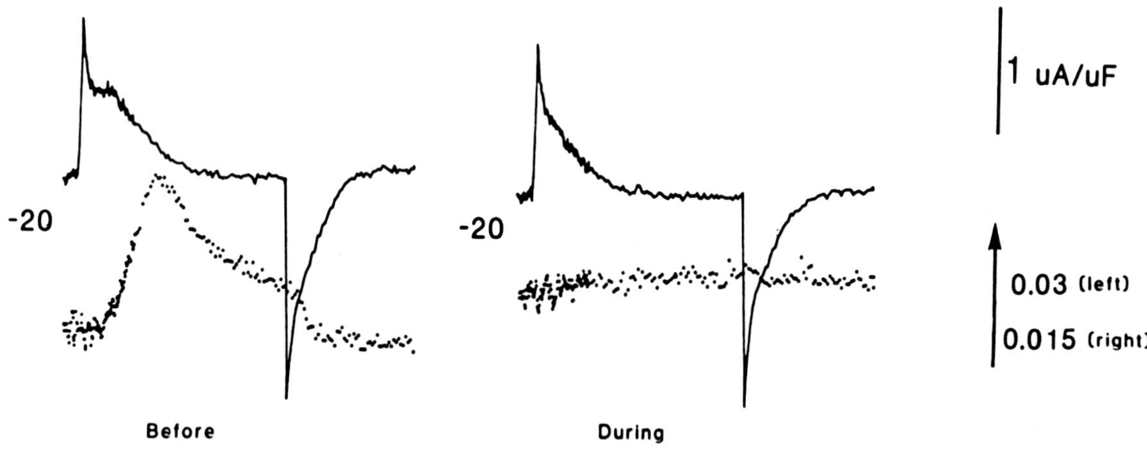

FIG. 14. Effect of 5 mM tetracaine charge movement and antipyrylazo III absorbance signal associated with voltage pulses to −20 mV. Voltage-clamped cut single muscle fiber of *Rana catesbeiana* (154). *Left*: controls. *Right*: obtained after addition of drug. Charge movement trace obtained by subtracting 4 traces associated with voltage steps of P/4 amplitude (applied from holding potential of −130 mV) from trace generated by voltage step of amplitude P (applied from holding potential of −100 mV). Charge movement records normalized with membrane capacity calculated by integration of current records of long duration and small amplitude. *Arrow*, absorbance increase of 0.03 or 0.015, referred to $\Delta A/A = (\Delta A_{710} - \Delta A_{790})/A_{550}$. Temperature, 9°C. (From J. Vergara and C. Caputo, unpublished observations.)

of these responses, abolishing the characteristic plateau and causing a much faster relaxation phase without affecting the contracture peak tension (271). This faster relaxation explains the discrepancy with whole muscle, since in this case the more peripheral fibers relaxing before the high K solution reaches those in the muscle core may cause the diminished contracture tension. This also explains why in whole muscles dantrolene appears to affect peak tension of tetanuses and K contractures differently.

The relationship between tension and K concentration shifts toward a higher K concentration, thus with lower K concentrations, submaximal contracture tension decreases (270). A contractile threshold shift may indicate that a less efficient coupling mechanism in the presence of dantrolene causes the twitch-tension reduction. The inactivation curve, obtained by exposing the fiber to high K conditioning solutions before applying the test contracture medium (122), shifts toward lower K concentrations, indicating that the fiber inactivates at more negative membrane potentials in the presence of dantrolene.

Dantrolene effects are potentiated in the absence of external Ca^{2+} or in the presence of procaine (235, 271). None of these effects are accompanied by gross ultrastructural changes at the level of the tubules or SR (271). In barnacle muscle fibers injected with aequorin (76) dantrolene reduces the resting light emission appreciably and reversibly, indicating a lowering of the myoplasmic free-Ca^{2+} content. This effect is independent of external Ca^{2+}. Dantrolene also reduces the mechanical response and the aequorin-Ca transient induced by electrical stimulation. In frog muscle fibers, however, dantrolene decreases the Ca entry associated with K-induced membrane depolarization; in barnacle muscle such an effect is not observed. Recently Hui (163a) reported that dantrolene, like tetracaine, effectively abolishes the nonexponentially decaying component of charge movement, or Q_Y.

In frog muscle fibers injected with aequorin dantrolene markedly reduces light emission during tetanic stimulation even though it does not greatly reduce tetanic tension (273). Unfortunately dantrolene is almost insoluble and thus it is difficult to test whether higher drug concentrations would completely block Ca release.

DEUTERIUM OXIDE. Deuterium oxide has been used as a tool to study phenomena related to ECC (23, 24, 30). Substituting D_2O for H_2O in Ringer's solutions causes a large depression in the rate of spontaneous beating and in the contractile force of isolated frog atria (182). It produces negligible changes in the resting and action potentials of frog skeletal muscle, affecting only the outward conductance and causing a prolonged action potential (178).

Twitch tension in frog sartorius muscle is almost completely abolished; tetanic tension is reduced by about half (254). In single muscle fibers K contractures are also markedly depressed, but not abolished, with large shifts of the activation curve toward high K concentrations (295). These effects are not caused by interactions with contractile proteins, since D_2O does not decrease the ATP-induced contraction in glycerinated fibers (182) and slightly increases (10%) the maximal response of skinned fibers activated by Ca (132). Furthermore caffeine-contracture maximal tension is not diminished in the presence of D_2O (295). In both barnacle (183) and frog (132) muscle fibers injected with aequorin the light signal and force generation decrease a similar extent; therefore the main effect of D_2O is on the mechanism of Ca release from the SR induced by membrane depolarization. The coupling mechanism seems to work less efficiently without being completely blocked because twitches are affected in larger proportions than tetanuses.

FORMALDEHYDE. Formaldehyde produces lengthening of the action potential plateau in cardiac Purkinje fibers (118) followed by an action potential and then a failure of the membrane to repolarize. Skeletal muscle action potentials are similarly affected (77). Later studies show that the action of formaldehyde on the K-conductance sytem of the muscle fiber membrane was the main cause of these effects (164). This compound almost completely abolishes the inward (anomalous) rectifier (168), which accounts for most of the K conductance in permanently depolarized (186) or normally polarized (165) resting mucles. In these studies the contractile response to electrical stimulation was abolished after exposure to formaldehyde. This treatment did not affect caffeine contractures of whole muscles (164). This observation is important because it distinguishes depolarization-induced from chemically (caffeine-) induced Ca release in intact fibers. Preliminary experiments with single muscle fibers (C. Caputo, unpublished observations), however, have shown that after the loss of K contractures caused by formaldehyde, caffeine contractures are also abolished.

Recently it has been shown that although formaldehyde completely blocks ECC it does not completely abolish charge movement, indicating that this substance acts during a later step in ECC (10, 11).

Other Treatment

EFFECTS OF PH CHANGE. Contractile activity of muscle fibers appears relatively insensitive to pH changes between 5 and 10 (114, 199). In fact membrane resting and action potentials, twitch, and contracture peak tension of whole muscles are not much affected in this range. The membrane conductance of frog muscle fibers to Cl^- is very sensitive to pH changes between 5 and 10, increasing in alkaline and decreasing in acid solution (167). Changes in this range appear to modify the time course of the K contractures of single muscle fibers, however (48). In solutions where Cl^- is the principal anion, the contractile threshold measured by visual observation of muscle fiber movement under current-clamp conditions appears to be pH independent between 6.5 and 8.5. Between 8.5 and 10.5 the threshold shifts toward more negative potentials; a shift in the opposite direction occurs between 6.5 and 4.5 (78). These effects appear to depend largely on the presence of divalent cations and have been explained in terms of changes in surface-charge density at the level of the fiber membrane. In media prepared with methanesulfonate as the main anion, moderate pH changes also shift the curve relating contracture tension to K concentration (199).

Large variations in pH impair contractility; thus at pH 4 and 11 both K contractures and twitch tension are almost completely abolished. Interestingly substituting ClO_4^- for Cl^- at pH 4 restores the twitch (114); the same substitution at pH 11 causes a transient contracture followed by twitch restoration; likewise increases in the external Ca concentration restore contractility at these extreme pH values. Intracellular pH appears well controlled when the external pH is moderately changed (230). At extreme values of external pH for long exposures, however, intracellular pH may also vary. Reduction in intracellular pH by exposing barnacle muscle fibers to CO_2 causes the intracellular Ca^{2+} to increase. Increased light emission by aequorin that is not caused by stimulation of Ca^{2+} influx demonstrates this (197). These results suggest that regulation of free-Ca^{2+} concentration by pH is possible, which could be particularly important, considering the pH changes during contractile activity (210). On the other hand pH modifications could be induced by increased free-Ca^{2+} levels during activity (7).

FATIGUE. Under normal conditions, when a muscle fiber is stimulated at low frequencies (about 1 Hz), twitch tension often increases at the beginning of the stimulation period (64) after which a constant tension value is maintained for a relatively long time. The number of undiminished twitches may vary from fiber to fiber but is normally larger than 1,000. After about 5,000–10,000 twitches at room temperature, tension declines to 10%–20% of the original value (83, 136, 202). Metabolic poisoning and low temperatures cause a much earlier twitch fatigue [after about 100 undiminished twitches (108, 136)]. In a fatigued fiber when the resting membrane potential is not diminished, although the magnitude of the action potential may not be affected, its duration is prolonged and the size of the negative afterpotential increased (136). Similar changes occur after shorter periods of stimulation at higher frequencies (139). Contractile activity in an exhausted fiber does not cease because of depletion of energy stores, since K and caffeine contractures of near maximal amplitude can be produced and twitch tension can be reactivated by caffeine. Under these conditions, however, the curve relating contracture tension to external K concentration shifts toward higher K concentrations as if the fibers had become partially inactivated. In mechanically exhausted and metabolically poisoned fibers the membrane resistance appears to be considerably lower, mainly because of an increase in the K conductance that seems to be related to a higher concentration of internal free Ca^{2+} since it can be suppressed by Ca EGTA injection and obtained in the presence of external caffeine (108, 291).

When stimulated at higher frequencies (>100 Hz) the amplitude of fiber action potentials diminishes before tension is affected. Interestingly this fatigue does not appear in exhausted fibers nor in fibers poisoned with cyanide and iodoacetate (202). In fibers fatigued after prolonged tetanic stimulation the ATP content is not lowered by more than 10%–15% although the phosphocreatine content falls to 10% of the normal concentration value (220). These results combined with those showing the ability of mechanically exhausted fibers to develop caffeine and K contractures indicate that the Ca-release mechanism is affected in the fatigued state, either by an inactivation-type mechanism or by accumulation of substances like H^+ or lactate.

REFERENCES

1. ADRIAN, R. H., AND W. ALMERS. Charge movement in the membrane of striated muscle. *J. Physiol. London* 254: 339–360, 1976.
2. ADRIAN, R. H., W. K. CHANDLER, AND A. L. HODGKIN. The kinetics of mechanical activation in frog muscle. *J. Physiol. London* 204: 207–230, 1969.
3. ADRIAN, R. H., W. K. CHANDLER, AND A. L. HODGKIN. Voltage clamp experiments in striated muscle fibres. *J. Physiol. London* 208: 607–644, 1970.
4. ADRIAN, R. H., W. K. CHANDLER, AND R. F. RAKOWSKI. Charge movement and mechanical repriming in skeletal muscle. *J. Physiol. London* 254: 361–388, 1976.
5. ADRIAN, R. H., AND A. PERES. Charge movement and membrane capacity in frog muscle. *J. Physiol. London* 289: 83–97, 1979.
6. AHMED, K., AND J. J. LEWIS. The influence of drugs which stimulate skeletal muscle and of their antagonist on flux of calcium, potassium and sodium ions. *J. Pharmacol. Exp. Ther.* 136: 298–304, 1962.
7. AHMED, Z., AND J. A. CONNOR. Intracellular pH changes induced by calcium influx during electrical activity in molluscan neurons. *J. Gen. Physiol.* 75: 403–426, 1980.
8. ALMERS, W. Differential effects of tetracaine on delayed potassium channels and displacement currents in frog skeletal muscle. *J. Physiol. London* 262: 613–637, 1976.
9. ALMERS, W. Gating currents and charge movements in excitable membranes. *Rev. Physiol. Biochem. Pharmacol.* 82: 96–190, 1978.
10. ALMERS, W., R. H. ADRIAN, AND S. R. LEVINSON. Some dielectric properties of muscle membrane and their possible importance for excitation-contraction coupling. *Ann. NY Acad. Sci.* 264: 278–292, 1975.
11. ALMERS, W., AND P. M. BEST. Effects of tetracaine on displacement currents and contraction of frog skeletal muscle. *J. Physiol. London* 262: 583–611, 1976.

11a. ALMERS, W., AND P. T. PALADE. Slow calcium and potassium currents across frog muscle membrane: measurements with a Vaseline-gap technique. *J. Physiol. London* 312: 159–176, 1981.

12. ANDERSSON, K. E. Effects of chlorpromazine, imipramine and quinidine on the mechanical activity of single skeletal muscle fibres of the frog. *Acta Physiol. Scand.* 85: 532–546, 1972.
13. ANDERSSON, K. E., AND K. A. P. EDMAN. Effects of lanthanum on the coupling between membrane excitation and contraction of isolated frog muscle fibres. *Acta Physiol. Scand.* 90: 113–123, 1974.
14. ANDERSSON, K. E., AND K. A. P. EDMAN. Effects of lanthanum on potassium contractures of isolated twitch muscle fibres of the frog. *Acta Physiol. Scand.* 90: 124–131, 1974.
15. APRIL, E., P. W. BRANDT, J. P. REUBEN, AND H. GRUNDFEST. Muscle contraction: the effect of ionic strength. *Nature London* 220: 182–184, 1968.
16. ARMSTRONG, C. M., F. M. BEZANILLA, AND P. HOROWICZ. Twitches in the presence of ethylene glycol bis (β-aminoethyl ether)-*N*, *N'*-tetraacetic acid. *Biochim. Biophys. Acta* 267: 605–608, 1972.
17. ASHLEY, C. C., AND E. B. RIDGWAY. On the relationships between membrane potential, calcium transient and tension in single barnacle muscle fibres. *J. Physiol. London* 209: 105–130, 1970.
18. AXELSSON, J., AND S. THESLEFF. Activation of the contractile mechanism in striated muscle. *Acta Physiol. Scand.* 44: 55–66, 1958.
19. BAKER, P. F., AND A. H. V. SCHAPIRA. Anaesthetics increase light emission from aequorin at constant ionized calcium. *Nature London* 284: 168–169, 1980.
20. BARRETT, J. N., AND E. F. BARRET. Excitation-contraction coupling in skeletal muscle: blockade by high extracellular concentrations of calcium buffers. *Science* 200: 1270–1272, 1978.
21. BATRA, S. The effects of zinc and lanthanum on calcium uptake by mitochondrial and fragmented sarcoplasmic reticulum of frog skeletal muscle. *J. Cell. Physiol.* 82: 245–256, 1973.
22. BAYLOR, S. M., W. K. CHANDLER, AND M. W. MARSHALL. Arsenazo III signals in frog muscle (Abstract). *Biophys. J.* 25: 141a, 1979.
23. BAYLOR, S. M., AND H. OETLIKER. A large birefringence signal preceding contraction in single twitch fibres of the frog. *J. Physiol. London* 264: 141–162, 1977.
24. BAYLOR, S. M., AND H. OETLIKER. The optical properties of birefringence signals from single muscle fibres. *J. Physiol. London* 264: 163–198, 1977.
25. BAYLOR, S. M., AND H. OETLIKER. Birefringence signals from surface and T-system membrane of frog single muscle fibres. *J. Physiol. London* 264: 199–213, 1977.
26. BEATY, G. N., AND E. F. STEFANI. Calcium dependent electrical activity in twitch muscle fibres of the frog. *Proc. R. Soc. London Ser. B* 194: 141–150, 1976.
27. BENOIT, P. H., N. CARPENI, AND J. PRYZBYSLAWSKI. Sur la contracture provoqueé par la quinine chez le muscle strié de Grenouille. *J. Physiol. Paris* 56: 289–290, 1964.
28. BEZANILLA, F., C. CAPUTO, AND P. HOROWICZ. Voltage clamp activation of contraction in short striated fibres of the frog. *Acta Cient. Venez.* 22: 72–74, 1971.
29. BEZANILLA, F., C. CAPUTO, AND P. HOROWICZ. Voltage activation of contraction in single fibers of frog striated muscle. *J. Phys. Soc. Jpn.* 34: 1, 1972.
30. BEZANILLA, F., AND P. HOROWICZ. Fluorescence intensity changes associated with contractile activation in frog muscle stained with Nile Blue A. *J. Physiol. London* 246: 709–735, 1975.
31. BIANCHI, C. P. The effect of caffeine on radiocalcium movement in frog sartorius. *J. Gen. Physiol.* 44: 845–858, 1961.
32. BIANCHI, C. P. Kinetics of radiocaffeine uptake and release in frog sartorius. *J. Pharmacol. Exp. Ther.* 138: 41–47, 1962.
33. BIANCHI, C. P. Action on calcium movements in frog sartorius muscles by drugs producing rigor. *J. Cell. Comp. Physiol.* 61: 255–263, 1963.
34. BIANCHI, C. P. Pharmacological actions on excitation-contraction coupling in striated muscle. *Federation Proc.* 27: 126–131, 1968.
35. BIANCHI, C. P., AND T. C. BOLTON. Action of local anesthetics on coupling systems in muscle. *J. Pharmacol. Exp. Ther.* 157: 388–405, 1967.
36. BIANCHI, C. P., AND A. M. SHANES. Calcium influx in skeletal muscle at rest, during activity, and during potassium contracture. *J. Gen. Physiol.* 42: 803–815, 1959.
37. BIRKS, R. I., AND D. F. DAVEY. Osmotic responses demonstrating the extracellular character of the sarcoplasmic reticulum. *J. Physiol. London* 202: 171–188, 1969.
38. BIRKS, R. I., AND D. F. DAVEY. An analysis of volume changes in the T-tubes of frog skeletal muscle exposed to sucrose. *J. Physiol. London* 222: 95–111, 1972.
39. BLINKS, J. R. Influence of osmotic strength on cross section and volume of isolated single muscle fibres. *J. Physiol. London* 177: 42–57, 1965.
40. BLINKS, J. R., F. G. PRENDERGAST, AND D. G. ALLEN. Photoproteins as biological indicators. *Pharmacol. Rev.* 28: 1–93, 1976.
41. BLINKS, J. R., R. RUDEL, AND S. R. TAYLOR. Calcium transients in isolated amphibian skeletal muscle fibres: detection with aequorin. *J. Physiol. London* 277: 291–323, 1978.
42. BLUM, J. J., R. CREESE, D. J. JENDEN, AND N. W. SCHOLES. The mechanism of action of ryanodine on skeletal muscle. *J. Pharmacol. Exp. Ther.* 121: 477–486, 1957.
43. BONDANI, A., AND R. KARLER. Interaction of calcium and local anesthetics with skeletal muscle microsomes. *J. Cell. Physiol.* 75: 199–211, 1970.
44. BORYS, H. K., AND R. KARLER. Effects of caffeine on the intracellular distribution of calcium in frog sartorius muscle. *J. Cell. Physiol.* 78: 387–404, 1971.
45. BRIGGS, F. N., AND M. FLEISHMAN. Calcium binding by particle-free supernatants of homogenates of skeletal muscle. *J. Gen. Physiol.* 49: 131–149, 1965.
46. BRUST, M. Combined effects of nitrate and caffeine on contractions of skeletal muscles. *Am. J. Physiol.* 208: 431–435, 1965.
47. CAPUTO, C. Caffeine- and potassium-induced contractures of frog striated muscle fibers in hypertonic solutions. *J. Gen. Physiol.* 50: 129–139, 1966.
48. CAPUTO, C. The role of calcium on the processes of excitation and contraction in skeletal muscle. *J. Gen. Physiol.* 51: 180–187, 1968.
49. CAPUTO, C. Volume and twitch tension changes in single muscle fibers in hypertonic solutions. *J. Gen. Physiol.* 52: 793–809, 1968.
50. CAPUTO, C. The effect of low temperature on the excitation-contraction coupling phenomena of frog single muscle fibres. *J. Physiol. London* 223: 461–482, 1972.
51. CAPUTO, C. The time course of potassium contractures of single muscle fibres. *J. Physiol. London* 223: 483–505, 1972.
52. CAPUTO, C. The effect of caffeine and tetracaine on the time course of potassium contractures of single muscle fibres. *J. Physiol. London* 255: 191–207, 1976.
52a. CAPUTO, C. Nickel substitution for calcium and the time course of potassium contractures of single muscle fibers. *J. Muscle Res. Cell Motab.* 2: 167–182, 1981.
53. CAPUTO, C., AND P. FERNANDEZ DE BOLAÑOS. Membrane potential, contractile activation and relaxation rates in voltage clamped short muscle fibres of the frog. *J. Physiol. London* 289: 175–189, 1979.
53a. CAPUTO, C., P. DE BOLAÑOS, AND M. E. VELAZ. Effect of barium ions in depolarization contraction coupling. *Biophys. J.* 37: 107a, 1982.
54. CAPUTO, C., AND M. GIMENEZ. Effects of external calcium deprivation on single muscle fibers. *J. Gen. Physiol.* 50: 2177–2195, 1967.
55. CAPUTO, C., J. VERGARA, AND F. BEZANILLA. Local anaesthetics inhibit tension development and Nile Blue fluorescence signals in frog muscle fibres. *Nature London* 277: 401–402, 1979.
56. CARTNILL, J. A., AND C. G. DOS REMEDIOS. Ionic radius specificity of cardiac muscle. *J. Mol. Cell. Cardiol.* 12: 219–223, 1980.

57. CARVALHO, A. P. Effects of potentiators of muscular contraction on binding of cations by sarcoplasmic reticulum. *J. Gen. Physiol.* 51: 427–442, 1968.
58. CHANDLER, W. K., R. F. RAKOWSKI, AND M. F. SCHNEIDER. Effects of glycerol treatment and maintained depolarization on charge movement in skeletal muscle. *J. Physiol. London* 254: 285–316, 1976.
59. CHIARANDINI, D. J., J. P. REUBEN, P. W. BRANDT, AND H. GRUNDFEST. Effects of caffeine on crayfish muscle fibers. I. Activation of contraction and induction of Ca spike electrogenesis. *J. Gen. Physiol.* 55: 640–664, 1970.
60. CHIARANDINI, D. J., J. P. REUBEN, L. GIRARDIER, G. M. KATZ, AND H. GRUNDFEST. Effects of caffeine on crayfish muscle fibers. II. Refractoriness and factors influencing recovery (repriming) of contractile responses. *J. Gen. Physiol.* 55: 665–687, 1970.
61. CHIARANDINI, D. J., J. A. SANCHEZ, AND E. STEFANI. Effect of calcium withdrawal on mechanical threshold in skeletal muscle fibres of the frog. *J. Physiol. London* 303: 153–163, 1980.
62. CHIARANDINI, D. J., AND E. STEFANI. Effects of manganese on the electrical and mechanical properties of frog skeletal muscle fibres. *J. Physiol. London* 232: 129–147, 1973.
63. COHEN, L. B., B. M. SALZBERG, H. V. DAVILA, W. N. ROSS, D. LANDOWNE, A. S. WAGGONER, AND C. H. WANG. Changes in axon fluorescence during activity: molecular probes of membrane potential. *J. Membr. Biol.* 19: 1–36, 1974.
64. COLOMO, F., AND P. ROCCHI. Staircase effect and posttetanic potentiation in frog nerve-single muscle fiber preparation. *Arch. Fisiol.* 64: 189–266, 1965.
65. COSTANTIN, L. L. The effect of calcium on contraction and conductance thresholds in frog skeletal muscle. *J. Physiol. London* 195: 119–132, 1968.
66. COSTANTIN, L. L. Contractile activation in frog skeletal muscle. *J. Gen. Physiol.* 63: 657–674, 1974.
67. COSTANTIN, L. L. Activation in striated muscle. In: *Handbook of Physiology. The Nervous System*, edited by J. M. Brookhart and V. B. Mountcastle. Bethesda, MD: Am. Physiol. Soc., 1977, sect. 1, vol. I, pt. 1, chapt. 7, p. 215–259.
68. COSTANTIN, L. L., C. FRANZINI-ARMSTRONG, AND R. J. PODOLSKY. Localization of calcium-accumulating structures in striated muscle fibers. *Science* 147: 158–160, 1965.
69. COSTANTIN, L. L., AND R. J. PODOLSKY. Calcium localization and the activation of striated muscle fibers. *Federation Proc.* 24: 1141–1145, 1965.
70. COSTANTIN, L. L., AND R. J. PODOLSKY. Evidence for depolarization of the internal membrane system in activation of frog semitendinosus muscle. *Nature London* 210: 483–486, 1966.
71. COSTANTIN, L. L., AND R. J. PODOLSKY. Depolarization of the internal membrane system in the activation of frog skeletal muscle. *J. Gen. Physiol.* 50: 1101–1124, 1967.
72. CURTIS, B. A. Some effects of Ca-free choline Ringer solution on frog skeletal muscle. *J. Physiol. London* 166: 75–86, 1963.
73. CURTIS, B. A. The recovery of contractile ability following a contracture in skeletal muscle. *J. Gen. Physiol.* 47: 953–964, 1964.
74. CURTIS, B. A. Ca fluxes in single twitch muscle fibers. *J. Gen. Physiol.* 50: 255–267, 1966.
75. DEL CASTILLO, J., AND G. ESCOLONA DE MOTTA. A new method for excitation-contraction uncoupling in frog skeletal muscle. *J. Cell Biol.* 78: 782–784, 1978.
76. DESMEDT, J. E., AND K. HAINAUT. Inhibition of the intracellular release of calcium by dantrolene in barnacle giant muscle fibres. *J. Physiol. London* 265: 565–585, 1977.
77. DOMINGUEZ, G., AND O. F. HUTTER. Changes in the action potential of skeletal muscle produced by formaldehyde. *J. Physiol. London* 204: 98P–100P, 1969.
78. DÖRRSCHEIDT-KÄFER, M. The action of Ca^{2+}, Mg^{2+}, and H^{+} on the contraction threshold of frog skeletal muscle. Evidence for surface charges controlling electro-mechanical coupling. *Pfluegers Arch.* 362: 33–41, 1976.
79. DÖRRSCHEIDT-KÄFER, M. Excitation-contraction coupling in frog sartorius and the role of the surface charge due to the carboxyl group of sialic acid. *Pfluegers Arch.* 380: 171–179, 1979.
80. DÖRRSCHEIDT-KÄFER, M. The interaction of ruthenium red with surface charges controlling excitation-contraction coupling in frog sartorius. *Pfluegers Arch.* 380: 181–187, 1979.
80a. DÖRRSCHEIDT-KÄFER, M. Comparison of the action of La^{3+} and Ca^{2+} on contraction threshold and other membrane parameters of frog skeletal muscle. *J. Membr. Biol.* 62: 95–103, 1981.
81. DYDYNSKA, M., AND D. R. WILKIE. The osmotic properties of striated muscle fibres in hypertonic solutions. *J. Physiol. London* 169: 312–329, 1963.
82. EBASHI, S. Excitation-contraction coupling. *Annu. Rev. Physiol.* 38: 293–313, 1976.
83. EBERSTEIN, A., AND A. SANDOW. Fatigue mechanism in muscle fibres. In: *The Effect of Use and Disuse on Neuromuscular Functions.* Prague: Caechoslovak Acad. Sci., 1963, p. 515–526.
84. EDMAN, K. A. P. The effect of zinc and certain other bivalent metal ions on the isometric tension development of glyceral-extracted muscle fibre bundles. *Acta Physiol. Scand.* 43: 275–291, 1958.
85. EDMAN, K. A. P. Depression of mechanical performance by active shortening during twitch and tetanus of muscle fibres. *Acta Physiol. Scand.* 109: 15–26, 1980.
86. EDMAN, K. A. P., AND D. W. GRIEVE. On the role of calcium in the excitation-contraction process of frog sartorius muscle. *J. Physiol. London* 170: 138–152, 1965.
87. EDMAN, K. A. P., AND A. KIESSLING. The time course of the active state in relation to sarcomere length and movement studied in single skeletal muscle fibres of the frog. *Acta Physiol. Scand.* 81: 182–196, 1971.
88. EDWARDS, C., J. M. RITCHIE, AND D. R. WILKIE. The effect of some cations on the active state of muscle. *J. Physiol. London* 133: 412–419, 1956.
89. EISENBERG, B., AND R. S. EISENBERG. Selective disruption of the sarcotubular system in frog sartorius muscle. A quantitative study with exogenous peroxidase as a marker. *J. Cell. Biol.* 39: 451–467, 1968.
89a. EISENBERG, B. R., AND R. S. EISENBERG. The T-SR junction in contracting single skeletal muscle fibers. *J. Gen. Physiol.* 79: 1–19, 1982.
90. EISENBERG, B. R., AND A. GILAI. Structural changes in single muscle of fibers after stimulation at a low frequency. *J. Gen. Physiol.* 74: 1–16, 1979.
91. EISENBERG, R. S., J. N. HOWELL, AND P. C. VAUGHAN. The maintenance of resting potentials in glycerol-treated muscle fibres. *J. Physiol. London* 215: 95–102, 1971.
92. ELLIS, K. O., AND S. H. BRYANT. Excitation-contraction uncoupling in skeletal muscle by dantrolene sodium. *Naunyn-Schmiedeberg's Arch. Pharmacol.* 274: 107–109, 1972.
93. ELLIS, K. O., AND J. F. CARPENTER. Studies on the mechanism of action of dantrolene sodium (a muscle relaxant). *Naunyn-Schmiedeberg's Arch. Pharmacol.* 275: 83–94, 1972.
94. ENDO, M. Calcium induced release of calcium from the sarcoplasmic reticulum of skinned skeletal muscle fibres. *Nature London* 228: 34–36, 1970.
95. ENDO, M. Conditions required for calcium-induced release of calcium from the sarcoplasmic reticulum. *Proc. Jpn. Acad.* 51: 467–472, 1975.
96. ENDO, M. Mechanism of action of caffeine on the sarcoplasmic reticulum of skeletal muscle. *Proc. Jpn. Acad.* 51: 479–484, 1975.
97. ENDO, M. Calcium release from the sarcoplasmic reticulum. *Physiol. Rev.* 57: 71–108, 1977.
98. ETZENSPERGER, J. Modifications du potentiel d'action de la fibre musculaire striée provoquées par la caféine et la quinine. *C. R. Soc. Biol.* 151: 587–590, 1957.
99. ETZENSPERGER, J. Etude des réponses électrique et mécanique de la fibre musculaire striée intoxiquée par la vératrine. Incidences sur le probléme du couplage excitation-contraction. *C. R. Soc. Biol.* 6: 1125–1131, 1962.

100. ETZENSPERGER, J. Effets des anesthésiques locaux sur le potentiel d'action et la secousse de la fibre musculaire squelettique de grenouille. *J. Physiol. Paris* 62: 315–325, 1970.
101. ETZENSPERGER, J., AND Y. BRETONNEAU. Potentiel consécutif et durée de l'état actif de la fibre musculaire striée. Action des ions NO_3^-, Br^- et I^-. *C. R. Soc. Biol.* 150: 1777–1781, 1956.
102. FABIATO, A., AND F. FABIATO. Calcium release from the sarcoplasmic reticulum. *Circ. Res.* 40: 119–129, 1977.
103. FAIRHURST, A. S., AND W. HASSELBACH. Calcium efflux from a heavy sarcotubular fraction. Effects of ryanodine, caffeine and magnesium. *Eur. J. Biochem.* 13: 504–509, 1970.
104. FAIRHURST, A. S., AND D. J. JENDEN. Effect of ryanodine on the calcium uptake system of skeletal muscle. *Proc. Natl. Acad. Sci. USA* 48: 807–813, 1962.
105. FAIRHUST, A. S., AND D. J. JENDEN. The distribution of a ryanodine sensitive calcium pump in skeletal muscle fractions. *J. Cell. Physiol.* 67: 233–238, 1966.
106. FALK, G. Electrical activity of skeletal muscle. In: *Biophysics of Physiological and Pharmacological Actions*, edited by A.M. Shanes. Washington, DC: AAAS, 1961, p. 259–280.
107. FEINSTEIN, M. B. Inhibition of caffeine rigor and radiocalcium movements by local anesthetics in frog sartorius muscle. *J. Gen. Physiol.* 47: 151–172, 1963.
108. FINK, R., AND H. C. LÜTTGAU. An evaluation of the membrane constants and the potassium conductance in metabolically exhausted muscle fibres. *J. Physiol. London* 263: 215–238, 1976.
109. FISCHMAN, D. A., AND R. C. SWAN. Nickel substitution for calcium in excitation-contraction coupling of skeletal muscle. *J. Gen. Physiol.* 50: 1709–1728, 1967.
110. FORD, L. E., AND R. J. PODOLSKY. Regenerative calcium release within muscle cells. *Science* 167: 58–59, 1970.
111. FORD, L. E., AND R. J. PODOLSKY. Calcium uptake and force development by skinned muscle fibres in EGTA buffered solutions. *J. Physiol. London* 223: 1–19, 1972.
112. FORD, L. E., AND R. J. PODOLSKY. Intracellular calcium movements in skinned muscle fibres. *J. Physiol. London* 223: 21–23, 1972.
113. FOULKS, J. G., AND F. A. PERRY. Some effects of organic anions on excitability and excitation-contraction coupling in frog skeletal muscle. *Can. J. Physiol. Pharmacol.* 55: 700–708, 1977.
114. FOULKS, J. G., AND F. A. PERRY. Effects of pH on excitation and contraction in frog twitch muscle. *Can. J. Physiol. Pharmacol.* 55: 709–723, 1977.
115. FOULKS, J. G., AND F. A. PERRY. Increased sensitivity of frog skeletal muscle to procaine in the presence of organic anions. *Can. J. Physiol. Pharmacol.* 56: 739–746, 1978.
116. FOULKS, J. G., F. A. PERRY, AND H. D. SANDERS. Augmentation of caffeine-contracture tension by twitch-potentiating agents in frog toe muscle. *Can. J. Physiol. Pharmacol.* 49: 889–900, 1971.
117. FOULKS, J. G., F. A. PERRY, AND P. TSANG. The influence of pH on the effects of organic anions in frog skeletal muscle. *Can. J. Physiol. Pharmacol.* 55: 1122–1134, 1977.
118. FOZZARD, H. A., AND G. DOMINGUEZ. Effect of formaldehyde and glutaraldehyde on electrical properties of cardiac Purkinje fibers. *J. Gen. Physiol.* 53: 530–540, 1969.
119. FRANK, G. B. Effects of changes in extracellular calcium concentration on the potassium-induced contracture of frog's skeletal muscle. *J. Physiol. London* 151: 518–538, 1960.
120. FRANK, G. B. Utilization of bound calcium in the action of caffeine and certain multivalent cations on skeletal muscle. *J. Physiol. London* 163: 254–268, 1962.
121. FRANKENHAEUSER, B., AND A. L. HODGKIN. The action of calcium on the electrical properties of squid axons. *J. Physiol. London* 137: 218–244, 1956.
122. FRANKENHAUSER, B., AND J. LANNERGREN. The effect of calcium on the mechanical response of single muscle fibres of *Xenopus laevis*. *Acta Physiol. Scand.* 69: 242–254, 1967.
123. FRANZINI-ARMSTRONG, C. Studies of the triad. I. Structure of the junction in frog twitch fibers. *J. Cell Biol.* 47: 488–499, 1970.
124. FRANZINI-ARMSTRONG, C. Membrane particles and transmission at the triad. *Federation Proc.* 34: 1382–1389, 1975.
124a. FRANZINI-ARMSTRONG, C. Structure of sarcoplasmic reticulum. *Federation Proc.* 39: 2403–2409, 1980.
125. FRANZINI-ARMSTRONG, C., J. E. HEUSSER, T. S. REESE, A. P. SOMLYO, AND A. V. SOMYLO. T-tubule swelling in hypertonic solutions: a freeze substitution study. *J. Physiol. London* 283: 133–140, 1978.
126. FRANZINI-ARMSTRONG, C., R. A. VENOSA, AND P. HOROWICZ. Morphology and accessibility of the "transverse" tubular system in frog sartorius muscle after glycerol treatment. *J. Membr. Biol.* 14: 197–212, 1973.
127. FRAZIER, D. T., T. NARAHASHI, AND M. YAMADA. The site of action and active form of local anesthetics. II. Experiments with quaternary compounds. *J. Pharmacol. Exp. Ther.* 171: 45–51, 1970.
128. FUJINO, S., AND M. FUJINO. Removal of the inhibitory effect of hypertonic solutions on the contractility in muscle cells and the excitation-contraction link. *Nature London* 201: 1331–1333, 1964.
129. GAGE, P. W., AND R. S. EISENBERG. Capacitance of the surface and transverse tubular membrane of frog sartorius muscle fibers. *J. Gen. Physiol.* 53: 265–278, 1969.
130. GAGE, P. W., AND R. S. EISENBERG. Action potentials, after potentials, and excitation-contraction coupling in frog sartorius fibers without transverse tubules. *J. Gen. Physiol.* 53: 298–310, 1969.
131. GEFFNER, E. S., S. R. TAYLOR, AND A. SANDOW. Contractures in partially depolarized muscle treated with caffeine or nitrate. *Am. J. Physiol.* 228: 17–22, 1975.
132. GODT, R. E., D. G. ALLEN, AND J. R. BLINKS. Effects of deuterium oxide (D_2O) on calcium transients and myofibrillar responses in frog skeletal muscle (Abstract). *Biophys. J.* 21: 17A, 1978.
133. GONZALEZ-SERRATOS, H. Graded activation of myofibrils and the effect of diameter on tension development during contractures in isolated skeletal muscle fibres. *J. Physiol. London* 253: 321–339, 1975.
134. GORDON, A. M., AND R. E. GODT. Some effects of hypertonic solutions on contraction and excitation-contraction coupling in frog skeletal muscles. *J. Gen. Physiol.* 55: 254–275, 1970.
135. GORDON, A. M., R. E. GODT, S. K. B. DONALDSON, AND C. E. HARRIS. Tension in skinned frog muscle fibers in solutions of varying ionic strength and neutral salt composition. *J. Gen. Physiol.* 62: 550–574, 1973.
136. GRABOWSKY, E. R., A. LOBSIGER, AND H. C. LÜTTGAU. The effect of repetitive stimulation at low frequencies upon the electrical and mechanical activity of single muscle fibres. *Pfluegers Arch.* 334: 222–239, 1972.
137. GUTMANN, E., AND A. SANDOW. Caffeine-induced contracture and potentiation of contraction in normal and denervated rat muscle. *Life Sci.* 4: 1149–1156, 1965.
138. HAMBLY, B. D., AND C. G. DOS REMEDIOS. Responses of skeletal muscle fibres to lanthanide ions. Dependence of the twitch response on ionic radii. *Experientia* 33: 1042–1044, 1977.
139. HANSON, J., AND A. PERSSON. Changes in the action potential and contraction of isolated frog muscle after repetitive stimulation. *Acta Physiol. Scand.* 81: 340–348, 1971.
140. HARVEY, A. M. The actions of quinine on skeletal muscle. *J. Physiol. London* 95: 45–67, 1939.
141. HASLETT, W. L., AND D. J. JENDEN. The influence of temperature on the kinetics of ryanodine contracture. *J. Cell. Comp. Physiol.* 54: 147–153, 1959.
142. HEGNAUER, A. H., W. O. FENN, AND D. M. COBB. The cause of the rise in oxygen consumption of frog muscles in excess potassium. *J. Cell. Comp. Physiol.* 4: 505–526, 1934.
143. HEILBRUNN, L. V. *An Outline of General Physiology* (2nd ed.). Philadelphia, PA: Saunders, 1943.
144. HEILBRUNN, L. V., AND F. WIERCINSKI. The action of various cations on muscle protoplasm. *J. Cell. Comp. Physiol.* 29: 15–32, 1947.

145. Heistracher, P., and C. C. Hunt. The relation of membrane changes to contraction in twitch muscle fibres. *J. Physiol. London* 201: 589–611, 1969.
146. Heistracher, P., and C. C. Hunt. Contractile repriming in snake twitch muscle fibres. *J. Physiol. London* 201: 613–626, 1969.
147. Heistracher, P., and C. C. Hunt. The effect of procaine on snake twitch muscle fibres. *J. Physiol. London* 201: 627–638, 1969.
148. Hellam, D. C., and R. J. Podolsky. Force measurements in skinned muscle fibres. *J. Physiol. London* 200: 807–819, 1969.
149. Hill, A. V. The abrupt transition from rest to activity in muscle. *Proc. R. Soc. London Ser. B* 136: 399–420, 1949.
150. Hill, A. V. On the time required for diffusion and its relation to processes in muscle. *Proc. R. Soc. London* 135: 446–453, 1952.
151. Hill, A. V., and L. MacPherson. The effect of nitrate, iodide and bromide on the duration of the active state in skeletal muscle. *Proc. R. Soc. London Ser. B* 143: 81–102, 1954.
152. Hill, D. K. Tension due to interaction between the sliding filaments in resting striated muscle. The effect of stimulation. *J. Physiol. London* 199: 637–684, 1968.
153. Hille, B. The pH-dependence rate of action of local anesthetics on the node of Ranvier. *J. Gen. Physiol.* 69: 475–496, 1977.
154. Hille, B., and D. T. Campbell. An improved vaseline gap voltage clamp for skeletal muscle fibers. *J. Gen. Physiol.* 67: 265–293, 1976.
155. Hodgkin, A. L., and P. Horowicz. The differential action of hypertonic solutions on the twitch and action potential of a muscle fibre. *J. Physiol. London* 136: 17P–18P, 1957.
156. Hodgkin, A. L., and P. Horowicz. The influence of potassium and chloride ions on the membrane potential of single muscle fibres. *J. Physiol. London* 148: 127–160, 1959.
157. Hodgkin, A. L., and P. Horowicz. Potassium contractures in single muscle fibres. *J. Physiol. London* 153: 386–403, 1960.
158. Hodgkin, A. L., and P. Horowicz. The effect of nitrate and other anions on the mechanical response of single muscle fibres. *J. Physiol. London* 153: 404–412, 1960.
159. Homsher, E., F. N. Briggs, and R. M. Wise. Effects of hypertonicity on resting and contracting frog skeletal muscles. *Am. J. Physiol.* 226: 855–863, 1974.
160. Horowicz, P. The effects of anions on excitable cells. *Pharmacol. Rev.* 16: 193–221, 1964.
161. Howarth, J. V. The behaviour of frog muscle in hypertonic solutions. *J. Physiol. London* 144: 167–175, 1958.
162. Howell, J. N. A lesion of the transverse tubules of skeletal muscle. *J. Physiol. London* 201: 515–533, 1969.
162a. Huang, C. L.-H. Dielectric components of charge movements in skeletal muscle. *J. Physiol. London* 313: 187–205, 1981.
162b. Huang, C. L.-H. Effects of local anesthetics on the relationship between charge movements and contractile thresholds in frog skeletal muscle. *J. Physiol. London* 320: 381–391, 1981.
163. Huddart, H. The effect of quinine on tension development, membrane potentials and excitation-contraction coupling of crab skeletal muscle fibres. *J. Physiol. London* 216: 641–657, 1971.
163a. Hui, C. S. Activation and inactivation properties of two charge species in frog skeletal muscle. *Biophys. J.* 37: 24A, 1982.
164. Hutter, O. F. Potassium conductance of skeletal muscle treated with formaldehyde. *Nature London* 224: 1215–1217, 1969.
165. Hutter, O. F., and D. Noble. The chloride conductance of frog skeletal muscle. *J. Physiol. London* 151: 89–102, 1960.
166. Hutter, O. F., and S. M. Padsha. Effect of nitrate and other anions on the membrane resistance of frog skeletal muscle. *J. Physiol. London* 146: 117–132, 1959.
167. Hutter, O. F., and A. E. Warner. The pH sensitivity of the chloride conductance of frog skeletal muscle. *J. Physiol. London* 189: 403–425, 1967.
168. Hutter, O. F., and T. L. Williams. A dual effect of formaldehyde on the inward rectifying potassium conductance in skeletal muscle. *J. Physiol. London* 286: 591–606, 1979.
169. Huxley, A. F., and R. E. Taylor. Local activation of striated muscle fibres. *J. Physiol. London* 144: 426–441, 1958.
170. Huxley, H. E. Evidence for continuity between the central elements of the triads and extracellular space in frog sartorius muscle. *Nature London* 202: 1967–1971, 1964.
171. Inoue, F., and G. B. Frank. Action of procaine on frog skeletal muscle. *J. Pharmacol. Exp. Ther.* 136: 190–196, 1962.
172. Isaacson, A., K. Jamaji, and A. Sandow. Quinine contractures and ^{45}Ca movements of frog sartorius muscles as affected by pH. *J. Pharmacol. Exp. Ther.* 171: 26–31, 1970.
173. Isaacson, A., and A. Sandow. Effects of zinc on responses of skeletal muscle. *J. Gen. Physiol.* 46: 655–677, 1963.
174. Isaacson, A., and A. Sandow. Quinine and caffeine effects on ^{45}Ca movements in frog sartorius muscle. *J. Gen. Physiol.* 50: 2109–2128, 1967.
175. Ishiko, N., and M. Sato. The effect of calcium ions on electrical properties of striated muscle fibres. *Jpn. J. Physiol.* 7: 51–63, 1957.
176. Jenden, D. J., and A. S. Fairhurst. The pharmacology of ryanodine. *Pharmacol. Rev.* 21: 1–25, 1969.
177. Jenden, D. J., and J. F. Reger. The role of resting potential changes in the contractile failure of frog sartorius muscle during calcium deprivation. *J. Physiol. London* 169: 889–901, 1963.
178. Jenerick, H. Action current of striated muscle in heavy water. *Am. J. Physiol.* 207: 944–946, 1964.
179. Jenerick, H. P., and R. W. Gerard. Membrane potential and threshold of single muscle fibers. *J. Cell. Comp. Physiol.* 42: 79–102, 1953.
180. Josse, M., J. A. Cerf, and G. Hulin. Effects of barium ions on the resting membrane potential of frog striated muscle fibres. *Life Sci.* 4: 77–81, 1965.
181. Kahn, A. J., and A. Sandow. Effects of bromide, nitrate, and iodine on responses of skeletal muscle. *Ann. NY Acad. Sci.* 62: 137–176, 1955.
182. Kaminer, B. Effect of heavy water on different types of muscle and on glycerol-extracted psoas fibres. *Nature London* 185: 172–173, 1960.
183. Kaminer, B., and J. Kimura. Deuterium oxide: inhibition of calcium release in muscle. *Science* 176: 406–407, 1972.
184. Kao, C. Y., and P. R. Stanfield. Actions of some anions on electrical properties and mechanical threshold of frog twitch muscle. *J. Physiol. London* 198: 291–309, 1968.
185. Kao, C. Y., and P. R. Stanfield. Actions of some cations on the electrical properties and mechanical threshold of frog sartorius muscle fibers. *J. Gen. Physiol.* 55: 620–639, 1970.
186. Katz, B. Les constantes electriques de la membrane du muscle. *Arch. Sci. Physiol.* 3: 285–299, 1949.
187. Katz, N. L., A. Ingenito, and L. Procita. Ryanodine induced contractile failure of skeletal muscle. *J. Pharmacol. Exp. Ther.* 171: 242–248, 1970.
188. Kovacs, L., E. Rios, and M. F. Schneider. Calcium transients and intramembrane charge movement in skeletal muscle fibres. *Nature London* 279: 391–396, 1979.
189. Kovacs, L., and M. F. Schneider. Contractile activation by voltage clamp depolarization of cut skeletal muscle fibres. *J. Physiol. London* 277: 483–506, 1978.
190. Krolenko, S. A. Changes in the T-system of muscle fibres under the influence of influx and efflux of glycerol. *Nature London* 221: 969–970, 1969.
191. Krolenko, S. A., and V. V. Fedorov. Recovery of isometric twitches after glycerol removal. *Experientia* 28: 424–425, 1972.
192. Kuffler, S. W. The relation of electrical potential changes to contracture in skeletal muscle. *J. Neurophysiol.* 9: 367–377, 1946.
193. Lammers, W., and J. M. Ritchie. The action of quinine and quinidine on the contractions of striated muscle. *J. Physiol. London* 129: 412–423, 1955.

194. LANGER, G. A. Events at the cardiac sarcolemma: localization and movement of contractile-dependent calcium. *Federation Proc.* 35: 1274–1278, 1967.
195. LANGLEY, J. N. On the contraction of muscle chiefly in relation to the presence of receptive substances. IV. The effect of curari and of some other substances on the nicotine response of the sartorius and gastrocnemius muscles of the frog. *J. Physiol. London* 39: 239–295, 1909.
196. LANNERGREN, J., AND J. NOTH. Tension in isolated frog muscle fibers induced by hypertonic solutions. *J. Gen. Physiol.* 61: 158–175, 1973.
197. LEA, T. J., AND C. C. ASHLEY. Increase in free Ca^{2+} in muscle after exposure to CO_2. *Nature London* 275: 236–238, 1978.
198. LOPEZ, J. R., L. A. WANEK, AND S. R. TAYLOR. Changes of intracellular Ca^{2+} during ECC in isolated muscle fibers treated with zinc (Abstract). *J. Gen. Physiol.* 68: 11a–12a, 1976.
199. LORKOVIĆ, H. The effect of pH on the mechanical activity of the frog toe muscle. *J. Gen. Physiol.* 50: 863–882, 1967.
200. LORKOVIĆ, H. Effects of some divalent cations on frog twitch muscles. *Am. J. Physiol.* 212: 623–628, 1967.
201. LÜTTGAU, H. C. The action of calcium ions on potassium contractures of single muscle fibres. *J. Physiol. London* 168: 679–697, 1963.
202. LÜTTGAU, H. C. The effect of metabolic inhibitors on the fatigue of the action potential in single muscle fibres. *J. Physiol. London* 178: 45–67, 1965.
203. LÜTTGAU, H. C., AND H. OETLIKER. The action of caffeine on the activation of the contractile mechanism in striated muscle fibres. *J. Physiol. London* 194: 51–74, 1968.
204. LÜTTGAU, H. C., AND W. SPIECKER. The effects of Ca deprivation upon mechanical and electrophysiological parameters in skeletal muscle fibres of the frog. *J. Physiol. London* 296: 411–429, 1979.
205. MASHIMA, H., AND M. MATSUMURA. Roles of external ions in the excitation contraction coupling of frog skeletal muscle. *Jpn. J. Physiol.* 12: 639–653, 1962.
206. MASHIMA, H., AND H. WASHIO. The effect of zinc on the electrical properties of membrane and the twitch tension in frog muscle fibres. *Jpn. J. Physiol.* 14: 538–550, 1964.
207. MATHIAS, R. T., R. A. LEVIS, AND R. S. EISENBERG. Electrical models of excitation contraction coupling and charge movement in skeletal muscle. *J. Gen. Physiol.* 76: 1–31, 1980.
208. MATSUMURA, M. Mode of action of caffeine on the twitch potentiation in the frog muscle fibre. *J. Phys. Soc. Jpn.* 29: 170–171, 1967.
209. MATSUSHIMA, T., M. FUJINO, AND T. NAGAI. Effects of anomalous anions on the caffeine contracture. *Jpn. J. Physiol.* 12: 106–112, 1962.
210. McDONALD, V. W., AND F. F. JÖBSIS. Spectrophotometric studies on the pH of frog skeletal muscle. pH change during and after contractile activity. *J. Gen. Physiol.* 68: 178–195, 1976.
211. MILEDI, R., I. PARKER, AND G. SCHALOW. Measurements of calcium transients in frog muscle by the use of arsenazo III. *Proc. R. Soc. London Ser. B* 198: 201–210, 1977.
212. MIYAMOTO, M., AND J. I. HUBBARD. On the inhibition of muscle contraction caused by exposure to hypertonic solutions. *J. Gen. Physiol.* 59: 689–700, 1972.
213. MIYAZAKI, E., H. YABU, AND M. TAKAHASHI. Increasing effect of caffeine on the oxygen consumption of the skeletal muscle. *Jpn. J. Physiol.* 12: 113–123, 1962.
214. MOISESCU, D. G., AND R. THIELECZEK. Calcium and strontium concentration changes within skinned muscle preparations following a change in the external bathing solution. *J. Physiol. London* 275: 241–262, 1978.
215. MOORE, L. E. Anion permeability of frog skeletal muscle. *J. Gen. Physiol.* 54: 33–52, 1969.
216. NAGAI, I., K. OBARA, I. OOTA, AND T. NAGAI. Effect of transverse tubule-disruption on ^{14}C-caffeine influx in frog skeletal muscle. *Jpn. J. Physiol.* 29: 275–281, 1979.
217. NAGAI, I., I. OOTA, AND T. NAGAI. Caffeine contracture in transverse tubules-disrupted fiber and effect of anomalous anions on the contracture in frog twitch fiber. *Jpn. J. Physiol.* 28: 783–798, 1978.
218. NARAHASHI, T., D. T. FRAZIER, AND M. YAMADA. The site of action and active form of local anesthetics. I. Theory and pH experiments with tertiary compounds. *J. Pharmacol. Exp. Ther.* 171: 32–44, 1970.
219. NARAHASHI, T., AND Y. YAMADA. Cationic forms of local anesthetics block action potential from inside the nerve membrane. *Nature London* 223: 748–749, 1969.
220. NASSAR-GENTINA, V., J. V. PASSONNEAU, J. L. VERGARA, AND S. I. RAPOPORT. Metabolic correlates of fatigue and of recovery in single frog muscle fibers. *J. Gen. Physiol.* 72: 593–606, 1978.
221. NATORI, R. Propagated contractions in isolated sarcolemma-free bundle of myofibrils. *Jikeikai Med. J.* 12: 214–221, 1965.
222. NICOLA SIRI, L., J. A. SANCHEZ, AND E. STEFANI. Effect of glycerol treatment on the calcium current of frog skeletal muscle. *J. Physiol. London* 305: 87–96, 1980.
223. NOVOTNY, I., AND F. VYSKOCIL. Possible role of Ca ions in the resting metabolism of frog sartorius muscle during potassium depolarization. *J. Cell. Physiol.* 67: 159–168, 1966.
224. NOVOTNY, K., F. VYSKOCIL, L. VYKLICKY, AND R. BERANEK. Potassium and caffeine induced increase of oxygen consumption in frog muscle and its inhibition by drugs. *Physiol. Bohemoslov.* 11: 277–283, 1962.
225. OETLIKER, H. Studies on the mechanism causing optical excitation-contraction coupling signals in skeletal muscle. *J. Physiol. London* 305: 26P–27P, 1980.
226. OETLIKER, H., AND R. A. SCHÜMPERLI. Birefringence signals and tension development in single frog muscle fibres at short stimulus intervals. *Experientia* 35: 496–498, 1979.
227. OGAWA, Y. Some properties of fragmented frog sarcoplasmic reticulum with particular reference to its response to caffeine. *J. Biochem. Tokyo* 67: 667–683, 1970.
228. OOTA, I., M. TAKAUJI, AND T. NAGAI. Effect of manganese ions on excitation-contraction coupling in frog sartorius muscle. *Jpn. J. Physiol.* 22: 379–392, 1972.
229. PAGALA, M. K. D. Effect of length and caffeine on isometric tetanus relaxation of frog sartorius muscles. *Biochim. Biophys. Acta* 591: 177–186, 1980.
230. PAILLARD, M. Direct intracellular pH measurement in rat and crab muscle. *J. Physiol. London* 223: 297–319, 1972.
232. PARSONS, R. L., AND W. L. NASTUK. Activation of contractile system in depolarized skeletal muscle fibers. *Am. J. Physiol.* 217: 364–369, 1969.
233. PEACHEY, L. D. The sarcoplasmic reticulum and transverse tubules of the frog's sartorius. *J. Cell Biol.* 25: 209–231, 1965.
234. POTREAU, D., AND G. RAYMOND. Slow inward barium current and contraction on frog single muscle fibres. *J. Physiol. London* 303: 91–109, 1980.
235. PUTNEY, J. W. JR., AND C. P. BIANCHI. Site of action of dantrolene in frog sartorius muscle. *J. Pharmacol. Exp. Ther.* 189: 202–212, 1974.
236. RAPOPORT, S. I., L. D. PEACHEY, AND D. A. GOLDSTEIN. Swelling of the transverse tubular system in frog sartorius. *J. Gen. Physiol.* 54: 166–177, 1969.
237. RAYMOND, G., AND D. POTREAU. Barium ions and excitation-contraction coupling of frog single muscle fibres under controlled current and voltage. *J. Physiol. Paris* 73: 617–631, 1977.
238. RITCHIE, J. M. The effect of nitrate on the active state of muscle. *J. Physiol. London* 126: 155–168, 1954.
239. ROME, E. X-ray diffraction studies of the filament lattice of striated muscle in various bathing media. *J. Mol. Biol.* 37: 331–334, 1968.
240. RUDEL, R., AND S. R. TAYLOR. Striated muscle fibers: facilitation of contraction at short lengths by caffeine. *Science* 172: 387–388, 1971.
241. RUDEL, R., AND S. R. TAYLOR. Aequorin luminiscence during contraction of amphibian skeletal muscle. *J. Physiol. London* 233: 5P–6P, 1973.
242. RUSSELL, J. T., T. BEELER, AND A. MARTONOSI. Optical probe

responses on sarcoplasmic reticulum. Oxacarbocyanines. *J. Biol. Chem.* 254: 2040–2046, 1979.

243. RUSSELL, J. T., T. BEELER, AND A. MARTONOSI. Optical probe responses on sarcoplasmic reticulum. Merocyanine and Oxonol dyes. *J. Biol. Chem.* 254: 2047–2053, 1979.
244. SAKAI, T., E. S. GEFFNER, AND A. SANDOW. Caffeine contracture in muscle with disrupted transverse tubules. *Am. J. Physiol.* 220: 712–717, 1970.
245. SAKAI, T., AND S. KURIHARA. A study on rapid cooling contracture from the view point of excitation-contraction coupling. *Jikeikai Med. J.* 21: 47–88, 1974.
246. SAKAI, T., S. KURIHARA, AND T. YOSHIOKA. Action of manganese ions on excitation-contraction coupling of frog skeletal muscle fibres. *Jpn. J. Physiol.* 24: 513–530, 1974.
247. SANCHEZ, J. A., AND E. STEFANI. Inward current in twitch muscle fibres of the frog. *J. Physiol. London* 283: 197–209, 1978.
248. SANDOW, A. Excitation-contraction coupling in muscular response. *Yale J. Biol. Med.* 176: 201, 1952.
249. SANDOW, A. Excitation-contraction coupling in skeletal muscle. *Pharmacol. Rev.* 17: 265–320, 1965.
250. SANDOW, A. Skeletal muscle. *Annu. Rev. Physiol.* 32: 87–138, 1970.
251. SANDOW, A., AND M. BRUST. Caffeine potentiation of twitch tension in frog sartorius muscle. *Biochem. Z.* 345: 232–247, 1966.
252. SANDOW, A., AND A. ISAACSON. Effects of methylene blue, acridine orange and zinc on muscular contraction. *Biochem. Biophys. Res. Commun.* 2: 455–458, 1960.
253. SANDOW, A., AND A. ISAACSON. Topochemical factors in potentiation of contraction by heavy metal cations. *J. Gen. Physiol.* 49: 937–962, 1966.
254. SANDOW, A., M. K. D. PAGALA, AND E. C. SPHICAS. Deuterium oxide effects on excitation-contraction coupling of skeletal muscle. *Biochim. Biophys. Acta* 440: 733–743, 1976.
255. SANDOW, A., S. R. TAYLOR, AND H. PREISER. Role of the action potential in excitation-contraction coupling. *Federation Proc.* 24: 1116–1123, 1965.
256. SCHNEIDER, M. F., AND W. K. CHANDLER. Voltage dependent charge movement in skeletal muscle: a possible step in excitation contraction coupling. *Nature London* 242: 244–246, 1973.
257. SERAYDARIAN, M. W., D. J. JENDEN, AND B. C. ABBOTT. The effect of ryanodine on relaxation of frog sartorius. *J. Pharmacol. Exp. Ther.* 135: 374–381, 1962.
258. SEVCIK, C., AND T. NARAHASHI. Electrical properties and excitation-contraction coupling in skeletal muscle treated with ethylene glycol. *J. Gen. Physiol.* 60: 221–236, 1972.
259. SHANES, A. M., AND C. P. BIANCHI. Radiocalcium release by stimulated and potassium-treated sartorius muscles of the frog. *J. Gen. Physiol.* 43: 481–493, 1960.
260. SHLEVIN, H. H., AND S. R. TAYLOR. Calcium transients in skeletal muscle: effect of hypertonic solutions on aequorin luminiscence (Abstract). *Biophys. J.* 25: 141A, 1979.
261. SOMLYO, A. V. Bridging structures spanning the junctional gap at the triad of skeletal muscle. *J. Cell Biol.* 80: 743–750, 1979.
262. SOMLYO, A. V., H. SHUMAN, AND A. P. SOMLYO. Elemental distribution in striated muscle and the effects of hypertonicity. *J. Cell Biol.* 74: 828–857, 1977.
263. SOMLYO, A. P., A. V. SOMLYO, H. SHUMAN, B. SLOANE, AND A. SCARPA. Electron probe analysis of calcium compartments in cryo sections of smooth and striated muscles. *Ann. NY Acad. Sci.* 307: 523–544, 1978.
264. SPERELAKIS, N., M. F. SCHNEIDER, AND E. J. HARRIS. Decreased K^+ conductance produced by Ba^{++} in frog sartorius fibers. *J. Gen. Physiol.* 50: 1565–1583, 1967.
265. STANFIELD, P. R. The effect of the tetraethylammonium ion on the delayed currents of frog skeletal muscle. *J. Physiol. London* 209: 209–229, 1970.
266. STANFIELD, P. R. The differential effects of tetraethylammonium and zinc ions on the resting conductance of frog skeletal muscle. *J. Physiol. London* 209: 231–256, 1970.
267. STEFANI, E., AND D. J. CHIARANDINI. Skeletal muscle: dependence of potassium contractures on extracellular calcium. *Pfluegers Arch.* 343: 143–150, 1973.
268. STEPHENSON, E. W., AND R. J. PODOLSKY. Regulation by magnesium of intracellular calcium movement in skinned muscle fibers. *J. Gen. Physiol.* 69: 1–16, 1977.
269. STEPHENSON, E. W., AND R. J. PODOLSKY. Influence of magnesium on chloride-induced calcium release in skinned muscle fibers. *J. Gen. Physiol.* 69: 17–35, 1977.
270. TAKAUJI, M., AND T. NAGAI. Effect of dantrolene sodium on the inactivation of excitation-contraction coupling in frog skeletal muscle. *Jpn. J. Physiol.* 27: 743–754, 1977.
271. TAKAUJI, M., N. TAKAHASHI, T. SUZUKI., AND T. NAGAI. Inhibitory action of dantrolene sodium on the activation of excitation-contraction coupling in frog skeletal muscle. *Jpn. J. Physiol.* 27: 731–741, 1977.
272. TAYLOR, R. E. Effect of procaine on electrical properties of squid axon membrane. *Am. J. Physiol.* 196: 1071–1078, 1959.
273. TAYLOR, S. R., J. R. LOPEZ, AND H. H. SHLEVIN. Calcium movement in relation to muscle contraction. *Proc. West. Pharmacol. Soc.* 22: 321–326, 1979.
274. TAYLOR, S. R., H. PREISER, AND A. SANDOW. Mechanical threshold as a factor in excitation-contraction coupling. *J. Gen. Physiol.* 54: 352–368, 1969.
275. TAYLOR, S. R., H. PREISER, AND A. SANDOW. Action potential parameters affecting excitation-contraction coupling. *J. Gen. Physiol.* 59: 421–436, 1972.
276. TAYLOR, S. R., R. RUDEL, AND J. R. BLINKS. Calcium transients in amphibian muscle. *Federation Proc.* 34: 1379–1381, 1975.
277. THESLEFF, S. The mode of neuromuscular block caused by acetylcholine, nicotine, decamethonium and succinylcholine. *Acta Physiol. Scand.* 34: 218–231, 1955.
278. THORENS, S., AND M. ENDO. Calcium-induced calcium release and "depolarization"-induced calcium release: their physiological significance. *Proc. Jpn. Acad.* 51: 473–478, 1975.
279. THORPE, W. R., AND P. SEEMAN. The site of action of caffeine and procaine in skeletal muscle. *J. Pharmacol. Exp. Ther.* 179: 324–330, 1971.
280. TRUBE, G., J. R. LOPEZ, L. A. WANEK, AND S. R. TAYLOR. Effects of the local anesthetic procaine on E-C Coupling in frog skeletal muscle (Abstract). *Federation Proc.* 39: 580a, 1980.
281. ULBRICHT, W. The effect of veratridine on excitable membranes of nerve and muscle. *Rev. Physiol.* 61: 18–71, 1969.
282. VARGA, E., L. KOVACS, AND I. GESZTELYI. Depolarizing effect of veratrine on frog skeletal muscle. *Acta Physiol. Acad. Sci. Hung.* 41: 81–93, 1972.
283. VERGARA, J., AND F. BEZANILLA. Fluorescence changes during electrical activity in frog muscle stained with merocyanine. *Nature London* 259: 684–686, 1976.
284. VERGARA, J., F. BEZANILLA, AND B. M. SALZBERG. Nile blue fluorescence signals from cut single muscle fibers under voltage or current clamp conditions. *J. Gen. Physiol.* 72: 775–800, 1978.
285. WASHIO, H., AND H. MASHIMA. Effects of some anions and cations on the membrane resistance and twitch tension of frog muscle fibre. *Jpn. J. Physiol.* 13: 617–629, 1963.
286. WEBER, A. The mechanism of the action of caffeine on sarcoplasmic reticulum. *J. Gen. Physiol.* 52: 760–772, 1968.
287. WEBER, A., AND R. HERZ. The relationship between caffeine contracture in intact muscle and the effect of caffeine on reticulum. *J. Gen. Physiol.* 52: 750–759, 1968.
288. WEISS, G. B. The effect of potassium on nicotine-induced contracture and Ca^{45} movements in frog sartorius muscle. *J. Pharmacol. Exp. Ther.* 154: 595–604, 1966.
289. WEISS, G. B. The effect of pH on nicotine-induced contracture and Ca^{45} movements in frog sartorius muscle. *J. Pharmacol. Exp. Ther.* 154: 605–612, 1966.
290. WEISS, G. B. On the site of action of lanthanum in frog sartorius muscle. *J. Pharmacol. Exp. Ther.* 174: 517–526, 1970.
291. WETTWER, E., S. HASE, AND H. C. LUTTGAU. The increase in potassium conductance in metabolically poisoned skeletal mus-

cle fibers (Abstract). In: *Proc. Int. Congr. Physiol. Sci., 28th, Budapest, 1980*, vol. 14, p. 3653.
292. WINEGRAD, S. Intracellular calcium movements in excitation-contraction coupling in skeletal muscle. *Federation Proc.* 24: 1146–1152, 1965.
293. WINEGRAD, S. Intracellular calcium movements of frog skeletal muscle during recovery from tetanus. *J. Gen. Physiol.* 51: 65–83, 1968.
294. WINEGRAD, S. The intracellular site of calcium activation of contraction in frog skeletal muscle. *J. Gen. Physiol.* 55: 77–88, 1970.
295. YAGI, S., AND M. ENDO. Effect of deuterium oxide (D_2O) on excitation-contraction coupling of skeletal muscle. *J. Phys. Soc. Jpn.* 38: 298–300, 1976.
296. YAMAGUCHI, T. Caffeine-induced potentiation of twitches in frog single muscle fiber. *Jpn. J. Physiol.* 25: 693–704, 1975.
297. YAMAGUCHI, T., T. MATSUSHIMA, M. FUJINO, AND T. NAGAI. The excitation-contraction coupling of the skeletal muscle and the "glycerol effect." *Jpn. J. Physiol.* 12: 129–142, 1962.
298. ZOETHOUT, W. D. The effects of various salts on the tonicity of skeletal muscles. *Am. J. Physiol.* 10: 211–221, 1904.

CHAPTER 15

Mechanism of Ca^{2+} transport by sarcoplasmic reticulum

ANTHONY N. MARTONOSI
TROY J. BEELER

Department of Biochemistry, State University of New York, Upstate Medical Center, Syracuse, New York

CHAPTER CONTENTS

SINCE THE DISCOVERY of adenosine triphosphate (ATP)-dependent Ca^{2+} uptake of muscle microsomes by Ebashi and Hasselbach about 20 years ago (138, 144, 189), our knowledge of the structure, composition, and function of the sarcoplasmic reticulum (SR) has expanded to such extent that a comprehensive review of the field is no longer practical.

In addition to the growing interest in the physiological role of SR in the regulation of excitation-contraction coupling in skeletal, cardiac, and smooth muscles, SR vesicles represent a nearly ideal model system for the analysis of the structural, kinetic, and thermodynamic requirements of ion translocation across cellular membranes. The impressive advances in these areas stimulated the recognition of the role of Ca^{2+} and Ca^{2+}-transport systems in nerve conduction, vision, hormone secretion, intercellular communication, metabolic regulation, and other cellular functions.

The main topic of this chapter is the mechanism of energy conversion during Ca^{2+} translocation across SR membranes (251). The discussion is based largely on the developments of the last decade.

For other points of view the reader is referred to the following reviews: 36, 42, 58, 64, 94, 122, 139–143, 147, 148, 157, 166, 183, 185–187, 213, 234–236, 245, 307, 332, 337–339, 374–376, 381, 475, 482, 489, 531, 579, 598, 648, 652, and 672.

Important collections of articles dealing with the mechanism of calcium transport have appeared [Carafoli et al. (63), Wasserman et al. (647), Scarpa and Carafoli (515), Mukohata and Packer (429), and Martonosi (381)].

STRUCTURE OF SARCOPLASMIC RETICULUM AND TRANSVERSE TUBULES

During excitation of muscle the depolarization of surface membrane (plasmalemma) spreads into the interior of muscle fiber through the transverse tubules (T tubules) (94, 221). At specialized junctions the action potential of the T tubules triggers the release of calcium from the SR (3, 62, 147, 155, 157, 332). Binding of calcium to the troponin-tropomyosin-actin complex or in certain muscles to the myosin light chain facilitates actin-myosin interaction, with activation of ATP hydrolysis and development of tension (146, 333). During relaxation the surface membrane and T tubules are repolarized. The active uptake of calcium by the SR lowers the cytoplasmic free-Ca^{2+} concentration to 10^{-7} M or below, where the troponin-tropomyosin system inhibits actin-myosin interaction (138–143).

The transmission of excitatory stimulus from the T tubules to the SR occurs at specialized junctions that link the two systems (172). The junctions assume different forms in different types of muscles. In vertebrate skeletal muscle, two elements of SR are connected with one T tubule; this is called the triad (Fig. 1). In myocardium, slow-twitch fibers, or invertebrate muscles, frequently one element of SR forms junctions with a T tubule (diad) or with the plasmalemma (peripheral coupling). The triads, diads, and peripheral couplings are structurally and functionally analogous; their role is to sense the electrical signal arriving through the T tubules and transmit it to the SR. The plasmalemma, T tubules, and SR show unique structural features that are related to their functions.

Structure of Plasmalemma and T Tubules

The surface membranes of muscles of fish, frog (171), chicken (595), and other animals contain particles of 6- to 13-nm diameter, which are visible after freeze fracture. The density of the particles is generally greater on the cytoplasmic than on the external leaflet, and in frog fast-twitch fibers it is estimated to be between 3,000 and 6,000/μm^2 (171). Lower particle densities were observed in the surface membrane of embryonic and adult chicken and adult human muscle (39, 518, 521, 595). In rat, rabbit, and human fast-twitch muscles, some of the particles form characteristic square arrays that are absent in surface membranes of slow-twitch muscles (518). The identification of freeze-fracture particles with the numerous protein components of the surface membrane is likely to be difficult.

The nonjunctional regions of T tubules in fish muscle have no particles in either the cytoplasmic or luminal leaflets. In frog muscle the luminal leaflet contains some particles, whereas the cytoplasmic leaflet is smooth (171). The transition between the particle-rich plasmalemma and the particle-poor T tubules occurs near the mouth of the T tubules, indicating a barrier to the free diffusion of surface membrane particles into the T tubules. The smaller indentations of the surface membrane called caveolae are also particle free.

In the junctional region of the T tubules, the cytoplasmic leaflet contains large (11- to 13-nm diam) particles. These are present in triads (171), diads (170), and peripheral couplings (315) and may have a role in the transmission of excitatory stimulus from the T tubules to the SR. In toadfish swim-bladder muscle, the particles appear in groups of four arranged in two parallel rows located in the same position as the two rows of junctional feet. The average distance between the groups in a row is approximately twice the distance between the feet (172). The functional significance of this arrangement is unknown.

Sarcoplasmic Reticulum

The SR is divided into free, prejunctional, and junctional regions, which differ morphologically and functionally.

FREE SARCOPLASMIC RETICULUM. The principal feature of freeze-fractured free SR is the presence of 85-

FIG. 1. Longitudinal section of toadfish swim-bladder muscle. Four triads are shown. T, T tubule; C, terminal cisternae. *Single arrow* points to a "foot" with a core of low density. *Double arrow,* foot that forms an apparent intermediate line in the junctional gap. Junctional sarcoplasmic reticulum is the portion of the lateral sacs that is located between *arrowheads.* × 110,000. [From Franzini-Armstrong (172).]

Å intramembranous particles, which are more numerous in the cytoplasmic than in the luminal fracture face (102, 342, 459, 595). The asymmetric distribution of the particles is common to all muscles examined so far and presumably reflects the polarity of the Ca^{2+}-transport ATPase within the membrane. The density of 85-Å freeze-etch particles roughly correlates with the Ca^{2+}-transport activity of SR and with the speed of contraction of various muscles (22, 38, 55, 124, 486, 595). Heart and smooth muscle SR have fewer particles than skeletal muscle (124, 486), and more particles were observed in the SR of fast-twitch skeletal muscle than in slow-twitch skeletal muscle (55).

The density of 85-Å freeze-etch particles in fast-twitch skeletal muscles is about 3,000–5,000/μm^2 surface area throughout the nonjunctional SR, which includes most of the lateral sac, the cisternae, the longitudinal tubules, and the fenestrated collar (56, 171). Similar freeze-etch particle densities were observed in SR vesicles isolated from fully developed fast-twitch skeletal muscle (102, 459, 595). The even distribution of Ca^{2+}-transport ATPase throughout the SR is consistent with free lateral diffusion and implies that the various segments of free SR are functionally homogeneous.

Negative staining of isolated SR vesicles with phosphotungstate reveals 40-Å particles on the outer surface that appear to be connected to the membrane with a stalk (232, 371). Similar particles cover the surface of reconstituted ATPase vesicles, which contain the Ca^{2+}-transport ATPase as the only major protein constituent (255, 556). Therefore the 40-Å surface particles presumably represent a portion of Ca^{2+}-transport ATPase molecule, which projects from the cytoplasmic membrane surface into the water phase. The number of 40-Å surface particles visualized by negative staining (15,000–25,000/μm^2), is 4–6 times greater than the number of 85-Å intramembranous particles revealed by freeze-etch electron microscopy (3,000–4,000/μm^2) (255, 378, 510). Two interpretations were proposed to account for the different density of intramembranous and surface particles: *1*) the intramembranous 85-Å particles represent clusters of several (probably 4) ATPase molecules, which appear as individual 40-Å particles after negative staining; and *2*) each 85-Å intramembranous particle corresponds to one ATPase molecule with several polypeptide chain segments projecting into the water phase, which are visible as 40-Å particles.

The ATPase polypeptide chain concentration determined by labeling the active sites with [^{32}P]ATP and by polyacrylamide gel electrophoresis (PAGE) is estimated to be 15,000–25,000/μm^2 surface area, i.e., it is close to the density of 40-Å surface particles. Therefore it is likely that the Ca^{2+}-transport ATPase is present in the membrane in the form of oligomers.

The existence of ATPase oligomers in SR is further supported by the following findings: *1*) the presence of 200,000- to 400,000-dalton oligomers in detergent-solubilized SR observed by ultracentrifugation and exclusion chromatography (263, 323), *2*) fluorescence energy transfer between ATPase molecules in reconstituted membranes (613), *3*) inhibition of Ca^{2+}-ATPase by 1 mol dicyclohexylcarbodiimide per four ATPase molecules (465), and *4*) immobilization of fatty acid spin labels covalently attached to the Ca^{2+}-ATPase (12).

Ultrastructural studies on the Na^+- and K^+-activated ATPase (Na^+-K^+-ATPase) of rabbit kidney, an enzyme closely related to the Ca^{2+}-ATPase (213), also support the oligomeric nature of intramembranous freeze-etch particles (109).

JUNCTIONAL SR. In the vicinity of the triad, the SR membrane changes in structure. In the cytoplasmic leaflet, the 85-Å particles of the Ca^{2+}-transport ATPase are replaced by larger and less densely packed particles. Two rows of pits are usually visible on the luminal surface separated in each row by a distance of about 300 Å. It is reasonable to assume that the large junctional particles are responsible for the pits on the luminal surface (171). Differences in surface particle distribution, which may be related to junctional and free SR, have also been observed by negative staining of isolated SR vesicles (371). The sharp transition between the two types of surface structure implies some barrier to free diffusion between free and junctional SR.

Junction Between T Tubules and SR

The triad junction is formed by the flattened junctional surfaces of a T tubule and the lateral sacs of the SR, which face each other at a distance of 120–140 Å. At intervals of about 300 Å, the SR forms projections (called feet) that connect the SR with the surface of the T tubules (Fig. 1). The feet are attached to the SR in two or more rows on both sides of the T tubule (167–172), as indicated by the following observations: in some muscle fibers feet are present on SR surfaces not covered by T tubules (252, 534, 681), and after disruption of the triad, the feet are still visible on the surface of the isolated SR elements (61). The relationship between the feet and the large intramembranous particles in the junctional regions of the T tubules and SR is not clear.

In addition to the feet or in association with it, a membranous bridge may span the junctional gap, in which the cytoplasmic leaflets of the T tubules and SR membranes are continuous (545). The luminal leaflets of the two membranes appear separate, making direct electrical coupling between the T system and SR during excitation unlikely. Earlier indirect evidence for communication between the lumina of T tubules and the SR may require revision (43).

MECHANISM OF EXCITATION-CONTRACTION COUPLING

The nature of signal transmission at the triad is not established. Several interesting possibilities are under consideration.

1. Voltage-dependent charge movement. An initial step in the coupling process may be a voltage-dependent movement of charge across some part of the surface membrane, presumably the junctional T tubule (3, 78, 220, 483, 519, 520). There is a rough correlation between the magnitude of the charge movement and the number of feet. The charge movement may be a form of gating current related to the opening and closing of Ca^{2+} channels in the junctional region of SR. In this view Ca^{2+} release is localized to the junctional region and propagative depolarization of SR is not required.

2. Conductance channels. According to Mathias et al. (401), the charge movement described by Chandler and co-workers (78, 520) may arise from the transient opening of a low-resistance pathway across the junction between T tubules and SR, with subsequent voltage-dependent increase in the permeability of SR to calcium.

It is usually assumed, without evidence, that the SR membrane is polarized in resting muscle. Although the Ca^{2+} transport through SR is electrogenic (30–32, 682), the generated potential is readily dissipated by compensating ion movements through cation and anion channels in the SR membrane (32, 33). X-ray electron-microprobe studies of ion concentrations in frozen muscle preparations do not indicate the existence of large K^+, Na^+, and Cl^- gradients across the SR membrane (544, 546–548) and therefore argue against significant membrane potential in the SR during rest.

3. Trigger substances. The coupling across the triad junction may involve the release of hypothetical trigger substances from the T tubules (41), which act on a receptor of the junctional SR membrane causing Ca^{2+} release. For example, the small transsarcolemmal influx of Ca^{2+} during action potential may serve as a trigger for Ca^{2+}-induced Ca^{2+} release from SR, with subsequent activation of contractile material (18, 147, 148, 155, 157). Although Ca^{2+}-induced Ca^{2+} release appears feasible in mammalian cardiac muscle (157), it is an unlikely mechanism in skeletal muscle, where twitches can be produced in the absence of extracellular calcium (16, 504, 552). No other trigger substances have been suggested.

For more detailed discussions of the mechanism of excitation-contraction coupling see the chapters by Baylor, Caputo, and R. S. Eisenberg in this *Handbook*.

ISOLATION OF SR, T TUBULES, AND SURFACE MEMBRANE ELEMENTS FROM SKELETAL MUSCLE

Biochemical analysis of excitation-contraction coupling requires the isolation, characterization, and eventual reassembly of the membrane systems involved in the process. Significant advances were made in recent years in all three areas.

Surface membranes of various cells, including muscle, are characterized by relatively high lipid:protein ratio and the presence of cholesterol and Na^+-K^+-ATPase activity. Since the T tubules are extensions of the surface membrane, they are expected to show similar composition. The presence of Na^+-K^+-ATPase in these fractions permits selective labeling with radioactive ouabain.

The SR of mammalian muscles consists of two morphologically distinct parts: the terminal cisterna with its content of electron-dense material and the slender longitudinal tubules with less visible content in their lumen. The membrane envelope of both regions is rich in proteins (primarily Ca^{2+}-ATPase) and contains little or no cholesterol or Na^+-K^+-ATPase.

Using [^{3}H]ouabain as a surface membrane and T-tubule marker, Caswell and his co-workers developed a sucrose-gradient centrifugation procedure that yields enriched fractions of the triads, terminal cisternae, longitudinal tubules, and T tubules (71, 73, 317–319).

Muscles were injected with [^{3}H]ouabain and the microsomal fraction was separated by sucrose-gradient centrifugation into two major bands located at 32% (light) and at 40% sucrose (heavy), respectively. These fractions are similar to those described previously by Meissner et al. (405, 408). The bound ouabain migrated largely in the heavy band with a shoulder at 32% sucrose concentration. It is assumed that the light fraction is derived primarily from the longitudinal tubules, whereas the heavy band contains vesicles of the terminal cisternae and some intact triad junctions (Fig. 2).

The T tubules can be detached from the terminal cisternae by French-press treatment of the heavy band and collected at 22%–25% sucrose concentration. The isolated T-tubule fractions contain elongated vesicles with an average length of 2,000 Å and a width of ≃ 200 Å that are characterized by unique protein and phospholipid composition, high cholesterol content, the presence of Na^+-K^+-ATPase (317–319), Ca^{2+}-transport ATPase (54), β-adrenergic receptors, and isoproterenol-stimulated adenylate cyclase activity (71). The concave fracture faces of the T-tubule vesicles are smooth, in contrast to vesicles derived from SR, which have a high particle density (318). The convex fracture face of T-tubule vesicles displays ridges formed by particle aggregates.

After French-press treatment of the heavy band, sucrose-gradient centrifugation separates the terminal cisternal vesicles into two layers. Vesicles from the lighter region appear empty in electron micrographs and contain, in addition to the Ca^{2+}-ATPase, the 55,000-dalton high-affinity Ca^{2+}-binding protein in relatively large amounts. The terminal cisternal vesicles from the denser region contain electron-dense deposits in their lumen, which are similar to those seen in the terminal cisternae in intact muscle (Fig. 3). The protein content of this fraction is characterized by the presence of the 45,000- and 42,000-dalton Ca^{2+}-binding proteins, in addition to the Ca^{2+}-ATPase.

Labeled T tubules incubated with microsomes or with purified terminal cisternal fractions combine with the terminal cisternae and sediment to the triad region

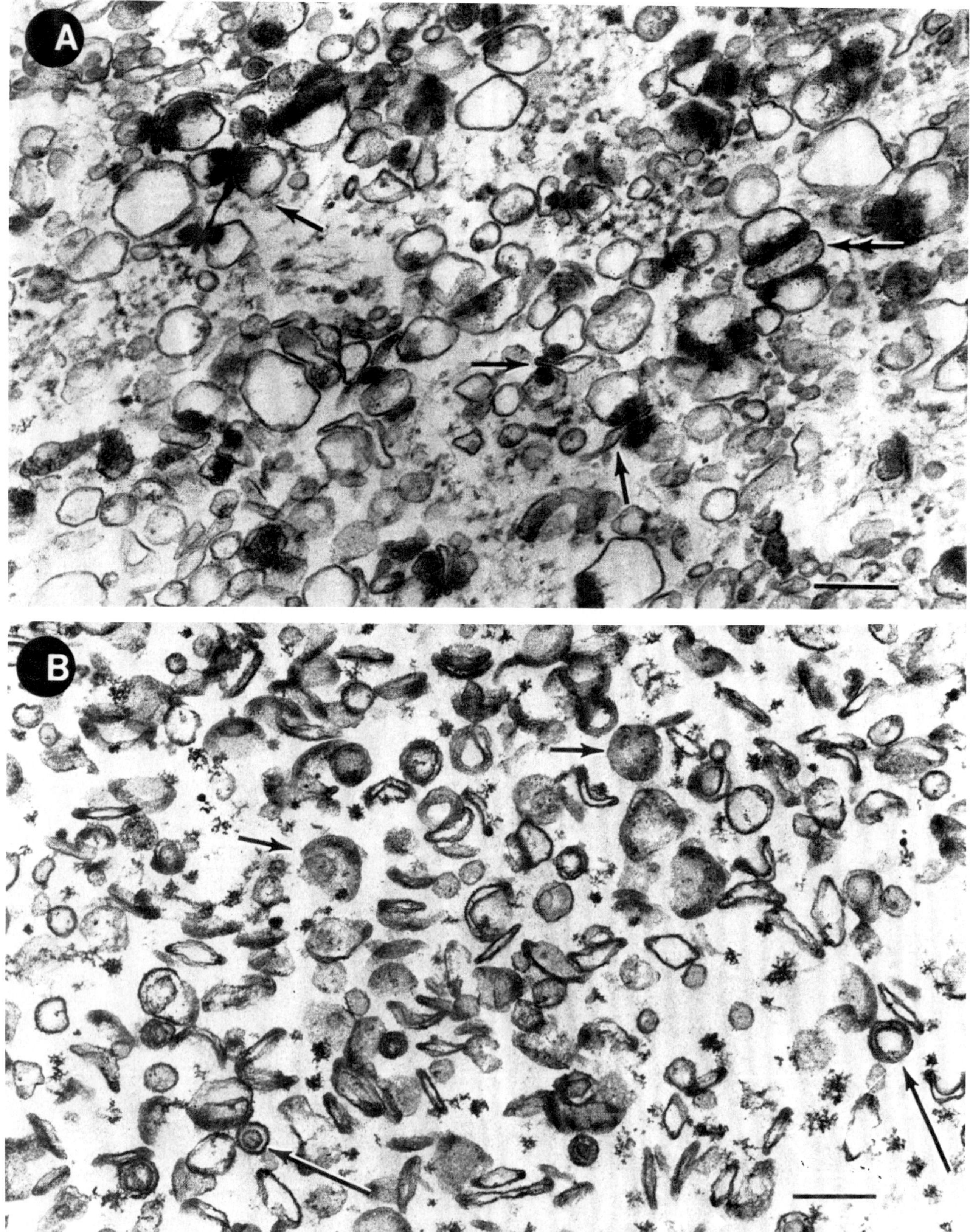

FIG. 2. *A*: heavy microsomal fraction obtained by sucrose-gradient centrifugation at 39%–41% sucrose. *Arrows*, triad junctions; *double arrow*, expanded T tubule. *Bar line*, 250 nm. *B*: ouabain-binding vesicles isolated from the heavy microsomal fraction, shown in *A*, by French-press treatment and sucrose-gradient centrifugation (22%–25% sucrose). *Long arrows*, vesicles with double profiles; *short arrows*, vesicles without clearly defined membranes. [From Lau et al. (317).]

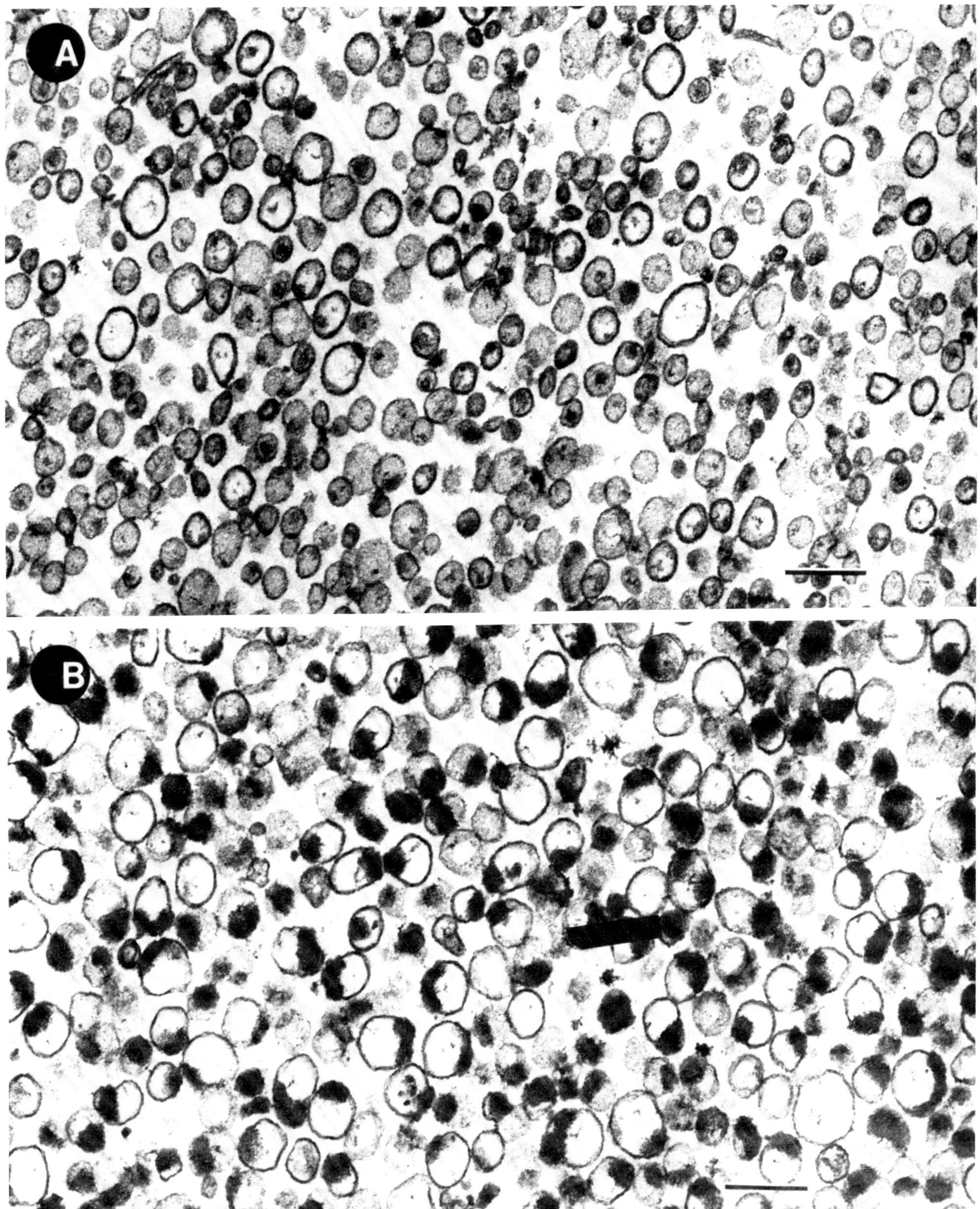

FIG. 3. *A*: terminal cisternae vesicles isolated from the heavy microsomal fraction by French-press treatment and sucrose-gradient centrifugation at 31%–33% sucrose concentration. *Bar*, 250 nm. *B*: terminal cisternae vesicles obtained as above but at 39%–41% sucrose concentration. Note electron-dense content, which is presumed to represent calsequestrin. *Bar*, 250 nm. [From Lau et al. (317).]

of the sucrose gradient (73). No attachment of T tubules to the longitudinal tubules of SR or to mitochondria was observed. The association between T tubules and terminal cisternae is promoted by 0.4–0.6 M K-cacodylate. The reformed junctions are usually diads. As the junctions formed from isolated T tubules and terminal cisternae are similar to natural diads, the surface structures required for this interaction apparently remain attached to the component vesicles.

The number of ouabain-binding sites in isolated T-tubule vesicles is about 37 pmol/mg protein, determined in 0.45% deoxycholate (319). Only about 10% of these sites are available for ouabain binding in "intact" T-tubule vesicles, indicating that the sites are primarily on the inside surface and the membranes are impermeable to ouabain. ATP-dependent accumulation of Na^+ and Cl^- and release of K^+ indicate that the system is capable of generating ion gradients. The Na^+ accumulation was inhibited by monensin or digitoxin but not by valinomycin or ouabain. The difference between digitoxin and ouabain is presumably related to the greater permeation of digitoxin into the intravesicular space. The existence of an ATP-dependent Na pump in isolated T tubules is consistent with earlier suggestions (93, 94) of propagative depolarization of T tubules during muscle contraction.

If isolated T tubules can generate membrane potential and isolated terminal cisternae are capable of accumulating Ca^{2+}, the possibility exists that in isolated or reconstituted triads the depolarization of T tubules can be experimentally linked to Ca^{2+} release.

Separation of Membrane Fractions by Calcium Oxalate or Calcium Phosphate Loading

After loading of crude microsomal fractions with Ca^{2+} in the presence of oxalate or phosphate as Ca^{2+}-precipitating agents, 30%–50% of the vesicles become sufficiently heavy to form pellets under a 20%–50% sucrose gradient (47, 48, 72, 410). The junctional T tubules cosediment with the calcium oxalate–loaded microsomes (72). After repeated calcium oxalate loading, 90%–95% of the vesicles in a crude SR preparation sediment into the pellet (511). The vesicles in the supernatant display the low freeze-fracture particle density commonly observed on the P face of the T tubule in whole muscle. Therefore the fraction was identified as purified T-tubule vesicles. It contained active Ca^{2+}-ATPase but only negligible amounts of Na^+-K^+-ATPase. Since according to Caswell et al. (72) much of the ouabain-binding T tubules sediment with the calcium oxalate–loaded fraction and contain Na^+-K^+ pump (319), the identity of the material obtained in the supernatant by Scales and Sabbadini (511) is uncertain. It may represent enriched free T-tubule vesicles or some other membranes with low particle density.

A preparation enriched in T tubules was obtained from rabbit skeletal muscle by sucrose-gradient centrifugation after removal of SR vesicles by loading them with calcium phosphate (495). These preparations are characterized by 20- to 30-fold enrichment of Mg^{2+}-activated ATPase, high cholesterol, sphingomyelin, and phosphatidylserine content, and unique protein composition. Immunofluorescence staining with antibodies against these membranes is localized at the boundary of the A and I bands, where the T tubules are located (495).

PROTEIN COMPOSITION OF SR

In SR vesicles isolated from rabbit, rat, mouse, chicken, or lobster muscle, the Ca^{2+}-transport ATPase represents 50%–80% of the total protein content. The molecular weight of the ATPase determined by sodium dodecyl sulfate (SDS)–PAGE, ultracentrifugation, and gel filtration ranges between 94,000 and 130,000 (321, 323, 334, 372, 390). The SDS-PAGE of SR yields a relatively simple protein profile with a major component of 100,000 daltons (Fig. 4). The identity of the 100,000-dalton protein with the Ca^{2+}-transport ATPase was established by covalent labeling

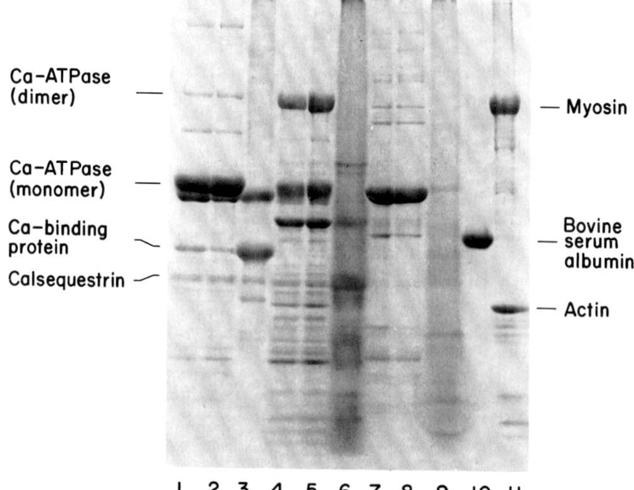

FIG. 4. Protein composition of rabbit, chicken, and lobster sarcoplasmic reticulum. Microsomes were prepared as described in ref. 47. For the removal of surface proteins microsomes were suspended in 0.25 M sucrose, 1 mM EGTA, 20 mM Tris-HCl, 2 mM dithiothreitol, pH 8.0, and 50 μg/ml phenylmethylsulfonylfluoride and incubated at 4°C for 30 min (129). After centrifugation at 145,000 g for 30 min, supernatant was carefully decanted and washing step was repeated. Combined supernatant was precipitated with 10% trichloroacetic acid (TCA) and sediments were neutralized with 0.1 *N* NaOH. Gel electrophoresis (5%–12% gradient gel) was carried out using 20- to 75-μg samples. Samples 1–3, rabbit microsomes; 4–6, chicken microsomes; 7–9, lobster microsomes; 10, bovine serum albumin; 11, rabbit skeletal muscle actomyosin. Samples 1, 4, 7, microsomes before EGTA washing. Samples 2, 5, 8, microsomes after EGTA washing (intrinsic membrane proteins). Samples 3, 6, 9, concentrated EGTA extract (surface proteins). [From Ohnoki and Martonosi (452), © 1980, with permission from Pergamon Press, Ltd.]

of the active site with [^{32}P]ATP or [^{32}P]acetylphosphate (372, 390).

The enzyme is solubilized by various detergents (370), with retention of activity, permitting the isolation of Ca^{2+}-ATPase in a relatively pure form (334). The deoxycholate-solubilized SR or purified ATPase readily reassembles into vesicular structures after removal of detergents, which actively transport Ca^{2+} at the expense of ATP hydrolysis (255, 370, 410, 470, 475, 478, 479, 482).

Fragmented SR membranes and reconstituted vesicles prepared from deoxycholate-solubilized SR (410) contain, in addition to the Ca^{2+}-ATPase, a proteolipid with an estimated molecular weight of 12,000 (344) and a glycoprotein of 53,000 daltons (416). Although there is a fairly constant relationship between the amount of glycoprotein and the amount of ATPase in the membrane, the glycoprotein is readily separated from the Ca^{2+}-ATPase (416), and it is probably not required for ATPase activity and Ca^{2+} transport.

The proteolipid copurified with the Ca^{2+}-ATPase (344). A possible role of proteolipid in Ca^{2+} transport was suggested (471, 472, 480), but its amount is too small in relationship to the Ca^{2+}-ATPase, and purified proteolipid is ineffective in potentiating the Ca^{2+}-transport activity of reconstituted ATPase vesicles.

Membranes of SR contain two water-soluble extrinsic membrane proteins, the calsequestrin and the high-affinity Ca^{2+}-binding protein (Fig. 4). Calsequestrin (mol wt 44,000) is enriched in the heavy microsomal fraction, which originates from the terminal cisternae of SR (317, 405); it may play a role in the sequestration of accumulated Ca^{2+}.

The high-affinity Ca^{2+}-binding protein (mol wt 55,000) is concentrated in the T-tubule fraction, which contains little or no 53,000-dalton glycoprotein (317, 416); its function is unknown.

In addition to these major proteins, SR membranes isolated from rabbit, chicken, and lobster muscle contain a large number of other proteins (452) that presumably represent the usual enzyme components of endoplasmic reticulum. The calsequestrin and the high-affinity Ca^{2+}-binding proteins are absent in lobster SR (Fig. 4), which also contains smaller amounts of the other accessory proteins and a correspondingly larger fraction of Ca^{2+}-ATPase. An 80,000-dalton protein is present frequently in chicken SR [Fig. 4; (452)] that may be identical with the component of embryonic microsomes that is phosphorylated by ATP (376) and the 80,000-dalton protein in cultured muscle cells whose synthesis is promoted by Ca^{2+} ionophores (497). The function of this protein is unknown.

The amino acid composition of the major protein components of rabbit SR is given in Table 1.

Structure of Ca^{2+}-Transport ATPase and Its Disposition in SR Membrane

The lipid:protein weight ratio in SR membranes is 0.5–0.6; this implies that the phospholipid content of the vesicles is sufficient to form a bilayer corresponding to only one-third of the membrane surface area (368). The remaining two-thirds is occupied largely by the polypeptide chains of the Ca^{2+}-transport ATPase.

The disposition of Ca^{2+}-transport ATPase in the membrane is asymmetric, with most of the protein mass exposed on the cytoplasmic surface of SR. This is supported by the following observations.

1. Negative staining by K phosphotungstate reveals 40-Å surface particles on the cytoplasmic surface of

TABLE 1. *Amino Acid Composition of Principal Protein Components of Rabbit Sarcoplasmic Reticulum*

Amino Acid	ATPase		Calsequestrin		54,000-Dalton Protein		Proteolipid	
	g/100 g protein	Residues/mol protein	g/100 g protein	Residues/mol protein	g/100 g protein	Residues/mol protein	g/100 g protein	Residues/mol protein
Lysine	6.47	51	7.53	26	11.75	51	1.25	1.10
Histidine	1.07	8	1.66	6	2.47	10	1.07	0.88
Arginine	8.09	53	2.43	7	3.65	13	13.90	10.00
Aspartic acid	9.67	85	19.40	74	15.12	73	5.25	5.12
Threonine	6.56	65	2.44	11	3.27	18	6.19	6.88
Serine	5.41	62	2.70	14	5.16	33	6.36	8.22
Glutamic acid	14.54	113	21.19	72	21.12	91	12.50	10.88
Proline	4.78	49	4.35	20	5.93	34	1.92	2.22
Glycine	4.35	76	1.87	15	4.62	45	1.46	2.88
Alanine	6.34	90	4.18	26	2.14	28	2.11	3.34
Cysteic acid	2.78	24	0.58	3	0.61	4	2.16	2.88
Valine	8.29	86	6.00	27	4.45	25	5.48	6.22
Methionine	4.09	32	1.70	6	1.18	5	2.33	2.00
Isoleucine	5.48	49	5.18	20	4.07	20	4.03	4.00
Leucine	11.96	108	8.90	35	5.33	26	17.24	17.12
Tyrosine	3.68	23	2.12	6	4.11	14	10.34	7.12
Phenylalanine	6.29	44	7.75	24	5.03	19	6.39	4.88

Source of data: ATPase, MacLennan et al. (342); calsequestrin, MacLennan and Wong (343); 54,000-dalton protein and proteolipid, MacLennan et al. (344). Two forms of calsequestrin isolated by MacLennan (335) differ only slightly in amino acid composition. The 54,000-dalton protein was recently resolved into 2 components by Michalak et al. (416).

microsomes (232, 238, 371). Similar surface particles are visible on reconstituted ATPase vesicles, which contain only the Ca^{2+}-transport ATPase. The number of surface particles is similar to the number of Ca^{2+}-ATPase molecules in the membrane (255, 510). Therefore the 40-Å particles represent a portion of ATPase polypeptide exposed on the cytoplasmic surface. Tryptic digestion of SR reduces the number of visible surface particles, but the Ca^{2+}-stimulated ATPase activity is still retained (371, 502, 557).

2. Freeze-etch electron microscopy reveals 85-Å intramembranous particles that are about 10 times more numerous on the cytoplasmic than on the luminal fracture face (102). The density of 85-Å particles is less than the concentration of ATPase polypeptide chains in the membrane, suggesting that the 85-Å particles are clusters of several (probably four) ATPase molecules (255, 510).

3. Tannic acid fixation. The trilaminar appearance of the membrane observed in thin sections after fixation with glutaraldehyde and 1% tannic acid is highly asymmetric. The outer electron opaque layer is appreciably wider (70 Å) than the inner layer (≃ 20 Å). This asymmetry is abolished by treatment of SR with trypsin, which cleaves the Ca^{2+}-ATPase and alters its distribution in the membrane (164, 502, 639).

4. X-ray–diffraction analysis of oriented multilayers of SR vesicles revealed marked asymmetry of the electron-density profiles (135, 206, 660). In accordance with electron microscopy, we may interpret that a major portion of the Ca^{2+}-ATPase resides on the exterior surface of the membrane with some penetration into the lipid hydrocarbon layer.

5. Reaction with side-specific, nonpenetrating reagents. The electron-dense thiol reagent mercuriazobenzene-ferritin reacts only with the cytoplasmic leaflet of nonvesicular membrane fragments (188), suggesting that essentially all reactive sulfhydryl (SH) groups are on the cytoplasmic surface. Similarly about 70% of the groups reacting with fluorescamine are accessible from the cytoplasmic surface (193, 195).

The Ca^{2+}-Mg^{2+}-ATPase is readily iodinated in sealed vesicles in the presence of free and immobilized lactoperoxidase introduced on the cytoplasmic side (81, 282, 329, 592, 602). The ATPase is digested by trypsin in sealed vesicles (248, 328, 371, 418, 556) and reacts with antibodies on the outer surface of the membrane (137, 389, 557).

By comparison there is little morphological or biochemical evidence relating to the portions of ATPase polypeptide exposed on the luminal surface.

Fragmentation of Ca^{2+}-ATPase With Proteolytic Enzymes

On exposure of SR to trypsin in the presence of 1 M sucrose, the Ca^{2+}-Mg^{2+}-ATPase is cleaved into a 55,000-dalton (A) and a 45,000-dalton (B) fragment (248, 418, 492–494, 556, 592–594). Both fragments remain attached to the membrane with retention of ATPase activity; the fragments are structurally dependent on each other and dissociate only after denaturation (340, 493).

Further digestion of the A fragment yields a 30,000-dalton (A_1) and a 20,000-dalton (A_2) subfragment. The A_1 fragment is assumed to be exposed on the cytoplasmic surface and contains the active-site aspartyl group that is phosphorylated by ATP (557). The A_2 fragment shows ionophoric activity in artificial bilayer membranes with a selectivity sequence of $P_{Ba} > P_{Ca} > P_{Sr} > P_{Mg} > P_{Mn}$ (526, 533). The fragment may represent the ionophoric portion of Ca^{2+}-Mg^{2+}-ATPase, which is partially immersed into the lipid phase of the membrane (531). The relatively hydrophobic 45,000-dalton (B) fragment is a nonselective ionophore at neutral pH (1, 527) when tested in oxidized cholesterol bilayer membranes.

Based on this information, Shamoo and Goldstein (528) proposed a model for calcium transport in which Ca^{2+} binding to the 55,000-dalton (A) portion of the Ca^{2+}-ATPase is followed by the phosphorylation of the active site located in the A_1 segment of the molecule by ATP; the energized system moves calcium through the ion channels contributed by the 20,000- (A_2) and 45,000-dalton (B) segments, followed by the release of Ca^{2+} on the luminal surface.

The hypothesis has an appealing plausibility, but the experimental evidence supporting it is open to several questions.

1. The conductance changes caused by the A_2 fragment are observed at millimolar Ca^{2+} concentrations, whereas the K_m for Ca^{2+} transport is 10^{-7} M. Relatively nonspecific ion leakage induced by millimolar concentrations of divalent cations through conformational changes in the protein may explain this conductance change without a necessary relationship to the postulated role in Ca^{2+} transport.

2. Proteolysis may generate ionophoric polypeptide artifacts, and the corresponding polypeptide segments may not possess ionophoric activity in the intact protein.

3. Whereas the intact ATPase and its proteolytic fragments (A_2 and B) enhance the permeability of bilayer membranes to Ca^{2+}, the selectivity between Ca^{2+} and Mg^{2+} is only twofold (529), in contrast to the 10^6-fold discrimination between Ca^{2+} and Mg^{2+} by the intact enzyme in the absence of ATP.

Clarification of these and other points is required before the specific features of the model can be accepted.

Primary Sequence of Ca^{2+}-Transport ATPase From Rabbit SR

Significant advances were made during the last decade in the analysis of the primary structure of Ca^{2+}-transport ATPase (5–11, 291).

The NH_2-terminal sequence of Ca^{2+}-transport ATPase from rabbit SR is *N*-acetylmethionine-Glu-Ala-Ala-His-Ser-Lys-Ser-Thr-Glx (5, 596, 597). The corresponding COOH-terminal sequence is Ile-Ala-Arg-Asn-Tyr-Leu-Glu-Gly (5, 10). In the Ca^{2+}-transport ATPase of chicken and lobster SR the COOH-terminal amino acids are Ala and Val, respectively (452).

The amino acid sequence in the vicinity of the active-site aspartyl residue is similar to that proposed for the Na^{+}-K^{+}-ATPase: Ile-Cys-Ser-*Asp*-Lys-Thr-Gly (5, 9).

Additional sequences, some of them tentative, have been established for about three-fourths of the molecule (Table 2), excluding the peptides that are aggregated in aqueous solutions (5–11).

TABLE 2. *Partial Amino Acid Sequence of Ca^{2+}-Transport ATPase of Rabbit Sarcoplasmic Reticulum*

Sequence 1 (NH_2-terminal)	X-Met-Glu-Ala-Ala-His-Ser-Lys-Ser-Thr-Glx-Glx-Cys-Leu-Ala-Tyr-Phe-Gly-Val-Ser-Glu -Thr-Thr-Gly-Leu-Thr-Pro-Asp-Gln-Val-Lys-Arg (His, Lys)
Sequence 2	10 20 Ile -Gly -Ile -Phe-Gly -Glu -Asn-Glu -Glu -Val -Ala -Asn -Arg -Ala -Tyr -Thr -Gly -Arg -Glx -Phe 30 40 -Asx -Asx -Leu -Pro -Leu -Ala -Glx -Glx -Arg -Glu -Ala -Cys -Arg -Arg -Ala -Cys -Cys -Phe -Ala -Arg 50 60 -Val -Glx -Pro -Ser -Lys -His -Ser -Lys -Ile -Val -Glx -Tyr -Leu -Glx -Ser -Tyr -Asx -Glx -Ile -Thr 70 80 -Ala -Met(Thr, Gly, Asx, Gly, Val, Asx, Asx, Ala, Pro, Ala) Leu -Lys -Lys -Ala -Glx -Ile -Gly -Ile 90 100 -Ala -Met-Gly -Ser -Gly -Thr -Ala -Val -Ala -Asx -Thr -Ala -Ser -Glx -Met -Val -Leu -Ala -Asx -Asx 110 120 -Asx -Phe -Ser -Thr -Ile -Val -Ala -Ala -Val -Glu -Glu -Gly -Arg -Ala -Ile -Tyr -Asx -Asx -Met -Lys -Glx -Phe
Sequence 3	10 20 Leu -Arg -Asn -Ala -Glu -Asn -Ala -Ile -Glx -Ala -Leu -Lys -Glu -Tyr -Glu -Pro -Glu -Met-Gly -Lys 30 40 -Val -Tyr -Arg -Ala -Asp -Arg -Lys -Ser -Val -Glx -Arg -Ile -Lys -Ala -Arg -Asp -Ile -Val -Pro -Gly 50 60 -Asp -Ile -Val -Glu -Val -Ala -Val -Gly -Asx -Lys -Val -Pro -Ala -Asx -Ile -Arg -Ile -Leu -Ser -Ile 70 80 -Lys -Ser -Thr -Thr -Leu -Arg -Val -Asx -Glx -Ser -Ile -Leu -Thr -Gly -Gln -Ser -Val -Ser -Val -Ile 90 -Lys -His -Thr -Glx -Pro -Val -Pro -Asx (Pro, Gly) Arg -Ala -Val -Asx -Glx -Asx -Lys
Sequence 4	10 20 Met-Ala -Lys -Lys -Asn -Ala -Ile -Val -Arg -Ser -Leu -Pro -Ser -Val -Glu -Thr -Leu -Gly -Cys -Thr 30 40 -Ser -Val -Ile -Cys -Ser -Asp -Lys -Thr -Gly -Thr -Leu -Thr -Thr -Asn -Gln -(Met, Ser, Val, Cys, Lys) 50 60 -Met-Phe -Ile -Ile -Asp -Lys -Val -Asx -Gly -Asx -Phe -Cys -Ser -Leu -Asx -Glx -Phe -Ile -Thr -Gly 70 80 -Ser -Thr -Tyr -Ala -Pro -Glx -Gly -Glx -Val -Leu -(Pro, Lys, Asx, Val, Asx, Asx) Ile -Arg -Ser -Gly 90 100 -Gln -Phe -Asp -Gly -Leu -Val -Glu -Leu -Ala -Thr -Ile -Cys -Ala -Leu -Cys -(Asx -Asx, Ser, Ser) Leu 110 120 -Asp -Phe -Asx -Glx -Thr -Lys -Gly -Val -Tyr -Glu -Lys -Val -Gly -Glx -Ala -Thr -Glx -Thr -Ala -Leu 130 140 -Thr -Thr -Leu -Val -Glx -Lys -Met-Asx -Val -Phe -Asx -Thr -Glx -Val -Arg -Asn -Leu -Ser -Lys -Val 150 160 -Glx -Arg -Ala -Asn -Ala -Cys -Asn -Ser -Val -Ile -Arg -Gln -Leu -Met-Lys -Lys -Glx -Phe -Thr -Leu 170 180 -Glx -Phe -Ser -Arg -Asp -Arg -Lys -Ser -Met -Ser -Val -Tyr -Cys -Ser -Pro -Ala -Lys -Ser -Ser -Arg 190 200 -Ala -Ala -Val -Gly -Asx -Lys -Met-Phe -Val -Lys -Gly -Ala -Pro -Glx -Gly -Val -Ile -Asx -Arg -Cys 210 220 -Asn -Tyr -Val -Arg -Val -Gly -Thr -Thr -Arg -Val -Pro -Met -Thr -Gly -Pro -Val -Lys -Glx -Lys -Ile 230 240 -Leu -Ser -Val -Ile -Lys -Glu -Trp -Gly -Thr -Gly -Arg -Asp -Thr -Leu -Arg -Cys -Leu -Ala -Leu -Ala 250 260 -Thr -Arg -Asn -Thr -Pro -Pro -Lys -Arg -Glx -Glx -Met -Val -Leu -Asx -Asx -Ser -Ser -Arg -Phe -Met
Sequence 5 (COOH-terminal)	Ile-Ala-Arg-Asn-Tyr-Leu-Glu-Gly

Preliminary sequence data on 5 regions of the primary structure of rabbit Ca^{2+}-ATPase are given that include the NH_2-terminal (sequence 1), the active-site aspartyl residue in position 26 (sequence 4), and the COOH-terminal peptide (sequence 5). Details of this work appeared recently (6–8, 11). [From Allen (5), © 1977, with permission from Pergamon Press, Ltd.]

The orientation of the COOH-terminal portion of the molecule with respect to the luminal and cytoplasmic membrane surfaces is unknown, and no information is available about the disposition of polypeptide chains in the lipid phase of the membrane. The following alignment of the major tryptic fragments has been suggested: NH_2-20,000-30,000-45,000-COOH (292). Since the 30 NH_2-terminal amino acids are relatively hydrophilic, the NH_2-terminal segment of the molecule may remain on the cytoplasmic side of the membrane (488). It is likely that the Ca^{2+}-ATPase crosses the membrane several times. The large intrinsic birefringence of SR (558) suggests structural domains arranged perpendicularly to the plane of the membrane, in a manner reminiscent of bacteriorhodopsin (205, 457). These structural domains may represent multiple α-helical segments of the Ca^{2+}-transport ATPase.

Structure of Proteolipids

The proteolipid was isolated from SR by extraction with acidified chloroform-methanol followed by purification either by thin-layer chromatography on Silica Gel-G and column chromatography on Sephadex LH 20 (336, 344) or by butanol extraction (541).

The purified proteolipid has an apparent 6,000 mol wt based on its mobility on SDS-polyacrylamide gels, but the minimum molecular weight from amino acid composition is 12,000 (336). It contains 2 mol covalently bound fatty acids per 12,000 daltons but no phospholipids. The amino acid composition of the proteolipid is relatively hydrophilic (451), and its lipid solubility may be due largely to the bound fatty acids.

The NH_2-terminal amino acid sequence of the proteolipid purified by the butanol extraction procedure is as follows (451): Met-Glx-Arg-Ser-Thr-Arg-Glx-Leu-Cys-Leu-Asp-Phe. The NH_2-terminal region is hydrophilic, and it is presumably exposed on the surface of the membrane. Tyrosine was identified as COOH-terminal amino acid by hydrazinolysis and by carboxypeptidase A digestion (451). The presence of unique NH_2- and COOH-terminal residues indicates that the proteolipid is composed of a single polypeptide chain, and the yield of NH_2- and COOH-terminal amino acids is consistent with the minimum 12,000 mol wt based on amino acid analysis.

The proteolipid is a highly α-helical protein that is distributed largely in the hydrocarbon phase of the membrane (312–314). The proteolipid content of SR is not known with certainty. Based on a yield of 2 mg proteolipid/g microsomal protein (i.e., about 700–800 mg ATPase) and a 12,000 mol wt, the estimate of proteolipid:ATPase molar ratio is 0.02. Therefore it is unlikely that the proteolipid and the ATPase would form stoichiometric complexes in the SR. The suggested role of proteolipid as a Ca^{2+} channel in the ATP-dependent Ca^{2+} uptake (472) seems unlikely, since the purified proteolipid has no influence on the Ca^{2+} transport of reconstituted ATPase vesicles (300). Although some proteolipid fractions had ionophoric activity in egg phosphatidylcholine vesicles, the relationship of this activity to Ca^{2+} transport or release is uncertain (300, 476).

Structure and Distribution of Calsequestrin and High-Affinity Ca^{2+}-Binding Protein in SR

Duggan and Martonosi (129) observed the presence of two extrinsic proteins in SR that were readily extracted with ethylene glycol-bis(β-aminoethyl-ether)-*N,N′*-tetraacetic acid (EGTA) solutions at slightly alkaline pH, whereas the ATPase remained attached to the membrane. MacLennan and his collaborators purified the two proteins and named them calsequestrin and high-affinity Ca^{2+}-binding protein, respectively (334, 336, 338, 339, 341, 343, 344, 455).

CALSEQUESTRIN. Calsequestrin occurs in two distinct molecular forms in rabbit skeletal muscle (335), with apparent molecular weights of 46,500 and 44,000, respectively, based on SDS-PAGE in Weber-Osborne gels (653) and as high as 63,000 in Laemmli gels (311). The variation of apparent molecular weight (226, 390, 408, 416) may in part be related to differences in pH between the two systems. Calsequestrin is a glycoprotein (262, 337) containing two glucosamine and three mannose residues per mole of protein. It is unlikely that the two forms of calsequestrin would arise from incomplete removal of a signal sequence since both have glutamate as the NH_2-terminal amino acid (337).

Calsequestrin is a highly acidic protein that is able to bind about 10 mol Ca/10,000 g with an approximate dissociation constant of 0.5 mM at physiological pH and ionic strength (455, 456). The circular dichroism, absorption, and fluorescence spectrum of both forms of calsequestrin change markedly on binding of cations, indicating a conformational change in the protein (226, 231, 456).

Calsequestrin is preferentially localized in the heavy microsome fraction obtained by sucrose-gradient centrifugation, which is probably derived from the terminal cisternae of SR (317, 405, 506, 512). This localization is consistent with the presence of electron-dense material and Ca^{2+} deposition in the lumen of terminal cisternae in intact muscle (95, 184, 544, 655–657). It is generally accepted that calsequestrin is an extrinsic membrane protein and its attachment to the membrane requires divalent cations (129). The uneven distribution of calsequestrin between the different regions of the SR may indicate that the calsequestrin network is anchored to some structural component of the membrane that is present only in the terminal cisternae.

A long debate is still in progress about the localization of calsequestrin on the internal or external surfaces of SR. An internal localization of calsequestrin within isolated SR vesicles is suggested by its resistance to trypsin (248, 556) and inaccessibility to antibodies (336, 389, 557), ^{125}I-diazotized diiodosulfanilic acid (680), fluorescamine cycloheptaamylose complex (210, 416), ^{35}S-diazotized sulfanilic acid (210), and under special conditions to iodination by Sepharose 4B–bound lactoperoxidase (602).

Iodination of calsequestrin by the lactoperoxidase reaction (81, 282, 329, 592) cannot be used as evidence for external localization because of the possibility of internal labeling by iodide radicals (344, 601). Labeling of calsequestrin by fluorescamine under conditions described by Hasselbach et al. (195) is accompanied by irreversible dissociation of calsequestrin from the membrane, leading to its extensive reaction (210). The release of calsequestrin from SR vesicles on treatment with chelating agents (129) is a slow process and is accompanied by increased permeability of the membrane, which may permit the passage of calsequestrin from the vesicle interior to the external medium.

Based on these considerations, the evidence is in favor of the localization of calsequestrin within the lumen of the SR. As calsequestrin represents about 7% of the protein content of rabbit SR, considering its Ca^{2+} affinity, it accounts for the binding of much of the accumulated Ca^{2+} (339).

The amount of calsequestrin in muscles of different species varies widely, and it is essentially absent in lobster SR (101, 452). Since lobster muscle microsomes have excellent Ca^{2+}-transport capacity (22), the binding of accumulated Ca^{2+} probably involves other Ca^{2+}-binding components. Light microsomes of rabbit skeletal muscle, which contain relatively small amounts of calsequestrin, accumulate Ca^{2+} as well or better than the heavy microsomes with relatively high calsequestrin content (405). These observations suggest that calsequestrin even in rabbit SR may not be the only major Ca^{2+}-binding component (609, 611) and raise the possibility that the principal function of calsequestrin is not the binding of accumulated Ca^{2+}. Varsanyi and Heilmeyer (622) observed a Ca^{2+}-insensitive protein kinase activity in purified calsequestrin preparations that is distinct from phosphorylase kinase.

HIGH-AFFINITY Ca^{2+}-BINDING PROTEIN. The second major acidic protein of SR is the high-affinity Ca^{2+}-binding protein. It has fewer acidic amino acids and about one-half of the Ca^{2+}-binding capacity of calsequestrin (336, 455). The molecular weight of the high-affinity Ca^{2+}-binding protein is 55,000 and in the presence of isotonic KCl binds about 1 mol Ca/mol with a dissociation constant of 3 μM, i.e., similar to that of troponin. The circular dichroism and the ultraviolet spectrum of the high-affinity Ca^{2+}-binding protein do not change upon Ca^{2+} binding (456). In intact SR vesicles the protein is not accessible to proteolytic enzymes and antibodies (344, 556); it does not react with fluorescamine-cycloheptaamylose (416), and no iodination is observed using Sepharose 4B–bound lactoperoxidase as catalyst (602). Therefore the protein is assumed to be localized in the interior of SR. The high-affinity Ca^{2+}-binding protein is released from its binding site after treatment of microsomes with EGTA at slightly alkaline pH, suggesting that divalent cations are required for its interaction with the membrane (129).

The 55,000-dalton band of SR proteins separated by SDS-PAGE also contains a glycoprotein of 53,000 daltons (416) in addition to the high-affinity Ca^{2+}-binding protein. The glycoprotein is nearly absent from the T tubules, whereas the high-affinity Ca^{2+}-binding protein is present both in T tubules and in the SR (416). Neither protein is required for Ca^{2+} transport or Ca^{2+}-dependent ATP hydrolysis, and their function is unknown.

LIPID COMPOSITION OF SR

The lipid composition of skeletal muscle and particularly of SR was discussed in an excellent recent review by Waku (632). Therefore only a brief summary is presented here.

The purified Ca^{2+}-transport ATPase and the SR contain about 0.6 mg lipid/mg protein, corresponding to about 90–100 mol phospholipid/mol Ca^{2+}-transport ATPase. Phospholipids account for about 90% of the total lipid content of SR, the remainder being cholesterol and some triglycerides.

The major phospholipid classes are phosphatidylcholine (53%–66%), phosphatidylethanolamine (17%–24%), phosphatidylinositol (8%–11%), phosphatidylserine (1%–3%), sphingomyelin ($\simeq$5%–10%), and cardiolipin (0.5%–2.5%). The relative amounts of the various lipids in rabbit, rat, chicken, and human muscle SR are given in Table 3 (365). These data are in general agreement with earlier observations from several laboratories (368, 385, 409, 458, 505, 632, 634, 638). The phospholipid composition of the purified Ca^{2+}-transport ATPase is similar to that of the SR [Table 4; (364)].

The fatty acid composition of SR phospholipids is unique compared with surface membranes, mitochondria, and the endoplasmic reticulum of other tissues (Table 5). The major fatty acid component of phosphatidylcholine and phosphatidylethanolamine is palmitate, which together with palmityl aldehyde makes up nearly 40% of the total fatty acid content. Other fatty acids are oleic and linoleic acid (40%), arachidonate (7.5%–10%), and stearate and polyunsaturated acids (3%–5%).

There are considerable differences in the distribution of the alk-1-enyl chains between phosphatidylcholine and phosphatidylethanolamine in the different species. In the rabbit SR, there is a higher proportion of plasmalogens in the phosphatidylethanolamine than in the phosphatidylcholine fraction, while the opposite is true in chicken SR. Rat liver microsomes contain no plasmalogens in phosphatidylcholine and

TABLE 3. *Lipid Content of Sarcotubular Vesicles of Skeletal Muscle of Selected Animal Species*

Lipid Classes	Rabbit	Rat	Chicken	Human
Total lipid	58.8 ± 3.6 (100)	55.4 ± 4.2 (100)	41.5 ± 3.8 (100)	31.4 ± 4.6 (100)
Phospholipid	52.2 ± 2.7 (88.7)	42.3 ± 3.2 (76.4)	30.7 ± 2.6 (74.0)	23.2 ± 3.1 (73.9)
Triglyceride	0.5 ± 0.2 (0.9)	2.3 ± 0.4 (4.1)	1.6 ± 0.5 (3.8)	1.9 ± 0.4 (6.0)
Free sterol	6.1 ± 0.7 (10.4)	10.8 ± 0.6 (19.5)	9.2 ± 0.7 (22.2)	6.3 ± 1.1 (20.1)
Sterol esters	Trace	Trace	Trace	Trace
Free fatty acids	0.5	0.5	0.5	0.5

Values are means of 2 determinations ± SD in milligrams of lipid per 100 mg of protein; numbers in parentheses are percent of total lipids. Total lipids were extracted with chloroform-methanol (2:1). After separation by thin-layer chromatography, neutral lipids and phospholipids were separately measured by gas chromatography of the fatty acid methyl esters with heptadecanoic acid as internal standard. Free sterols were estimated by gas chromatography in relation to tridecanoin as internal standard. [Adapted from Marai and Kuksis (365).]

TABLE 4. *Phospholipid Content of Sarcotubular Vesicles of Skeletal Muscle of Selected Animal Species*

Lipid Classes	Rabbit	Rat	Chicken	Human
Phosphatidylcholine	39.3 ± 2.0 (65.9)	29.0 ± 0.8 (62.1)	22.5 ± 1.6 (58.4)	14.1 ± 1.8 (53.0)
Diacyl	34.7	28.2	16.1	11.5
Alkenyl acyl	4.6	0.8	6.4	2.6
Phosphatidylethanolamine	10.4 ± 0.7 (17.4)	8.6 ± 1.2 (18.4)	7.5 ± 1.0 (19.5)	6.4 ± 1.2 (24.0)
Diacyl	3.2	7.1	6.9	3.3
Alkenyl acyl	7.2	1.5	0.6	3.1
Phosphatidylserine	0.5 ± 0.2 (0.8)	1.3 ± 0.4 (2.8)	0.4 ± 0.2 (1.0)	0.4 ± 0.2 (1.5)
Phosphatidylinositol	6.4 ± 0.4 (10.7)	4.1 ± 0.6 (8.8)	3.8 ± 0.5 (10.0)	2.3 ± 0.6 (8.6)
Sphingomyelin	2.8 ± 1.0 (4.7)	2.6 ± 0.5 (5.6)	3.4 ± 0.7 (8.8)	2.8 ± 0.8 (10.5)
Cardiolipin	0.3 ± 0.5 (0.4)	1.1 ± 0.3 (2.3)	0.9 ± 0.2 (2.3)	0.6 ± 0.2 (2.2)

Values are means of 3 determinations ± SD in micromoles of phospholipid per 100 mg of protein; numbers in parentheses are moles per 100 mols. Various phospholipid classes were isolated by thin-layer chromatography, and their quantities were estimated by gas chromatography of fatty acids and aldehydes with methyl heptadecanoate as internal standard. Diacyl and alkenyl acyl subfractions of the choline and ethanolamine phosphatides were obtained by gas-liquid chromatography of the neutral glyceride moieties isolated by thin-layer chromatography from phospholipase C hydrolysates. [Adapted from Marai and Kuksis (365).]

TABLE 5. *Composition and Positional Distribution of Fatty Acids of Phosphatidylcholines and Phosphatidylethanolamines of Sarcoplasmic Reticulum and Purified ATPase of Rabbit Skeletal Muscle*

	Phosphatidylcholines						Phosphatidylethanolamines					
Fatty Acids	Membrane			ATPase			Membrane			ATPase		
	Total	Pos. 1	Pos. 2	Total	Pos. 1	Pos. 2	Total	Pos. 1	Pos. 2	Total	Pos. 1	Pos. 2
14:0	0.2 ± 0.1	0.4	0.6	0.1 ± 0.1	0.3	0.5		2.3	0.5		2.9	Trace
16:0A	6.3 ± 1.4	10.6		5.4 ± 2.2	10.3		21.0 ± 0.8	44.6		21.4 ± 0.3	44.5	
16:0	34.0 ± 0.9	63.6	5.5	33.9 ± 1.7	64.4	5.5	4.6 ± 0.9	5.1	4.9	2.7 ± 0.3	5.3	2.7
16:1	0.8 ± 0.2	0.4	0.6	0.8 ± 0.1	0.5	1.0	1.4 ± 0.7	1.7	0.6	1.0 ± 0.1	1.8	1.7
18:0A	Trace				Trace		7.0 ± 0.8	13.8		6.9 ± 0.3	14.3	
18:0	3.7 ± 1.1	7.8	0.3	3.5 ± 0.4	7.5	0.7	7.7 ± 0.4	25.7	1.8	7.6 ± 0.7	24.5	4.9
18:1A	ND			ND			6.1 ± 0.7			6.4 ± 0.5		
18:1	16.8 ± 0.6	8.2	26.2	18.6 ± 1.6	8.4	27.0	13.6 ± 0.5	4.9	21.1	12.9 ± 1.9	4.8	22.0
18:2	24.7 ± 2.0	8.0	40.6	25.5 ± 0.4	7.6	41.1	6.0 ± 0.6	1.7	10.9	7.0 ± 0.7	1.2	9.1
20:1	0.6 ± 0.1	0.5	0.5	0.5 ± 0.2	0.5	0.5	0.7 ± 0.5	0.3	0.6	0.9 ± 0.2	0.7	0.9
20:2	0.4 ± 0.1	Trace	0.5	0.2 ± 0.1	Trace	0.6	Trace			Trace		
20:3	1.3 ± 0.2		3.3	1.3 ± 0.4		2.8	0.3 ± 0.1		1.0	0.7 ± 0.1		1.2
20:4	7.5 ± 1.1		14.8	7.3 ± 1.0		13.9	16.0 ± 0.5		26.8	15.8 ± 1.1		30.5
20:5	0.4 ± 0.1		0.1	0.4 ± 0.1		0.1	0.6 ± 0.2		0.9	0.6 ± 0.1		0.9
22:2	0.2 ± 0.1		0.5	0.2 ± 0.1		0.6	0.4 ± 0.2		0.2	0.5 ± 0.2		0.8
22:3	1.2 ± 0.0		2.2	1.2 ± 0.2		2.0	4.9 ± 0.6		9.4	5.6 ± 0.5		9.7
22:4	0.6 ± 0.2		0.8	0.8 ± 0.4		0.9	2.5 ± 0.6		6.1	2.9 ± 0.5		3.8
22:5	1.6 ± 0.1		2.8	1.3 ± 0.2		2.2	5.6 ± 0.7		10.9	5.2 ± 0.7		8.3
22:6	0.3 ± 0.1		0.5	0.3 ± 0.1		0.6	1.7 ± 0.4		3.8	1.7 ± 0.1		3.2

Values are means ± SD in moles per 100 mol. Total and positional composition of fatty acids was determined by gas chromatography of fatty acid methyl esters and dimethylacetals. Composition of the 2-position was obtained from the free fatty acids and composition of the 1-position from composition of the lysophosphatides released by phospholipase A_2. Free fatty acids and lysolecithins were resolved by thin-layer chromatography. Pos. 1, 1-position; Pos. 2, 2-position; ND, not determined. [From Marai and Kuksis (364).]

phosphatidylethanolamine (364). The SR and the purified Ca^{2+}-ATPase contain a small amount of glycolipid of unknown functional significance (375, 447).

The SR phospholipid composition is clearly different from that of the sarcolemma or mitochondria (163). The sarcolemma contains relatively high proportions of phosphatidylserine, sphingomyelin, and cholesterol, while the mitochondria contain more phosphatidylethanolamine and less phosphatidylcholine than SR.

Several key enzymes of lipid biosynthesis were identified in SR membranes. Among these are: acyl-CoA:glycerol-3-phosphate acyltransferase (507, 633); acyl-CoA:acyl *sn*-glycerol-3-phosphate acyltransferase (633); acyl-CoA:2-acyl-*sn*-glycero-3-phosphorylcholine acyltransferase (633); acyl-CoA:1-O-alkyl glycero-3-phosphorylcholine acyltransferase (636); acyl-CoA:1-alkenyl-glycero-3-phosphorylcholine acyltransferase (635). These enzymes play a role in the adjustment of the fatty acid composition of membrane phospholipids during development (507) and in adult animals.

The turnover rate of rat SR phospholipids (391, 637) is much slower than that of rat liver endoplasmic reticulum (454), in keeping with the generally slow rate of lipid biosynthesis in muscle.

Distribution of Phospholipids in Membrane Bilayer

The asymmetric distribution of phospholipids in the outer and inner leaflets of the bilayers of red blood cell membranes, various mammalian plasma membranes, microsomes, and bacterial and viral envelopes has been extensively investigated.

Each of the various techniques used in these studies [side-specific reagents, phospholipases, exchange proteins, and electron spin resonance (ESR) spectroscopy] perturbs the native membrane structure and may produce artifacts. This contributes a degree of uncertainty to the interpretation of most data and should be kept in mind in evaluating the data on SR.

DISTRIBUTION OF PHOSPHATIDYLCHOLINE. The distribution of phosphatidylcholine (110) in SR vesicles was studied by ^{13}C nuclear magnetic resonance (NMR) using the chemical shift reagent Dy^{3+}. Rats were fed a diet containing [*N*-Me_3-^{13}C]choline, leading to the labeling of 30% of the phosphatidylcholine in the SR. Titration of ^{13}C-enriched SR by Dy^{3+} (3 mM) abolished about 40% of the signal, suggesting that 60% of the phosphatidylcholine is in the internal leaflet of the bilayer, shielded from interaction with Dy^{3+}.

Incubation of ^{32}P-labeled SR with mitochondria and the phosphatidylcholine exchange protein results in the transfer of 80% of the [^{32}P]phosphatidylcholine to mitochondria. Since access of the exchange protein to the interior of the vesicles seems unlikely, these results indicate that there is a rapid transbilayer exchange of phosphatidylcholine between the inner and outer leaflet, which may be facilitated by the Ca^{2+}-transport ATPase.

About 42% of the lysophosphatidyl-*N*-[Me-^{13}C]-choline equilibrated with isolated SR vesicles in vitro is also inaccessible to Dy^{3+} and presumed to be located in the inner leaflet of the bilayer. A transbilayer movement of lysophosphatidylcholine is inferred because all lysophosphatidylcholine in the membrane is hydrolyzed by lysophospholipase II added to the external surface within 1 h at 25°C (612).

DISTRIBUTION OF PHOSPHATIDYLETHANOLAMINE. As much as 70%–80% of the phosphatidylethanolamine of rabbit SR is readily available for reaction with the nonpenetrating complex of fluorescamine and cycloheptaamylose (210), indicating that most of the phosphatidylethanolamine is present in the outer leaflet of the bilayer. Similar observations were made with diazotized [^{35}S]sulfanilic acid, trinitrobenzenesulfonate, and fluorodinitrobenzene (210, 608). By the same approaches phosphatidylserine was found to be enriched in the inside leaflet of the bilayer. These conclusions are subject to the assumptions that transbilayer exchange of phosphatidylethanolamine and phosphatidylserine does not take place and the reagents do not disturb the distribution of phospholipids in the membrane.

Reaction of SR vesicles with fluorescamine-cycloheptaamylose in the presence of ATP inhibits active Ca^{2+} translocation without inhibition of ATPase activity (209). The inhibition of Ca^{2+} transport is accompanied by a rapid reaction of phosphatidylethanolamine with the reagent and only a slight labeling of the Ca^{2+}-ATPase. These observations and earlier studies of Racker and his colleagues (296, 297, 299, 473, 481) emphasize the possible role of phosphatidylethanolamine in Ca^{2+} transport.

ROLE OF PHOSPHOLIPIDS IN ATPASE ACTIVITY AND CA^{2+} TRANSPORT

The ATPase and Ca^{2+}-transport activity of SR is absolutely dependent on membrane phospholipids. Depletion of membrane phospholipids by digestion with phospholipase C or A (367–369, 385, 386, 393, 410, 443) inhibits the ATPase activity and Ca^{2+} transport, without major change in the steady-state concentration of phosphoprotein intermediate. The inhibition of ATPase activity is accompanied by immobilization of spin-labeled fatty acids incorporated into the membrane (443, 524). Inhibition of ATPase activity and Ca^{2+} transport was also observed after extraction of membrane phospholipids with cholate or deoxycholate (104, 105, 370, 426, 644, 645).

The inhibited ATPase activity of lipid-depleted vesicles was reactivated after addition of micellar phospholipid dispersions of diverse fatty acid composition

(367, 368, 385). Lysolecithin, unsaturated fatty acids, and neutral or acidic detergents are all effective, indicating that the lipid specificity of the Ca^{2+} transport is rather broad (37, 104, 105, 161, 197, 207, 211, 212, 296, 367, 368, 385, 386, 439, 524, 587, 588, 644–646).

On the other hand the reactivation of Ca^{2+} transport in lipid-depleted vesicles specifically requires phospholipids (385). This is because in addition to the activation of Ca^{2+}-transport ATPase, the restoration of the normal permeability characteristics of the membrane is also important for the retention of accumulated Ca^{2+} (37, 106, 368, 370).

Addition of oleic acid to the lipid-depleted membranes reactivates the ATPase and restores the normal fluidity of the membrane environment as indicated by increased mobility of the fatty acid spin labels (524). These experiments support the assumption that the proper functioning of the Ca^{2+}-transport system depends on a unique arrangement of lipid molecules in the membrane. Whether the lipids required for enzymatic function are present in a bilayer arrangement or specifically interact with the enzyme protein is not known. A direct interaction between lipids and proteins is suggested by the rather polar environment of spin labels in the SR membrane (524) and the interaction of phospholipids with the Ca^{2+}-ATPase even in the presence of excess detergents (104, 105).

Although in most of these experiments nearly complete reactivation of ATPase and Ca^{2+}-transport activities was achieved with phosphatidylcholine alone, under certain conditions optimum Ca^{2+} accumulation may require mixtures of phosphatidylcholine and phosphatidylethanolamine (37, 296, 297, 299, 472, 481).

Boundary Lipids and the Problem of Lipid Annulus

Based on spin-label studies of cytochrome oxidase, Jost et al. (264, 265) proposed that a single layer of protein-bound phospholipid molecules forming an annulus around the protein may be essential for enzymatic activity. The existence of a similar lipid annulus surrounding the Ca^{2+}-transport ATPase of SR was suggested soon afterward by Metcalfe and his collaborators (207, 644–646) based on a set of observations that are now contested.

STOICHIOMETRY OF BOUND PHOSPHOLIPIDS. Native SR vesicles contain about 90–100 mol phospholipids/mol ATPase. Extraction of phospholipids with cholate did not influence the ATPase activity until about 30 mol phospholipids/mol ATPase remained. Further removal of phospholipids resulted in a rapid loss of enzymatic activity, and below 15 mol phospholipid/mol ATPase no significant ATPase activity remained (207, 296, 645). It was proposed that the lipid annulus surrounding the Ca^{2+}-ATPase consists of about 30 mol phospholipid/mol enzyme, and optimum enzymatic activity depends on the presence of a complete lipid annulus.

Although in the experiments of Warren et al. (645) the ATPase activity was relatively constant above 30 mol of phospholipid/mol ATPase, Martonosi et al. (385), Nakamura and Ohnishi (443), and Moore et al. (426) observed an appreciable decrease in enzymatic activity between 100 and 40 mol phospholipids/mol ATPase that is not expected on the basis of the lipid annulus model. A likely interpretation of these observations is that with decreasing lipid:protein ratio the ATPase molecules are progressively squeezed together in the membrane, which may interfere with the conformational changes required for ATPase activity and Ca^{2+} transport. At a lipid:protein ratio of 30 or less these effects may result in the observed dramatic drop of ATPase activity.

PHOSPHOLIPID ANNULUS DOES NOT UNDERGO NORMAL PHASE TRANSITIONS. Reconstituted dipalmitoyl phosphatidylcholine (DPPC)–ATPase vesicles retain significant ATPase activity as low as ~30°C, whereas the phase transition temperature in bilayers of DPPC is 41°C. With 5-deoxylstearate as spin probe, a well-defined phase transition was observed at 41°C in reconstituted ATPase vesicles at high DPPC:ATPase ratios that was absent in complexes containing only 25–30 DPPC molecules/mol ATPase. It was suggested that the phase transition that occurs in the lipid bilayer at 41°C has little influence on the enzymatic activity, whereas the decrease of fluidity of the annulus below 27°C–30°C is accompanied by ATPase inactivation (207).

However, significant changes in the mobility of spin labels were observed between 30°C and 40°C in pure DPPC vesicles, in the absence of proteins (453). Therefore the change in ATPase activity in reconstituted DPPC-ATPase vesicles could reflect such a pretransition change in the fluidity of bulk lipids. In fact there is a reasonable correlation between ATPase activity and the mobility of fluorescent and spin labels that respond to the microviscosity of bulk lipid environment (211, 212, 426, 590, 591).

CHOLESTEROL IS EXCLUDED FROM THE PHOSPHOLIPID ANNULUS. After titration of the Ca^{2+}-transport ATPase with an excess dioleoyl phosphatidylcholine or DPPC containing increasing proportion of cholesterol, the ATPase activity was unaffected by cholesterol even at cholesterol:phospholipid ratios as high as 1 (642, 643). These results seem to indicate that cholesterol is excluded from the lipid annulus. After the lipid annulus was stripped from the Ca^{2+}-ATPase in the presence of high concentrations of cholate, cholesterol apparently interacted with the enzyme, since ATPase activity was inhibited in proportion to the decrease in the amount of bound phospholipids (642, 643).

Recent experiments by Madden et al. (346) using cholesterol-enriched liposomes to modulate the cholesterol content of SR membranes indicate that the ATPase activity varies in proportion with the cholesterol content. Therefore if an annulus exists, cholesterol is apparently not excluded from it, in contrast to the suggestions of Warren et al. (643). Johannsson et al. (256) proposed an alternative interpretation of these data, which is more consistent with the original annulus model.

REACTIVATION OF ATPASE BY DETERGENTS. The ATPase activity of essentially phospholipid-free Ca^{2+}-ATPase can be reactivated using the detergent dodecyl octaethyleneglycol monoether (104, 105). These observations imply that if a lipid annulus is required for ATPase activity, detergents can readily substitute for phospholipids in forming this annulus. These new observations indicate that the physical properties of the bilayer lipids may be more important in the regulation of the ATPase and Ca^{2+}-transport activities of SR than previously realized. Further investigation of the properties and functional significance of the lipid annulus is necessary in the light of these observations.

Rate of ATP Hydrolysis and Physical Properties of the Lipid Phase

The activation of ATP hydrolysis by phospholipids, fatty acids, and detergents implies that the specific chemical structure of the activating lipid is less important in the enzyme activity than the general physical properties of the lipid environment.

Differential scanning calorimetry of SR membranes and extracted SR phospholipids provided the first indication that above 5°C the SR phospholipids are in a liquid crystalline state (377, 397). This conclusion is consistent with more recent X-ray–diffraction and proton NMR studies by Davis et al. (100), which indicate that at 1°C nearly all lipid hydrocarbon chains are in a disordered conformation. As the temperature is raised, the high-resolution NMR signals, indicating isotropic motion, increase in intensity, and at 35°C nearly all phosphatidylcholine-*N*-methyl protons and about 35% of the hydrocarbon-chain protons give high-resolution signals. The Arrhenius plots of ATPase and Ca^{2+}-transport activities parallel the changes in phospholipid molecular motions, suggesting a relationship between the physical state of the membrane lipids and the enzymatic activity. The break in the Arrhenius plot of ATPase activity at 20°C (247) corresponds to half-maximal intensity of the high-resolution signal of the *N*-methyl protons (100). The Arrhenius plots of enzyme activity and the microviscosity of the lipid environment measured by diphenylhexatriene fluorescence fit straight lines between 20°C and 40°C and both give activation energies of 7–9 kcal/mol, supporting the proposition that membrane fluidity is one of the rate-determining factors of enzyme activity (426). Surprisingly, incorporation of cholesterol into SR did not alter the temperature at which the discontinuity of the Arrhenius plots of enzyme activity appears, although it significantly reduced the fluidity of the membrane as measured by diphenylhexatriene fluorescence (347).

It is not possible to tell whether the thermotropic changes in the lipid phase arise from breakdown of lipid clusters (320), changes in fluid-fluid phase separations (664), melting of the lipid annulus surrounding the protein (207), or from a critical change in lipid fluidity due to increased isotropic motion (100).

The discontinuity of the Arrhenius plot of ATPase activity at 20°C may well be a property of the ATPase protein, since incorporation of cholesterol (347) or complete replacement of membrane phospholipids with dodecyl octaethyleneglycol monoether, dioleoyl phosphatidylcholine, or egg yolk phosphatidylcholine left the break at 18°C–20°C unaltered (14, 105). The transition in the temperature dependence of enzyme activity is associated with a change in the rotational motion of the ATPase protein, suggesting either a change in protein conformation or a change in protein-protein interaction around 15°C–20°C (14, 59, 212, 214, 288, 289, 591). Whether this change is an intrinsic response of the protein to temperature or whether it is triggered by changes in the microviscosity of the environment remains unresolved.

A closer insight into the mode of involvement of phospholipids in ATP hydrolysis was obtained by analysis of the elementary reaction steps of ATP hydrolysis using steady-state and rapid kinetic techniques (211, 373, 386, 393, 439).

The hydrolysis of ATP can be represented in the following two consecutive steps

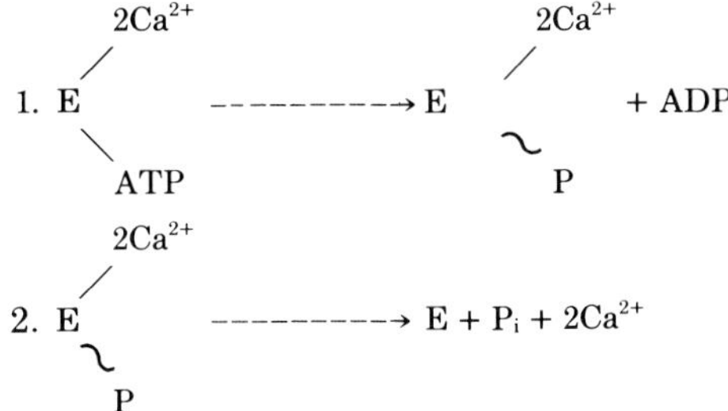

Step 1 is the formation of the aspartylphosphate enzyme intermediate (E~P) from ATP in the presence of Mg^{2+} and Ca^{2+}. The rate of this reaction is 1–2 orders of magnitude greater than the overall rate of ATP hydrolysis. Step 2 combines all reactions leading to the transfer of Ca^{2+} across the membrane and the eventual hydrolysis of the phosphoprotein intermediate. The rate of step 2 is similar to the overall rate of ATP hydrolysis and therefore it includes the rate-limiting step.

Depletion of membrane phospholipids by detergent extraction or by treatment with phospholipase C inhibits ATP hydrolysis without major change in the concentration of phosphoprotein intermediate [(211, 373, 386, 393, 410, 439, 443); see, however, ref. 161]. These observations imply a relatively selective requirement for phospholipids in step 2, the hydrolysis of phosphoprotein (373, 386). Measurement of the rate of formation and decomposition of phosphoprotein

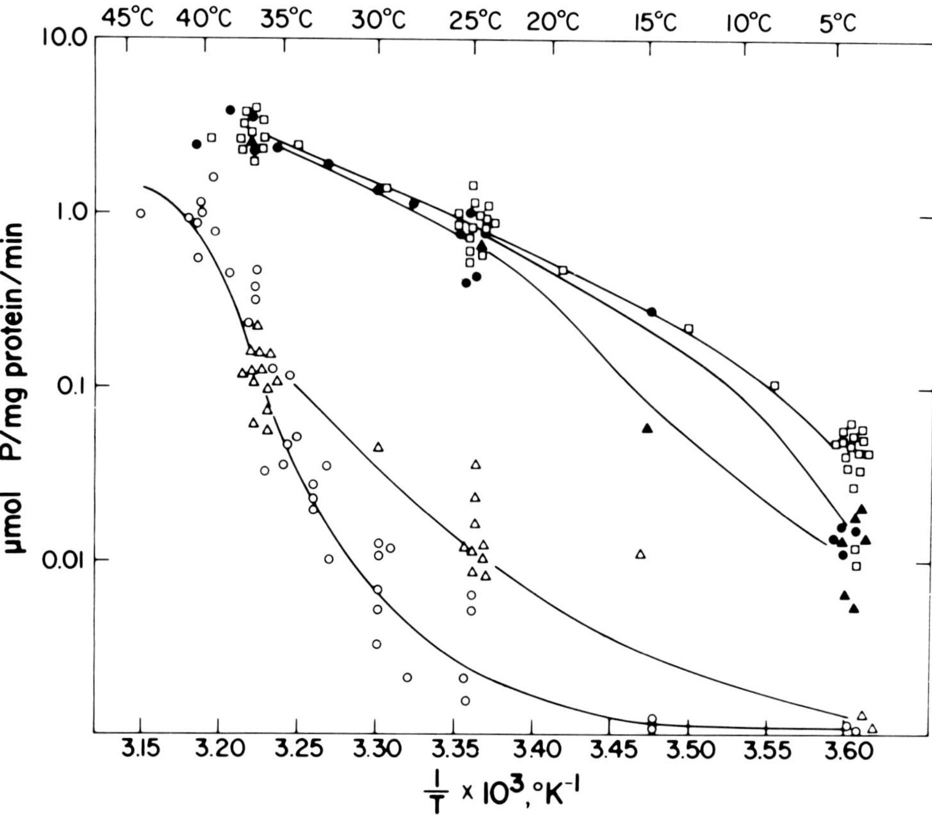

FIG. 5. Temperature dependence of the ATPase activity of microsomes, purified ATPase, and reconstituted vesicles containing dipalmitoyl, dimyristoyl, and dioleoyl lecithin. Enzyme preparations were obtained as described by Nakamura et al. (439). Mixing ratio of protein, phospholipid, and cholate was usually 1:4:1. ATPase activities were measured in a medium of 0.5 m KCl, 10 mM imidazole, 5 mM $MgCl_2$, 5 mM ATP, 0.5 mM EGTA, and 0.45 mM $CaCl_2$. Time of incubation and concentration of enzyme were varied in order to define reaction velocity from the linear portion of the time curve at each temperature. ○—○, Dipalmitoyl lecithin–ATPase; △—△, dimyristoyl lecithin–ATPase; ▲—▲, dioleyl lecithin–ATPase; □—□, microsomes; ●—●, purified ATPase without added lipid. [From Nakamura et al. (439).]

intermediate in native and phospholipase C–treated microsomes by rapid-quenching technique provided direct evidence supporting this conclusion (393). The rate of phosphoprotein hydrolysis in phospholipase C–treated microsomes was 8–10 times slower than in control microsomes, without major change in the rate of phosphoprotein formation (393).

The relationship between the "microviscosity" of the lipid phase and the ATPase activity was further studied on reconstituted ATPase vesicles in which the native phospholipids were exchanged with synthetic dipalmitoyl, dioleoyl, or dimyristoyl phosphatidylcholine (211, 212, 439). Substitution of microsomal phospholipids with DPPC inhibits ATP hydrolysis by decreasing the rate of hydrolysis of phosphoprotein intermediate. Much of the change in the ATPase activity of DPPC-ATPase vesicles occurs in the pretransition temperature range between 30°C and 40°C (Fig. 5), and the ATPase activity reaches control levels below the phase-transition temperature of pure DPPC at 41°C (207, 211, 212, 439, 642, 644). There is a good correlation between ATPase activity and the "microviscosity" of the lipid environment of DPPC-ATPase vesicles, as indicated by the mobility of spin labels and fluorescence probes over a wide range of temperatures (211, 212, 439, 618). The ATPase activity of dioleoyl lecithin–ATPase vesicles is greater than that of DPPC-ATPase vesicles or native SR at 25°C, in accord with the low microviscosity of dioleoyl phosphatidylcholine at this temperature.

Based on these observations the phospholipid requirement of ATP hydrolysis is presumed to be related to the reaction step(s) leading to the hydrolysis of phosphoprotein intermediate (step 2). This step presumably involves a conformational change of the enzyme, which is expected to be sensitive to the "microviscosity" of the lipid environment. It is unfortunate that the precise meaning of "microviscosity" must still be left undefined.

Mobility of Phospholipids and Ca^{2+}-Transport ATPase in SR

The SR membranes are dynamic structures in which the phospholipids (513, 524) and the Ca^{2+}-transport

ATPase molecules (14, 59, 212, 214, 288, 289, 363, 591) move rapidly.

Saturation-transfer ESR measurements with maleimide spin label covalently attached to the Ca^{2+}-transport ATPase yielded a rotational correlation time of 60 μs for the Ca^{2+}-transport ATPase (591). Similar (≃30 μs) rotational correlation time was obtained by Hoffman et al. (214), based on the rate of dichroism decay of a covalently attached triplet probe eosinethiocyanate, and by Bürkli and Cherry (59), using 5-iodoacetamidoeosine. These motions are much faster than the motions required to account for the enzymatic activity, and it is not known to what extent the motion of the probe reflects the segmental motion of the polypeptide chain to which it is attached. The Arrhenius plot for the rotational mobility of the triplet probe (59, 214) indicates two discontinuities at 15°C and at 35°C. Only the discontinuity at 15°C is accompanied by a change in ATPase activity.

Transition was also observed at 15°C by saturation-transfer ESR spectroscopy (289). The discontinuities in the temperature dependence of enzyme mobility were rationalized in terms of conformational changes in the enzyme (289) or a shift in the monomer-oligomer equilibrium of Ca^{2+}-transport ATPase in the temperature range of 15°C–35°C (214). The activation energies for rotational motion and enzymatic activity below 15°C were estimated to be 33.6 and 34 kcal/mol, respectively (214), as compared with 27–30 kcal/mol obtained by Inesi et al. (247).

Substitution of microsomal phospholipids with DPPC decreased the mobility of the short-chain maleimide spin label 4-maleimido 2,2,6,6-tetramethyl piperidinooxyl covalently bound to the Ca^{2+}-ATPase, parallel with inhibition of ATPase activity and a decrease in the fluidity of the lipid phase (211, 212, 440, 441) but without major change in enzyme phosphorylation. These results indicate that after replacement of endogenous lipids by DPPC the protein is in a conformation that permits the phosphorylation of the active site but does not possess the required motional freedom to complete the cycle leading to the hydrolysis of phosphoprotein.

The covalently attached long-chain maleimide spin label 3{[2-(2-maleimidoethoxy-)ethyl] carbamoyl}2,-2,5,5-tetramethyl-1-pyrrolidinyloxyl was less sensitive to changes in the lipid environment (440). If both short- and long-chain maleimide spin labels are attached to the same site on the ATPase, the increase in the distance between the attachment site and the nitroxide group from 9 Å to 14 Å removes the nitroxide from the range of influence of phospholipids. Inclusion of 20%–40% glycerol in the water phase caused a sharp decrease in the amplitude of the weakly immobilized component, supporting this interpretation (441).

The mobility of Ca^{2+}-ATPase is reduced in the presence of 10 mM Ca^{2+} with inhibition of enzyme activity but without a change in the microviscosity of the lipid phase (212, 591). These results suggest that the molecular motion that is essential for phosphoprotein hydrolysis is an intrinsic property of the enzyme protein and can be controlled either by Ca^{2+} or by the associated phospholipids.

In all experiments with fluorescent and spin-labeled ATPase preparations the site of attachment of the probe, its independent mobility, and the relationship between the probe and the active site(s) of the enzyme is unknown. Therefore further work is required before a precise correlation between enzymatic activity and the mobility of certain polypeptide segments of the ATPase is established.

An alternative interpretation of the effects of phospholipid substitution on the temperature dependence of enzyme activity is that replacement of membrane phospholipids with DPPC or exposure of the membranes to low temperature causes a redistribution of the Ca^{2+}-ATPase molecules in the membrane, with the formation of patches of ATPase aggregates. This may be accompanied by inhibition of ATPase activity and a restriction of the mobility of covalently bound spin labels due to protein-protein interactions (440). Clustering of ATPase molecules in artificial membranes was in fact observed by Kleeman and McConnell (290). Until this possibility is excluded, the significance of the relationship between the mobility of ATPase-bound spin labels and the viscosity of lipid microenvironment remains uncertain.

SUMMARY. The studies on the relationship between membrane lipids and the activity of Ca^{2+}-transport ATPase lead to these conclusions. Phospholipids are required for the activity of Ca^{2+}-transport ATPase. This phospholipid requirement is connected with the rate-limiting step of the reaction leading to the hydrolysis of phosphoprotein intermediate. In addition, phospholipids are necessary in the barrier function of the membrane that permits the retention of accumulated Ca^{2+} within the vesicles.

The phospholipid requirement in the enzymatic activity is relatively nonspecific and may be satisfied in addition to phosphatidylcholine by lysophosphatidylcholine, fatty acids, and detergents. The enzymatic activity is influenced by the microviscosity of the lipid environment. The properties of the bulk lipid phase may provide a satisfactory explanation for the correlation between lipid composition and enzymatic activity. The existence and the functional role of the lipid annulus are undergoing reevaluation. The discontinuities in the Arrhenius plots of enzymatic activity and the rotational motion of the Ca^{2+}-transport ATPase cannot be explained entirely by the properties of the bulk lipid phase or the lipid annulus, and temperature-dependent changes in the ATPase protein itself must be invoked. Further studies are required to correlate the information obtained from the motion of spin labels and fluorescence probes covalently linked to the Ca^{2+}-transport ATPase and the assumed motion of polypeptide chains related to Ca^{2+} translocation.

MECHANISM OF ATP HYDROLYSIS AND CA^{2+} TRANSPORT

Introduction of Reaction Sequence

The accumulation of Ca^{2+} by SR is coupled to the hydrolysis of ATP. For each mole of ATP hydrolyzed, usually two Ca^{2+} ions are transferred across the membrane (185–187, 236, 579, 672). The process involves the following elementary reaction steps (122)

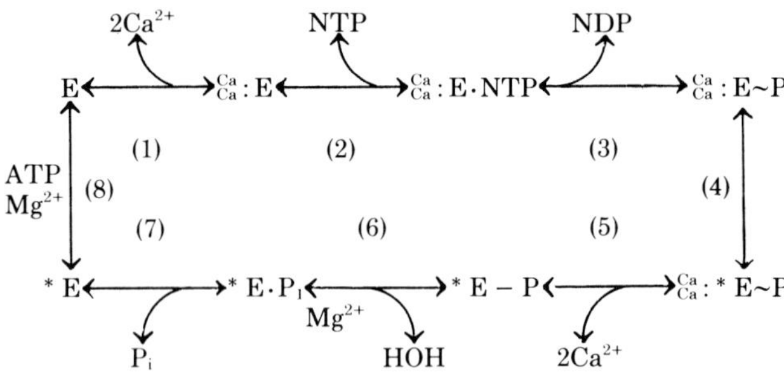

where NTP is nucleoside triphosphate, NDP is nucleoside diphosphate. The interaction of Ca^{2+} and ATP with the Ca^{2+}-transport ATPase is a kinetically random process (272) that leads to the formation of the enzyme-ATP-Ca_2 complex (steps 1–2). Rapid phosphorylation of the enzyme follows (174, 175, 354, 369, 373, 673, 674) and adenosine diphosphate (ADP) is released on the cytoplasmic side (step 3). The formation of phosphoprotein intermediate (E~P-Ca_2) is dependent on Ca^{2+} and is modulated by Mg^{2+}. The relationship between the rate of enzyme phosphorylation and the extravesicular Ca^{2+} concentration is cooperative, with a Hill coefficient close to 2 (87, 175, 272). The maximum steady-state concentration of phosphoprotein intermediate with ATP as substrate is usually close to 0.5 mol/mol ATPase, suggesting "half-of-the-sites" reactivity (175, 378, 393). The phosphate is covalently attached to the enzyme through an active-site aspartyl residue and has the characteristics of an acylphosphate (108).

Kinetic evidence indicates the formation of a series of phosphorylated enzyme intermediates (174, 175, 581, 666, 668, 669) with decreasing Ca^{2+} affinity (step 4), followed by the eventual release of Ca^{2+} (step 5) on the membrane interior (223, 224).

The hydrolysis of the phosphorylated intermediate is promoted by Mg^{2+} (246, 272, 373), requires membrane phospholipids (211, 369, 373, 386, 393, 439, 443), and yields inorganic phosphate (P_i) on the outside surface of the membrane [steps 6–7; (298)]. There is no direct evidence implicating Mg^{2+} as a counterion in Ca^{2+} transport, although such a role seems plausible in view of the kinetic data. In intact SR (30–32) and in reconstituted ATPase vesicles (682) active Ca^{2+} transport generates positive membrane potential, which indicates that the charge compensation is at best partial.

The Ca^{2+} transport is reversible (122, 186, 187) and permits the synthesis of 1 mol ATP from ADP and P_i for each two Ca^{2+} ions released across the membrane. The ATP synthesis is not absolutely dependent on a transmembrane gradient of Ca^{2+} but occurs even in soluble ATPase systems if the conditions are met for converting the energy of substrate binding into the chemical energy of ATP synthesis (122). An excellent analysis of this problem was provided recently by Jencks (251).

The various steps of this reaction sequence are discussed in detail below. The process was extensively reviewed in recent years (122, 186, 187, 236, 251, 579, 672), and therefore the discussion concentrates on recent developments.

Ca^{2+} Binding to SR

The rate of Ca^{2+} uptake by SR in the presence of saturating concentrations of MgATP rises with Ca^{2+} concentration and reaches a maximum at ~1 μM Ca^{2+} (189–191, 360). The K_m of the Ca^{2+}-transport ATPase for Ca^{2+} is in the range of 0.1–0.3 μM (187, 236, 338, 579, 672). Kinetic studies suggest that the reaction of Ca^{2+} and ATP occurs by a random mechanism (272, 404), and for each mole of ATP, two Ca^{2+} ions interact with the Ca^{2+}-ATPase. At Ca^{2+} concentrations exceeding 0.1 mM the rate of ATP hydrolysis is inhibited (649, 650, 652) due to Ca^{2+} binding to low-affinity sites on the Ca^{2+}-ATPase.

Under optimum conditions, SR vesicles are capable of accumulating about 0.15 μmol Ca^{2+}/mg protein against a large electrochemical gradient and lowering the Ca^{2+} concentration of the reaction medium to 10^{-8} M or less (144, 189–191). Much of the accumulated Ca^{2+} is bound to low-affinity sites in the vesicle interior (68, 69, 648–650, 652).

Equilibrium studies of Ca^{2+} binding to SR and to the purified Ca^{2+}-transport ATPase indeed revealed two high-affinity Ca^{2+} sites per mole of Ca^{2+}-ATPase, with a dissociation constant $K = 0.1–4.0$ μM, that bind Ca^{2+} selectively, even in the presence of an excess of Mg^{2+} (79, 88, 162, 222–224, 243, 404, 408).

There are also low-affinity Ca^{2+}-binding sites that bind about 0.10–0.15 μmol Ca^{2+}/mg SR protein (68, 69) and represent contributions from the Ca^{2+}-ATPase (222–224), calsequestrin (343, 455), the high-affinity Ca^{2+}-binding protein (344, 455, 456), and other components of the SR (424).

Binding of Ca^{2+} to Ca^{2+}-Transport ATPase

Ikemoto observed that at 0°C there are three classes of Ca^{2+}-binding sites (α, β, γ) on the Ca^{2+}-transport ATPase (222–224). The association constants (K) and the maximum number of sites (n) in each set are as follows: α-sites ($K = 3 \times 10^6$ M^{-1}, $n = 1$); β-sites ($K = 5 \times 10^4$ M^{-1}, $n = 1$); γ-sites ($K = 10^3$ M^{-1}, $n = 3$). Similar measurements at 22°C gave two α-sites, no β-sites, and three γ-sites per mol ATPase, with affinity constants similar to those observed at 0°C. Binding of

Ca^{2+} to the α-sites was accompanied by activation of ATP hydrolysis and enzyme phosphorylation, while Ca^{2+} binding to the γ-sites inhibited ATPase activity. The β-sites were apparently not involved in the reaction (223). The temperature-dependent increase in the number of α-sites is in accord with the observations of Sumida and Tonomura (564) that the molar ratio of Ca^{2+} transported per mole of ATP hydrolyzed increases from 1 at 0°C to 2 at 22°C.

The high-affinity Ca^{2+}-binding sites are located on the outside surface of the vesicles (424). The relationship between α- and γ-sites is not clear. If during Ca^{2+} translocation across the membrane the affinity of Ca^{2+}-binding sites decreases, leading to Ca^{2+} release (224), some of the Ca^{2+}-binding sites titrated at high Ca^{2+} concentration may arise by conversion of high-affinity (α-) into low-affinity (γ-) sites.

The binding of Ca^{2+} to the high-affinity sites of the Ca^{2+}-ATPase induces a conformational change in the protein that is reflected in increased tryptophan fluorescence (130, 132, 136, 180, 445), changes in ultraviolet absorbance (445), and altered mobility of spin labels covalently attached to the Ca^{2+}-ATPase (76, 83–85, 243, 438).

The conformation change of the protein caused by Ca^{2+} binding is also reflected in altered reactivity of sulfhydryl (SH) groups to *N*-ethylmaleimide (665), 5,5′-dithiobis-(2-nitrobenzoate) (13, 431, 433, 594), 5-mercuric *N*-dansylcysteine (225, 230), and by changes in the reactivity of lysine residues to 2,4,6-trinitrobenzenesulfonate (675, 676) and pyridoxal-5′-phosphate (281).

The relationships among enzyme conformation, Ca^{2+} binding, and the overall process of Ca^{2+} transport are illustrated by the fluorescence changes that follow the interaction of Ca^{2+} with the high-affinity Ca^{2+}-binding sites of the Ca^{2+}-ATPase (136). Addition of Ca^{2+} to SR vesicles increases the tryptophan fluorescence, and the change is reversed after the addition of EGTA. The dependence of fluorescence intensity and ATPase activity on Ca^{2+} concentration are similar and inhibition of ATPase activity with 2-chloromercury-4-nitrophenol inhibited the Ca^{2+}-induced fluorescence response (130, 180). Therefore the Ca^{2+}-induced conformation change may be related to one of the rate-limiting steps of the ATPase reactions. The rate of fluorescence change after addition of calcium to Ca^{2+}-free membranes in the absence of ATP is surprisingly slow (5/s at 22°C) even at saturating (1 μM) Ca^{2+} concentration, suggesting that Ca^{2+} binding is followed by a slow conformation change of the protein leading to the high fluorescence state (${}^{Ca}_{Ca}E$). This transition may be involved in the delay of enzyme phosphorylation by ATP, when ATP and Ca^{2+} are added together to enzyme preincubated with EGTA (243, 485, 565).

The decrease of fluorescence intensity that follows the release of Ca^{2+} from the high-affinity binding site of the enzyme in the presence of EGTA is faster (15–30/s at 22°C). This transition may explain the brief lag phase in enzyme phosphorylation by P_i in the presence of Mg^{2+}, when the reaction is started by simultaneous addition of EGTA and P_i to the ${}^{Ca}_{Ca}E$ form (75, 484) and the slow decline in the enzyme phosphorylation by ATP after addition of EGTA to microsomes equilibrated with Ca^{2+} (485, 523, 565).

The relationship between Ca^{2+} binding and enzyme conformation was further investigated by Inesi et al. (243). The Ca^{2+} binding to the high-affinity site is cooperative, with a Hill coefficient of 1.82 (243). The positive cooperativity was not observed in previous studies of Ca^{2+} binding to the Ca^{2+}-ATPase (187, 222–224, 404, 677), presumably because the binding studies were not extended to very low (10^{-7} M) Ca^{2+} concentrations. In the range of 0.1–1.0 μM medium Ca^{2+} concentration, about 8 nmol Ca^{2+} is bound per mg SR protein. Since the concentration of phosphoprotein intermediate is 4 nmol/mg protein, there are 2 mol Ca^{2+} bound per mole of ATP at the active site. A spectral change of the protein-bound iodoacetamide spin label accompanies Ca^{2+} binding to the high-affinity site, indicating a conformation change of the protein (84, 243). In this system the conformational change requires the presence of nucleotides and shows the same cooperativity with respect to medium Ca^{2+} as the Ca^{2+} binding. These observations were rationalized in terms of a mechanism in which the $E''Ca_2$ complex arises by two successive Ca^{2+}-binding steps, which precede and follow the binding of ATP, respectively (243)

1. $E + Ca^{2+}_{out} \longleftrightarrow E \cdot Ca$
2. $ATP + E \cdot Ca \longleftrightarrow ATP \cdot E \cdot Ca$
3. $ATP \cdot E \cdot Ca \longleftrightarrow ATP \cdot E' \cdot Ca$
4. $ATP \cdot E' \cdot Ca + Ca \longleftrightarrow ATP \cdot E'' \cdot Ca_2$
5. $ATP \cdot E'' \cdot Ca_2 \longleftrightarrow ADP \cdot E'' \sim P \cdot Ca_2$
6. $ADP \cdot E'' \sim P \cdot Ca_2 \longleftrightarrow ADP \cdot E''' \sim P \cdot Ca_2$
7. $ADP \cdot E''' \sim P \cdot Ca_2 \longleftrightarrow ADP \cdot E''' \sim P \cdot Ca + Ca^{2+}_{in}$
8. $ADP \cdot E''' \sim P \cdot Ca \longleftrightarrow ADP \cdot E''' \sim P + Ca^{2+}_{in}$
9. $ADP \cdot E''' \sim P \longleftrightarrow ADP + E''' \sim P$
10. $E''' \sim P \longleftrightarrow E - P$
11. $E - P \longleftrightarrow E \cdot P_i$
12. $E \cdot P_i \longleftrightarrow E + P_i$

The rapid binding of the first Ca (step 1) and ATP (step 2) to the enzyme causes a conformational change (step 3), which facilitates the binding of the second Ca^{2+} to the active site (step 4). This accounts for the cooperativity of Ca^{2+} binding. The phosphorylation of the enzyme by ATP (step 5) reduces the affinity of the Ca^{2+}-binding sites (step 6) with sequential release of two Ca^{2+} from the enzyme into the vesicle interior (steps 7, 8). The reaction is completed by the hydrolysis of phosphoprotein and a return of the enzyme to the E state (steps 9–12).

After addition of ATP to the E″Ca_2 form, the phosphorylation proceeds at rates as high as 150/s at 22°C. In a Ca^{2+}-free system the enzyme is in the E form. The phosphorylation of the Ca^{2+}-free ATPase initiated by the simultaneous addition of ATP and Ca^{2+} is slow because the formation of E″Ca_2 complex proceeds through a slow isomerization step [step 3; (243, 442, 485, 565)].

An effect of ATP on the rate of conversion of the enzyme from one form (E) into the other (E″) is suggested by the following observations: *1)* The rate of enzyme phosphorylation initiated by simultaneous addition of ATP and Ca^{2+} to the Ca^{2+}-free enzyme was faster (243, 485) than the rate of fluorescence change after addition of Ca^{2+} in the absence of ATP (136). *2)* The presence of 5′-adenylylimidodiphosphate [AMPP(NH)P] was required for the conformation change detected by protein-bound spin labels to occur on the binding of calcium to the high-affinity Ca^{2+}-binding site of the ATPase (243).

The presumed retention of ADP on the enzyme throughout the cycle conflicts with the observations of Takisawa and Tonomura (581).

The specificity of the high-affinity Ca^{2+}-binding site is best illustrated by the fact that Ca^{2+} transport continues at free-Ca^{2+} concentrations as low as 10^{-8} M in media containing 5–10 mM Mg^{2+}. Therefore the discrimination between Ca^{2+} and Mg^{2+} is close to a millionfold. At higher Mg^{2+} concentrations (20–50 mM), inhibition of Ca^{2+} transport and ATP synthesis occurs (272), suggesting competition by Mg^{2+} for the Ca^{2+}-binding sites.

Sr^{2+} can substitute for Ca^{2+} in ATPase activity and Ca^{2+} transport (415, 652, 669), although its affinity for the enzyme is about 80–100 times lower than that of Ca^{2+}. Due to the low affinity of Sr^{2+} for the internal inhibitory sites (γ-sites), SR vesicles can accumulate 1.5 μmol Sr^{2+}/mg protein, i.e., 10–20 times the maximum amount of calcium (415). The corresponding internal Sr^{2+} concentration would amount to 0.3 M, if most of the accumulated Sr^{2+} is free in the vesicle interior. The ratio of Sr^{2+}-transported:ATP-hydrolyzed was reported to be 1 throughout the uptake period (415), raising the possibility that the binding of Sr^{2+} to the high-affinity site is not cooperative.

La^{3+} (79, 305, 669) and Gd^{3+} (555) inhibit the Ca^{2+}-ATPase at concentrations close to 10 μM. The inhibition of phosphoenzyme formation by Gd^{3+} is presumably explained by tight binding of Gd^{3+} to the high-affinity Ca^{2+} sites (for Gd K_d = 3.5 × 10^{-8} M). Interactions among the enzyme bound Gd^{3+}, Li, and CrATP may permit the mapping of the active site with spectroscopic methods (555).

Binding of Mg^{2+} to Ca^{2+}-ATPase

MgATP is the substrate of the enzyme in the forward reaction (186, 272, 358, 359, 627, 652, 673, 677), although CaATP (373, 393), CoATP, and MnATP can also be used to phosphorylate the enzyme (666). In addition, there are indications of a separate Mg "activator" site (177, 358, 359, 404) in the nonphosphorylated form of the enzyme.

The phosphate acceptor in the reverse reaction is Mg-free ADP (358, 359), and the involvement of a second activator Mg^{2+} in the process is very likely. The binding of Mg^{2+} to the enzyme in the absence of ATP is promoted by 0.02 mM Ca^{2+} (358, 359), suggesting an interaction between the Ca^{2+}- and Mg^{2+}-binding sites. In agreement with these observations, the K_m of Mg ($\simeq$0.1 mM) for gradient-dependent phosphorylation of enzyme by P_i (187) is much lower than the Mg^{2+} concentrations required for gradient-independent phosphorylation in the absence of Ca^{2+} (398).

Four sets of Mg^{2+}-binding sites were derived from competition by Mg^{2+} for the binding of Mn^{2+} to SR (266). The association constants (K, in M^{-1}) and the number of sites (n) in each group are as follows: I_1, K = 2.3 × 10^2, n = 2; I_2, K = 6 × 10^3, n = 1; I_3, K = 8.5 × 10^2, n = 23; C, K = 5.8 × 10^2, n = 2. The C sites are highly cooperative, with a Hill coefficient of 4.

About 60 kcal of heat are released per mole of enzyme on addition of Mg^{2+}, suggesting that a major conformational change occurs on interaction of the enzyme with divalent cations (152). Such heat changes may provide important clues to the molecular mechanism of Ca^{2+} translocation (476).

Binding of ATP to Ca^{2+}-ATPase

The Ca^{2+}-transport ATPase of intact SR vesicles displays a complex dependence on ATP. The ATPase activity increases at low ATP concentration in a hyperbolic fashion, reaching a plateau around 0.1 mM ATP, followed by a secondary activation of the enzyme at higher ATP concentration (118, 131, 145, 174, 242, 496, 584, 625, 652, 673). This results in a downward curve of the double reciprocal plot of steady-state ATPase activity at high ATP concentrations (272), yielding two distinct K_m values of 2–3 μM and 500 μM, respectively.

The results are more varied on solubilized microsome preparations, indicating that some solubilization procedures may disrupt the protein-protein and protein-lipid interactions that are necessary for the activation at high ATP concentrations. The secondary activation of ATP hydrolysis was lost after solubilization of microsomes in studies reported by Yamada et al. (670), Takisawa and Tonomura (581), Inesi et al. (240), and Dean and Tanford (105). Others have observed the activation at high ATP concentration even in solubilized preparations that had no Ca^{2+}-transport activity (425, 448, 549, 587, 589, 627).

The complex kinetic behavior is explained by the presence of two distinct ATP-binding sites in the Ca^{2+}-ATPase. The high-affinity site (K_d = 2–3 μM) binds MgATP and is identified as the catalytic site (131). The SR vesicles bind 4.4 nmol ATP/mg protein at the high-affinity sites; this represents 50% occupancy of the ATPase molecules, consistent with half-of-the-sites reactivity. The maximum amount of Ca^{2+} bound to the enzyme at the high-affinity Ca^{2+} sites is about 9 nmol/mg protein. Therefore the bound Ca^{2+}:ATP ratio of the enzyme saturated with both substrates is 2.

At millimolar ATP concentrations, a second set of ATP-binding sites was detected with a dissociation constant $K_d \simeq 500$ μM (131). The activation of ATP hydrolysis at high substrate concentrations is probably related to the effect of ATP binding to these low-affinity regulatory sites. Adenosine 5′-(α-β-methylene)triphosphate (AMPPCP) or inorganic pyrophosphate (PP_i) readily displace ATP from the low-affinity sites. Although these two analogues are not cleaved by the enzyme to a significant extent, they are capable of activating the hydrolysis of micromolar concentrations of ATP, presumably by interacting with the low-affinity sites (131). These observations eliminate the possibility that the activation at high ATP concentration is due to a distinct ATPase. The low-affinity ATP binding apparently promotes interaction between a regulatory site and the high-affinity catalytic site of the enzyme. This results in increased rate of ATP hydrolysis (131, 625), without significant change in the concentration of phosphoenzyme intermediate [see, however, Inesi et al. (246)], which implies an increased turnover (625).

Dupont (131) suggested that the low-affinity ATP-binding site may be responsible for the slow, Mg-activated ATP hydrolysis of SR (basic ATPase). The K_m for ATP is similar to the dissociation constant of the low-affinity site (≃500 μM), and AMPP(NH)P, which binds to the low-affinity site, is a strong inhibitor of basic ATPase.

Although MgATP is the substrate of the Ca^{2+}-transport ATPase (272, 358, 359, 387, 627, 652, 673, 677), significant ATP binding occurs at the high-affinity site even in the presence of EDTA, i.e., at a very low concentration of free divalent metal ions (237, 462). Addition of Mg^{2+} increases the affinity of ATP binding (237, 404, 677).

The affinity of ADP binding to the enzyme depends on its functional state. From the inhibition of Ca^{2+}-dependent ATP hydrolysis and from the activation of ATP synthesis coupled to Ca^{2+} release, the affinity of ATP and ADP for the active site appears to be similar (187), although binding experiments under equilibrium conditions indicate a significantly lower affinity of MgADP than MgATP for the catalytic site.

Aderem et al. (2) observed the presence of tightly bound ATP and ADP in SR vesicles. Mild acid treatment of the vesicles or exposure to EGTA inactivates Ca^{2+} transport without inhibition of ATP hydrolysis, and under these conditions the tightly bound nucleotide pool is lost. The tightly bound nucleotides may be of interest in considering the alternating site mechanism of ATP synthesis (50, 52), but their mode of involvement in ATP hydrolysis and Ca^{2+} transport is unknown.

Binding of Various Substrates to Ca^{2+}-ATPase

The Ca^{2+}-Mg^{2+}-ATPase of SR catalyzes the hydrolysis of a wide range of phosphate compounds. In addition to the physiological substrate ATP, these include inosine 5′-triphosphate (ITP), guanosine 5′-triphosphate (GTP), cytidine 5′-triphosphate (CTP), uridine 5′-triphosphate (UTP) (118, 362, 387, 388), formycin triphosphate, 6-mercaptoinosine-5′-triphosphate, adenosine 5′-(3-thio)triphosphate (677), acetylphosphate (111, 112, 117, 119, 468), carbamylphosphate (468), *p*-nitrophenylphosphate (233, 444), dinitrophenylphosphate, methylumbelliferylphosphate, and furoylacryloylphosphate (496). The hydrolysis of most substrates is coupled to Ca^{2+} transport, although the reported coupling ratios vary (496). The relative velocity of hydrolysis of various nucleoside triphosphates is ATP (1.0), ITP (0.8), GTP (0.7), CTP (0.55), UTP (0.25).

The K_m for most nonnucleotide substrates is in the millimolar range. The hydrolysis of *p*-nitrophenylphosphate, dinitrophenylphosphate, furoylacryloylphosphate, acetylphosphate, and carbamylphosphate follows simple dependence on substrate concentration.

The ratio of Ca^{2+} transported to substrate hydrolyzed is usually 2 Ca:1 NTP for the various nucleoside triphosphates (362). A stoichiometry of 2 Ca:1 substrate was also suggested for *p*-nitrophenylphosphate (233) and acetylphosphate (173), but recently Rossi et al. (496) found a ratio of 1. In view of the observed fluctuation of Ca:ATP ratio with temperature (564), ATP concentration (496), Ca^{2+} concentration (183), and pH (496), the fixed Ca:ATP ratio of 2 may not be valid for all conditions and should be carefully evaluated in each case. An Sr:ATP ratio of 1 was reported during Sr^{2+} transport by Mermier and Hasselbach (415). Activation of carbamylphosphate hydrolysis by Ca^{2+} was not observed during Ca^{2+} transport induced by carbamylphosphate (468, 326), suggesting that the rate-limiting step of the reaction is independent of external Ca^{2+}.

Influence of ATP on Mobility and Reactivity of Protein Side-Chain Groups

The blocking of thiol groups of the Ca^{2+}-transport ATPase inhibits the ATPase activity and Ca^{2+} transport; ATP protects against the reaction of several SH groups and prevents or markedly reduces the loss of enzymatic activity in the presence of thiol reagents (13, 196, 225, 379, 431, 433, 460, 594). The protective effect of ATP extends to a large number of SH groups (379, 594), suggesting that it is caused by a conformational change in the enzyme molecule induced by the nucleotide binding. Therefore protection by ATP may be a difficult approach for the selective identification of active-site SH groups involved in ATP binding or enzymatic activity.

Major effort is directed at the analysis of the conformational changes that accompany or follow the binding of ATP to the Ca^{2+}-transport ATPase, by analyzing the reactivity of various side-chain groups in different phases of the Ca^{2+}-transport cycle.

Changes in SH group reactivity connected with different states of the enzyme were observed by Champeil et al. (76), Yamada and Ikemoto (665), Ikemoto et al. (225, 230), Murphy (431, 433), Yoshida and Tonomura (678), Andersen and Møller (13), Martonosi (379), and Thorley-Lawson and Green (594). The effect of ATP on the reactivity of lysyl groups was reported by Murphy (432) and by Yamamoto and Tonomura (675, 676). Although the involvement of histidine residues in ATPase activity was suggested by several investigators (382, 679), ATP or *p*-nitrophenylphosphate did not protect against the loss of ATPase activity during ethoxyformylation of the Ca^{2+}-ATPase (586).

Changes induced by ATP in the mobility of spin labels covalently attached to SH groups of Ca^{2+}-ATPase were reported by Nakamura et al. (438), Pang et al. (463), and Coan and Inesi et al. (84, 85, 243). Changes in the spectrum of protein-bound spin labels were also found in the presence of acetylphosphate (83). The observations of Coan et al. (85) indicate that the Ca^{2+}-induced changes in the spectral parameter of protein-bound 2,2,6,6-tetramethyl-4-amino (*N*-iodoacetamide) nitroxide occur between 10^{-7} and 10^{-8} M [Ca^{2+}] in the presence of AMPP(NH)P, but shift to 10^{-3}–10^{-2} M Ca^{2+} in the presence of ATP. The two ranges of Ca^{2+} concentrations correspond to the activation and inhibition of ATPase activity, respectively. The relationship of conformational change and enzyme activity to Ca^{2+} concentration is highly cooperative with Hill coefficients close to 2. The nonhydrolyzable ATP analogue AMPP(NH)P binds to the high-affinity site and presumably induces a conformation characteristic for the E^{ATP}_{2Ca} complex. In the presence of ATP the reaction proceeds through phosphorylation followed by a conformational change and reduction of the Ca^{2+} affinity of the enzyme. Under these conditions, the vesicles are filled with Ca^{2+}, saturating all internal binding sites. Therefore with ATP as substrate the probe samples a conformational state(s) of low Ca^{2+} affinity. A small Ca^{2+} response with ATP at 10^{-7}–10^{-6} M Ca^{2+} indicates that a small fraction of the enzyme retains high-affinity Ca^{2+}-binding sites.

The spectral change caused by Ca^{2+} requires the presence of nucleotide on the enzyme. Since ATP and ADP produce similar spectral changes and ATP is rapidly cleaved during the early part of the Ca^{2+}-transport cycle, it is assumed (85) that the predominant form of enzyme in the system is the ${}^{Ca\cdot}_{Ca\cdot}E^{\cdot ADP}_{\sim P}$ complex. With solubilized ATPase, however, the main reaction intermediates do not contain bound ADP (581).

Analogous ligand-induced conformational changes were also observed on the Na^+-K^+-ATPase (213, 308).

Formation of Enzyme-Substrate Complex

The formation of phosphoprotein intermediate (E∼P) requires Ca^{2+} and MgATP as substrates, and it is markedly accelerated by $MgCl_2$. Lineweaver-Burk plots of the initial rate of E∼P formation at low ATP concentration (below 5 μM) yield straight lines (272). The maximum velocity (V_{max}) of the reaction decreases with decreasing Ca^{2+} concentration in the external medium, whereas the K_m for ATP (≃1 μM) remains unchanged. A linear relationship exists between the maximum velocity of E∼P formation and the square of the external Ca^{2+} concentration (87, 272). These observations suggest that the Michaelis complex is formed by the random reaction of the enzyme with 2 Ca^{2+} and MgATP yielding a ${}^{Ca}_{Ca}E$-MgATP complex (272). This is consistent with the 2 Ca:1 ATP stoichiometry of the Ca^{2+} transport.

The cooperativity of Ca^{2+} binding (243) implies that the addition of one Ca^{2+} ion to the enzyme facilitates the binding of the second. An interaction between Ca^{2+} and nucleotide-binding sites is indicated by the recent observation of Coan et al. (85) that the Ca^{2+}-induced change in the mobility of spin labels covalently bound to SH groups on the enzyme requires the presence of 5′-adenylimidodiphosphate (AMPPNP), a nonhydrolyzable analogue of ATP. Previous steady-state kinetic studies of Yamamoto and Tonomura (673) suggested an ordered sequence of reactions, in which MgATP binds first to the enzyme with subsequent addition of Ca^{2+}, yielding ${}^{Ca}_{Ca}E$-MgATP. This may be followed by the dissociation of Mg^{2+} to give ${}^{Ca}_{Ca}E$-ATP (272).

As the ATP concentration is increased above 10 μM, a plateau of ATPase activity is reached, followed by a secondary activation at ATP concentrations higher than 100 μM (242, 648, 652, 673). The activation of ATPase activity and Ca^{2+} transport at high ATP concentrations was also reflected in increased velocity of E∼P formation (272). The reciprocal plots of the initial velocity of E∼P formation against ATP concentration show a downward curve at ATP concentrations higher than 5 μM (272). The secondary activation by ATP probably involves ATP binding to a regulatory site. Similar activation of ATP hydrolysis is produced by the binding of the nonhydrolyzable ATP analogues, AMPPCP and PP_i, to the enzyme (131, 584).

In early studies the steady-state concentration of E∼P increased parallel with the ATPase activity (246, 272), and the v/E∼P was constant over a wide range of ATP concentrations. Therefore Kanazawa et al. (272) suggested that ATP activates by accelerating the formation of E∼P. To account for the increased rate of E∼P formation at high ATP concentration, they proposed the existence of two E-ATP-Ca_2 complexes; ^{o} denotes outside (cytoplasmic), ^{i} denotes inside (tubular)

$$ {}_1E^{\cdot Ca_2^o}_{\cdot MgATP^o} \rightleftharpoons {}_2E^{\cdot Ca_2^o}_{\cdot ATP^o} + Mg^o $$

$$_{2}E^{\cdot Ca_2^o}_{\cdot ATP^o} \rightleftharpoons E^{\cdot Ca_2^i}_{\sim P} + ADP^o$$

and assumed that at high ATP concentration the equilibrium shifts in favor of $_{2}E^{Ca_2^o}_{ATP}$.

Later a number of investigators observed an increase in v/E~P during activation of ATP hydrolysis at high ATP concentration, which implies that the secondary activation may be due to activation of the hydrolysis of phosphoprotein (118, 174, 625).

The experimental evidence about the effect of ATP on phosphoprotein hydrolysis is conflicting. Although Inesi et al. (246) found an increase in the steady-state concentration of E~P at high ATP concentrations, more recent studies from the same laboratory suggest an activation of E~P turnover without a change in E~P concentration (625). De Meis and de Mello (118) found severalfold activation of phosphoprotein hydrolysis in the absence of K^+ by 10 μM ATP, whereas 1 mM ATP had no effect on the E~P hydrolysis in the presence of 0.1 M KCl in the experiments of Kanazawa et al. (272), Martonosi et al. (393), and Sumida et al. (562). Since K^+ may alter the rate-limiting step of the reaction and thereby modify the effect of ATP on E~P decomposition (537), clearly further experiments are needed to settle this question.

Formation and Properties of Phosphoproteins

The existence of a high-energy phosphorylated intermediate on the pathway of ATP-dependent Ca^{2+} transport was first suggested by the rapid Ca^{2+}-dependent ATP-ADP exchange reaction catalyzed by SR vesicles (144, 190, 353, 606, 607). The phosphoprotein intermediate was identified by phosphorylation of the enzyme with [γ-^{32}P]ATP followed by quenching with trichloroacetic acid (TCA) and measurement of the protein-bound radioactivity (354, 369, 373, 673, 674). The phosphoprotein is acid stable and alkaline labile, and it is decomposed by hydroxylamine or hydrazine (246, 354, 369, 373, 674), suggesting that it is an acylphosphate. Reductive cleavage of the acylphosphate bond with sodium [^{3}H]borohydride followed by acid hydrolysis of the protein yielded radioactive homoserine, indicating that the phosphoryl group is covalently attached to the β-carboxyl group of an aspartyl residue (108).

The tryptic peptide that contains the phosphate acceptor region of the protein was isolated and its sequence determined (5)

> Ser-Leu-Pro-Ser-Val-Glu-Thr-Leu-Gly-Cys-Thr-Ser-Val-Ile-Cys-Ser-Asp-Lys (Thr-Thr-Gly) Leu-Thr-Thr-Asn-Gln-Val-(Cys-Met-Ser-Lys)

The sequence next to the functional aspartyl residue, Ser-Asp-Lys, is apparently identical to that found in the Na^+-K^+-ATPase of kidney microsomes (24), suggesting some similarity between the two enzymes in the structure of the active site (213, 279).

In comparison with TCA-denatured membranes, the phosphoprotein of native SR is less sensitive to hydroxylamine (373) or sodium borohydride (87). The difference may be due to environmental effects or altered access of reagents to the active site. Phosphorylation of chemically distinct sites in native membranes with phosphate migration from an initial acceptor to secondary sites during acid denaturation has not been excluded.

Kinetics of E~P Formation

The formation of E~P initiated by addition of ATP to SR vesicles equilibrated with micromolar Ca^{2+} (Fig. 6) occurs without a lag phase (174, 175, 272). Therefore the rate of formation of $^{Ca}_{Ca}$E-ATP complex is relatively fast compared with the rate of enzyme phosphorylation.

At ATP concentrations up to 1 μM the steady-state concentration of E~P is reached within 80 ms at 22°C and its level is defined by the ATP concentration (Fig. 6.) The release of P_i shows a lag phase followed by an increase in rate that coincides with the increase in E~P concentration. This behavior is consistent with the simple scheme

$$E + S \rightleftharpoons E \cdot S \rightleftharpoons E{\sim}P \rightleftharpoons E + P_i$$

Lag in P_i production implies that P_i release follows the formation of E~P.

At higher ATP concentration (5–100 μM), the rate of formation of E~P continues to rise and an "overshoot" in E~P concentration is observed, followed by a decline and a slow adjustment to a steady state (Fig. 6). A "burst" in P_i production occurs with a time course similar to the decline in E~P following the overshoot.

The overshoot and the P_i burst at 5–100 μM ATP can be explained by the following scheme

$$E + S \rightleftharpoons E \cdot S \rightleftharpoons E{\sim}P \rightleftharpoons E \cdot P_i \rightleftharpoons E + P_i$$

According to this scheme, P_i is released from a hypothetical TCA-labile enzyme·phosphate compound (E·P), which in turn arises from the TCA-stable E~P intermediate (174). A TCA-labile E·P intermediate was earlier proposed by Yamamoto and Tonomura (673) on different grounds.

Both E~P overshoot and the early P_i burst were absent after solubilization of SR vesicles with Triton X-100 (175, 581). No overshoot was seen when the reaction was initiated by the addition of ATP to Ca^{2+}-loaded microsomes (581) or when ATP and Ca^{2+} were added together to microsomes preincubated in Mg-EGTA (581). The initial burst of P_i production was also observed in the absence of Ca^{2+} (175), although under these conditions no E~P was formed. It was suggested that the Ca^{2+}-independent ATPase is an alternate pathway of the transport enzyme in which E~P does not accumulate.

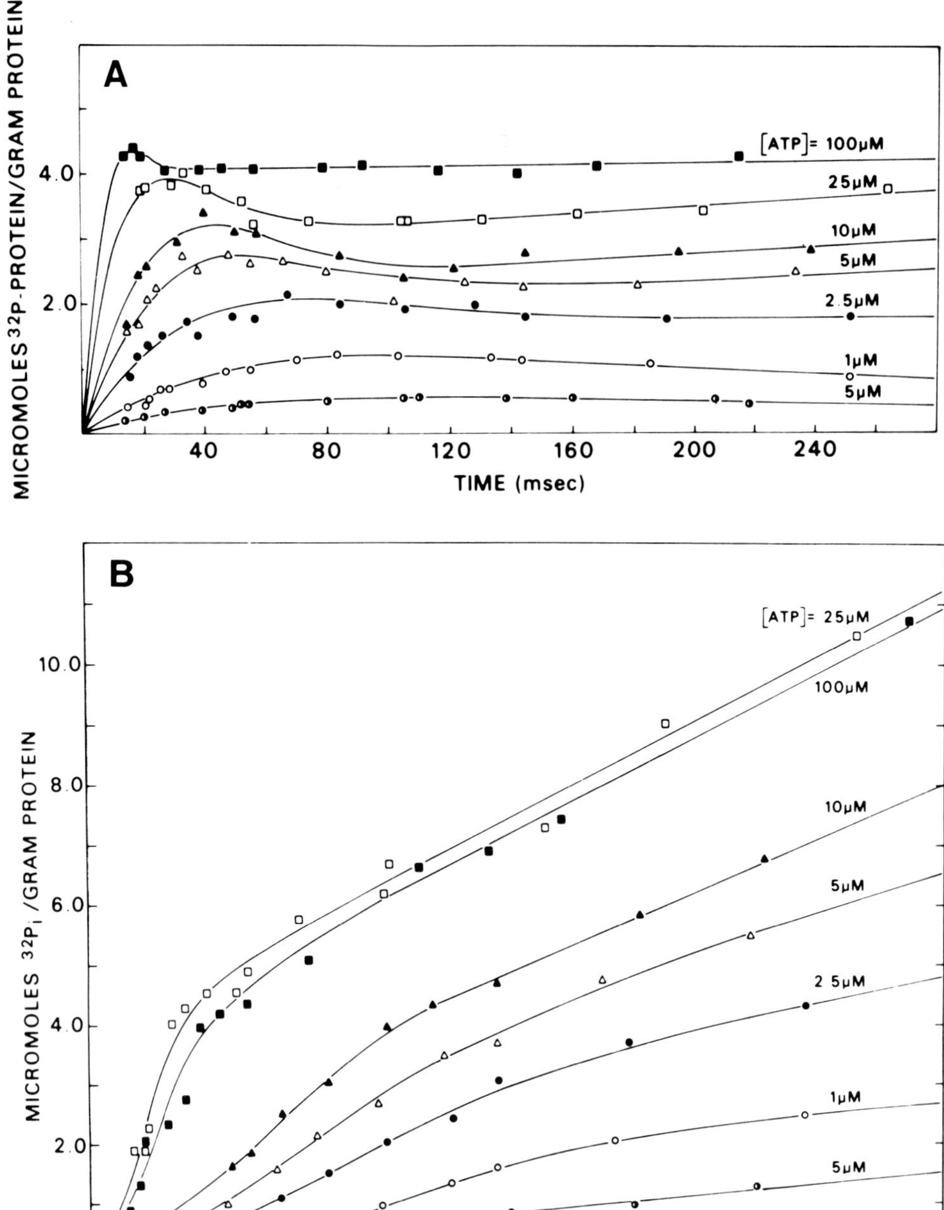

FIG. 6. Dependence on ATP concentration of transient enzyme phosphorylation (*A*) and transient inorganic phosphate (P_i) liberation (*B*) by sarcoplasmic reticulum vesicles. Final ATP concentration in μM: ◑—◑, 0.5; ○—○, 1; ●—●, 2.5; △—△, 5; ▲—▲, 10; □—□, 25; ■—■, 100. [From Froehlich and Taylor (174).]

The existence of E·P is based entirely on the kinetic evidence outlined above. The early burst of phosphate liberation and the overshoot in E~P may arise by several alternative mechanisms (672).

Relationship Between Enzyme Phosphorylation and Translocation of Calcium

Kanazawa et al. (272) suggested that the formation of E~P is connected with Ca^{2+} translocation across the membrane, since the reaction of the enzyme with ATP requires external calcium, while the reverse reaction, the formation of ATP from E~P and ADP, depends on Ca^{2+} inside the vesicles. Direct evidence for Ca^{2+} translocation connected with enzyme phosphorylation was provided by Sumida and Tonomura (564). The time courses of E~P formation and Ca^{2+} translocation were compared at 0°C in the absence of Mg^{2+} and at low Ca^{2+} concentration to minimize the hydrolysis of E~P. Ca^{2+} uptake was measured by adding EGTA to a suspension of vesicles followed by Millipore filtration, utilizing the observation (129) that EGTA removes external Ca^{2+} but leaves the intravesicular Ca^{2+} unaffected. The time course of Ca^{2+} uptake determined by this method showed a fast initial phase, which correlated with the rate of E~P formation, and a slow steady phase, which followed the course of slow P_i liberation. During both phases the Ca:E~P ratio was 1. If the stopping solution contained EGTA + ADP, only the slow steady phase of Ca^{2+} uptake was detected. These data suggest that Ca^{2+} bound to the enzyme substrate complex ($^{Ca}_{Ca}$E-ATP) is rapidly translocated on phosphorylation of the enzyme, yielding the rapid burst of Ca^{2+} uptake in the first cycle of the reaction, followed by a slower steady-state Ca^{2+} accumulation.

The correlation between E~P formation and Ca^{2+} uptake was further analyzed in greater detail using rapid kinetic techniques (239, 244, 309, 310, 565, 625, 626). The initial burst of Ca^{2+} uptake after ATP addition was clearly resolved at ATP concentrations less than 5 μM, and its time course was identical to that of enzyme phosphorylation ($k \simeq 85$/s) (Fig. 7). The magnitude of the Ca^{2+}-uptake burst is related with a 2:1 stoichiometry to the level of phosphoenzyme intermediate (625). At saturating ATP concentration the level of phosphoenzyme is about 4 nmol/mg protein, i.e., about one-half of the estimated number of active sites. Under these conditions the initial burst of Ca^{2+} uptake is about 8 nmol Ca/mg protein. The initial rapid Ca^{2+} uptake was attributed to the first cycle of enzyme phosphorylation and Ca^{2+} translocation. After the initial burst, Ca^{2+} transport continues at a slower velocity (5–6/s), its rate being limited by the turnover of the enzyme.

In these experiments ^{45}Ca "translocated" across the membrane is defined as the amount of ^{45}Ca radioactivity that remains bound to the microsomes after EGTA treatment; EGTA is assumed to remove all Ca^{2+} attached to binding sites on the outside surface of microsomes. Recent experiments by Dupont (134) and by Waas and Hasselbach (629) suggest, however, that the rapid burst of Ca^{2+} uptake that accompanies enzyme phosphorylation may represent "occlusion" of Ca^{2+} by the Ca^{2+}-ATPase on the outside surface of microsomes so that it is not released in the presence of EGTA. According to these studies, the translocation of occluded Ca^{2+} across the membrane may follow enzyme phosphorylation in a relatively slow reaction step that could be rate limiting under certain conditions.

The initial and the steady-state velocities of Ca^{2+} uptake are doubled by increasing the concentration of ATP to 50 μM or above, without significant change in the level of phosphoenzyme or in the magnitude of the initial rapid Ca^{2+} uptake. Therefore the activation of ATP hydrolysis and Ca^{2+} transport at millimolar ATP concentrations was attributed to an increase in enzyme turnover [(625); see, however, ref. 672].

The maximum velocity of enzyme phosphorylation with ITP as substrate is only 16/s, i.e., about one-fifth of that obtained with ATP (626). Furthermore after enzyme phosphorylation by ITP, the initial burst of Ca^{2+} uptake occurs after a considerable lag, which indicates that the rate constant of Ca^{2+} translocation or occlusion is slower using ITP as compared with ATP as phosphate donor (Fig. 7). The difference suggests either that the nucleoside diphosphate remains attached to the enzyme after phosphorylation or that another nucleotide molecule binds to a regulatory site, which modulates the kinetics of Ca^{2+} translocation. As no ADP binding to the phosphoenzyme could be detected (581), the latter explanation appears more plausible. In fact the secondary activation of Ca^{2+} transport observed at high ATP concentration can be achieved by millimolar concentrations of nonhydrolyzable ATP analogues (AMPPNP or PP_i) in the presence of micromolar concentrations of ATP (131). These observations indicate an ATP effect at or beyond step 4 of the transport scheme given on p. 436.

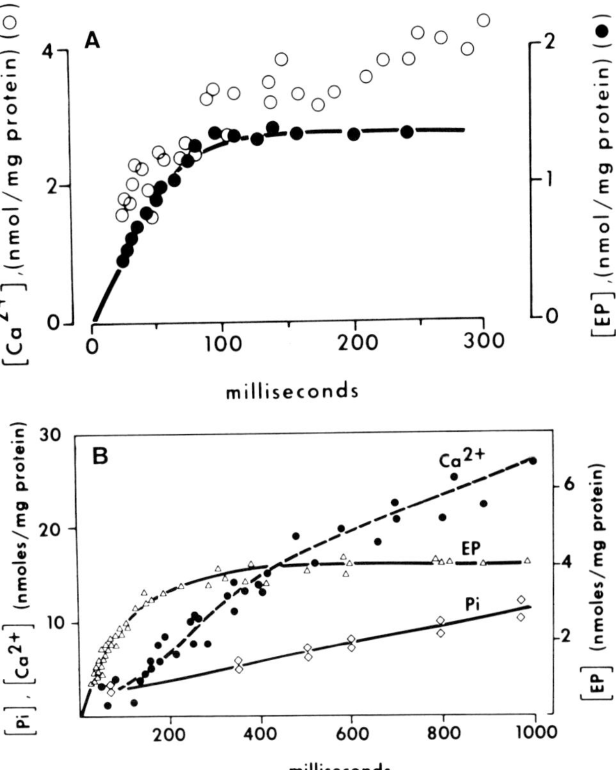

FIG. 7. *A*: time resolution of the Ca^{2+} translocation burst with ATP as substrate. Phosphoenzyme (EP) was measured by acid quenching (●) and Ca^{2+} uptake by the EGTA-quenching method (○). The reaction medium contained 20 mM morpholinopropane sulfonic acid (MOPS), pH 6.8, 80 mM KCl, 5 mM $MgCl_2$, 0.4 mg of protein/ml, 35 μM $CaCl_2$, and 2 μM [γ-^{32}P]ATP (●) or 35 μM $^{45}CaCl_2$ and 2 μM ATP (○). *B*: enzyme phosphorylation by ITP, Ca^{2+} uptake and P_i production during the transient state. [ITP] = 1 mM. Phosphoenzyme (△) and P_i (◇) were assayed by acid-quenching method, and Ca^{2+} uptake (●) by EGTA-quenching method. [*A* from Verjovski-Almeida and Inesi (625), *B* from Verjovski-Almeida et al. (626), reprinted with permission from *Biochemistry*, © 1978 American Chemical Society.]

Changes in Ca^{2+} Affinity of Phosphoenzyme During Ca^{2+} Translocation

In order to generate a Ca^{2+} gradient of 1,000 or greater across the membrane, the Ca^{2+} affinity of the carrier is expected to decrease during Ca^{2+} translocation from 10^6 M^{-1} to $\sim 10^3$ M^{-1}. Since Ca^{2+} release in the vesicle interior precedes the hydrolysis of phosphoenzyme (357), the affinity change must occur during transition between two or more states of the phosphoenzyme intermediates.

Rapid kinetic measurements of the rate of enzyme phosphorylation by the acid-quench technique and of the Ca^{2+} binding with arsenazo III as Ca^{2+} indicator provided conclusive evidence that phosphorylation of the purified Ca^{2+}-transport ATPase occurs with a decrease in the Ca^{2+} affinity of the transport sites [Fig. 8; (223, 224)]. The formation of 0.1 mol phosphorylated intermediate per mole enzyme was accompanied by the release of 0.24 mol Ca^{2+} into the medium. The release of Ca^{2+} follows E-P formation with a lag time of about 15 ms. The maximum of Ca^{2+} release is reached about 250 ms after addition of ATP or about 100 ms later than full phosphorylation. During most of this time the Ca^{2+}-release/E~P stoichiometry is less than 2, suggesting sequential formation of acid-stable intermediates of differing Ca^{2+} affinities.

The amount of released Ca^{2+} (0.24 mol/mol) exceeds the expected amount (0.2 mol/mol enzyme), suggesting that some acid-labile intermediate may also con-

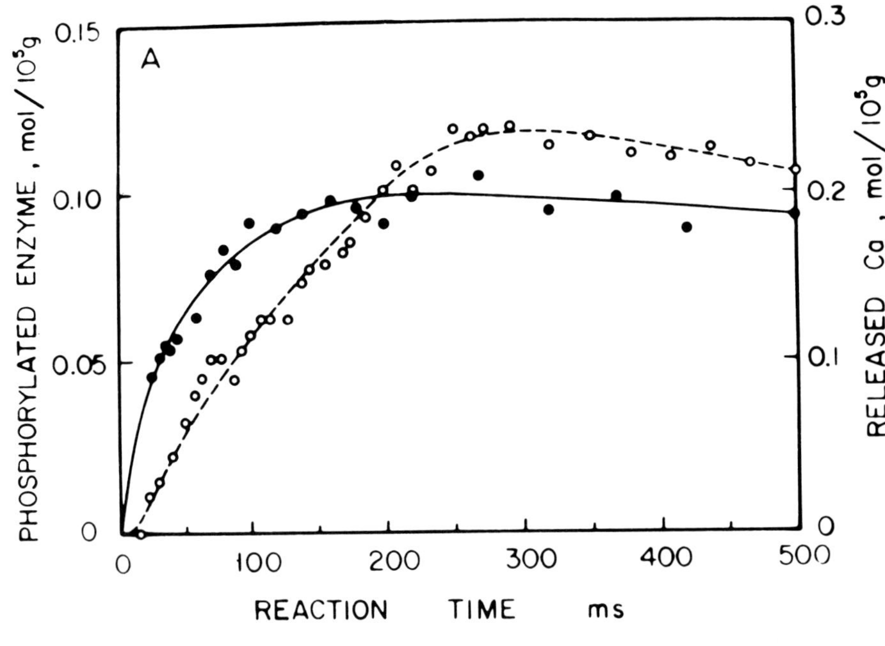

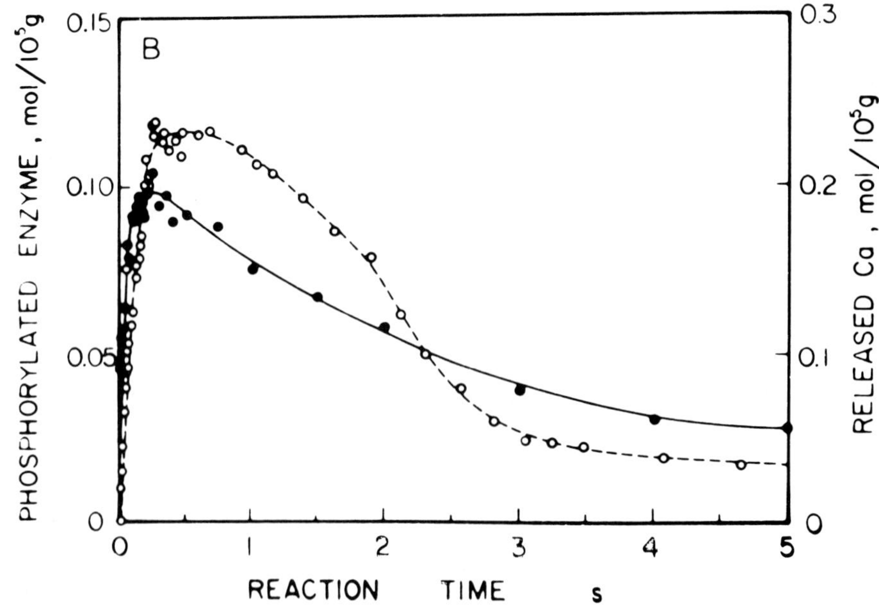

FIG. 8. Relation between Ca^{2+} release and rebinding, and formation and decay of the phosphorylated enzyme. Final concentration of [γ-^{32}P]ATP was 5 μM. For other details see Ikemoto (224). Note that the ordinates are drawn in a 2:1 ratio to facilitate comparison of the amount of phosphorylated intermediate with that of the released Ca^{2+}. ○, Amount of released Ca^{2+}; ●, phosphorylated enzyme. [From Ikemoto (224).]

tribute to the Ca^{2+} binding. The data do not permit the quantitative assessment of the affinity change causing this Ca^{2+} release.

Decomposition of the phosphoenzyme intermediate leads to rebinding of the Ca^{2+} to the enzyme. Surprisingly the Ca^{2+} rebinding occurs faster than the dephosphorylation of the enzyme, raising the possibility that interaction between phosphorylated and nonphosphorylated subunits of the Ca^{2+}-ATPase oligomer (613) could affect the Ca^{2+} affinity. Recent observations by Ikemoto et al. (227, 228) suggest the existence of two types of ATPase subunits that differ with respect to the rate of Ca^{2+} release after addition of EGTA. The ratio of the two types of molecules is 1:1 under various conditions.

Yamada and Tonomura (669) measured the rate of E~P formation over a wide range of Mg^{2+} and Ca^{2+} concentrations using purified Ca^{2+}-ATPase. The Ca^{2+}-dependent E~P formation was competitively inhibited by Mg. The apparent dissociation constants of the Ca^{2+} and Mg^{2+} complexes of the enzyme were 0.35 μM (K_{Ca}) and 10.5 mM (K_{Mg}), respectively. Therefore the affinity of the purified ATPase was 30,000 times greater for Ca^{2+} than for Mg^{2+} in the E state. From the competitive inhibition by calcium of the Mg^{2+}-dependent phosphorylation of the enzyme, a K_{Ca}:K_{Mg} ratio of about 2.5 was obtained, which indicates that E~P barely discriminates between Ca^{2+} and Mg^{2+}. It is likely, therefore, that the decrease in the Ca^{2+} affinity of the enzyme on phosphorylation is accompanied by an increase in its affinity for Mg^{2+}.

ADP-Sensitive and ADP-Insensitive Phosphoprotein Intermediates

The rate of ATP-ADP exchange under optimum conditions is about 10 times greater than the rate of ATP hydrolysis and Ca^{2+} transport (190). Therefore in the presence of ADP there is a greater than even chance that the phosphoprotein transfers its phosphate to ADP, forming ATP, than that it participates in Ca^{2+} translocation, with eventual hydrolysis to P_i.

The transfer of phosphate from E~P to ADP was first demonstrated by Kanazawa et al. (271). To SR vesicles phosphorylated with [^{32}P]ATP in the presence of 0.16 M KCl, 1.1 mM Mg, and 55 μM Ca, solutions containing EGTA or EGTA + 2.2 mM ADP were added (Fig. 9). EGTA lowers the external Ca^{2+} concentration below 10^{-8} M and inhibits further phosphorylation of the enzyme by ATP.

The concentration of E~P decreases exponentially after the addition of EGTA, accompanied by the liberation of P_i. The dephosphorylation of E~P requires Mg^{2+}. The rate of E~P disappearance was accelerated by ADP, with the formation of nearly stoichiometric amounts of ATP and very little P_i. The formation of ATP was independent of external Ca^{2+} concentration but required high Ca^{2+} concentration in the vesicle interior (272). These results indicate that in the presence of 0.165 M KCl essentially all E~P can be converted into ATP by simultaneous addition of EGTA and ADP to the phosphorylated and Ca^{2+}-loaded vesicles (ADP-sensitive E~P).

The reaction of E~P with ADP decreases markedly if addition of ADP is delayed 5–10 s after the addition of EGTA (272). Under these conditions the ADP-sensitive E~P is converted into an ADP-insensitive form. The formation of ATP from insensitive E~P and ADP was reactivated after the addition of 7 mM Ca^{2+} to the incubation medium. Under similar conditions but in the absence of ADP, 7 mM Ca^{2+} slightly inhibited the rate of E~P decomposition. Based on these observations, Sumida and Tonomura (564) and Takisawa and Tonomura (582) proposed the following reaction scheme

$$E + ATP + 2Ca^{2+} \rightleftarrows {}^{Ca}_{Ca}\cdot E - ATP \xleftrightarrow[(2)]{\;\to ADP\;} {}^{Ca}_{Ca}\cdot E\underset{1}{\sim}P \rightarrow$$

(1) (2) (ADP-sensitive E~P)

$$\rightarrow {}^{Ca}_{Ca}\cdot {}^{*}E - P \xleftrightarrow[(3)\;\to Ca]{Mg \to} {}^{Mg\cdot}_{Mg\cdot}E\underset{2}{\sim}P \xleftrightarrow[(4)]{} E + 2Mg^{2+} + P_i$$

(3) (4)

Ca (ADP-insensitive E~P)

The ADP-sensitive phosphoenzyme (E_1P) is formed first, followed by conversion into ADP-insensitive phosphoenzyme (E_2P). The conversion is promoted by the loss of intravesicular Ca^{2+}. The noncompetitive inhibition of ATPase activity by ADP indicates that a portion of E~P reacts with ADP before Ca^{2+} translocation.

The relationship between ADP-sensitive and ADP-insensitive phosphorylated enzyme intermediates was further investigated (580, 582) with a solubilized ATPase preparation (321). With 2 mM Ca^{2+} present essentially all the E~P reacted with ADP to form ATP (ADP-sensitive E~P). After removal of Ca^{2+} with EGTA, only 40% of the E-^{32}P remained ADP sensitive. The ratio of the two kinds of E~P depends on the relative concentration of $MgCl_2$ and $CaCl_2$ in the system. From the relationships among Ca^{2+}, Mg^{2+}, and E~P concentrations, the ADP-sensitive E~P binds two Ca^{2+}, whereas the ADP-insensitive E~P binds two Mg^{2+}/mol enzyme.

At pH 9.0, 10°C, the conversion of E_1P into E_2P is much faster than the rate of decomposition of E_2P into E + P_i and therefore E_1P and E_2P are in equilibrium. At physiological pH the $E_1P \rightarrow E_2P$ conversion may be rate limiting in the presence of 0.1 M K (536, 537). The conversion of ADP-sensitive into ADP-insensitive E~P is inhibited by treatment of the enzyme with *N*-ethylmaleimide.

Further resolution of the various forms of E~P was obtained by Yamada and Ikemoto (666). Reaction of

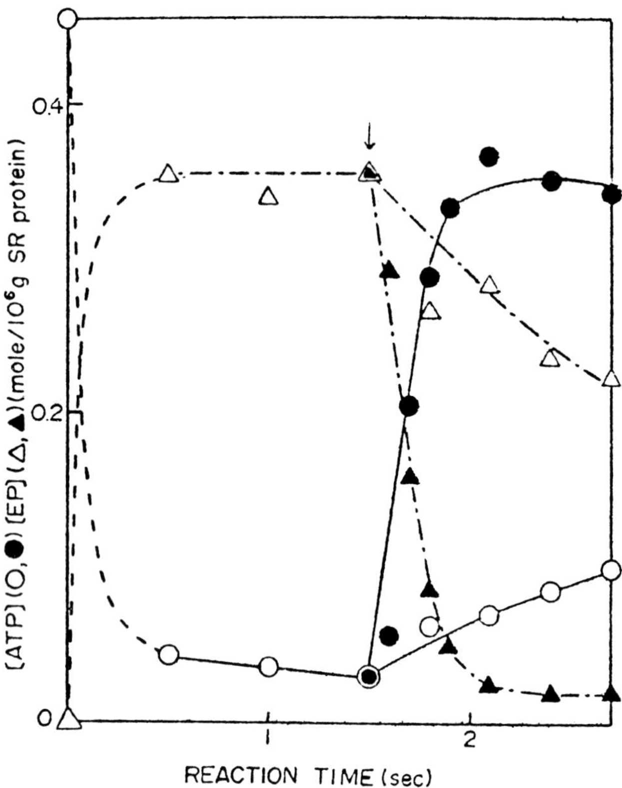

FIG. 9. Formation of ATP from E-P and ADP. Sarcoplasmic reticulum (11 mg/ml protein) was phosphorylated with 5.0 μM [^{32}P]ATP in 0.909 ml of reaction medium containing 1.1 mM $MgCl_2$, 55 μM $CaCl_2$, 165 mM KCl, and 110 mM Tris-HCl at pH 8.8 and 15°C. After 1.5 s, the phosphorylation reaction was stopped by addition (↓) of 0.091 ml of solution containing 366 mM EGTA and 2.2 mM ADP at pH 8.8 (●, ▲), or of 366 mM EGTA alone at pH 8.8 (○, △). At intervals after the start of phosphorylation, SR was denatured with perchloric acid, and the concentrations of [^{32}P]ATP (●, ○) and EP (▲, △) were measured. [From Kanazawa et al. (271).]

the purified Ca^{2+}-transport ATPase with ATP in the presence of 0.11 mM Ca^{2+} at pH 7.0 yields stable ADP-sensitive phosphoenzyme, which does not decompose spontaneously (E-P_{D+}). Chelation of calcium with EGTA converts E-P_{D+} into an ADP-insensitive intermediate (E-P_{D-}) in agreement with Takisawa and Tonomura (582). Addition of Mg^{2+} after EGTA causes rapid hydrolysis of a small portion of E-P_{D-} with the formation of P_i. For this reaction K_{Mg} is 3.3×10^3 M^{-1}. The fraction of E-P_{D-} that is Mg sensitive (E-P_{D-Mg+}) increases at a slower rate after EGTA addition than the Mg^{2+}-insensitive portion of E-P_{D-} (E-P_{D-Mg-}). The results suggest the sequential formation of E-P_{D+} $\rightleftarrows$ E-P_{D-Mg-} $\rightleftarrows$ E-P_{D-Mg+}. The terminal intermediate E-P_{D-Mg+} is presumably identical with the $^{Mg}_{Mg}$ E$\underset{2}{\sim}$P intermediate of Takisawa and Tonomura (582). The E-P_{D-Mg+} intermediate may be the initial product of gradient-dependent or gradient-independent phosphorylation of the enzyme by P_i in the reverse reaction.

Effect of Potassium on ATPase Activity and Ca^{2+} Transport

The ATP hydrolysis and Ca^{2+} transport of SR are activated by low concentrations of monovalent cations [(125–128, 279, 370, 540, 671); for review see ref. 128].

The effect of K^+ on the elementary steps of the reaction was investigated in detail by Shigekawa and his collaborators (535–538). Even in the absence of alkali metal ions the ADP-sensitive (E_1P) intermediate forms first, followed by conversion into the ADP-insensitive (E_2P) form. The $E_1P \rightarrow E_2P$ conversion is promoted by a low concentration of Mg (20 μM), whereas the reverse reaction ($E_2P \rightarrow E_1P$) requires a relatively high concentration of Ca^{2+} ($\simeq$1 mM). The inhibition of P_i liberation from E_2P at high Ca^{2+} concentration (2 mM) may be due to the accumulation of the E_1P form, which depletes the E_2P pool.

The rate of hydrolysis of E_2P into E + P_i is accelerated by MgATP, Mg^{2+}, and Ca^{2+}, and under all conditions the rate of E~P hydrolysis is similar to the steady-state rate of the overall process. Therefore it was suggested that in the absence of alkali metal ions the hydrolysis of E_2P limits the rate of overall ATP hydolysis. This explains why the ADP-insensitive E_2P is the dominant phosphoenzyme form in the absence of K^+ at high Mg^{2+} (2 mM) and low Ca^{2+} (20 μM) concentration.

In the presence of 2 mM Mg^{2+}, 93 mM KCl accelerates the hydrolysis of E_2P about 14-fold, whereas the K^+ stimulation of overall ATP hydrolysis is only about 4-fold. Since at 93 mM K^+ concentration the predominant phosphoenzyme form in steady state is E_1P, the rate-limiting step in the presence of K^+ is probably the $E_1P \rightarrow E_2P$ conversion. This explains the low steady-state concentration of E_2P in the presence of 0.1 M KCl. The K^+ stimulation of ATPase activity is slight at low Mg^{2+} and high Ca^{2+} concentrations, which shift the equilibrium greatly in favor of the E_1P form.

Large activation E-P hydrolysis by ATP was reported by de Meis and de Mello (118), although Kanazawa et al. (272) observed no ATP effect and Martonosi et al. (393) found only a slight activation. A possible explanation of these differences is that the experiments of de Meis and de Mello (118) were carried out in the absence of added alkali metal salts where E_2P is the dominant phosphoenzyme form and ATP activates E_2P decomposition. In assay systems that contain 0.1 M KCl (272, 393), ATP activation is not expected, since the rate-limiting step may be the conversion of E_1P into the E_2P form.

The observations indicate that the steady-state concentrations of various enzyme intermediates and the rate-limiting step of the overall reaction are subject to large variations, depending on the experimental conditions.

In media containing 2 mM MgATP and low Ca^{2+} (0.44 μM), Na^+ and K^+ inhibit the ATPase activity,

Ca^{2+} transport, and membrane phosphorylation. The inhibition is probably related to competition between K^+ or Na^+ and Ca^{2+} at the Ca^{2+}-binding site of the Ca^{2+}-transport ATPase (178, 491, 538, 540). Inhibition by Na^+ and K^+ was also observed at low ATP concentration (113, 114). The physiological significance of these effects is not clear.

REVERSAL OF THE CA^{2+} PUMP

The subject was recently reviewed (51, 122, 185–187, 672), and the brief discussion here is confined to selected aspects of the problem.

Ca^{2+} Release Induced by ADP + P_i

The rate of passive Ca^{2+} release from Ca^{2+}-loaded vesicles after transfer into media containing EGTA and Mg^{2+} is rather slow, about 1% of the initial rate of ATP-mediated Ca^{2+} uptake (375). The rate of Ca^{2+} release is accelerated 10- to 50-fold by the addition of ADP and inorganic orthophosphate (P_i) to the release medium (17). At pH 7.0 the Ca^{2+} outflux is optimally activated by 0.05 mM ADP and ~3 mM P_i. In the absence of Mg^{2+}, ADP + P_i are ineffective. Na^+ inhibits Ca^{2+} release (399).

The Ca^{2+} release is inhibited by ionized Ca^{2+} in the medium with a K_I of about 0.2 μM, which is similar to the apparent K_m of Ca^{2+} in the ATP-mediated Ca^{2+}-uptake reaction. The inhibition of ADP + P_i–induced Ca^{2+} release by micromolar Ca^{2+} concentration in the medium suggests the involvement of the same Ca^{2+}-binding site on the outside surface of the microsomes where the ATP-dependent Ca^{2+} transport is activated by calcium. Therefore it was suggested that the Ca^{2+} efflux represents a reversal of the ATP-dependent Ca^{2+} transport (17).

Ca^{2+} Gradient–Dependent Phosphorylation of ATPase by P_i

The ADP + P_i–induced Ca^{2+} release is accompanied by the formation of an acylphosphate enzyme intermediate from P_i (355, 356) that can donate its phosphate to ADP, yielding 1 mol ATP for two Ca^{2+} ions released across the membrane (356, 361, 667, 668). The pH stability and hydroxylamine sensitivity of the phosphoenzyme formed from P_i is identical to the phosphorylated intermediate formed from ATP (356, 667).

The formation of phosphoenzyme from P_i by Ca^{2+}-loaded microsomes is inhibited competitively by the binding of ATP on the outside surface of the membrane (667), and only medium phosphate serves as substrate for enzyme phosphorylation (117). These observations indicate that P_i interacts with the ATPase on the external surface.

The level of enzyme phosphorylation by P_i depends on the magnitude of the Ca^{2+}-concentration gradient (667). Abolition of the Ca^{2+} gradient by treatment of the vesicles with ether, phospholipases, detergents, and Ca^{2+} ionophores inhibits the synthesis of ATP (361, 611). The relationship between the steady-state concentration of phosphoenzyme and the Ca^{2+} gradient suggests the binding of 2 mol Ca^{2+}/mol ATPase, in agreement with the 2 Ca:1 ATP stoichiometry of Ca^{2+} release (667).

These observations led to the conclusion that the energy required for ATP synthesis during the ADP + P_i-induced Ca^{2+} release is derived from the Ca^{2+} gradient across the membrane (17, 186, 187, 355, 356, 361, 667). The calculated free-energy change for chemiosmotic coupling ($\simeq -12$ kcal/mol) is sufficient for the synthesis of the high-energy acylphosphate intermediate and ATP (187, 667). Under appropriate conditions, Ca^{2+} gradient–dependent formation of PP_i from P_i was also observed (194).

The Ca^{2+} gradient-dependent phosphorylation of the ATPase in a medium containing EGTA, Mg, and P_i but no ADP yields 2–4 nmol phosphoprotein/mg protein, which represents about one-half of the calculated concentration of ATPase-active sites. Phosphorylation of the enzyme in the absence of the ADP does not induce Ca^{2+} release. The subsequent addition of ADP to the phosphorylated microsomes decreases the level of phosphoprotein, with synthesis of ATP and enhancement of the rate of Ca^{2+} efflux (115, 356, 667). Therefore the fast release of calcium accompanies the transfer of phosphate from the phosphoenzyme to ADP (361). The ATP synthesized during reversal of Ca^{2+} transport is released from the microsomes into the outside medium (121, 298, 361).

Arsenate-Induced Ca^{2+} Release

A rapid release of calcium from Ca^{2+}-loaded microsomes was observed in media containing EGTA, Mg, and 0.5–5 mM arsenate. The K_m for arsenate was ~8 mM. The Ca^{2+} release induced by arsenate suggests the transient formation of an arsenylated enzyme intermediate that by spontaneous hydrolysis allows Ca^{2+} efflux (192). Mg^{2+} is apparently required for the arsenylation of the enzyme. The Ca^{2+} release is inhibited noncompetitively by ADP and P_i. The maximum rate of arsenate-induced Ca^{2+} release is similar to that obtained with ADP + P_i. These observations are consistent with the view that ADP promotes Ca^{2+} release from the vesicles by increasing the rate of dephosphorylation of ADP-sensitive phosphoenzyme intermediate, yielding ATP.

Mechanism of Ca^{2+} Release Induced by ADP + P_i

The reaction steps involved in the reversal of Ca^{2+} transport are most conveniently discussed in terms of the minimum reaction mechanism given in the scheme on p. 436 (122, 523). Two functional states of the enzyme are distinguished: E and *E.

FORWARD REACTION. The E form of the enzyme binds Ca^{2+} (step 1) on the outside surface with high affinity ($K_m \simeq 0.2$–$2.0\ \mu M$), followed by phosphorylation with NTPs (steps 2–3) but not with P_i. Phosphorylation of the enzyme initiates the translocation of Ca^{2+} from the outside to the inside surface (step 4) and its eventual release into the lumen (step 5). Mg^{2+}-dependent hydrolysis of *E-P (steps 6–7) and the conversion of *E to E (step 8) complete the cycle. The interconversion between *E and E (step 8) may be one of the rate-limiting steps during Ca^{2+} transport (75, 625). The reaction sequence in the forward direction, which leads to the ATP-dependent accumulation of calcium, was discussed in the section on MECHANISM OF ATP HYDROLYSIS AND CA^{2+} TRANSPORT, p. 436.

REVERSE REACTIONS. The Ca^{2+}-binding site of the *E form faces the interior [(70); see, however, ref. 180], and it is characterized by low Ca^{2+} affinity ($K_m \simeq 1$ mM). The *E form can be phosphorylated with P_i but not by NTP.

The reverse reactions, which contribute to the ADP + P_i–induced Ca^{2+} release, are initiated by the phosphorylation of the *E form of the enzyme with P_i in the absence of external Ca^{2+} (steps 7 and 6), followed by binding of internal Ca^{2+} (step 5) and the conversion of an ADP-insensitive $^{Ca}_{Ca}{*E}{\sim}P$ intermediate into an ADP-sensitive $^{Ca}_{Ca}E{\sim}P$ form (step 4). The $^{Ca}_{Ca}E{\sim}P$ donates its phosphoryl group to ADP (step 3) with synthesis of ATP (step 2) and the release of Ca^{2+} (step 1) on the outside.

The inhibition of gradient-dependent enzyme phosphorylation with P_i at high Ca^{2+} concentration in medium is related to the accumulation of the $^{Ca}_{Ca}E$ form of the enzyme and a corresponding decrease in the concentration of the *E form, which serves as phosphate acceptor. Similarly the inhibition by ATP may involve the accumulation of E·ATP complex with a decrease in *E. High internal Ca^{2+} concentration is required to convert the ADP-insensitive *E-P complex into the ADP-sensitive $^{Ca}_{Ca}E{\sim}P$ form.

Ca^{2+} Gradient–Independent Phosphorylation of Ca^{2+}-ATPase by P_i

The Ca^{2+}-ATPase can also be phosphorylated by P_i in the absence of a transmembrane Ca^{2+} gradient with the formation of a phosphoenzyme intermediate (267, 268, 270, 298, 398, 611). Under optimum conditions (pH 6.0, 2–4 mM P_i, 10 mM Mg, 1 mM EGTA) the steady-state concentration of phosphoenzyme (2–3 nmol/mg protein) is similar to that obtained by gradient-dependent phosphorylation (115). The phosphoenzyme formation is inhibited by Ca^{2+} and to a lesser extent by Na^+ and K^+. ATP and ADP compete with P_i for the phosphorylation site (115, 398). The Ca^{2+} concentration required for half-maximal activation of the enzyme phosphorylation by ATP is close to the Ca^{2+} concentration that produced 50% inhibition of the $E{\sim}P$ formation from P_i. The pH of the medium influences the affinity of the enzyme for Ca^{2+}, P_i, and ATP. The pH optimum for membrane phosphorylation by P_i is 6.0. At pH 5.7 the Ca^{2+} concentration required for 50% inhibition of enzyme phosphorylation is 100 μM, whereas at pH 7.0 it is 1 μM. As the pH is increased from 6 to 7.5 the affinity of the enzyme for P_i decreases and for ATP increases, irrespective of the transmembrane Ca^{2+} gradient (115). The pH optima for ATP synthesis and for enzyme phosphorylation are slightly different. The Mg and P_i randomly bind to the enzyme to form Mg·E·P ternary complex, which eventually yields a Mg-phosphoprotein (301, 436, 469).

The steady-state concentration of gradient-independent phosphoenzyme increases markedly with increasing temperature (34, 267, 484, 610), yielding an apparent standard enthalpy change of 15.9 kcal/mol and an entropy change of 50.2 eu/mol. Therefore the phosphorylated enzyme is stabilized by a great increase in entropy (267, 270).

A high intravesicular Ca^{2+} concentration (Ca^{2+} gradient) increases the affinity of the enzyme for medium P_i, particularly at pH 7.0 (34, 115, 467). When a saturating concentration of P_i is added to vesicles that were preincubated with EGTA, the phosphorylation of the enzyme by P_i is a rapid process ($k \simeq 30$/s). The rate of phosphorylation is much slower ($k = 2$/s) using Ca^{2+}-loaded vesicles after brief incubation with EGTA (34, 75). Therefore the Ca^{2+} concentration inside the vesicles exerts great influence on the kinetics of phosphorylation and on the affinity of the enzyme for P_i, suggesting the predominance of different enzyme forms in Ca^{2+}-loaded and -unloaded vesicles.

If the phosphorylation reaction is started by the simultaneous addition of EGTA and P_i to vesicles preincubated with Ca^{2+}, a lag period of 30–50 ms precedes the increase in phosphoenzyme concentration (75, 484). At low and high intravesicular Ca^{2+} concentrations the lag period is similar and reflects the slow removal of Ca^{2+} from the high-affinity Ca^{2+}-binding sites on the outside surface of the microsomes (136, 484, 485). The removal of Ca^{2+} initiates the slow transformation of E to the *E form, which is the presumed acceptor for phosphorylation.

The rate constant of hydrolysis of gradient-dependent and gradient-independent phosphoenzymes measured by dilution of phosphate at pH 6.2 is 8–11/s, i.e., similar to the turnover of the enzyme operating with ATP as substrate (75). Much slower dephosphorylation rates were obtained when the decay of $E{\sim}P$ was initiated by Ca^{2+} alone (500 μM) (75, 121, 484, 628). Simultaneous addition of Ca^{2+} and ADP results in rapid phosphate transfer from $^{Ca}_{Ca}E{\sim}P$ to ADP, yielding ATP.

The gradient-dependent phosphorylation of microsomes by P_i yields a phosphoenzyme that reacts with

ADP to form ATP (ADP-sensitive phosphoenzyme). On the other hand the gradient-independent phosphoenzyme obtained by phosphorylation of Ca^{2+}-free microsomes or purified ATPase cannot synthesize ATP (ADP-insensitive phosphoenzyme) (34, 115). These observations raised the question (186, 187) whether the ADP-sensitive and ADP-insensitive phosphoenzymes are intermediates of the same reaction sequence or parts of parallel or branched pathways.

Knowles and Racker (298) observed that phosphorylation of purified Ca^{2+}-transport ATPase by P_i in media containing EGTA and Mg^{2+} at pH 6.3 yields ADP-insensitive phosphoenzyme, which after addition of ADP and 3–10 mM Ca^{2+} transfers its phosphate to ADP, yielding ATP. The formation of ATP and the disappearance of phosphoenzyme are fast processes with half times of the order of 20–40 ms (121). The ATP is released from the enzyme and it is free in solution available to hexokinase. Ca^{2+} gradient–dependent formation of pyrophosphate was also observed (194).

These experiments suggest that the ADP-insensitive phosphoenzyme is the precursor of the ADP-sensitive form and acquires the ability to synthesize ATP when the internal low-affinity Ca^{2+}-binding sites of the ATPase are saturated with calcium. As the synthesis of ADP takes place without an ion gradient across the membrane, the energy for ATP synthesis is probably derived from ion-protein interactions.

Role of Ca^{2+}-Protein Interactions in ATP Synthesis

Significant gradient-independent phosphorylation of the Ca^{2+}-ATPase by P_i occurs at 0.6 mM medium Ca^{2+} concentration at pH 5.0, since at low pH the Ca^{2+} binding to the high-affinity binding sites is minimized. At pH 8.0 the affinity of Ca^{2+}-binding sites increases, and the same Ca^{2+} concentration provides sufficient saturation of the internal low-affinity binding sites to allow the transfer of phosphate from $*E{\sim}P$ to ADP (121). Therefore phosphorylation of the enzyme by P_i at pH 5.0 in the presence of 0.6 mM Ca^{2+} followed by the addition of ADP and sufficient KOH to adjust the pH to 8.0 should lead to significant ATP synthesis. This was in fact observed (121). Under these conditions, ATP synthesis occurs in the absence of a Ca^{2+} gradient; the pH jump is used merely to modify the Ca^{2+} affinity of the low- and high-affinity Ca^{2+}-binding sites. These experiments emphasize the importance of Ca^{2+}-protein interactions as the source of energy for ATP synthesis.

Vale et al. (611) observed that on release of membrane-bound Ca^{2+} by EGTA in the presence of X-537A, which is presumed to abolish Ca^{2+} gradients, synthesis of ATP occurs.

In the absence of a Ca^{2+} gradient, the driving force for the incorporation of phosphate into the protein is the high P_i concentration and the removal of Ca^{2+} from the high-affinity site of the Ca^{2+}-ATPase (187). While these conditions favor the accumulation of the *E enzyme form, this is barely sufficient to form a high-energy acylphosphate bond. In contrast plentiful energy is available for enzyme phosphorylation when at low external Ca^{2+} concentration the intravesicular Ca^{2+} concentration is 1–10 mM.

$P_i \leftrightarrows$ HOH Exchange

Kanazawa, Boyer, and Ariki (51, 268) observed that gradient-independent phosphorylation of SR vesicles by P_i in the presence of Mg^{2+} and EGTA at pH 7.0 is accompanied by a rapid incorporation of water oxygen atoms into P_i ($P_i \leftrightarrows$ HOH exchange). The bridge oxygen in the acylphosphate intermediate is provided by the carboxyl group. The acylphosphate is cleaved by water oxygen attack on the phosphorus atom, and it is re-formed by attack of carboxylate oxygen on the phosphorus atom, with displacement of a hydroxyl group (15, 51, 98). The $P_i \leftrightarrows$ HOH exchange was inhibited by medium Ca^{2+}; half-maximal inhibition was obtained at a medium Ca^{2+} concentration of 2 μM. The Hill coefficient for the Ca^{2+} effect was 1.8. Although only a small amount of phosphoenzyme was formed under these conditions, the rate of oxygen exchange was 10–15 times greater than the maximum rate of Ca^{2+}-activated ATP cleavage, indicating that the turnover rate of phosphoenzyme is approximately 300/s. The $P_i \leftrightarrows$ HOH exchange is also observed on SR membranes solubilized by Triton X-100 (267).

The oxygen exchange results from dynamic reversal of steps 6 and 7 of the scheme on p. 436 (53). At pH 6.0 in the absence of external Ca^{2+} the *E-P enzyme form accumulates. The rate of labeling of the phosphoenzyme by $^{32}P_i$ is sufficiently rapid ($t_{1/2}$ = 30–40 ms) to explain the rate of $P_i \leftrightarrows$ HOH exchange. The inhibition of $P_i \leftrightarrows$ HOH exchange by Ca^{2+} is explained by reactions 1, 7, and 8, which leads to the accumulation of ${}^{Ca}_{Ca}E$ form and a decrease of *E concentration, with inhibition of phosphorylation by P_i.

NTP $\leftrightarrows$ P_i Exchange

The Ca^{2+} gradient-dependent and gradient-independent enzyme phosphorylations are inhibited when the high-affinity Ca^{2+}-binding sites of the Ca^{2+}-ATPase are saturated with Ca^{2+} (122). The Ca^{2+} inhibition is relieved by various NTPs (70, 116, 118, 120, 355, 357, 400, 466, 600, 628).

Vesicles incubated in the presence of ATP, ADP, Mg, $^{32}P_i$, and 0.2 mM Ca^{2+} actively accumulate Ca^{2+} with the hydrolysis of ATP until a steady state is reached. The rapid $^{45}Ca^{2+}$ exchange through the membrane at steady state is accompanied by incorporation of $^{32}P_i$ into ATP (355, 357). Therefore, simultaneously with ATP hydrolysis, ATP synthesis from ADP + P_i takes place. Under these conditions enzyme phosphorylation by P_i occurs at high Ca^{2+} concentrations in medium, because the forward reaction of ATP-mediated Ca^{2+} transport generates sufficient *E enzyme form to react with P_i. Similar observations were made using various NTPs or acetylphosphate as energy donors for Ca^{2+} transport instead of ATP (120). The inhibition of $P_i \leftrightarrows$ HOH exchange by medium Ca^{2+} is also reduced by NTPs (116) or acetylphosphate (268) by the same mechanism.

Under these conditions the enzyme is simultaneously phosphorylated by P_i and by NTP or acetylphosphate; the portion of enzyme phosphorylated by P_i depends on the relative affinity, concentration, and kinetic properties of the various substrates, which define the concentration of enzyme intermediates in the cycle (122). For example, the relatively low rate of $P_i \leftrightarrows$ ATP as compared with $P_i \leftrightarrows$ ITP exchange is presumably due to more effective competition by ATP for the binding site of P_i and the increased conversion of *E to E in the presence of ATP (70).

PHYSICAL BASIS OF CA^{2+} TRANSLOCATION

Two main classes of mechanisms were considered for the ATP-energized transfer of Ca^{2+} across the membrane (553). In the *rotating carrier mechanisms* the transport protein rotates or diffuses through the membrane carrying the bound Ca^{2+} from one surface to the other (393, 599, 672). This mechanism implies massive reorientation of the transport protein in the membrane connected with each transport cycle. In various types of *pore mechanisms* the transport protein or its oligomers form a channel that spans the thickness of the membrane. In one state the active site is exposed to the outside, while in the other state to the inside, and the translocation of Ca^{2+} occurs by transition between the two states. The energy level of the two states is not very different, and the conversion from the lower- to the higher-energy state may be driven by the free energy of ligand binding, the energy of ATP hydrolysis, or the membrane potential (250, 393, 474, 527, 543, 554, 672). These mechanisms require only minor changes in the conformation of the protein.

Distinction between the two types of models may be made by testing the effect of antibodies directed against the Ca^{2+}-transport ATPase on the rate of ATP hydrolysis and Ca^{2+} transport. If a rotating carrier mechanism operates, attachment of antibody to the Ca^{2+}-transport ATPase is expected to reduce the rate of Ca^{2+} transport, since passage of the attached antibody through the membrane would involve a prohibitively large change in free energy.

The Ca^{2+}-activated ATPase and Ca^{2+}-transport activities of rabbit skeletal muscle microsomes were not inhibited in the absence of complement by sheep or guinea pig antisera or immunoglobulin G directed against the Ca^{2+}-ATPase (389). Similarly no inhibition of ATPase activity and Ca^{2+} transport was observed on binding of anti-2,4-dinitrophenyl antibodies to SR membranes covalently tagged with dinitrophenylcadaverine (137). The inhibition of the Ca^{2+} transport of chicken skeletal muscle SR by rabbit antiserum against chicken Ca^{2+}-transport ATPase occurred without an effect on the Ca^{2+}-dependent ATP hydrolysis (563) and therefore does not indicate inhibition of the Ca^{2+} pump. On the basis of these observations, a major reorientation of the Ca^{2+}-transport ATPase is not required for Ca^{2+} translocation. Together with thermodynamic considerations (543), this fact suggests that carrier rotation is an unlikely mechanism for Ca^{2+} transport.

Tonomura and Morales (599) measured the rate of reduction of maleimide spin labels covalently attached to SR by externally added ascorbate. The time course of reduction indicated two components. The fast component was assigned to spin labels on the outside and the slow component to spin labels on the inside surface of SR. The ratio of the fast to the slow components decreased under conditions that favor E-P formation and Ca^{2+} transport. This was attributed to rotation of the transport protein, with relocation of externally bound spin label to the vesicle interior. A more likely explanation is that the biphasic reduction of spin labels by ascorbate indicates two populations of different reactivity. The following evidence argues in favor of this interpretation:

1. Ascorbate rapidly penetrates across SR membranes. Because the vesicles are unable to maintain significant membrane potential in the presence of 80 mM KCl (33), the concentration of ascorbate on the two sides of the membrane is expected to be equal during much of the reaction time of ascorbate reduction measurements. Therefore the biphasic kinetics of reduction cannot be attributed to different ascorbate concentrations on the outside and inside of the vesicles.
2. When the slowly penetrating nickel and ferricyanide ions were used as line-broadening agents for signals arising from spin labels located on the outside, no significant differences were observed, which could be attributed to rotation of the carrier during the formation of E-ATP and E-P enzyme complexes (77).
3. The spin-labeled SH groups are apparently located only on the outside of the vesicles (77), in agreement with the highly asymmetric distribution of Hg-azoferritin in sonicated microsomes (188).
4. The biphasic quenching kinetics with ascorbate is still observed after solubilization of the membranes by deoxycholate or Triton X-100 (437).

In the light of these observations a more likely interpretation of the ascorbate reduction data of Tonomura and Morales (599) is that the reactivity of spin labels attached to the outside surface of microsomes is altered by conformational changes of the enzyme during transition between the different enzyme states, without transmembrane reorientation of major portions of the molecule (77).

As a rotary motion of the Ca^{2+}-ATPase is not supported by immunological and ESR data, the attention of most investigators now turns toward various channel mechanisms. These involve relatively minor, localized conformational changes of the Ca^{2+}-ATPase that may be linked to specific steps of the Ca^{2+}-transport cycle. The conformational changes are reflected in changes of ESR signals, tryptophan fluorescence, the fluorescence of extrinsic fluorophores, and in altered reactivity of SH, lysine, arginine, and histidine residues in various phases of the transport cycle (see MECHANISM OF ATP HYDROLYSIS AND CA^{2+} TRANSPORT, p 436.)

Several speculative channel mechanisms of Ca^{2+} translocation were proposed that vary in detail (137, 471, 474, 476, 528, 585, 672). Relevant experimental evidence is lacking, however, and the physical basis of Ca^{2+} translocation remains essentially unknown.

PROTEIN-PROTEIN INTERACTIONS IN SR AND THEIR FUNCTIONAL SIGNIFICANCE

Interactions between lipoprotein complexes are common in biological membranes and presumably contribute to the wide range of cooperative phenomena expressed in excitability, transport processes, receptor functions, and enzymatic activity. Recent evidence obtained by enzyme kinetic, electron-microscopic, ultracentrifuge, and fluorescence-energy transfer techniques indicates that the Ca^{2+}-transport ATPase of SR may also represent a self-associating system in which oligomers (dimers, trimers, and tetramers) of the enzyme are present in equilibrium with monomers. The estimated concentration of Ca^{2+}-transport ATPase in SR membranes of adult animals is about 3–6 mM, which is expected to promote such interactions.

This section points out the strengths and weaknesses of the evidence and analyzes the physiological perspectives that may give relevance to the existence of ATPase oligomers.

Electron Microscopy

The density of 85-Å intramembrane particles seen by freeze-etch electron microscopy in native SR membranes and in reconstituted ATPase vesicles (2,500–4,000/μm^2) is 4–6 times less than the density of 40-Å surface particles (13,000–16,000/μm^2) observed by negative staining (255, 378). Both sets of particles are associated with the Ca^{2+}-transport ATPase. In favorably oriented regions of the negatively stained SR membrane the 40-Å surface particles frequently appear in clusters, which can be resolved into four subunits (394, 613) by image enhancement techniques (366). The arrays of clustered subunits occur only on portions of the surface and their analysis requires some selection. On the basis of these observations we suggested that the 85-Å intramembranous particles may represent ATPase tetramers, which are resolved as individual 40-Å particles after negative staining (255, 378, 613). The calculated concentration of ATPase polypeptide chains in the membrane (12,000–17,000/μm^2) is close to the observed density of 40-Å particles, supporting this proposition. These observations were confirmed by Scales and Inesi (510) with deep etching in addition to negative staining for the visualization of 40-Å surface particles. An essentially identical relationship between intramembranous and surface particles was found in the case of Na^+-K^+-ATPase (109).

Because the particle clusters obtained on SR membranes and on reconstituted ATPase vesicles (which do not contain accessory proteins) were similar, the minor protein components of SR are not likely to contribute to the visible particle counts (255, 378).

The observations with the electron microscope imply that under conditions of freeze-fracture essentially all ATPase molecules are present in the form of oligomers.

The properties of interacting protein systems are sharply dependent on protein concentration, raising the possibility that in membranes of low ATPase content, dissociation of oligomers may lead to changes in function. In early phases of embryonic development the ATPase content of SR is 10–20 times less than in adult animals (47, 376, 595). Yet even under these conditions the density of 85-Å freeze-etch particles is proportional to the ATPase content of the membrane, as judged by the ATPase activity, the rate of Ca^{2+} transport, and the concentration of Ca^{2+}-transport sites determined by labeling with [^{32}P]ATP and by PAGE. The increase in 85-Å freeze-etch particle density during subsequent development parallels the changes in Ca^{2+}-transport activity. Therefore there is no indication from electron-microscopic and transport data that a 10- to 20-fold change in the ATPase concentration would significantly alter either the equilibrium between monomers and oligomers or the transport properties of the ATPase membrane. The same conclusions apply to reconstituted ATPase vesicles of varied ATPase:lipid ratio, although the range of ATPase content in this case is limited (255, 639).

The interpretation of data from the electron microscope is subject to the usual limitations. We have no information about the extent of redistribution of ATPase molecules in the membrane during specimen preparations. Uncertainties in the calculation of the surface area and ATPase content may have led to overestimation of the ATPase polypeptide chain density in the membrane; this raises the possibility that each 85-Å particle may correspond to one ATPase molecule with several polypeptide segments projecting into the water phase, which are visualized by negative staining as 40-Å particles. Stronger evidence in favor of the oligomer structure of 85-Å particles would be provided by their resolution into component subunits using rotary shadowing.

Fluorescence-Energy Transfer

Resonance-energy transfer between pairs of fluorophores of appropriate excitation and emission characteristics proved useful for distance measurements within protein molecules (559). We employed this method for the assessment of distances between Ca^{2+}-transport ATPase molecules in reconstituted membranes (394, 613). The experiments were performed as follows: one portion of a Ca^{2+}-transport ATPase preparation was labeled with *N*-iodoacetyl-*N*′-(5-sulfo-1-naphthyl) ethylenediamine (IAEDANS) as fluorescence-energy donor and another portion with iodoacetamidofluorescein (IAF) as fluorescence-energy acceptor. In reconstituted vesicles containing both donor- and acceptor-labeled ATPase molecules, fluorescence-energy transfer was observed, as judged by the ratio of donor and acceptor fluorescence intensities and by the effect of acceptor ATPase molecules on the rate of decay of donor fluorescence. The observed energy transfer was not influenced by a 10-fold dilution of the lipid phase of the membrane with egg lecithin or by changes in the temperature between 6°C and 37°C, but it was abolished by the addition of unlabeled ATPase. Although the data obtained so far support the idea that a major part of the energy transfer occurs within oligomers containing several ATPase molecules, which do not dissociate measurably after 10-fold dilution of the lipid phase, further experiments at widely different ATPase:lipid ratios are necessary to assess accurately the contribution of collision between ATPase molecules in the membrane to the observed energy transfer (153). The abolition of energy transfer within a few minutes after addition of unlabeled ATPase indicates a relatively rapid exchange between unlabeled and labeled ATPase molecules in the oligomers.

It is not possible to predict from these experiments the size of the oligomers or the average distance between donor and acceptor fluorophores, but the method promises to be useful for following dynamic changes in the equilibrium between monomers and oligomers during ATP-mediated Ca^{2+} transport or Ca^{2+} release.

Electron Spin Resonance Studies

Immobilization of a spin-labeled fatty acid chain covalently attached to the Ca^{2+}-ATPase also suggests an interaction between ATPase molecules (12, 123). The percentage of the immobilized component decreased with increasing temperature. Partial dissociation of the hypothetical ATPase oligomers was observed on perturbation of membrane structure with a low concentration of detergent (12). Alternative interpretations of the data are different conformational states of the ATPase and partitioning of the probe between different lipid layers (12).

ATPase-ATPase Interactions in Detergent Solutions

Enzymatically active molecular dispersions of Ca^{2+}-ATPase can be obtained by solubilization with anionic and nonionic detergents. These preparations should permit an accurate evaluation of the role of protein-protein interactions in the regulation of enzymatic activity (104, 105, 263, 321–323, 425, 492–494, 583).

In early reports (104, 323), with Tween 80 and dodecyl octaoxyethyleneglycol monoether ($C_{12}E_8$) used for solubilization of ATPase, the enzymatic activity was found to be associated with the oligomers; more recent reports generally emphasize that a major part of the ATPase activity is in the monomer fraction (105, 263, 321, 322, 425). The tentative conclusion at this stage is that although the ATPase activity does not require an oligomeric structure, the self-association of the ATPase is promoted to such extent by phospholipids that it is likely to exist in the native membranes in the form of oligomers. Radiation-inactivation data support this conclusion (623).

The ATPase activity of the monomer fraction differs with respect to cooperative kinetic features and stability from the ATPase of native membranes. The deoxycholate solubilized monomers require 0.4 M KCl and 0.3 M sucrose to maintain activity (263). The Ca^{2+} dependence of ATPase activity was similar to that of the vesicular ATPase with half-maximal activation at 0.01 μM Ca^{2+} (pH 8.0) and a Hill coefficient of 1.5. The K_m for MgATP at the high-affinity sites was also the same as in control microsomes (16 μM), but the secondary activation at high ATP concentrations was absent.

The monomeric ATPase preparations obtained by solubilization with $C_{12}E_8$ required Ca^{2+} or MgATP/MgADP for stability and rapidly lost activity after exposure to EGTA (425). The K_m for Ca^{2+} and ATP at the high-affinity sites and the secondary activation by ATP at concentrations higher than 100 μM, however, were similar in monomer and in vesicular preparations. The negative cooperativity of ATP hydrolysis at 2–50 μM ATP concentration was absent in the monomers. Oligomeric ATPase preparations derived from the monomers by DEAE cellulose chromatography reacquired the negative cooperativity and became more resistant to inactivation by EGTA, compared with the $C_{12}E_8$ solubilized monomers. These observations suggest that modulation by ATP and the resistance to inactivation by EGTA are properties that may arise from protein-protein interactions. There is no information about the role of protein-protein interactions in the regulation of Ca^{2+} transport.

Incorporation of Ca^{2+}-transport ATPase into phospholipid vesicles increases their passive Ca^{2+} permeability by several orders of magnitude (254, 255, 377). This raised the possibility that the Ca^{2+}-transport ATPase, in addition to its generally accepted role in Ca^{2+} transport, may also participate in the regulation of the passive Ca^{2+} permeability of the membrane. It was proposed that the oligomers of the Ca^{2+}-transport ATPase may represent a Ca^{2+} channel, and the equilibrium between monomers and oligomers would define the Ca^{2+} permeability (378, 380, 394). Further experiments are needed to test the validity of this suggestion.

Chemical Cross-Linking

Stabilization of interactions by cross-linking with bifunctional reagents followed by isolation and characterization of the covalently cross-linked complexes appears, in principle, a useful method for demonstrating the existence of ATPase oligomers in SR. In practice these methods rarely yield satisfactory results. The concentration of ATPase in the membrane is about 50 mg/ml and random cross-linking between ATPase molecules is likely to occur. Cross-linking of SR with different reagents led to the demonstration of dimers (331), tetramers (430), or hexamers (229). The stabilization of ATPase tetramers by cross-linking with Cu phenanthroline (430), however, could not be confirmed (81, 201, 330). Massive accumulation of high-molecular-weight aggregates during cross-linking with various reagents and loss of enzyme activity, even when significant amount of monomer was still present, raises the possibility that cross-linking with the reagents routinely used so far causes denaturation of the enzyme and may not reflect naturally occurring interactions. The problem should be reinvestigated with modern photoactivated cross-linking reagents (253), under conditions where random cross-linking is minimized (low temperature, millisecond reaction time, reconstituted ATPase vesicles of low protein:lipid ratio).

Effects of Inhibitors on ATPase Activity

In the presence of Ca^{2+}-chelating agents, dicyclohexylcarbodimide (DCCD) inhibits the Ca^{2+}-ATPase activity and Ca^{2+} transport (465). Ca^{2+} at micromolar concentrations specifically protects against DCCD inhibition, suggesting that DCCD may react with the Ca^{2+}-binding site of the ATPase. Much of the bound DCCD appears in the 20,000-dalton fragment of the ATPase, after tryptic hydrolysis.

Complete inhibition of ATPase activity is accompanied by the binding of 0.44 mol DCCD/mol enzyme, compared with binding of 0.2 mol DCCD/mol ATPase without inhibition in the presence of Ca^{2+}. Therefore the inhibition of ATPase activity is related to the binding of 0.24 mol DCCD/mol enzyme, which implies that 1 mol DCCD inhibits 4 mol ATPase. This is surprising, because in detergent-solubilized systems the ATPase monomers are enzymatically active; therefore side reactions of DCCD must be excluded (66) before the implied requirement for tetramers in ATP hydrolysis is accepted.

Fluorescein isothiocyanate (FITC) inhibits completely Ca^{2+} transport at FITC concentration one-half that of the ATPase protein, suggesting that the active ATPase unit may be a dimer (464). Because ATP protects specifically against FITC inhibition, FITC may react with a lysine residue at the nucleotide-binding site of the ATPase. After tryptic hydrolysis, the bound FITC was located in the 45,000-dalton subfragment, suggesting its involvement in the nucleotide binding.

Possibility of Subunit Heterogeneity

Madeira (348, 352) observed that isoelectric focusing of detergent-solubilized Ca^{2+}-transport ATPase yields several components with isoelectric points in the range of pH 5–6. The suggestion was made that these represent isoenzyme forms of the Ca^{2+}-transport ATPase with some differences in their primary structure. Although this possibility still exists, recent observations of Melgunov and Akimova (414) do not indicate subunit heterogeneity by isoelectric focusing after solubilization of SR in 10% Triton X-100.

The existence of two types of ATPase molecules was inferred by Ikemoto et al. (227, 228) from the observation that EGTA releases the Ca^{2+} bound to high-affinity binding sites much faster from about one-half of the ATPase molecules than from the other half. Whether this is due to the constraint imposed by the structure of the oligomer or represents chemical heterogeneity of the molecules is not known.

There are major differences in the specific Ca^{2+}-transport activity of SR isolated from fast, slow, and cardiac muscles (257, 375), so the likelihood for the presence of muscle-specific Ca^{2+}-ATPase isoenzymes is great (640). Immunological differences between cardiac and skeletal Ca^{2+}-transport ATPases have in fact been observed (107). The presence of chemically distinct Ca^{2+}-ATPase isoenzymes in muscles containing mixed fiber types could explain some of the observed heterogeneity.

Conclusion

In summary, evidence from kinetic, electron-microscopic, ultracentrifuge, fluorescence energy-transfer, and inhibition studies suggests the existence of ATPase oligomers in SR membranes and in systems containing the purified Ca^{2+}-transport ATPase. None of this evidence is conclusive if taken independently. Since ATPase monomers are active in ATP cleavage, oligomer formation may have significance in the allosteric regulatory aspects of ATP hydrolysis. The possible role of oligomers in Ca^{2+} translocation and in the regulation of the Ca^{2+} permeability of the membrane remains to be established.

PERMEABILITY OF SR

The permeability of rabbit SR vesicles to various solutes, determined by isotope exchange, increases as follows: sucrose, Ca^{2+}, Mn^{2+} < gluconate$^-$, choline$^+$, Tris$^+$, < methanesulfonate$^-$ < urea, glycerol, K^+, Na^+, Li^+, Cl^- (255, 411). Although the permeability to Ca^{2+} is relatively low, it is still 4–6 orders of magnitude greater than the Ca^{2+} permeability of phospholipid bilayers (106, 255, 375, 392, 617). The permeability to

K^+, Na^+, and Cl^- is so high that it is difficult to measure by isotope exchange and Millipore filtration (129, 255, 276, 277, 402, 403).

A better kinetic resolution is obtained by measuring the volume changes of SR vesicles equilibrated in 5 mM 2-amino-2-hydroxymethyl-1,3-propanediol-maleate (Tris-maleate, pH 6.5) and 2 mM KCl after dilution with buffer solutions containing the various penetrant molecules at the concentrations indicated in Table 6 (273, 275, 302). The volume change was followed by monitoring the 90° light scattering in a stopped-flow spectrophotometer. The permeation time (τ) is defined as the time required to reach half-maximal change in light-scattering intensity. The permeability coefficient $P = 0.231\ (r/\tau)$, where r is the average radius of the vesicles (275). The permeability of cations seems to be related to their hydrated ionic radii. The permeability of Cl^- is 50 times greater than that of K^+, indicating the presence of anion channels, which may be similar to those of red blood cell membranes (19–21, 293–295).

Monovalent-Cation Channels in SR

The isotope spaces of SR vesicles for [^3H]choline, ^{22}Na, and ^{86}Rb were measured after equilibration with the isotope and dilution into unlabeled medium of identical composition. The efflux of the radioactive compounds monitored by Millipore filtration (255, 277, 402, 403) yielded a choline space of 3 μl/mg protein that is close to the internal space of the vesicles (129). The apparent isotope space for Na^+ and Rb^+ was about one-third of the choline space; this implies that two-thirds of the ^{22}Na and ^{86}Rb were rapidly lost from the vesicles within 20–30 s after dilution into the isotope-free medium (402, 403). The remaining $^{22}Na^+$ and $^{86}Rb^+$ were released from the vesicles at a rate similar to that of choline. The SR preparations are therefore likely to contain two types of vesicles (402, 403). Type I, which represents about two-thirds of the vesicle population, is highly permeable to Na^+ and Rb^+, whereas in type II vesicles the permeability of the membrane for Na^+, Rb^+ and choline is similar (402, 403). These findings suggest that SR membranes contain channels for small cations like Na^+ and K^+. The unequal distribution of these channels among type I and II vesicles may be due to low channel density in the membrane, which results in the formation of significant numbers of channel-free vesicles or to preferential localization of cation channels in some elements of sarcoplasmic reticulum. The role of these channels may be to minimize osmotic and charge effects during Ca^{2+} transport and release.

The K^+ channels in SR were further investigated by Sergeeva et al. (525) and by Miller and his co-workers (92, 419, 422, 423) in planar phospholipid bilayer membranes (BLM). On addition of SR vesicles and 0.5 mM Ca^{2+} to one side of a bilayer made of 30% phosphatidylserine and 70% phosphatidylethanolamine, the membrane conductance increases due to Ca^{2+}-induced fusion of SR vesicles with the BLM (420, 421). The process is aided by osmotic swelling of the vesicles during fusion. The conductance change is quantal, and each jump in conductance may reflect the fusion of a single SR vesicle. It is estimated that in a usual experiment only 1 out of 10^9 vesicles fuses over a 10-min period (421). This raises the possibility that the vesicles that fuse may not originate from the SR. The conductance channels are incorporated into the membrane irreversibly with uniform orientation (419, 423). The channels can be blocked with Ca^{2+} on the *cis* (cytoplasmic) side (419), with transition metals on the *trans* (luminal) side, and with SH-group reagents on both sides (423). The single-channel K^+ conductance is 3–5 times greater than the Na^+ conductance. The K^+ conductance is blocked in a voltage-dependent manner by Cs^+ (92).

In membranes containing a large number of channels, the K^+ conductance is voltage dependent, but the open-state conductance of individual channels is not influenced by potential (419, 422). An alkaline proteinase B isolated from pronase of *Streptomyces griseus* reduced the voltage dependence of K^+ conductance when added to the *trans* side of the membrane (422). The kinetics of the proteinase effect was voltage dependent, suggesting that the enzyme can react only with the open state of the channel. The results imply that proteinase treatment reduces the gating charge that regulates the transition between the open and closed states of the channel, perhaps by cleaving lysine and arginine residues from the gating polypeptide (422). These elegant experiments raise

TABLE 6. *Permeability Properties of Sarcoplasmic Reticulum Membrane*

Species	Final Concn, mM	Permeation Time (τ), s	$\Delta I/I_0$
KCl	50	10	0.45
K acetate	50	10	0.45
K propionate	50	10	0.45
K butyrate	50	10	0.45
K_2 oxalate	35	90	0.51
K methanesulfonate	50	50	0.48
Na methanesulfonate	50	50	0.48
NaCl	50	13	0.45
LiCl	50	18	0.48
RbCl	50	8	0.45
Choline-Cl	50	360	0.69
Tris-Cl	50	600	0.73
$MgCl_2$	33	1,800	0.75
$CaCl_2$	33	6,000	0.75
K_2-EDTA	20	3,000	0.51
Tris-maleate	50	900	0.71
$K_2HPO_4 + KH_2PO_4$	14	25	0.26
Thiourea	100	0.6	0.69
Urea	100	1.2	0.69
Ethylene glycol	100	0.6	0.69
Glycerol	100	1.8	0.69
Glucose	100	1,500	0.69
H_2O		0.1	

[From Kometani and Kasai (302).]

important questions about the localization of K^+ channels within the sarcotubular system and their physiological significance.

The role of the K^+ channels, provided they are genuine components of the SR, may be to maintain the even distribution of Na^+ and K^+ across the two sides of the membrane (544). As depolarization of SR is not likely to contribute to Ca^{2+} release (33) and in the resting state SR membranes probably do not maintain a transmembrane potential (544), it is unlikely that K^+ channels would participate in the primary processes of muscle activation. The contribution of T tubules that are capable of propagative depolarization (93, 94, 96) to the observed cation channels is unknown.

Anion Channels in SR

The Ca^{2+}-storage capacity of SR increases 50- to 100-fold in the presence of Ca^{2+}-precipitating anions, like oxalate, phosphate, pyrophosphate, and fluoride (189, 387, 388). The enhanced Ca^{2+}-storage capacity is best explained by assuming that anions follow passively the active accumulation of Ca^{2+}, as their Ca^{2+} salts precipitate within the SR.

Beil et al. (35) observed that in Ca^{2+}-uptake media containing both phosphate and oxalate, phosphate may compete with oxalate uptake and cause an inhibition of oxalate-potentiated Ca^{2+} transport. They suggested the existence of a highly cooperative anion-gating mechanism in SR, which may be an integral part of the Ca^{2+}-transport system (35, 198). This conclusion is consistent with the high permeability of SR to various anions (129, 275, 411).

In analogy with the anion channel of erythrocytic membranes (19–21, 60, 293–295), the permeability of SR for Cl, P_i, and methanesulfonate is inhibited by 4-acetamido 4′-isothiocyanostilbene-2,2′-disulfonate (SITS), with a slight increase in the permeability of Na^+, K^+, choline$^+$, and glycerol (274). The inhibition of anion penetration requires 5 μmol SITS/g protein, and most of the inhibitor was found covalently attached to a protein of ~100,000 daltons, which may be the Ca^{2+}-transport ATPase.

Carley and Racker (65) solubilized the anion transport complex of SR, but no detailed characterization of its properties is available (477).

The probable significance of anion channels in SR is to permit the exchange of metabolic anions, phosphate, and chloride across the membrane, which may contribute to the buffering of the large osmotic and electrical effects connected with the transport and release of Ca^{2+} during muscle activity. It is also likely that SR contains some enzyme systems that require free penetration of anionic substrates and products across the membrane (375). The anion channels are not permeable for ATP and ADP (652).

Sucrose-gradient fractionation of microsomes loaded with Ca^{2+} in the presence of oxalate indicates that only about 30%–40% of the vesicles are readily loaded with Ca-oxalate, whereas the remainder either do not accumulate Ca^{2+} or accumulate Ca^{2+} only after prolonged incubation (511). These observations suggest a heterogeneity of the vesicle population in Ca^{2+}-ATPase content, passive Ca^{2+} permeability, or in the density of anion channels, which facilitates the entry of oxalate into the vesicles.

Effect of Membrane Proteins on Permeability of SR Membranes

The permeability of isolated SR vesicles for anions, cations, and neutral molecules is far greater (129, 255, 375) than that of mitochondria (64, 413) and surface membranes from muscle and other cells (44, 181, 489).

Because the ion permeability of artificial phospholipid bilayers formed from SR lipids is very small, the relatively high anion and cation permeability of SR probably reflects the contribution of membrane proteins (106, 254, 255, 392).

ROLE OF CA^{2+}-ATPASE IN THE REGULATION OF CA^{2+} PERMEABILITY. Incorporation of the Mg^{2+}-Ca^{2+}-ATPase into artificial phospholipid bilayers increased the Ca^{2+} permeability to levels approaching that of SR (255, 377, 384). The permeability of the vesicles for sucrose, Na^+, choline, and SO_4 also increased, indicating that the Ca^{2+}-transport ATPase did not act as a specific Ca^{2+} channel. The high-affinity Ca^{2+}-binding protein and calsequestrin had no effect on the Ca^{2+} permeability (255). The conductance of planar BLM also increased on the addition of succinylated Ca^{2+}-ATPase (529). The hypothetical Ca^{2+} channel may be intramolecular or may arise from interaction among several Ca^{2+}-ATPase molecules in the membrane (378, 380, 394).

Tryptic cleavage of the Ca^{2+}-ATPase produces a 55,000- and a 45,000-dalton fragment. Further hydrolysis of the 55,000-dalton unit gives a 30,000-dalton fragment containing the phosphorylation site of the Ca^{2+}-ATPase and a 20,000-dalton fragment without enzymatic activity (533, 557).

An ionophore effect on planar BLM was associated with the 55,000- and 20,000-dalton proteolytic fragments of the Ca^{2+}-ATPase (530–533, 557). The selectivity sequence for divalent cations was identical for intact succinylated Ca^{2+}-ATPase and for the 20,000-dalton subfragment: $P_{Ba} > P_{Ca} > P_{Sr} > P_{Mg} > P_{Mn}$.

The suggestion was made that the active site of the Ca^{2+}-ATPase and the polypeptide segment that serves as a Ca^{2+} channel are separated in the 30,000-dalton and in the 20,000-dalton regions of the 55,000-dalton component (526, 530–533). The 45,000-dalton tryptic fragment has a nonselective divalent-cation ionophoric activity (1, 531).

Because the ionophore effect of the 20,000- and 45,000-dalton tryptic fragments is relatively nonspecific and the Ca^{2+}-induced conductance changes are observed only at high Ca^{2+} concentrations, the relationship between ATP-mediated Ca^{2+} transport and the conductance effects of the proteolytic fragments is uncertain. It would be interesting to know whether conductance changes are produced by proteolytic fragments obtained from proteins that are not expected to have ion transport function.

EFFECT OF PROTEOLIPID ON MEMBRANE PERMEABILITY. Purified preparations of the Ca^{2+}-transport ATPase contain a proteolipid that is soluble in acidified chloroform-methanol and has an estimated molecular weight of 12,000 (336, 344). Racker suggested the possible involvement of the proteolipid as an ion channel in ATP-dependent Ca^{2+} transport (472, 473, 480). This suggestion was based on the observation that addition of crude "proteolipid" to reconstituted Ca^{2+}-ATPase vesicles improved the coupling efficiency between ATP hydrolysis and Ca^{2+} transport without significant change in ATPase activity. Purified proteolipid preparations were found to be less effective or inactive (300, 472).

The proteolipid has a relatively high α-helix content (312). It is presumed to be located in the hydrocarbon interior of the bilayer because it decreases the motional freedom of the alkyl chains of stearic acid spin labels but leaves the glycerol backbone relatively unaffected (313). As a result of this effect, instead of serving as an ion channel, proteolipid reduced the nonspecific ion and water permeability of planar phospholipid bilayers (314), with only transient and minor increases in conductance immediately after the formation of the bilayer (529).

The slightly improved coupling efficiency of Ca^{2+} transport in reconstituted ATPase vesicles after the addition of proteolipid may be due to the condensing effect of proteolipid, which reduces the passive Ca^{2+} leak across the reconstituted membrane. So far there is no indication of a direct interaction between the Ca^{2+}-ATPase and the proteolipid that could be implicated in Ca^{2+} transport or ATP hydrolysis.

RELATIONSHIP BETWEEN MEMBRANE POTENTIAL AND CALCIUM FLUXES ACROSS SR MEMBRANE

The regulation of the cytoplasmic Ca^{2+} concentration during excitation and relaxation of muscle cells involves large Ca^{2+} fluxes across the SR membrane. It is expected that these fluxes produce and are in turn influenced by changes in the membrane potential of the SR.

Probes as Indicators of SR Membrane Potential

To establish the relationship between membrane potential and the rate of Ca^{2+} uptake and release, methods are needed to monitor membrane potential changes. Due to the small size of the SR, direct measurement of the membrane potential with electrodes is not feasible, but voltage-sensitive optical probes can be used (89, 631).

Dyes that respond to changes in the membrane potential fall into two general classes (Fig. 10). First, oxacarbocyanines, oxadicarbocyanines, thiadicarbocyanines, thiacarbocyanines, and indodicarbocyanines are characterized by a delocalized charge making them relatively permeant through lipid bilayers (542, 630). These dyes accumulate in vesicles under the influence of membrane potential, and fluorescence or absorbance changes result when an increase in the internal dye concentration causes the formation of dye dimers and aggregates. Binding of the dye to membrane sites may also contribute to the optical response (32, 500, 501).

The second class of voltage-sensitive dyes, such as 8-anilino-1-naphthalenesulfonic acid (ANS) and merocyanines, contain localized charges and are relatively impermeant through lipid bilayers. Their response to membrane potential is complex but involves primarily the redistribution of bound dye within the membrane (89, 91).

The positive cyanine dyes, 3,3′-dipentyloxacarbocyanine (403), diethyloxodicarbocyanine (33), 3,3′-dipropylthiadicarbocyanine (133), and 3,3′-diethylthiadicarbocyanine (30, 31), have been shown to respond to changes in the membrane potential of SR vesicles generated by ion gradients across the vesicle membrane. Within a specific range, the response of these dyes shows a linear relationship with potential as defined by the Nernst equation. In addition, all of the above dyes respond in varying degrees to changes in the surface potential caused by the binding of cations (Na^+, K^+, Ca^{2+}, Mg^{2+}, La^{2+}) and anions (such as Cl^-, and ATP^{3-}) to the membrane (32, 33, 500, 501). The responses related to changes in membrane diffusion potential and surface potential can be distinguished by a suitable choice of experimental conditions.

Influence of SR Membrane Potential on Calcium Permeability

The existence of voltage-regulated Ca^{2+} channels in the surface membrane of excitable cells raises the possibility that similar channels in the SR membrane are activated during excitation-contraction coupling.

The transfer of Ca^{2+}-loaded SR vesicles (276, 277) or skinned muscle fibers (94, 96, 147, 165, 435) equilibrated in a medium containing a slowly penetrating anion into KCl solution induces the release of accumulated Ca^{2+}. It was proposed that the influx of Cl^- produces an inside-negative membrane potential, which causes Ca^{2+} channels in the membrane to open, permitting Ca^{2+} release. An alternative explanation is that the influx of KCl causes osmotic swelling of the SR, increasing the permeability of the membrane to Ca^{2+} (411).

Using voltage-sensitive fluorescent dyes, Beeler et al. (33) studied the relationship between the membrane potential and the rate of Ca^{2+} efflux, after diluting SR vesicles equilibrated in 0.3 M K methanesulfonate into media of different ionic composition. Only dilution of the vesicles into NaCl or KCl stimulated Ca^{2+} release, even though the change in membrane

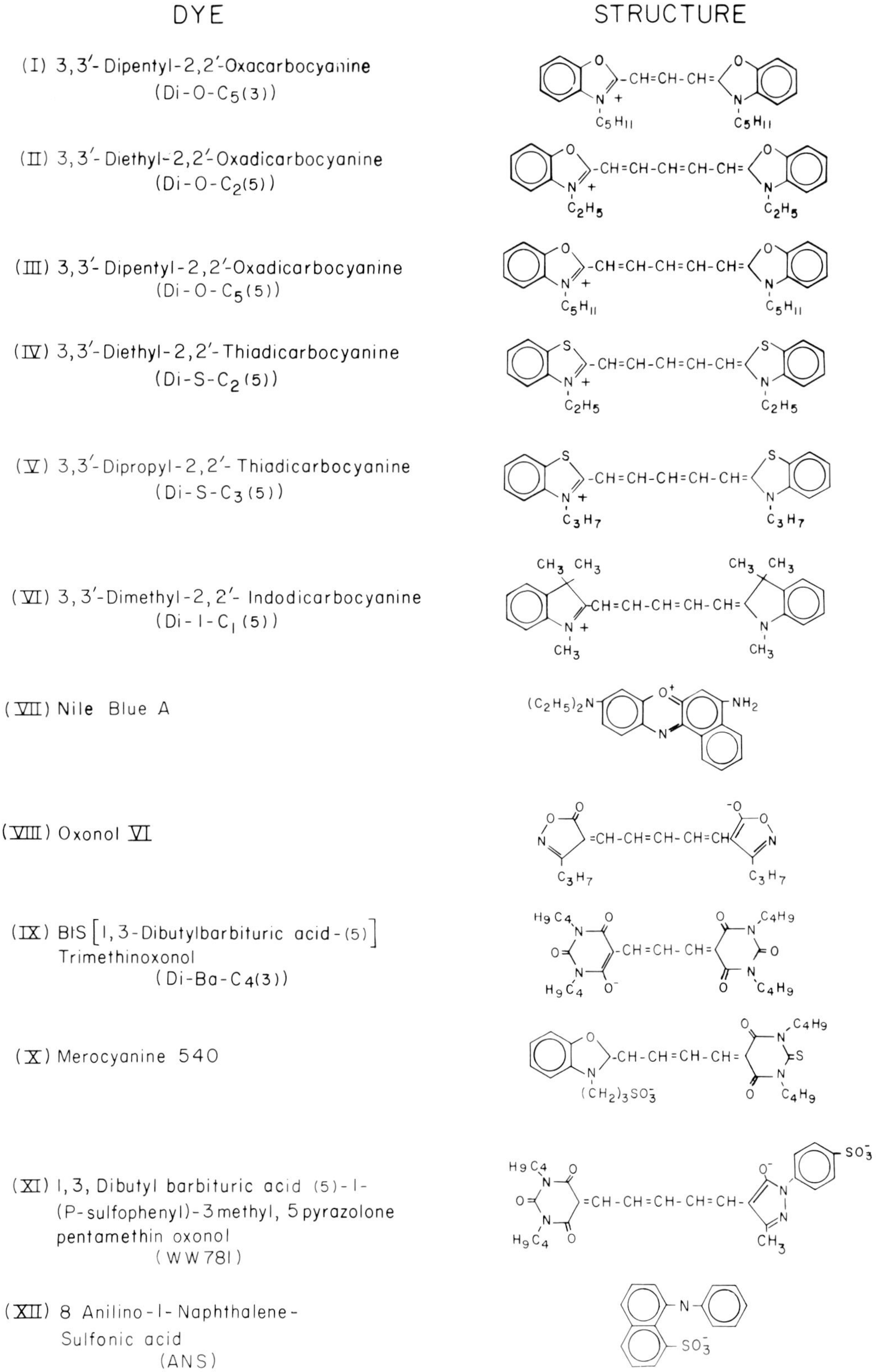

DYE

STRUCTURE

(I) 3,3′-Dipentyl-2,2′-Oxacarbocyanine (Di-O-C_5(3))

(II) 3,3′-Diethyl-2,2′-Oxadicarbocyanine (Di-O-C_2(5))

(III) 3,3′-Dipentyl-2,2′-Oxadicarbocyanine (Di-O-C_5(5))

(IV) 3,3′-Diethyl-2,2′-Thiadicarbocyanine (Di-S-C_2(5))

(V) 3,3′-Dipropyl-2,2′-Thiadicarbocyanine (Di-S-C_3(5))

(VI) 3,3′-Dimethyl-2,2′-Indodicarbocyanine (Di-I-C_1(5))

(VII) Nile Blue A

(VIII) Oxonol VI

(IX) BIS [1,3-Dibutylbarbituric acid-(5)] Trimethinoxonol (Di-Ba-C_4(3))

(X) Merocyanine 540

(XI) 1,3, Dibutyl barbituric acid (5)-1-(P-sulfophenyl)-3 methyl, 5 pyrazolone pentamethin oxonol (WW781)

(XII) 8 Anilino-1-Naphthalene-Sulfonic acid (ANS)

FIG. 10. Structure of dyes used as membrane potential indicators. Oxacarbocyanine (I), oxadicarbocyanine (II, III), thiadicarbocyanine (IV, V), and indodicarbocyanine (VI) have delocalized positive charges. Nile blue A (VII) contains one localized positive charge. Oxonol VI (VIII) and Di-Ba-C_4 (3) (IX) have delocalized negative charges, whereas merocyanine 540 (X), WW781 (XI), and ANS (XII) contain a localized negative charge. Dyes with delocalized charges penetrate across membranes, while those with localized charges are relatively impermeant. Mechanisms of dye response to potential are different in each class (630, 631).

potential generated under these conditions was small. Larger negative membrane potentials (≃ −80 mV) were generated by dilution into media containing slowly penetrating anions such as Tris methanesulfonate and valinomycin, or Na methanesulfonate and valinomycin, without any stimulated Ca^{2+} release. Similar results were obtained by Ohnishi (450). The KCl-induced Ca^{2+} release can be inhibited by the addition of sucrose or other relatively nonpermeant solutes to the KCl dilution medium, indicating that osmotic swelling is an important factor in the KCl-stimulated Ca^{2+} release (33, 276, 277, 411, 450).

These observations indicate that the passive Ca^{2+} permeability of isolated SR vesicles is not influenced by membrane potential. As there is no clear indication for the existence of membrane potential across the SR membrane in intact muscle (544), propagative depolarization of SR is not likely to contribute to the mechanism of Ca^{2+} release during excitation.

Influence of Membrane Potential on Active Calcium Transport

The membrane potential of the SR could influence the transport of Ca^{2+} in several ways. First, the free energy change of the reaction would be dependent on the membrane potential. Second, membrane potential may alter the movement of ions, dipoles, or other charged constituents involved in the Ca^{2+} uptake. In addition, conformational changes of the ATPase induced by electrical fields across the membrane may modify the activity of the ATPase. If one of the rate-limiting intermediate reactions is voltage sensitive, the overall rate of Ca^{2+} transport could be influenced by membrane potential.

Zimniak and Racker (682) reported that the rate of Ca^{2+} uptake by reconstituted ATPase-phosphatidylcholine vesicles is dependent on the membrane potential established with K^+ gradients and valinomycin. An imposed membrane potential of 61 mV (inside positive) had little effect on the rate of Ca^{2+} transport, whereas more negative potentials increased the Ca^{2+}-uptake rate. It was suggested that the 61-mV (inside-positive) membrane potential represented the equilibrium potential of Ca^{2+} transport (682). Inside-negative potentials caused a maximum of a twofold increase in the rate of calcium uptake when the reconstitution of the ATPase was carried out with phosphatidylcholine, but only minor activation was observed on ATPase vesicles reconstituted with asolectin or soy phosphatidylethanolamine. In these experiments, no effect of potential was found on the Ca^{2+} uptake of native SR vesicles (682).

Beeler et al. (30–32) found that the Ca^{2+} transport of SR vesicles can be activated by K^+-diffusion potentials if the medium contains relatively nonpermeant anions such as glutamate. The rate of ATP-dependent Ca^{2+} uptake in a glutamate medium increased in a roughly linear manner with K^+-diffusion potentials in the range of 0 to 97 mV (Fig. 11). In the absence of ATP, changes in the membrane potential had little influence on Ca^{2+} binding to SR vesicles. The increased rate of Ca^{2+} uptake caused by inside-negative membrane potential was accompanied by a proportional increase in the rate of Ca^{2+}-dependent ATP hydrolysis, indicating that the activation of Ca^{2+} uptake is due to an increased rate of Ca^{2+} transport by the Ca^{2+}-Mg^{2+}-ATPase, rather than a decrease in the rate of Ca^{2+} efflux. The steady-state level of the phosphoenzyme intermediate and the coupling ratio between Ca^{2+} transport and ATP hydrolysis are not significantly influenced by the membrane potential (30, 31).

Because the phosphorylation rate of the enzyme by ATP is orders of magnitude faster than the overall rate of ATP hydrolysis, the rate-limiting step of Ca^{2+} transport is assumed to be the hydrolysis of the phosphoenzyme intermediate or some other step following enzyme phosphorylation. The influence of membrane potential on the rate of Ca^{2+} transport is probably exerted at one of these rate-limiting steps.

Effect of Calcium Uptake on Membrane Potential of SR

The magnitude of the membrane potential generated during Ca^{2+} uptake by the Ca^{2+}-Mg^{2+}-ATPase is dependent on the turnover rate of the ATPase, the density of the transport sites in the membrane, and the ability of other ions to compensate for the positive charges of the Ca^{2+} translocated across the membrane. The turnover number of the ATPase is of the order of 8/s at 25°C (249), with two Ca^{2+} transported per cycle. The concentration of ATPase in the membrane is estimated to be 16,000–23,000 ATPase molecules per μm^2 surface area (255). Assuming a membrane capacitance of 1 $\mu F/cm^2$ and the transfer of four charges per cycle, each turnover would generate a membrane potential of approximately 1.25 V, if no compensating ion fluxes occur during Ca^{2+} uptake. Under these conditions, only one turnover would be necessary to reach inhibitory levels of membrane potential.

There are indications, however, that the Ca^{2+} transport is at least partially counterbalanced by the movement of Mg^{2+}, K^+, or H^+ across the membrane (32, 407, 412, 604, 605).

The involvement of Mg^{2+} in Ca^{2+} transport is suggested by the following observations: *1)* $Mg^{2+}$is required for the decomposition of the phosphoenzyme intermediate (272, 373). *2)* The Mg^{2+}-binding site involved in dephosphorylation appears to be located on the inner side of the membrane (272). *3)* Ca^{2+} competes with Mg^{2+} for the binding site regulating dephosphorylation. This suggests that Mg^{2+} may replace Ca^{2+} bound to the enzyme and could be transported out of the SR during dephosphorylation of E~P (669). *4)* The decrease in Ca^{2+} affinity of the transport site during Ca^{2+} translocation is accompanied by an increase in Mg^{2+} affinity.

There is, however, no direct experimental evidence

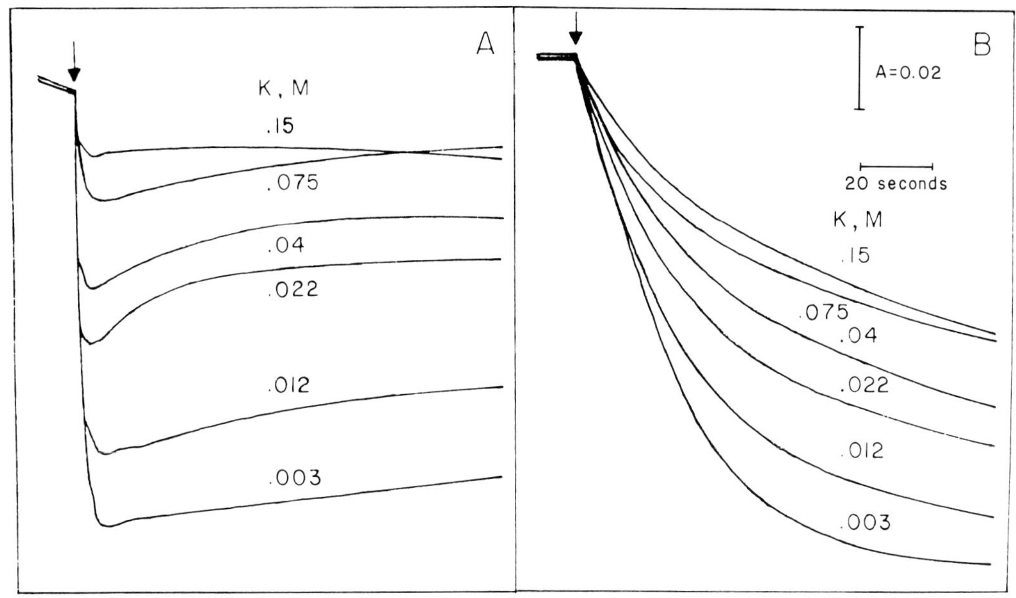

FIG. 11. Correlation between membrane potential and the rate of Ca^{2+} uptake. *A*: generation of membrane potential. Microsomes (4 mg protein/ml) suspended in 0.15 M K-glutamate, 10.0 mM imidazole, 5.0 mM Mg^{2+}-maleate were diluted 50-fold into media containing 5 mM Mg^{2+}-maleate, 10 mM imidazole, 0.1 mM Ca^{2+}-maleate, 10 μM 3,3′-diethylthiodicarbocyanine and 1 μM valinomycin, with glycine and K-glutamate at the following concentrations: *1*) 0.150 M K-glutamate, no glycine; *2*) 0.075 M K-glutamate, 0.150 M glycine; *3*) 0.040 M K-glutamate, 0.225 M glycine; *4*) 0.022 M K-glutamate, 0.262 M glycine; *5*) 0.012 M K-glutamate, 0.281 M glycine; *6*) no K-glutamate, 0.300 M glycine. Absorbance change of 3,3′-diethylthiodicarbocyanine at 660 mm was monitored using 600 nm as a reference wavelength. Temperature, 15°C. *B*: effect of membrane potential on Ca^{2+} uptake. Experiment was similar to that described in *A* except that microsome concentration was 10 times greater, and dilution medium contained 1 mM ATP (diNa) as energy source for Ca^{2+} transport and arsenazo III (50 μM) instead of 3,3′-diethylthiodicarbocyanine to monitor Ca^{2+} transport. Absorbance response of arsenazo III to Ca^{2+} (10–100 μM), measured at 660 nm using 685 nm as a reference wavelength, was 20% less in 0.15 M K-glutamate than in 0.3 M glycine. [Adapted from Beeler (31).]

for Mg^{2+} countertransport. Although Carvalho and Leo (69) measured release of Mg^{2+} from SR vesicles during Ca^{2+} uptake, it was not determined whether the Mg^{2+} efflux resulted from Mg^{2+} countertransport or from competition between Ca^{2+} and Mg^{2+} for the low-affinity cation-binding sites within the SR. Recently, Ueno and Sekine (603) reported that Ca^{2+} uptake in the absence of added Mg^{2+}, K^+, or Na^+ occurs without release of any of these cations.

The role of Mg^{2+} as a counterion during Ca^{2+} transport is placed in further doubt by recent observations that the passive permeability of SR vesicles to Mg^{2+} is similar to that of Ca^{2+} (434). If Mg^{2+} is required as a counterion, then after the internal Mg^{2+} is depleted, further transport of Ca^{2+} would be limited by the slow Mg^+ influx. Since SR vesicles are able to accumulate large amounts of Ca^{2+} in the presence of oxalate faster than the apparent Mg^{2+} influx, it is unlikely that Mg^{2+} countertransport is required for Ca^{2+} uptake.

The activation of E~P decomposition by K^+ (536–538) raises the possibility that K^+ serves as a counterion for Ca^{2+} transport. Although Haynes (199) reported that for activation of Ca^{2+} transport, K^+ is required inside the SR vesicles, there is no direct experimental evidence linking K^+ countertransport to Ca^{2+} uptake.

Proton countertransport has been proposed by Madeira (349–351) and Chiesi et al. (80) based on measurements that indicate a net release of protons from SR during Ca^{2+} uptake. The proton release cannot be attributed to protons produced by ATP hydrolysis. It was proposed that proton efflux is mediated by the Ca^{2+}-Mg^{2+}-ATPase through a specific proton pump (349) or by proton release from the high-affinity Ca^{2+}-binding site (80). An alternative explanation is that protons are released from internal Ca^{2+}-binding sites and passively equilibrate across the membrane (69). Consistent with this interpretation, proton ionophores do not influence either the rate of H^+ release during Ca^{2+} uptake (80, 351) or the rate of Ca^{2+} uptake (80, 103, 387, 514).

The formation of membrane potential during Ca^{2+} uptake is so severely limited by compensating ion movements through cation and anion channels that the detection of potential changes in the presence of 0.1 M KCl is difficult. In fact the physiological role of these ion channels may be to minimize potential changes during Ca^{2+} fluxes.

A Critical Analysis of Experimental Findings on Effects of Ca^{2+} Transport on Membrane Potential

The generation of inside-positive membrane potential during Ca^{2+} uptake in reconstituted ATPase-phosphatidylcholine vesicles was first demonstrated by Zimniak and Racker (682) using ANS as a potentiometric probe. When added to one side of the membrane, ANS fluorescence was proportional to inside-positive membrane potential from 0 to 90 mV. The membrane potential change calculated from the increase in the ANS fluorescence during Ca^{2+} uptake was 51 mV. The effects of Ca^{2+} binding on the fluorescence signal were minimized by precipitation of the accumulated Ca^{2+} with phosphate and by using solutions of high ionic strength that reduce surface potential effects.

Electrogenic transport of Ca^{2+} was subsequently observed on SR vesicles by Meissner (406) and Beeler (30, 31). Artificially imposed inside-negative membrane potential generated by ion gradients and monitored with 3,3′-dipentyloxacarbocyanine (406) or 3,3′-diethylthiadicarbocyanine (30, 31) was sharply diminished during ATP-induced Ca^{2+} uptake. A membrane potential of approximately −97 mV was dissipated within 30 s on initiation of Ca^{2+} transport (31); during this time at least nine turnovers of the Ca^{2+}-Mg^{2+}-ATPase had occurred. A quantitative evaluation of these experiments requires precise knowledge of the effect of intravesicular Ca^{2+} on the optical response of the dyes to potential (32).

Effect of Calcium on Optical Response of Positive Cyanine Dyes

The fluorescence and absorbance changes of 3,3′-dipentyloxadicarbocyanine (349), 3,3′-dipropylthiadicarbocyanine (133, 603), 3,3′-dipropyloxacarbocyanine (500), and 3,3′-diethyloxadicarbocyanine (33) that accompany ATP-induced Ca^{2+} uptake by SR may be due to the generation of transmembrane potentials, to changes in the membrane surface charge caused by the binding of accumulated Ca^{2+} to the membrane, and to the screening of membrane charges by Ca^{2+}.

For example, the fluorescence enhancement of 3,3′-dipropylthiadicarbocyanine during Ca^{2+} transport was attributed by Dupont (133) to an increase in inside-positive membrane potential, whereas Ueno and Sekine (603) interpreted their results in terms of the displacement of dye bound to the vesicles by increase in internal Ca^{2+} concentration. Because the fluorescence of 3,3′-dipropylthiadicarbocyanine is quenched when the dye binds to the SR, release of bound dye from the membrane due to Ca^{2+} binding would be expected to cause an increase in dye fluorescence.

Changes in the fluorescence intensity caused by transmembrane potential should be eliminated by ionophores and highly permeant ions without significantly altering Ca^{2+} transport. Although the addition of 100 mM Cl^- to the Ca^{2+}-uptake medium decreased the fluorescence change of dipropylthiadicarbocyanine only by one-third, oxalate (5 mM) completely reversed the optical response (133). This behavior is difficult to explain in terms of transmembrane potential, because the Cl^- permeability is several orders of magnitude greater than that of oxalate (302). It is therefore likely that much of the observed response is due to Ca^{2+} binding and that oxalate, by precipitating the accumulated Ca^{2+}, minimizes the contribution of internal Ca^{2+} to the optical response.

The absorbance change of 3,3′-diethyloxadicarbocyanine during Ca^{2+} accumulation by SR is also attributable to Ca^{2+} binding rather than changes in transmembrane potential for the following reasons (32, 33, 500, 501).

1. The wavelength dependence of the absorbance change induced by Ca^{2+} uptake is identical to that observed on increasing the Ca^{2+} concentration of the medium to millimolar levels and different from the effect of inside-negative membrane potential generated with K^+ gradients in the presence of valinomycin. The wavelength dependence of the absorbance change of the oxacarbocyanine and oxadicarbocyanine dyes caused by Ca^{2+} accumulation presumably reflects changes in the amount of dye bound to the membrane, whereas the optical change induced by negative potential is consistent with the formation of dye dimers and aggregates, along with changes in the amount of bound dye due to increased internal dye concentration.
2. The optical response to Ca^{2+} uptake reached a maximum when the SR vesicles were saturated with Ca^{2+} and held constant until Ca^{2+} release was induced by Ca^{2+} ionophores or by pump reversal. Under similar conditions, potentials generated by ion gradients were transient with lifetimes of only 10–30 s.
3. Reducing the internal free-Ca^{2+} concentration by oxalate precipitation inhibited the optical response to Ca^{2+} uptake, although Ca^{2+} transport continued at a high rate. Oxalate (5 mM) did not inhibit the formation of membrane potentials by artificially imposed ion gradients.
4. The time course of the optical response was very similar to that of Ca^{2+} uptake measured with arsenazo III.
5. Inclusion of valinomycin, a potassium ionophore, into the Ca^{2+}-uptake medium containing K^+ did not affect the optical response of the probe during Ca^{2+} uptake, although the formation of membrane potentials would have been inhibited by the movement of K^+ across the membrane.

Similar considerations may apply to the observations of Madeira (349) on the transient changes in the absorbance and fluorescence of 3,3′-dipentyloxadicarbocyanine during Ca^{2+} uptake. Although Madeira attributed this optical change to the formation of inside-positive membrane potential, the response of 3,3′-dipentyloxadicarbocyanine to artificially imposed inside-positive potentials was not defined, nor was the effect of Ca^{2+} on the dye response considered.

Response of Negatively Charged Dyes to Calcium Transport by SR Vesicles

Ca^{2+} uptake by SR vesicles is accompanied by changes in the absorbance and fluorescence of ANS (200, 603, 614–616, 618), merocyanines (501, 503), and oxonols (4, 501).

The enhancement of ANS and merocyanine fluorescence during Ca^{2+} uptake is attributed to the effect of increased internal Ca^{2+} concentration on the dye binding to the membrane (501, 615, 616). The amount of dye bound and the location of the bound dye within the membrane depend on the surface potential, which is altered by Ca^{2+} binding (32).

Although Åkerman and Wolff (4) attributed the absorbance changes of oxonol VI during Ca^{2+} uptake to the formation of inside-positive membrane potential, addition of valinomycin, nigericin, or highly permeant anions such as Cl^- or SCN^- to the Ca^{2+}-uptake system caused only a small decrease in the response. Since the oxonol VI response to K^+-diffusion gradients was not calibrated, it is not certain how much of the optical change resulted from membrane potential changes and how much from the Ca^{2+} accumulated in the vesicles.

Membrane Potential of SR In Vivo

Analysis of the ionic composition of the SR lumen and the surrounding cytoplasm by electron X-ray microprobe on thin slices of rapidly frozen resting, tetanized, and fatigued muscle did not reveal a significant Cl^- or K^+ gradient across the SR (544, 546–548). Therefore it is unlikely that a sustained resting potential is generated by Ca^{2+} uptake in vivo. The data do not rule out transient membrane potential changes due to rapid Ca^{2+} fluxes during relaxation or contraction.

Effect of Ca^{2+} Release on Membrane Potential of SR

A Ca^{2+} gradient equivalent to a diffusion potential of approximately 120 mV exists across the SR membrane in the resting muscle, but little of this is expressed electrically since the permeability of the membrane to Ca^{2+} is much lower than that of many other ions found in the cytoplasm. But if Ca^{2+} is released selectively from the SR following depolarization of the T system, large inside-negative membrane potentials may develop. These potentials could influence both the rate of the Ca^{2+} release and the subsequent rate of Ca^{2+} uptake during relaxation.

Unfortunately no subcellular system has been devised to study activated Ca^{2+} release from the SR vesicles. Consequently changes in the SR membrane potential must be measured using fiber bundles and single-fiber or skinned-fiber preparations. Absorbance and fluorescence changes of the potentiometric probes, Nile blue A (25, 40, 449, 624), indodicarbocyanine (25, 449), WW 781, a pentamethinoxonol (25), and changes in the birefringence signal of muscle (25–29) have been correlated with Ca^{2+} release after excitation of muscle fibers.

There is no direct experimental evidence that these optical signals arise from changes in the membrane potential of SR. The optical signals may indicate conformational changes in the contractile proteins or the Ca^{2+}-Mg^{2+}-ATPase induced by Ca^{2+} binding or changes in the surface potential of SR caused by Ca^{2+} release. Indeed, the birefringence signal attributed to depolarization of the SR is eliminated by injection of EGTA into the muscle cytoplasm (560). Baylor et al. (25) have recently reported that the signals previously thought to monitor the SR membrane potential consist of several components with distinct time courses, and it is difficult to know which, if any, of the signals reflect changes in the membrane potential of the SR.

Of five dyes tested in vitro, Nile blue A appeared to produce the cleanest signal to inside-negative potentials, with least interference from Ca^{2+} (32). Therefore the Nile blue A fluorescence signals obtained during muscle activation may represent the best evidence to date for the generation of inside-negative potential in SR during activating Ca^{2+} release (40, 624). As binding of Nile blue A to SR vesicles was accompanied by an increase in fluorescence intensity, the results in living muscle suggest that activation promotes the entry of Nile blue A into the SR, with subsequent binding to the membrane. Conformational changes in contractile proteins may also influence the dye response if Nile blue A, like dihexyloxacarbocyanine, is bound to myofibrils.

If the Nile blue A signal during muscle activation indicates a negative potential in SR, this potential change during a single twitch lasts only for ~50 ms (40). The Nile blue A signal coexists during part of its course with the Ca^{2+} transient measured by calcium indicators, raising the possibility that the membrane potential of SR regulates the rate of Ca^{2+} transport. As shown in Figure 11, the rate of Ca^{2+} uptake by isolated SR vesicles is enhanced by negative potential; in turn the potential signal is attenuated during Ca^{2+} uptake. It is plausible to assume that the negative potential generated in living muscle during activation facilitates the subsequent reabsorption of Ca^{2+}, which, in turn, accelerates the disappearance of negative potential. This possibility may be tested in two ways.

1. Inhibition of Ca^{2+} uptake by injection of EGTA into living muscle fibers should prolong the Nile blue A signal, since the dissipation of negative potential under these conditions would depend only on the passive ion fluxes across the SR. The presence of EGTA should abolish the Nile blue A signal if it arises from interaction of Ca^{2+} with myofibrils or the Ca^{2+}-ATPase on the outer surface of SR, or if EGTA interferes with the Ca^{2+} release.

2. The rate of Ca^{2+} reabsorption into SR should be faster after a depolarizing pulse of short duration while

the negative potential still exists, compared with depolarizing pulses lasting several seconds, which may allow the dissipation of negative potential.

TRANSPORT OF CA^{2+} BY CARDIAC SR

Calcium plays a similar role in the regulation of contraction and relaxation in cardiac and skeletal muscles, and the mechanism of Ca^{2+} transport by SR is also similar in the two systems. Cardiac microsomes accumulate Ca^{2+} against a concentration gradient coupled to the hydrolysis of ATP (67, 159, 241, 651). The ATP hydrolysis occurs by transient phosphorylation of the enzyme (160, 446, 461, 539, 561, 566), yielding an acylphosphate enzyme intermediate with very similar characteristics to those observed in skeletal muscle microsomes. The maximum steady-state concentration of phosphoenzyme intermediate is 0.6–1.5 nmol/mg protein in cardiac microsomes isolated from various animals, i.e., about 20%–25% of the maximum phosphoenzyme content of microsomes obtained from skeletal muscle. The formation of phosphoenzyme requires Ca^{2+} in the external medium. Half-maximal activation of the phosphoprotein formation and ATP-ADP exchange is reached at an ionized Ca^{2+} concentration of about 0.3 μM (561).

The Ca^{2+}-transport ATPase of cardiac SR, like its skeletal counterpart, is a lipoprotein of 100,000 daltons. Although the amino acid composition of dog cardiac ATPase is similar to that of rabbit skeletal SR (579), immunologically the cardiac and skeletal Ca^{2+}-transport ATPases are clearly different (107).

The slower Ca^{2+} transport and Ca^{2+}-dependent ATPase activity of cardiac muscle SR, compared with skeletal muscle SR, arises largely from the low density of Ca^{2+}-transport sites in cardiac microsomes (539). In addition, recent rapid kinetic studies reveal significant differences in the rates of several reaction steps of the Ca^{2+}-transport cycle between cardiac and fast-twitch or slow-twitch skeletal muscle microsomes (57, 565, 566, 640).

The time course of phosphoenzyme formation at 21°C is characterized by a rapid rise to a maximum level (overshoot) followed by a decline. During the rising phase of phosphoenzyme formation, the time courses of phosphorylation of rabbit cardiac and skeletal microsomes coincide, although there is a large difference in the maximum amount of phosphoenzyme formed (4 nmol/mg in rabbit skeletal and 0.6 nmol/mg in rabbit cardiac microsomes) (566). The release of P_i occurs with a distinct lag phase during the accumulation of phosphoenzyme, followed by a rapid burst of P_i liberation that coincides with a decay of the phosphoprotein. The half time of phosphorylation (10 ms at 10 μM ATP) is independent of Ca^{2+}, Mg^{2+}, and enzyme concentration but decreases to about 4 ms by increasing the ATP concentration to 50 μM. These observations suggest that the reactions leading to enzyme phosphorylation occur at similar rates in cardiac and skeletal microsomes.

Significant differences were observed between cardiac and skeletal enzymes in the rate of decomposition of E~P (565) and in the calculated rates of some of the reaction steps that follow E~P decomposition (566). Rapidly and slowly hydrolyzing phosphoenzymes were detected in cardiac and skeletal microsomes during dephosphorylation in the presence of EGTA. The initial rate of phosphoenzyme decay was monophasic in cardiac microsomes (8–9/s), whereas in skeletal muscle microsomes the decay was faster (12–15/s) and showed an early biphasic pattern. It appears that the rate of reaction in the cardiac system is more influenced by the step involving the conversion of *E to E, whereas in skeletal muscle the P_i-release step ($*E \cdot P_i \rightarrow *E + P_i$) is rate limiting. This is consistent with the observation that the overshoot of phosphoenzyme formation is more pronounced with cardiac than with skeletal enzymes.

In the presence of 10^{-5} M Ca^{2+}, K^+ (100 mM) increases the rate of Ca^{2+}-dependent ATP hydrolysis 3- to 5-fold at 37°C (258–260). Under similar conditions the steady-state concentration of phosphoenzyme is not affected by K^+ over a wide range of ATP concentrations (0.02–1 mM), suggesting that K^+ stimulates enzyme activity by increasing the rate of hydrolysis of phosphoenzyme intermediate. Indeed phosphoenzyme decay rates measured at 5°C in the presence of 3 mM ATP and various monovalent cations correlated qualitatively with the stimulation of ATPase activity. These observations imply that in cardiac (259, 260) and in skeletal systems (536, 537), K^+ affects the rate-limiting step of ATP hydrolysis.

KINETIC DIFFERENCES BETWEEN SR OF FAST-TWITCH AND SLOW-TWITCH SKELETAL MUSCLES

The Ca^{2+}-ATPase and Ca^{2+}-transport activity of SR isolated from fast-twitch skeletal muscle is greater than that of slow-twitch muscle (202, 204, 375, 551).

Some of this difference is attributable to the lower concentration of Ca^{2+}-transport sites in SR of slow-twitch as compared with fast-twitch skeletal muscles, but distinct differences in the rate of elementary reaction steps of ATP hydrolysis suggest that the Ca^{2+}-transport ATPases in muscles of different fiber types may be chemically distinct isoenzymes (99). For example, the initial rate of E-P formation in cat caudofemoralis (fast) SR is 0.46 $nmol \cdot mg^{-1} \cdot 10\ ms^{-1}$ compared with 0.25 $nmol \cdot mg^{-1} \cdot 10\ ms^{-1}$ in cat soleus SR (640). The corresponding values for the steady-state concentrations of phosphoenzyme are 1.47 nmol/mg and 0.75 nmol/mg for fast and slow SR, respectively. The rate constants (k_d) of E-P decomposition were 11.0/s for fast and 5.7/s for slow muscle SR.

Taking into consideration the concentration of Ca^{2+}-transport sites derived from the steady-state concentration of E~P, the differences in k_d account for the differences in the maximum velocity (V_{max}) of steady-state ATP hydrolysis (90 μmol $P_i \cdot mg^{-1} \cdot h^{-1}$ for fast SR and 20 μmol $P_i \cdot mg^{-1} \cdot h^{-1}$ for slow SR, respectively) (640).

REGULATION OF CA^{2+} TRANSPORT BY MEMBRANE PHOSPHORYLATION

Catecholamines increase the rate of tension development, the maximum tension, and the rate of relaxation of heart and slow-twitch skeletal muscles (for review see ref. 278), whereas in fast-twitch skeletal muscle only a slight change in tension is observed, due to prolongation of the active state. The involvement of adenosine 3,5′-cyclic monophosphate (cAMP) in the positive inotropic response of the heart to catecholamines was first suggested by Sutherland and his colleagues (567, 568). After the recognition of the role of protein kinases in the mediation of cAMP effects (90, 306), it soon became apparent that cAMP-dependent phosphorylation of protein receptors involved in the regulation of Ca^{2+} fluxes through the surface membrane (490) and SR (577, 578) may contribute significantly to the effect of catecholamines.

Kirchberger et al. (287) observed that the Ca^{2+} uptake of dog cardiac microsomes is stimulated by cAMP in the presence of protein kinase. Similar observations were made independently by Wollenberger (658), La Raia and Morkin (316), and Wray et al. (662). The relationship between membrane phosphorylation and Ca^{2+} transport became the subject of intense investigation in the intervening years (278, 283–287, 570–579, 619, 659).

The stimulation of Ca^{2+} uptake and Ca^{2+}-dependent ATP hydrolysis of cardiac microsomes in the presence of cAMP and protein kinases isolated from bovine heart or rabbit skeletal muscle (286, 573) is apparently related to the Mg^{2+}-dependent phosphorylation of a 22,000-dalton component of cardiac SR, which is named phospholamban (570, 571). Under similar conditions little or no phosphorylation of the Ca^{2+}-ATPase was observed (304, 571). Over a wide range of protein-kinase concentrations, the phosphorylation of phospholamban paralleled the increase in Ca^{2+}-transport activity (286). Slow phosphorylation of phospholamban also occurs without added protein kinase due to the presence of adenylate cyclase (280) and endogenous cAMP-dependent protein kinases in SR (662). The endogenous protein kinase is not inhibited by heat-stable protein kinase inhibitor and is relatively insensitive to guanosine 3,5′-cyclic monophosphate (cGMP).

A phosphate-acceptor protein of 22,000 daltons was also phosphorylated with increase in Ca^{2+}-transport activity in skeletal muscle microsomes of the slow-twitch rabbit soleus muscle (285), while no effect was observed on fast-twitch skeletal muscle microsomes. There may be a relationship between the relaxation-promoting effect of epinephrine in cardiac and slow-twitch skeletal muscles and the cAMP-dependent changes in SR Ca^{2+} transport (285).

The phospholamban is phosphorylated primarily at serine (80%) and threonine (20%) residues (286); the total amount of phosphate incorporated into the 22,000-dalton component of cardiac microsomes isolated from dog, cat, rabbit, and guinea pig is 0.75, 0.25, 0.30, and 0.14 nmol/mg protein, respectively (285); this is only slightly less than the estimated concentration of Ca^{2+}-ATPase in the membrane (283, 286), suggesting a 1:1 stoichiometry between phospholamban and the Ca^{2+}-transport ATPase.

In mixtures of ionic and nonionic detergents the 22,000-dalton phospholamban apparently dissociates into two presumably identical polypeptide chains of 11,000 daltons (325). Therefore the phospholamban of 22,000 daltons may be a dimer. Le Peuch et al. (325) proposed a model in which each ATPase monomer interacts with a phospholamban monomer of 11,000 daltons. On the basis of this model the molar ratio of the ATPase:phospholamban dimer in the membrane is expected to be 2.

No satisfactory method was reported so far for the isolation of pure phospholamban, and therefore no information is available concerning its amino acid composition and sequence.

In addition to phospholamban, pigeon heart microsomes contain two phosphate acceptor proteins of 15,000 and 11,000 daltons, respectively (654). The 11,000-dalton component sedimented with the lightest fractions, which contained largely vesicles of sarcolemmal origin. The 15,000-dalton protein is probably a component of SR; it is phosphorylated nearly evenly at threonine and serine residues and can be extracted from the membrane by acidified chloroform-methanol.

In addition to the cAMP-stimulated phosphorylation of cardiac microsomes through cAMP-dependent protein kinase, a Ca^{2+}-calmodulin–dependent phosphorylation was also observed (325). This is mediated by a membrane-bound protein kinase that is not inhibited by cAMP–protein kinase inhibitor. The calmodulin-dependent protein kinase requires Ca^{2+} for activity and incorporates phosphate into phospholamban at a distinct site, which is of prime importance in the stimulation of Ca^{2+} transport. In fact, in purified cardiac SR preparations, phosphorylation of phospholamban by the pure catalytic subunit of cAMP-dependent protein kinase has no effect on Ca^{2+} transport. The stimulation of Ca^{2+} uptake by Ca^{2+}-calmodulin–dependent kinase is amplified by cAMP-dependent phosphorylation of phospholamban. This is in accord with previous observations of Wray and Gray (661) on the effects of Ca^{2+} on the stimulation of Ca^{2+}-ATPase by cAMP.

Dephosphorylation of phospholamban by phosphoprotein phosphatase causes inhibition of Ca^{2+} transport, which is viewed as the reversal of the effect of phosphorylation (284, 572).

During stimulation of Ca^{2+} transport by membrane phosphorylation the $2Ca^{2+}$:1ATP stoichiometry of the transport process is maintained (573). Over the range of free-Ca^{2+} concentrations between 0.1 and 10 μM, the steady-state level of phosphoenzyme is significantly lower, whereas the rate of P_i liberation is greater in phosphorylated than in control microsomes. Therefore, the v/E-P ratio, while independent of Ca^{2+} concentration, increases more than twofold upon phosphorylation of phospholamban (577, 578). As suggested by these observations, the rate of hydrolysis of E-P measured in the presence of 2 mM EGTA between 0°C–30°C is enhanced about twofold in phosphorylated, as compared with control, microsomes (577, 578). The Arrhenius plots of the hydrolysis rate constant indicate a transition at 18°C, with activation energies of 11.4 and 19.2 kcal/mol at high and low temperatures, respectively (577, 578).

At pH 6.8, phosphorylation of the membrane had no effect on the rate of formation of E~P (304, 577). At pH 6.0, where the rate of E~P formation is slow and the steady-state concentration of E~P is depressed, cAMP-dependent phosphorylation increased the rate of E~P formation with increase in steady-state E~P concentration (304). These observations indicate that cAMP-dependent phosphorylation of phospholamban can compensate for the effect of acidosis on E~P.

The dependence of the ATPase activity of cardiac microsomes on external Ca^{2+} concentration yields a K for Ca of 2.4 μM for nonphosphorylated and 1.1 μM for phosphorylated membranes, indicating that phosphorylation increases the apparent Ca^{2+} affinity of the enzyme (208). The dependence of ATPase activity on Ca^{2+} concentration in nonphosphorylated membranes is cooperative with a Hill coefficient of 1.81. The cooperativity decreases after phosphorylation, yielding a Hill coefficient of 1.27. These observations led to the hypothesis that nonphosphorylated phospholamban interacts with the Ca^{2+}-ATPase to form a highly cooperative, constrained conformation with diminished Ca^{2+} affinity at low Ca^{2+} concentration. Phosphorylation reduces the affinity of phospholamban for the ATPase, resulting in a relaxed conformation with increased apparent Ca^{2+} affinity (208). Phosphorylation of phospholamban makes it *less* dissociable from the membrane by treatment with 0.1 mg deoxycholate/mg protein (578) and increases its resistance to tryptic digestion.

Role of Protein Kinase-Dependent Membrane Phosphorylation in Regulation of Ca^{2+} Transport by Skeletal Muscle SR

Treatment of SR prepared from fast-twitch skeletal muscle of rabbit with cAMP and protein kinase had no effect on the initial rate of Ca^{2+} uptake, and no radioactivity attributable to protein kinase–catalyzed phosphorylation of microsomes was apparent after SDS-PAGE (285). Under similar conditions, microsomes isolated from the slow-twitch muscles of rabbit soleus or dog biceps femoris or from heart responded with phosphorylation of phospholamban and stimulation of Ca^{2+} transport. The amount of ^{32}P incorporated into phospholamban ranged between 0.005–0.16 nmol/mg protein in dog biceps femoris microsomes compared with 0.14–0.75 nmol/mg protein in heart microsomes isolated from dog, cat, rabbit, and guinea pig. Thus it was suggested (285) that the relaxation-promoting effects of epinephrine may be related to the presence of phospholamban in cardiac and slow-twitch skeletal muscle microsomes, whereas the absence of such effects in fast-twitch skeletal muscle is due to the absence of phospholamban.

Most of these observations were confirmed by Schwartz et al. (522) and by Galani-Kranias et al. (176), except that a stimulation of Ca^{2+} uptake was found in skeletal muscle microsomes treated with cAMP-dependent protein kinase or with phosphorylase *b* kinase, together with ^{32}P incorporation into components of 95,000 and 100,000 daltons, but without phosphorylation of phospholamban (522). It appears that SR preparations from different sources contain a number of protein kinases and protein phosphatases that may modulate Ca^{2+} transport by phosphorylation of various membrane components, including the Ca^{2+}-ATPase (49, 176, 218, 219, 620, 621). Some of these enzymes may be associated with the glycogen complex that cosediments with the SR under certain conditions (149–151, 619, 641), and others may be components of the SR membrane. In most instances the relationship between the phosphorylation of various membrane components and their influence on the Ca^{2+} transport is unclear.

Physiological Significance of Phospholamban Phosphorylation

The effects of catecholamines on cardiac muscle may be explained by regulation of Ca^{2+} fluxes across the surface membranes (490) and the SR (154, 156) or by a direct effect on contractile proteins (427).

Because the level of phospholamban phosphorylation in living muscle is unknown and phosphorylation of other proteins may also contribute to the modulation of tension, an accurate assessment of the role of phospholamban phosphorylation in the catecholamine response is not possible.

BIOSYNTHESIS OF SR

During early embryonic development, skeletal muscles perform little work and the microsomes isolated from them possess the low ATPase and Ca^{2+}-transport activities that characterize the endoplasmic reticulum of nonmuscle cells. In late embryonic and postnatal

TABLE 7. *Developmental Changes in ATPase Activity, Ca^{2+} Transport, Ca^{2+}-Transport ATPase Concentration in the Chicken Pectoralis Muscle Sarcoplasmic Reticulum Membrane*

Days of Development	Ca^{2+}-Transport Activity, μmol $Ca \cdot mg^{-1} \cdot min^{-1}$	Ca^{2+}-Modulated ATPase, μmol $P_i \cdot mg^{-1} \cdot min^{-1}$	Phosphorylated Intermediate (E~P), nmol/mg protein	ATPase Content From Gel Electrophoresis, % of total protein	85-Å-Diam Freeze-Etch Particle Density/ μm^2 Surface Area	
					In isolated microsomes	In whole muscle
10	0.015	0.02	0.12	2	186	212
12	0.025	0.03	0.18			
14	0.034		0.22	6	352	462
16	0.060	0.08	0.31		405	
18	0.089			12		826
21	0.120	0.15	0.50			
22	0.200	0.19	0.87		1,257	
26	0.32	0.35	1.35	55		3,800
33	0.41	0.42	1.86	62		
46	0.60	0.70	2.20	65	2,750	4,330

For details see Boland et al. (47) and Tillack et al. (595). [From Martonosi et al. (396).]

development, the Ca^{2+}-activated ATPase and Ca^{2+}-transport activity of SR sharply increases, together with the deposition of contractile proteins and the appearance of contractile function (158, 215, 382, 569).

The evolution of the highly specialized SR with its characteristic protein and phospholipid composition from the phospholipid-rich primitive endoplasmic reticulum involves regulation of protein and phospholipid biosynthesis at several levels. The process was extensively studied in vivo (23, 45–47, 97, 376, 382, 395, 396, 507–509), in tissue culture (182, 217, 261, 262, 327, 345, 417, 683), and in cell-free translation systems (82, 179, 428, 663).

The results of these studies suggest that during development the SR of skeletal muscle evolves from the rough endoplasmic reticulum of myoblasts and myotubes by cotranslational insertion of ATPase molecules synthesized on membrane-bound polysomes into the membrane. The process is accompanied by characteristic changes in phospholipid composition and is subject to regulation by myogenic as well as neurogenic mechanisms.

Studies on SR Development In Vivo

CHANGES IN CA^{2+}-ATPASE CONTENT. In microsomes isolated from pectoralis or leg muscles of 10-day-old chicken embryos, the Ca^{2+}-transport ATPase, identified as a protein of 100,000 daltons by SDS-PAGE, is only about 2% of the total protein. The Ca^{2+}-transport and Ca^{2+}-modulated ATPase activities are low, and the steady-state concentration of phosphoprotein, which is a measure of the concentration of Ca^{2+}-ATPase, is only 0.12 nmol/mg microsomal protein (47, 382, 395).

Within a few weeks of development the Ca^{2+}-transport ATPase content of isolated microsomes increases more than 20-fold and constitutes 50%–60% of the total protein content of the membrane; parallel changes were observed in ATPase activity, Ca^{2+} transport, and the steady-state concentration of phosphoprotein intermediate [Table 7; (47, 382, 395)].

The density of 85-Å freeze-etch particles, characteristic of the Ca^{2+}-ATPase, increased from $212/\mu m^2$ in 10-day-old embryos to $4{,}300/\mu m^2$ after 46 days of development, both in intact muscles and in isolated SR vesicles (595). Corresponding changes in the density of 40-Å surface particles were observed after negative staining with K phosphotungstate [Table 7; (376, 508)].

As the 85-Å intramembranous particles probably represent clusters of about four ATPase molecules (255, 510), the approximate density of Ca^{2+}-ATPase molecules in the SR is about $800/\mu m^2$ in 10-day-old embryos and close to $16{,}000/\mu m^2$ in fully differentiated muscle.

These observations imply successive insertion of Ca^{2+}-ATPase molecules into the primitive, phospholipid-rich endoplasmic reticulum membrane until its concentration approaches physical saturation.

FATTY ACID COMPOSITION OF PHOSPHOLIPIDS. The fatty acid composition of phospholipids in microsomes isolated from 10-day-old chicken embryos is characterized by relatively high concentrations of palmitate (46, 47). As development proceeds, the concentration of palmitate decreases with increase in linoleate content. The increasing unsaturation of membrane phospholipids during development is reflected in a slight decrease in the transition temperature of membrane lipids detected by differential scanning calorimetry (376). The developmental changes in fatty acid composition are not of sufficient magnitude to cause detectable functional changes, since the specific Ca^{2+}-transport activity per mole of ATPase remains constant throughout the investigated range of development.

EXTRINSIC MEMBRANE PROTEINS. Membranes of SR contain, in addition to the Ca^{2+}-transport ATPase, two extrinsic proteins: the calsequestrin and the high-affinity Ca^{2+}-binding protein (129, 343, 416). The concentration of calsequestrin and the high-affinity Ca^{2+}-binding proteins in SR is already high at early stages of embryonic development, when only traces of Ca^{2+}-transport ATPase are present (376, 382, 508), and changes only slightly as the Ca^{2+}-transport ATPase accumulates. These observations, together with similar evidence obtained in rat skeletal muscle cultures (417, 683), suggest that the synthesis and insertion of intrinsic and extrinsic proteins of SR are independently regulated.

Assembly of SR in Cultured Skeletal and Cardiac Muscle

The major conclusions derived from studies of SR development in vivo were confirmed in tissue culture (182, 217, 395, 417, 683) with some additional insight into the mechanism of regulation of the synthesis of the major SR proteins.

In cultured chicken pectoralis or rat muscle the synthesis of Ca^{2+}-ATPase sharply increases parallel with the fusion of myoblasts into multinucleated myotubes (182, 217, 395). The synthesis of calsequestrin (683) and the high-affinity Ca^{2+}-binding protein (417) is initiated well before fusion and precedes the synthesis of Ca^{2+}-transport ATPase. In chicken muscle cultures grown in low-Ca^{2+} media, which inhibit fusion, the synthesis of Ca^{2+}-transport ATPase is also inhibited (182). In rat muscle cultures grown for 44 h in normal media, transfer into low-Ca^{2+} medium delayed, but did not inhibit, the accumulation of Ca^{2+}-ATPase (217).

The temporal relationship between the synthesis of Ca^{2+}-ATPase and calsequestrin was confirmed by immunofluorescence studies using antibodies against the Ca^{2+}-ATPase and calsequestrin (262). In mononucleated cells, calsequestrin was detected well before fusion (after ~45 h of development) localized at discrete perinuclear regions, which may represent the Golgi apparatus. As development progressed, the calsequestrin became distributed throughout the myotubes. The Ca^{2+}-ATPase appeared after 60 h of growth in granular patches throughout the cytoplasm of all fused and some unfused cells (262).

In rat skeletal muscle the calsequestrin is preferentially localized at the interface between the A and I bands; the ATPase is distributed throughout the I band and stains only very weakly in some of the A bands of the sarcomere (261). Such distribution conforms with the expected localization of calsequestrin in the terminal cisternae of SR and the more uniform distribution of ATPase throughout the terminal cisternae and the longitudinal tubules (171). The rather weak staining with anti-ATPase antibodies in the A zone is unexpected and may require further investigation as this region contains significant amounts of SR. The ATPase and calsequestrin were present in higher concentrations in fast than in slow muscle fibers.

In cardiac muscle culture, the synthesis of Ca^{2+}-transport ATPase increases steadily during the entire culture period, accompanied by cell proliferation, without the initial lag phase seen in skeletal muscle (216). It is known that contracting cardiac muscle cells, with cross-striated myofibrils, may undergo mitosis to yield spontaneously beating daughter cells (74); undividing heart cells may also show an increase in myosin content (86). Therefore cessation of cell proliferation is not a required prelude to differentiation and Ca^{2+}-ATPase synthesis in cardiac muscle (216).

Synthesis of Ca^{2+}-Transport ATPase in Cell-Free Systems and Its Insertion into the Membrane

The translation of Ca^{2+}-ATPase polypeptide and its incorporation into the membrane were studied in cell-free translation systems using membrane-bound and free polysomes isolated from 14- to 16-day-old chicken embryo muscles (82) or from leg muscles of neonatal rats (179).

The synthesis of Ca^{2+}-transport ATPase, measured by immunoprecipitation with anti-ATPase antibodies, occurred only on membrane-bound polysomes or rough microsomes. Although capable of the synthesis of a large number of proteins with a molecular weight of up to 200,000, free polysomes were essentially inactive in the synthesis of Ca^{2+}-transport ATPase.

The electrophoretic mobilities, isoelectric points, and tryptic peptide maps (Fig. 12) of the immunoprecipitated ATPases translated in cell-free systems from rough microsomes or membrane-bound polysomes were identical with the properties of mature ATPases isolated from microsomal membranes of adult chicken muscle or from chicken pectoralis muscle cultures (82).

The ATPase polypeptide synthesized on rough microsomes was directly incorporated into the membrane, as it was not released from the microsomes by washing with 0.5 M KCl and 10 mM EGTA or with 0.05–0.1 mg deoxycholate/mg protein, which remove loosely attached proteins. Only conditions leading to the solubilization of the membrane (0.5–1.0 mg deoxycholate/mg protein) released substantial amounts of Ca^{2+}-ATPase into the supernatant (82). Further evidence for cotranslational insertion of the ATPase was reported recently (428).

It is unlikely that cleavage of a major fragment or glycosylation of the Ca^{2+}-transport ATPase accompanies its insertion into the membrane, because *1)* the tryptic peptide map and the electrophoretic mobility of the ATPase translated on membrane-bound polysomes are similar to the properties of mature ATPase obtained from microsomes (82, 487); and *2)* the ATPase isolated by immunoprecipitation from cultured muscle cells grown in the presence of [^{3}H]glucosamine, [^{3}H]mannose, or [^{14}C]galactosamine contains only trace amounts of sugars.

The data obtained in vivo and in the cell-free translation systems are consistent with cotranslational insertion of the Ca^{2+}-transport ATPase synthesized on bound polysomes into the membranes of rough endo-

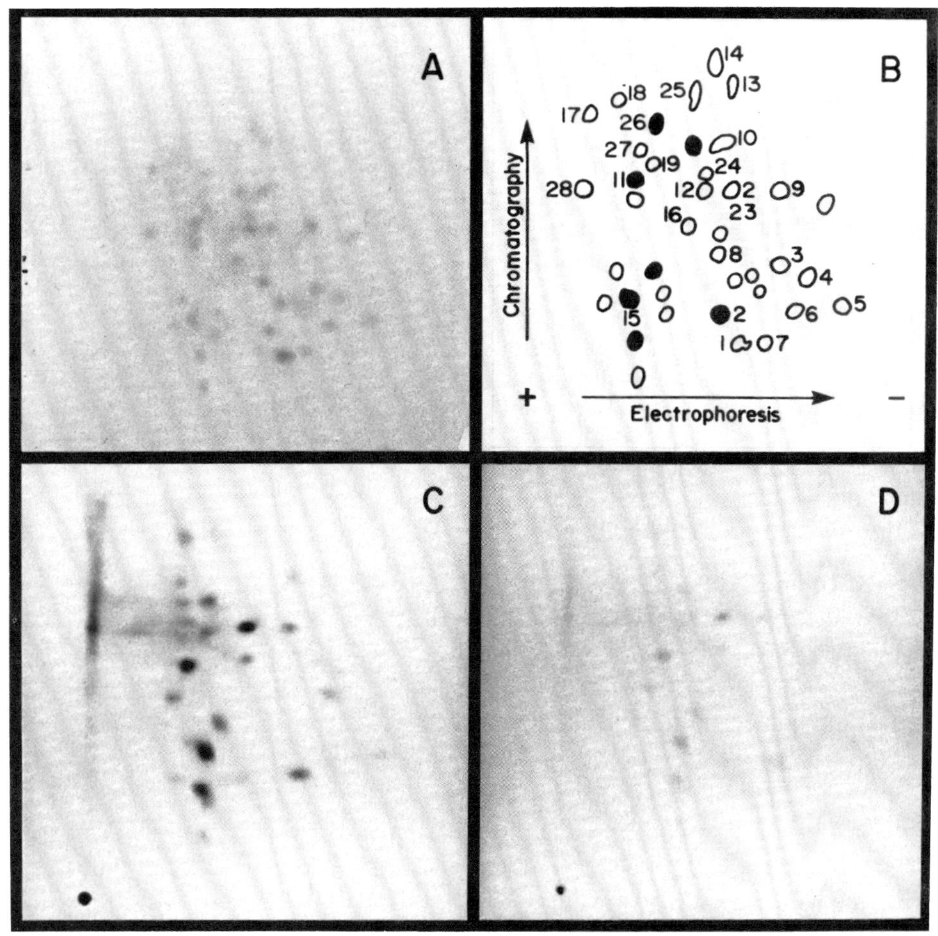

FIG. 12. Tryptic peptide maps of [^{35}S]methionine-labeled Ca^{2+}-transport ATPases. Maps were prepared from tryptic digests of reduced and carboxymethylated ATPases isolated from muscle or synthesized in vitro. Plates were sprayed with 7% 2,5-diphenyloxazole in acetone and exposed on X-ray film at −70°C for fluorography. *A*: ninhydrin-stained peptide map of Ca^{2+}-transport ATPase purified from adult chicken pectoralis muscle. *B*: diagram of the peptide pattern in *A*; positions of the principal [^{35}S]methionine-labeled peptides of *C* are indicated by filled circles. *C*: autoradiogram of [^{35}S]methionine-labeled peptides in tryptic digests of Ca^{2+}-transport ATPase from 5-day-old cultured chicken muscle cells, labeled for 24 h in a culture medium containing 50 μCi of [^{35}S]methionine/ml. ATPase was isolated by immunoprecipitation and purified by gel electrophoresis. *D*: autoradiogram of [^{35}S]methionine-labeled peptides in tryptic digests of ATPase synthesized in vitro by bound polysomes. ATPase was isolated by immunoprecipitation and purified by gel electrophoresis. [From Chyn et al. (82).]

plasmic reticulum (47, 82, 179, 345, 376, 428). The mode of insertion of Ca^{2+}-ATPase into the membrane and the location of the NH_2- and COOH-terminal groups with respect to the internal and external surface are unknown.

The symmetrical arrangement of SR in the two halves of the sarcomere and its precise relationship to the contractile filaments suggest that the synthesis of Ca^{2+}-transport ATPase may be confined to central growth regions of the membrane. The newly synthesized ATPase molecules are symmetrically distributed over the surface of endoplasmic reticulum by lateral diffusion. The precise alignment of membrane elements and contractile filaments may imply some interaction between them.

Synthesis of Calsequestrin

Calsequestrin is also synthesized on membrane-bound polysomes (179). Since it is a glycoprotein (262, 345), it is assumed that the NH_2-terminal of the growing polypeptide chain crosses the membrane of the rough endoplasmic reticulum and is transported to the Golgi apparatus like many secretory proteins (262). The mechanism of its subsequent distribution in SR is unknown.

Calsequestrin occurs in two molecular forms, which differ in molecular weight (335). As the NH_2-terminal amino acid of both forms is glutamyl, it is unlikely that one of them would represent a processing intermediate (337).

Regulation of Synthesis of Ca^{2+}-Transport ATPase

The maintenance of intracellular free-Ca^{2+} concentration depends on a balance between regulatory systems located in the surface membrane, mitochondria, SR, and a number of Ca^{2+}-binding proteins, which control muscle contraction and key metabolic processes (381).

The concentration and activity of the various systems must be accurately matched, which requires coordinate regulation of their synthesis and degradation. Some aspects of this regulation are the properties of muscle cells; others are under neural control.

Myogenic Regulation

Membrane-bound polysomes isolated from 11- to 12-day-old chicken embryo skeletal muscles were less active in the translation of Ca^{2+}-ATPase than corresponding preparations from 16-day-old embryos. This suggests that the increase in the rate of synthesis of Ca^{2+}-transport ATPase in the late prenatal and early postnatal periods may be due to an increase in the concentration of translatable Ca^{2+}-ATPase messenger ribonucleic acid (mRNA) in the cell. Therefore the synthesis of Ca^{2+}-ATPase is probably regulated at the transcriptional level or at some stage of the processing of mRNA.

The increase in the concentration of Ca^{2+}-transport ATPase in chicken pectoralis muscle cells during development in vivo or in tissue culture is initiated about the time of the fusion of myoblasts into multinucleated myotubes (395, 396) and roughly follows the time course of accumulation of myofibrillar proteins and ATP–creatine phosphotransferase. Inhibition of fusion by lowering the Ca^{2+} concentration in medium below 150 μM prevents the accumulation of Ca^{2+}-ATPase (182) and other muscle-specific proteins, suggesting coordinate regulation of their concentration in the cell.

A hypothesis was proposed in which changes in intracellular free-Ca^{2+} concentration are assumed to influence the rate of synthesis of Ca^{2+}-ATPase, by Ca^{2+}-dependent regulation of the concentration of relevant classes of translatable mRNAs (383). The effect of cytoplasmic Ca^{2+} concentration may be mediated through nuclear Ca^{2+}-binding proteins serving as inducers or repressors of gene transcription. The existence of nuclear Ca^{2+}-binding proteins was recently demonstrated (516, 517). There are several indications that favor this hypothesis.

1. The total Ca^{2+} content of muscle cells is high just before the increased synthesis of Ca^{2+}-ATPase begins and decreases with age both in vivo and in tissue culture as development proceeds (395). In view of the small amount of SR (376) and parvalbumin (324) in embryonic muscle and the rapid Ca^{2+} fluxes across the surface membrane of undifferentiated muscle cells (499), if a major part of this Ca^{2+} is intracellular, the free-Ca^{2+} concentration in the cytoplasm of embryonic muscle is likely to be elevated.

2. Continuous exposure of culture muscle cells to low concentration (10^{-8} M) A23187 increases the steady-state concentration of Ca^{2+}-sensitive, hydroxylamine-labile phosphoprotein, which is assumed to reflect the concentration of Ca^{2+}-ATPase (395). Brief exposure (2–4 h) to 10^{-6} M ionomycin or A23187 produced a selective increase in the incorporation of [^{35}S]methionine into two proteins of 100,000 and 80,000 daltons (497, 499, 663). The 100,000-dalton protein is tentatively identified as the Ca^{2+}-ATPase, but firm evidence on this point is not available. The 80,000-dalton component may be identical with the 80,000-dalton phosphoprotein earlier observed in microsomes isolated from embryonic muscle (376). Its relation to the 84,000-dalton subunit of alkaline phosphatase is being investigated.

3. In chicken embryos between 13 and 19 days of development, the action potential is largely due to Ca^{2+} current, indicating the presence of Ca^{2+} channels in the surface membrane (550). The influx of Ca^{2+} causes spontaneous contractions. This is the time period when the accumulation of Ca^{2+}-ATPase begins. During subsequent development the contribution of Ca^{2+} channels to the action potential gradually decreases and the Ca^{2+}-ATPase concentration reaches a steady level.

Direct analysis of cytoplasmic free Ca^{2+} during development of muscle cells is required to fully substantiate its role in the regulation of SR biosynthesis.

Neural Influence on Concentration of Ca^{2+}-ATPase in Muscle Cells

Much of the increase in the Ca^{2+}-ATPase content of chicken muscle cells occurs around and after the time of hatching and coincides with the onset of muscle activity. Several indications favor the suggestion that the nerve impulses connected with muscle activity promote the synthesis and accumulation of Ca^{2+}-ATPase (257). *1)* The concentration of Ca^{2+}-transport ATPase in cultured muscle cells is only one-fourth to one-third of their innervated in vivo counterparts (395, 396). *2)* Chronic denervation of muscle decreases the Ca^{2+}-transport activity of SR (257, 375). *3)* Functional denervation of muscles by daily injection of curare into the chorioallantois sac of chicken embryos between the 7th and 14th days of development decreases the concentration of Ca^{2+}-ATPase in pectoralis and leg muscles (498). *4)* Cross innervation or chronic stimulation of fast-twitch and slow-twitch muscles changes the Ca^{2+}-transport activity of SR (203, 204).

Neural influence on muscle phenotype may explain the rough correlation between the speed of contraction and relaxation and the Ca^{2+}-transport activity of SR in red and white skeletal, cardiac, and smooth muscles (204, 551, 640). Some of these differences are only quantitative as the relative amount of SR is less in red than in white skeletal muscles and the density of 85-Å particles on fracture faces of SR is also lower in slow-twitch than in fast-twitch fibers (55, 257). It is important, however, to consider the possibility that structurally distinct Ca^{2+}-ATPase isoenzymes may be present in different muscles of the same animal (99) and the neural influence selectively promotes the synthesis of certain muscle-specific isoenzymes.

REFERENCES

1. Abramson, J. J., and A. E. Shamoo. Purification and characterization of the 45,000 dalton fragment from tryptic digestion of (Ca^{2+} + Mg^{2+})-adenosine triphosphatase of sarcoplasmic reticulum. *J. Membr. Biol.* 44: 233–257, 1978.
2. Aderem, A. A., D. B. McIntosh, and M. C. Berman. Occurrence and role of tightly bound adenine nucleotides in sarcoplasmic reticulum of rabbit skeletal muscle. *Proc. Natl. Acad. Sci. USA* 76: 3622–3626, 1979.
3. Adrian, R. H. Charge movement in the membrane of striated muscle. *Annu. Rev. Biophys. Bioeng.* 7: 85–112, 1978.
4. Åkerman, K. E. O., and C. H. J. Wolff. Charge transfer during Ca^{2+} uptake by rabbit skeletal muscle sarcoplasmic reticulum vesicles as measured with oxonol VI. *FEBS Lett.* 100: 291–295, 1979.
5. Allen, G. On the primary structure of the Ca^{2+}-ATPase of sarcoplasmic reticulum. In: *Membrane Proteins*, edited by P. Nicholls, J. V. Møller, P. L. Jørgensen, and A. J. Moody. New York: Pergamon, 1977, p. 159–168. (Proc. FEBS, 11th, Copenhagen, 1977.)
6. Allen, G. The primary structure of the calcium-transporting adenosine triphosphatase of rabbit skeletal sarcoplasmic reticulum. Soluble tryptic peptides from the succinylated carboxymethylated protein. *Biochem. J.* 187: 545–563, 1980.
7. Allen, G. Primary structure of the calcium ion-transporting adenosine triphosphatase of rabbit skeletal sarcoplasmic reticulum. Soluble peptides from the α-chymotryptic digest of the carboxymethylated protein. *Biochem. J.* 187: 565–575, 1980.
8. Allen, G., R. C. Bottomley, and B. J. Trinnaman. Primary structure of the calcium ion-transporting adenosine triphosphatase from rabbit skeletal sarcoplasmic reticulum. Some peptic, thermolytic, tryptic and staphylococcal-proteinase peptides. *Biochem. J.* 187: 577–589, 1980.
9. Allen, G., and N. M. Green. A 31-residue tryptic peptide from the active site of the [Ca^{++}]-transporting adenosine triphosphatase of rabbit sarcoplasmic reticulum. *FEBS Lett.* 63: 188–192, 1976.
10. Allen, G., and N. M. Green. Primary structures of cysteine containing peptides from the calcium ion transporting adenosine triphosphatase of rabbit sarcoplasmic reticulum. *Biochem. J.* 173: 393–402, 1978.
11. Allen, G., B. J. Trinnaman, and N. M. Green. The primary structure of the calcium ion-transporting adenosine triphosphatase protein of rabbit skeletal sarcoplasmic reticulum. Peptides derived from digestion with cyanogen bromide, and the sequences of three long extramembranous segments. *Biochem. J.* 187: 591–616, 1980.
12. Andersen, J. P., P. Fellmann, J. V. Møller, and P. F. Devaux. Immobilization of a spin-labeled fatty acid chain covalently attached to Ca^{2+}-ATPase from sarcoplasmic reticulum suggests an oligomeric structure. *Biochemistry* 20: 4928–4936, 1981.
13. Andersen, J. P., and J. V. Møller. Reaction of sarcoplasmic reticulum Ca^{2+}-ATPase in different functional states with 5,5′-dithiobis (2-nitrobenzoate). *Biochim. Biophys. Acta* 485: 188–202, 1977.
14. Anzai, K., Y. Kirino, and H. Shimizu. Temperature-induced change in the Ca^{2+}-dependent ATPase activity and in the state of the ATPase protein of sarcoplasmic reticulum membrane. *J. Biochem. Tokyo* 84: 815–821, 1978.
15. Ariki, M., and P. D. Boyer. Characterization of medium inorganic phosphate-water exchange catalyzed by sarcoplasmic reticulum vesicles. *Biochemistry* 19: 2001–2004, 1980.
16. Armstrong, C. M., F. M. Bezanilla, and P. Horowicz. Twitches in the presence of ethylene glycol bis(β-aminoethyl ether)-N,N′-tetraacetic acid. *Biochim. Biophys. Acta* 267: 605–608, 1972.
17. Barlogie, B., W. Hasselbach, and M. Makinose. Activation of calcium efflux by ADP and inorganic phosphate. *FEBS Lett.* 12: 267–268, 1971.
18. Barrett, J. N., and E. F. Barrett. Excitation-contraction coupling in skeletal muscle: blockade by high extracellular concentrations of calcium buffers. *Science* 200: 1270–1272, 1978.
19. Barzilay, M., and Z. I. Cabantchik. Anion transport in red blood cells. II. Kinetics of reversible inhibition by nitroaromatic sulfonic acids. *Membr. Biochem.* 2: 255–281, 1979.
20. Barzilay, M., and Z. I. Cabantchik. Anion transport in red blood cells. III. Sites and sidedness of inhibition by high-affinity reversible binding probes. *Membr. Biochem.* 2: 297–322, 1979.
21. Barzilay, M., S. Ship, and Z. I. Cabantchik. Anion transport in red blood cells. I. Chemical properties of anion recognition sites as revealed by structure-activity relationships of aromatic sulfonic acids. *Membr. Biochem.* 2: 227–254, 1979.
22. Baskin, R. J. Ultrastructure and calcium transport in crustacean muscle microsomes. *J. Cell Biol.* 48: 49–60, 1971.
23. Baskin, R. J. Ultrastructure and calcium transport in microsomes from developing muscle. *J. Ultrastruct. Res.* 49: 348–371, 1974.
24. Bastide, F., G. Meissner, S. Fleischer, and R. L. Post. Similarity of the active site of phosphorylation of the adenosine triphosphate for transport of sodium and potassium ions in kidney to that for transport of calcium ions in the sarcoplasmic reticulum of muscle. *J. Biol. Chem.* 248: 8385–8391, 1973.
25. Baylor, S. M., W. K. Chandler, and M. W. Marshall. Studies in the skeletal muscle using the optical probes of membrane potential. In: *Regulation of Muscle Contraction: Excitation-Contraction Coupling*, edited by A. D. Grinnell and M. A. B. Brazier. New York: Academic, 1981, p. 97–130. (UCLA Forum Med. Sci. 22.)
26. Baylor, S. M., and H. Oetliker. Birefringence experiments on isolated skeletal muscle fibres suggest a possible signal from the sarcoplasmic reticulum. *Nature London* 253: 97–101, 1975.
27. Baylor, S. M., and H. Oetliker. A large birefringence signal preceding contraction in single twitch fibres of the frog. *J. Physiol. London* 264: 141–162, 1977.
28. Baylor, S. M., and H. Oetliker. The optical properties of birefringence signals from single muscle fibres. *J. Physiol. London* 264: 163–198, 1977.
29. Baylor, S. M., and H. Oetliker. Birefringence signals from surface and T-system membranes of frog single muscle fibres. *J. Physiol. London* 264: 199–213, 1977.
30. Beeler, T. J. Relationship between calcium uptake and membrane potential of the sarcoplasmic reticulum. *Federation Proc.* 39: 1663, 1980.
31. Beeler, T. J. Ca^{2+} uptake and membrane potential in sarcoplasmic reticulum vesicles. *J. Biol. Chem.* 255: 9156–9161, 1980.
32. Beeler, T. J., R. H. Farmen, and A. N. Martonosi. The mechanism of voltage-sensitive dye responses on sarcoplasmic reticulum. *J. Membr. Biol.* 62: 113–137, 1981.
33. Beeler, T. J., J. T. Russell, and A. Martonosi. Optical probe responses on sarcoplasmic reticulum: oxacarbocyanines as probes of membrane potential. *Eur. J. Biochem.* 95: 579–591, 1979.
34. Beil, F. U., D. Chak, and W. Hasselbach. Phosphorylation from inorganic phosphate and ATP synthesis of sarcoplasmic membranes. *Eur. J. Biochem.* 81: 151–164, 1977.
35. Beil, F. U., D. Chak, W. Hasselbach, and H. H. Weber. Competition between oxalate and phosphate during active

calcium accumulation by sarcoplasmic vesicles. *Z. Naturforsch. Teil C* 32: 281–287, 1977.

36. Bennett, J. P., K. A. McGill, and G. B. Warren. The role of lipids in the functioning of a membrane protein: the sarcoplasmic reticulum calcium pump. *Curr. Top. Membr. Transp.* 14: 127–164, 1980.
37. Bennett, J. P., G. A. Smith, M. D. Houslay, T. R. Hesketh, J. C. Metcalfe, and G. B. Warren. The phospholipid headgroup specificity of an ATP-dependent calcium pump. *Biochim. Biophys. Acta* 513: 310–320, 1978.
38. Beringer, T. A freeze fracture study of sarcoplasmic reticulum from fast and slow muscle of the mouse. *Anat. Rec.* 184: 647–664, 1976.
39. Bertaud, W. S., D. G. Rayns, and F. O. Simpson. Freeze-etch studies on fish skeletal muscle. *J. Cell Sci.* 6: 537–557, 1970.
40. Bezanilla, F., and P. Horowicz. Fluorescence intensity changes associated with contractile activation in frog muscle stained with Nile Blue A. *J. Physiol. London* 246: 709–735, 1975.
41. Bianchi, C. P., and T. C. Bolton. Action of local anesthetics on coupling systems in muscle. *J. Pharmacol. Exp. Ther.* 157: 388–405, 1967.
42. Biltonen, R. L., and E. Freire. Thermodynamic characterization of conformational states of biological macromolecules using differential scanning calorimetry. *Crit. Rev. Biochem.* 5: 85–124, 1978.
43. Birks, R. I., and D. F. Davey. Osmotic responses demonstrating the extracellular character of the sarcoplasmic reticulum. *J. Physiol. London* 202: 171–188, 1969.
44. Blaustein, M. P. The ins and outs of calcium transport in squid axons: internal and external ion activation of calcium efflux. *Federation Proc.* 35: 2574–2578, 1976.
45. Boland, R., T. Chyn, D. Roufa, E. Reyes, and A. Martonosi. The lipid composition of muscle cells during development. *Biochim. Biophys. Acta* 489: 349–359, 1977.
46. Boland, R., and A. Martonosi. The lipid composition and Ca transport function of sarcoplasmic reticulum (SR) membranes during development in vivo and in vitro. In: *Function and Biosynthesis of Lipids*, edited by N. G. Bazan, R. R. Brenner, and N. M. Guisto. New York: Plenum, 1976, p. 233–239.
47. Boland, R., A. Martonosi, and T. W. Tillack. Developmental changes in the composition and function of sarcoplasmic reticulum. *J. Biol. Chem.* 249: 612–623, 1974.
48. Bonnet, J. P., M. Galante., D. Brethes, J. C. Dedieu, and J. Chevallier. Purification of sarcoplasmic reticulum vesicles through their loading with calcium phosphate. *Arch. Biochem. Biophys.* 191: 32–41, 1978.
49. Bornet, E. P., M. L. Entman, W. B. Van Winkle, A. Schwartz, D. C. Lehotay, and G. S. Levey. Cyclic AMP modulation of calcium accumulation by sarcoplasmic reticulum from fast skeletal muscle. *Biochim. Biophys. Acta* 468: 188–193, 1977.
50. Boyer, P. D. A model for conformational coupling of membrane potential and proton translocation to ATP synthesis and to active transport. *FEBS Lett.* 58: 1–6, 1975.
51. Boyer, P. D., and M. Ariki. ^{18}O probes of phosphoenzyme formation and cooperativity with sarcoplasmic reticulum ATPase. *Federation Proc.* 39: 2410–2421, 1980.
52. Boyer, P. D., B. Chance, L. Ernster, P. Mitchell, E. Racker, and E. C. Slater. Oxidative phosphorylation and photophosphorylation. *Annu. Rev. Biochem.* 46: 955–1026, 1977.
53. Boyer, P. D., L. de Meis, M. da G. C. Carvalho, and D. D. Hackney. Dynamic reversal of enzyme carboxyl group phosphorylation as the basis of the oxygen exchange catalyzed by sarcoplasmic reticulum adenosine triphosphatase. *Biochemistry* 16: 136–140, 1977.
54. Brandt, N. R., A. H. Caswell, and J.-P. Brunschwig. ATP-energized Ca^{2+} pump in isolated transverse tubules of skeletal muscle. *J. Biol. Chem.* 255: 6290–6298, 1980.
55. Bray, D. F., and D. G. Rayns. A comparative freeze-etch study of the sarcoplasmic reticulum of avian fast and slow muscle fibers. *J. Ultrastruct. Res.* 57: 251–259, 1976.
56. Bray, D. F., D. G. Rayns, and E. B. Wagenaar. Intramembrane particle densities in freeze fractured sarcoplasmic reticulum. *Can. J. Zool.* 56: 140–145, 1978.
57. Briggs, F. N., R. M. Wise, and J. A. Hearn. The effect of lithium and potassium on the transient state kinetics of the (Ca + Mg)-ATPase of cardiac sarcoplasmic reticulum. *J. Biol. Chem.* 253: 5884–5885, 1978.
58. Brinley, F. J., Jr. Calcium buffering in squid axons. *Annu. Rev. Biophys. Bioeng.* 7: 363–392, 1978.
59. Bürkli, A., and R. J. Cherry. Rotational motion and flexibility of Ca^{2+}, Mg^{2+} dependent adenosine 5′-triphosphatase in sarcoplasmic reticulum membranes. *Biochemistry* 20: 138–145, 1981.
60. Cabantchik, Z. I., P. A. Knauf, and A. Rothstein. The anion transport system of the red blood cell. The role of membrane protein evaluated by the use of 'probes.' *Biochim. Biophys. Acta* 515: 239–302, 1978.
61. Campbell, K. P., C. Franzini-Armstrong, and A. E. Shamoo. Further characterization of light and heavy sarcoplasmic reticulum vesicles. Identification of the "sarcoplasmic reticulum feet" associated with heavy sarcoplasmic reticulum vesicles. *Biochim. Biophys. Acta* 602: 97–116, 1980.
62. Caputo, C. Excitation and contraction processes in muscle. *Annu. Rev. Biophys. Bioeng.* 7: 63–83, 1978.
63. Carafoli, E., F. Clementi, W. Drabikowski, and A. Margreth (editors). *Calcium Transport in Contraction and Secretion.* Amsterdam: North-Holland, 1975.
64. Carafoli, E., and M. Crompton. The regulation of intracellular calcium. *Curr. Top. Membr. Transp.* 10: 151–216, 1978.
65. Carley, W. W., and E. Racker. ATP dependent phosphate transport in sarcoplasmic reticulum, and reconstituted proteoliposomes. *J. Membr. Biol.* In press.
66. Carraway, K. L., and D. E. Koshland, Jr. Carbodiimide modification of proteins. *Methods Enzymol.* 25: 616–623, 1972.
67. Carsten, M. E. The cardiac calcium pump. *Proc. Natl. Acad. Sci. USA* 52: 1456–1462, 1964.
68. Carvalho, A. P. Effects of potentiators of muscular contraction on binding of cations by sarcoplasmic reticulum. *J. Gen. Physiol.* 51: 427–442, 1968.
69. Carvalho, A. P., and B. Leo. Effects of ATP on the interaction of Ca^{++}, Mg^{++}, and K^{+}, with fragmented sarcoplasmic reticulum isolated from rabbit skeletal muscle. *J. Gen. Physiol.* 50: 1327–1352, 1967.
70. Carvalho, M. da G. C., D. G. de Souza, and L. de Meis. On a possible mechanism of energy conservation in sarcoplasmic reticulum membrane. *J. Biol. Chem.* 251: 3629–3636, 1976.
71. Caswell, A. H., S. P. Baker, H. Boyd, L. T. Potter, and M. Garcia. β-Adrenergic receptor and adenylate cyclase in transverse tubules of skeletal muscle. *J. Biol. Chem.* 253: 3049–3054, 1978.
72. Caswell, A. H., Y. H. Lau, and J.-P. Brunschwig. Ouabain binding vesicles from skeletal muscle. *Arch. Biochem. Biophys.* 176: 417–430, 1976.
73. Caswell, A. H., Y. H. Lau, M. Garcia, and J. P. Brunschwig. Recognition and junction formation by isolated transverse tubules and terminal cisternae of skeletal muscle. *J. Biol. Chem.* 254: 202–208, 1979.
74. Chacko, S. DNA synthesis, mitosis, and differentiation in cardiac myogenesis. *Dev. Biol.* 35: 1–18, 1973.
75. Chaloub, R. M., H. Guimaraes-Motta, S. Verjovski-Almeida, L. de Meis, and G. Inesi. Sequential reactions in P_i utilization for ATP synthesis by sarcoplasmic reticulum. *J. Biol. Chem.* 254: 9464–9468, 1979.
76. Champeil, P., S. Bushlen-Boucly, F. Bastide, and C. Gary-Bobo. Sarcoplasmic reticulum ATPase. Spin labeling detection of ligand-induced changes in the relative reactivities of certain sulfhydryl groups. *J. Biol. Chem.* 253: 1179–1186, 1978.
77. Champeil, P., J. L. Rigaud, and C. M. Gary-Bobo. Calcium

translocation mechanism in sarcoplasmic reticulum vesicles, deduced from location studies of protein-bound spin labels. *Proc. Natl. Acad. Sci. USA* 77: 2405–2409, 1980.

78. Chandler, W. K., R. F. Rakowski, and M. F. Schneider. A non-linear voltage dependent charge movement in frog skeletal muscle. *J. Physiol. London* 254: 245–283, 1976.
79. Chevallier, J., and R. A. Butow. Calcium binding to the sarcoplasmic reticulum of rabbit skeletal muscle. *Biochemistry* 10: 2733–2737, 1971.
80. Chiesi, M., D. Lewis, and G. Inesi. Ca^{2+}-H^+ exchange mechanism in sarcoplasmic reticulum (SR) vesicles. *Federation Proc.* 39: 2037, 1980.
81. Chyn, T., and A. N. Martonosi. Chemical modification of sarcoplasmic reticulum membranes. *Biochim. Biophys. Acta* 468: 114–126, 1977.
82. Chyn, T. L., A. N. Martonosi, T. Morimoto, and D. D. Sabatini. In vitro synthesis of the Ca^{2+} transport ATPase by ribosomes bound to sarcoplasmic reticulum membranes. *Proc. Natl. Acad. Sci. USA* 76: 1241–1245, 1979.
83. Coan, C. R., and G. Inesi. Ca^{2+} dependent effect of acetylphosphate on spin-labeled sarcoplasmic reticulum. *Biochem. Biophys. Res. Commun.* 71: 1283–1288, 1976.
84. Coan, C. R., and G. Inesi. Ca^{2+}-dependent effect of ATP on spin-labeled sarcoplasmic reticulum. *J. Biol. Chem.* 252: 3044–3049, 1977.
85. Coan, C., S. Verjovski-Almeida, and G. Inesi. Ca^{2+} regulation of conformational states in the transport cycle of spin-labeled sarcoplasmic reticulum ATPase. *J. Biol. Chem.* 254: 2968–2974, 1979.
86. Coetzee, G. A., and W. Gevers. Myosin in primary cultures of hamster heart cells. *Dev. Biol.* 63: 128–138, 1978.
87. Coffey, R. L., E. Lagwinska, M. Oliver, and A. N. Martonosi. The mechanism of ATP hydrolysis by sarcoplasmic reticulum. *Arch. Biochem. Biophys.* 170: 37–48, 1975.
88. Cohen, A., and Z. Selinger. Calcium binding properties of sarcoplasmic reticulum membranes. *Biochim. Biophys. Acta* 183: 27–35, 1969.
89. Cohen, L. B., and B. M. Salzberg. Optical measurement of membrane potential. *Rev. Physiol. Biochem. Pharmacol.* 83: 35–88, 1978.
90. Cohen, P. The role of cyclic AMP dependent protein kinase in the regulation of glycogen metabolism in mammalian skeletal muscle. *Curr. Top. Cell. Regul.* 14: 117–196, 1978.
91. Conti, F. Fluorescent probes in nerve membranes. *Annu. Rev. Biophys. Bioeng.* 4: 287–310, 1975.
92. Coronado, R., and C. Miller. Voltage-dependent caesium blockade of a cation channel from fragmented sarcoplasmic reticulum. *Nature London* 280: 807–810, 1979.
93. Costantin, L. L. The role of sodium current in the radial spread of contraction in frog muscle fibers. *J. Gen. Physiol.* 55: 703–715, 1970.
94. Costantin, L. L. Contractile activation in skeletal muscle. *Prog. Biophys. Mol. Biol.* 29: 197–224, 1975.
95. Costantin, L. L., C. Franzini-Armstrong, and R. J. Podolsky. Localization of calcium-accumulating structures in striated muscle fibers. *Science* 147: 158–160, 1965.
96. Costantin, L. L., and R. J. Podolsky. Depolarization of the internal membrane system in the activation of frog skeletal muscle. *J. Gen. Physiol.* 50: 1101–1124, 1967.
97. Crowe, L. M., and R. J. Baskin. Stereological analysis of developing sarcotubular membranes. *J. Ultrastruct. Res.* 58: 10–22, 1977.
98. Dahms, A. S., T. Kanazawa, and P. D. Boyer. Source of the oxygen in the C-O-P linkage of the acyl phosphate in transport adenosine triphosphatases. *J. Biol. Chem.* 248: 6592–6595, 1973.
99. Damiani, E., R. Betto, S. Salvatori, P. Volpe, G. Salviati, and A. Margreth. Polymorphism of sarcoplasmic-reticulum adenosine triphosphatase of rabbit skeletal muscle. *Biochem. J.* 197: 245–248, 1981.
100. Davis, D. G., G. Inesi, and T. Gulik-Krzywicki. Lipid molecular motion and enzyme activity in sarcoplasmic reticulum membrane. *Biochemistry* 15: 1271–1276, 1976.
101. Deamer, D. W. Isolation and characterization of a lysolecithin-adenosinetriphosphatase complex from lobster muscle microsomes. *J. Biol. Chem.* 248: 5477–5485, 1973.
102. Deamer, D. W., and R. J. Baskin. Ultrastructure of sarcoplasmic reticulum preparations. *J. Cell Biol.* 42: 296–307, 1969.
103. Deamer, D. W., and R. J. Baskin. ATP synthesis in sarcoplasmic reticulum. *Arch. Biochem. Biophys.* 153: 47–54, 1972.
104. Dean, W. L., and C. Tanford. Reactivation of lipid depleted Ca^{2+} ATPase by nonionic detergent. *J. Biol. Chem.* 252: 3551–3553, 1977.
105. Dean, W. L., and C. Tanford. Properties of a delipidated detergent-activated Ca^{2+}-ATPase. *Biochemistry* 17: 1683–1690, 1978.
106. De Boland, A. R., R. L. Jilka, and A. N. Martonosi. Passive Ca^{2+} permeability of phospholipid vesicles and sarcoplasmic reticulum membranes. *J. Biol. Chem.* 250: 7501–7510, 1975.
107. De Foor, P. H., D. Levitsky, T. Biryukova, and S. Fleischer. Immunological dissimilarity of the calcium pump protein of skeletal and cardiac muscle sarcoplasmic reticulum. *Arch. Biochem. Biophys.* 200: 196–205, 1980.
108. Degani, C., and P. D. Boyer. A borohydride reduction method for characterization of the acyl phosphate linkage in proteins and its application to sarcoplasmic reticulum adenosine triphosphatase. *J. Biol. Chem.* 248: 8222–8226, 1973.
109. Deguchi, N., P. L. Jørgensen, and A. B. Maunsbach. Ultrastructure of the sodium pump. Comparison of thin sectioning, negative staining and freeze fracture of purified membrane bound (Na^+, K^+) ATPase. *J. Cell Biol.* 75: 619–634, 1977.
110. De Kruijff, B., A. M. H. P. van den Besselaar, H. van den Bosch, and L. L. M. van Deenen. Inside-outside distribution and diffusion of phosphatidylcholine in rat sarcoplasmic reticulum as determined by ^{13}C NMR and phosphatidylcholine exchange protein. *Biochim. Biophys. Acta* 555: 181–192, 1979.
111. De Meis, L. Activation of Ca^{2+} uptake by acetyl phosphate in muscle microsomes. *Biochim. Biophys. Acta* 172: 343–344, 1969.
112. De Meis, L. Ca^{2+} uptake and acetyl phosphatase of skeletal muscle microsomes. Inhibition by Na^+, K^+, Li^+ and adenosine triphosphate. *J. Biol. Chem.* 244: 3733–3739, 1969.
113. De Meis, L. Allosteric inhibition by alkali ions of the Ca^{2+} uptake and adenosine triphosphatase activity of skeletal muscle microsomes. *J. Biol. Chem.* 246: 4764–4773, 1971.
114. De Meis, L. Phosphorylation of the membranous protein of the sarcoplasmic reticulum; inhibition by Na^+ and K^+. *Biochemistry* 11: 2460–2465, 1972.
115. De Meis, L. Regulation of steady state level of phosphoenzyme and ATP synthesis in sarcoplasmic reticulum vesicles during reversal of the Ca^{2+} pump. *J. Biol. Chem.* 251: 2055–2062, 1976.
116. De Meis, L., and P. D. Boyer. Induction by nucleotide triphosphate hydrolysis of a form of sarcoplasmic reticulum ATPase capable of medium phosphate-oxygen exchange in presence of calcium. *J. Biol. Chem.* 253: 1556–1559, 1978.
117. De Meis, L., and M. da G. C. Carvalho. On the sidedness of membrane phosphorylation by P_i and ATP synthesis during reversal of the Ca^{2+} pump of sarcoplasmic reticulum vesicles. *J. Biol. Chem.* 251: 1413–1417, 1976.
118. De Meis, L., and M. C. F. de Mello. Substrate regulation of membrane phosphorylation and of Ca^{2+} transport in the sarcoplasmic reticulum. *J. Biol. Chem.* 248: 3691–3701, 1973.
119. De Meis, L., and W. Hasselbach. Acetyl phosphate as substrate for Ca^{2+} uptake in skeletal muscle microsomes. Inhibition by alkali ions. *J. Biol. Chem.* 246: 4759–4763, 1971.
120. De Meis, L., and H. Masuda. Phosphorylation of the sarcoplasmic reticulum membrane by orthophosphate through two different reactions. *Biochemistry* 13: 2057–2062, 1974.
121. De Meis, L., and R. K. Tume. A new mechanism by which an H^+ concentration gradient drives the synthesis of adenosine triphosphate, pH jump, and adenosine triphosphate synthesis by the Ca^{2+}-dependent adenosine triphosphatase of sarcoplasmic reticulum. *Biochemistry* 16: 4455–4463, 1977.

122. De Meis, L., and A. L. Vianna. Energy interconversion by the Ca^{2+}-dependent ATPase of the sarcoplasmic reticulum. *Annu. Rev. Biochem.* 48: 275–292, 1979.
123. Devaux, P. F., and J. Davoust. Current views on boundary lipids deduced from electron-spin resonance studies. In: *Membranes and Transport*, edited by A. Martonosi. New York: Plenum, 1982, vol. 1, p. 125–133.
124. Devine, C. E., and D. G. Rayns. Freeze fracture studies of membrane systems in vertebrate muscle. II. Smooth muscle. *J. Ultrastruct. Res.* 51: 293–306, 1975.
125. Duggan, P. F. Some properties of the monovalent-cation-stimulated adenosine triphosphatase of frog sartorius microsomes. *Biochim. Biophys. Acta* 99: 144–155, 1965.
126. Duggan, P. F. Potassium-activated adenosinetriphosphatase and calcium uptake by sarcoplasmic reticulum. *Life Sci.* 6: 561–567, 1967.
127. Duggan, P. F. The monovalent cation-stimulated calcium pump in frog skeletal muscle. *Life Sci.* 7: 913–919, 1968.
128. Duggan, P. F. Calcium uptake and associated adenosine triphosphatase activity in fragmented sarcoplasmic reticulum. Requirement for potassium ions. *J. Biol. Chem.* 252: 1620–1627, 1977.
129. Duggan, P. F., and A. Martonosi. Sarcoplasmic reticulum. IX. The permeability of sarcoplasmic reticulum membranes. *J. Gen. Physiol.* 56: 147–167, 1970.
130. Dupont, Y. Fluorescence studies of the sarcoplasmic reticulum calcium pump. *Biochem. Biophys. Res. Commun.* 71: 544–550, 1976.
131. Dupont, Y. Kinetics and regulation of sarcoplasmic reticulum ATPase. *Eur. J. Biochem.* 72: 185–190, 1977.
132. Dupont, Y. Mechanism of the sarcoplasmic reticulum calcium pump. Fluorometric study of the phosphorylated intermediates. *Biochem. Biophys. Res. Commun.* 82: 893–900, 1978.
133. Dupont, Y. Electrogenic calcium transport in the sarcoplasmic reticulum membrane. In: *Cation Flux Across Biomembranes*, edited by Y. Mukohata and L. Packer. New York: Academic, 1979, p. 141–160.
134. Dupont, Y. Occlusion of divalent cations in the phosphorylated calcium pump of sarcoplasmic reticulum. *Eur. J. Biochem.* 109: 231–238, 1980.
135. Dupont, Y., S. C. Harrison, and W. Hasselbach. Molecular organization in the sarcoplasmic reticulum membrane studied by X-ray diffraction. *Nature London* 244: 555–558, 1973.
136. Dupont, Y., and J. B. Leigh. Transient kinetics of sarcoplasmic reticulum Ca^{2+} + Mg^{2+} ATPase studied by fluorescence. *Nature London* 273: 396–398, 1978.
137. Dutton, A., E. D. Rees, and S. J. Singer. An experiment eliminating the rotating carrier mechanism for the active transport of Ca ion in sarcoplasmic reticulum membranes. *Proc. Natl. Acad. Sci. USA* 73: 1532–1536, 1976.
138. Ebashi, S. Calcium binding activity of vesicular relaxing factor. *J. Biochem.* 50: 236–244, 1961.
139. Ebashi, S. Excitation-contraction coupling. *Annu. Rev. Physiol.* 38: 293–313, 1976.
140. Ebashi, S. Muscle contraction and pharmacology. *Trends Pharmacol. Sci.* 1: 29–31, 1979.
141. Ebashi, S. Ca ion and muscle contraction. In: *Advances in Pharmacology and Therapeutics. Ions-Cyclic Nucleotides-Cholinergy*, edited by J. C. Stoclet. Oxford, UK: Pergamon, 1979, vol. 3, p. 81–98.
142. Ebashi, S., and M. Endo. Calcium ion and muscle contraction. *Prog. Biophys. Mol. Biol.* 18: 123–183, 1968.
143. Ebashi, S., M. Endo, and I. Ohtsuki. Control of muscle contraction. *Q. Rev. Biophys.* 2: 351–384, 1969.
144. Ebashi, S., and F. Lipmann. Adenosine triphosphate-linked concentration of calcium ions in a particulate fraction of rabbit muscle. *J. Cell Biol.* 14: 389–400, 1962.
145. Eckert, K., R. Grosse, D. O. Levitski, A. V. Kuzmin, V. N. Smirnov, and K. R. H. Repke. Determination and functional significance of low affinity nucleotide sites of Ca^{2+} + Mg^{2+}-dependent ATPase of sarcoplasmic reticulum. *Acta Biol. Med. Ger.* 36: K1–K10, 1977.
146. Eisenberg, E., and L. E. Greene. The relation of muscle biochemistry to muscle physiology. *Annu. Rev. Physiol.* 42: 293–309, 1980.
147. Endo, M. Calcium release from the sarcoplasmic reticulum. *Physiol. Rev.* 57: 71–108, 1977.
148. Endo, M., Y. Kakuta, and T. Kitazawa. A further study of the Ca-induced Ca release mechanism. In: *Regulation of Muscle Contraction: Excitation-Contraction Coupling*, edited by A. D. Grinnell and M. A. B. Brazier. New York: Academic, 1981, p. 181–195. (UCLA Forum Med. Sci., 22.)
149. Entman, M. L., E. P. Bornet, A. J. Garber, A. Schwartz, G. S. Levey, D. C. Lehotay, and L. A. Bricker. The cardiac sarcoplasmic reticulum-glycogenolytic complex. A possible effector site for cyclic AMP. *Biochim. Biophys. Acta* 499: 228–237, 1977.
150. Entman, M. L., M. A. Goldstein, and A. Schwartz. The cardiac sarcoplasmic reticulum-glycogenolytic complex, an internal beta adrenergic receptor. *Life Sci.* 19: 1623–1630, 1976.
151. Entman, M. L., K. Kaniike, M. A. Goldstein, T. E. Nelson, E. P. Bornet, T. W. Futch, and A. Schwartz. Association of glycogenolysis with cardiac sarcoplasmic reticulum. *J. Biol. Chem.* 251: 3140–3146, 1976.
152. Epstein, M., Y. Kuriki, R. Biltonen, and E. Racker. Calorimetric studies of ligand-induced modulation of calcium adenosine 5′-triphosphatase from sarcoplasmic reticulum. *Biochemistry* 19: 5564–5568, 1980.
153. Estep, T. N., and T. E. Thompson. Energy transfer in lipid bilayers. *Biophys. J.* 26: 195–208, 1979.
154. Fabiato, A., and F. Fabiato. Relaxing and inotropic effects of cyclic AMP on skinned cardiac cells. *Nature London* 253: 556–558, 1975.
155. Fabiato, A, and F. Fabiato. Calcium-induced release of calcium from the sarcoplasmic reticulum of skinned cells from adult human, dog, cat, rabbit, rat, and frog hearts and from fetal and new-born rat ventricles. *Ann. NY Acad. Sci.* 307: 491–522, 1978.
156. Fabiato, A., and F. Fabiato. Cyclic AMP-induced enhancement of calcium accumulation by the sarcoplasmic reticulum with no modification of the sensitivity of the myofilaments to calcium in skinned fibres from a fast skeletal muscle. *Biochim. Biophys. Acta* 539: 253–260, 1978.
157. Fabiato, A., and F. Fabiato. Calcium and cardiac excitation-contraction coupling. *Annu. Rev. Physiol.* 41: 473–484, 1979.
158. Fanburg, B. L., D. B. Drachman, and D. Moll. Calcium transport in isolated sarcoplasmic reticulum during muscle maturation. *Nature London* 218: 962–964, 1968.
159. Fanburg, B., R. M. Finkel, and A. Martonosi. The role of calcium in the mechanism of relaxation of cardiac muscle. *J. Biol. Chem.* 239: 2298–2306, 1964.
160. Fanburg, B. L., and S. Matsushita. Phosphorylated intermediate of ATPase of isolated cardiac sarcoplasmic reticulum. *J. Mol. Cell. Cardiol.* 5: 111–115, 1973.
161. Fiehn, W., and W. Hasselbach. The effect of phospholipase A on the calcium transport and the role of unsaturated fatty acids in ATPase activity of sarcoplasmic vesicles. *Eur. J. Biochem.* 13: 510–518, 1970.
162. Fiehn, W., and A. Migala. Calcium binding to sarcoplasmic membranes. *Eur. J. Biochem.* 20: 245–248, 1971.
163. Fiehn, W., J. B. Peter, J. F. Mead, and M. Gan-Elepano. Lipids and fatty acids of sarcolemma, sarcoplasmic reticulum, and mitochondria from rat skeletal muscle. *J. Biol. Chem.* 246: 5617–5620, 1971.
164. Fleischer, S., C. T. Wang, A. Saito, M. Pilarska, and J. T. McIntyre. Structural studies of sarcoplasmic reticulum in vitro and in situ. In: *Cation Flux Across Biomembranes*, edited by Y. Mukohata and L. Packer. New York: Academic, 1979, p. 193–205.
165. Ford, L. E., and R. J. Podolsky. Regenerative calcium release within muscle cells. *Science* 167: 58–59, 1970.
166. Fozzard, H. A. Heart excitation-contraction coupling. *Annu. Rev. Physiol.* 39: 201–220, 1977.
167. Franzini-Armstrong, C. Studies of the triad. I. Structure of

the junction in frog twitch fibers. *J. Cell Biol.* 47: 488–499, 1970.

168. FRANZINI-ARMSTRONG, C. Studies of the triad. II. Penetration of tracers into the junctional gap. *J. Cell Biol.* 49: 196–203, 1971.
169. FRANZINI-ARMSTRONG, C. Studies of the triad. IV. Structure of the junction in frog slow fibers. *J. Cell Biol.* 56: 120–128, 1973.
170. FRANZINI-ARMSTRONG, C. Freeze fracture of skeletal muscle from the tarantula spider. Structural differentiations of sarcoplasmic reticulum and transverse tubular system membranes. *J. Cell Biol.* 61: 501–513, 1974.
171. FRANZINI-ARMSTRONG, C. Membrane particles and transmission at the triad. *Federation Proc.* 34: 1382–1389, 1975.
172. FRANZINI-ARMSTRONG, C. Structure of sarcoplasmic reticulum. *Federation Proc.* 39: 2403–2409, 1980.
173. FRIEDMAN, Z., AND M. MAKINOSE. Phosphorylation of skeletal muscle microsomes by acetylphosphate. *FEBS Lett.* 11: 69–72, 1970.
174. FROEHLICH, J. P., AND E. W. TAYLOR. Transient state kinetic studies of sarcoplasmic reticulum adenosine triphosphatase. *J. Biol. Chem.* 250: 2013–2021, 1975.
175. FROEHLICH, J. P., AND E. W. TAYLOR. Transient state kinetic effects of calcium ion on sarcoplasmic reticulum adenosine triphosphatase. *J. Biol. Chem.* 251: 2307–2315, 1976.
176. GALANI-KRANIAS, E., R. BICK, AND A. SCHWARTZ. Phosphorylation of a 100,000 dalton component and its relationship to calcium transport in sarcoplasmic reticulum from rabbit skeletal muscle. *Biochim. Biophys. Acta* 628: 438–450, 1980.
177. GARRAHAN, P. J., A. F. REGA, AND G. L. ALONSO. The interaction of magnesium ions with the calcium pump of sarcoplasmic reticulum. *Biochim. Biophys. Acta* 448: 121–132, 1976.
178. GATTASS, C. R., AND L. DE MEIS. Ca^{2+} dependent inhibitory effects of Na^+ and K^+ on Ca^{2+} transport in sarcoplasmic reticulum vesicles. *Biochim. Biophys. Acta* 389: 506–515, 1975.
179. GREENWAY, D. C., AND D. H. MACLENNAN. Assembly of the sarcoplasmic reticulum. Synthesis of calsequestrin and the Ca^{2+} + Mg^{2+}-adenosine triphosphatase on membrane-bound polyribosomes. *Can. J. Biochem.* 56: 452–456, 1978.
180. GUILLAIN, F., M. P. GINGOLD, S. BUSCHLEN, AND P. CHAMPEIL. A direct fluorescence study of the transient steps induced by calcium binding to sarcoplasmic reticulum ATPase. *J. Biol. Chem.* 255: 2072–2076, 1980.
181. GUNN, R. B. Co- and counter-transport mechanisms in cell membranes. *Annu. Rev. Physiol.* 42: 249–259, 1980.
182. HA, D. B., R. BOLAND, AND A. MARTONOSI. Synthesis of the calcium transport ATPase of sarcoplasmic reticulum and other muscle proteins during development of muscle cells in vivo and in vitro. *Biochim. Biophys. Acta* 585: 165–187, 1979.
183. HASSELBACH, W. Relaxing factor and the relaxation of muscle. *Prog. Biophys. Mol. Biol.* 14: 167–222, 1964.
184. HASSELBACH, W. Relaxation and the sarcotubular calcium pump. *Federation Proc.* 23: 909–912, 1964.
185. HASSELBACH, W. Sarcoplasmic membrane ATPases. In: *The Enzymes*, edited by P. D. Boyer. New York: Academic, 1974, vol. X, p. 431–467.
186. HASSELBACH, W. The reversibility of the sarcoplasmic calcium pump. *Biochim. Biophys. Acta* 515: 23–53, 1978.
187. HASSELBACH, W. The sarcoplasmic calcium pump. A model of energy transduction in biological membranes. *Top. Curr. Chem.* 78: 1–56, 1979.
188. HASSELBACH, W., AND L. G. ELFVIN. Structural and chemical asymmetry of the calcium-transporting membranes of the sarcotubular system as revealed by electron microscopy. *J. Ultrastruct. Res.* 17: 598–622, 1967.
189. HASSELBACH, W., AND M. MAKINOSE. Die Calciumpumpe der "Erschlaffungsgrana" des Muskels und ihre Abhängigkeit von der ATP-Spaltung. *Biochem. Z.* 333: 518–528, 1961.
190. HASSELBACH, W., AND M. MAKINOSE. ATP and active transport. *Biochem. Biophys. Res. Commun.* 7: 132–136, 1962.
191. HASSELBACH, W., AND M. MAKINOSE. Über den Mechanismus des Calciumtransportes durch die Membranen des Sarkoplasmatischen Reticulums. *Biochem. Z.* 339: 94–111, 1963.
192. HASSELBACH, W., M. MAKINOSE, AND A. MIGALA. The arsenate induced calcium release from sarcoplasmic vesicles. *FEBS Lett.* 20: 311–315, 1972.
193. HASSELBACH, W., AND A. MIGALA. Arrangement of proteins and lipids in the sarcoplasmic membrane. *Z. Naturforsch. Teil C* 30: 681–683, 1975.
194. HASSELBACH, W., AND A. MIGALA. Calcium gradient dependent pyrophosphate formation by sarcoplasmic vesicles. *Z. Naturforsch. Teil C* 32: 993–996, 1977.
195. HASSELBACH, W., A. MIGALA, AND B. AGOSTINI. The location of the calcium precipitating protein in the sarcoplasmic membrane. *Z. Naturforsch. Teil C* 30: 600–607, 1975.
196. HASSELBACH, W., AND K. SERAYDARIAN. The role of sulfhydryl groups in calcium transport through the sarcoplasmic membranes of skeletal muscle. *Biochem. Z.* 345: 159–172, 1966.
197. HASSELBACH, W., J. SUKO, M. H. STROMER, AND R. THE. Mechanism of calcium transport in sarcoplasmic reticulum. *Ann. NY Acad. Sci.* 264: 335–349, 1976.
198. HASSELBACH, W., AND H. H. WEBER. Anion specific carriers in the sarcoplasmic membranes. In: *Membrane Proteins in Transport and Phosphorylation*, edited by G. F. Azzone, M. E. Klingenberg, E. Quagliariello, and N. Siliprandi. Amsterdam: North-Holland, 1974, p. 103–111.
199. HAYNES, D. Rapid kinetics of active Ca^{2+} transport by skeletal sarcoplasmic reticulum monitored by a fluorescent probe. *Federation Proc.* 39: 1663, 1980.
200. HAYNES, D. H., AND V. C. K. CHIU. 1-anilino-8-naphthalenesulfonate as a fluorescent probe of calcium transport: application to skeletal sarcoplasmic reticulum. *Ann. NY Acad. Sci.* 307: 217–220, 1978.
201. HEBDON, G. M., L. W. CUNNINGHAM, AND N. M. GREEN. Cross-linking experiments with the adenosine triphosphatase of sarcoplasmic reticulum. *Biochem. J.* 179: 135–139, 1979.
202. HEILMANN, C., D. BRDICZKA, E. NICKEL, AND D. PETTE. ATPase activities, Ca^{2+} transport and phosphoprotein formation in sarcoplasmic reticulum subfractions of fast and slow rabbit muscles. *Eur. J. Biochem.* 81: 211–222, 1977.
203. HEILMANN, C., W. MULLER, AND D. PETTE. Correlation between ultrastructural and functional changes in sarcoplasmic reticulum during chronic stimulation of fast muscle. *J. Membr. Biol.* 59: 143–149, 1981.
204. HEILMANN, C., AND D. PETTE. Molecular transformations in sarcoplasmic reticulum of fast-twitch muscle by electro-stimulation. *Eur. J. Biochem.* 93: 437–446, 1979.
205. HENDERSON, R., AND P. N. T. UNWIN. Three-dimensional model of purple membrane obtained by electron microscopy. *Nature London* 257: 28–32, 1975.
206. HERBETTE, L., J. MARQUARDT, A. SCARPA, AND J. K. BLASIE. A direct analysis of lamellar x-ray diffraction from hydrated oriented multilayers of fully functional sarcoplasmic reticulum. *Biophys. J.* 20: 245–272, 1977.
207. HESKETH, T. R., G. A. SMITH, M. D. HOUSLAY, K. A. MCGILL, N. J. M. BIRDSALL, J. C. METCALFE, AND G. B. WARREN. Annular lipids determine the ATPase activity of a calcium transport protein, complexed with dipalmitoyllecithin. *Biochemistry* 15: 4145–4151, 1976.
208. HICKS, M. J., M. SHIGEKAWA, AND A. M. KATZ. Mechanism by which cyclic adenosine 3′:5′-monophosphate-dependent protein kinase stimulates calcium transport in cardiac sarcoplasmic reticulum. *Circ. Res.* 44: 384–391, 1979.
209. HIDALGO, C. Inhibition of calcium transport in sarcoplasmic reticulum after modification of highly reactive amino groups. *Biochem. Biophys. Res. Commun.* 92: 757–765, 1980.
210. HIDALGO, C., AND N. IKEMOTO. Disposition of proteins and aminophospholipids in the sarcoplasmic reticulum membrane. *J. Biol. Chem.* 252: 8446–8454, 1977.
211. HIDALGO, C., N. IKEMOTO, AND J. GERGELY. Role of phospholipids in the calcium-dependent ATPase of the sarcoplasmic reticulum. Enzymatic and ESR studies with phospholipid-replaced membranes. *J. Biol. Chem.* 251: 4224–4232, 1976.
212. HIDALGO, C., D. D. THOMAS, AND N. IKEMOTO. Effect of the

lipid environment on protein motion and enzymatic activity of the sarcoplasmic reticulum calcium ATPase. *J. Biol. Chem.* 253: 6879–6887, 1978.

213. HOBBS, A. S., AND R. W. ALBERS. The structure of proteins involved in active membrane transport. *Annu. Rev. Biophys. Bioeng.* 9: 259–291, 1980.

214. HOFFMANN, W., M. G. SARZALA, AND D. CHAPMAN. Rotational motion and evidence for oligomeric structures of sarcoplasmic reticulum Ca activated ATPase. *Proc. Natl. Acad. Sci. USA* 76: 3860–3864, 1979.

215. HOLLAND, D. L., AND S. V. PERRY. The adenosine triphosphatase and calcium ion-transporting activities of the sarcoplasmic reticulum of developing muscle. *Biochem. J.* 114: 161–170, 1969.

216. HOLLAND, P. C. Biosynthesis of the Ca^{2+} and Mg^{2+}-dependent adenosine triphosphatase of sarcoplasmic reticulum in cell cultures of embryonic chick heart. *J. Biol. Chem.* 254: 7604–7610, 1979.

217. HOLLAND, P. C., AND D. H. MACLENNAN. Assembly of sarcoplasmic reticulum. Biosynthesis of the adenosine triphosphatase in rat skeletal muscle cell culture. *J. Biol. Chem.* 251: 2030–2036, 1976.

218. HÖRL, W. H., AND L. M. G. HEILMEYER, JR. Evidence for the participation of a Ca^{2+}-dependent protein kinase and protein phosphatase in the regulation of Ca^{2+} transport ATPase of the sarcoplasmic reticulum. 2. Effect of phosphorylase kinase and phosphorylase phosphatase. *Biochemistry* 17: 766–772, 1978.

219. HÖRL, W. H., H. P. JENNISSEN, AND L. M. G. HEILMEYER. Evidence for the participation of a Ca^{2+}-dependent protein kinase and a protein phosphatase in the regulation of the Ca^{2+} transport ATPase of the sarcoplasmic reticulum. 1. Effect of inhibitors of the Ca^{2+}-dependent protein kinase and protein phosphatase. *Biochemistry* 17: 759–766, 1978.

220. HUI, C. S., AND W. F. GILLY. Mechanical activation and voltage-dependent charge movement in stretched muscle fibres. *Nature London* 281: 223–225, 1979.

221. HUXLEY, A. F., AND R. E. TAYLOR. Local activation of striated muscle fibres. *J. Physiol. London* 144: 426–441, 1958.

222. IKEMOTO, N. The calcium binding sites involved in the regulation of the purified adenosine triphosphatase of the sarcoplasmic reticulum. *J. Biol. Chem.* 249: 649–651, 1974.

223. IKEMOTO, N. Transport and inhibitory Ca^{2+} binding sites on the ATPase enzyme isolated from the sarcoplasmic reticulum. *J. Biol. Chem.* 250: 7219–7224, 1975.

224. IKEMOTO, N. Behavior of the Ca^{2+} transport sites linked with the phosphorylation reaction of ATPase purified from the sarcoplasmic reticulum. *J. Biol. Chem.* 251: 7275–7277, 1976.

225. IKEMOTO, N. Conformation of various reaction intermediates of sarcoplasmic reticulum Ca^{2+}-ATPase. In: *Cation Flux Across Biomembranes*, edited by Y. Mukohata and L. Packer. New York: Academic, 1979, p. 77–87.

226. IKEMOTO, N., G. M. BHATNAGAR, B. NAGY, AND J. GERGELY. Interaction of divalent cations with the 55,000-dalton protein component of the sarcoplasmic reticulum. Studies of fluorescence and circular dichroism. *J. Biol. Chem.* 247: 7835–7837, 1972.

227. IKEMOTO, N., A. M. GARCIA, AND Y. KUROBE. Nonequivalent subunits in the calcium pump of sarcoplasmic reticulum (Abstract). *Federation Proc.* 39: 1663, 1980.

228. IKEMOTO, N., A. M. GARCIA, Y. KUROBE, AND T. L. SCOTT. Nonequivalent subunits in the calcium pump of sarcoplasmic reticulum. *J. Biol. Chem.* 256: 8593–8601, 1981.

229. IKEMOTO, N., A. M. GARCIA, P. A. O'SHEA, AND J. GERGELY. New structural aspects of proteins (ATPase, calsequestrin) of the sarcoplasmic reticulum. *J. Cell Biol.* 67: 187a, 1975.

230. IKEMOTO, N., J. F. MORGAN, AND S. YAMADA. Ca^{2+} controlled conformational states of the Ca^{2+} transport enzyme of sarcoplasmic reticulum. *J. Biol. Chem.* 253: 8027–8033, 1978.

231. IKEMOTO, N., B. NAGY, G. M. BHATNAGAR, AND J. GERGELY. Studies on a metal-binding protein of the sarcoplasmic reticulum. *J. Biol. Chem.* 249: 2357–2365, 1974.

232. IKEMOTO, N., F. A. SRÉTER, A. NAKAMURA, AND J. GERGELY. Tryptic digestion and localization of calcium uptake and ATPase activity in fragments of sarcoplasmic reticulum. *J. Ultrastruct. Res.* 23: 216–232, 1968.

233. INESI, G. p-Nitrophenylphosphate hydrolysis and calcium ion transport in fragmented sarcoplasmic reticulum. *Science* 171: 901–903, 1971.

234. INESI, G. Active transport of calcium ion in sarcoplasmic membranes. *Annu. Rev. Biophys. Bioeng.* 1: 191–210, 1972.

235. INESI, G. The sarcoplasmic reticulum: structure, function and development. In: *Aging*, edited by G. Kaldor and W. J. Di-Battista. New York: Raven, 1978, vol. 6, p. 159–177.

236. INESI, G. Transport across sarcoplasmic reticulum in skeletal and cardiac muscle. In: *Membrane Transport in Biology*, edited by G. Giebisch, D. C. Tosteson, and H. H. Ussing. Berlin: Springer-Verlag, 1979, p. 357–393.

237. INESI, G., AND J. ALMENDARES. Interaction of fragmented sarcoplasmic reticulum with ^{14}C-ADP, ^{14}C-ATP, and ^{32}P-ATP. Effect of Ca and Mg. *Arch. Biochem. Biophys.* 126: 733–735, 1968.

238. INESI, G., AND H. ASAI. Trypsin digestion of fragmented sarcoplasmic reticulum. *Arch. Biochem. Biophys.* 126: 469–477, 1968.

239. INESI, G., C. COAN, S. VERJOVSKI-ALMEIDA, M. KURZMACK, AND D. E. LEWIS. Mechanism of free energy utilization for active transport of calcium ions. In: *Frontiers of Biological Energetics: From Electrons to Tissues*, edited by P. L. Dutton, J. S. Leigh, and A. Scarpa. New York: Academic, 1978, vol. II, p. 1212–1219.

240. INESI, G., J. A. COHEN, AND C. R. COAN. Two functional states of sarcoplasmic reticulum ATPase. *Biochemistry* 15: 5293–5298, 1976.

241. INESI, G., S. EBASHI, AND S. WATANABE. Preparation of vesicular relaxing factor from bovine heart tissue. *Am. J. Physiol.* 207: 1339–1344, 1964.

242. INESI, G., J. J. GOODMAN, AND S. WATANABE. Effect of diethyl ether on the adenosine triphosphatase activity and the calcium uptake of fragmented sarcoplasmic reticulum of rabbit skeletal muscle. *J. Biol. Chem.* 242: 4637–4643, 1967.

243. INESI, G., M. KURZMACK, C. COAN, AND D. E. LEWIS. Cooperative calcium binding and ATPase activation in sarcoplasmic reticulum vesicles. *J. Biol. Chem.* 255: 3025–3031, 1980.

244. INESI, G., M. KURZMACK, AND S. VERJOVSKI-ALMEIDA. ATPase phosphorylation and calcium ion translocation in the transient state of sarcoplasmic reticulum activity. *Ann. NY Acad. Sci.* 307: 224–227, 1978.

245. INESI, G., AND N. MALAN. Mechanisms of calcium release in sarcoplasmic reticulum. *Life Sci.* 18: 773–780, 1976.

246. INESI, G., E. MARING, A. J. MURPHY, AND B. H. MCFARLAND. A study of the phosphorylated intermediate of sarcoplasmic reticulum ATPase. *Arch. Biochem. Biophys.* 138: 285–294, 1970.

247. INESI, G., M. MILLMAN, AND S. ELETR. Temperature induced transitions of function and structure in sarcoplasmic reticulum membranes. *J. Mol. Biol.* 81: 483–504, 1973.

248. INESI, G., AND D. SCALES. Tryptic cleavage of sarcoplasmic reticulum protein. *Biochemistry* 13: 3298–3306, 1974.

249. INESI, G., AND A. SCARPA. Fast kinetics of adenosine triphosphate dependent Ca^{2+} uptake by fragmented sarcoplasmic reticulum. *Biochemistry* 11: 356–359, 1972.

250. JARDETZKY, O. Simple allosteric model for membrane pumps. *Nature London* 211: 969–970, 1966.

251. JENCKS, W. P. The utilization of binding energy in coupled vectorial processes. In: *Advances in Enzymology and Related Areas of Molecular Biology*, edited by A. Meister. New York: Wiley, 1980, vol. 51, p. 75–106.

252. JEWETT, P. H., J. R. SOMMER, AND E. A. JOHNSON. Cardiac muscle. Its ultrastructure in the finch and hummingbird with special reference to the sarcoplasmic reticulum. *J. Cell Biol.* 49: 50–65, 1971.

253. JI, T. H. The application of chemical crosslinking for studies on cell membranes and the identification of surface receptors. *Biochim. Biophys. Acta* 559: 39–69, 1979.

254. JILKA, R. L., AND A. N. MARTONOSI. The effect of calcium ion transport ATPase upon the passive calcium ion permeability

of phospholipid vesicles. *Biochim. Biophys. Acta* 466: 57–67, 1977.

255. JILKA, R. L., A. N. MARTONOSI, AND T. W. TILLACK. Effect of the purified [Mg^{2+} + Ca^{2+}]-activated ATPase of sarcoplasmic reticulum upon the passive Ca^{2+} permeability and ultrastructure of phospholipid vesicles. *J. Biol. Chem.* 250: 7511–7524, 1975.
256. JOHANNSSON, A., C. A. KEIGHTLEY, G. A. SMITH, AND J. C. METCALFE. Cholesterol in sarcoplasmic reticulum and the physiological significance of membrane fluidity. *Biochem. J.* 196: 505–511, 1981.
257. JOLESZ, F., AND F. A. SRÉTER. Development, innervation, and activity-pattern induced changes in skeletal muscle. *Annu. Rev. Physiol.* 43: 531–552, 1981.
258. JONES, L. R. Mg^{2+} and ATP effects on K^+ activation of the Ca^{2+}-transport ATPase of cardiac sarcoplasmic reticulum. *Biochim. Biophys. Acta* 557: 230–242, 1979.
259. JONES, L. R., H. R. BESCH, AND A. M. WATANABE. Monovalent cation stimulation of Ca^{2+} uptake by cardiac membrane vesicles. Correlation with stimulation of Ca^{2+}-ATPase activity. *J. Biol. Chem.* 252: 3315–3323, 1977.
260. JONES, L. R., H. R. BESCH, AND A. M. WATANABE. Regulation of the calcium pump of cardiac sarcoplasmic reticulum. Interactive roles of potassium and ATP on the phosphoprotein intermediate of the (K^+, Ca^{2+})-ATPase. *J. Biol. Chem.* 253: 1643–1653, 1978.
261. JORGENSEN, A. O., V. KALNINS, AND D. H. MACLENNAN. Localization of sarcoplasmic reticulum proteins in rat skeletal muscle by immunofluorescence. *J. Cell Biol.* 80: 372–384, 1979.
262. JORGENSEN, A. O., V. I. KALNINS, E. ZUBRZYCKA, AND D. H. MACLENNAN. Assembly of the sarcoplasmic reticulum. Localization by immunofluorescence of sarcoplasmic reticulum proteins in differentiating rat skeletal muscle cell cultures. *J. Cell Biol.* 74: 287–298, 1977.
263. JØRGENSEN, K. E., K. E. LIND, H. RØIGAARD-PETERSEN, AND J. V. MØLLER. The functional unit of calcium-plus-magnesium-ion-dependent adenosine triphosphatase from sarcoplasmic reticulum. The aggregational state of the deoxycholate-solubilized protein in an enzymically active form. *Biochem. J.* 169: 489–498, 1978.
264. JOST, P., O. H. GRIFFITH, R. A. CAPALDI, AND G. VANDERKOOI. Identification and extent of fluid bilayer regions in membranous cytochrome oxidase. *Biochim. Biophys. Acta* 311: 141–152, 1973.
265. JOST, P. C., O. H. GRIFFITH, R. A. CAPALDI, AND G. VANDERKOOI. Evidence for boundary lipid in membranes. *Proc. Natl. Acad. Sci. USA* 70: 480–484, 1973.
266. KALBITZER, H. R., D. STEHLIK, AND W. HASSELBACH. The binding of calcium and magnesium to sarcoplasmic reticulum vesicles as studied by manganese electron paramagnetic resonance. *Eur. J. Biochem.* 82: 245–255, 1978.
267. KANAZAWA, T. Phosphorylation of solubilized sarcoplasmic reticulum by orthophosphate and its thermodynamic characteristics. The dominant role of entropy in the phosphorylation. *J. Biol. Chem.* 250: 113–119, 1975.
268. KANAZAWA, T., AND P. D. BOYER. Occurrence and characteristics of a rapid exchange of phosphate oxygens catalyzed by sarcoplasmic reticulum vesicles. *J. Biol. Chem.* 248: 3163–3172, 1973.
269. KANAZAWA, T., M. SAITO, AND Y. TONOMURA. Formation and decomposition of a phosphorylated intermediate in the reaction of Na^+ + K^+ dependent ATPase. *J. Biochem. Tokyo* 67: 693–711, 1970.
270. KANAZAWA, T., Y. TAKAKUWA, AND F. KATABAMI. Entropy-driven phosphorylation with Pi of the transport ATPase of sarcoplasmic reticulum. In: *Cation Flux Across Biomembranes,* edited by Y. Mukohata and L. Packer. New York: Academic, 1979, p. 127–128.
271. KANAZAWA, T., S. YAMADA, AND Y. TONOMURA. ATP formation from ADP and a phosphorylated intermediate of Ca^{2+}-dependent ATPase in fragmented sarcoplasmic reticulum. *J. Biochem. Tokyo* 68: 593–595, 1970.
272. KANAZAWA, T., S. YAMADA, T. YAMAMOTO, AND Y. TONOMURA. Reaction mechanism of the Ca^{2+}-dependent ATPase of sarcoplasmic reticulum from skeletal muscle. V. Vectorial requirements for calcium and magnesium ions of three partial reactions of ATPase: formation and decomposition of a phosphorylated intermediate and ATP-formation from ADP and the intermediate. *J. Biochem. Tokyo* 70: 95–123, 1971.
273. KASAI, M., T. KANEMASA, AND S. FUKUMOTO. Determination of reflection coefficients for various ions and neutral molecules in sarcoplasmic reticulum vesicles through osmotic volume change studied by stopped flow technique. *J. Membr. Biol.* 51: 311–324, 1979.
274. KASAI, M., AND T. KOMETANI. Inhibition of anion permeability of sarcoplasmic reticulum vesicles by 4-acetoamido-4′-isothiocyanostilbene-2,2′-disulfonate. *Biochim. Biophys. Acta* 557: 243–247, 1979.
275. KASAI, M., AND T. KOMETANI. Ionic permeability of sarcoplasmic reticulum membrane. In: *Cation Flux Across Biomembranes,* edited by Y. Mukohata and L. Packer. New York: Academic, 1979, p. 167–177.
276. KASAI, M., AND H. MIYAMOTO. Depolarization-induced calcium release from sarcoplasmic reticulum fragments. I. Release of calcium taken up upon using ATP. *J. Biochem. Tokyo* 79: 1053–1066, 1976.
277. KASAI, M., AND H. MIYAMOTO. Depolarization-induced calcium release from sarcoplasmic reticulum fragments. II. Release of calcium incorporated without ATP. *J. Biochem. Tokyo* 79: 1067–1076, 1976.
278. KATZ, A. M. Role of the contractile proteins and sarcoplasmic reticulum in the response of the heart to catecholamines: an historical review. In: *Advances in Cyclic Nucleotide Research, New Assay Methods for Cyclic Nucleotides,* edited by P. Greengard, R. Paoletti, and G. A. Robison. New York: Raven, 1979, vol. 11, p. 303–343.
279. KATZ, A. M., AND D. I. REPKE. Sodium and potassium sensitivity of calcium uptake and calcium binding by dog cardiac microsomes. *Circ. Res.* 21: 767–775, 1967.
280. KATZ, A. M., M. TADA, D. I. REPKE, J. M. IORIO, AND M. A. KIRCHBERGER. Adenylate cyclase: its probable localization in sarcoplasmic reticulum as well as sarcolemma of the canine heart. *J. Mol. Cell. Cardiol.* 6: 73–78, 1974.
281. KAWAKITA, M., K. YASUOKA, AND Y. KAZIRO. Effect of Ca^{2+} ions on the reactivity of the nucleotide binding site of sarcoplasmic reticulum Ca^{2+}, Mg^{2+}-adenosine triphosphatase. In: *Cation Flux Across Biomembranes,* edited by Y. Mukohata and L. Packer. New York: Academic, 1979, p. 119–124.
282. KING, I. A., AND C. F. LOUIS. The location of membrane components in sarcoplasmic reticulum membranes by using free and immobilized lactoperoxidase. *Biochem. Soc. Trans.* 4: 245–248, 1976.
283. KIRCHBERGER, M. A., AND G. CHU. Correlation between protein kinase mediated stimulation of calcium transport by cardiac sarcoplasmic reticulum and phosphorylation of a 22,000 dalton protein. *Biochim. Biophys. Acta* 419: 559–562, 1976.
284. KIRCHBERGER, M. A., AND A. RAFFO. Decrease in calcium transport associated with phosphoprotein phosphatase-catalyzed dephosphorylation of cardiac sarcoplasmic reticulum. *J. Cyclic Nucleotide Res.* 3: 45–53, 1977.
285. KIRCHBERGER, M. A., AND M. TADA. Effects of adenosine 3′,5′-monophosphate-dependent protein kinase on sarcoplasmic reticulum isolated from cardiac and slow and fast contracting skeletal muscles. *J. Biol. Chem.* 251: 725–729, 1976.
286. KIRCHBERGER, M. A., M. TADA, AND A. M. KATZ. Adenosine 3′:5′-monophosphate-dependent protein kinase-catalyzed phosphorylation reaction and its relationship to calcium transport in cardiac sarcoplasmic reticulum. *J. Biol. Chem.* 249: 6166–6173, 1974.
287. KIRCHBERGER, M. A., M. TADA, D. I. REPKE, AND A. M. KATZ. Cyclic adenosine 3′,5′-monophosphate-dependent protein kinase stimulation of calcium uptake by canine cardiac microsomes. *J. Mol. Cell. Cardiol.* 4: 673–680, 1972.
288. KIRINO, Y., K. ANZAI, H. SHIMIZU, S. OHTA, M. NAKANISHI, AND M. TSUBOI. Thermotropic transition in the states of

proteins in sarcoplasmic reticulum vesicles. *J. Biochem. Tokyo* 82: 1181–1184, 1977.

289. KIRINO, Y., T. OHKUMA, AND H. SHIMIZU. Saturation transfer electron spin resonance study on the rotational diffusion of calcium and magnesium dependent adenosine triphosphatase in sarcoplasmic reticulum membranes. *J. Biochem. Tokyo* 84: 111–115, 1978.
290. KLEEMANN, W., AND H. M. MCCONNELL. Interactions of proteins and cholesterol with lipids in bilayer membranes. *Biochim. Biophys. Acta* 419: 206–222, 1976.
291. KLIP, A., AND D. H. MACLENNAN. Zeroing in on the ionophoric site of the (Ca^{2+} + Mg^{2+})-ATPase. In: *Frontiers in Biological Energetics: From Electrons to Tissues*, edited by L. Dutton, J. Leigh, and A. Scarpa. New York: Academic, 1978, vol. II, p. 1137–1147.
292. KLIP, A., R. A. F. REITHMEIER, AND D. H. MACLENNAN. Alignment of the major tryptic fragments of the adenosine triphosphatase from sarcoplasmic reticulum. *J. Biol. Chem.* 255: 6562–6568, 1980.
293. KNAUF, P. A., W. BREUER, L. MCCULLOCH, AND A. ROTHSTEIN. *N*-(4-Azido-2-Nitrophenyl)-2-aminoethylsulfonate (NAP-taurine) as a photoaffinity probe for identifying membrane components containing the modifier site of the human red blood cell anion exchange system. *J. Gen. Physiol.* 72: 631–649, 1978.
294. KNAUF, P. A., G. P. FUHRMANN, S. S. ROTHSTEIN, AND A. ROTHSTEIN. The relationship between anion exchange and net anion flow across the human red blood cell membrane. *J. Gen. Physiol.* 69: 363–386, 1977.
295. KNAUF, P. A., S. SHIP, W. BREUER, L. MCCULLOCH, AND A. ROTHSTEIN. Asymmetry of the red cell anion exchange system. Different mechanisms of reversible inhibition by *N*-(4-azido-2-nitrophenyl)-2-aminoethylsulfonate (NAP-taurine) at the inside and outside of the membrane. *J. Gen. Physiol.* 72: 607–630, 1978.
296. KNOWLES, A. F., E. EYTAN, AND E. RACKER. Phospholipid-protein interactions in the Ca^{2+}-adenosine triphosphatase of sarcoplasmic reticulum. *J. Biol. Chem.* 251: 5161–5165, 1976.
297. KNOWLES, A. F., A. KANDRACH, E. RACKER, AND H. G. KHORANA. Acetyl phosphatidylethanolamine in the reconstitution of ion pumps. *J. Biol. Chem.* 250: 1809–1813, 1975.
298. KNOWLES, A. F., AND E. RACKER. Formation of adenosine triphosphate from P_i and adenosine diphosphate by purified Ca^{2+}-adenosine triphosphatase. *J. Biol. Chem.* 250: 1949–1951, 1975.
299. KNOWLES, A. F., AND E. RACKER. Properties of a reconstituted calcium pump. *J. Biol. Chem.* 250: 3538–3544, 1975.
300. KNOWLES, A., P. ZIMNIAK, M. ALFONZO, A. ZIMNIAK, AND E. RACKER. Isolation and characterization of proteolipids from sarcoplasmic reticulum. *J. Membr. Biol.* 55: 233–239, 1980.
301. KOLASSA, N., C. PUNZENGRUBER, J. SUKO, AND M. MAKINOSE. Mechanism of calcium-independent phosphorylation of sarcoplasmic reticulum ATPase by orthophosphate. Evidence of magnesium-phosphoprotein formation. *FEBS Lett.* 108: 495–500, 1979.
302. KOMETANI, T., AND M. KASAI. Ionic permeability of sarcoplasmic reticulum vesicles measured by light scattering method. *J. Membr. Biol.* 41: 295–308, 1978.
303. KONDO, M., AND M. KASAI. Photodynamic inactivation of sarcoplasmic reticulum vesicle membranes by xanthene dyes. *Photochem. Photobiol.* 19: 35–41, 1974.
304. KRANIAS, E. G., F. MANDEL, AND A. SCHWARTZ. Involvement of cAMP-dependent protein kinase and pH on the regulation of cardiac sarcoplasmic reticulum. *Biochem. Biophys. Res. Commun.* 92: 1370–1376, 1980.
305. KRASNOW, N. Effects of lanthanum and gadolinium on cardiac sarcoplasmic reticulum. *Biochim. Biophys. Acta* 282: 187–194, 1972.
306. KREBS, E. G., AND J. A. BEAVO. Phosphorylation-dephosphorylation of enzymes. *Annu. Rev. Biochem.* 48: 923–959, 1979.
307. KRETSINGER, R. H. Calcium binding proteins. *Annu. Rev. Biochem.* 45: 239–266, 1976.
308. KURIKI, Y., J. HALSEY, R. BILTONEN, AND E. RACKER. Calorimetric studies of the interaction of magnesium and phosphate with (Na^+, K^+) ATPase. Evidence for a ligand-induced conformational change in the enzyme. *Biochemistry* 15: 4956–4961, 1976.
309. KURZMACK, M., AND G. INESI. The initial phase of Ca^{2+} uptake and ATPase activity of sarcoplasmic reticulum vesicles. *FEBS Lett.* 74: 35–37, 1977.
310. KURZMACK, M., S. VERJOVSKI-ALMEIDA, AND G. INESI. Detection of an initial burst of Ca^{2+} translocation in sarcoplasmic reticulum. *Biochem. Biophys. Res. Commun.* 78: 772–776, 1977.
311. LAEMMLI, U. K. Cleavage of structural proteins during the assembly of the head of bacteriophage T4. *Nature London* 227: 680–685, 1970.
312. LAGGNER, P. A highly α-helical structure protein in sarcoplasmic reticulum membranes. *Nature London* 255: 427–428, 1975.
313. LAGGNER, P., AND M. D. BARRATT. The interaction of a proteolipid from sarcoplasmic reticulum membranes with phospholipids. A spin label study. *Arch. Biochem. Biophys.* 170: 92–101, 1975.
314. LAGGNER, P., AND D. E. GRAHAM. The effect of a proteolipid from sarcoplasmic reticulum on the physical properties of artificial phospholipid membranes. *Biochim. Biophys. Acta* 433: 311–317, 1976.
315. LANDIS, D. M. D., M. HENKART, AND T. S. REESE. Similar arrays of plasma membrane particles at subsurface cisterns in striated muscle and neurons. *J. Cell Biol.* 59: 184a, 1973.
316. LA RAIA, P. J., AND E. MORKIN. Adenosine 3′,5′-monophosphate-dependent membrane phosphorylation: a possible mechanism for the control of microsomal calcium transport in heart muscle. *Circ. Res.* 35: 298–306, 1974.
317. LAU, Y. H., A. H. CASWELL, AND J.-P. BRUNSCHWIG. Isolation of transverse tubules by fractionation of triad junctions of skeletal muscle. *J. Biol. Chem.* 252: 5565–5574, 1977.
318. LAU, Y. H., A. H. CASWELL, J.-P. BRUNSCHWIG, R. J. BAERWALD, AND M. GARCIA. Lipid analysis and freeze fracture studies on isolated transverse tubules and sarcoplasmic reticulum subfractions of skeletal muscle. *J. Biol. Chem.* 254: 540–546, 1979.
319. LAU, Y. H., A. H. CASWELL, M. GARCIA, AND L. LETELLIER. Ouabain binding and coupled sodium, potassium, and chloride transport in isolated transverse tubules of skeletal muscle. *J. Gen. Physiol.* 74: 335–349, 1979.
320. LEE, A. G., N. J. M. BIRDSALL, J. C. METCALFE, P. A. TOON, AND G. B. WARREN. Clusters in lipid bilayers and the interpretation of thermal effects in biological membranes. *Biochemistry* 13: 3699–3705, 1974.
321. LE MAIRE, M., K. E. JØRGENSEN, H. RØIGAARD-PETERSEN, AND J. V. MØLLER. Properties of deoxycholate solubilized sarcoplasmic reticulum Ca^{2+}-ATPase. *Biochemistry* 15: 5805–5812, 1976.
322. LE MAIRE, M., K. E. LIND, K. E. JØRGENSEN, H. RØIGAARD, J. V. MØLLER. Enzymatically active Ca^{2+} ATPase from sarcoplasmic reticulum membranes, solubilized by nonionic detergents. Role of lipid for aggregation of the protein. *J. Biol. Chem.* 253: 7051–7060, 1978.
323. LE MAIRE, M., J. V. MØLLER, AND C. TANFORD. Retention of enzyme activity by detergent-solubilized sarcoplasmic Ca^{2+}-ATPase. *Biochemistry* 15: 2336–2342, 1976.
324. LE PEUCH, C. J., C. FERRAZ, M. P. WALSH, J. G. DEMAILLE, AND E. H. FISCHER. Calcium and cyclic nucleotide dependent regulatory mechanisms during development of chick embryo skeletal muscle. *Biochemistry* 18: 5267–5273, 1979.
325. LE PEUCH, C. J., J. HAIECH, AND J. G. DEMAILLE. Concerted regulation of cardiac sarcoplasmic reticulum calcium transport by cyclic adenosine monophosphate dependent and calcium-calmodulin-dependent phosphorylations. *Biochemistry* 18: 5150–5157, 1979.
326. LIGURI, G., M. STEFANI, A. BERTI, P. NASSI, AND G. RAMPONI. Effect of acylphosphates on Ca^{2+} uptake by sarcoplasmic reticulum vesicles. *Arch. Biochem. Biophys.* 200: 357–363, 1980.
327. LOUGH, J. W., M. L. ENTMAN, E. H. BOSSEN, AND J. L. HANSEN. Calcium accumulation by isolated sarcoplasmic retic-

ulum of skeletal muscle during development in tissue culture. *J. Cell. Physiol.* 80: 431–436, 1972.

328. LOUIS, C. F., R. BUONAFFINA, AND B. BINKS. Effect of trypsin on the proteins of skeletal muscle sarcoplasmic reticulum. *Arch. Biochem. Biophys.* 161: 83–92, 1974.
329. LOUIS, C. F., AND A. M. KATZ. Lactoperoxidase-coupled iodination of cardiac sarcoplasmic reticulum proteins. *Biochim. Biophys. Acta* 494: 255–265, 1977.
330. LOUIS, C. F., M. J. SAUNDERS, AND J. A. HOLROYD. The cross-linking of rabbit skeletal muscle sarcoplasmic reticulum protein. *Biochim. Biophys. Acta* 493: 78–92, 1977.
331. LOUIS, C. F., AND E. M. SHOOTER. The proteins of rabbit skeletal muscle sarcoplasmic reticulum. *Arch. Biochem. Biophys.* 153: 641–655, 1972.
332. LUTTGAU, H. C., AND G. D. MOISESCU. Ion movements in skeletal muscle in relation to the activation of contraction. In: *Physiology of Membrane Disorders*, edited by T. E. Andreoli, J. F. Hoffman, and D. D. Fanestil. New York: Plenum, 1978, p. 493–515.
333. LYMN, R. W. Kinetic analysis of myosin and actomyosin ATPase. *Annu. Rev. Biophys. Bioeng.* 8: 145–163, 1979.
334. MACLENNAN, D. H. Purification and properties of an adenosine triphosphatase from sarcoplasmic reticulum. *J. Biol. Chem.* 245: 4508–4518, 1970.
335. MACLENNAN, D. H. Isolation of a second form of calsequestrin. *J. Biol. Chem.* 249: 980–984, 1974.
336. MACLENNAN, D. H. Resolution of the calcium transport system of sarcoplasmic reticulum. *Can. J. Biochem.* 53: 251–261, 1975.
337. MACLENNAN, D. H., AND K. P. CAMPBELL. Structure, function and biosynthesis of sarcoplasmic reticulum proteins. *Trends Biochem. Sci.* 4: 148–151, 1979.
338. MACLENNAN, D. H., AND P. C. HOLLAND. Calcium transport in sarcoplasmic reticulum. *Annu. Rev. Biophys. Bioeng.* 4: 377–404, 1975.
339. MACLENNAN, D. H., AND P. C. HOLLAND. The calcium transport ATPase of sarcoplasmic reticulum. In: *The Enzymes of Biological Membranes*, edited by A. Martonosi. New York: Plenum, 1976, vol. 3, p. 221–259.
340. MACLENNAN, D. H., V. K. KHANNA, AND P. S. STEWART. Restoration of calcium transport in the trypsin-treated (Ca^{2+} + Mg^{2+})-dependent adenosine triphosphatase of sarcoplasmic reticulum exposed to sodium dodecyl sulfate. *J. Biol. Chem.* 251: 7271–7274, 1976.
341. MACLENNAN, D. H., T. J. OSTWALD, AND P. S. STEWART. Structural components of the sarcoplasmic reticulum membrane. *Ann. NY Acad. Sci.* 227: 527–536, 1974.
342. MACLENNAN, D. H., P. SEEMAN, G. H. ILES, AND C. C. YIP. Membrane formation by the adenosine triphosphatase of sarcoplasmic reticulum. *J. Biol. Chem.* 246: 2702–2710, 1971.
343. MACLENNAN, D. H., AND P. T. S. WONG. Isolation of a calcium-sequestering protein from sarcoplasmic reticulum. *Proc. Natl. Acad. Sci. USA* 68: 1231–1235, 1971.
344. MACLENNAN, D. H., C. C. YIP, G. H. ILES, AND P. SEEMAN. Isolation of sarcoplasmic reticulum proteins. *Cold Spring Harbor Symp. Quant. Biol.* 37: 469–477, 1972.
345. MACLENNAN, D. H., E. ZUBRZYCKA, A. O. JORGENSEN, AND V. I. KALNINS. Assembly of the sarcoplasmic reticulum. In: *The Molecular Biology of Membranes*, edited by S. Fleischer, Y. Hatefi, D. H. MacLennan, and A. Tzagoloff. New York: Plenum, 1978, p. 309–320.
346. MADDEN, T. D., D. CHAPMAN, AND P. J. QUINN. Cholesterol modulates activity of the calcium dependent ATPase of the sarcoplasmic reticulum. *Nature London* 279: 538–540, 1979.
347. MADDEN, T. D., AND P. J. QUINN. Arrhenius discontinuities of Ca^{2+} ATPase activity are unrelated to changes in membrane lipid fluidity of sarcoplasmic reticulum. *FEBS Lett.* 107: 110–112, 1979.
348. MADEIRA, V. M. C. Subunits of the calcium ion-pump system of sarcoplasmic reticulum. *Biochim. Biophys. Acta* 464: 583–588, 1977.
349. MADEIRA, V. M. C. Proton gradient formation during transport of Ca^{2+} by sarcoplasmic reticulum. *Arch. Biochem. Biophys.* 185: 316–325, 1978.
350. MADEIRA, V. M. C. Alkalinization within sarcoplasmic reticulum during the uptake of calcium ions. *Arch. Biochem. Biophys.* 193: 22–27, 1979.
351. MADEIRA, V. M. C. Proton movements across the membranes of sarcoplasmic reticulum during the uptake of calcium ions. *Arch. Biochem. Biophys.* 200: 319–325, 1980.
352. MADEIRA, V. M. C., AND M. C. ANTUNES-MADEIRA. Resolution of Ca^{++}-ATPase of sarcoplasmic reticulum into subunits. *Experientia* 33: 188–190, 1977.
353. MAKINOSE, M. Die Nucleosidtriphosphat-Nucleosiddiphosphat-Transphosphorylase-Aktivitat der Vesikel des sarkoplasmatischen Reticulums. *Biochem. Z.* 345: 80–86, 1966.
354. MAKINOSE, M. The phosphorylation of the membranal protein of the sarcoplasmic vesicles during active calcium transport. *Eur. J. Biochem.* 10: 74–82, 1969.
355. MAKINOSE, M. Calcium efflux dependent formation of ATP from ADP and orthophosphate by the membranes of the sarcoplasmic vesicles. *FEBS Lett.* 12: 269–270, 1971.
356. MAKINOSE, M. Phosphoprotein formation during osmo-chemical energy conversion in the membrane of the sarcoplasmic reticulum. *FEBS Lett.* 25: 113–115, 1972.
357. MAKINOSE, M. Possible functional states of the enzyme of the sarcoplasmic calcium pump. *FEBS Lett.* 37: 140–143, 1973.
358. MAKINOSE, M., AND W. BOLL. Reaction sequence in the sarcoplasmic calcium transport (II)—binding sequence of Ca, Mg, ATP and ADP. In: *Function and Molecular Aspects of Biomembrane Transport*, edited by E. M. Klingenberg, F. Palmieri, and E. Quagliariello. Amsterdam: Elsevier/North-Holland, 1979, p. 115–117. (Proc. Symp. Bari, Italy, 1979.)
359. MAKINOSE, M., AND W. BOLL. The role of magnesium on the sarcoplasmic calcium pump. In: *Cation Flux Across Biomembranes*, edited by Y. Mukohata and L. Packer. New York: Academic, 1979, p. 89–100.
360. MAKINOSE, M., AND W. HASSELBACH. Der Einfluss von Oxalat auf den Calcium-Transport isolierter Vesikel des sarkoplasmatischen Reticulum. *Biochem. Z.* 343: 360–382, 1965.
361. MAKINOSE, M., AND W. HASSELBACH. ATP synthesis by the reverse of the sarcoplasmic calcium pump. *FEBS Lett.* 12: 271–272, 1971.
362. MAKINOSE, M., AND R. THE. Calcium-Akkumulation und Nucleosidtriphosphat-Spaltung durch die Vesikel des sarkoplasmatischen Reticulum. *Biochem. Z.* 343: 383–393, 1965.
363. MANUCK, B. A., AND B. D. SYKES. Rapid anisotropic motion of the Ca^{2+}-transport ATPase of the rabbit skeletal muscle sarcoplasmic reticulum. *Can. J. Biochem.* 55: 587–596, 1977.
364. MARAI, L., AND A. KUKSIS. Molecular species of glycerolipids of adenosine triphosphatase and sarcotubular membranes of rabbit skeletal muscle. *Can. J. Biochem.* 51: 1248–1261, 1973.
365. MARAI, L., AND A. KUKSIS. Comparative study of molecular species of glycerolipids in sarcotubular membranes of skeletal muscle of rabbit, rat, chicken, and man. *Can. J. Biochem.* 51: 1365–1379, 1973.
366. MARKHAM, R., S. FREY, AND G. J. HILLS. Methods for the enhancement of image detail and accentuation of structure in electron microscopy. *Virology* 20: 88–102, 1963.
367. MARTONOSI, A. The activating effect of phospholipids on the ATP-ase activity and Ca^{++} transport of fragmented sarcoplasmic reticulum. *Biochem. Biophys. Res. Commun.* 13: 273–278, 1963.
368. MARTONOSI, A. Role of phospholipids in ATPase activity and Ca^{2+} transport of fragmented sarcoplasmic reticulum. *Federation Proc.* 23: 913–921, 1964.
369. MARTONOSI, A. The role of phospholipids in the ATP-ase activity of skeletal muscle microsomes. *Biochem. Biophys. Res. Commun.* 29: 753–757, 1967.
370. MARTONOSI, A. Sarcoplasmic reticulum. IV. Solubilization of microsomal adenosine triphosphatase. *J. Biol. Chem.* 243: 71–81, 1968.
371. MARTONOSI, A. Sarcoplasmic reticulum. V. The structure of sarcoplasmic reticulum membranes. *Biochim. Biophys. Acta* 150: 694–704, 1968.

372. Martonosi, A. The protein composition of sarcoplasmic reticulum membranes. *Biochem. Biophys. Res. Commun.* 36: 1039–1044, 1969.
373. Martonosi, A. Sarcoplasmic reticulum. VII. Properties of a phosphoprotein intermediate implicated in calcium transport. *J. Biol. Chem.* 244: 613–620, 1969.
374. Martonosi, A. The structure and function of sarcoplasmic reticulum membranes. In: *Biomembranes*, edited by L. A. Manson. New York: Plenum, 1971, vol. 1, p. 191–256.
375. Martonosi, A. Biochemical and clinical aspects of sarcoplasmic reticulum function. In: *Current Topics in Membranes and Transport*, edited by F. Bronner and A. Kleinzeller. New York: Academic, 1972, vol. 3, p. 83–197.
376. Martonosi, A. Membrane transport during development in animals. *Biochim. Biophys. Acta* 415: 311–333, 1975.
377. Martonosi, A. Some recent observations on the structure and function of sarcoplasmic reticulum. In: *Biomembranes-Lipids, Proteins and Receptors*, edited by R. M. Burton and L. Packer. Webster Groves, MO: BI Sci. Publ. Div. 1975, p. 369–390. (Proc. NATO Adv. Study Inst. 1974.)
378. Martonosi, A. The mechanism of calcium transport in sarcoplasmic reticulum. In: *Calcium Transport in Contractions and Secretion*, edited by E. Carafoli, F. Clementi, W. Drabikowski, and A. Margreth. Amsterdam: North-Holland, 1975, p. 313–327.
379. Martonosi, A. The effect of ATP upon the reactivity of SH groups in sarcoplasmic reticulum membranes. *FEBS Lett.* 67: 153–155, 1976.
380. Martonosi, A. Protein-protein interaction in sarcoplasmic reticulum: functional significance. In: *Membrane Proteins*, edited by P. Nicholls, J. V. Møller, P. L. Jørgensen, and A. J. Moody. Oxford: Pergamon, 1977, p. 135–140. (Proc. FEBS 11th, Copenhagen, 1977.)
381. Martonosi, A. N. Calcium pumps (Introduction). *Federation Proc.* 39: 2401–2402, 1980.
382. Martonosi, A., R. Boland, and R. A. Halpin. The biosynthesis of sarcoplasmic reticulum membranes and the mechanism of calcium transport. *Cold Spring Harbor Symp. Quant. Biol.* 37: 455–468, 1972.
383. Martonosi, A. N., T. L. Chyn, and A. Schibeci. The calcium transport of sarcoplasmic reticulum. *Ann. NY Acad. Sci.* 307: 148–159, 1978.
384. Martonosi, A., A. R. De Boland, R. Boland, J. M. Vanderkooi, and R. A. Halpin. The mechanism of Ca transport and the permeability of sarcoplasmic reticulum membranes. In: *Myocardial Biology. Recent Advances in Studies on Cardiac Structure and Metabolism*, edited by N. Dhalla. Baltimore, MD: University Park, 1974, vol. 4, p. 473–494.
385. Martonosi, A., J. Donley, and R. A. Halpin. Sarcoplasmic reticulum. III. The role of phospholipids in the adenosine triphosphatase activity and Ca^{++} transport. *J. Biol. Chem.* 243: 61–70, 1968.
386. Martonosi, A., J. R. Donley, A. G. Pucell, and R. A. Halpin. Sarcoplasmic reticulum. XI. The mode of involvement of phospholipids in the hydrolysis of ATP by sarcoplasmic reticulum membranes. *Arch. Biochem. Biophys.* 144: 529–540, 1971.
387. Martonosi, A., and R. Feretos. Sarcoplasmic reticulum. I. The uptake of Ca^{++} by sarcoplasmic reticulum fragments. *J. Biol. Chem.* 239: 648–658, 1964.
388. Martonosi, A., and R. Feretos. Sarcoplasmic reticulum. II. Correlation between adenosine triphosphatase activity and Ca^{++} uptake. *J. Biol. Chem.* 239: 659–668, 1964.
389. Martonosi, A., and F. Fortier. The effect of anti-ATPase antibodies upon the Ca^{++} transport of sarcoplasmic reticulum. *Biochem. Biophys. Res. Commun.* 60: 382–389, 1974.
390. Martonosi, A., and R. A. Halpin. Sarcoplasmic reticulum. X. The protein composition of sarcoplasmic reticulum membranes. *Arch. Biochem. Biophys.* 144: 66–77, 1971.
391. Martonosi, A., and R. A. Halpin. Sarcoplasmic reticulum. XVII. The turnover of proteins and phospholipids in sarcoplasmic reticulum membranes. *Arch. Biochem. Biophys.* 152: 440–450, 1972.
392. Martonosi, A., R. L. Jilka, and F. Fortier. The permeability of sarcoplasmic reticulum membranes. In: *Membrane Proteins in Transport and Phosphorylation*, edited by G. F. Azzone, E. M. Klingenberg, E. Quagliariello, and N. Siliprandi. Amsterdam: North-Holland, 1974, p. 113–124.
393. Martonosi, A., E. Lagwinska, and M. Oliver. Elementary processes in the hydrolysis of ATP by sarcoplasmic reticulum membranes. *Ann. NY Acad. Sci.* 227: 549–567, 1974.
394. Martonosi, A., H. Nakamura, R. L. Jilka, and J. M. Vanderkooi. Protein-protein interactions and the functional states of sarcoplasmic reticulum membranes. In: *Biochemistry of Membrane Transport*, edited by G. Semenza and E. Carafoli. Berlin: Springer-Verlag, 1977, p. 401–415.
395. Martonosi, A., D. Roufa, R. Boland, E. Reyes, and T. W. Tillack. Development of sarcoplasmic reticulum in cultured chicken muscle. *J. Biol. Chem.* 252: 318–332, 1977.
396. Martonosi, A., D. Roufa, D.-B. Ha, and R. Boland. The biosynthesis of sarcoplasmic reticulum. *Federation Proc.* 39: 2415–2421, 1980.
397. Martonosi, M. A. Thermal analysis of sarcoplasmic reticulum membranes. *FEBS Lett.* 47: 327–329, 1974.
398. Masuda, H., and L. de Meis. Phosphorylation of the sarcoplasmic reticulum membrane by orthophosphate. Inhibition by calcium ions. *Biochemistry* 12: 4581–4585, 1973.
399. Masuda, H., and L. de Meis. Calcium efflux from sarcoplasmic reticulum vesicles. *Biochem. Biophys. Acta* 332: 313–315, 1974.
400. Masuda, H., and L. de Meis. Effect of temperature on the Ca^{2+} transport ATPase of sarcoplasmic reticulum. *J. Biol. Chem.* 252: 8567–8571, 1977.
401. Mathias, R. T., R. A. Levis, and R. S. Eisenberg. Electrical models of excitation-contraction coupling and charge movement in skeletal muscle. *J. Gen. Physiol.* 76: 1–31, 1980.
402. McKinley, D., and G. Meissner. Sodium and potassium ion permeability of sarcoplasmic reticulum vesicles. *FEBS Lett.* 82: 47–50, 1977.
403. McKinley, D., and G. Meissner. Evidence for a K^+, Na^+ permeable channel in sarcoplasmic reticulum. *J. Membr. Biol.* 44: 159–186, 1978.
404. Meissner, G. ATP and Ca^{2+} binding by the Ca^{2+} pump protein of sarcoplasmic reticulum. *Biochim. Biophys. Acta* 298: 906–926, 1973.
405. Meissner, G. Isolation and characterization of two types of sarcoplasmic reticulum vesicles. *Biochim. Biophys. Acta* 389: 51–68, 1975.
406. Meissner, G. Effects of Ca^{2+} transport on a membrane potential in sarcoplasmic reticulum. *Biophys. J.* 25: 108a, 1979.
407. Meissner, G. Calcium transport and monovalent cation and proton fluxes in sarcoplasmic reticulum vesicles. *J. Biol. Chem.* 256: 636–643, 1981.
408. Meissner, G., G. E. Conner, and S. Fleischer. Isolation of sarcoplasmic reticulum by zonal centrifugation and purification of Ca^{2+}-pump and Ca^{2+}-binding proteins. *Biochim. Biophys. Acta* 298: 246–269, 1973.
409. Meissner, G., and S. Fleischer. Characterization of sarcoplasmic reticulum from skeletal muscle. *Biochim. Biophys. Acta* 241: 356–378, 1971.
410. Meissner, G., and S. Fleischer. The role of phospholipid in Ca^{2+} stimulated ATPase activity of sarcoplasmic reticulum. *Biochim. Biophys. Acta* 255: 19–33, 1972.
411. Meissner, G., and D. McKinley. Permeability of sarcoplasmic reticulum membrane. The effect of changed ionic environments on Ca^{2+} release. *J. Membr. Biol.* 30: 79–98, 1976.
412. Meissner, G., and R. C. Young. Proton permeability of sarcoplasmic reticulum vesicles. *J. Biol. Chem.* 255: 6814–6819, 1980.
413. Mela, L. Mechanism and physiological significance of calcium transport across mammalian mitochondrial membranes. *Curr. Top. Membr. Transp.* 9: 321–366, 1977.
414. Melgunov, V. I., and E. I. Akimova. On subunit structure of Ca^{2+} dependent ATPase of sarcoplasmic reticulum. *FEBS Lett.*

111: 197-200, 1980.
415. MERMIER, P., AND W. HASSELBACH. Comparison between strontium and calcium uptake by the fragmented sarcoplasmic reticulum. *Eur. J. Biochem.* 69: 79-86, 1976.
416. MICHALAK, M., K. P. CAMPBELL, AND D. H. MACLENNAN. Localization of the high affinity calcium binding protein and an intrinsic glycoprotein in sarcoplasmic reticulum membranes. *J. Biol. Chem.* 255: 1317-1326, 1980.
417. MICHALAK, M., AND D. H. MACLENNAN. Assembly of the sarcoplasmic reticulum. Biosynthesis of the high affinity calcium binding protein in rat skeletal muscle cell cultures. *J. Biol. Chem.* 255: 1327-1334, 1980.
418. MIGALA, A., B. AGOSTINI, AND W. HASSELBACH. Tryptic fragmentation of the calcium transport system in the sarcoplasmic reticulum. *Z. Naturforsch. Teil C* 28: 178-182, 1973.
419. MILLER, C. Voltage-gated cation conductance channel from fragmented sarcoplasmic reticulum: steady-state electrical properties. *J. Membr. Biol.* 40: 1-23, 1978.
420. MILLER, C., P. ARVAN, J. N. TELFORD, AND E. RACKER. Ca^{++} induced fusion of proteoliposomes: dependence on transmembrane osmotic gradient. *J. Membr. Biol.* 30: 271-282, 1976.
421. MILLER, C., AND E. RACKER. Ca^{++} induced fusion of fragmented sarcoplasmic reticulum with artificial planar bilayers. *J. Membr. Biol.* 30: 283-300, 1976.
422. MILLER, C., AND R. L. ROSENBERG. Modification of a voltage gated K^+ channel from sarcoplasmic reticulum by a pronase-derived specific endopeptidase. *J. Gen. Physiol.* 74: 457-478, 1979.
423. MILLER, C., AND R. L. ROSENBERG. A voltage gated cation conductance channel from fragmented sarcoplasmic reticulum. Effects of transition metal ions. *Biochemistry* 18: 1138-1145, 1979.
424. MIYAMOTO, H., AND M. KASAI. Asymmetric distribution of calcium binding sites of sarcoplasmic reticulum fragments. *J. Biochem. Tokyo* 85: 765-773, 1979.
425. MØLLER, J. V., K. E. LIND, AND J. P. ANDERSEN. Enzyme kinetics and substrate stabilization of detergent solubilized and membraneous (Ca^{2+} + Mg^{2+}) activated ATPase from sarcoplasmic reticulum. Effects of protein-protein interactions. *J. Biol. Chem.* 255: 1912-1920, 1980.
426. MOORE, B. M., B. R. LENTZ, AND G. MEISSNER. Effects of sarcoplasmic reticulum Ca^{2+}-ATPase on phospholipid bilayer fluidity: boundary lipid. *Biochemistry* 17: 5248-5255, 1978.
427. MOPE, L., G. B. MCCLELLAN, AND S. WINEGRAD. Calcium sensitivity of the contractile system and phosphorylation of troponin in hyperpermeable cardiac cells. *J. Gen. Physiol.* 75: 271-282, 1980.
428. MOSTOV, K. E., P. DEFOOR, S. FLEISCHER, AND G. BLOBEL. Co-translational membrane integration of calcium pump protein without signal sequence cleavage. *Nature London* 292: 87-88, 1981.
429. MUKOHATA, Y., AND L. PACKER (editors). *Cation Flux Across Biomembranes*. New York: Academic, 1979.
430. MURPHY, A. J. Cross-linking of the sarcoplasmic reticulum ATPase protein. *Biochem. Biophys. Res. Commun.* 70: 160-166, 1976.
431. MURPHY, A. J. Sulfhydryl group modification of sarcoplasmic reticulum membranes. *Biochemistry* 15: 4492-4496, 1976.
432. MURPHY, A. J. Sarcoplasmic reticulum adenosine triphosphatase: labeling of an essential lysyl residue with pyridoxal-5'-phosphate. *Arch. Biochem. Biophys.* 180: 114-120, 1977.
433. MURPHY, A. J. Effects of divalent cations and nucleotides on the reactivity of the sulfhydryl groups of sarcoplasmic reticulum membranes. Evidence for structural changes occurring during the calcium transport cycle. *J. Biol. Chem.* 253: 385-389, 1978.
434. NAGASAKI, K., AND M. KASAI. Magnesium permeability of sarcoplasmic reticulum vesicles monitored in terms of chlortetracycline fluorescence. *J. Biochem. Tokyo* 87: 709-716, 1980.
435. NAKAJIMA, Y., AND M. ENDO. Release of calcium induced by "depolarization" of the sarcoplasmic reticulum membrane. *Nature London New Biol.* 246: 216-218, 1973.
436. NAKAMARU, Y., AND K. NOMURA. Two types of sarcoplasmic reticulum-orthophosphate interactions observed with dye probe. *J. Biochem. Tokyo* 81: 321-328, 1977.
437. NAKAMURA, H. Spin-labeling of adenosine triphosphatase in sarcoplasmic reticulum membrane and change in the state of the spin labels induced by deoxycholate. *J. Biochem. Tokyo* 82: 923-930, 1977.
438. NAKAMURA, H., H. HORI, AND T. MITSUI. Conformational change in sarcoplasmic reticulum induced by ATP in the presence of magnesium ion and calcium ion. *J. Biochem. Tokyo* 72: 635-646, 1972.
439. NAKAMURA, H., R. L. JILKA, R. BOLAND, AND A. N. MARTONOSI. Mechanism of ATP hydrolysis by sarcoplasmic reticulum and the role of phospholipids. *J. Biol. Chem.* 251: 5414-5423, 1976.
440. NAKAMURA, H., AND A. N. MARTONOSI. Effect of phospholipid substitution on the mobility of protein-bound spin labels in sarcoplasmic reticulum. *J. Biochem. Tokyo* 87: 525-534, 1980.
441. NAKAMURA, H., AND A. N. MARTONOSI. Effect of phospholipid substitution on the mobility of spin labels bound to the ATPase of sarcoplasmic reticulum. *J. Biochem. Tokyo* 89: 21-28, 1981.
442. NAKAMURA, J., Y. ENDO, AND K. KONISHI. The formation of phosphoenzyme of sarcoplasmic reticulum. Requirement for membrane-bound Ca^{2+}. *Biochim. Biophys. Acta* 471: 260-272, 1977.
443. NAKAMURA, M., AND S. OHNISHI. Organization of lipids in sarcoplasmic reticulum membrane and Ca^{2+}-dependent ATPase activity. *J. Biochem. Tokyo* 78: 1039-1045, 1975.
444. NAKAMURA, Y., AND Y. TONOMURA. Reaction mechanism of *p*-nitrophenylphosphatase of sarcoplasmic reticulum: evidence for two kinds of phosphorylated intermediates with and without bound *p*-nitrophenol. *J. Biochem. Tokyo* 83: 571-583, 1978.
445. NAKAMURA, Y., Y. TONOMURA, AND B. HAGIHARA. Change in the ultraviolet spectrum of solubilized Ca^{2+}-dependent ATPase from sarcoplasmic reticulum due to binding with Ca^{2+} ions. *J. Biochem. Tokyo* 86: 443-446, 1979.
446. NAMM, D. H., E. L. WOODS, AND J. L. ZUCKER. Incorporation of the terminal phosphate of ATP into membranal protein of rabbit cardiac sarcoplasmic reticulum. Correlation with active calcium transport and study of the effects of cyclic AMP. *Circ. Res.* 31: 308-316, 1972.
447. NARASIMHAN, R., R. K. MURRAY, AND D. H. MACLENNAN. Presence of glycosphingolipids in the sarcoplasmic reticulum fraction of rabbit skeletal muscle. *FEBS Lett.* 43: 23-26, 1974.
448. NEET, K. E., AND N. M. GREEN. Kinetics of the cooperativity of the Ca^{2+} transporting adenosine triphosphatase of sarcoplasmic reticulum and the mechanism of the ATP interaction. *Arch. Biochem. Biophys.* 178: 588-597, 1977.
449. OETLIKER, H., S. M. BAYLOR, AND W. K. CHANDLER. Simultaneous changes in fluorescence and optical retardation in single muscle fibres during activity. *Nature London* 257: 693-696, 1975.
450. OHNISHI, S. T. A method for studying the depolarization-induced calcium ion release from fragmented sarcoplasmic reticulum. *Biochim. Biophys. Acta* 587: 121-128, 1979.
451. OHNOKI, S., AND A. MARTONOSI. Purification and characterization of the proteolipid of rabbit sarcoplasmic reticulum. *Biochim. Biophys. Acta* 626: 170-178, 1980.
452. OHNOKI, S., AND A. MARTONOSI. Structural differences between Ca^{2+} transport ATPases isolated from sarcoplasmic reticulum of rabbit, chicken and lobster muscle. *Comp. Biochem. Physiol. B* 65: 181-189, 1980.
453. OLDFIELD, E., K. M. KEOUGH, AND D. CHAPMAN. The study of hydrocarbon chain mobility in membrane systems using spin-label probes. *FEBS Lett.* 20: 344-346, 1972.
454. OMURA, T., P. SIEKEVITZ, AND G. E. PALADE. Turnover of constituents of the endoplasmic reticulum membranes of rat hepatocytes. *J. Biol. Chem.* 242: 2389-2396, 1967.
455. OSTWALD, T. J., AND D. H. MACLENNAN. Isolation of a high affinity calcium-binding protein from sarcoplasmic reticulum. *J. Biol. Chem.* 249: 974-979, 1974.
456. OSTWALD, T. J., D. H. MACLENNAN, AND K. J. DORRINGTON.

Effects of cation binding on the conformation of calsequestrin and the high affinity calcium-binding protein of sarcoplasmic reticulum. *J. Biol. Chem.* 249: 5867–5871, 1974.

457. OVCHINNIKOV, Y. A. Physico-chemical basis of ion transport through biological membranes: ionophores and ion channels. *Eur. J. Biochem.* 94: 321–336, 1979.

458. OWENS, K., R. C. RUTH, AND W. B. WEGLICKI. Lipid composition of purified fragmented sarcoplasmic reticulum of the rabbit. *Biochim. Biophys. Acta* 288: 479–481, 1972.

459. PACKER, L., C. W. MEHARD, G. MEISSNER, W. L. ZAHLER, AND S. FLEISCHER. The structural role of lipids in mitochondrial and sarcoplasmic reticulum membranes. Freeze-fracture electron microscopy studies. *Biochim. Biophys. Acta* 363: 159–181, 1974.

460. PANET, R., AND Z. SELINGER. Specific alkylation of the sarcoplasmic reticulum ATPase by N-ethyl-[1-^{14}C]maleimide and identification of the labeled protein in acrylamide gel-electrophoresis. *Eur. J. Biochem.* 14: 440–444, 1970.

461. PANG, D. C., AND F. N. BRIGGS. Reaction mechanism of the cardiac sarcotubule calcium(II) dependent adenosine triphosphatase. *Biochemistry* 12: 4905–4911, 1973.

462. PANG, D. C., AND F. N. BRIGGS. Effect of calcium and magnesium on binding of β,γ-methylene ATP to sarcoplasmic reticulum. *J. Biol. Chem.* 252: 3262–3266, 1977.

463. PANG, D. C., F. N. BRIGGS, AND R. S. ROGOWSKI. Analysis of the ATP-induced conformational changes in sarcoplasmic reticulum. *Arch. Biochem. Biophys.* 164: 332–340, 1974.

464. PICK, U., AND S. J. D. KARLISH. Indications for an oligomeric structure and for conformational changes in sarcoplasmic reticulum Ca^{2+}-ATPase labeled selectively with fluorescein. *Biochim. Biophys. Acta* 626: 255–261, 1980.

465. PICK, U., AND E. RACKER. Inhibition of the (Ca^{2+}) ATPase from sarcoplasmic reticulum by dicyclohexylcarbodiimide. Evidence for location of the Ca^{2+} binding site in a hydrophobic region. *Biochemistry* 18: 108–113, 1979.

466. PLANK, B., G. HELLMANN, C. PUNZENGRUBER, AND J. SUKO. ATP-P_i and ITP-P_i exchange by cardiac sarcoplasmic reticulum. *Biochim. Biophys. Acta* 550: 259–268, 1979.

467. PRAGER, R., C. PUNZENGRUBER, N. KOLASSA, F. WINKLER, AND J. SUKO. Ionized and bound calcium inside isolated sarcoplasmic reticulum of skeletal muscle and its significance in phosphorylation of adenosine triphosphatase by orthophosphate. *Eur. J. Biochem.* 97: 239–250, 1979.

468. PUCELL, A., AND A. MARTONOSI. Sarcoplasmic reticulum. XIV. Acetylphosphate and carbamylphosphate as energy sources for Ca^{++} transport. *J. Biol. Chem.* 246: 3389–3397, 1971.

469. PUNZENGRUBER, C., R. PRAGER., N. KOLASSA, F. WINKLER, AND J. SUKO. Calcium gradient-dependent and calcium gradient-independent phosphorylation of sarcoplasmic reticulum by orthophosphate. The role of magnesium. *Eur. J. Biochem.* 92: 349–359, 1978.

470. RACKER, E. Reconstitution of a calcium pump with phospholipids and a purified Ca^{++}-adenosine triphosphatase from sarcoplasmic reticulum. *J. Biol. Chem.* 247: 8198–8200, 1972.

471. RACKER, E. Reconstitution, mechanism of action and control of ion pumps. *Biochem. Soc. Trans.* 3: 785–802, 1975.

472. RACKER, E. *A New Look at Mechanisms in Bioenergetics.* New York: Academic, 1976.

473. RACKER, E. Structure and function of ATP-driven ion pumps. *Trends Biochem. Sci.* 1: 244–247, 1976.

474. RACKER, E. Proposal for a mechanism of Ca^{2+} transport. In: *Calcium-Binding Proteins and Calcium Function*, edited by R. H. Wasserman, R. A. Corradino, E. Carafoli, R. H. Kretsinger, D. H. MacLennan, and F. L. Siegel. Amsterdam: Elsevier/North-Holland, 1977, p. 155–163.

475. RACKER, E. Transport of ions. *Acc. Chem. Res.* 12: 338–344, 1979.

476. RACKER, E. Fluxes of Ca^{2+} and concepts. *Federation Proc.* 39: 2422–2426, 1980.

477. RACKER, E., J. A. BELT, W. W. CARLEY, AND J. H. JOHNSON. Studies on anion transporters. *Ann. NY Acad. Sci.* 341: 27–36, 1980.

478. RACKER, E., T.-F. CHIEN, AND A. KANDRACH. A cholate-dilution procedure for the reconstitution of the Ca^{++} pump, $^{32}P_i$-ATP exchange, and oxidative phosphorylation. *FEBS Lett.* 57: 14–18, 1975.

479. RACKER, E., AND E. EYTAN. Reconstitution of an efficient calcium pump without detergents. *Biochem. Biophys. Res. Commun.* 55: 174–178, 1973.

480. RACKER, E., AND E. EYTAN. A coupling factor from sarcoplasmic reticulum required for the translocation of Ca^{2+} ions in a reconstituted Ca^{2+} ATPase pump. *J. Biol. Chem.* 250: 7533–7534, 1975.

481. RACKER, E., A. F. KNOWLES, AND E. EYTAN. Resolution and reconstitution of ion-transport systems. *Ann. NY Acad. Sci.* 264: 17–33, 1975.

482. RACKER, E., B. VIOLAND, S. O'NEAL, M. ALFONZO, AND J. TELFORD. Reconstitution, a way of biochemical research; some new approaches to membrane-bound enzymes. *Arch. Biochem. Biophys.* 198: 470–477, 1979.

483. RAKOWSKI, R. F. Inactivation and recovery of membrane charge movement in skeletal muscle. In: *Regulation of Muscle Contraction: Excitation-Contraction Coupling*, edited by A. D. Grinnell and M. A. B. Brazier. New York: Academic, 1981, p. 23–38. (UCLA Forum Med. Sci. 22.)

484. RAUCH, B., D. CHAK, AND W. HASSELBACH. Phosphorylation by inorganic phosphate of sarcoplasmic membranes. *Z. Naturforsch. Teil C* 32: 828–834, 1977.

485. RAUCH, B., D. V. CHAK, AND W. HASSELBACH. An estimate of the kinetics of calcium binding and dissociation of the sarcoplasmic reticulum transport ATPase. *FEBS Lett.* 93: 65–68, 1978.

486. RAYNS, D. G., C. E. DEVINE, AND C. L. SUTHERLAND. Freeze fracture studies of membrane systems in vertebrate muscle. I. Striated muscle. *J. Ultrastruct. Res.* 50: 306–321, 1975.

487. REITHMEIER, R. A. F., S. DE LEON, AND D. H. MACLENNAN. Assembly of the sarcoplasmic reticulum. Cell-free synthesis of the Ca^{2+} + Mg^{2+}-adenosine triphosphatase and calsequestrin. *J. Biol. Chem.* 255: 11839–11846, 1980.

488. REITHMEIER, R. A. F., AND D. H. MACLENNAN. The NH_2 terminus of the (Ca^{2+} + Mg^{2+})-adenosine triphosphatase is located on the cytoplasmic surface of the sarcoplasmic reticulum membrane. *J. Biol. Chem.* 256: 5957–5960, 1981.

489. REQUENA, J., AND L. J. MULLINS. Calcium movement in nerve fibres. *Q. Rev. Biophys.* 12: 371–460, 1979.

490. REUTER, H., AND H. SCHOLZ. The regulation of the calcium conductance of cardiac muscle by adrenaline. *J. Physiol. London* 264: 49–62, 1977.

491. RIBEIRO, J. M. C., AND A. L. VIANNA. Allosteric modification by K^+ of the (Ca^{2+} + Mg^{2+})-dependent ATPase of sarcoplasmic reticulum. Interaction with Mg^{2+}. *J. Biol. Chem.* 253: 3153–3157, 1978.

492. RIZZOLO, L. J., M. LE MAIRE, J. A. REYNOLDS, AND C. TANFORD. Molecular weights and hydrophobicity of the polypeptide chain of sarcoplasmic reticulum calcium(II) adenosine triphosphatase and of its primary tryptic fragments. *Biochemistry* 15: 3433–3437, 1976.

493. RIZZOLO, L. J., AND C. TANFORD. Denaturation of the tryptic fragments of the calcium(II) adenosine triphosphatase from sarcoplasmic reticulum by guanidinium hydrochloride. *Biochemistry* 17: 4044–4048, 1978.

494. RIZZOLO, L. J., AND C. TANFORD. Behavior of fragmented calcium(II) adenosine triphosphatase from sarcoplasmic reticulum in detergent solution. *Biochemistry* 17: 4049–4055, 1978.

495. ROSEMBLATT, M., C. HIDALGO, C. VERGARA, AND N. IKEMOTO. Immunological and biochemical properties of transverse tubule membranes isolated from rabbit skeletal muscle. *J. Biol. Chem.* 256: 8140–8148, 1981.

496. ROSSI, B., F. DE ASSIS LEONE, C. GACHE, AND M. LAZDUNSKI. Pseudosubstrates of the sarcoplasmic Ca^{2+}-ATPase as tools to study the coupling between substrate hydrolysis and Ca^{2+} transport. *J. Biol. Chem.* 254: 2302–2307, 1979.

497. ROUFA, D., AND A. N. MARTONOSI. The effect of Ca^{2+} iono-

phores upon the synthesis of muscle proteins in normal and fusion blocked cultured skeletal muscle. *Federation Proc.* 39: 954, 1980.

498. ROUFA, D., AND A. N. MARTONOSI. Effect of curare on the development of chicken embryo skeletal muscle *in ovo*. *Biochem. Pharmacol.* 30: 1501–1505, 1981.
499. ROUFA, D., F. S. WU, AND A. N. MARTONOSI. The effect of Ca^{2+} ionophores upon the synthesis of proteins in cultured skeletal muscle. *Biochim. Biophys. Acta* 674: 225–237, 1981.
500. RUSSELL, J. T., T. BEELER, AND A. MARTONOSI. Optical probe responses on sarcoplasmic reticulum. Oxacarbocyanines. *J. Biol. Chem.* 254: 2040–2046, 1979.
501. RUSSELL, J. T., T. BEELER, AND A. MARTONOSI. Optical probe responses on sarcoplasmic reticulum: merocyanine and oxonol dyes. *J. Biol. Chem.* 254: 2047–2052, 1979.
502. SAITO, A., C. T. WANG, AND S. FLEISCHER. Membrane asymmetry and enhanced ultrastructural detail of sarcoplasmic reticulum revealed with use of tannic acid. *J. Cell Biol.* 79: 601–616, 1978.
503. SALAMA, G., AND A. SCARPA. Optical signals of merocyanine dyes bound to sarcoplasmic reticulum during Ca^{++} transport. *Biophys. J.* 21: 12a, 1978.
504. SANDOW, A., M. K. D. PAGALA, AND E. C. SPHICAS. Excitation-contraction coupling: effects of 'zero'-Ca^{2+} medium. *Biochim. Biophys. Acta* 404: 157–163, 1975.
505. SANSLONE, W. R., H. A. BERTRAND, B. P. YU, AND E. J. MASORO. Lipid components of sarcotubular membranes. *J. Cell. Physiol.* 79: 97–102, 1972.
506. SARZALA, M. G., AND M. MICHALAK. Studies on the heterogeneity of sarcoplasmic reticulum vesicles. *Biochim. Biophys. Acta* 513: 221–235, 1978.
507. SARZALA, M. G., AND M. PILARSKA. Phospholipid biosynthesis in sarcoplasmic reticulum membrane during development. *Biochim. Biophys. Acta* 441: 81–92, 1976.
508. SARZALA, M. G., M. PILARSKA, E. ZUBRZYCKA, AND M. MICHALAK. Changes in the structure, composition and function of sarcoplasmic reticulum membrane during development. *Eur. J. Biochem.* 57: 25–34, 1975.
509. SARZALA, M. G., E. ZUBRZYCKA, AND M. MICHALAK. Comparison of some features of undeveloped and mature sarcoplasmic reticulum vesicles. In: *Calcium Transport in Contraction and Secretion*, edited by E. Carafoli, F. Clementi, W. Drabikowski, and A. Margreth. Amsterdam: Elsevier/North-Holland, 1975, p. 329–338.
510. SCALES, D., AND G. INESI. Assembly of ATPase protein in sarcoplasmic reticulum membranes. *Biophys. J.* 16: 735–751, 1976.
511. SCALES, D. J., AND R. A. SABBADINI. Microsomal T system. A stereological analysis of purified microsomes derived from normal and dystrophic skeletal muscle. *J. Cell Biol.* 83: 33–46, 1979.
512. SCALES, D., R. SABBADINI, AND G. INESI. The involvement of sarcotubular membranes in genetic muscular dystrophy. *Biochim. Biophys. Acta* 465: 535–549, 1977.
513. SCANDELLA, C. J., P. DEVAUX, AND H. M. MCCONNELL. Rapid lateral diffusion of phospholipids in rabbit sarcoplasmic reticulum. *Proc. Natl. Acad. Sci. USA* 69: 2056–2060, 1972.
514. SCARPA, A., J. BALDASSARE, AND G. INESI. The effects of calcium ionophores on fragmented sarcoplasmic reticulum. *J. Gen. Physiol.* 60: 735–749, 1972.
515. SCARPA, A., AND E. CARAFOLI (editors). Calcium transport and cell function. *Ann. NY Acad. Sci.* 307: 1–655, 1978.
516. SCHIBECI, A., AND A. MARTONOSI. Ca^{2+} binding to muscle and liver nuclei. *Federation Proc.* 38: 494, 1979.
517. SCHIBECI, A., AND A. MARTONOSI. Ca^{2+}-binding proteins in nuclei. *Eur. J. Biochem.* 113: 5–14, 1980.
518. SCHMALBRUCH, H. 'Square arrays' in the sarcolemma of human skeletal muscle fibres. *Nature London* 281: 145–146, 1979.
519. SCHNEIDER, M. F. Membrane charge movement and depolarization-contraction coupling. *Annu. Rev. Physiol.* 43: 507–517, 1981.
520. SCHNEIDER, M. F., AND W. K. CHANDLER. Voltage dependent charge movement in skeletal muscle: a possible step in excitation-contraction coupling. *Nature London* 242: 244–246, 1973.
521. SCHOTLAND, D. L., E. BONILLA, AND Y. WAKAYAMA. Application of the freeze-fracture technique to the study of human neuromuscular disease. *Muscle Nerve* 3: 21–27, 1980.
522. SCHWARTZ, A., M. L. ENTMAN, K. KANIIKE, L. K. LANE, W. B. VAN WINKLE, AND E. P. BORNET. The rate of calcium uptake into sarcoplasmic reticulum of cardiac muscle and skeletal muscle. Effects of cyclic AMP-dependent protein kinase and phosphorylase β kinase. *Biochim. Biophys. Acta* 426: 57–72, 1976.
523. SCOFANO, H. M., A. VIEYRA, AND L. DE MEIS. Substrate regulation of the sarcoplasmic reticulum ATPase. Transient kinetic studies. *J. Biol. Chem.* 254: 10227–10231, 1979.
524. SEELIG, J., AND W. HASSELBACH. A spin label study of sarcoplasmic vesicles. *Eur. J. Biochem.* 21: 17–21, 1971.
525. SERGEEVA, N. S., A. F. POGLAZOV, AND Y. A. VLADIMIROV. Investigation of permeability of planar lipid membranes in presence of vesicles of sarcoplasmic reticulum. *Biofizika* 20: 1029–1032, 1975.
526. SHAMOO, A. E. Ionophorous properties of the 20,000 dalton fragment of (Ca^{2+} + Mg^{2+})-ATPase in phosphatidylcholine:cholesterol membranes. *J. Membr. Biol.* 43: 227–242, 1978.
527. SHAMOO, A. E., AND J. J. ABRAMSON. Ca^{2+} ionophore from Ca^{2+} + Mg^{2+} ATPase. In: *Calcium-Binding Proteins and Calcium Function*, edited by R. H. Wasserman, R. A. Corradino, E. Carafoli, R. H. Kretsinger, D. H. MacLennan, and F. L. Siegel. Amsterdam: Elsevier/North-Holland, 1977, p. 173–180.
528. SHAMOO, A. E., AND D. A. GOLDSTEIN. Isolation of ionophores from ion transport systems and their role in energy transduction. *Biochim. Biophys. Acta* 472: 13–53, 1977.
529. SHAMOO, A. E., AND D. H. MACLENNAN. A Ca^{++}-dependent and -selective ionophore as part of the Ca^{++} + Mg^{++}-dependent adenosinetriphosphatase of sarcoplasmic reticulum. *Proc. Natl. Acad. Sci. USA* 71: 3522–3526, 1974.
530. SHAMOO, A. E., AND D. H. MACLENNAN. Separate effects of mercurial compounds on the ionophoric and hydrolytic functions of the (Ca^{++} + Mg^{++})-ATPase of sarcoplasmic reticulum. *J. Membr. Biol.* 25: 65–74, 1975.
531. SHAMOO, A. E., AND T. J. MURPHY. Ionophores and ion transport across natural membranes. *Curr. Top. Bioenerg.* 9: 147–177, 1979.
532. SHAMOO, A. E., AND T. E. RYAN. Isolation of ionophores from ion transport systems. *Ann. NY Acad. Sci.* 264: 83–97, 1975.
533. SHAMOO, A. E., T. E. RYAN, P. S. STEWART, AND D. H. MACLENNAN. Localization of ionophore activity in a 20,000-dalton fragment of the adenosine triphosphatase of sarcoplasmic reticulum. *J. Biol. Chem.* 251: 4147–4154, 1976.
534. SHERMAN, R. G., AND A. R. LUFF. Structural features of the tarsal claw muscles of the spider *Eurypelma marxi* Simon. *Can. J. Zool.* 49: 1549–1556, 1971.
535. SHIGEKAWA, M., AND A. A. AKOWITZ. On the mechanism of Ca^{2+}-dependent adenosine triphosphatase of sarcoplasmic reticulum. Occurrence of two types of phosphoenzyme intermediates in the presence of KCl. *J. Biol. Chem.* 254: 4726–4730, 1979.
536. SHIGEKAWA, M., AND J. P. DOUGHERTY. Reaction mechanism of Ca^{2+}-dependent ATP hydrolysis by skeletal muscle sarcoplasmic reticulum in the absence of added alkali metal salts. II. Kinetic properties of the phosphoenzyme formed at the steady state in high Mg^{2+} and low Ca^{2+} concentrations. *J. Biol. Chem.* 253: 1451–1457, 1978.
537. SHIGEKAWA, M., AND J. P. DOUGHERTY. Reaction mechanism of Ca^{2+}-dependent ATP hydrolysis by skeletal muscle sarcoplasmic reticulum in the absence of added alkali metal salts. III. Sequential occurrence of ADP-sensitive and ADP-insensitive phosphoenzymes. *J. Biol. Chem.* 253: 1458–1464, 1978.
538. SHIGEKAWA, M., J. P. DOUGHERTY, AND A. M. KATZ. Reaction mechanism of Ca^{2+}-dependent ATP hydrolysis by skeletal muscle sarcoplasmic reticulum in the absence of added alkali

metal salts. I. Characterization of steady state ATP hydrolysis and comparison with that in the presence of KCl. *J. Biol. Chem.* 253: 1442–1450, 1978.
539. SHIGEKAWA, M., J. M. FINEGAN, AND A. M. KATZ. Calcium transport ATPase of canine cardiac sarcoplasmic reticulum. A comparison with that of rabbit fast skeletal muscle sarcoplasmic reticulum. *J. Biol. Chem.* 251: 6894–6900, 1976.
540. SHIGEKAWA, M., AND L. J. PEARL. Activation of calcium transport in skeletal muscle sarcoplasmic reticulum by monovalent cations. *J. Biol. Chem.* 251: 6947–6952, 1976.
541. SIGRIST, H., K. SIGRIST-NELSON, AND C. GITLER. Single-phase butanol extraction: a new tool for proteolipid isolation. *Biochem. Biophys. Res. Commun.* 74: 178–184, 1977.
542. SIMS, P. J., A. S. WAGGONER, C.-H. WANG, AND J. F. HOFFMAN. Studies on the mechanism by which cyanine dyes measure membrane potential in red blood cells and phosphatidylcholine vesicles. *Biochemistry* 13: 3315–3330, 1974.
543. SINGER, S. J. The molecular organization of membranes. *Annu. Rev. Biochem.* 43: 805–833, 1974.
544. SOMLYO, A. P., A. V. SOMLYO , H. SHUMAN, B. SLOANE, AND A. SCARPA. Electron probe analysis of calcium compartments in cryo sections of smooth and striated muscles. *Ann. NY Acad. Sci.* 307: 523–544, 1978.
545. SOMLYO, A. V. Bridging structures spanning the junctional gap at the triad of skeletal muscle. *J. Cell Biol.* 80: 743–750, 1979.
546. SOMLYO, A. V., H. GONZALEZ-SERRATOS, H. SHUMAN, G. MCCLELLAN, AND A. P. SOMLYO. Calcium release and ionic changes in the sarcoplasmic reticulum of tetanized muscle: an electron-probe study. *J. Cell Biol.* 90: 577–594, 1981.
547. SOMLYO, A. V., H. SHUMAN, AND A. P. SOMLYO. Composition of sarcoplasmic reticulum *in situ* by electron probe X-ray microanalysis. *Nature London* 268: 556–558, 1977.
548. SOMLYO, A. V., A. P. SOMLYO, ᵗ. GONZALEZ-SERRATOS, H. SHUMAN, AND G. MCCLELLAN. Sarcoplasmic reticulum and mitochondria in excitation-contraction (E-C) coupling in smooth and striated muscle. In: *Regulation of Muscle Contraction: Excitation-Contraction Coupling*, edited by A. D. Grinnell and M. A. B. Brazier. New York: Academic, 1981, p. 199–214. (UCLA Forum Med. Sci. 22.)
549. SOUZA, D. O. G., AND L. DE MEIS. Calcium and magnesium regulation of phosphorylation by ATP and ITP in sarcoplasmic reticulum vesicles. *J. Biol. Chem.* 251: 6355–6359, 1976.
550. SPITZER, N. C. Ion channels in development. *Annu. Rev. Neurosci.* 2: 363–397, 1979.
551. SRÉTER, F. A. Temperature, pH and seasonal dependence of Ca-uptake and ATPase activity of white and red muscle microsomes. *Arch. Biochem. Biophys.* 134: 25–33, 1969.
552. STEFANI, E., AND D. J. CHIARANDINI. Skeletal muscle: dependence of potassium contractures on extracellular calcium. *Pfluegers Arch.* 343: 143–150, 1973.
553. STEIN, W. D. *The Movement of Molecules Across Cell Membranes.* New York: Academic, 1967.
554. STEIN, W. D., Y. EILAM, AND W. R. LIEB. Active transport of cations across biological membranes. *Ann. NY Acad. Sci.* 227: 328–336, 1974.
555. STEPHENS, E. M., AND C. M. GRISHAM. Lithium-7 nuclear magnetic resonance, water proton nuclear magnetic resonance, and gadolinium electron paramagnetic resonance studies of the sarcoplasmic reticulum calcium ion transport adenosine triphosphatase. *Biochemistry* 18: 4876–4885, 1979.
556. STEWART, P. S., AND D. H. MACLENNAN. Surface particles of sarcoplasmic reticulum membranes. Structural features of the adenosine triphosphatase. *J. Biol. Chem.* 249: 985–993, 1974.
557. STEWART, P. S., D. H. MACLENNAN, AND A. E. SHAMOO. Isolation and characterization of tryptic fragments of adenosine triphosphatase of sarcoplasmic reticulum. *J. Biol. Chem.* 251: 712–719, 1976.
558. STROMER, M., AND W. HASSELBACH. Fusion of isolated sarcoplasmic reticulum membranes. *Z. Naturforsch. Teil C* 31: 703–707, 1976.
559. STRYER, L. Fluorescence energy transfer as a spectroscopic ruler. *Annu. Rev. Biochem.* 47: 819–846, 1978.
560. SUAREZ-KURTZ, G., AND I. PARKER. Birefringence signals and calcium transients in skeletal muscle. *Nature London* 270: 746–748, 1977.
561. SUKO, J., AND W. HASSELBACH. Characterization of cardiac sarcoplasmic reticulum ATP-ADP phosphate exchange and phosphorylation of the calcium transport adenosine triphosphatase. *Eur. J. Biochem.* 64: 123–130, 1976.
562. SUMIDA, M., T. KANAZAWA, AND Y. TONOMURA. Reaction mechanism of the Ca^{2+}-dependent ATPase of sarcoplasmic reticulum from skeletal muscle. XI. Re-evaluation of the transition of ATPase activity during the initial phase. *J. Biochem. Tokyo* 79: 259–264, 1976.
563. SUMIDA, M., AND S. SASAKI. Inhibition of Ca^{2+} uptake into fragmented sarcoplasmic reticulum by antibodies against purified Ca^{2+}, Mg^{2+}-dependent ATPase. *J. Biochem. Tokyo* 78: 757–762, 1975.
564. SUMIDA, M., AND Y. TONOMURA. Reaction mechanism of the Ca^{2+}-dependent ATPase of sarcoplasmic reticulum from skeletal muscle. X. Direct evidence for Ca^{2+} translocation coupled with formation of a phosphorylated intermediate. *J. Biochem. Tokyo* 75: 283–297, 1974.
565. SUMIDA, M., T. WANG, F. MANDEL, J. P. FROEHLICH, AND A. SCHWARTZ. Transient kinetics of Ca^{2+} transport of sarcoplasmic reticulum. A comparison of cardiac and skeletal muscle. *J. Biol. Chem.* 253: 8772–8777, 1978.
566. SUMIDA, M., T. WANG, A. SCHWARTZ, C. YOUNKIN, AND J. P. FROEHLICH. The Ca^{2+}-ATPase partial reactions in cardiac and skeletal sarcoplasmic reticulum. A comparison of transient state kinetic data. *J. Biol. Chem.* 255: 1497–1503, 1980.
567. SUTHERLAND, E. W., AND T. W. RALL. The relation of adenosine-3′,5′-phosphate and phosphorylase to the actions of catecholamines and other hormones. *Pharmacol. Rev.* 12: 265–299, 1960.
568. SUTHERLAND, E. W., G. A. ROBISON, AND R. W. BUTCHER. Some aspects of the biological role of adenosine 3′,5′-monophosphate (cyclic AMP). *Circulation* 37: 279–306, 1968.
569. SZABOLCS, M., A. KOVER, AND L. KOVACS. Studies on the postnatal changes in the sarcoplasmatic reticular fraction of rabbit muscle. *Acta Biochim. Biophys. Acad. Sci. Hung.* 2: 409–415, 1967.
570. TADA, M., AND M. A. KIRCHBERGER. Regulation of calcium transport by cyclic AMP. A proposed mechanism for the beta-adrenergic control of myocardial contractility. *Acta Cardiol.* 30: 231–237, 1975.
571. TADA, M., M. A. KIRCHBERGER, AND A. M. KATZ. Phosphorylation of a 22,000 dalton component of the cardiac sarcoplasmic reticulum by adenosine 3′,5′-monophosphate-dependent protein kinase. *J. Biol. Chem.* 250: 2640–2647, 1975.
572. TADA, M., M. A. KIRCHBERGER, AND H. C. LI. Phosphoprotein phosphatase-catalyzed dephosphorylation of the 22,000 dalton phosphoprotein of cardiac sarcoplasmic reticulum. *J. Cyclic Nucleotide Res.* 1: 329–338, 1975.
573. TADA, M., M. A. KIRCHBERGER, D. I. REPKE, AND A. M. KATZ. The stimulation of calcium transport in cardiac sarcoplasmic reticulum by adenosine 3′,5′-monophosphate-dependent protein kinase. *J. Biol. Chem.* 249: 6174–6180, 1974.
574. TADA, M., F. OHMORI, N. KINOSHITA, AND H. ABE. Significance of two classes of phosphoproteins in the function of cardiac sarcoplasmic reticulum: phosphorylation of Ca^{2+}-dependent ATPase and phospholamban. In: *Calcium-Binding Proteins and Calcium Function*, edited by R. H. Wasserman, R. A. Corradino, E. Carafoli, R. H. Kretsinger, D. H. MacLennan, and F. L. Siegel. Amsterdam: Elsevier/North-Holland, 1977, p. 200–202.
575. TADA, M., F. OHMORI, N. KINOSHITA, AND H. ABE. Cyclic-AMP regulation of active calcium transport across membranes of sarcoplasmic reticulum: role of the 22,000 dalton protein phospholamban. *Adv. Cyclic Nucleotide Res.* 9: 355–369, 1978.
576. TADA, M., F. OHMORI, N. KINOSHITA, M. KADOMA, H. MATSUO, H. SAKAKIBARA, Y. NIMURA, AND H. ABE. Effects of protein kinase modulator on cAMP- and cGMP-dependent protein kinase-catalyzed phosphorylation and the rate of cal-

cium uptake by cardiac microsomes. *J. Mol. Cell. Cardiol.* 9, Suppl.: 45–46, 1977.

577. TADA, M., F. OHMORI, M. YAMADA, AND H. ABE. Mechanism of the stimulation of Ca^{2+}-dependent ATPase of cardiac sarcoplasmic reticulum by adenosine 3′,5′-monophosphate-dependent protein kinase. Role of the 22,000-dalton protein. *J. Biol. Chem.* 254: 319–326, 1979.
578. TADA, M., M. YAMADA, F. OHMORI, T. KUZUYA, AND H. ABE. Mechanism of cyclic AMP regulation of active calcium transport by cardiac sarcoplasmic reticulum. In: *Cation Flux Across Biomembranes*, edited by Y. Mukohata and L. Packer. New York: Academic, 1979, p. 179–190.
579. TADA, M., T. YAMAMOTO, AND Y. TONOMURA. Molecular mechanism of active calcium transport by sarcoplasmic reticulum. *Physiol. Rev.* 58: 1–79, 1978.
580. TAKAKUWA, Y., AND T. KANAZAWA. Slow transition of phosphoenzyme from ADP-sensitive to ADP-insensitive forms in solubilized Ca^{2+}, Mg^{2+}-ATPase of sarcoplasmic reticulum: evidence for retarded dissociation of Ca^{2+} from the phosphoenzyme. *Biochem. Biophys. Res. Commun.* 88: 1209–1216, 1979.
581. TAKISAWA, H., AND Y. TONOMURA. Factors affecting the transient phase of the Ca^{2+} + Mg^{2+} dependent ATPase reaction of sarcoplasmic reticulum from skeletal muscle. *J. Biochem. Tokyo* 83: 1275–1284, 1978.
582. TAKISAWA, H., AND Y. TONOMURA. ADP-sensitive and -insensitive phosphorylated intermediates of solubilized Ca^{2+}, Mg^{2+}-dependent ATPase of the sarcoplasmic reticulum from skeletal muscle. *J. Biochem. Tokyo* 86: 425–441, 1979.
583. TANFORD, C. The hydrophobic effect and the organization of living matter. *Science* 200: 1012–1018, 1978.
584. TAYLOR, J. S., AND D. HATTAN. Biphasic kinetics of ATP hydrolysis by calcium dependent ATPase of the sarcoplasmic reticulum of skeletal muscle. *J. Biol. Chem.* 254: 4402–4407, 1979.
585. TENU, J. P., A. DUPAIX, J. YON, F. J. SEYDOUX, AND J. CHEVALLIER. A plausible model for calcium transport in sarcoplasmic reticulum. *Biol. Cell.* 33: 219–224, 1978.
586. TENU, J. P., C. GHELIS, D. S. LEGER, J. CARRETTE, AND J. CHEVALLIER. Mechanism of an active transport of calcium. Ethoxyformylation of sarcoplasmic reticulum vesicles. *J. Biol. Chem.* 251: 4322–4329, 1976.
587. THE, R., AND W. HASSELBACH. Properties of the sarcoplasmic ATPase reconstituted by oleate and lysolecithin after lipid depletion. *Eur. J. Biochem.* 28: 357–363, 1972.
588. THE, R., AND W. HASSELBACH. Unsaturated fatty acids as reactivators of the calcium-dependent ATPase of delipidated sarcoplasmic membranes. *Eur. J. Biochem.* 39: 63–68, 1973.
589. THE, R., AND W. HASSELBACH. Stimulatory and inhibitory effects of dimethyl sulfoxide and ethylene glycol on ATPase activity and calcium transport of sarcoplasmic membranes. *Eur. J. Biochem.* 74: 611–621, 1977.
590. THOMAS, D. D. Large scale rotational motions of proteins detected by electron paramagnetic resonance and fluorescence. *Biophys. J.* 24: 439–462, 1978.
591. THOMAS, D. D., AND C. HIDALGO. Rotational motion of the sarcoplasmic reticulum Ca^{2+}-ATPase. *Proc. Natl. Acad. Sci. USA* 75: 5488–5492, 1978.
592. THORLEY-LAWSON, D. A., AND N. M. GREEN. Studies on the location and orientation of proteins in the sarcoplasmic reticulum. *Eur. J. Biochem.* 40: 403–413, 1973.
593. THORLEY-LAWSON, D. A., AND N. M. GREEN. Separation and characterization of tryptic fragments from the adenosine triphosphatase of sarcoplasmic reticulum. *Eur. J. Biochem.* 59: 193–200, 1975.
594. THORLEY-LAWSON, D. A., AND N. M. GREEN. The reactivity of the thiol groups of the adenosine triphosphatase of sarcoplasmic reticulum and their location on tryptic fragments of the molecule. *Biochem. J.* 167: 739–748, 1977.
595. TILLACK, T. W., R. BOLAND, AND A. N. MARTONOSI. The ultrastructure of developing sarcoplasmic reticulum. *J. Biol. Chem.* 249: 624–633, 1974.
596. TONG, S. W. The acetylated NH_2 terminus of Ca-ATPase from rabbit skeletal muscle sarcoplasmic reticulum: a common NH_2 terminal acetylated methionyl sequence. *Biochem. Biophys. Res. Commun.* 74: 1242–1248, 1977.
597. TONG, S. W. Studies on the structure of the calcium-dependent adenosine triphosphatase from rabbit skeletal muscle sarcoplasmic reticulum. *Arch. Biochem. Biophys.* 203: 780–791, 1980.
598. TONOMURA, Y. *Muscle Proteins, Muscle Contraction and Cation Transport.* Tokyo: Univ. of Tokyo Press, 1972.
599. TONOMURA, Y., AND M. F. MORALES. Change in state of spin labels bound to sarcoplasmic reticulum with change in enzymic state, as deduced from ascorbate-quenching studies. *Proc. Natl. Acad. Sci. USA* 71: 3687–3691, 1974.
600. TROTTA, E. E., AND L. DE MEIS. Adenosine 5′-triphosphate orthophosphate exchange catalyzed by the Ca^{2+}-transport ATPase of brain. Activation by a small transmembrane Ca^{2+} gradient. *J. Biol. Chem.* 253: 7821–7825, 1978.
601. TSAI, C. M., C. C. HUANG, AND E. S. CANELLAKIS. Iodination of cell membranes. I. Optimal conditions for the iodination of exposed membrane components. *Biochim. Biophys. Acta* 332: 47–58, 1973.
602. TUME, R. K. Iodination of calsequestrin in the sarcoplasmic reticulum of rabbit skeletal muscle: a reexamination. *Austr. J. Biol. Sci.* 32: 177–185, 1979.
603. UENO, T., AND T. SEKINE. Study on calcium transport by sarcoplasmic reticulum vesicles using fluorescence probes. *J. Biochem. Tokyo* 84: 787–794, 1978.
604. UENO, T., AND T. SEKINE. A role of H^+ flux in active Ca^{2+} transport into sarcoplasmic reticulum vesicles. I. Effect on an artificially imposed H^+ gradient on Ca^{2+} uptake. *J. Biochem. Tokyo* 89: 1239–1246, 1981.
605. UENO, T., AND T. SEKINE. A role of H^+ flux in active Ca^{2+} transport into sarcoplasmic reticulum vesicles. II. H^+ ejection during Ca^{2+} uptake. *J. Biochem. Tokyo* 89: 1247–1252, 1981.
606. ULBRECHT, M. Beruht der Phosphat-Austausch zwischen Adenosin-triphosphat und Adenosin [^{32}P]-diphosphate in gereinigten Fibrillen und Actomyosin Praparaten auf einer Verunreinigung durch Muskel-grana? *Biochim. Biophys. Acta* 57: 438–454, 1962.
607. ULBRECHT, M. Der Austausch und die Abspaltung des γ-Phosphats des Adenosin-Triphosphates durch Sarkosomen und kleine Grana des Kaninchen-Muskels. *Biochim. Biophys. Acta* 57: 455–474, 1962.
608. VALE, M. G. P. Localization of the amino phospholipids in sarcoplasmic reticulum membranes revealed by trinitrobenzenesulfonate and fluorodinitrobenzene. *Biochim. Biophys. Acta* 471: 39–48, 1977.
609. VALE, M. G. P., AND A. P. CARVALHO. Utilization of X-537A to distinguish between intravesicular and membrane-bound calcium ions in sarcoplasmic reticulum. *Biochim. Biophys. Acta* 413: 202–212, 1975.
610. VALE, M. G. P., AND A. P. CARVALHO. Effect of temperature on the reversal of the calcium ion pump in sarcoplasmic reticulum. *Biochem. J.* 186: 461–467, 1980.
611. VALE, M. G. P., V. R. OSÓRIO, E. CASTRO, AND A. P. CARVALHO. Synthesis of adenosine triphosphate during release of intravesicular and membrane-bound calcium ions from passively loaded sarcoplasmic reticulum. *Biochem. J.* 156: 239–244, 1976.
612. VAN DEN BESSELAAR, A. M. P. H., B. DE KRUIJFF, H. VAN DEN BOSCH, AND L. L. M. VAN DEENEN. Transverse distribution and movement of lysophosphatidylcholine in sarcoplasmic reticulum membranes as determined by ^{13}C NMR and lysophospholipase. *Biochim. Biophys. Acta* 555: 193–199, 1979.
613. VANDERKOOI, J. M., A. IEROKOMOS, H. NAKAMURA, AND A. MARTONOSI. Fluorescence energy transfer between Ca^{2+} transport ATPase molecules in artificial membranes. *Biochemistry* 16: 1262–1267, 1977.
614. VANDERKOOI, J., AND A. MARTONOSI. Sarcoplasmic reticulum. VIII. Use of 8-anilino-1-naphthalene sulfonate as conformational probe on biological membranes. *Arch. Biochem. Biophys.* 133: 153–163, 1969.
615. VANDERKOOI, J. M., AND A. MARTONOSI. Sarcoplasmic reticulum. XII. The interaction of 8-anilino-1-naphthalene sulfo-

nate with skeletal muscle microsomes. *Arch. Biochem. Biophys.* 144: 87–98, 1971.

616. VANDERKOOI, J. M., AND A. MARTONOSI. Sarcoplasmic reticulum. XIII. Changes in the fluorescence of 8-anilino-1-naphthalene sulfonate during Ca^{2+} transport. *Arch. Biochem. Biophys.* 144: 99–106, 1971.
617. VANDERKOOI, J. M., AND A. MARTONOSI. Sarcoplasmic reticulum. XVI. The permeability of phosphatidyl choline vesicles for calcium. *Arch. Biochem. Biophys.* 147: 632–646, 1971.
618. VANDERKOOI, J. M., AND A. MARTONOSI. Use of 8-anilino-1-naphthalene sulfonate as conformational probe on biological membranes. In: *Probes of Structure and Function of Macromolecules and Membranes*, edited by B. Chance, C. P. Lee, and J. K. Blasie. New York: Academic, 1971, vol. I, p. 293–301.
619. VAN WINKLE, W. B., AND M. L. ENTMAN. Mini review. Comparative aspects of cardiac and skeletal muscle sarcoplasmic reticulum. *Life Sci.* 25: 1189–1200, 1979.
620. VARSANYI, M., U. GRÖSCHEL-STEWART, AND L. M. G. HEILMEYER, JR. Characterization of a Ca^{2+}-dependent protein kinase in skeletal muscle membranes of I-strain and wild-type mice. *Eur. J. Biochem.* 87: 331–340, 1978.
621. VARSANYI, M., AND L. M. G. HEILMEYER, JR. Ca^{2+} regulation of sarcoplasmic reticular protein phosphatase activity. *Biochemistry 18:* 4869–4875, 1979.
622. VARSANYI, M., AND L. M. G. HEILMEYER. The protein kinase properties of calsequestrin. *FEBS Lett.* 103: 85–88, 1979.
623. VEGH, K., P. SPIEGLER, C. CHAMBERLAIN, AND W. F. H. M. MOMMAERTS. The molecular size of the calcium transport ATPase of sarcotubular vesicles estimated from radiation inactivation. *Biochim. Biophys. Acta* 163: 266–268, 1968.
624. VERGARA, J., F. BEZANILLA, AND B. M. SALZBERG. Nile blue fluorescence signals from cut single muscle fibers under voltage or current clamp conditions. *J. Gen. Physiol.* 72: 775–800, 1978.
625. VERJOVSKI-ALMEIDA, S., AND G. INESI. Fast kinetic evidence for an activating effect of ATP on the Ca^{2+} transport of sarcoplasmic reticulum ATPase. *J. Biol. Chem.* 254: 18–21, 1979.
626. VERJOVSKI-ALMEIDA, S., M. KURZMACK, AND G. INESI. Partial reactions in the catalytic and transport cycle of sarcoplasmic reticulum ATPase. *Biochemistry* 17: 5006–5013, 1978.
627. VIANNA, A. L. Interaction of calcium and magnesium in activating and inhibiting the nucleoside triphosphatase of sarcoplasmic reticulum vesicles. *Biochim. Biophys. Acta* 410: 389–406, 1975.
628. VIEYRA, A., H. M. SCOFANO, H. GUIMARAES-MOTTA, R. K. TUME, AND L. DE MEIS. Transient state kinetic studies of phosphorylation by ATP and Pi of the calcium dependent ATPase from sarcoplasmic reticulum. *Biochim. Biophys. Acta* 568: 437–445, 1979.
629. WAAS, W., AND HASSELBACH, W. Interference of nucleoside diphosphates and inorganic phosphate with NTP-dependent calcium fluxes and calcium dependent NTP hydrolysis in vesicular sarcoplasmic reticulum membranes. *Eur. J. Biochem.* 116: 601–608, 1981.
630. WAGGONER, A. Optical probes of membrane potential. *J. Membr. Biol.* 27: 317–334, 1976.
631. WAGGONER, A. S. Dye indicators of membrane potential. *Annu. Rev. Biophys. Bioeng.* 8: 47–58, 1979.
632. WAKU, K. Skeletal muscle. In: *Lipid Metabolism in Mammals*, edited by F. Snyder. New York: Plenum, 1977, vol. 2, p. 189–208.
633. WAKU, A., F. HAYAKAWA, AND Y. NAKAZAWA. Regulation of the fatty acid pattern of phospholipids in rabbit sarcoplasmic reticulum. Specificity of glycerophosphate, 1-acylglycerophosphate and 2-acylglycerophosphorylcholine acyltransferase systems. *J. Biochem. Tokyo* 82: 671–677, 1977.
634. WAKU, K., H. ITO, T. BITO, AND Y. NAKAZAWA. Fatty chains of acyl, alkenyl, and alkyl phosphoglycerides of rabbit sarcoplasmic reticulum. The metabolic relationship considered on the basis of structural analyses. *J. Biochem. Tokyo* 75: 1307–1312, 1974.
635. WAKU, K., AND W. E. M. LANDS. Acyl coenzyme A: 1-alkenyl-glycero-3-phosphoryl choline acyltransferase action in plasmalogen biosynthesis. *J. Biol. Chem.* 243: 2654–2659, 1968.
636. WAKU, K., AND Y. NAKAZAWA. Acyltransferase activity to 1-0-alkyl-glycero-3-phosphorylcholine in sarcoplasmic reticulum. *J. Biochem. Tokyo* 68: 459–466, 1970.
637. WAKU, K., AND Y. NAKAZAWA. The rates of incorporation of inorganic orthophosphate, glycerol, and acetate into phospholipids of rabbit sarcoplasmic reticulum. *J. Biochem. Tokyo* 73: 497–504, 1973.
638. WAKU, K., Y. UDA, AND Y. NAKAZAWA. Lipid composition in rabbit sarcoplasmic reticulum and occurrence of alkyl ether phospholipids. *J. Biochem. Tokyo* 69: 483–491, 1971.
639. WANG, C. T., S. SAITO, AND S. FLEISCHER. Correlation of ultrastructure of reconstituted sarcoplasmic reticulum membrane vesicles with variation in phospholipid to protein ratio. *J. Biol. Chem.* 254: 9209–9219, 1979.
640. WANG, T., A. O. GRASSI DE GENDE, AND A. SCHWARTZ. Kinetic properties of calcium adenosine triphosphatase of sarcoplasmic reticulum isolated from cat skeletal muscles. A comparison of caudofemoralis (fast), tibialis (mixed), and soleus (slow). *J. Biol. Chem.* 254: 10675–10678, 1979.
641. WANSON, J. C., AND P. DROCHMANS. Role of the sarcoplasmic reticulum in glycogen metabolism. Binding of phosphorylase, phosphorylase kinase, and primer complexes of the sarcovesicles of rabbit skeletal muscle. *J. Cell Biol.* 54: 206–224, 1972.
642. WARREN, G. B., J. P. BENNETT, T. R. HESKETH, M. D. HOUSLAY, G. A. SMITH, AND J. C. METCALFE. The lipids surrounding a calcium transport protein: their role in calcium transport and accumulation. *Proc. FEBS Meet., 10th* 41: 3–15, 1975.
643. WARREN, G. B., M. D. HOUSLAY, J. C. METCALFE, AND N. J. M. BIRDSALL. Cholesterol is excluded from the phospholipid annulus surrounding an active calcium transport protein. *Nature London* 255: 684–687, 1975.
644. WARREN, G. B., P. A. TOON, N. J. M. BIRDSALL, A. G. LEE, AND J. C. METCALFE. Complete control of the lipid environment of membrane-bound proteins: application to a calcium transport system. *FEBS Lett.* 41: 122–124, 1974.
645. WARREN, G. B., P. A. TOON, N. J. M. BIRDSALL, A. G. LEE, AND J. C. METCALFE. Reversible lipid titrations of the activity of pure adenosine triphosphatase-lipid complexes. *Biochemistry* 13: 5501–5507, 1974.
646. WARREN, G. B., P. A. TOON, N. J. M. BIRDSALL, A. G. LEE, AND J. C. METCALFE. Reconstitution of a calcium pump using defined membrane components. *Proc. Natl. Acad. Sci. USA* 71: 622–626, 1974.
647. WASSERMAN, R. H., R. A. CORRADINO, E. CARAFOLI, R. H. KRETSINGER, D. H. MACLENNAN, AND F. L. SIEGEL (editors). *Calcium-Binding Proteins and Calcium Function.* New York: Elsevier/North-Holland, 1977.
648. WEBER, A. Energized calcium transport and relaxing factors. In: *Current Topics in Bioenergetics*, edited by A. Sanadi. New York: Academic, 1966, vol. 1, p. 203–254.
649. WEBER, A. Regulatory mechanisms of the calcium transport system of fragmented rabbit sarcoplasmic reticulum. I. The effect of accumulated calcium on transport and adenosine triphosphate hydrolysis . *J. Gen. Physiol.* 57: 50–63, 1971.
650. WEBER, A. Regulatory mechanisms of the calcium transport system of fragmented rabbit sarcoplasmic reticulum. II. Inhibition of outflux in calcium-free media. *J. Gen. Physiol.* 57: 64–70, 1971.
651. WEBER, A., R. HERZ, AND I. REISS. The regulation of myofibrillar activity by calcium. *Proc. R. Soc. London Ser. B* 160: 489–501, 1964.
652. WEBER, A., R. HERZ, AND I. REISS. Study of the kinetics of calcium transport by isolated fragmented sarcoplasmic reticulum. *Biochem. Z.* 345: 329–369, 1966.
653. WEBER, K., AND M. OSBORN. The reliability of molecular weight determinations by dodecyl sulfate-polyacrylamide gel electrophoresis. *J. Biol. Chem.* 244: 4406–4412, 1969.
654. WILL, H., T. S. LEVCHENKO, D. O. LEVITSKY, V. N. SMIRNOV, AND A. WOLLENBERGER. Partial characterization of protein kinase-catalyzed phosphorylation of low molecular weight pro-

teins in purified preparations of pigeon heart sarcolemma and sarcoplasmic reticulum. *Biochim. Biophys. Acta* 543: 175–193, 1978.

655. WINEGRAD, S. Autoradiographic studies of intracellular calcium in frog skeletal muscle. *J. Gen. Physiol.* 48: 455–479, 1965.
656. WINEGRAD, S. The location of muscle calcium with respect to the myofibrils. *J. Gen. Physiol.* 48: 997–1002, 1965.
657. WINEGRAD, S. Intracellular calcium movements of frog skeletal muscle during recovery from tetanus. *J. Gen. Physiol.* 51: 65–83, 1968.
658. WOLLENBERGER, A. Cyclic nucleotides and the regulation of heart beat. *Int. Congr. Pharmacol., 5th, Abstracts of Invited Presentations, 1972,* p. 231–233.
659. WOLLENBERGER, A., AND H. WILL. Protein kinase-catalyzed membrane phosphorylation and its possible relationship to the role of calcium in the adrenergic regulation of cardiac contraction. *Life Sci.* 22: 1159–1178, 1978.
660. WORTHINGTON, C. R., AND S. C. LIU. Structure of sarcoplasmic reticulum membranes at low resolution (17Å). *Arch. Biochem. Biophys.* 157: 573–579, 1973.
661. WRAY, H. L., AND R. R. GRAY. Cyclic AMP stimulation of membrane phosphorylation and Ca^{2+}-activated, Mg^{2+} dependent ATPase in cardiac sarcoplasmic reticulum. *Biochim. Biophys. Acta* 461: 441–459, 1977.
662. WRAY, H. L., R. R. GRAY, AND R. A. OLSSON. Cyclic adenosine 3′,5′-monophosphate-stimulated protein kinase and a substrate associated with cardiac sarcoplasmic reticulum. *J. Biol. Chem.* 248: 1496–1498, 1973.
663. WU, F. S., Y.-C. PARK, D. ROUFA, AND A. MARTONOSI. Selective stimulation of the synthesis of an 80,000 dalton protein by calcium ionophores. *J. Biol. Chem.* 256: 5309–5312, 1981.
664. WU, S. H., AND H. M. MCCONNELL. Phase separations in phospholipid membranes. *Biochemistry* 14: 847–854, 1975.
665. YAMADA, S., AND N. IKEMOTO. Distinction of thiols involved in the specific reaction steps of the Ca^{2+}-ATPase of the sarcoplasmic reticulum. *J. Biol. Chem.* 253: 6801–6807, 1978.
666. YAMADA, S., AND N. IKEMOTO. Reaction mechanism of calcium ATPase of sarcoplasmic reticulum. Substrates for phosphorylation reaction and back reaction, and further resolution of phosphorylated intermediates. *J. Biol. Chem.* 255: 3108–3119, 1980.
667. YAMADA, S., M. SUMIDA, AND Y. TONOMURA. Reaction mechanism of the Ca^{2+}-dependent ATPase of sarcoplasmic reticulum from skeletal muscle. VIII. Molecular mechanism of the conversion of osmotic energy to chemical energy in the sarcoplasmic reticulum. *J. Biochem. Tokyo* 72: 1537–1548, 1972.
668. YAMADA, S., AND Y. TONOMURA. Phosphorylation of the Ca^{2+}-Mg^{2+}-dependent ATPase of the sarcoplasmic reticulum coupled with cation translocation. *J. Biochem. Tokyo* 71: 1101–1104, 1972.
669. YAMADA, S., AND Y. TONOMURA. Reaction mechanism of the Ca^{2+}-dependent ATPase of sarcoplasmic reticulum from skeletal muscle. VII. Recognition and release of Ca^{2+} ions. *J. Biochem. Tokyo* 72: 417–425, 1972.
670. YAMADA, S., T. YAMAMOTO, T. KANAZAWA, AND Y. TONOMURA. Reaction mechanism of the Ca^{2+}-dependent ATPase of sarcoplasmic reticulum from skeletal muscle. VI. Co-operative transition of ATPase activity during the initial phase. *J. Biochem. Tokyo* 70: 279–291, 1971.
671. YAMADA, S., T. YAMAMOTO, AND Y. TONOMURA. Reaction mechanism of the Ca^{2+}-dependent ATPase of sarcoplasmic reticulum from skeletal muscle. III. Ca^{2+}-uptake and ATP-splitting. *J. Biochem. Tokyo* 67: 789–794, 1970.
672. YAMAMOTO, T., H. TAKISAWA, AND Y. TONOMURA. Reaction mechanisms for ATP hydrolysis and synthesis in the sarcoplasmic reticulum. *Curr. Top. Bioenerg.* 9: 179–236, 1979.
673. YAMAMOTO, T., AND Y. TONOMURA. Reaction mechanism of the Ca^{2+}-dependent ATPase of sarcoplasmic reticulum from skeletal muscle. I. Kinetic studies. *J. Biochem. Tokyo* 62: 558–575, 1967.
674. YAMAMOTO, T., AND Y. TONOMURA. Reaction mechanism of the Ca^{2+}-dependent ATPase of sarcoplasmic reticulum from skeletal muscle. II. Intermediate formation of phosphoryl protein. *J. Biochem. Tokyo* 64: 137–145, 1968.
675. YAMAMOTO, T., AND Y. TONOMURA. Chemical modification of the Ca^{2+}-dependent ATPase of sarcoplasmic reticulum from skeletal muscle. II. Use of 2,4,6-trinitrobenzenesulfonate to show functional movements of the ATPase molecule. *J. Biochem. Tokyo* 79: 693–707, 1976.
676. YAMAMOTO, T., AND Y. TONOMURA. Chemical modification of the Ca^{2+}-dependent ATPase of sarcoplasmic reticulum from skeletal muscle. III. Changes in the distribution of exposed lysine residues among subfragments with change in enzymatic state. *J. Biochem. Tokyo* 82: 653–660, 1977.
677. YATES, D. W., AND V. C. DUANCE. The binding of nucleotides and bivalent cations to the calcium and magnesium ion dependent adenosine triphosphatase from rabbit muscle sarcoplasmic reticulum. *Biochem. J.* 159: 719–728, 1976.
678. YOSHIDA, H., AND Y. TONOMURA. Chemical modification of the Ca^{2+}-dependent ATPase of sarcoplasmic reticulum from skeletal muscle. I. Binding of N-ethylmaleimide to sarcoplasmic reticulum: evidence for sulfhydryl groups in the activity site of ATPase and for conformational changes induced by adenosine tri- and diphosphate. *J. Biochem. Tokyo* 79: 649–654, 1976.
679. YU, B. P., E. J. MASORO, AND H. A. BERTRAND. The functioning of histidine residues of sarcoplasmic reticulum in Ca^{2+} transport and related activities. *Biochemistry* 13: 5083–5087, 1974.
680. YU, B. P., E. J. MASORO, AND T. F. MORLEY. Analysis of the arrangement of protein components in the sarcoplasmic reticulum of rat skeletal muscle. *J. Biol. Chem.* 251: 2037–2043, 1976.
681. ZEBE, E., AND W. RATHMAYER. Elektronenmikroskopische Untersuchungen an Spinnenmuskeln. *Z. Zellforsch. Mikrosk. Anat.* 92: 377–387, 1968.
682. ZIMNIAK, P., AND E. RACKER. Electrogenicity of Ca^{2+} transport catalyzed by the Ca^{2+}-ATPase from sarcoplasmic reticulum. *J. Biol. Chem.* 253: 4631–4637, 1978.
683. ZUBRZYCKA, E., AND D. H. MACLENNAN. Assembly of the sarcoplasmic reticulum. Biosynthesis of calsequestrin in rat skeletal muscle cell cultures. *J. Biol. Chem.* 251: 7733–7738, 1976.

CHAPTER 16

Physiology of insect flight muscle

RICHARD T. TREGEAR | *Biophysics Unit, Agricultural Research Council Institute of Animal Physiology, Babraham, Cambridge, United Kingdom*

CHAPTER CONTENTS

INSECT FLIGHT MUSCLE has fascinated many people. Each has applied his own discipline to solve the problem it presents and each has, in turn, rephrased the problem in fresh terms to pass it on to another discipline. In the present article I have sought to outline the searches that they undertook, the ideas that they proposed, and the blocks over which they stumbled.

The story started with the aeronautical problem of how motion of an insect's wings enables it to fly. As soon as the requirements for wing motion were established the problem changed to the physiological one of how such motion can be produced by the animal's muscles. This problem naturally subdivides into the provision of the necessary timing, speed, and power of contraction, which are each readily considered relative to their vertebrate skeletal counterparts. The comparative approach encompasses all the flight muscle's properties except for the extremely frequent activation necessary to support the high wingbeat frequency of these small animals.

Pursuit of the cause of insect flight muscle activation has led observers through a veritable dance of disciplines. Cellular dissection showed that the activation was not a membrane phenomenon but was a direct mechanical effect on the contractile machinery. The mechanical response of the dissected muscle fiber to applied strains was therefore minutely examined and expressed in terms of the behavior of model components. The models were at first empirical but were later applied to the steps of the actomyosin reaction sequence, as these emerged from the study of the isolated vertebrate proteins.

These ideas are attractive, but they cannot be fully tested unless they are directly related to the muscle structure. The searches of protein chemists have revealed a series of novel proteins in the insect flight muscle, and immunological localization has indicated the possible involvement of some of them in the activation mechanism. The activated system, the filamentous actin and myosin of the muscle, is organized in a particular way in the insect flight muscle and has also been examined for clues indicating its mechanism of activation. X-ray diffraction of the filament architecture does indicate a possible matching mechanism, whereas electron microscopy of the myosin cross bridges shows that actin selection is strongly developed.

At several places along the structural search for the basis of flight muscle activation the observations have uncovered clues to other problems. Some of the novel proteins discovered in the flight muscle may be involved in the apparatus of motile cells, the thick-filament architecture of the muscle appears to be a special case of a general form of myosin filament assembly, and the cross-bridge interaction seen in rigor flight muscle may represent the end state of the normal active cross-bridge stroke. Because it is relatively easy to visualize cross bridges, the cross-bridge mechanism has been comprehensively studied in insect flight muscle and is the subject of the final section of this chapter.

DESIGN PARAMETERS

Contraction Timing

The flight of an insect poses a particular aerodynamic problem. For a wing to generate lift, it must produce vortices in the adjacent air. To do so it must move through the air at greater than a critical velocity: the smaller the wing, the greater is this velocity (86, 119). Insect wings are small and move only a short distance in each wingbeat, so they must move many times a second to exceed the critical velocity demanded by aerodynamic theory. Flight has been experimentally analyzed in the locust and shown to follow normal aerodynamic principles (54). Steady-state theory accounts for most of the observed lift (134), but the rapid accelerations inherent in insect flight may also produce part of the lift (32, 143).

The solution of the aerodynamic problem raises a physiological one. The wingbeat frequency of smaller insects exceeds 100 s^{-1} and is sometimes as high as 1,000 s^{-1} (112); therefore flight muscles must contract at the right phase within a repeat period of less than 10 ms. In terms of the conventional calcium-activation system this requires an exactly timed nerve impulse followed by a release of calcium to the myofibril and regain from it, all completed within a few milliseconds. Such requirements are met elsewhere in the animal kingdom, for example, in the antennal nerve of the lobster where an astonishing network of reticulum surrounds narrow myofibrils (100). The conditions for rapid cyclic calcium activation are met in the flight muscle of many of the larger insects with a wingbeat of lower frequency, such as the locust, and a few of the smaller insects (144). In these insects electrical recording shows a nerve impulse for each muscle contraction (86) and electron microscopy reveals a sheath of sarcoplasmic reticulum around narrow myofibrils (111). In most of the small insects with rapid wingbeats and some of the larger ones with slower wingbeats, the picture is entirely different. The motor nerve impulses are usually much less frequent than the muscle contractions and occur at a random phase relative to contraction (86), whereas the sarcoplasmic reticulum is much reduced and does not enclose the broad myofibrils (8, 111).

The two types of muscle are quite distinct, and an intensive search of Hemiptera has not revealed structural intermediates (33). They are variously dichotomized as asynchronous or synchronous, fibrillar or nonfibrillar, myogenic or neurogenic, and oscillatory or nonoscillatory. As far as is known, these divisions are all equivalent. The terms are all unsatisfactory: asynchronous muscle is synchronous to stretch activation, nonfibrillar muscle contains small myofibrils, myogenic muscle requires nerve activity to work, and nonoscillatory muscles will oscillate under experimental conditions! The asynchronous/synchronous dichotomy is used here.

The detailed skeletal anatomy of insects allows an exact description of their phylogeny, so it is possible to pinpoint the evolution of the specialized asynchronous muscle from the general, synchronous type. The groups in which asynchronous muscles occur separate before the evolution of asynchrony; distinct synchronous ancestral lines may be distinguished for the several asynchronous families. This has been worked out in particular detail for the Hemiptera (Fig. 1). Asynchronous muscle has evolved many times, and the similarity of form and function in the various asynchronous muscles is an example of convergent evolution. Asynchronous muscle appears to be evolutionarily stable, once attained, because it is present in many large insects whose low wingbeat frequencies do not demand it (33, 89).

Contraction Extent and Speed

The contraction of the flight muscle of a small insect must be complete within a few milliseconds for the animal to fly. Mammalian skeletal muscle commonly contracts efficiently when shortening at less than 1%/ms (31). Thus insect flight muscle must either be able to contract efficiently much faster than mammalian muscles or shorten over only a small fraction of its length. The contraction velocity of insect flight muscle, where studied, has not proved very fast (19), so this does not seem to be a major adaptive factor. The second factor certainly is: in bees, flies, and locusts the shortening during normal flight is only 1%, 3%, and 5%, respectively (16, 134). These are functional limits; experimentally both synchronous and asynchronous muscles can be made to shorten more than they do in life (135, 149).

Since the muscle shortens only a small amount, no great length of free thick or thin filament is required for its function. Synchronous muscle has a short but distinguishable I band (135), whereas asynchronous muscle has filaments that overlap almost completely (8). All synchronous and some asynchronous muscles studied can be extended to give lesser overlap of the filaments (18, 39), so this is also a functionally rather than a structurally enforced state. However, some asynchronous muscles disrupt on extension, even when relaxed, as if the functional state had become a structural necessity.

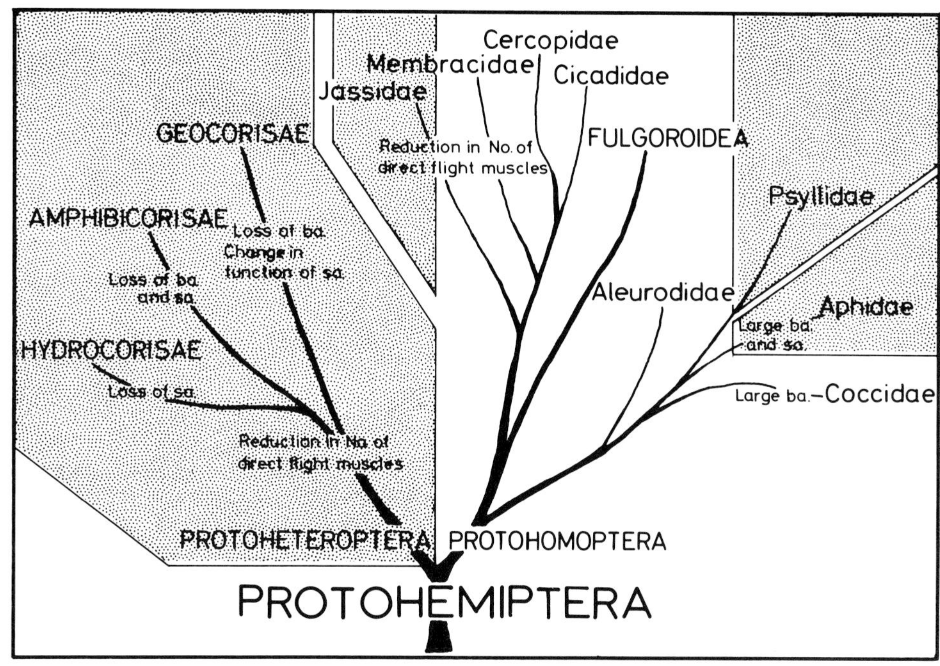

FIG. 1. Schematic representation of evolutionary distribution of asynchronous flight muscles (*shaded areas*) within the order Hemiptera. Note that Aphidae and Psyllidae probably separated before asynchrony evolved and that fibrillar muscle also appears in the sound-producing mechanism of certain Cicadidae. [Adapted from Cullen (33).]

Energy Storage

Insect flight uses a lot of energy; it is a major metabolic load to the animal and thus must be as efficient as possible. The wingbeat is an oscillatory motion of the system formed by the combination of wing, thorax, and muscle action (Fig. 2*A*). To maintain efficiency such a system must contain minimal damping; the elastic components should be as perfect as possible. Some of the energy is stored in specialized cuticle formed of resilin (a remarkably perfect rubber), some in the hard cuticle of the thorax (55), and the remainder in the muscle itself. Since the working stroke of the muscle is very short, the elasticity in parallel with the active contractile system must be high. Thus relaxed flight muscle, whether synchronous or asynchronous, has an elasticity not much less than its activated value and greatly in excess of that of relaxed vertebrate striated muscle (6, 65, 135).

The combination of an inertial wing with combined elasticity constitutes a resonant system (Fig. 2*A*) that must be driven at a frequency close to that of resonance for efficient operation. The wingbeat frequency is therefore not a free variable for an insect. It is neurogenically controlled in insects with synchronous muscles (99) but is a structural characteristic of those with asynchronous muscle, shown by the way the frequency rises when the wings are clipped (36).

The mechanical resonance condition determines that the actomyosin kinetics of the muscle must be matched in speed to the optimal frequency of the wingbeat for the system to operate efficiently. This can only occur at one temperature, since the biochemical reactions involved have high temperature coefficients, whereas the mechanical elasticities do not (5, 67). Many insects fly at a constant intrathoracic temperature of around 40°C (48), and most warm up their muscles to the desired temperature before taking off (49).

Energy Transduction

The power produced in flight is high; the power-weight ratio of an insect flight muscle exceeds that of most other muscles (83). It can only be efficiently fueled by aerobic respiration, and the aerobic system is hypertrophied in all insect flight muscles. The muscle cells are sometimes 1 mm or more wide (123), but this does not represent an aqueous diffusion barrier for oxygen because the air-filled tracheae penetrate deep into the fibers (98).

The mitochondria in which the oxygen is metabolized are different shapes and form different arrangements in the various orders of insects (110, 111). They constitute a large part of cell volume and protein mass (133), and their adenosine triphosphate (ATP) output determines the permitted continuous energy usage by the tissue. The ATP produced by the mitochondria diffuses into the myofibrils. No diffusional limitation is expected in this process because the myofibril can be crossed by a large flux at the cost of a drop in concentration of a few millimoles per liter provided that the diffusivity is maintained close to that of water; some of the most active muscles have the widest

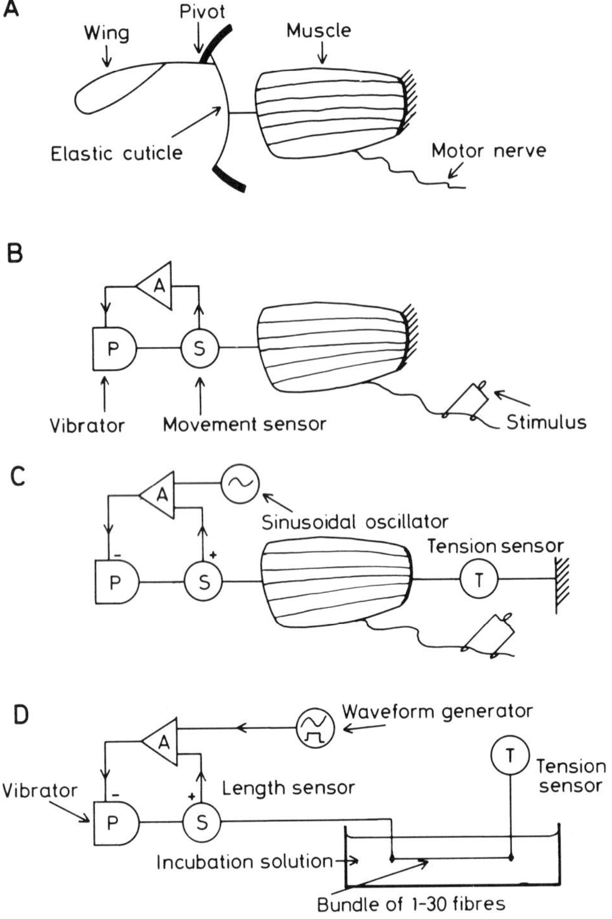

FIG. 2. Methods of investigating mechanism of asynchronous muscle. *A*: operation in vivo: muscle pulls rhythmically on the thorax elastic cuticle and the distortion moves the wings up and down (87). *B*: same muscle detached from the thorax and attached to position sensor (S) that drives the vibrator (P) to resist motion in the muscle. By adjustment of the amplifier (A) characteristics the mechanical system can simulate any desired elasticity, viscosity, and inertia. Motor nerve to muscle is stimulated electrically, and when artificial viscosity is low the system vibrates in "free oscillation" (65). *C*: same muscle during driven oscillation. Position drive from S to P is adjusted to strongly resist any movement unless a further electrical signal is injected into P, when the fixed point of the system changes. Sinusoidal oscillation applied to amplifier (A) therefore imposes a sinusoidal length change on the muscle independent of the tension within it (66). *D*: demembranated muscle in an apparatus similar to that shown in *C*. [Adapted from Tregear (124).]

myofibrils (33). In all muscles ATP is finally hydrolyzed to produce mechanical energy at the myosin ATPase site on the thick filaments of the myofibril, which are present along the entire length of each filament except for the bare zone in the center (122). The myosin concentration is very high in insect flight muscle (71).

The net result of the large energy throughput is a large internal heat flux, in addition to the mechanical energy expended in flight (83). This allows a large temperature drop between the thorax and the air surrounding it and hence the maintenance of a constant high intrathoracic temperature during flight as well as rapid heating during preflight maneuvers; temperature rises of up to 8°C/min have been recorded (49).

Interactions Between Factors

The factors affecting the function of insect flight muscle interact in the design of the tissue, sometimes in the same and sometimes in opposing directions. Where factors act in the same direction the resultant specialization usually appears complete; where they act in opposition the structure may be considered in balance between the opposing conditions.

Several factors converge to promote near-complete overlap between the thick and thin filaments in the flight muscle. First, the muscle only contracts by a small fraction of its length, so a long I band is not needed. Second, high elasticity demands that there be no weak link along the tension-bearing chain of the relaxed muscle; this can most obviously be arranged by the provision of a structure in series with either the thick or the thin filaments. Third, such a structure provides a basis on which strain of the filaments can activate asynchronous muscle. Fourth, volumetric economy for power production favors total overlap of the myosin heads with their activator, actin.

Optimizing energy transfer through the tissue implies a balance of mitochondria versus myofibrillar mass and may exclude the use of the high-frequency calcium-activation specialization, since this demands that a large volume fraction of the muscle be sarcoplasmic reticulum. Economy may account for the retention of the asynchronous mode, once evolved, in relatively large insects. Maximizing power may also be the reason for the high myosin concentration within the myofibrils.

The enzyme kinetics of the myosin ATPase sites are defined by the contraction velocity, which is itself determined by the overall flight system's resonant frequency and amplitude. This means that a certain temperature of operation must be chosen. The large power output of the system predicates that the temperature chosen should be high to allow both heat dissipation and the rapid operation of all the enzyme systems involved. The myosin kinetics are further restricted in asynchronous muscle by the separate condition that the muscle be activated at the right timing to match the system's resonance.

FLIGHT MUSCLE PREPARATIONS

To analyze a general situation it is desirable to choose a particular preparation and work on it intensively. The properties of vertebrate skeletal muscle have been studied most in intact frog sartorius and semitendinosus fibers and in demembranated rabbit psoas fibers. In the insect the chosen preparations have been the dorsal longitudinal muscles of the locust, the basalar muscle of the rhinoceros beetle *Oryctes*, and the dorsal longitudinal muscle of the tropical waterbug *Lethocerus*; the first two have been studied intact, the last when demembranated.

Intact Muscles

Insect flight muscle is permeated by the tracheae, so it is impossible to separate out fibers without impairing their oxygen supply. Therefore measurements have been made on the intact muscle in situ, perfused with gaseous oxygen via the tracheae. Painstaking work was needed to establish good preparations: Weis-Fogh and his associates became known for their work on the locust (134), Pringle and his group for their work on the rhinoceros beetle (66).

Buchthal and Weis-Fogh (18) found that the relaxed locust muscle could be only slightly extended before it began to resist strongly. Empty sarcolemma tubes could bear only a very small force, so they concluded that the passive elasticity was mainly due to the muscle and not its sheath.

Stimulation of locust flight muscle yielded a short twitch contraction. The duration of twitch was originally found to be too long to account for efficient flight (19), but careful repetition of the experiments showed that at the thoracic temperature of 40°C the twitch was over in 25 ms, within the wing's stroke time (84). A frequency of stimulation in excess of 40 s^{-1} was needed to obtain appreciable tetanic tension, and there was no staircase effect (84). During shortening at an optimal velocity, much of the work was performed on an external load rather than on an internal load (19), so the system is efficient if correctly loaded. There is no indication of any contractile peculiarity in locust flight muscle (135), a normal muscle contracting a short distance in a short time at frequent intervals.

Machin and Pringle (65) found that relaxed *Oryctes* muscle was also resistant to extension. As in locust muscle, activation had only a slight effect on the tension-length curve. They examined the mechanical properties of the muscle by sinusoidal analysis, a method in which the muscle is forcibly vibrated and the amplitude and phase of the resultant tension is recorded (Fig. 2*C*). They found that the elasticity of the relaxed muscle contained a small viscous component. Neither elasticity nor viscosity was much affected by a temperature variation in the range of 15°–43°C (67).

Oryctes flight muscle did not produce a twitch on nerve stimulation. In contrast to the results on locust muscle, repetitive nerve stimulation produced a pronounced staircase effect and a smooth tetanic contraction, maximal by a stimulation frequency of 40 Hz (65). These properties are consistent with maintenance of a near-constant free-calcium level during the interval between stimuli.

Forced vibration of the tetanized muscle exposed its mode of operation. At a certain vibration frequency the muscle behaved as if it contained a negative viscosity (66). In other words the tension rose in the time after the muscle was extended, so that at an appropriate vibration frequency the muscle was exerting greater tension during shortening than during extension. The process is best exemplified by an experiment in which the muscle was not forcibly vibrated (as described above) but was instead connected to an electronically adjusted resonant load close to the resonance of the natural system (Fig. 2*B*). On tetanic excitation the muscle built up an internally powered vibration, driving energy into each cycle of oscillation by pulling back harder than it was pulled out.

The response to a forced vibration (Fig. 2*C*) showed that positive work was only produced within a wave band of oscillation frequency. The optimal frequency for work production at the thoracic temperature was close to its wingbeat frequency (67). Below the operating wave band the preparation appeared almost totally elastic; above it showed a normal viscosity (66). Such a performance is not readily explained in terms of a mechanical model and hence is very intriguing.

Demembranated Muscle

Demembranation of muscle is a powerful technique; it allows alteration at will of the internal constituents of the muscle fiber. Vertebrate fibers have been demembranated mechanically (mechanical skinning), by surfactant (chemical skinning), or by osmotic shock (glycerol extraction). Only glycerol extraction has been employed on asynchronous insect flight muscle fibers, because in the tropical waterbug *Lethocerus* there is the additional requirement that the demembranated muscle last through periods of storage. *Lethocerus* has proved impossible to breed in captivity (34) and is difficult to maintain alive in the laboratory. High concentrations of glycerol that freeze only at very low temperatures can be used to preserve the muscle after its removal from the animal. Routinely such muscle has been held at −20°C in 50% glycerol and can be used for several weeks or even months, although there is some evidence of gradual deterioration. Storage in higher concentrations of glycerol at lower temperatures may provide a more permanent preparation (30).

Demembranated *Lethocerus* flight muscle fibers are easy to handle. They have little connective tissue between them and so can be cleanly separated, whereas the low level of their activation by calcium alone reduces the tendency of one part of the muscle to contract relative to another when activated. Single-fiber preparations are usually employed, because this reduces the problems of fiber attachment and ATP starvation.

Demembranated *Lethocerus* flight muscle fibers behave differently from their vertebrate striated counterparts. In the absence of calcium they relax but remain elastic, like intact flight muscle. Addition of calcium only partially activates the muscle; even at high calcium concentrations the tension produced is low. For the muscle to be fully activated it must vibrate as in life (90). If the muscle is connected to a resonant load in which optimal frequency of vibration is similar to that of the wingbeat and is given an adequate supply of ATP and calcium, it goes into spontaneous and maintained oscillation (56) like the intact beetle muscle. Again, forced motion of the muscle allows analysis of its properties. Two methods have been employed: *1*) oscillation of the muscle by a particular amplitude and at a range of frequencies or *2*) rapid extension of the muscle by a fixed amount and observation of the consequent time course of tension change (Fig. 2*D*). These two methods are formally equivalent. Both show that the demembranated muscle fiber will perform work at a range of oscillation frequency similar to that of the wingbeat in life.

Glycerol storage disrupts *Lethocerus* muscle fiber membrane systems without causing their loss (10). Poisoning of the mitochondria with oligomycin or sodium azide and further disruption of the membrane systems with detergent do not affect the work done by the muscle (3), so neither sarcoplasmic reticulum nor mitochondria are needed for the system's operation. Split fibers will also do work, so the lateral organization of the fiber is not essential either (121). The capacity for vibrational work therefore appears to be a property of the individual myofibrils.

OSCILLATORY RESPONSE OF ASYNCHRONOUS MUSCLE

Full Mechanical Performance

It proved difficult to achieve the full flight performance of *Lethocerus* muscle in the isolated preparation. Eventually maximal work was obtained from the preparation when it was forcibly vibrated at an amplitude of 4%–8% (90), which is comparable to the amplitude achieved by other asynchronous flight muscles in flight. Under this strain the isolated muscle produced up to 8 J/liter of work in each cycle of vibration, measured from the area of the tension-length loop produced. Since there are some 0.2 mM myosin enzymatic sites in the muscle (71), the work delivered represented 40 kJ/mol enzymatic site, almost all of the energy available from ATP hydrolysis if each site worked once in each vibration. Therefore probably most of the myosin in the preparation is in working order and capable of synchronized activation.

The ATP hydrolyzed by muscle fibers can be measured by their release of phosphate or adenosine diphosphate (ADP), provided that the incubating volume is kept small and a sensitive assay for the product is used (64, 91, 103, 108). The methodology of these assays has been improved over the years and has culminated in a direct continuous assay that responds in approximately 10 s to a change in the rate of ATP hydrolysis (63). Even this is too slow to follow the time course of tension generation in vibration or after a sudden change in length, so that only average values of ATP hydrolysis rate can be obtained. By vibrating the muscle at different frequencies, Steiger and Rüegg (118) showed that when the muscle produced work the ATP hydrolysis rate increased greatly (Fig. 3*A*). At its best the preparation is quite efficient: values of 12 kJ work done per mole ATP hydrolyzed have been recorded (91); note the distinction between work per ATP hydrolyzed cited here and work per enzymatic site cited in the previous paragraph. This is equivalent to an efficiency of approximately 30%.

Flight is therefore reasonably well simulated by the demembranated preparation, because a large fraction of the muscle is activated by a mechanical disturbance similar to that of flight and reacts by efficiently driving energy into the simulated flight mechanism.

Specification of the Mechanical Response

The reason for work production in asynchronous insect flight muscle is that on stretch the muscle generates greater tension after a delay. If this delay matches the time between extension and shortening of the muscle—for a vibration, half the period of the oscillation—then the muscle will do work (Fig. 4*A*, *B*). This statement is independent of the mechanism proposed; in general terms the question "how does the insect muscle do work in flight?" can be translated into "how does the flight muscle generate delayed tension after being stretched?"

STIFFNESS AND TENSION. There are two obvious alternative effects that might generate tension: either more myosin might attach to actin or attached myosin might change state (rotate) to create more tension (109, 137). The demonstration by Ford, Huxley, and Simmons (37, 52) that in frog muscle the number of attached cross bridges can be measured by the instantaneous change in tension when a rapid length change is applied has been used to settle the question. If the cross bridge rotated, the stiffness, as defined by the response to a rapid length change, would not be expected to alter as the tension rose, whereas if more cross bridges attached it would become greater. Initially it appeared that stiffness did not rise (109), but later observations showed that it did and that unless the length change generating the delayed tension was very large it rose linearly with the tension (50, 101, 137). Thus the delayed tension apparently is due primarily to recruitment of additional cross bridges rather than to their rotation.

Although the stiffness is linearly related to tension in these experiments, the extrapolated line to zero tension does not pass through the origin; White et al. (140) have shown that the stiffness predicted at zero tension is the same as the stiffness of the relaxed muscle (Fig. 3*B*). This result also occurs in the synchronous dragonfly muscle, whereas in rabbit psoas muscle the two variables are truly proportional to one

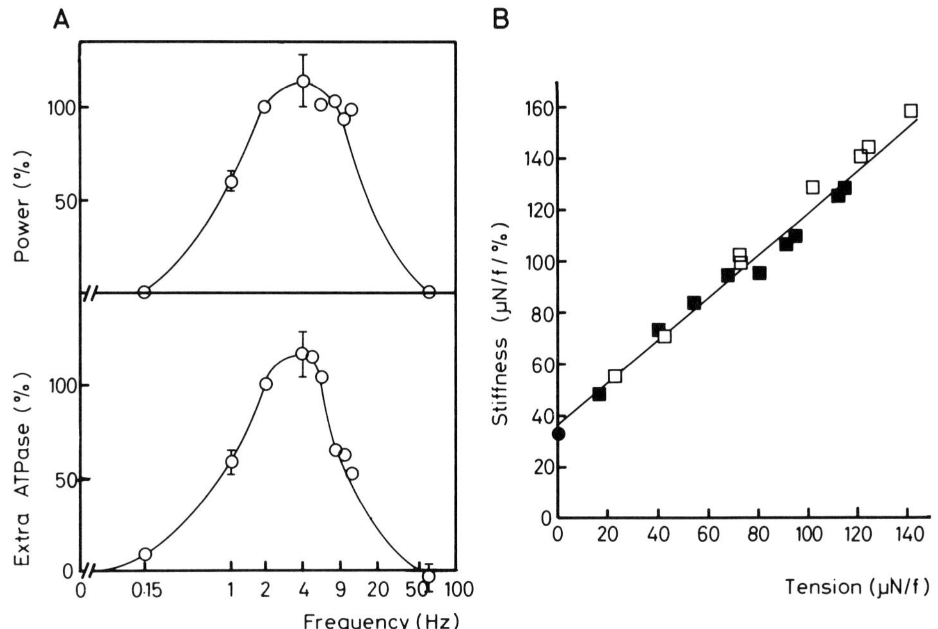

FIG. 3. *A*: relation between power output and ATPase in a bundle of demembranated oscillating *Lethocerus* flight muscle fibers. Effect of varying frequency of applied vibration is shown. *B*: linear relation between stiffness and tension during development of activation in isometric demembranated *Lethocerus* fibers. Activation by calcium (■) or stretch (□). Relation between stiffness and tension extrapolates close to stiffness of muscle in relaxation (●). Stiffness was measured from tension change occurring during application of rapid change in length. [*A*, adapted from Steiger and Rüegg (118). *B*, adapted from White et al. (140).]

another. They therefore deduced that the structure producing the relaxed stiffness of both forms of insect flight muscle is still operative in activity. It appears functionally desirable to retain on activation the relaxed stiffness of synchronous muscle, otherwise energy would be lost in each vibration.

EMPIRICAL DESCRIPTION OF THE RATE PROCESS. The rate at which tension equilibrates after stretch is the factor determining optimal vibration frequency for a muscle. To estimate the rate the results must be put into a formal framework. One method is to reduce the amplitude of the test vibration until the response obtained is linear, i.e., of amplitude proportional to the vibration amplitude and of phase invariant with amplitude.

Jewell and Rüegg (56), in their pioneer observations, obtained linear mechanical responses of the muscle to vibration amplitudes less than 0.1% and established the frequency response of the muscle at this low range of amplitude. Abbott (1) made more detailed observations of the same sort and extracted a single major exponential delay from the data. By independent variation of the length and calcium concentration he showed that the rate constant of the exponential delay rose sharply with calcium concentration but that it did not vary with extension of the muscle at a given calcium concentration.

Other observers have studied the small-signal response of *Lethocerus* flight muscle and found that, in addition to calcium, the concentration of substrate and products of the reaction affect it. Adenosine triphosphate raises the optimal frequency (138); ADP reduces it (4). The effect of phosphate is undecided; it either raises the optimal frequency (91) or does not affect it (138). The temperature coefficient of the rate constant of the delayed tension, which is the equivalent of this optimal frequency, is also high (117).

The idea of a single rate constant for the rise of delayed tension is extremely attractive because it suggests that the process generating the tension might be simple. Before proceeding to analysis based on this idea, however, it must be noted that recent observations have cast doubt on its experimental basis. Cuminetti and Rossmanith (35) found that in the absence of phosphate there were considerable harmonic components in response to a 0.1% vibration, particularly at and close to the optimal vibration frequency (Fig. 5*A*). They sought conditions under which the harmonics were reduced and found that at very low amplitudes (0.02%–0.04%) the response was indeed linear because the fundamental amplitude was proportional to vibration amplitude and its harmonics were negligible (Fig. 5*A*). In this truly linear range the fundamental response to frequency was very different from the response observed at higher amplitudes both by Cuminetti and Rossmanith and by previous workers (Fig. 5*B*, *C*). Its variation in phase and amplitude with frequency was much greater and occurred over a shorter frequency range than at the higher amplitude.

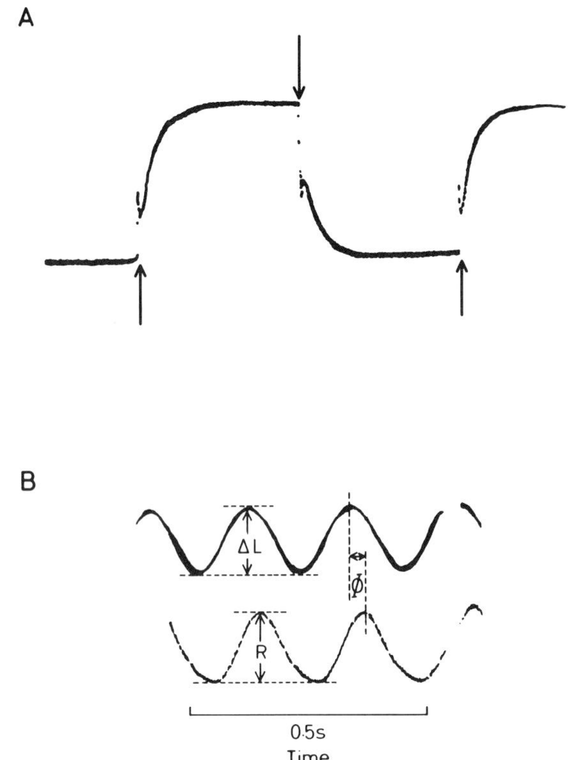

FIG. 4. Form of *Lethocerus* flight muscle mechanical response. *A*: tension response to abrupt stretch and release by 0.1% of muscle length. Note near-exponential rise and fall of delayed tension after stretch and release. *B*: tension response (*lower record*) to a forced sinusoidal vibration of muscle (*upper record*). Response is specified by its gain ($G_o = R/\Delta L$) and phase (ϕ). At this frequency (5 Hz) muscle tension lagged behind length (L); thus ϕ was negative and work was done by muscle on apparatus. [Adapted from Tregear (124).]

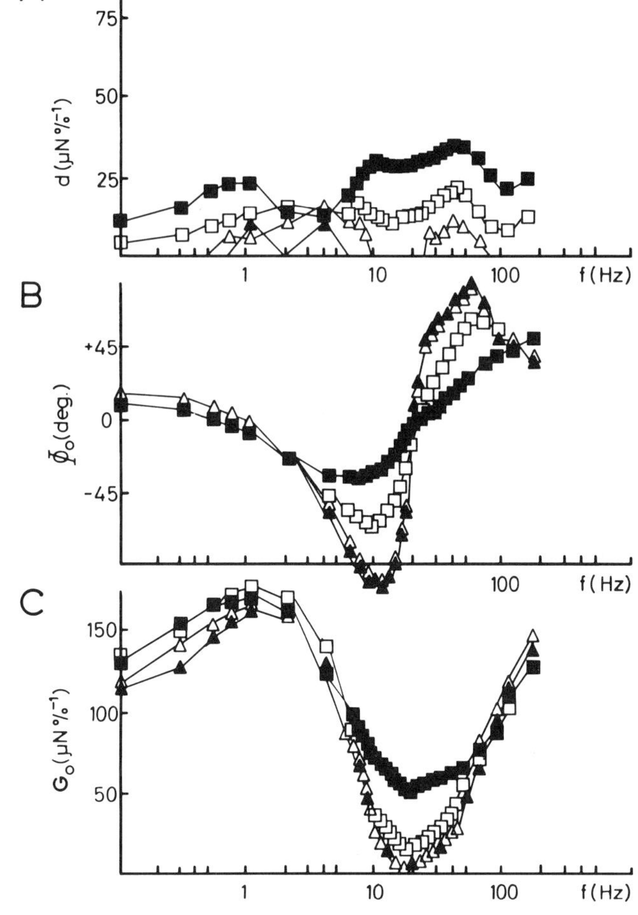

FIG. 5. Search for linearity in mechanical response. Response of single *Lethocerus* flight muscle fiber to vibration of amplitude 0.02% (▲), 0.04% (△), 0.8% (□), or 0.14% (■). In these experiments the various Fourier components of mechanical response were separated. *A*: total distortion ($d = \sum_{i=1}^{n} G_i$); summated gain of all except fundamental component. *B*: phase angle of fundamental component. *C*: gain of fundamental component (G_o). All data are plotted against frequency of forced vibration. Note low values of *A* and constancy of *B* and *C* with amplitude at lowest values of this parameter, indicating linearity of muscle response. [Adapted from Cuminetti and Rossmanith (35).]

At the center of this frequency range the response was almost null, as if the active element had canceled the passive elasticity (Fig. 5*C*).

These results indicate that the elementary process may be complex, and the apparently simple first-order response seen at higher vibration amplitudes may be a summation of a set of the more complex elementary processes. If so, the following analysis, which was devised before Cuminetti and Rossmanith's results, will have to be revised.

Simulation of the Mechanical Response

MODELING THE FIRST-ORDER PROCESS. Thorson and White (120) showed that two states of the cross bridge, attached to and detached from actin, were enough to explain the first-order delayed tension rise, provided that the rate constant of actomyosin attachment rose with muscle extension (Fig. 6*A*). In this model the rate constant of the delayed tension rise is equal to the sum of the attachment and detachment rate constants. Since the mechanical rate constant is invariant with muscle extension, it is necessary to assume that the variable rate constant (of attachment) is a lot less than the other. Thus on this model the attachment rate determines overall cycling rate, whereas the detachment rate determines the optimal frequency of oscillation (120).

Thorson and White's model is testable. In an isometric muscle it predicts that the ratio of ATP hydrolysis rate to mean tension (tension cost) should be proportional to the mechanical rate constant; both are proportional to the detachment rate constant of the cross bridges. The critical data have been slow to acquire because the technique is difficult. Schädler (108) showed that tension and ATPase rose in parallel as calcium was added to insect flight (or other) muscles; this was prima facie evidence against the hypothesis, because the mechanical rate constant rose sharply with calcium (1). Loxdale (64) improved the ATPase

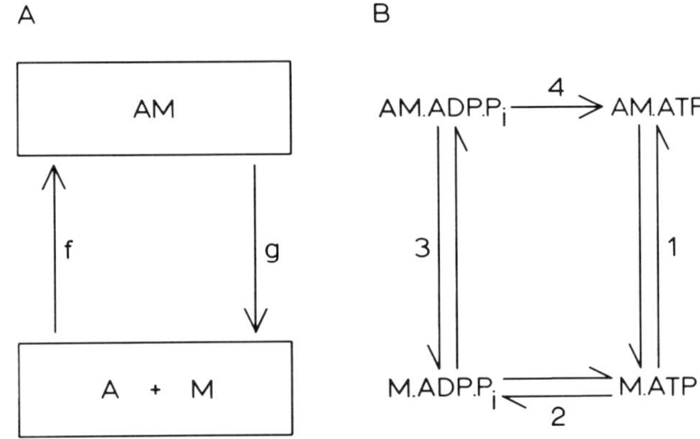

FIG. 6. Cross-bridge models of mechanical response. A, actin; M, myosin; AM, actomyosin. *A*: 2-state model. Attachment rate constant (f) is assumed to be proportional to muscle extension and detachment rate constant (g) to be independent of extension. Rate constant of delayed tension, $r = f + g$, and tension cost, $c \propto g$. *B*: 4-state model. Reactions 1 and 3 are rapid equilibria; reaction 4 is relatively slow and irreversible. [*A*, adapted from Thorson and White (120). *B*, adapted from Steiger and Abbott (117).]

assay so that accurate measurements could be made on static preparations, and he established definitely that the tension cost does not rise with calcium concentration; if anything, it falls. The two-state hypothesis is therefore wrong; there must be other states involved.

Steiger and Abbott (117) have pointed out that these results can be simulated by separation of the cross bridges into two groups, each in equilibrium between attachment and detachment, and connected by an irreversible step (Fig. 6*B*). If one of the equilibria is speeded up without change in its equilibrium constant, the mechanical rate constant can be raised without changing the tension cost.

MODELING THE FULL MECHANICAL PERFORMANCE. White and Thorson (138) remeasured the response of the muscle to large-amplitude step functions in length. They found large nonlinearities when phosphate was absent, which they termed *phosphate-starvation transients*, that had contributed largely to previous observations (90). Discounting the phosphate-starvation transients, which should be absent in the phosphate-containing live muscle, they were able to account for many observations in terms of cross-bridge distortion and its distribution along the strained array of cross bridges within the sarcomere (138). To explain the phosphate-starvation transients they invoked a further attached state (139).

Rüegg and his collaborators (109) showed that a rapid stretch of high amplitude induced an isometric oscillation in which frequency parallels that of the optimal vibration frequency for work production. Linear models, even when elaborated by the factors mentioned above, do not predict such oscillation (117).

With this exception, it appears probable that cross-bridge models can, in principle, account for the flight performance of the muscle. They do not, however, indicate what causes cross-bridge activation. For this one must examine the muscle structure.

MYOFIBRILLAR PROTEINS

Asynchronous insect flight muscle contains all the major proteins of a striated muscle and a large number of other components as well. The search for further myofibrillar protein components has been motivated by the physiologist's desire to find the critical factor in producing delayed tension, but actual progress has been achieved by the painstaking work of protein chemists. The field has been illuminated by the work of Bullard and her collaborators, who have successfully detected, isolated, and localized many myofibrillar proteins (Table 1). Some proteins contribute to the Z line, others to the A or I filaments, whereas at least one appears to lie in the short A-Z gap. The results of this work are most simply considered structure by structure.

Proteins of the Thick Filament

Insect myosin has a molecular weight similar to that of rabbit myosin and has the same complement of heavy and light chains. The light chains have a different molecular weight from the rabbit ones, at least as judged by sodium dodecyl sulfate–polyacrylamide gel electrophoresis (SDS-PAGE); the heaviest has a molecular weight of 30,000 (22).

TABLE 1. *Myofibrillar Proteins of Lethocerus Flight Muscle*

Location and Name	Peptide MW on SDS-PAGE*	Comment	Ref.
Thick filament			
Myosin	200,000 30,000 15,000	Phosphorylated; calcium sensitive	22, 62, 142
Paramyosin	105,000	Readily proteolyzed	21–24
Thin filament			
Actin	42,000	Normal properties	22
Arthrin	55,000	Similar to actin except for MW	20
Tropomyosin	35,000	Normal properties	22
Troponin	18,000 27,000	Apparently normal C and I components, T not identified	22
Z line			
α-Actinin	95,000	Normal properties	27, 41, 46
Zeelin	35,000 25,000	Found in vertebrates	25, 27, 106
C region			
"Connecting protein"	180,000	Only found in asynchronous muscle (to date)	21, 23
Overall			
Connectin	Cross linked	Small content	75

* MW, molecular weight; SDS-PAGE, sodium dodecyl sulfate–polyacrylamide gel electrophoresis.

In general the enzymatic properties appeared qualitatively similar to those of rabbit smooth muscle myosin. Early work indicated a low degree of calcium activation for crude insect actomyosin (132), and a more elaborate trial showed that this low activation was restricted to asynchronous flight muscle; both locust flight and *Lethocerus* leg muscle showed a much higher degree of activation by calcium than did *Lethocerus* flight muscle myosin (78), as if the asynchronous myosin was intrinsically less activable by calcium.

Later work showed that this conclusion may not be valid. Synthetic actomyosin made with *Lethocerus* myosin required tropomyosin for activity; when troponin was added its regulation was as strong, and its activity as great, as that of rabbit myosin (22). This myosin preparation, made by protein precipitation, was only calcium sensitive when the thin filaments contained troponin and tropomyosin. A later preparation, made without precipitation of the protein, was controlled by calcium even when pure actin was used as the cofactor (62). Thus *Lethocerus* flight myosin, like other invertebrate myosins, is directly controlled by calcium. The calcium control requires that the regulatory light chains with a molecular weight of 30,000 of the myosin be phosphorylated (142).

Taken together these observations show that native, phosphorylated *Lethocerus* flight myosin probably has a much greater calcium sensitivity than did the early preparations, so that the low calcium activation of the glycerol-extracted muscle fibers (103) could well be due to the organization of the myosin in the sarcomere rather than to the properties of the individual molecules of myosin.

Paramyosin has been isolated from many invertebrate muscles (141) and in particular from asynchronous flight muscle of four different insect species (24). In *Lethocerus* flight muscle there is about one-eighth as much paramyosin as myosin (24). *Lethocerus* paramyosin, like its myosin, is readily degraded in preparation; unless ethylenediaminetetraacetic acid is employed the molecule is slightly shortened and its solubility altered (21). Insect paramyosin is structurally similar to other paramyosins: it is highly α-helical and forms two-chain rods that aggregate into regular tactoids of 15-nm or 75-nm periodicity (22). In mollusks, paramyosin fills the core of the thick filaments, but in some insects the mass available is insufficient for this (21). Even when sufficient paramyosin is available, as in *Lethocerus*, antibodies to insect paramyosin bind only at the center of the myofibril. Myosin extraction did not extend this staining (21), and antibody binding to the ends of the filaments proved to be due to an impurity (23). The area of exposable paramyosin thus appeared to be limited to the center of the thick filaments, although its mass is too great to fit within this volume. The location appears to exclude it as a candidate for the cause of stretch activation.

No other components of the thick filaments have been isolated, although M-line proteins certainly must exist because the structures are highly developed.

Proteins of the Thin Filament

Lethocerus actin is of the same molecular weight as rabbit actin, polymerizes into the normal two-stranded filaments, and activates both rabbit and insect myosin in a similar manner (22). It has no known abnormalities. It is, however, accompanied by a protein with a molecular weight of 55,000 named arthrin, initially confused with tubulin. Arthrin's characteristics are those of a heavy actin: it also polymerizes into two-stranded filaments and activates myosin (20). Arthrin is a major component, making up approximately 25% of the total actin in the muscle. Its function is unknown.

Thin-filament regulation occurs in both synchronous and asynchronous insect flight muscles (62). When troponin is extracted from *Lethocerus* muscle in alkali, the muscle is permanently activated (79). Both tropomyosin and troponin have been isolated from asynchronous flight muscles (22). Tropomyosin reactivated the insect actomyosin system as if it exposed the actin to reaction with the myosin, whereas troponin restored calcium sensitivity and produced additional density along the thin filaments at 40-nm intervals (22). Two components of insect troponin have been identified as C (calcium binding), with a molecular weight of 18,000, and I (inhibitory), with a molecular weight of 27,000 (22); the T component has not yet been established. The system appears similar to that of vertebrate striated muscle.

The two insect regulatory systems together produce an extremely powerful regulation; at low calcium concentrations locust actomyosin is switched off as in life (62).

Z-Line Proteins

α-Actinin is a constituent of asynchronous flight muscle (46). On purification it appears very similar in solubility, amino acid composition, and molecular weight (95,000) to the vertebrate protein (41). Antibody reaction to the highly purified protein is restricted to the Z line, and in separated I-Z-I brushes, which are assemblies of thin filaments attached to Z disks, α-actinin extraction removes many of the I filaments (41). α-Actinin is a major component of the isolated Z disk (27).

Z disks can be isolated intact, but with attached filament stubs, by solution of asynchronous myofibrils in acid (105) or high salt (27). The isolated disks contain a large number of proteins, some of which are filamentous contaminants, but in addition to α-actinin two have been shown to be specific to the Z line (106). The heavier of these two, a peptide with a molecular weight of 35,000 called zeelin, was initially confused with tropomyosin (27) but on isolation proved to be a separate proline-rich peptide. Antibody to this protein bound to vertebrate Z lines as well as the insect ones, so it is a general Z-line component (25). The lighter protein, with a molecular weight of 25,000, is also proline rich. On digestion of these proteins with calcium-activated protease, the isolated Z disks disintegrate, so the proteins are probably integral to the Z-line structure.

Again there is no obvious difference between the proteins of Z lines from asynchronous flight muscle and those of other muscles, although detailed study of Z lines from synchronous flight muscle has not yet been possible since the Z lines do not separate out in the same way.

Connecting Proteins

There is a long-standing hypothesis of mechanical connection between the thick filaments and the Z lines of fibrillar muscle; paramyosin was once considered as the connecting protein. Recently a new candidate has been detected. This protein, or group of proteins, known at present simply as "connecting protein," was found as a contaminant in *Lethocerus* paramyosin (21, 23). Absorption of the antibody to impure paramyosin on purified paramyosin left an antibody that specifically bound to the short region between the thick filaments and the Z line (21). In honeybee muscle (but not *Lethocerus*) this region could be extended without breaking the thin filaments off the Z line, and when this was done the antibody binding also extended (21). Dissolving away myosin from the myofibrils did not expose more antigenic sites, so the connecting protein apparently does not continue along the thick filaments (21, 23). In muscle extracts, the antibody binds to a peptide with a molecular weight of 180,000 (not myosin), the present candidate for the connecting protein. It has not yet been isolated and other peptides may be involved.

Connecting protein must be distinguished from connectin, a highly insoluble protein found by Maruyama et al. (76, 77) in the residue after exhaustive extraction of myofibrils from vertebrate and invertebrate muscles. It could be solubilized in SDS but did not enter SDS-PAGE. It is believed to form an elastic net around myofibrils and to provide the elasticity that prevents their easy extension above the nonoverlap length. Small amounts of connectin are present in asynchronous flight muscle but are unlikely to be responsible for the stiffness of the relaxed muscle, because the stiffness is abolished on dissolving myosin from the tissue, whereas the connectin remains (75).

MACROMOLECULAR ASSEMBLY

All insect flight muscles are cross striated. There are three thin filaments to each thick filament in the array, arranged so that each thin filament has thick filament on either side (Fig. 7*A*). In asynchronous

A

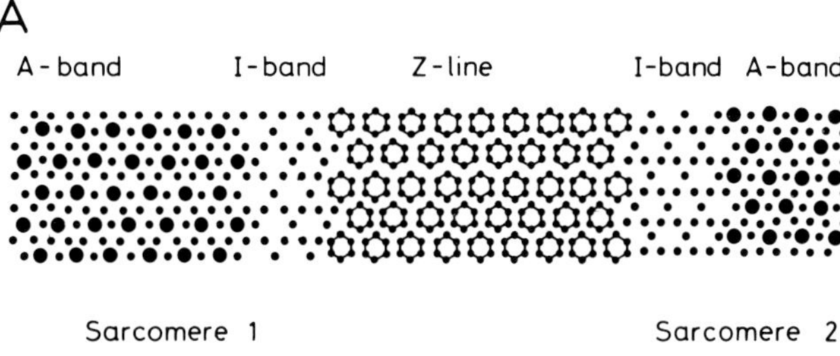

B

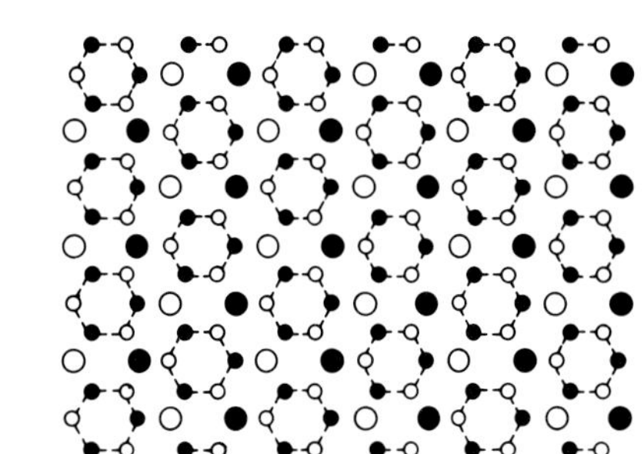

FIG. 7. Diagrams illustrating interdigitation of filament lattices of adjacent sarcomeres within Z line. *A*: interdigitation of I filaments. *B*: superimposition of complete filament lattices of 2 sarcomeres. *Open circles* represent filaments from 1 sarcomere, *closed circles* from the next. *Smaller circles* represent I filaments, whose formation of hexagonal groups within Z line is indicated. *Larger circles* represent A filaments, whose relative position in their hypothetical extension into the Z line is thus illustrated. [Adapted from Ashhurst (12).]

flight muscle this array reaches a crystalline regularity that is evident both in transverse sections of the tissue and X-ray–diffraction patterns from it. The axial regularity of the fibrillar sarcomere is also great. The thin filaments are connected to each other by a precise Z-line structure and the thick filaments by a precise M-line structure. The overlap of the two filament sets is almost complete.

The structure of the flight muscle sarcomere has intrigued electron microscopists and X-ray diffractionists alike. Three features revealed by their work are of special interest in relation to theories of the oscillatory mechanism: the thick filament's connection to the Z line, the pattern of the myosin heads on the thick-filament surface, and the pattern of attachment of the myosin heads to the thin filaments. Technically the three subjects are quite distinct: the first is an exercise in electron microscopy, the second in X-ray diffraction, and the third in the marriage of the two techniques.

Thick-Filament Connections

The structure of the Z line of asynchronous insect flight muscle is different from that of the vertebrate. The actin filaments from each side of the Z line enter it, without gross deviation, in the hexagonal lattice formed by their overlap with the thick filaments. These two hexagonal lattices overlap by interdigitation (Fig. 7*A*). The interdigitated double array creates smaller, shared hexagons (9). Adjacent actin filaments within these hexagons come from opposed sarcomeres; optical analysis of isolated Z disks shows that the hexagons are deformed so that pairs of opposed actin are closer together with links between them (107). The gaps between these hexagons are the positions occupied by the thick filaments (Fig. 7*B*). There is thus no direct continuity of either thick or thin filaments across the Z line (11).

There is evidence that the Z line is directly connected to the thick filaments in asynchronous muscle. First, when a muscle was stretched in rigor (or in many cases even when relaxed), causing the thin filaments to break away from the Z line and leaving a clear area, this region was crossed by thin filaments that could be traced from the ends of the thick filaments through into the Z line (139). Second, when fresh bee muscle was stretched reversibly so that the thin filaments did not break away from the Z line and a clear area formed between thick and thin filaments rather than between thick filaments and Z line, connecting filaments again crossed the clear area from the tips of the thick ones (40). Thus under these unphysiological conditions it is clear that connecting filaments do occur. Evidence for their occurrence in unstretched or mildly stretched muscle is equivocal. Longitudinal sections have frequently shown an apparent connection between thick filament and Z line (129), but Ashhurst (12) has pointed out how easily such images arise due to superposition of thin and thick filaments within the section. Counting filaments in cross sections indicated the presence of connections (104, 131), but the irregularity of the array makes their significance uncertain.

In sum, connecting filaments may be present all the time but may only form an extension as from orientation of a gel (88). They connect the thick filament and Z line but cannot directly interconnect thick filaments on opposite sides of the Z line because these are not in line.

Thick-Filament Structure

Many of the layer lines of X-ray–diffraction patterns from a relaxed muscle come from the helical array of myosin heads (detached cross bridges) on the surface of the thick filaments. The axial spacing of these layer lines is the pitch of this surface helix (p) divided by the number of helical tracks on the surface (n); n must be determined independently for the pitch to be known. The myosin heads protrude from the filament at 14-nm axial intervals (exactly 14.5 nm; all spacings are given here to the nearest nm) so n also defines the filament mass, since provided the surface array is unitary there are n myosin molecules per 14-nm length of the filament, excluding the central smooth zone. Measurements of the filament mass taken in conjunction with the X-ray–diffraction pattern therefore define the surface geometry of the thick filament.

The X-ray–diffraction pattern of relaxed *Lethocerus* flight muscle gave a 38-nm layer line and other layer lines that were at 38-nm spacing from the 14-nm meridional reflection (81); the latter, being part of a regularity derived from the surface protrusion of the heads each 14 nm along the filament, proved that the 38-nm periodicity comes from the thick-filament surface array as well (113).

The mass of the thick filaments has been a matter of much measurement and debate. Measurements of myofibrillar extracts on SDS-PAGE showed a very high mass ratio of myosin heavy chain to actin (26, 127) and hence a value of $n = 5$–5.5 for the number of myosin molecules per 14-nm interval. Quantitative light and electron microscopy gave $n = 6$ (94). A value of 6 was hence adopted for several years, but recent measurements of single thick filaments on the scanning transmission electron microscope have favored $n = 4$ (97); the presence of arthrin would also lower values of n deduced from SDS-PAGE densitometry.

The surface lattice of myosin heads arises from the internal order of the tails within the filament. Transverse electron micrographs show that the center of invertebrate thick filaments contains a protein that stains less than the surface does, so general models have been devised in which the myosin tails pack as an annulus around a hypothetical core protein. Squire (114) proposed a model in which the tails were packed individually at a nearly uniform density within the annulus. Wray (145) detected further layer lines in patterns from various arthropod muscles, which he attributed to regularity within the annulus. He devised a model containing groups of tails (subfilaments) within the annulus. The numerical relation between the axial spacing of the myosin head helices and the subfilament helices showed that there were three subfilaments to each head strand, whereas the equatorial spacing of the subfilament reflection gave its diameter as 4 nm. For *Lethocerus* flight muscle the filament diameter is 20 nm, so there should be about 12 subfilaments around its periphery and four helical tracks of myosin heads on the surface (145). This deduction agrees with the evidence from the scanning transmission electron microscope.

It is therefore probable that the surface lattice of the *Lethocerus* flight muscle thick filament is a four-start helix of pitch 152 nm and that there are four myosin molecules protruding from the filament at 14-nm intervals along it (Fig. 9*B*), although results from interference microscopy are incompatible with this view.

Cross-Bridge Interaction

Rigor is a state of maximum cross-bridge formation. It can be produced in glycerol-extracted muscle by withdrawing the substrate, ATP; tension rises and the muscle becomes stiff (136). *Lethocerus* flight muscle in rigor develops a particularly regular array of cross bridges that has been described in detail by Reedy and his collaborators (93, 95, 96). The cross bridges formed in groups at 38-nm intervals along each thin filament, spanning the gap between the thin filament and the two adjacent thick filaments (Fig. 8*A*). The internal structure of the groups was very exact. They angled across the interfilament gap both axially and azimuthally (93). Each group was split into two, and the azimuthal forms of the two groups were distinct [Fig. 8*A*; (95)].

X-ray diffraction from *Lethocerus* flight muscle in rigor showed an intense series of layer lines produced by this cross-bridge interaction. They were caused by the regularity of form of the individual myosin head's interaction with the actin monomers (81). Analysis showed that these heads must be grouped at each half turn of the two-start actin helix to account for the reflections near the meridian of the diagram (51). The pitch of the actin helix is 76 nm, so that these model groups correspond to Reedy's observations of groups at 38-nm intervals. Similar X-ray–diffraction patterns have been obtained and analyzed from other arthropod muscles (68, 82, 147).

X-ray diffraction of relaxed crab muscle indicated that arthropod troponin was located at 38-nm intervals along the thin filaments (69) and could be the cause of the grouping of myosin attachments (68). X-ray–diffraction patterns from vertebrate-striated muscle, however, also indicated a grouping of the attached cross bridges at the half-pitch of the actin helix, 36 nm, rather than the 38-nm repeat of the troponin (115). Therefore the grouping is probably caused by the twist of the actin in vertebrate muscle and, by inference, also in insect flight muscle.

Model building indicates that at most half of the total orientations of the actin monomers toward the thick filament are available for attachment (113). If the cross bridges are also assumed to have considerable axial range of search, then the splitting of the 38-nm groups is achieved, since some of the cross bridges reach up and some down the filament toward the available actin region [Fig. 8*B*; (47)].

It has generally been assumed that the two heads of a single myosin molecule attach to adjacent actin monomers on a thin filament. Offer and Elliott (85) have challenged this assumption and supposed that the two heads spread out to attach to adjacent actin filaments (Fig. 8*C*). The idea is presently being tested (17, 38, 128); if it is correct the geometrical constraints for attachment are tighter and the number of cross bridges formed less than previously assumed.

A

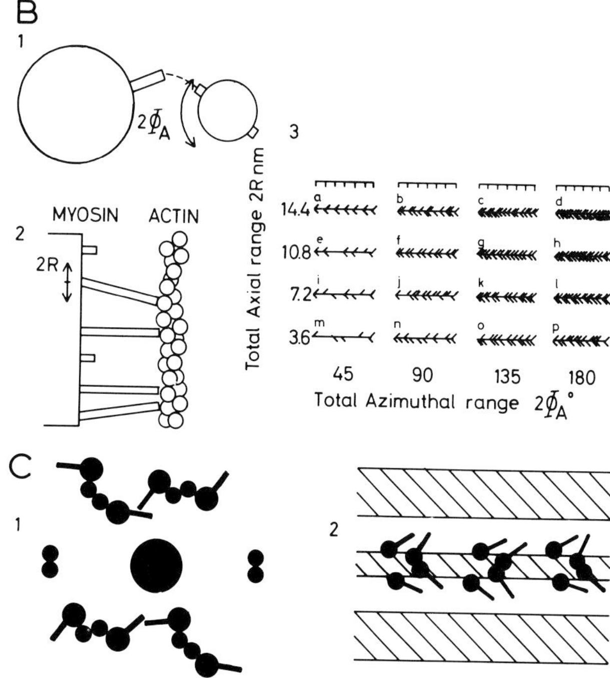

FIG. 8. Pattern of cross-bridge attachment to thin filaments of *Lethocerus* flight muscle in rigor (absence of nucleotide). *A*: thin longitudinal section of overlap zone through a plane connecting thin and thick filaments (cf. Fig. 7). Note angled chevrons crossing interfilament gap at 38-nm intervals. Many of these chevrons appear double. (Original micrograph supplied by Dr. M. K. Reedy.) *B*: explanation of double-chevron formation by restriction of rotation and axial range of the cross bridges. *1*, Subunit azimuthal orientation of actin (ϕ_A) defined relative to interfilament axis; *2*, axial displacement of cross bridge (R) at its contact with actin; *3*, cross-bridge attachment arrays for different degrees of rotational and axial freedom (cases *b* and *f* resemble Reedy's observations). *C*: explanation of double-chevron formation by attachment of the 2 heads of 1 myosin molecule to adjacent thin filaments. *1*, Angles of actin helix at which 2-filament attachment is expected; *2*, resultant longitudinal cross-bridge array. [*B*, adapted from Haselgrove and Reedy (47). *C*, adapted from Offer and Elliott (85).]

CAUSE OF STRETCH ACTIVATION

The oscillatory response of asynchronous insect flight muscle is due to the phenomenon of stretch activation, by which the muscle tension rises gradually after it is stretched. For the evidence that this process represents an increase in the speed of attachment of the myosin-product complex to actin see *Specification of the Mechanical Response*, p. 492. The question is, what could cause such a change?

Calcium Binding

Stretch could cause an increase in the amount of calcium bound, either by troponin or by the calcium-sensitive myosin itself. Early results (28) showed such an increase, but a repeat of the experiments showed no change in calcium binding on muscle extension (73). Furthermore flight muscle could still be activated by stretch in very high calcium concentrations (103), and calcium affected the rate constant of the delayed tension, whereas extension did not (1). It is therefore unlikely that stretch activates asynchronous muscle by increasing the amount of calcium bound to the regulatory proteins.

Filament Match

A second possible change is that stretching the muscle brings the myosin heads closer to the optimal actin monomers for attachment. In the asynchronous *Lethocerus* flight muscle, but not in the synchronous dragonfly flight muscle, the helices of the myosin head origins on the thick-filament surface and the actin monomers on the thin filament are integrally related; both are multiples of 38 nm (81). Wray (146) further pointed out that if the myosin filament had four tracks of myosin heads then extension of the muscle would alter the distance between cross bridge and preferred actin, with a cyclic effect every 38 nm, or 3.2% of extension (Fig. 9). Abbott and Cage (2) found evidence of such a cyclic effect; the mechanical response to small-amplitude vibration waxed and waned with a spatial period of approximately 3% as the muscle was extended. Filament match on stretch therefore probably occurs, but its functional significance remains uncertain.

Filament Strain

Stretch activation is shown by many muscles. In particular, vertebrate striated (102) and vertebrate heart (116) muscle preparations have both been induced to produce good delayed tension and to do work in forced vibration. These muscles have incommensurate actin and myosin helices and therefore cannot operate by filament match.

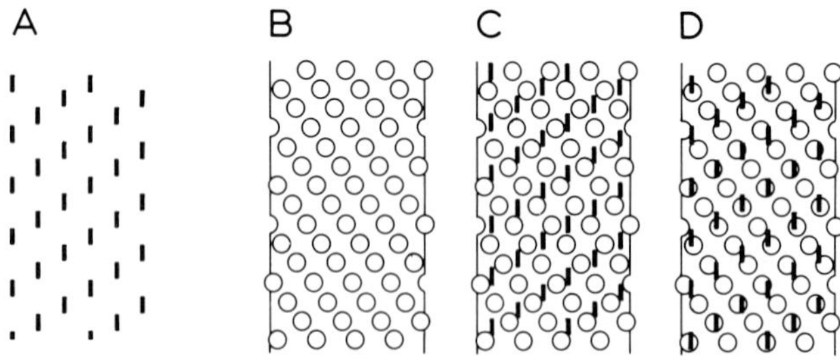

FIG. 9. Diagram illustrating possible filament match in *Lethocerus* flight muscle. All diagrams are radial projections centered on axis of a single thick filament. *A*: actin envelope about 1 thick filament. Each thin filament is represented by vertical *double line*, and *solid bars* represent regions of thin filaments accessible to cross-bridge attachment. *B*: lattice of cross-bridge origins on thick-filament surface. Each circle represents a single myosin molecule, bearing 2 potential cross bridges. *C*, *D*: extreme mismatch and match positions of arrays shown in *A* and *B*. The 2 diagrams differ only in vertical shift of *A* vs. *B*. [Adapted from Wray (146).]

High stress appears to promote stretch activation. Vertebrate heart and striated fibers required high calcium activation to show it, whereas insect flight muscle needed to be stretched above a critical stress to produce a large response (90).

Lethocerus flight muscle can be stretch activated by extension before calcium is added (29, 90). Provided that the stress produced by such extension is carried by the connecting protein and not by hypothetical long-lived cross bridges [which would have to have very unusual properties (87)], it follows that the critical strain is in the insect thick filaments rather than the cross bridges or thin filaments. The strain on the thick filaments is small; X-ray–diffraction patterns of stretched *Lethocerus* flight muscle showed that the 14-nm spacing was unchanged within limits of 0.4% (7).

Stress-induced strain, possibly of different types in separate phyla, seems the most likely cause of stretch activation.

Evolution of Stretch Activation

Although delayed tension after stretch is a general characteristic of striated muscle preparations, it is well developed in only a few of them. Delayed tension may promote the timing or raise the amplitude of the vertebrate heartbeat (88), but its only certain function is that of asynchronous activation in insect flight.

Aidley and White (6) discovered pronounced asynchronous properties in fibers from a synchronously activated timbal muscle in a cicada; both the relaxed stiffness of the muscle and the delayed tension response to stretch were large. They proposed that stretch activation combined with a mechanical switch (click) mechanism promotes the speed of response and hence is advantageous before the loss of synchrony. Thus a quantitative evolution of asynchrony could occur and may account for its independent appearance in different insect groups (33). Quantitative evolution of filament strain is easy to imagine, but filament match would have to be precise to ensure that averaging effects along the sarcomere did not negate its effectiveness (146). Comparative study of closely related synchronous and asynchronous muscles is a possible way of deciding between the two proposed mechanisms (89).

CROSS-BRIDGE MECHANISM

Study of stretch activation led workers to use the *Lethocerus* flight muscle preparation to study the general mechanism of force generation in muscle. The preparation's principal advantages are that it retains structural order when activated by calcium because it has little tendency for one sarcomere to shorten and pull out another and that in rigorlike states the cross bridges form regular arrays that can be studied. Its disadvantages are that the high stiffness of the relaxed muscle enforces a large and uncertain subtraction in analyzing the transient mechanical response, and the specialization of the cross-bridge array means that conclusions drawn from structural studies must be verified with studies on other muscles.

Mechanical Transients

Abbott and Steiger (5) were the first to analyze the early changes in tension after a quick stretch of *Lethocerus* muscle. They subdivided their data into exponential components and found that at low temperatures the drop in tension, after the initial rise on stretch and before the delayed tension, required splitting into two components. The fastest of the two components showed no variation in rate with temperature, whereas the second did. Hence they concluded that the two components represented different processes. Neither component's speed changed with the extent and direction of motion in the manner demanded by the theory of Huxley and Simmons (52) of rotating cross bridges. Steiger and Abbott (117) proposed a model to explain these and other observations based on the idea that each enzymatic intermediate of myosin is in a relatively rapid equilibrium of attachment and detachment to actin. The first, temperature-insensitive, phase of tension decay was assigned to a change in the actomyosin ATP/myosin ATP equilibrium, rather than to a head rotation or change between attached states.

Guth and colleagues (45) also measured the response of activated *Lethocerus* muscle to quick stretches, using an apparatus capable of more rapid response. With stretches greater than 0.5% they found an irreversible rapid drop in tension that they interpreted as cross-bridge "slippage" (detachment and reattachment to a different actin). During smaller stretches they found that all the changes were reversible and that there was no change in the slope of the instantaneous tension-length curve after stretch or release. They concluded that the number of attached cross bridges remained constant and that Huxley and Simmons' model held. They also confirmed Abbott and Steiger's finding of two exponential phases but did not analyze them. They later found that the initial tension rise upon stretch was nonlinearly related to stretch amplitude and that the form of the nonlinearity changed when the temperature was raised (61). They attributed this phenomenon to a rapid rotation of the myosin head that reduced the elastic effect of large extensions and fitted these data, plus data on the steady-state parameters, to the model of Huxley and Simmons. Hence they defined the temperature variation of both free and activation energy between hypothetical rapidly equilibrating attached states. Although the interpretations presented by these two groups appear mutually exclusive, this is not necessarily so. An extremely rapid head rotation could be temporally enclosed within a moderately rapid detachment equilibrium.

The study of mechanical transients is at present concentrated particularly on frog muscle, because good skinned frog fiber preparations have now been made (43) and transient X-ray-diffraction observations are being performed on frog muscle (53).

Steady-State Intermediates

POPULATION DISTRIBUTION. If the stiffness of an active muscle is a measure of the number of cross bridges attached (52, 140), then the ratio of tension to stiffness is a measure of the average tension produced by those attached cross bridges. The incremental ratio of tension to stiffness is constant in *Lethocerus* flight muscle when the muscle is activated by calcium or stretch (cf. Fig. 3*B*). There is therefore no indication of relative alteration of hypothetical cross-bridge populations generating different tensions under these conditions.

If this is so, the tension cost, or ratio of ATP hydrolysis rate to tension, is a measure of the average lifetime of the tension-generating cross bridges. It also varies only slightly as the muscle is activated by calcium or stretch (64), as if the lifetimes of steady-state actomyosin intermediates do not change greatly under these conditions. If the substrate itself is changed, this invariance is lost: when Mg^{2+} is excluded, a state of low tension and ATPase but high stiffness is reached, reminiscent of rigor (44). Such cross bridges presumably attach for a long time without generating much tension.

PHOSPHATE EXCHANGE. Phosphate (^{32}P) incorporation into MgATP is speeded up by isometric tension in *Lethocerus* muscle and still more by stretch activation (70, 130). The simplest interpretation of this result is that the enzymatic site allows a more rapid exchange of phosphate into the tight product complex when tension is generated.

CROSS-BRIDGE STRUCTURE. The X-ray-diffraction patterns of calcium- and stretch-activated *Lethocerus* muscle show a reduction in the intensities of the layer lines derived from the thick-filament origins of the myosin heads. The 14-nm meridional intensity drops by up to 40% at the peak of tension generation during vibration, as if at least 20% of the cross bridges had moved away from their origins (Fig. 10*B*). This is accompanied by only a very small change in the inner equatorial intensities (Fig. 10*A*) and little if any increase in actin-based layer lines (Fig. 10*C*). There is thus definite evidence of cross-bridge movement away from the relaxed, detached position but no convincing evidence of attachment in a regular rigorlike form.

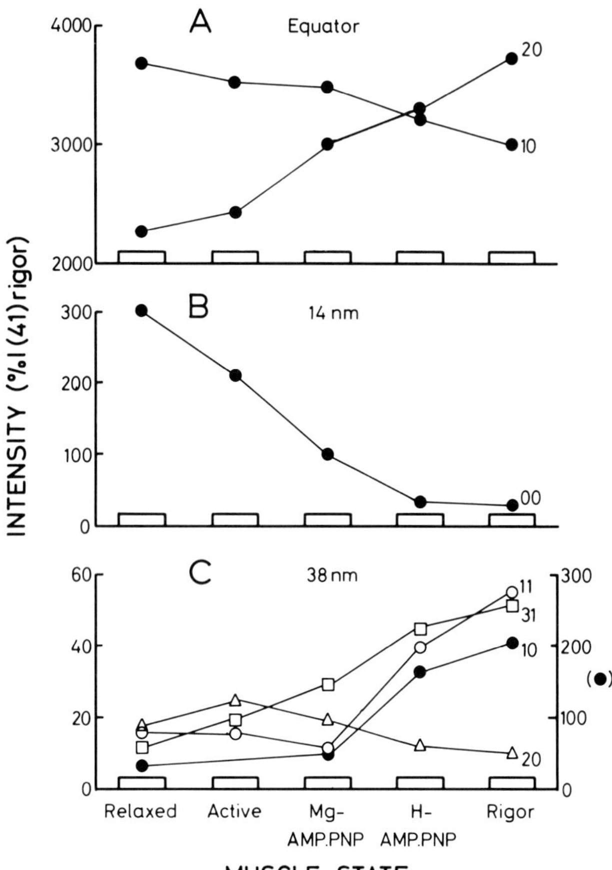

FIG. 10. X-ray diffraction from *Lethocerus* flight muscle in different steady-state or equilibrium conditions. Intensities of various lattice-sampled diffraction reflections are given as percentage of a particular reflection (4, 1 of the equator) in rigor. *A*: 2 major inner equatorial reflections that depend on movement of cross bridges between filaments. *B*: 14-nm meridional reflection that arises from regularity of cross bridges on thick filament. *C*: 38-nm layer-line reflections. Most of the intensity of these reflections arises from regular attachment of cross bridges to thin filaments. The 2, 0 reflection is an exception; it is prohibited from the cross-bridge attachment lattice by phase cancelation (51). [Adapted from Tregear et al. (126).]

Equilibrium States

The standard biochemical approach to a problem is to apply a competitive inhibitor to the reaction. This can be done with muscle; the compound β,γ-imido-ATP, commonly known as AMPPNP, acts in such a way on the enzymatic site of myosin (148). It presumably fits well into the enzymatic site, but the NH group at the β,γ-junction is not hydrolyzed.

Going into rigor from relaxation, *Lethocerus* muscle generated a high isometric tension (136) that it maintained for a long period (59). When AMPPNP was added it bound to the myosin enzymatic site (72), and the isometric tension fell to a lower equilibrium value without loss of muscle stiffness (57, 72). On removal of the inhibitor the tension reverted to its initial value. By allowing the muscle to shorten in rigor and then reextending it in AMPPNP the muscle could be made to do work against the dilution of the nucleotide (57); vice versa extension of the muscle raised its affinity for nucleotide (74) so that extension-shortening cycles could be used to separate nucleotide concentrations (58). The thermodynamic nature of these "teinochemical" relationships has been developed by Kuhn (60).

In rigor the muscle maintained a constant tension over periods much greater than the detachment rate constant of actomyosin in solution (59), indicating an effect of the structure on the rates of intermolecular events.

These mechanical observations are not specific either to AMPPNP or to insect muscle; ADP had a qualitatively similar effect on insect muscle, and AMPPNP a similar effect on rabbit muscle (72, 74).

Since AMPPNP acts as a competitive inhibitor to ATP at myosin's enzymatic site (148), it may reasonably be supposed that its binding favors a protein structure like that when either the productive complex of ATP or its tightly bound products are in place. The mechanical behavior is consistent with this idea: the lower-tension state with AMPPNP bound could represent an earlier enzymatic state than the rigor one (125) and thus provide the necessary coupling between free energy of dilution and mechanical free energy.

Because of the intrinsic interest in such a change, the structural correlates of AMPPNP binding have been investigated in detail. The X-ray-diffraction pattern of *Lethocerus* muscle in rigor showed that the long axes of the cross bridges were bent by ~30° relative to the filament axis (51, 81), and electron microscopy showed that this bend stresses their tails (93). Adding AMPPNP changed the X-ray-diffraction pattern (14). The inner equatorial intensities changed in proportion to the expected binding of AMPPNP (42) as if the centers of gravity of the cross bridges moved away from the thin filaments when the inhibitor bound. The intensities of the actin-based layer lines fell as if the regularity of the cross bridges relative to the actin monomers was reduced without great change in their overall form (13). The 14-nm meridional reflection, characteristic of the myosin head regularity on the thick filament itself, increased. All these effects were greater in MgAMPPNP than in the absence of magnesium (126). Electron microscopy has shown similar changes, from a 38-nm to a 14-nm periodicity, in both insect (72, 92) and crayfish filament arrays (80). Individual cross bridges appeared to lie more directly across the filament axes than they do in rigor (15).

These changes show that in AMPPNP the cross bridges are partially ordered relative to their thick-filament origins as well as to the helix of the actin monomers. Whether the cross bridges that are ordered relative to the thick filament are attached to the actin is uncertain. Cross bridges ordered to the thick filament appear to contact the actin in actively contracting frog muscle (53). If they also do in the AMPPNP-treated *Lethocerus* muscle, their closer fit to the actin when the AMPPNP is removed would provide the tension rise, and hence chemomechanical coupling, in Kuhn's dilution-energy machine.

Both the rigor and AMPPNP equilibrium states are structurally different from active muscle: the cross bridges are closer to the thin filaments, their regular actin attachment is more marked, and their regular thick-filament attachment is less marked than that in active muscle (126). The equilibrium states do, however, belong to a regular sequence of states that may be placed in the order relaxation, activation, Mg-AMPPNP, HAMPPNP, and rigor (Fig. 10) as if all of the conditions, whether steady state or equilibrium, were related. If so, the explanation of chemomechanical coupling proposed in the preceding paragraph may also apply to active contraction.

CONCLUSIONS

Research on this subject has progressed over the last 20 years by accretion and deletion: the adoption of a new outlook or technique, followed by the construction of a theoretical edifice, its demolition by the next innovator, and so on. At present there are few certainties, even on the major points. The form of the elementary mechanical response of asynchronous muscle to stretch is in doubt because of the latest results; hence, naturally, its interpretation may have to be reconsidered. Its cause, for many years thought to be filament strain, has also recently been questioned: the match between filaments may well be a significant factor in stretch activation. The only reasonable candidate for the origin of filament strain still appears to be the connecting protein.

The debates continue; if past experience is any guide, the subject has plenty of delights to offer to the inquiring mind.

I thank Dr. M. K. Reedy for kindly allowing me to reproduce one of his unpublished electron micrographs.

REFERENCES

1. Abbott, R. H. The effects of fibre length and calcium ion concentration on the dynamic response of glycerol-extracted insect fibrillar muscle. *J. Physiol. London* 231: 195–208, 1973.
2. Abbott, R. H., and P. E. Cage. Periodicity in insect flight muscle stretch activation. *J. Physiol. London* 289: 32P–33P, 1979.
3. Abbott, R. H., and R. A. Chaplain. Preparation and properties of the contractile element of insect fibrillar muscle. *J. Cell Sci.* 1: 311–330, 1966.
4. Abbott, R. H., and H. G. Mannherz. Activation by ADP and the correlation between tension and ATPase activity in insect fibrillar muscle. *Pfluegers Arch.* 321: 223–232, 1970.
5. Abbott, R. H., and G. J. Steiger. Temperature and amplitude dependence of tension transients in glycerinated skeletal and insect fibrillar muscle. *J. Physiol. London* 266: 13–42, 1977.
6. Aidley, D. J., and D. C. S. White. Mechanical properties of glycerinated fibres from the tymbal muscles of a Brazilian cicada. *J. Physiol. London* 205: 179–192, 1969.
7. Armitage, P. M., R. T. Tregear, and A. Miller. Effect of activation by calcium on the X-ray diffraction pattern from insect flight muscle. *J. Mol. Biol.* 92: 39–53, 1975.
8. Ashhurst, D. E. The fibrillar flight muscles of giant waterbugs: an electron-microscope study. *J. Cell Sci.* 2: 435–444, 1967.
9. Ashhurst, D. E. Z-line of the flight muscle of belostomatid water bugs. *J. Mol. Biol.* 27: 385–389, 1967.
10. Ashhurst, D. E. The effect of glycerination on the fibrillar flight muscles of Belostomatid waterbugs. *Z. Zellforsch. Mikrosk. Anat.* 93: 36–44, 1969.
11. Ashhurst, D. E. The Z-line in insect flight muscle. *J. Mol. Biol.* 55: 283–285, 1971.
12. Ashhurst, D. E. The Z-line: its structure and evidence for the presence of connecting filaments. In: *Insect Flight Muscle*, edited by R. T. Tregear. Amsterdam: North-Holland, 1977, p. 57–73.
13. Barrington-Leigh, J., R. S. Goody, W. Hofmann, K. Holmes, H. G. Mannherz, G. Rosenbaum, and R. T. Tregear. The interpretation of X-ray diffraction from glycerinated flight muscle fibre bundles: new theoretical and experimental approaches. In: *Insect Flight Muscle*, edited by R. T. Tregear. Amsterdam: North-Holland, 1977, p. 137–146.
14. Barrington-Leigh, J., K. C. Holmes, H. G. Mannherz, G. Rosenbaum, F. Eckstein, and R. Goody. Effects of ATP analogs on the low-angle X-ray diffraction pattern of insect flight muscle. *Cold Spring Harbor Symp. Quant. Biol.* 37: 443–448, 1973.
15. Beinbrech, G. Electron micrography of *Lethocerus* muscle in the presence of nucleotides. In: *Insect Flight Muscle*, edited by R. T. Tregear. Amsterdam: North-Holland, 1977, p. 147–160.
16. Boettiger, E. G. The machinery of insect flight. In: *Recent Advances in Invertebrate Physiology*, edited by B. T. Scheer. Eugene: Univ. of Oregon Press, 1957, p. 117–142.
17. Borejdo, J., and A. Oplatka. Heavy meromyosin cross-links thin filaments in striated muscle myofibrils. *Nature London* 291: 322–323, 1981.
18. Buchthal, F., and T. Weis-Fogh. Contribution of the sarcolemma to the force exerted by resting muscle of insects. *Acta Physiol. Scand.* 35: 345–364, 1956.
19. Buchthal, F., T. Weis-Fogh, and P. Rosenfalck. Twitch contractions of isolated flight muscle of locusts. *Acta Physiol. Scand.* 39: 246–276, 1957.
20. Bullard, B., J. L. Bell, R. Craig, and K. Leonard. An actinlike protein from insect muscle. *J. Muscle Res. Cell Motil.* 1: 194–195, 1980.
21. Bullard, B., J. L. Bell, and B. M. Luke. Immunological investigation of proteins associated with thick filaments of insect flight muscle. In: *Insect Flight Muscle*, edited by R. T. Tregear. Amsterdam: North-Holland, 1977, p. 41–52.
22. Bullard, B., R. Dabrowska, and L. Winkelman. The contractile and regulatory proteins of insect flight muscle. *Biochem. J.* 135: 277–286, 1973.
23. Bullard, B., K. S. Hammond, and B. M. Luke. The site of paramyosin in insect flight muscle and the presence of an unidentified protein between myosin filaments and Z-line. *J. Mol. Biol.* 115: 417–440, 1977.
24. Bullard, B., B. M. Luke, and L. Winkelman. The paramyosin of insect flight muscle. *J. Mol. Biol.* 75: 359–367, 1973.
25. Bullard, B., J. W. S. Pringle, and G. M. Sainsbury. Localization of a new protein in the Z-discs of insect flight and vertebrate striated muscle. *J. Physiol. London* 317: 25P–26P, 1981.
26. Bullard, B., and M. K. Reedy. How many myosins per cross-bridge? II. Flight muscle myosin from the blowfly, *Sarcophaga bullata*. *Cold Spring Harbor Symp. Quant. Biol.* 37: 423–428, 1973.
27. Bullard, B., and G. M. Sainsbury. The proteins in the Z-line of insect flight muscle. *Biochem. J.* 161: 399–403, 1977.
28. Chaplain, R. A. The effect of Ca^{2+} and fibre elongation on the activation of the contractile mechanism of insect fibrillar flight muscle. *Biochim. Biophys. Acta* 131: 385–392, 1967.
29. Chaplain, R. A. Changes of adenosine triphosphatase activity

and tension with fibre elongation in glycerinated insect fibrillar flight muscle. *Pfluegers Arch.* 307: 120–126, 1969.
30. CLARKE, M. L., AND R. T. TREGEAR. Supercooling as a method for storing glycerol-extracted muscle fibres. *J. Physiol. London* 308: 104–105, 1980.
31. CLOSE, R. I. Dynamic properties of mammalian skeletal muscles. *Physiol. Rev.* 52: 129–197, 1972.
32. CLOUPEAU, M., J. F. DEVILLIERS, AND D. DEVEZEAUX. Direct measurements of instantaneous lift in desert locust; comparison with Jensen's experiments on detached wings. *J. Exp. Biol.* 80: 1–15, 1979.
33. CULLEN, M. J. The distribution of asynchronous muscle in insects with particular reference to the Hemiptera: an electron microscope study. *J. Entomol. Ser. A* 49: 17–41, 1974.
34. CULLEN, M. J. The breeding of giant waterbugs in the laboratory. In: *Insect Flight Muscle*, edited by R. T. Tregear. Amsterdam: North-Holland, 1977, p. 357–366.
35. CUMINETTI, R., AND A. ROSSMANITH. Small amplitude nonlinearities in the mechanical response of an asynchronous flight muscle. *J. Muscle Res. Cell Motil.* 1: 345–356, 1980.
36. DANZER, A. The flight mechanism of Diptera considered as a resonant system. *Z. Vgl. Physiol.* 38: 259–283, 1956.
37. FORD, L. E., A. F. HUXLEY, AND R. M. SIMMONS. The relation between stiffness and filament overlap in stimulated frog muscle fibres. *J. Physiol. London* 311: 219–249, 1981.
38. FREUNDLICH, A., P. K. LUTHER, AND J. M. SQUIRE. High-voltage electron microscopy of crossbridge interactions in striated muscle. *J. Muscle Res. Cell Motil.* 1: 321–343, 1980.
39. GARAMVOLGYI, N. The arrangement of myofilaments in insect flight muscle. *J. Ultrastruct. Res.* 13: 409–424, 1965.
40. GARAMVOLGYI, N. The structural basis of the elastic properties in the flight muscle of the bee. *J. Ultrastruct. Res.* 27: 462–471, 1969.
41. GOLL, D. E., M. H. STROMER, R. M. ROBSON, B. M. LUKE, AND K. S. HAMMOND. Extraction, purification, and localization of α-actinin from asynchronous insect flight muscle. In: *Insect Flight Muscle*, edited by R. T. Tregear. Amsterdam: North-Holland, 1977, p. 15–40.
42. GOODY, R. S., J. BARRINGTON-LEIGH, H. G. MANNHERZ, R. T. TREGEAR, AND G. ROSENBAUM. X-ray titration of binding of β,γ-imido-ATP to myosin in insect flight muscle. *Nature London* 262: 613–615, 1976.
43. GRIFFITHS, P. J., K. GUTH, H. J. KUHN, AND J. C. RÜEGG. Cross bridge slippage in skinned frog muscle fibres. *Biophys. Struct. Mech.* 7: 107–124, 1980.
44. GRIFFITHS, P. J., H. J. KUHN, AND J. C. RÜEGG. Activation of the contractile system of insect fibrillar muscle at very low concentrations of Mg^{2+} and Ca^{2+}. *Pfluegers Arch.* 382: 155–163, 1979.
45. GUTH, K., H. J. KUHN, B. DREXLER, W. BERBERICH, AND J. C. RÜEGG. Stiffness and tension during and after sudden length changes of glycerinated single insect fibrillar muscle fibres. *Biophys. Struct. Mech.* 5: 255–276, 1979.
46. HAMMOND, K. S., AND D. E. GOLL. Purification of insect myosin and α-actinin. *Biochem. J.* 151: 189–192, 1975.
47. HASELGROVE, J. C., AND M. K. REEDY. Modeling rigor crossbridge patterns in muscle. I. Initial studies of the rigor lattice of insect flight muscle. *Biophys. J.* 24: 713–728, 1978.
48. HEINRICH, B. Temperature regulation of the sphinx moth. *J. Exp. Biol.* 54: 141–152, 1971.
49. HEINRICH, B., AND G. A. BARTHOLOMEW. An analysis of preflight warm-up in the sphinx moth. *J. Exp. Biol.* 55: 223–239, 1971.
50. HERZIG, J. W. A model of stretch activation based on stiffness measurements in glycerol extracted insect fibrillar muscle. In: *Insect Flight Muscle*, edited by R. T. Tregear. Amsterdam: North-Holland, 1977, p. 209–219.
51. HOLMES, K. C., R. T. TREGEAR, AND J. BARRINGTON-LEIGH. Interpretation of the low angle X-ray diffraction from insect flight muscle in rigor. *Proc. R. Soc. London Ser. B* 207: 13–33, 1980.
52. HUXLEY, A. F., AND R. M. SIMMONS. Proposed mechanism of force generation in muscle. *Nature London* 233: 533–538, 1971.
53. HUXLEY, H. E., R. M. SIMMONS, A. R. FARUQI, M. KRESS, J. BORDAS, AND M. H. J. KOCH. Millisecond time-resolved changes in X-ray reflections from contracting muscle during rapid mechanical transients, recorded using synchrotron radiation. *Proc. Natl. Acad. Sci. USA* 78: 2297–2301, 1981.
54. JENSEN, M. The aerodynamics of locust flight. *Philos. Trans. R. Soc. London Ser. B* 239: 511–552, 1956.
55. JENSEN, M., AND T. WEIS-FOGH. The physics of locust cuticle. *Philos. Trans. R. Soc. London Ser. B* 245: 137–169, 1962.
56. JEWELL, B. R., AND J. C. RÜEGG. Oscillatory contraction of insect fibrillar muscle after glycerol-extraction. *Proc. R. Soc. London Ser. B* 164: 429–459, 1966.
57. KUHN, H. J. Transformation of chemical into mechanical energy by glycerol-extracted fibres of insect flight muscles in the absence of nucleosidetriphosphate-hydrolysis. *Experientia* 29: 1086–1088, 1973.
58. KUHN, H. J. Reversible transformation of mechanical work into chemical free energy by stretch dependent binding of AMP-PNP in glycerinated fibrillar muscle fibres. In: *Insect Flight Muscle*, edited by R. T. Tregear. Amsterdam: North-Holland, 1977, p. 307–315.
59. KUHN, H. J. Cross bridge slippage induced by the ATP analogue AMPPNP and stretch in glycerol-extracted fibrillar muscle fibres. *Biophys. Struct. Mech.* 4: 159–168, 1978.
60. KUHN, H. J. The mechanochemistry of force production in muscle. *J. Muscle Res. Cell Motil.* 2: 7–44, 1981.
61. KUHN, H. J., K. GUTH, B. DREXLER, W. BERBERICH, AND J. C. RÜEGG. Investigation of the temperature dependence of the cross bridge parameters for attachment, force generation and detachment as deduced from mechano-chemical studies in glycerinated single fibres from the dorsal longitudinal muscle of *Lethocerus maximus*. *Biophys. Struct. Mech.* 6: 1–29, 1979.
62. LEHMAN, W., B. BULLARD, AND K. HAMMOND. Calcium-dependent myosin from insect flight muscles. *J. Gen. Physiol.* 63: 553–563, 1974.
63. LOXDALE, H. D. A method for the continuous assay of picomole quantities of ADP released from glycerol-extracted skeletal muscle fibres on MgATP activation. *J. Physiol. London* 260: 4P, 1977.
64. LOXDALE, H. D. Molecular Parameters of Diverse Muscle Systems. Oxford, UK: Univ. of Oxford, 1980. Dissertation.
65. MACHIN, K. E. W., AND J. W. S. PRINGLE. Mechanical properties of a beetle flight muscle. *Proc. R. Soc. London Ser. B* 151: 204–225, 1959.
66. MACHIN, K. E. W., AND J. W. S. PRINGLE. The effect of sinusoidal changes of length on a beetle flight muscle. *Proc. R. Soc. London Ser. B* 152: 311–330, 1960.
67. MACHIN, K. E. W., J. W. S. PRINGLE, AND M. TAMASIGE. The effect of temperature on a beetle muscle. *Proc. R. Soc. London Ser. B* 155: 493–499, 1962.
68. MAEDA, Y. Arrangement of troponin and cross-bridges around the thin filaments in crab leg striated muscle. In: *Cross-Bridge Mechanism in Muscle Contraction*, edited by H. Sugi and G. H. Pollack. Tokyo: Univ. of Tokyo Press, 1979, p. 457–470.
69. MAEDA, Y., I. MATSUBARA, AND N. YAGI. Structural changes in thin filaments of crab striated muscle. *J. Mol. Biol.* 127: 191–201, 1979.
70. MANNHERZ, H. G. On the reversibility of the biochemical reactions of muscular contraction during the absorption of negative work. *FEBS Lett.* 10: 233–236, 1970.
71. MARSTON, S. B. The nucleotide complexes of myosin in glycerol-extracted muscle fibres. *Biochim. Biophys. Acta* 305: 397–412, 1973.
72. MARSTON, S. B., C. D. RODGER, AND R. T. TREGEAR. Changes in muscle crossbridges when β,γ-imido-ATP binds to myosin. *J. Mol. Biol.* 104: 263–276, 1976.
73. MARSTON, S. B., AND R. T. TREGEAR. Calcium binding and the activation of fibrillar insect flight muscle. *Biochim. Biophys. Acta* 347: 311–318, 1974.
74. MARSTON, S. B., R. T. TREGEAR, C. D. RODGER, AND M. L. CLARKE. Coupling between the enzymatic site of myosin and

the mechanical output of muscle. *J. Mol. Biol.* 128: 111–126, 1979.

75. Maruyama, K., P. E. Cage, and J. L. Bell. The role of connectin in elastic properties of insect flight muscle. *Comp. Biochem. Physiol. A* 61: 623–627, 1978.
76. Maruyama, K., S. Matsubara, R. Natori, Y. Nonomura, and S. Kimura. Connectin, an elastic protein of muscle. Characterization and function. *J. Biochem. Tokyo* 82: 317–337, 1977.
77. Maruyama, K., F. Murakami, and K. Ohashi. Connectin, an elastic protein of muscle. Comparative biochemistry *J. Biochem. Tokyo* 82: 339–345, 1977.
78. Maruyama, K., J. W. S. Pringle, and R. T. Tregear. The calcium sensitivity of ATPase activity of myofibrils and actomyosins from insect flight and leg muscles. *Proc. R. Soc. London Ser. B* 169: 229–240, 1968.
79. Meinrenken, W. Calciumionen-unabhangige Kontraktion und ATPase bei glycerinierten Muskelfasern nach alkalischer Extraktion von Troponin. *Pfluegers Arch.* 311: 243–255, 1969.
80. Meisner, D., and G. Beinbrech. Alterations of crossbridge angle induced by β,γ-imido-adenosine-triphosphate. Electron microscope and optical diffraction studies on myofibrillar fragments of abdominal muscles of the crayfish *Orconectes limosus. Eur. J. Cell Biol.* 19: 189–195, 1979.
81. Miller, A., and R. T. Tregear. Structure of insect fibrillar flight muscle in the presence and absence of ATP. *J. Mol. Biol.* 70: 85–104. 1972.
82. Namba, K., K. Watkabayashi, and T. Mitsui. The structure of thin filament of crab striated muscle in the rigor state. In: *Cross-Bridge Mechanism in Muscle Contraction*, edited by H. Sugi and G. H. Pollack. Tokyo: Univ. of Tokyo Press, 1979, p. 445–456.
83. Neville, A. C. Energy and economy in insect flight. *Sci. Prog. London* 54: 203–219, 1965.
84. Neville, A. C., and T. Weis-Fogh. The effect of temperature on locust flight muscle. *J. Exp. Biol.* 40: 111–121, 1963.
85. Offer, G., and A. Elliott. Can a myosin molecule bind to two actin filaments? *Nature London* 271: 325–329, 1978.
86. Pringle, J. W. S. *Insect Flight.* London: Cambridge Univ. Press, 1956.
87. Pringle, J. W. S. The mechanical characteristics of insect fibrillar muscle. In: *Insect Flight Muscle*, edited by R. T. Tregear. Amsterdam: North-Holland, 1977, p. 177–196.
88. Pringle, J. W. S. The Croonian Lecture, 1977. Stretch activation of muscle: function and mechanism. *Proc. R. Soc. London Ser. B* 201: 107–130, 1978.
89. Pringle, J. W. S. The evolution of fibrillar muscle in insects. *J. Exp. Biol.* 94: 1–14, 1981.
90. Pringle, J. W. S., and R. T. Tregear. Mechanical properties of insect fibrillar muscle at large amplitudes of oscillation. *Proc. R. Soc. London Ser. B* 174: 33–50, 1969.
91. Pybus, J., and R. T. Tregear. The relationship of ATP activity to tension and power output of insect flight muscle. *J. Physiol. London* 247: 71–89, 1975.
92. Reedy, M., M. K. Reedy, and R. S. Goody. Crossbridge structure in rigor and AMPPNP states of insect flight muscle. *Biophys. J.* 33: 22a, 1981.
93. Reedy, M. K. Ultrastructure of insect flight muscle. I. Screw sense and structural grouping in the rigor cross-bridge lattice. *J. Mol. Biol.* 31: 155–176, 1968.
94. Reedy, M. K., G. F. Bahr, and D. A. Fischman. How many myosins per cross-bridge? I. Flight muscle myofibrils from the blowfly, *Sarcophaga bullata. Cold Spring Harbor Symp. Quant. Biol.* 37: 397–422, 1973.
95. Reedy, M. K., and W. E. Garrett, Jr. Electron microscope studies of *Lethocerus* flight muscle in rigor. In: *Insect Flight Muscle*, edited by R. T. Tregear. Amsterdam: North-Holland, 1977, p. 115–136.
96. Reedy, M. K., K. C. Holmes, and R. T. Tregear. Induced changes in orientation of the cross-bridges of glycerinated insect flight muscle. *Nature London* 207: 1276–1280, 1965.
97. Reedy, M. K., K. R. Leonard, R. Freeman, and T. Arad. Thick myofilament mass determination by electron scattering measurements with the scanning transmission electron microscope. *J. Muscle Res. Cell Motil.* 2: 45–64, 1981.
98. Reger, J. F., and D. P. Cooper. Wing and leg muscles in a lepidopteran. *J. Cell Biol.* 33: 531–542, 1967.
99. Roeder, K. C. Movements of the thorax and potential changes in the thoracic muscles of insects during flight. *Biol. Bull. Woods Hole, Mass.* 100: 95–106, 1951.
100. Rosenbluth, J. Sarcoplasmic reticulum of an unusually fast-acting crustacean muscle. *J. Cell Biol.* 42: 534–547, 1969.
101. Rüegg, J. C., K. Guth, H. J. Kuhn, J. W. Herzig, P. J. Griffiths, and T. Yamamoto. Muscle stiffness in relation to tension development of skinned striated muscle fibres. In: *Cross-Bridge Mechanism in Muscle Contraction*, edited by H. Sugi and G. H. Pollack. Tokyo: Univ. of Tokyo Press, 1979, p. 125–143.
102. Rüegg, J. C., G. J. Steiger, and M. Schadler. Mechanical activation of the contractile system in skeletal muscle. *Pfluegers Arch.* 319: 139–145, 1970.
103. Rüegg, J. C., and R. T. Tregear. Mechanical factors affecting the ATPase activity of glycerol-extracted insect fibrillar flight muscle. *Proc. R. Soc. London Ser. B* 165: 497–512, 1966.
104. Saide, J. D., and W. C. Ullrick. Fine structure of the honeybee Z-disc. *J. Mol. Biol.* 79: 329–337, 1973.
105. Saide, J. D., and W. C. Ullrick. Purification and properties of the isolated honeybee Z-disc. *J. Mol. Biol.* 87: 671–683, 1974.
106. Sainsbury, G., and B. Bullard. New proline-rich proteins in isolated insect Z-discs. *Biochem. J.* 191: 333–339, 1980.
107. Sainsbury, G. M., and D. Hulmes. Notes on the structure of the Z-disc of insect flight muscle. In: *Insect Flight Muscle*, edited by R. T. Tregear. Amsterdam: North-Holland, 1977, p. 75–78.
108. Schädler, M. Proportionale Aktivierung von ATPase-Aktivität und Kontrakionsspannung durch Calciumionen in isolierten contractilen Strukturen verschiedenet Muskelarten. *Pfluegers Arch.* 296: 70–90, 1967.
109. Schädler, M., G. J. Steiger, and J. C. Rüegg. Mechanical activation and isometric oscillation in insect fibrillar muscle. *Pfluegers Arch.* 330: 217–229, 1971.
110. Smith, D. S. The organization of a flight muscle in a dragonfly. *J. Biophys. Biochem. Cytol.* 11: 119–145, 1961.
111. Smith, D. S. The organization and function of the sarcoplasmic reticulum and T-system of muscle cells. *Prog. Biophys. Mol. Biol.* 16: 107–142, 1966.
112. Sotavalta, O. The wingbeat frequency of insects. *Acta Entomol. Fenn.* 4: 1–117, 1947.
113. Squire, J. M. General model of myosin filament structure. II. Myosin filaments and cross-bridge interactions in vertebrate striated and insect flight muscles. *J. Mol. Biol.* 72: 125–138, 1972.
114. Squire, J. M. General model of myosin filament structure. III. Molecular packing arrangements in myosin filaments. *J. Mol. Biol.* 77: 291–323, 1973.
115. Squire, J. M. Actin target area labelling in rigor striated muscles (Abstract). *J. Muscle Res. Cell Motil.* 1: 450, 1980.
116. Steiger, G. J. Stretch activation and tension transients in cardiac, skeletal and insect flight muscle. In: *Insect Flight Muscle*, edited by R. T. Tregear. Amsterdam: North-Holland, 1977, p. 221–268.
117. Steiger, G. J., and R. H. Abbott. Biochemical interpretation of tension transients produced by a four state mechanical model. *J. Muscle Res. Cell Motil.* 2: 245–260, 1981.
118. Steiger, G. J., and J. C. Rüegg. Energetics and efficiency in the isolated contractile machinery of an insect fibrillar muscle. *Pfluegers Arch.* 307: 1–21, 1969.
119. Thom, A., and P. Scuart. The forces on an aerofoil at very low speeds. *J. R. Aeronaut. Soc.* 44: 761–770, 1940.
120. Thorson, J., and D. C. S. White. Distributed representations for actin-myosin interaction in the oscillatory contraction of muscle. *Biophys. J.* 9: 360–390, 1969.
121. Thorson, J., and D. C. S. White. Dynamic force measurements at the microgram level with application to myofibrils of striated muscle. *IEEE Trans. Biomed. Eng.* 4: 293–299, 1975.

122. TICE, L. W., AND D. S. SMITH. Localization of myofibrillar ATPase activity in the flight muscles of the blowfly. *J. Cell Biol.* 25: 121–135, 1965.
123. TIEGS, O. W. The flight muscles of insects. *Philos. Trans. R. Soc. London Ser. B* 238: 221–348, 1955.
124. TREGEAR, R. T. The biophysics of insect flight muscle. In: *Insect Muscle,* edited by P. N. R. Usherwood. New York: Academic, 1975, p. 357–403.
125. TREGEAR, R. T., AND S. B. MARSTON. The crossbridge theory. *Annu. Rev. Physiol.* 41: 723–736, 1979.
126. TREGEAR, R. T., J. R. MILCH, R. S. GOODY, K. C. HOLMES, AND C. D. RODGER. The use of some novel X-ray diffraction techniques to study the effect of nucleotides on cross-bridges in insect flight muscle. In: *Cross-Bridge Mechanism in Muscle Contraction,* edited by H. Sugi and G. H. Pollack. Tokyo: Univ. of Tokyo Press, 1979, p. 407–423.
127. TREGEAR, R. T., AND J. M. SQUIRE. Myosin content and filament structure in smooth and striated muscle. *J. Mol. Biol.* 77: 279–290, 1973.
128. TRINICK, J., AND G. OFFER. Cross-linking of actin filaments by heavy meromyosin. *J. Mol. Biol.* 133: 549–556, 1979.
129. TROMBITAS, C., AND A. TIGYI-SEBES. Fine structure and mechanical properties of insect muscle. In: *Insect Flight Muscle,* edited by R. T. Tregear. Amsterdam: North-Holland, 1977, p. 79–90.
130. ULBRICH, M., AND J. C. RÜEGG. Stretch induced formation of ATP-^{32}P in glycerinated fibres of insect flight muscle. *Experientia* 27: 45–46, 1971.
131. ULLRICK, W. C., P. A. TOSELLI, D. CHASE, AND K. DASSE. Are there extensions of thick filaments to the Z-line in vertebrate and invertebrate striated muscle? *J. Ultrastruct. Res.* 60: 263–271, 1977.
132. VOM BROCKE, H. H. The activating effects of calcium ions on the contractile systems of insect fibrillar flight muscle. *Pfluegers Arch. Gesamte Physiol. Menschen Tiere* 290: 70–79, 1966.
133. VOM BROCKE, H. H., AND J. C. RÜEGG. Fractionation of the ATPase of fibrillar insect flight muscle. *Helv. Physiol. Pharmacol. Acta* 23: c79–c81, 1965.
134. WEIS-FOGH, T. Flight performance of the desert locust. *Philos. Trans. R. Soc. London Ser. B* 239: 459–510, 1956.
135. WEIS-FOGH, T. Tetanic force and shortening in locust flight muscle. *J. Exp. Biol.* 33: 668–684, 1956.
136. WHITE, D. C. S. Rigor contraction and the effect of various phosphate compounds on glycerinated insect flight and vertebrate muscle. *J. Physiol. London* 208: 583–605, 1970.
137. WHITE, D. C. S., M. M. K. DONALDSON, G. E. PEARCE, AND M. G. A. WILSON. The resting elasticity of insect fibrillar flight muscle and properties of the crossbridge cycle. In: *Insect Flight Muscle,* edited by R. T. Tregear. Amsterdam: North-Holland, 1977, p. 197–208.
138. WHITE, D. C. S., AND J. THORSON. Phosphate starvation and the non-linear dynamics of insect fibrillar flight muscle. *J. Gen. Physiol.* 60: 307–336, 1972.
139. WHITE, D. C. S., AND J. THORSON. The kinetics of muscle contraction. In: *Progress in Biophysics and Molecular Biology,* edited by J. A. V. Butler and D. Nobel. Oxford, UK: Pergamon, 1973, vol. 27, p. 173–255.
140. WHITE, D. C. S., M. G. A. WILSON, AND J. THORSON. What does insect flight muscle tell us about the mechanism of active contraction? In: *Crossbridge Mechanism in Muscle Contraction,* edited by H. Sugi and G. H. Pollack. Tokyo: Univ. of Tokyo Press, 1979, p. 193–210.
141. WINKELMAN, L. Comparative studies of paramyosins. *Comp. Biochem. Physiol.* B 55: 391–397, 1976.
142. WINKELMAN, L., AND B. BULLARD. Phosphorylation of a locust myosin light chain and its effect on calcium regulation. *J. Muscle Res. Cell Motil.* 1: 221–222, 1980.
143. WOOD, J. An experimental determination of the relationship between lift and aerodynamic power in *Calliphora erythrocephala* and *Phormia regina. J. Exp. Biol.* 56: 31–36, 1972.
144. WOOTTON, R. J., AND D. J. S. NEWMAN. Whitefly have the highest contraction frequencies yet recorded in non-fibrillar flight muscles. *Nature London* 280: 402–403, 1979.
145. WRAY, J. S. Filament geometry and the activation of insect flight muscles. *Nature London* 280: 325–326, 1979.
146. WRAY, J. S. Structure of the backbone in myosin filaments of muscle. *Nature London* 277: 37–40, 1979.
147. WRAY, J., P. VIBERT, AND C. COHEN. Actin filaments in muscle: pattern of myosin and tropomyosin/troponin attachments. *J. Mol. Biol.* 124: 501–521, 1978.
148. YOUNT, R. G., D. OJALA, AND D. BABCOCK. Interaction of P-N-P and P-C-P analogs of adenosine triphosphate with heavy meromyosin, myosin and actomyosin. *Biochemistry* 10: 2490–2495, 1971.
149. ZEBE, E., W. MEINRENKEN, AND J. C. RÜEGG. Supercontraction of glycerol-extracted insect flight muscles in the presence of ITP. *Z. Zellforsch. Mikrosk. Anat.* 87: 603–621, 1968.

CHAPTER 17

Emergence of specialization in skeletal muscle

ALAN M. KELLY | *Department of Pathology, School of Veterinary Medicine, University of Pennsylvania, Philadelphia, Pennsylvania*

CHAPTER CONTENTS

MAMMALIAN MUSCLES can be broadly subdivided into fast- and slow-twitch types based on differences in the intrinsic speed of shortening, immunologic (4, 60, 61) and biochemical distinctions in the contractile proteins [especially myosin (111, 159)], as well as on the levels of actomyosin ATPase (8) and its stability at alkaline and acid pH (23, 169). Most muscles are not composed of pure populations of one type of fiber; they have mixed populations of fast- and slow-twitch fibers with a predominance of the fiber type characterizing the contractile properties of the whole muscle. For example, the slow-twitch soleus muscle in adult rats is composed of approximately 80% slow fibers and 20% fast fibers, whereas the fast-twitch extensor digitorum longus (EDL) of the rat has about 94% fast-twitch and only 4% slow-twitch fibers (3). These specialized types of fiber are distributed in a mosaic throughout muscles. This reflects the intermingling of fast and slow motor units, since it is now clearly established that within a single unit all fibers have uniform metabolic and contractile properties (32, 57, 126).

These properties (metabolic and contractile) can be correlated with the structural and physiological characteristics of the innervating motoneurons (28, 32, 74). Slow-twitch fibers are fatigue resistant and are innervated by small motoneurons that are readily excited and discharge for long periods with comparatively low firing rates. Investigators claim that a normally slow muscle increases its speed of contraction as a result of intermittent high-frequency stimulation (100 Hz), and conversely it decreases its twitch time as a result of continuous low-frequency stimulation (10 Hz).

The correlation between the properties of motoneurons and the muscle fibers they innervate suggests that neural activity patterns regulate gene expression within myofibers. This has been convincingly demonstrated in a number of elegant studies (73, 135, 137, 157, 158, 167, 178) showing, for example, that chronic neural stimulation of a fast-twitch muscle with a frequency pattern resembling the firing rate of a slow motoneuron ultimately effects a complete transformation from fast to slow, most dramatically with respect to conversion toward the slow phenotype. Consistent with the classic cross-reinnervation studies of Buller et al. (29), virtually complete transformation of twitch properties, contractile proteins, metabolic enzymes, and capillary density was observed [see Jolesz and Sréter (89)]. Surprisingly, however, changes in each of these properties take place independently of one another (135). Immunologic and biochemical studies reveal that both fast and slow myosin isozymes are present within single fibers during the conversion (136, 154), indicating that the transformation occurs within the preexisting set of fibers and that the muscle phenotype is not rigidly determined.

Using differing patterns of chronic stimulation imposed directly on denervated muscle, Lømo and his colleagues (110) have shown that transformation can occur in the absence of the nerve and that a wide variety of both fast and slow muscle phenotypes can be obtained, depending on the pattern of impulse activity. They claim that a normally slow muscle increases its speed of contraction as a result of intermittent high-frequency stimulation (100 Hz), and conversely it decreases its twitch time as a result of continuous low-frequency stimulation (10 Hz). This research, which in many respects complements classic cross-reinnervation studies (9, 27, 29, 31, 55, 65, 92, 120), emphasizes the central role of the nerve's electrical activity in the specialization of mature muscle. Although the development of characteristic nerve impulse patterns in fast and slow muscles is certainly important to the final maturation of specialized muscle properties, results obtained by imposing extreme patterns of activation cannot conclusively prove that comparable conversions occur during normal development or as a result of training. Indeed in a recent review Salmons and Henriksson (156) noted that the contractile characteristics of myofibers are remarkably stable during exercise. They observed that to date there is no good evidence for interconversion between slow (type I) and fast (type II) fibers in human muscle. Consequently the high percentage of type I fibers in muscles of endurance athletes and the low percentage of this fiber type in sprinters may be determined genetically.

Literature on the control of muscle metabolism has been dominated by work on the mechanisms of neural regulation, and only recently have scientists recognized the influence of the entire milieu in which muscle differentiates. In particular the involvement of endocrine secretions such as the sex hormones and T_4 has been acknowledged. Such a delayed recognition of their importance is surprising, however, because the influences of testosterone on fiber growth were described in the mouse levator ani muscle (40) and the temporalis muscle of the guinea pig (67, 102) over a decade ago. In the male rat (A. M. Kelly, unpublished observations) and in man (56) testosterone appears to have a selective effect: type II fibers are significantly larger in the male than in the female. The presence of cytosolic androgen-binding sites in rat skeletal muscle implies that the hormone directly mediates fiber size, although it may not be the only factor. In *Xenopus laevis* Erulkar et al. (58) have found that when testosterone is administered to the mature male, it produces sexual activity, and the motoneurons supplying the clasping muscles fire at faster repetitive rates. Hence testosterone can influence the function of motoneurons in *Xenopus*, and this is reflected in the properties of muscle.

Treatment of mature rats with thyroid hormones [T_3 + T_4] is reported to cause an increase in mitochondrial enzymes, but there are differences between muscle types in their magnitude of response: in both innervated and denervated forms (194) fast muscles increased their oxidative enzyme activity about 40% compared with a 150% increase in slow muscles. Ianuzzu et al. (82) reported a dramatic increase in type II fibers of the soleus after 6 wk of hyperthyroidism and a parallel increase in myosin ATPase activity. Conversely hypothyroidism is believed to cause a decrease in the proportion of type II cells and an increase in type I cells in the soleus. In the soleus there is a marked slowing of isometric twitch times accompanying the change in fiber type (88). Transformation toward type I cells in hypothyroid rats is prevented by denervation, suggesting that in contrast to the oxidative enzyme change, this is a cooperative neurohormonal response. It is not known whether or not these hormonally regulated effects, though comparable to the cross-reinnervation experiments in magnitude of change, are caused by alterations in the firing pattern of the motoneuron.

The greater responsiveness of slow muscle to T_4 control appears to be related to the peripheral T_3-generating process studied by Jansen et al. (85). They report that mean T_4 levels are approximately the same in red as in white muscles of mature rats but that T_3 levels are significantly higher in the red. Thus formation of T_3 from T_4 occurs in skeletal muscle, probably to a greater extent in red than in white muscle.

This review discusses some of the processes involved in the emergence of specialized fast- and slow-twitch muscles, particularly in the rat. Muscle evolution is highly ordered and complex: myofibers undergo differentiation and motoneurons synapse with and organize fibers into functional motor units. The stage at which selective neural control is imposed upon differentiating myofibers is uncertain, as is the extent to which intrinsic properties of muscle fibers themselves contribute to the development of specialized biochemical and physiological properties. Although these aspects of neuromuscular development are considered in detail here, the contributions of endocrine secretions to the evolution of diversity are not discussed. Although the latter are undoubtedly important, particularly thyroid hormone, they are not considered because of lack of information on the subject.

MUSCLE HISTOGENESIS

One of the features that most clearly distinguishes in vivo from in vitro myogenesis is the pattern of muscle assembly. In vitro myoblasts proliferate rapidly, fusing in very large numbers into irregularly branched myotubes, whereas in vivo the rate of proliferation and fusion is lower (19). Nevertheless in the embryo these two cellular events—replication and fusion—generate the precise complement of muscle cells for each muscle at a comparatively early stage of development and also continuously supplement the numbers of nuclei within myofibers during the entire period of growth. Unfortunately comparatively little is known about the mechanisms controlling these highly ordered morphogenic processes.

For over 100 years histologists have recognized that muscle is progressively built up from successive orders of cells (6, 39, 44, 99, 116, 122). At the inception of myogenesis, myoblasts in the primary muscle mass replicate and fuse to form small numbers of myotubes called primary-generation myotubes [Fig. 1; (99)]. Initially these cells lie in close proximity to one another, and their juxtaposed membranes are interconnected by various forms of specialized membrane, including gap junctions (91, 99, 141, 164) that mediate electrical coupling (22, 47, 48, 91, 104).

What role gap junctions play in early muscle histogenesis is not known, but it seems likely that the segregation of myotubes from the primary muscle mass into specific muscle primordia involves these structures. Gap junctions also facilitate electrical coupling throughout muscle primordia and are sufficiently strong in intercostal muscles of 16-day fetal rats that an action potential initiated in one cell can propagate laterally between fibers across the entire muscle (48).

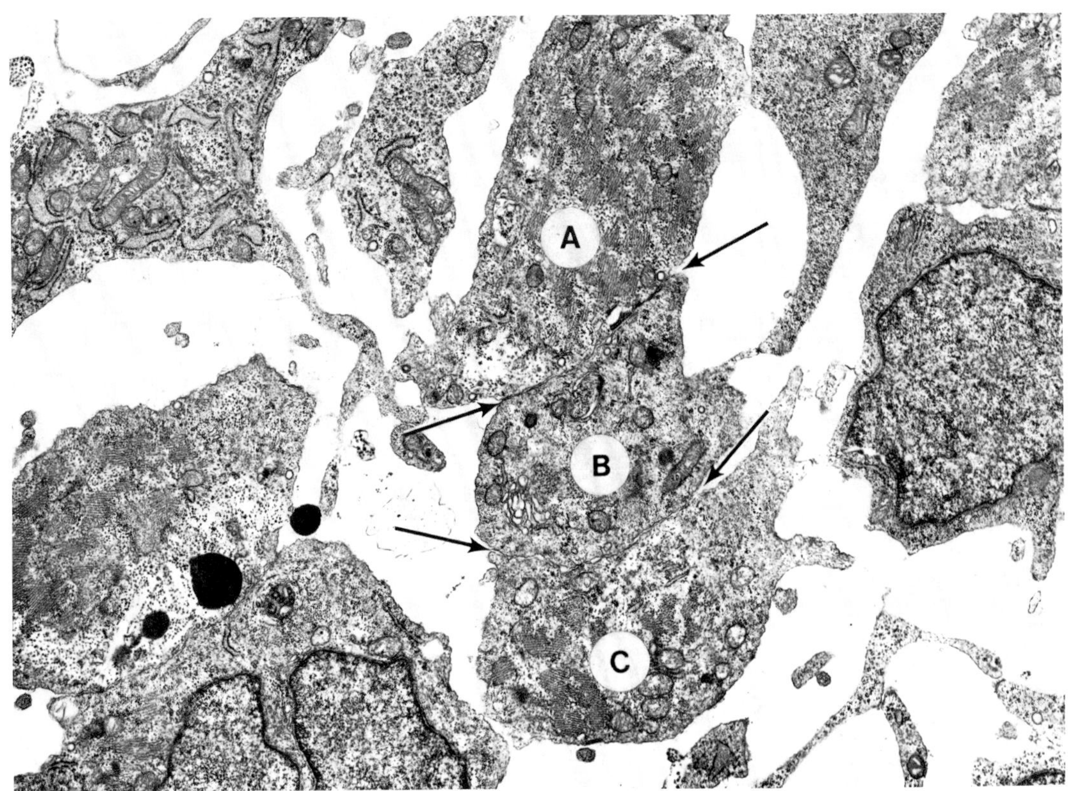

FIG. 1. Rat intercostal muscle, 16 days of gestation, with large extracellular space. *A*, *B*, and *C*: 3 small primary-generation myotubes aggregated in a group, their membranes intimately apposed. Gap junctions are commonly found interconnecting these cells at this stage of development. In the surrounding tissue there are several undifferentiated cells. × 10,000.

Thus the early muscle primordium is organized to respond as a single unit when stimulated, generating a contraction of optimal force. These early contractions are probably required to flex the initially straight limb primordium and induce normal joint formation (54), as well as to obtain the correct fetal posture to ensure that muscles grow under appropriate tension. Dennis (47) has suggested that small organic molecules (both inhibitory and inductive) generated in a more mature cell may diffuse via gap junctions to influence the development of less differentiated fibers, particularly in the early stages of fiber specialization. In vitro metabolic coupling between chick embryo myoblasts has been demonstrated by use of [^{3}H]-uridine (91).

As with electrical coupling in general, very little is known about the controls over gap junction formation during myogenesis. The fact that gap junctions persist in paralyzed fetal muscle (71) suggests that muscular activity may, in part, bring about their elimination. Breakdown of these junctions coincides with the separation of primary cells into independent units of contraction (each surrounded by its own basal lamina) and with the early differentiation of motor end plates on the walls of primary cells (99, 100). Because the primordium may no longer necessarily respond to stimulation as a single unit after primary fibers separate into individual entities, this event can be viewed as an essential step in the development of discrete motor unit control and the evolution of graded movements.

In the intercostal muscles of the rat, primary myotubes separate between 16 and 18 days of gestation. Coincidentally a replicating population of myoblasts congregates around and attaches to the walls of the primary cell by various forms of membrane junction. These cells undergo further muscle growth in one of two interrelated ways. Those that fuse with differentiating myotubes and myofibers in maturing muscle to complement their multinuclearity and growth (1, 34, 39, 95, 99, 162) are termed *satellite cells* (115). Kelly and Zacks (99) originally proposed that membrane junctions are necessary to stabilize membranes together prior to fusion, and Rash et al. (140, 141) have implicated the formation of gap junctions and electrical coupling as essential components in the progression of fusion (Fig. 2). Their studies have significantly advanced the understanding of fusion, but because electrical coupling is prevalent early in myogenesis it seems unlikely that all cells connected by gap junctions must necessarily fuse. The work of Kalderon et al. (91) supports this conclusion: they showed that in fusion-arrested myoblasts in vitro, gap junction communication is present and virtually identical to that

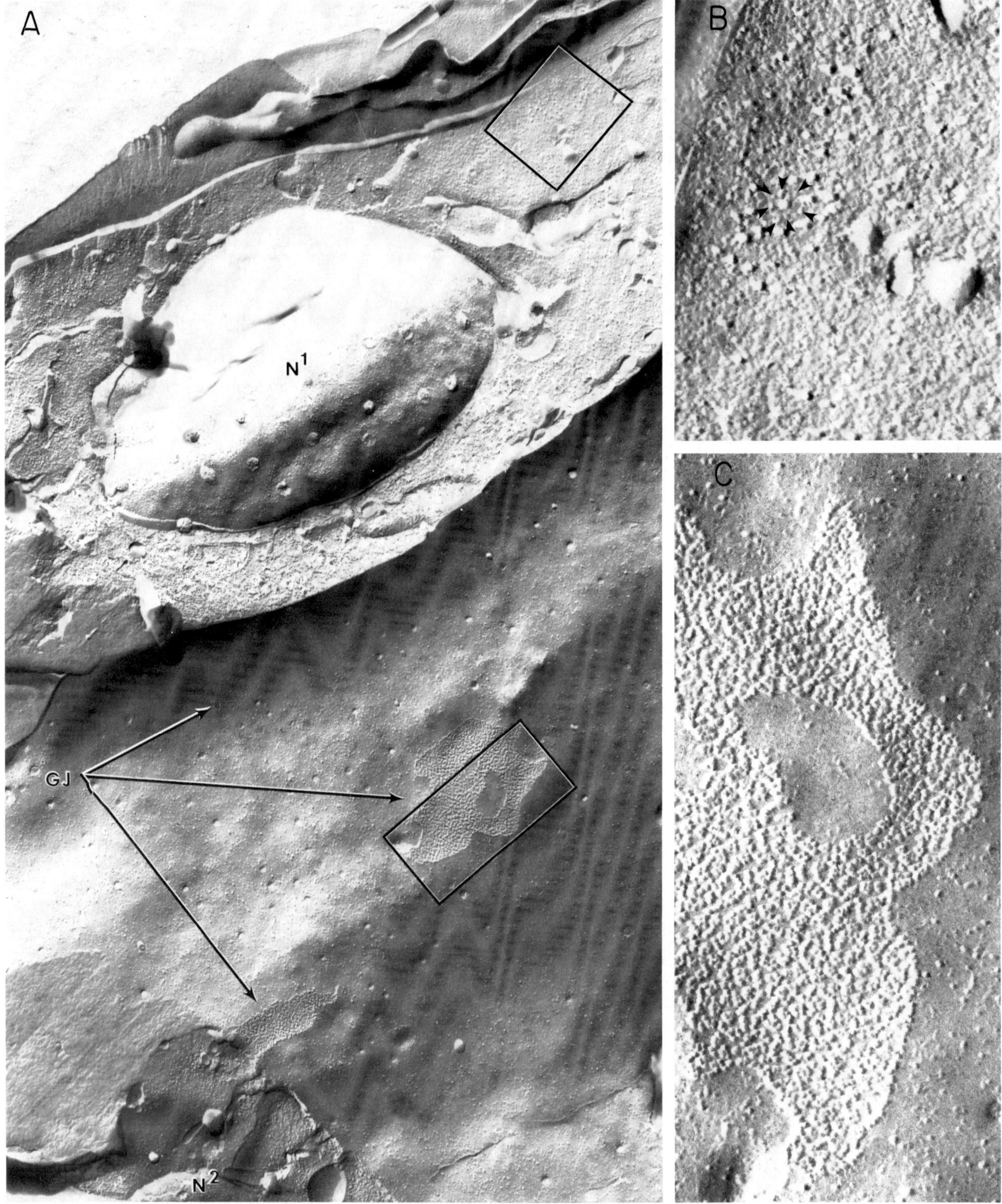

FIG. 2. Rat hindlimb, 19-day fetus. *A*: 3 gap junctions (*GJ*) may be recognized as arrays of particles on A face of plasmalemma. × 21,000. *Upper inscribed area* and *B*, rudimentary myofibril observed in the limited area of cleaved cytoplasm. Characteristic 400-Å hexagonal array of thick filaments and faint hexagonal array of thin filaments (*circle*) are partially obscured by very low, local shadowing angle. × 68,000. *C*: portion of 1 gap junction, *lower inscribed area of A*, is enlarged to reveal 8- to 9-nm subunit particles in cluster configuration. × 81,000. N^1 and N^2, multinuclei. [From Rash and Staehelin (141).]

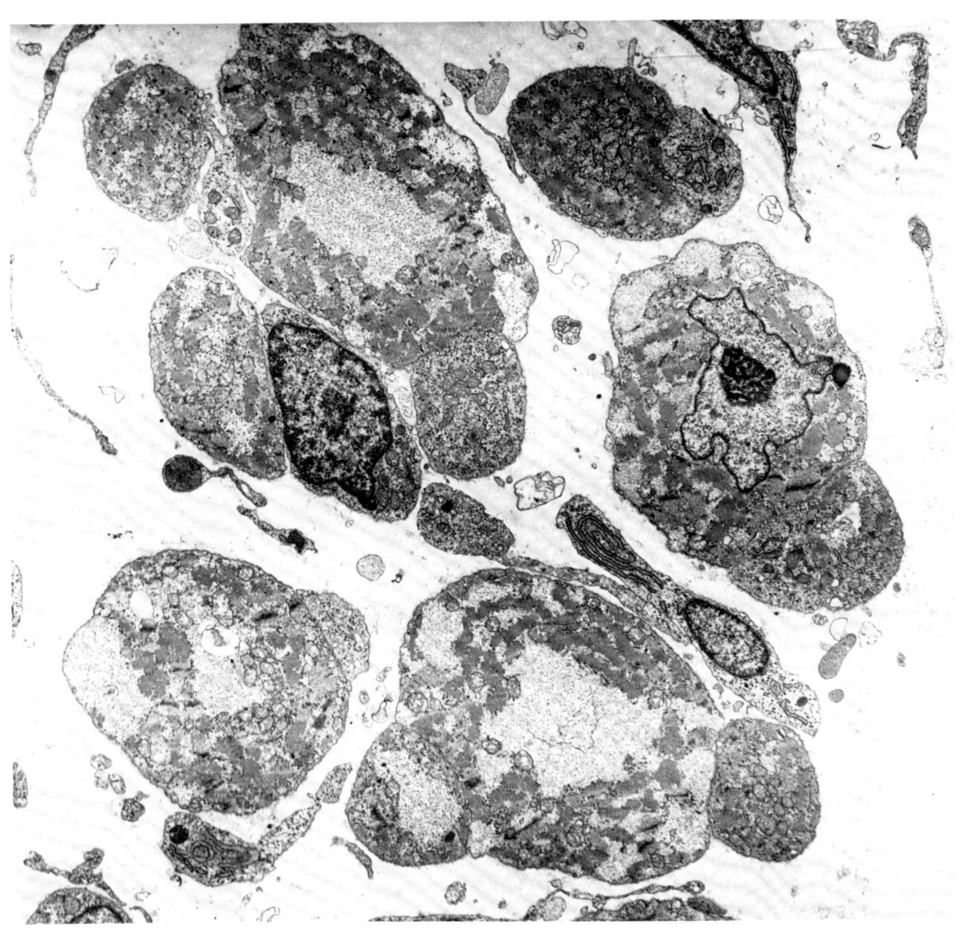

FIG. 3. Rat intercostal muscle, 18 days of gestation. Large primary-generation myotubes, containing much glycogen and peripherally dispersed myofibrils, dominate cell groups. Undifferentiated cells and small secondary-generation myotubes are intimately applied to their walls. Each muscle cell group is peripherally ensheathed by a basement membrane. × 6,000.

detected in fusion-competent myoblasts. Hence electrical coupling must be involved in some more general way in the progression of myogenesis.

Instead of fusing with primary-generation muscle cells, the replicating myoblasts may fuse with one another to form new, secondary-generation cells. In most animals these new orders of cells preferentially form along the walls of primary myotubes; de novo fiber formation is uncommon [Fig. 3; (130, 131)]. Initially, secondary cell membranes form complex interdigitations with the primary myotubes to which they are attached by small membrane junctions, including gap junctions (Fig. 4). These membrane specializations interconnect primary and secondary cells within groups so that each cell complex almost certainly contracts and relaxes as a single unit.

With further development the incidence of membrane junctions between primary and secondary cells precipitously declines (99), and concurrently the strength of electrical coupling is diminished (47). Primary and secondary cells segregate to become independent units of contraction, each surrounded by its own basal lamina (Fig. 5). This is a necessary prelude to discrete motor unit control over primary- and secondary-generation fibers and is a further step in the evolution of finely tuned movements. The result of this piggyback pattern of histogenesis is that each muscle bundle is composed of primary and secondary cells distributed in a mosaic (Fig. 5). Actually both the environmental milieu and the type of neuromuscular interaction under which primary cells are initiated differ from those in which secondary cells later form.

Harris (71, 72), who investigated the regulation of formation of primary and secondary fibers in the embryonic rat diaphragm, has recently addressed the question of whether these temporal differences are in some way correlated with the patterns of gene expression in primary and secondary cells. Influences of nerve on this process were examined in 14- to 21-day rat fetuses that had been individually, chronically paralyzed by insertion of diffusion capsules containing tetrodotoxin or had been chemically denervated by direct injection of β-bungarotoxin. In the normal fetus the primary cells form at between 14 and 17 days in

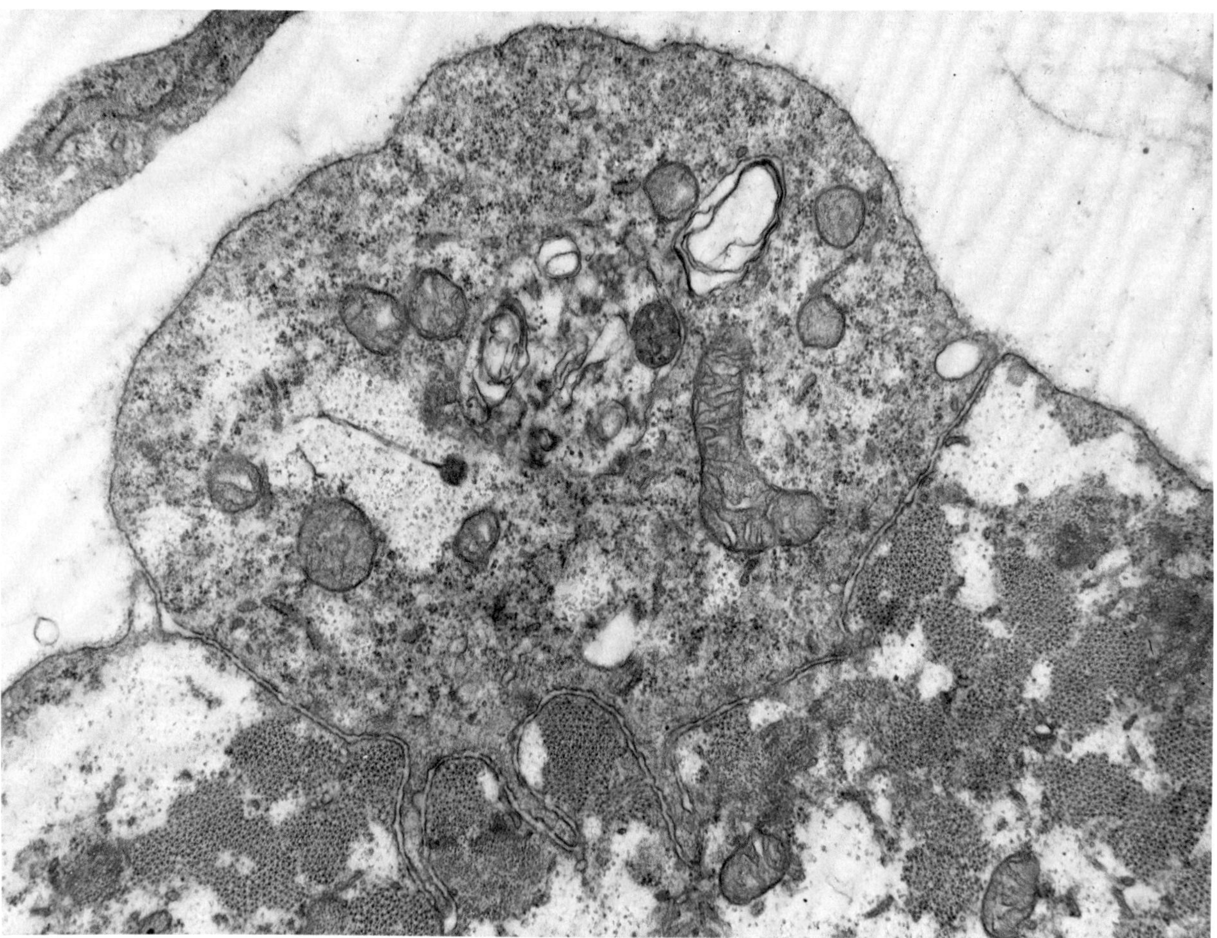

FIG. 4. Rat intercostal muscle, 18 days of gestation. Small secondary-generation myotube lies in a shallow depression of the wall of a large primary myotube. Processes protrude from the secondary cell into invaginations of the wall of the large myotube; invaginations are probably developing T tubules. Intercellular space between cells measures 80–100 Å. The presence of these complex membrane relations implies coordinate function of the 2 cells. × 30,000. [From Kelly and Zacks (99).]

utero. Harris concluded that the initiation of these cells is relatively autonomous because their development is little affected by either paralysis or denervation. Secondary myotubes normally form after 17 days of gestation and give rise to the majority of fibers in the developing muscle. It is significant that Harris found their generation to be crucially dependent on both innervation and muscle contraction: in denervated muscles and in innervated muscles that failed to contract, formation of secondary cells was promptly halted (Fig. 6). These studies therefore reveal intrinsic differences between primary and secondary cells and suggest that nerves regulate the absolute size of a muscle by their electrical activity and probably also by the tension this activity generates.

The dual prerequisite of innervation and contraction for formation of secondary fibers implies that muscle must be innervated to produce the necessary contractions. Initially these contractions must come from primary cells, since the latter dominate the anlage at 17 and 18 days of gestation (Figs. 3 and 7) and end-plate differentiation is limited to the primary cells at this stage. Separate innervation of secondary fibers is unusual; structural studies of 18-day intercostal muscle reveal that the clusters of primary and secondary cells are mutually innervated by a single end plate formed on the walls of the primary cell [(100); see Fig. 7]. Thus neurally mediated contractions of primary cells are thought to induce formation of secondary myotubes. This supports the previous observation that the membranes of primary and secondary cells are coupled and must function coordinately. Furthermore it suggests that the inductive influences of the nerve on formation of secondary fibers are indirectly mediated, at least in part, via the primary cell. Determining whether this involves electrical transmission between primary and secondary cells or whether metabolic coupling is also involved requires further study, particularly since primary myotubes predominantly become slow type I fibers whereas secondary myotubes

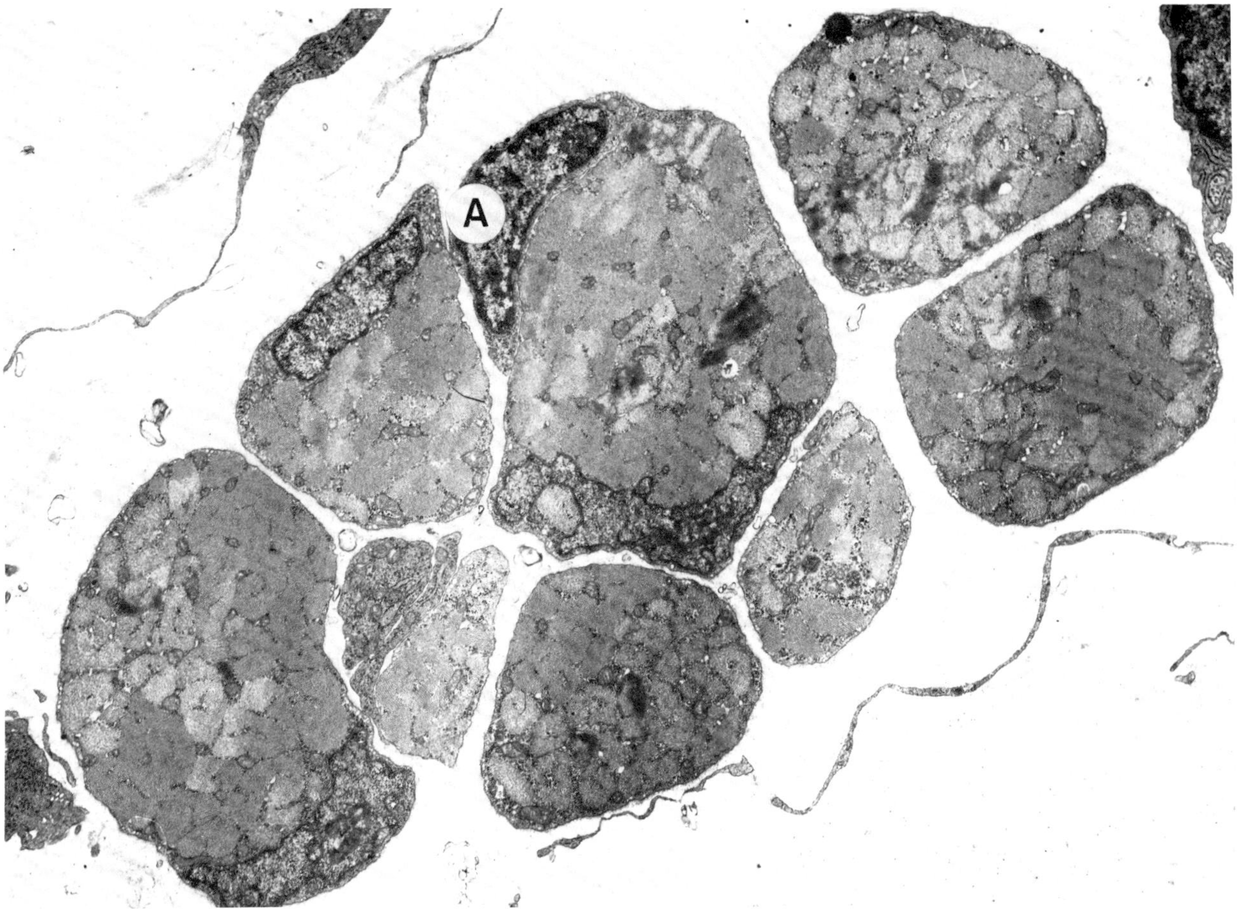

FIG. 5. Rat intercostal muscle at birth. Myofibers, packed with myofibrils, compose a muscle bundle. Myofibers vary greatly in size and intermingle in a checkerboard pattern. Small myofibers are interpreted to be secondary-generation cells that have developed on the walls of large primary cells. *A*, satellite cell abuts wall of large myofiber. × 6,000. [From Kelly and Zacks (99).]

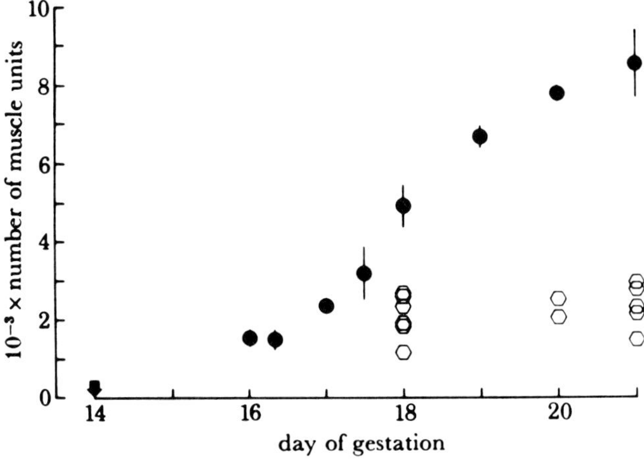

FIG. 6. Neural control of muscle cell formation in the rat embryo. *Open hexagons*, number of muscle units in aneural muscles from rat embryos injected with β-bungarotoxin on day 14 and examined at later times. *Filled circles*, muscle unit formation in control animals (mean ± SD). [From Harris (71).]

become fast type II fibers (6, 98, 152, 153). Similar indirect neural control is observed postpartum when satellite cells divide and then fuse with hypertrophying myofibers (20) instead of forming new myotubes: these myoblasts abruptly cease replication when the limb is immobilized by denervation (95).

Betz and his colleagues (16) have also investigated neural involvement in controlling fiber formation in developing muscle. Their analysis of neural contributions to this process are in many respects complemented by Harris's studies, but their deduction of the nature of neural control over fiber formation differs from that of Harris. Betz et al. investigated the relationship between the number of muscle fibers and the number of motor units within the developing IVth lumbrical muscle from birth to 30 days postpartum in the rat. This muscle increases its complement of fibers from 600 at birth to a mature value of about 950 by 10 days (Fig. 8). It is innervated by approximately 12 motor units, although this number can be selectively

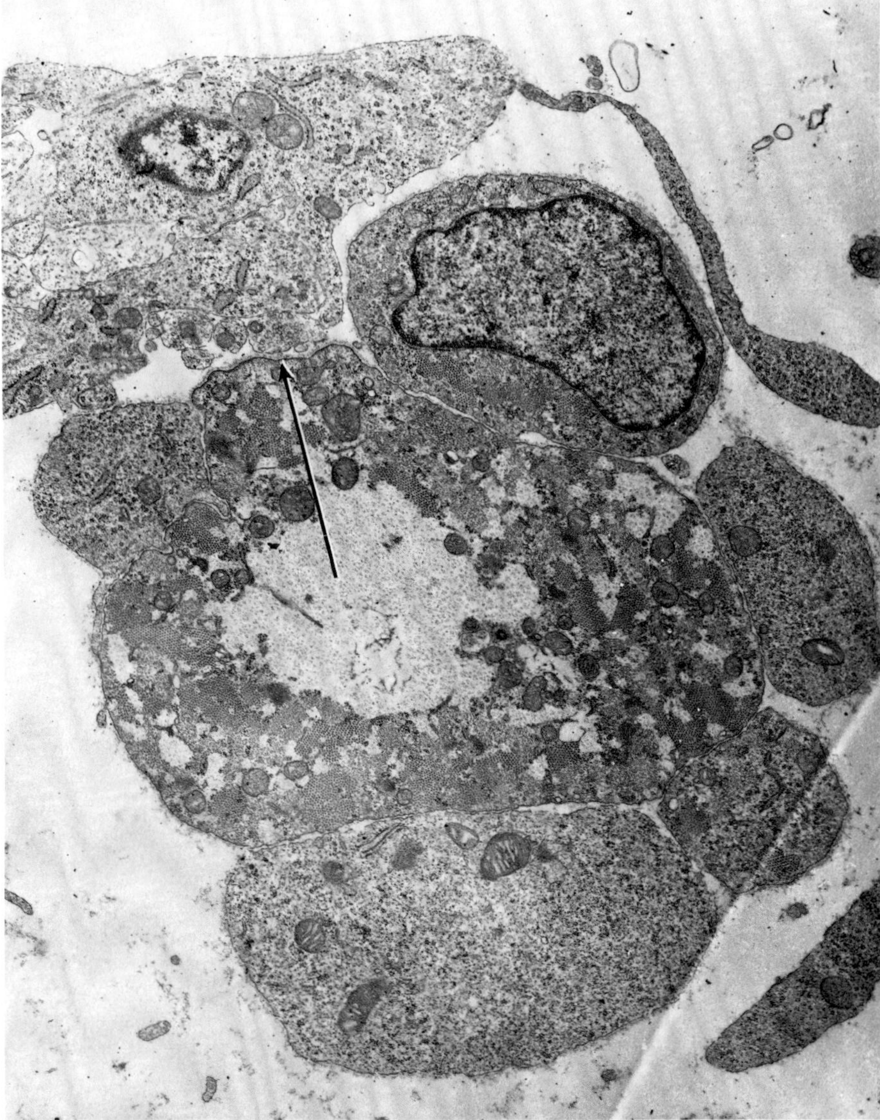

FIG. 7. Rat intercostal muscle, 18 days of gestation. Large primary-generation myotube containing much glycogen is surrounded by new generations of secondary cells. *Arrow*, group of axon sprouts approaching large myotube membrane. In this area of contact primary cell membranes have increased electron density, indicating early differentiation of postsynaptic membrane. This configuration suggests that the primary-secondary cell complex is innervated as a single unit. [From Kelly and Zacks (100).]

reduced to a single innervating axon by partial denervation. Muscle that was completely denervated at birth and examined at 4–5 wk of age had the average 600 fibers, which is very similar to the number at birth. Since necrotizing fibers were not seen, investigators concluded that postnatal production of muscle fibers depends on the presence of a nerve supply. This was supported by the finding of an additive effect on numbers of muscle fibers as fewer and fewer motor axons were severed during partial denervation. The full complement of 950 fibers was obtained when eight motor axons innervated the muscle; beyond this, additional motor axons did not further augment the number of muscle fibers, thus establishing an upper limit to the number of muscle fibers produced irrespective of the number of innervating motoneurons. Betz et al. concluded that the postnatal role of the nerve is permissive rather than instructive, promoting production of muscle fibers within limits established prenatally.

PERIPHERAL NERVE DEVELOPMENT

From an early stage of myogenesis the precise growth and differentiation of muscle is skillfully orchestrated in the presence of motor axons (48, 69, 70, 79, 105–108) that impose almost continual direction and probably have multiple regulative influences on muscle differentiation. In addition to electrically mediated effects, a variety of remote influences of nerve on muscle have been described. These imply that the motor nerve may influence muscle differentiation prior to synaptogenesis. Podleski et al. (139), for example, have shown that spinal cord extracts added to cultures of rat myotubes produce increased clustering of acetylcholine receptors. These results raise the possibility that this "trophic factor" may condition the muscle for subsequent innervation. Many other studies reveal mitogenic or growth-promoting effects of neural extracts on muscle cultures. Oh and Markelonis (129) have purified a protein from chick sciatic nerve that

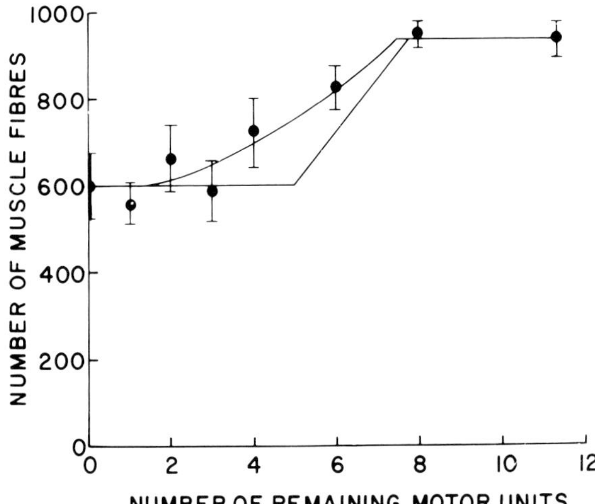

FIG. 8. Motor units and muscle cell development in the rat lumbrical muscle. Number of muscle fibers plotted as a function of number of remaining motor units in muscles 4–5 wk old that had been partially or completely denervated at birth. Point at 12 motor units is from control muscles. *Points*, mean ± SD. [From Betz et al. (16).]

they believe exerts trophic influences on cultured muscle cells. Gospodarowicz et al. (64) have described a central nervous system polypeptide that increases the rate of proliferation of cultured myoblasts among other mesodermally derived tissues. Comparable studies by Singer (163) indicated that an extractable protein from nerve stimulates the absolute rate of protein synthesis in regenerating newt limb.

Virtually all skeletal muscles are innervated by discrete pools of motoneurons occurring in characteristic locations in the central nervous system. There have been a number of studies, particularly in the chick embryo, on the specificity with which these motoneuron pools innervate the primordium of muscle from the inception of neuromuscular contact. From the very beginning of development, innervation is highly selective and nonrandom; this was demonstrated in electrophysiological recordings from chick embryo spinal cord and specific limb muscles, as well as by retrograde tracing of innervation after injection of horseradish peroxidase into selected muscles (105–107). Landmesser (107) found that motoneurons very rarely send axons to inappropriate muscles; they appear to connect in a precisely specified pattern at an extraordinarily early stage of ontogeny. Prior to penetrating the limb, axons already appear to possess identity: they traverse other axons during plexus formation in pursuit of their particular muscle target. Within the limb they may be able to use environmental cues to reach their prescribed target with little error (107).

From the initiation of synaptogenesis, motor axons have the capacity to secrete acetylcholine (13, 107). Bekoff (11) has shown that very soon after functional neuromuscular contacts are formed in the chick leg, neural circuitry for generating patterned motor activity of synergists and antagonists is laid down. Thus Bekoff demonstrates that very soon after innervation, muscles begin to function in a cooperative way that closely simulates their activity in the adult. That this occurs at such early stages of development implies that most motoneurons that have made functional peripheral synapses with a specific muscle have also made specific central connections appropriate to the function of that muscle. Studies of the evolution of motility in the rat embryo (124), though less critical than those in the chick (11), suggest a similar predetermined sequence of development.

Histogenesis of peripheral nerve is an asynchronous process. It has been described in a number of studies, the first being Weiss's (184) classic description of nerve growth from pioneering and later differentiating, trailing axons. As noted previously neuromuscular contact occurs at a very early stage of myogenesis (13, 48, 109). In the rat intercostal muscle a single axon makes contact and initiates innervation at about 14 days of gestation. At 18 days of gestation a progressive increase in the number of axons to an average of three per fiber (48) takes place as polyneural innervation develops. On contact the initial innervating axon (pioneer axon) determines where on the primitive myotube the single end plate forms, and it inhibits further neuromuscular junction development by other axons. Consequently all of the multiple axons that innervate rat intercostal fibers by 18 days of gestation are constrained to one synaptic area apparently determined by the inaugural neuromuscular contacts (see also refs. 13, 25, 109, 144). As previously noted, synaptic areas are localized on primary-generation cells with the result that each of the primary-secondary complexes appears to be mutually innervated as a single unit at 18 days in utero [Fig. 7; (100)].

Although electrical coupling between muscle cells declines with development and the cells move apart to become independent units of contraction, many of them remain functionally linked in large motor units and are supplied by branches of more than one axon (7, 13, 48, 128, 142, 144). This design presumably increases the contraction strength of developing muscle and complements the effects of electrical coupling between muscle cells. Polyneural innervation persists after cell segregation but is then eliminated during the first 2–3 wk postpartum in an animal such as the rat (16, 25, 144, 145). Not surprisingly investigators have considerable interest in the process of elimination and in how an axon from one motoneuron comes to dominate a differentiating end plate. This is a significant problem, since it has been widely accepted that the reorganization defines the size of motor units in mature muscle. Elimination of multiple innervation involves axonal competition (15, 21, 25) and, like gap junction elimination, is influenced by muscle activity: it can be delayed by reduced activity either as the result of tenotomy (14) or nerve block (176). Conversely O'Brien et al. (128) found that elimination of polyneural innervation can be accelerated by stimulation of early postnatal muscle for 2–4 days at a frequency of 8 Hz over a 4- to 6-h period per day (128).

They have attributed the elimination of superfluous axons to the release of a proteolytic factor at the end plate.

In a study of synapse elimination in the neonatal and juvenile rat soleus, Brown et al. (25) made the interesting observation that although the total spread of motor unit sizes was considerably greater in the young than in the adult, some motor units were within the adult range at all ages examined. They believe that the shrinkage of motor unit territories in this muscle is not accomplished simply by the synchronous withdrawal of a fixed percentage of terminal axons from each motoneuron. Rather there is either considerable variability in the times at which different motor units reach their peak size or, alternatively, the early spread of motor unit territories involves some but not all motoneurons.

These observations correlate with recent studies by Miyata and Yoshioka (119), who found that in early postnatal development about 50% of soleus myofibers were singly innervated by the L_5 ventral root and that this nerve-to-fiber relation did not change throughout development. In contrast the L_4 root innervated all the muscle fibers polyneurally at 6 days postpartum, and at 16 days the remaining 50% of the fibers were singly innervated by motor axons from L_4. Hence this study indicates that elimination of motor nerve terminals in the soleus involves the L_4 but not the L_5 ventral nerves. The program of elimination in this muscle is therefore selective and follows a predetermined sequence.

Miyata and Yoshioka (119) speculate that this pattern of innervation and remodeling may be partially related to the early events of neuromuscular contact. As previously discussed, primary myotubes are initially innervated by only one axon directing the original events of synaptogenesis; further axons then grow into this end plate. All the reasons why this occurs are not understood, but one factor seems to involve the succession of new fibers that form on the walls of primary myotubes. It is possible that the most stable neuromuscular contacts are established by the first axons to innervate primary myotubes, whereas successive axons establish more labile contacts. Then as secondary myotubes develop they may be innervated by the successive orders of axons that subsequently migrate off the primary cell. This hypothetical scheme (see Fig. 18) implies that the initial distribution of terminal axons from each motor axon is not entirely random. Consistent with the work of Kelly and Zacks (100) and Harris (71), it proposes that there is a sequence of innervation following the progression of muscle assembly from primary and secondary cells.

Betz's (15) studies of polyneural innervation in neonatal rat lumbrical muscle can be correlated with this analysis. In the lumbrical muscle approximately one-half of the adult population of fibers is present at birth, and the full complement is generated during the first 10 days postpartum. All of the initial fibers are multiply innervated at birth, and because Brown et al. (25) have observed that the total number of motor units remains constant in the rat soleus after birth, it seems probable that the mature set of motor axons is already present at the onset, awaiting and influencing the completion of muscle histogenesis. As additional secondary-generation fibers are formed in the lumbrical muscle, selected axons apparently withdraw their terminals from the primary cells, simultaneously forming new, multiple synapses with the recently generated fibers (Fig. 9). Production of additional fibers ceases in the lumbrical muscle between 10 and 20 days postpartum, and in the final stages of neuromuscular maturation superfluous synapses are eliminated from the secondary fibers. Thus the adult pattern of a single innervating axon per muscle fiber is achieved.

The proposed mechanism also finds confirmation in previous studies by Riley (145). He observed that in the soleus muscle of 13- to 15-day-old rats the majority of multiply innervated fibers were small, whereas most singly innervated fibers were larger. At these stages small fibers are almost all type II and larger fibers are type I (151). Thus patterns of phenotypic expression and of innervation appear to be correlated in this developing muscle and, as Riley observed, the results show that histochemical fiber differentiation precedes elimination of polyneural innervation.

MYOFIBER SPECIALIZATION

Limb muscles of most mammals have slow contractile characteristics at birth (29, 41, 42, 68, 80). Animals such as the guinea pig are an exception: they have a long gestation, are delivered in a remarkably mature state, and at birth have differentiated rates of contraction (68). In the rat, more typically, isometric contraction and half-relaxation times are prolonged in both the soleus and EDL at birth [Fig. 10; (41, 42)]. Even at this stage of development, though, these properties are not identical in the two muscles; portending its future specialization, EDL reacts slightly faster than soleus, and significant differences in myosin ATPase in the two have also been reported (174). A progressive increase in speed of shortening and decrease in twitch times then take place in EDL, which attains its mature values by 3 wk postpartum. During the same period in the soleus a less pronounced increase in the twitch characteristics occurs. The reaction of this muscle slows with further development, and prolongation of contraction and half-relaxation times continues even after 4 mo. However, these times do not return to the slow values of the neonate (41). According to Brown (26), sciatic neurectomy at birth interferes with this progression of differentiation, revealing that specialization is under neural influence even at this early stage. The normal progressive increase in speed of contraction developed incompletely in the neonatally

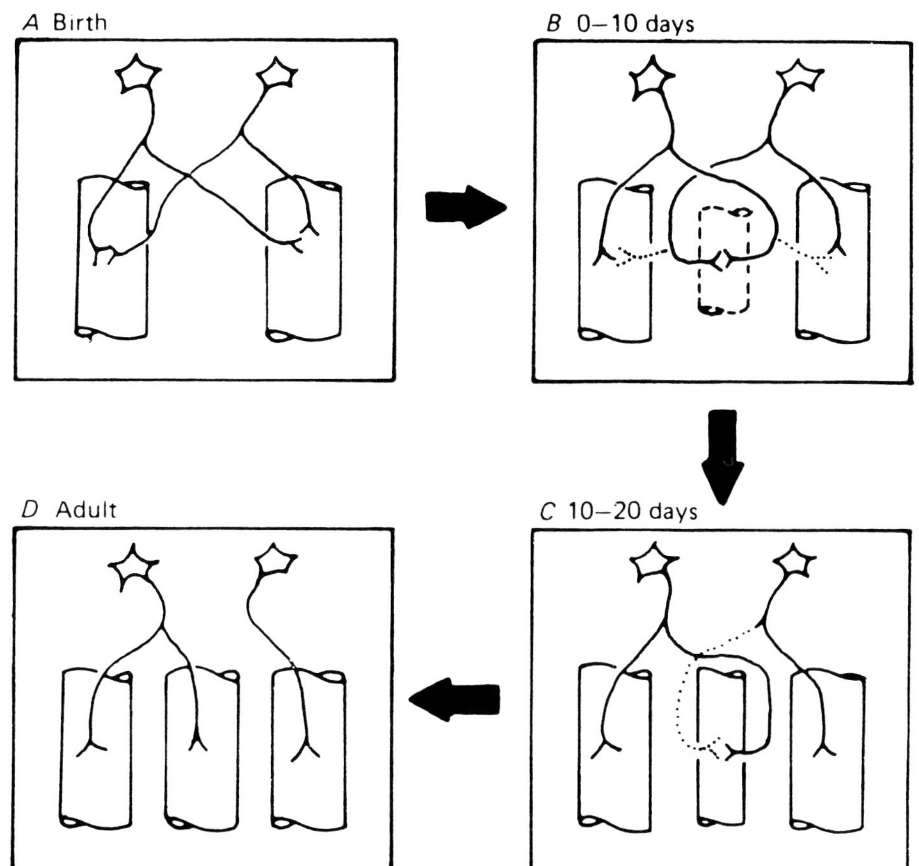

FIG. 9. Schematic diagrams illustrating postnatal development of rat lumbrical muscle. *A*: at birth all muscle fibers are polyneuronally innervated. *B*: during the first 10 days postpartum motoneurons lose some of their terminals (*dotted lines*) through synapse elimination, but the same motoneurons form new synapses on newly produced muscle fibers (*dashed lines*). New muscle fibers probably become polyneuronally innervated. Synapse elimination and synapse formation balance one another so that there is little change in the number of synapses made by each motoneuron, and thus motor unit size remains approximately constant. *C*: between 10 and 20 days postpartum muscle fiber production ceases, but elimination of synapses from polyneuronally innervated fibers (*dotted line*) continues. Average motor unit size decreases. *D*: at about 20 days postpartum, adult pattern of innervation is reached, where each muscle fiber is singly innervated. [From Betz et al. (15).]

denervated EDL, but surprisingly the speed of shortening of the neonatally denervated soleus increased significantly.

Changes in physiological properties of normal developing muscles correspond to postnatal functional maturation of motoneurons. Sato et al. (160) have shown that during this period there is differential growth of motoneurons supplying the soleus and the fast-twitch, medial gastrocnemius muscle of the cat. This can be correlated with the development of their size-dependent electrophysiological properties. In the same period, α-motoneurons to fast and slow muscles in kittens differentiate in terms of the duration of after-hyperpolarization (80), but how well this is correlated with differentiative changes in the contractile properties of muscle is uncertain. Ridge (143) showed that in the newborn kitten the conduction velocity of α-axons to all muscles was slow, but that even at this time the mean conduction velocity of axons to fast-twitch muscle was higher than in axons to slow-twitch muscle. This distinction remained proportionately the same from birth to maturity. How well conduction velocity of α-axons is correlated with speed of muscle contraction has been questioned by Huizar et al. (80).

In studies on motor units of neonatal and adolescent rats, Bursian and Sviderskaya (33) described the frequency of discharge as uniformly low at birth but increasing more than fivefold during the ensuing 3 wk. They found small differences in amplitude or discharge frequency in successively recruited motor units in neonatal rats, and they concluded that functional differences between units developed during the postnatal period and were probably correlated with maturation of both suprasegmental and afferent control. Threshold differences between motor units do exist at birth in the rat, however, as Redfern (142) revealed when first describing polyneural innervation. In a recent study on motor unit maturation in the juvenile rat (7–25 days postpartum) Navarrete and Vrbová (125) reported that a considerable proportion of units fire at low frequency in the EDL during the 2nd wk after birth. The proportion of those firing at low rates declines during the 3rd wk after birth and reciprocally, the proportion of units firing at higher frequencies increases. Thus the fast motor unit apparently evolves from one with a low firing frequency. Although the firing frequency of motor units in the soleus is also low at 7 days postpartum, the muscle is activated only phasically; the continuous, tonic activity seen in mature animals is established only after 25 days. These observations imply that although contraction times of the period between birth and 25 days are significantly slower in the soleus than in the EDL, the development of these slow properties is not directly correlated with

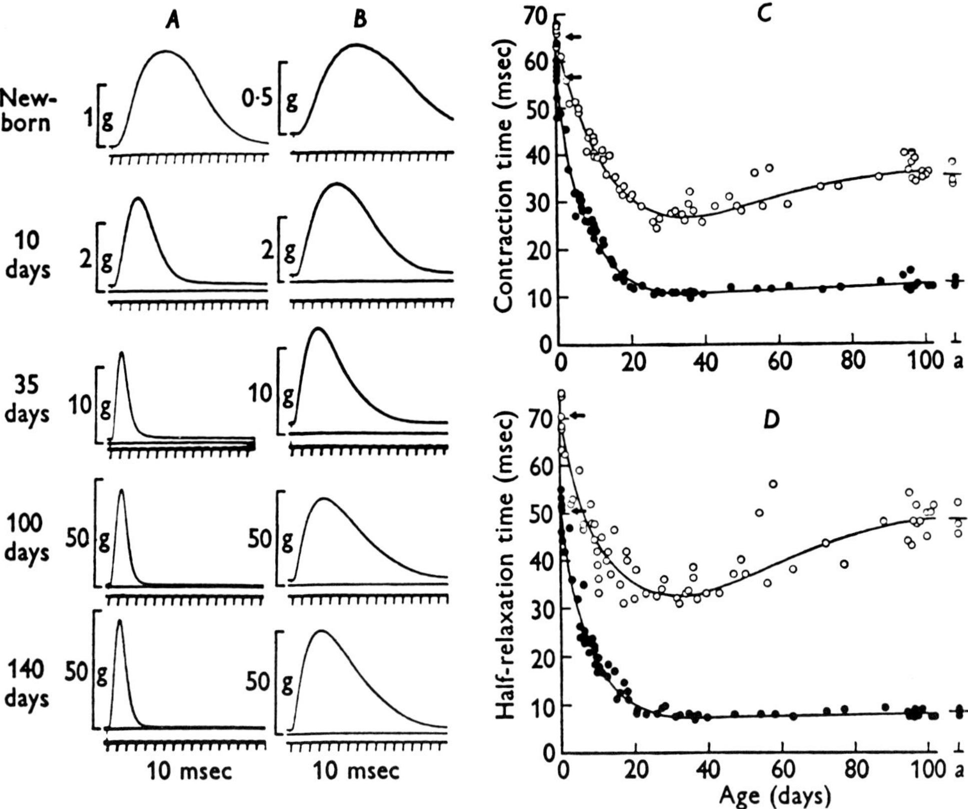

FIG. 10. Time relations of isometric twitch contractions of extensor digitorum longus (EDL) and soleus muscles at various times during development. Representative records of tension: time curves of isometric twitch contractions of EDL and soleus shown in *A* and *B*, respectively. Age of animal indicated in vertical column (*left*). *C* and *D*: times for contraction and half relaxation for EDL (*filled circles*) and soleus (*open circles*) plotted against animal age. *Points* above *a* on abscissas for muscles from animals aged 140 days or more. *Arrows* on graphs in *C* and *D* indicate mean values for contraction and half-relaxation times of soleus (*upper arrows*) and EDL (*lower arrows*) from newborn animals. [From Close (41).]

generation of continuous, tonic patterns of neural activity. The results obtained have yet to be corroborated but are consistent with other studies by Vrbová (179) and with the behavioral activity of baby rats, which do not commence hindlimb postural activity until approximately 8 days postpartum. At that time the duration of antigravity movements is brief, progressively increasing as the animal learns to stand and to run. Because differentiation of fast and slow muscles in the rat hindlimb is clearly evident at birth, specialization must precede and prepare muscle for mature function rather than be the result of imposed demands for support and locomotion. The degree of specialization achieved by the guinea pig in utero (68) amplifies this conclusion. Differentiation into fast and slow muscles thus appears to be a programmed event related to the general maturity of the animal, anticipating and preparing the muscle for future locomotor behavior. Movements of the fetus are probably important in the initiation of diversity, but why an animal requires distinct muscle types in utero is presently obscure.

Histochemical and immunochemical studies also show differential postnatal development of fast and slow muscles (24, 62, 97, 98, 152, 153). Based on histochemical myosin ATPase activity at acid and alkaline pH, adult myofibers are presently classified as slow type I or fast type IIA or IIB, the latter two corresponding to fast red and fast white fibers, respectively. In developing and in injured muscle, type IIC fibers also occur; these are not differentiated by preincubation in acid or alkaline media. In fetal rats all fibers are type IIC. Distinctions between type I and II fibers are clearly evident by 1–2 days postpartum (24, 98), although all type II fibers are IIC and differentiation into type I is incomplete at this time. In future fast muscles Brooke et al. (24) observed differentiation of IIC to IIB fibers by 7 days and of IIC to IIA fibers by approximately 3 wk postpartum.

Rat soleus can be clearly defined with myosin ATPase stains at 2 days postpartum by the comparatively large numbers of developing type I fibers. At this time approximately 50% are differentiating type I and the remainder are type IIC fibers (151); between 2 and 7 days postpartum IIC fibers become IIA. The prolonged yet progressive transformation of IIA to type I fibers (103, 151) is interpreted as a response to the increased weight-bearing demands imposed on the soleus as the animal matures. Kugelberg (103) described the relative proportions of muscle fibers in the 600-g male rat as 90% type I and only 10% type II. Complete transformation to type I fibers occurs in the guinea pig soleus (93). Thus, although the adult guinea pig soleus has uniform metabolic properties, it is—like the rat soleus—derived from a heterogeneous population of cells. This heterogeneous origin is consistent with observed variations in the pattern of cellular response after perturbation.

The localization of myosin ATPase in differentiating fibers can be correlated with staining patterns produced with highly purified antibodies to adult fast and slow muscle myosin. Gauthier et al. (62), for example, found that all of the constitutive type IIC fibers in the diaphragm and EDL of fetal and neonatal rats stain with both antifast and antislow myosin. This pattern persisted until 3 wk postpartum, although the intensity of staining with antislow myosin progressively declined in most fibers. Only in a minority of fibers, presumably differentiating type I fibers, did strong reactivity to antislow myosin remain. Gauthier et al. interpreted the dual affinity for fast and slow myosin to indicate that fast and slow isozymes, or the precursors thereof, coexist within individual fibers; they become segregated into specialized populations as differentiation progresses and polyneural innervation is eliminated. Subsequent recognition of embryonic and neonatal forms of myosin in differentiating rat and rabbit muscle (185) suggests the alternative possibility that these precursors share common antigenic determinants with the mature form (78). Therefore type IIC fibers that stain with both antifast and antislow myosin probably contain either the fetal or neonatal isozyme. These are gradually eliminated and replaced by the specialized mature isozyme as development proceeds (190).

All of these studies document the extensive postnatal maturational changes that occur in muscles of the rat and cat. However, in view of the fundamental differences in structure, function, and metabolism between fast and slow muscles, one is led intuitively to the idea that neuromuscular distinctions already exist in the embryo and slowly unfold postpartum in response to appropriate environmental cues. The specificity of initial neural projections to muscle (69, 70, 79, 105–108) and the early development of central connections appropriate to the integrated function of embryonic muscles (11) strongly support this postulate. Groups of neurons penetrating muscle primordia thus appear to be specified and to anticipate their future function. In addition the studies of Betz et al. (16) and Harris (71, 72) suggest that neural activity is responsible for matching the size of individual muscles with the volume of innervating nerve.

Although myofiber specialization in the rat can be demonstrated postpartum, development of these properties in the prenatal animal has been less easily resolved. Figure 11 includes serial transverse sections of the entire distal limb of a 19-day rat fetus. The sections were stained by the immunoperoxidase method with purified antibodies to fast and slow muscle. All fibers in the soleus and EDL stain equivalently

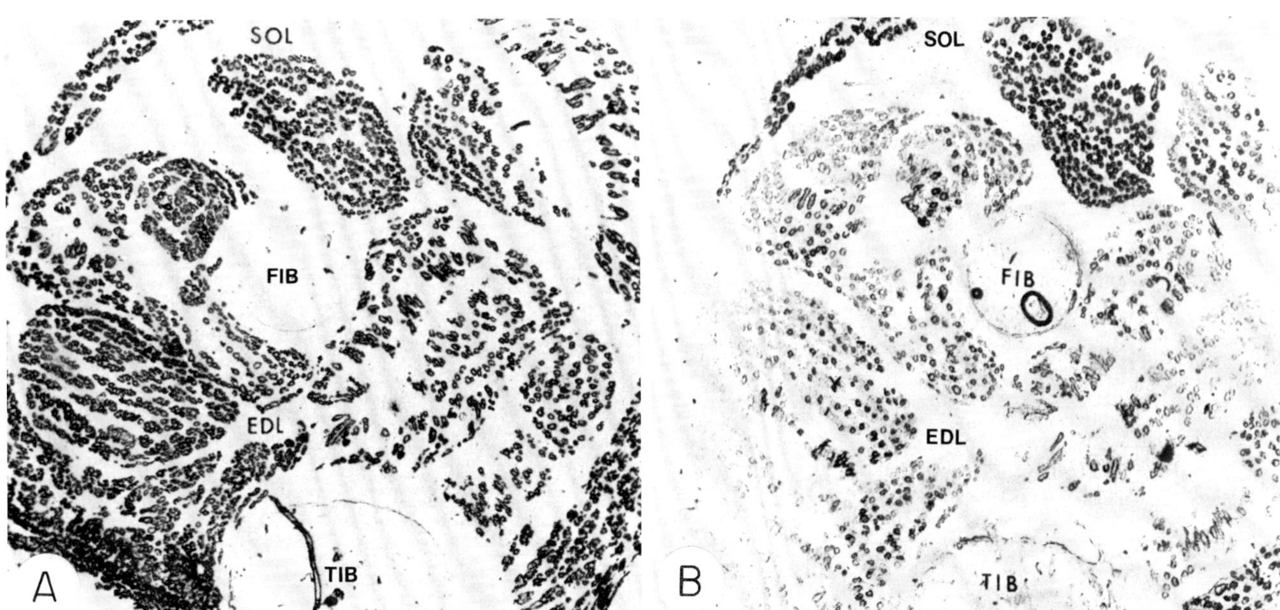

FIG. 11. Serial transverse sections through calf muscles of 19-day fetal rat hindlimb. *FIB*, fibula; *TIB*, tibia. Sections are stained by the indirect peroxidase-antiperoxidase method with antibodies specific to adult fast (*A*) and adult slow (*B*) myosin. By this method positively stained fibers are dark. All fibers in the soleus (*SOL*) and extensor digitorum longus (*EDL*) react positively with antifast myosin, probably reflecting cross-reactivity with an embryonic form of myosin. With antislow myosin almost all soleus fibers stain well, but in *EDL* only a select population of fibers stain well. They are arranged in a nonrandom fashion through the muscle, and their distribution simulates that of slow fibers in the more mature *EDL*.

with antifast antibody, but with antislow antibody there is a differential pattern of staining. Most fibers in the EDL stain weakly with antislow myosin, although a small population of myotubes, interspersed nonrandomly in the EDL, have a strong affinity for antislow myosin. This distribution closely simulates that of differentiating slow fibers in the EDL at 2 and 14 days postpartum (Figs. 12 and 13). All 19-day

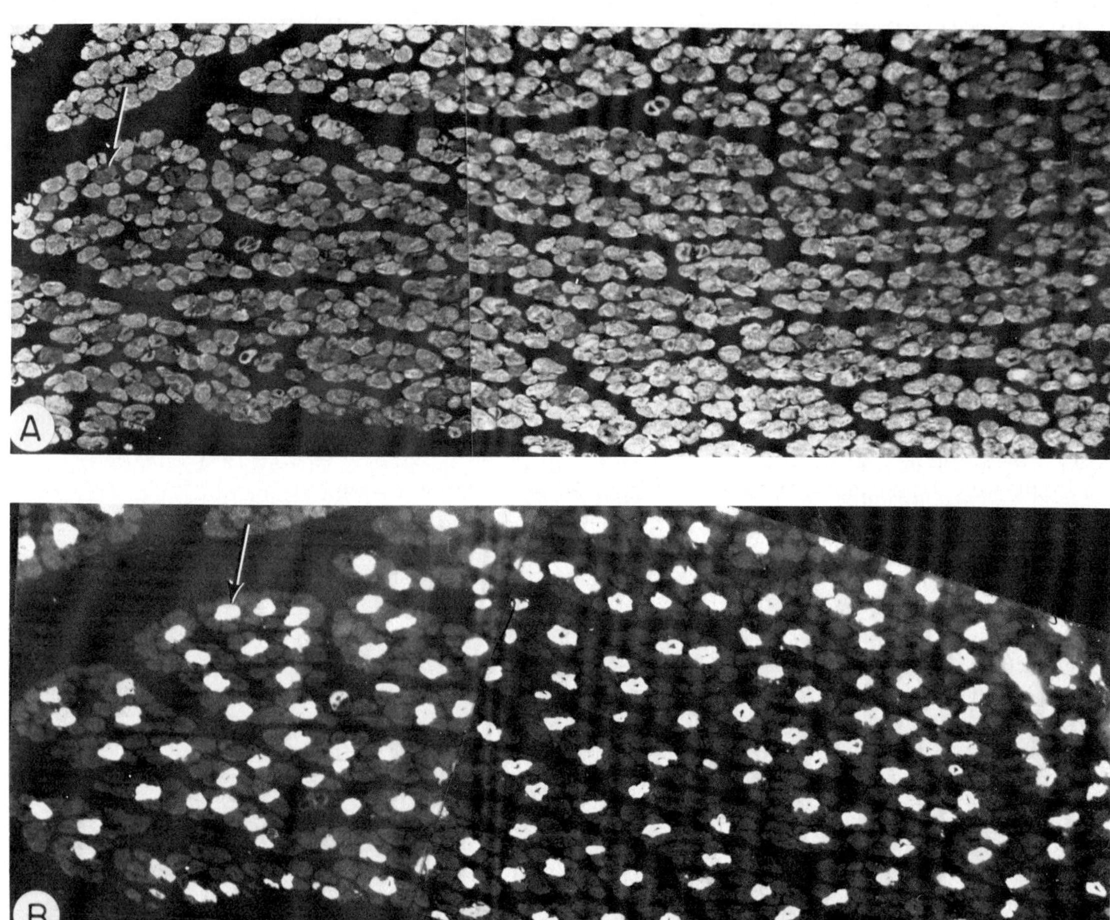

FIG. 12. Rat EDL, 2 days postpartum. Serial, transverse sections stained by direct fluorescence with AF (antifast myosin; *A*) and AS (antislow myosin; *B*). Positively stained fibers are light. Almost all fibers stain well with AF, although a few, widely distributed fibers stain weakly. The latter stain intensely with AS and are thus interpreted to be developing slow fibers.

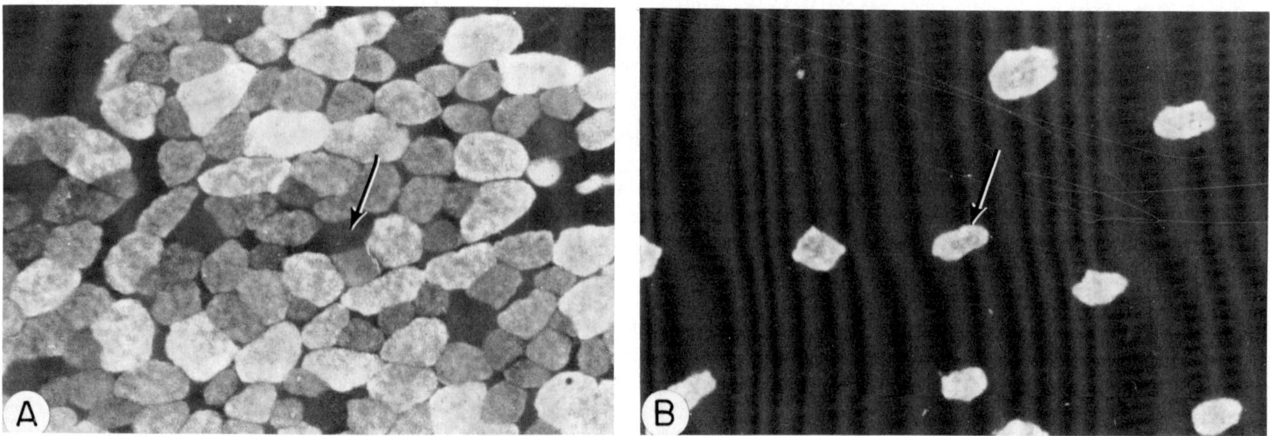

FIG. 13. Rat EDL, 14 days postpartum. Serial, transverse sections stained by direct fluorescence with AF (*A*) and AS (*B*). Adult pattern of myosin staining has been approached. Most but not all fibers are positive with AF; those that do not react with AF now react with AS.

primordial soleus fibers, by contrast, stain with antislow myosin, thus portending their future evolution. Differential characteristics of these future fast and slow muscles therefore are expressed in the rat before parturition and may contribute to the distinction between the contractile properties of these two muscles at birth.

These observations of early neuromuscular specificity contrast with those of Gauthier et al. (62) but correlate with immunochemical studies by Rowlerson (146, 147) and Dhoot and Perry (51). Rowlerson examined developing rat hindlimb muscle by using homologous antibodies prepared against adult rat slow muscle and detected fiber differentiation by 19 days of gestation. Dhoot and Perry used monospecific antibodies to the fast and slow forms of troponin I to study fiber differentiation in the rat hindlimb. In the 18-day fetal limb they found that all fibers stained with antifast troponin I but that only a select population of fibers stained with antislow troponin I. The latter they termed presumptive slow fibers.

What determines these differences? If they are regulated by the nerve then the distinctions in the forms of myosin and in those of the troponin complex of 18-day fetal rats must indicate differences in the motor units innervating the muscles at this stage (97, 134). Because of the importance of fetal movements for normal limb development—particularly the generation of secondary fibers (71, 72)—this possibility cannot be excluded. However, if this specialization is controlled by the nervous system, then selected axons must have obtained dominance over these fetal myotubes despite the presence of multiple innervation. Presently it is not known whether the diversity of the primordial pattern reflects distinctions in impulse activity patterns of nerves innervating prospective fast and slow fibers, but this would be surprising in view of the immaturity of the system and the prevalence of electrical coupling between myotubes at this stage of development. Alternatively Perry and Dhoot (134) speculate that there may be other mechanisms involved in the initiation of muscle specialization.

This question has been approached by several researchers who have concluded that the temporal sequence of muscle assembly from primary- and secondary-generation cells contributes to the evolution of specialized muscle fiber types (5, 6, 97, 98, 153, 195). Though further work is required, these studies conclude that primary cells preferentially develop into slow type I fibers, whereas the majority of secondary myotubes become fast type II fibers (5, 6, 97, 98, 152, 153). Figure 14 is from the EDL of an 18-day rat fetus stained by the peroxidase method with affinity-purified antibodies to adult fast and slow myosin. Most of the large primary fibers stain intensely with both antifast and antislow myosin. These cells are distributed throughout the primordium, and each is intimately surrounded by numerous secondary cells that stain well with antifast but weakly with antislow myosin. Thus there is a quantitative difference in antibody affinity between the primary and secondary cells, and it seems probable that this reflects the presence of both slow and embryonic myosins within the same cell. As development progresses (Figs. 11–13) secondary cells persistently stain well only with antifast myosin, and affinity for antislow myosin gradually diminishes as they differentiate into fast type II myofibers. By contrast the affinity of primary cells for antifast myosin progressively declines, and in the postnatal animal they stain well only with antislow myosin. As in Dhoot and Perry's analysis these are interpreted as emerging type I cells (97, 153).

In 18-day fetal soleus all myotubes stain with both antifast and antislow myosin, and in contrast to EDL there appears to be little evidence of heterogeneity (Fig. 15). One reason for this is the relative paucity of secondary cells in the primordium. They form later and apparently in fewer numbers than in the EDL. When they do form, however, their staining properties are comparable to those of EDL (Fig. 16). Indeed the relation between primary "slow" and secondary "fast" fibers is most clearly seen in the soleus at birth. The population of fast fibers observed in the soleus at 14 days postpartum (Fig. 17) thus almost certainly arises from secondary myotubes. Early in ontogeny, therefore, distinct architectural and antigenic identities can be recognized between the primordia of the soleus and EDL; furthermore these can be correlated with the destiny of these muscles in the mature limb.

There is an analogy between this pattern of development of extrafusal fibers and the sequence of intrafusal fiber assembly in the fetal and neonatal rat. Milburn (118) describes the first fibers formed in the evolving spindle as nuclear bag fibers that resemble slow, tonic, extrafusal fibers. New secondary generations develop by appositional growth around their walls; these are the intermediate fibers that are most comparable to extrafusal, slow-twitch fibers. Finally nuclear chain fibers develop by appositional growth on the nuclear bag and intermediate fibers. Nuclear chain fibers have properties resembling fast-twitch muscle.

Figure 18 is a hypothetical model summarizing some of the data on neuromuscular histogenesis and specialization discussed here. It proposes that the temporal sequence of assembly is important in determining the initial expression of diversity. Primary-generation cells are depicted as receiving the first neural contacts (shown as permanent synapses) from pioneering axons. The primary cells are thought to be organized into fundamental motor units responsible for generating the earliest fetal movements (97). These cells develop into slow fibers, though the forms of myosin they contain in the fetus and neonate is uncertain. The rise of secondary-generation cells on the walls of primary myotubes is correlated with the intrusion of new orders of axons. The cells become fast fibers, at least initially, and their innervation is derived from branches of the multiple axons that transiently synapse with the primary cell.

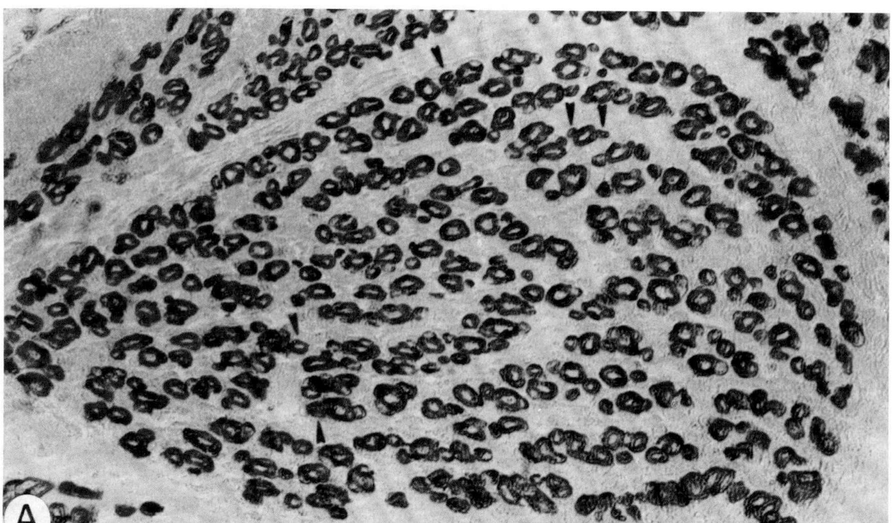

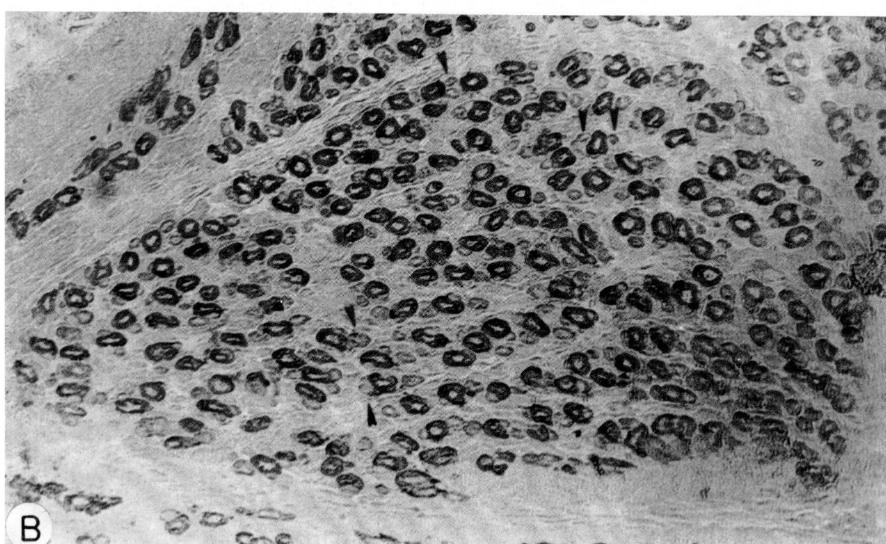

FIG. 14. Rat EDL, 18 days of gestation. Serial, transverse sections stained by the peroxidase-antiperoxidase (PAP) method with AF (*A*) and AS (*B*). Muscle primordium is composed mainly of large primary-generation myotubes, most of which stain well with both AF and AS. *Arrows*, a few secondary-generation cells attached to the walls of primary myotubes. All of these react strongly with AF and weakly with AS. [From Rubinstein and Kelly (153).]

The model, however, is a simplistic one: it is unlikely that a single mechanism such as sequence of fiber formation moderates the whole developmental order of specialization. Many factors are involved in this complex and dynamic process, and the initial model is clearly modified as the animal matures. As previously discussed, secondary type II fibers of the neonatal rat soleus undergo an adaptive transformation to type I cells, apparently as the demands for weight bearing increase in the maturing animal (103). Not all primary fibers become type I cells, however, as evidenced in studies by Beermann et al. (10) and A. M. Kelly and N. A. Rubinstein (unpublished observations) of the fetal pig and guinea pig, respectively. Hence primary cells are not all endogenously programmed to be slow fibers; other factors, possibly related to positional distribution in the limb, contribute to the initial pattern of gene expression. The data thus suggest an initial pattern of specificity that is expressed very early in myogenesis and reflects an intrinsic program of neuromuscular development. This program predicts future muscle function. It is then finely adjusted in the maturing animal for optimal locomotor activity. The inherent program may also define the physiological limits of muscle plasticity.

CONTRACTILE PROTEINS

Myosin

A decade ago there appeared to be little mystery or ambiguity surrounding the contractile proteins of developing muscle. A variety of studies showed that the time course of contraction and relaxation was slow in both future fast and slow muscles (29, 30, 41, 42, 63). Despite the fact that twitch times were slower than in mature slow muscle, researchers believed that fast fibers formed from a muscle akin to that of adult slow

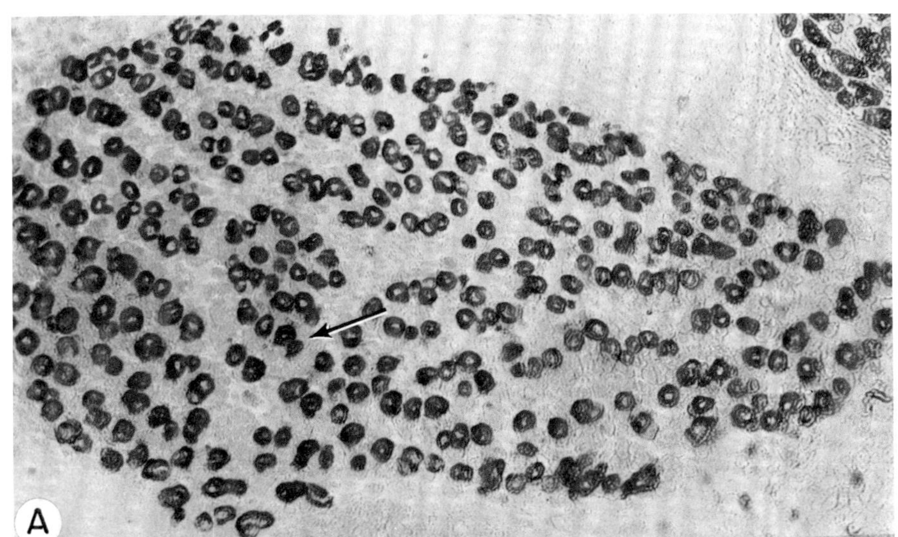

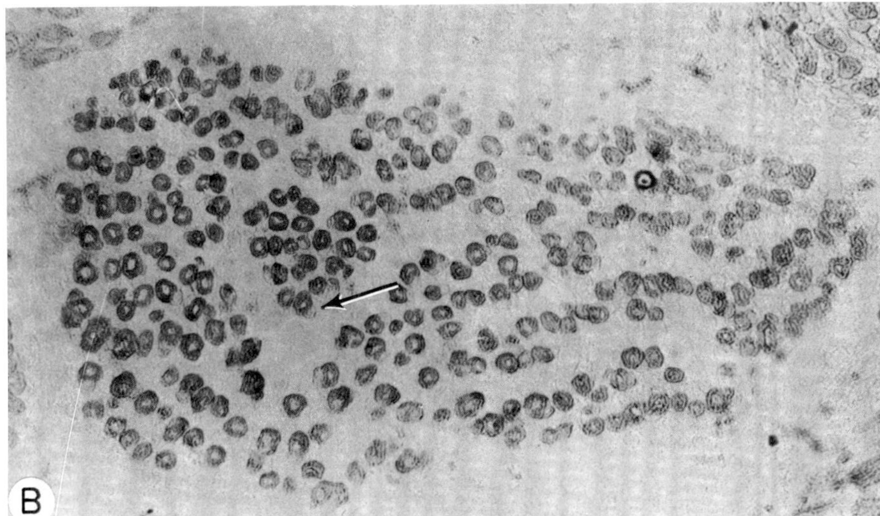

FIG. 15. Rat soleus, 18 days of gestation. Serial, transverse sections stained by the PAP method with AF (*A*) and AS (*B*). All primary- and secondary-generation fibers react strongly with AF. Unlike EDL, most soleus fibers are primary cells; there are very few secondary cells. Like EDL, however, most primary fibers additionally react with AS, whereas few of the secondary fibers bind this antibody well. *Arrow*, secondary cells reacting strongly with AF but weakly with AS. [From Rubinstein and Kelly (153).]

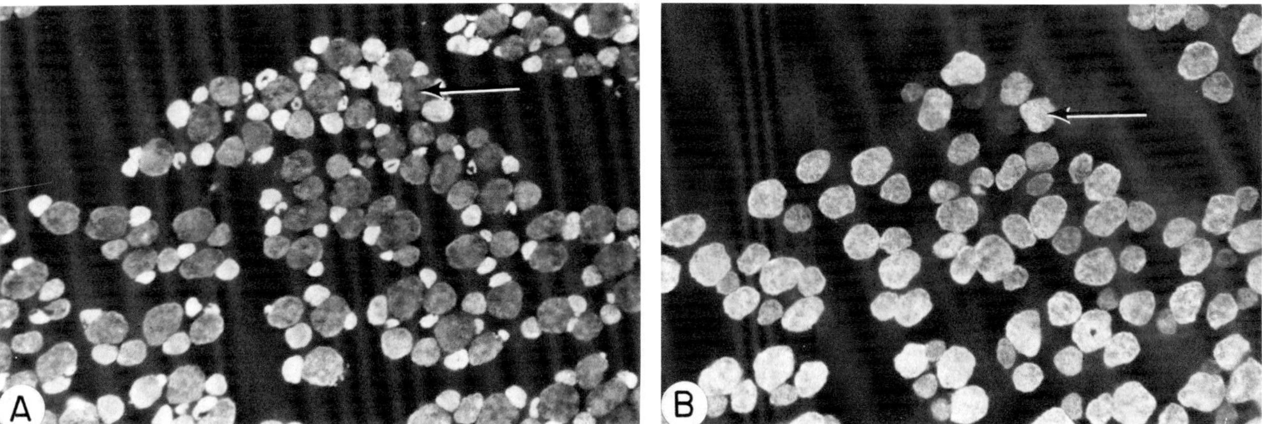

FIG. 16. Rat soleus, 2 days postpartum. Serial, transverse sections stained with AF (*A*) and AS (*B*) by direct fluorescence. By this stage most soleus fibers react weakly with AF but continue to stain well with AS. A number of smaller secondary-generation fibers are seen closely apposed to larger fibers. These stain well with AF but weakly with AS.

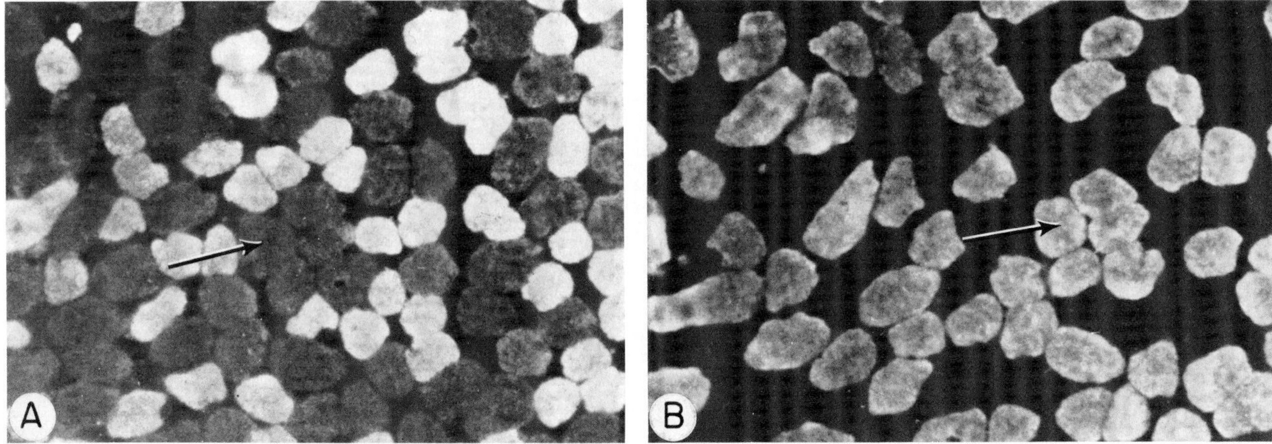

FIG. 17. Rat soleus, 14 days postpartum. Serial, transverse sections stained with AF (*A*) and AS (*B*) by direct fluorescence. Fifty percent of the fibers react intensely with AF and not at all with AS. These are usually comparatively small and are interpreted to be secondary-generation cells. The other 50% react well with AS and not with AF. These are the larger cells of the muscle and are interpreted to be primary-generation, slow fibers.

muscle. Investigations of the biochemical characteristics of myosin in differentiating muscle, particularly in the rabbit, appeared consistent with this interpretation. Initial estimates claimed that Ca^{2+}-activated ATPase activity in fetal rabbits was low and that the myosin also lacked 3-methylhistidine residues (177); these properties were seen in adult slow-twitch but not in adult fast-twitch muscle. Methylated histidine emerged gradually during the 1st mo postpartum in developing rabbit muscle and at about 5 wk approached the amount present in the adult. Huszar (81) subsequently showed that this change was not a result of a lack of histidine residues but more likely was caused by a deficiency of the methylating enzyme system in fetal muscle. More importantly Huszar also discovered differences in amino acid sequences in the three methylhistidine peptides obtained from fetal compared with adult myosins. This was the first demonstration of developmental differences in the primary structure of myosin. Interest in the isomeric forms of myofibrillar protein as markers of differentiation has expanded in recent years largely because of the development of suitable analytic probes, particularly polyacrylamide gel electrophoresis. The isozymes of myosin are a primary research focus because of the correlation in adult muscle between the pattern of neural control, the speed of shortening, and the rate at which myosin hydrolyzes ATP (8). There is further evidence of developmental variation in the forms of myosin light chains and heavy chains, as well as in those of the regulatory proteins tropomyosin and troponin. Surprisingly, although the entire complex array of contractile proteins is coordinately assembled into the myofilaments of early myotubes (49), the polymorphic forms of these proteins vary independently during the course of differentiation. For example, the fast light chains LC1F and LC2F in adult human muscle are associated with distinct heavy chains in fast red and fast white fibers, respectively (17). These light chains are prominent in differentiating muscle (180) where they associate with embryonic and neonatal forms of heavy chain (190). Even hybrids of fast and slow myosin subunits (including the light-chain subunits) have been seen within single fibers of normal adult muscle, adding further to the complexity of the system (17, 84, 196).

The levels of actomyosin ATPase activity in developing muscle also present a confusing picture. Differentiating muscles have significantly slower speeds of contraction than their mature counterparts. In the neonatal rat, actomyosin ATPase activity is low but increases with development in both fast and slow muscles, although much less conspicuously in the latter (53, 123, 174). Paradoxically the levels of ATPase enzyme activity are high in the embryonic chick—comparable to those in mature fast muscles (12, 38, 52, 165, 168). Hence the correlation between speed of contraction and level of actomyosin ATPase activity, though valid for the adult, may be subject to species variation and may not apply in all developing muscles.

These diverse results have caused a great deal of confusion and controversy in understanding the forms of contractile protein in differentiating muscle. Because a unified summary of pertinent literature is not possible, results of various studies in the field are discussed under three separate headings, more or less in the chronological order in which they have appeared in the literature.

DIFFERENTIATING MUSCLE INITIALLY CONTAINS A FORM OF FAST MUSCLE MYOSIN. Because of their size (mol wt 200,000) the myosin heavy chains do not readily penetrate sodium dodecyl sulfate (SDS) polyacrylamide gels, and until recently information on

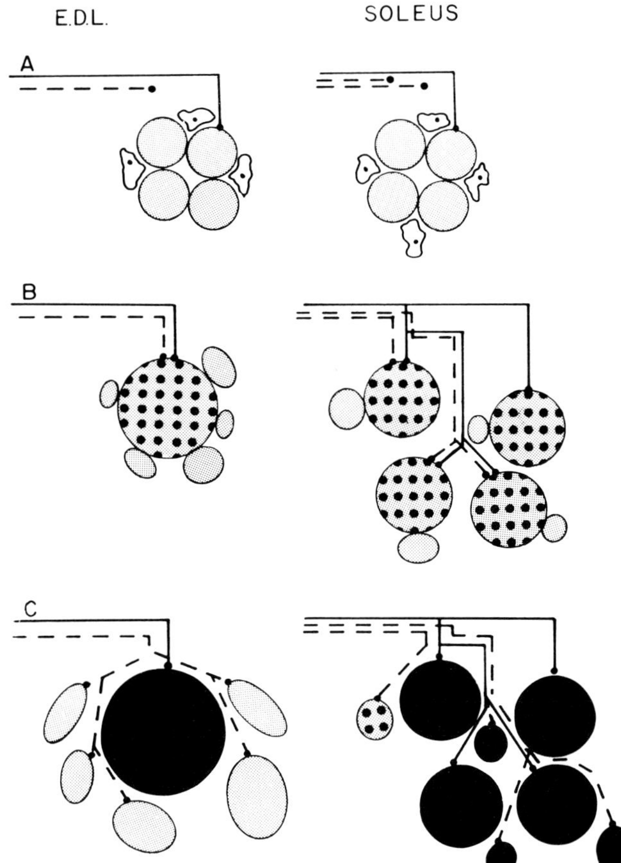

FIG. 18. Possible sequence of events leading to muscle fiber diversity. *Light area*, appreciable reaction of cells only with AF; *dotted area*, significant reaction with both AF and AS; *dark area*, appreciable reaction only with AS. *A*: group of primary-generation fibers, surrounded by replicating mononucleated myoblasts, are being innervated by a pathfinder motoneuron (*solid line*). *B*: small, secondary-generation cells have formed and are attached to primary cell walls. Successive cohorts of motoneurons (*broken lines*) are constrained to innervate the primary cell at the neuromuscular junction determined by the pathfinder motoneuron. Separate innervation of secondary cells is unusual at this time. Primary cells stain heavily with antibody to slow as well as to fast myosin; secondary cells stain heavily only with AF. *C*: secondary cells have relinquished their intimate connections with primary cells and have become independently innervated; their innervation is apparently derived from the multiple innervation of primary cells. At this point a major difference between developing fast and slow muscles is seen. While practically all secondary cells in fast muscle mature as type II fibers, most secondary soleus cells slowly convert to type I fibers during the 1st yr after birth (25). Generation of type I fibers from secondary cells postpartum may depend on the pattern of muscle usage, whereas initial formation of type I fibers from primary cells may have a different cause. [From Rubinstein and Kelly (153).]

these subunits has been lacking. The myosin light chains, however, are readily resolved by one- and two-dimensional SDS gel electrophoresis, and a number of studies on myogenesis have concentrated on these subunits.

In most adult fast muscles there are three light chains: the alkali light chains LC1F and LC3F with molecular weights of 25,000 and 16,000, respectively (182), and LC2F—also known as the 5′, 5′-dithiobis(2-nitrobenzoate) or DTNB light chain—with a molecular weight of 18,000. In mature muscle the amount of LC1F plus LC3F is approximately equal to the amount of LC2F. In most adult slow muscle, by comparison, there are only two light chains, LC1S and LC2S, present in equal proportions and having molecular weights of 27,000 and 19,000, respectively (111, 159, 181).

Because of the physiological characteristics of developing muscle, it was anticipated that the light-chain complement of fetal muscle would be analogous to that of adult slow myosin. Thus it came as a surprise when Sréter et al. (168) demonstrated that the light chains of embryonic chicken muscle both in vivo and in vitro were identical to those of adult fast muscle (Fig. 19). The one distinction was that LC3F was present in much lower proportions in the embryo than in the adult, a finding that was consistent with previous studies by Dow and Stracher (52). These observations have since been confirmed both in the chicken and in a variety of mammals (38, 87, 127, 138, 148, 149, 151, 154, 173–175), and it is indisputable that the

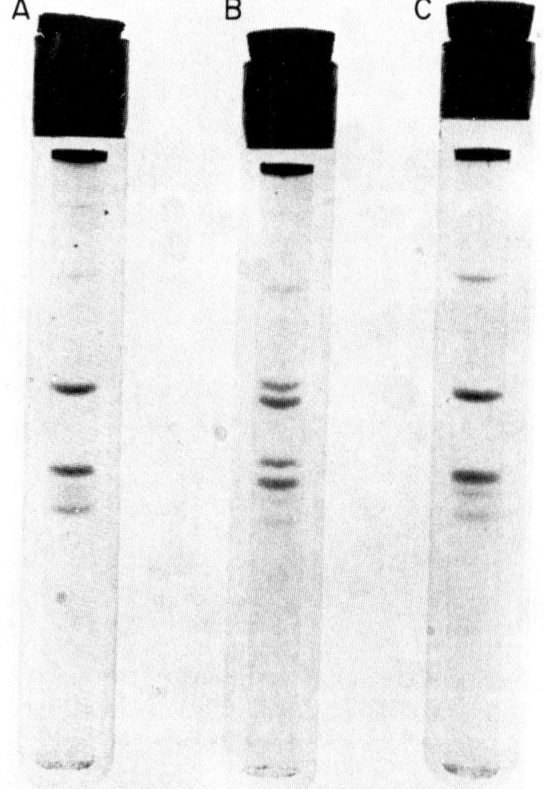

FIG. 19. Coelectrophoresis of embryonic and adult myosin samples in 12.5% polyacrylamide gels. *A*: myosins from embryonic chicken muscle (15 μg) and adult fast-twitch muscle (15 μg). *B*: myosins from embronic chicken muscle (20 μg) and adult slow tonic muscle (30 μg). *C*: embryonic chicken twitch muscle myosin (30 μg). [From Sréter et al. (168).]

primordia of both fast and slow muscles contain significant proportions of fast light chains having the same charge and molecular weight as those in adult fast muscle.

Syrovy (173) and Roy et al. (148, 149) have studied the stoichiometry of the three fast light chains at successive stages of development in the rabbit and chicken. Early in development LC3F is either absent or present in very small proportions, and the major species are LC1F and LC2F. As development proceeds the relative proportions of LC2F remain constant, but the proportions of LC1F decline and reciprocally those of LC3F increase (Fig. 20). Using pyrophosphate gels of native myosin, Hoh (76) and Hoh and Yeoh (78) have produced results that compare with these findings, and they led Hoh (76) to observe that the myosin with the greatest relative amounts of LC3F has the highest actin-activated ATPase activity. Thus the developing muscle's progressive increase in speed can be correlated with the distribution of myosin isozymes. Julian et al. (90) have since raised questions about such a correlation: in skinned single fibers from neonatal and adult rabbit fast- and slow-twitch muscle, they found no consistent relation between the maximum velocity of shortening (V_{max}), tension development, and the relative amounts of light chains. These researchers conclude that, whereas the particular complement of light chains correlates with mature muscle type, fast or slow, the relative amounts of these light chains do not directly determine V_{max}. Consistent with this and equally surprising are their results showing that V_{max} values for the newborn and adult fast-twitch rabbit psoas fibers do not differ significantly and are constantly above those obtained for adult soleus fibers.

The light-chain complement of developing fast muscles in the fetal rat predominantly contains LC1F and LC2F (Fig. 21). Small proportions of LC1S are also present for a short time early in differentiation (A. M. Kelly and N. A. Rubinstein, unpublished observations). In early stages of slow muscle development in the rabbit, rat, and chicken (132, 138, 154), light chains with electrophoretic mobilities identical to adult LC1S, LC2S, LC1F, and LC2F are present. The relative proportions of slow light chains progressively increase with development and concomitantly those of fast light chains decline (Fig. 21). Whether the initial synthesis of fast light chains is suppressed in developing slow muscle or is simply eclipsed by the progressively increasing proportions of slow subunits is unclear: in the adult guinea pig soleus, which is a muscle uniformly composed of type I slow-twitch fibers, small proportions of the fast light chain LC1F coexist with the predominant slow light chains (A. M. Kelly and N. A. Rubinstein, unpublished observations). A recent corroborative finding by Billeter et al. (17) and Ishiura et al.(84) was that LC1F is present in a significant proportion of mature slow fibers of human muscle. Both groups of authors speculate that this is associated with transformation from fast to slow muscle, and Ishiura et al. conclude that it is an expression of LC1F resistance to change.

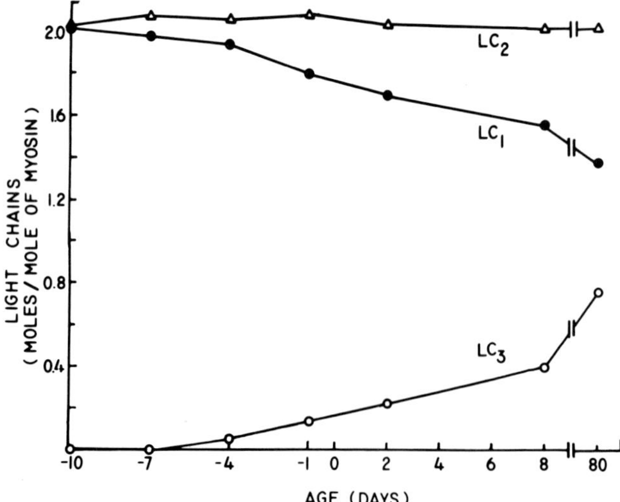

FIG. 20. Time course of developmental changes of the 3 fast light chains in chicken breast muscle. [From Roy et al. (149).]

Conventional gel electrophoresis studies on the light-chain pattern from cultured presumptive fast and slow muscles of the chicken were initially reported to contain light chains only of the fast type (150). Rubinstein and Holtzer (150) thus hypothesized that all muscles originate from fibers that exclusively synthesize fast muscle myosin, whereas slow myosin is induced through physiological activity imposed by the nerve (150, 151, 154). Subsequent work requires reevaluation of this analysis, but the endogenous programming of fast-myosin synthesis and the neural dependence of slow-myosin synthesis are key concepts supported by numerous studies.

Rat hindlimbs denervated at birth and examined at 14 days show that the light-chain composition of fast-twitch EDL is virtually unaltered compared with the soleus, where significant proportions of fast light chains persist (151). Morphologically these results correlate with the persistence of large numbers of fibers that stain intensely with myofibrillar ATPase, whereas in normal innervated muscle there is a gradual transition of such fibers toward the type I phenotype (103). Margreth et al. (112) have described changes very similar to those of neonatal denervation in rats that were cordotomized at birth and examined at age 3 mo. In addition Carraro et al. (35, 36) have shown in adult rat diaphragm and gastrocnemius muscles denervated for 6 mo that a fast type of myosin heavy and light chain is selectively preserved and that no evidence of slow myosin, normally present in these mixed muscles, can be detected.

If the hindlimbs of adult rats are rendered electrically silent by spinal cord transection at the level of T_{13}-L_1, the light chains of the immobilized EDL are unaltered; in the soleus, however, significant proportions of fast light chains are evident in addition to slow

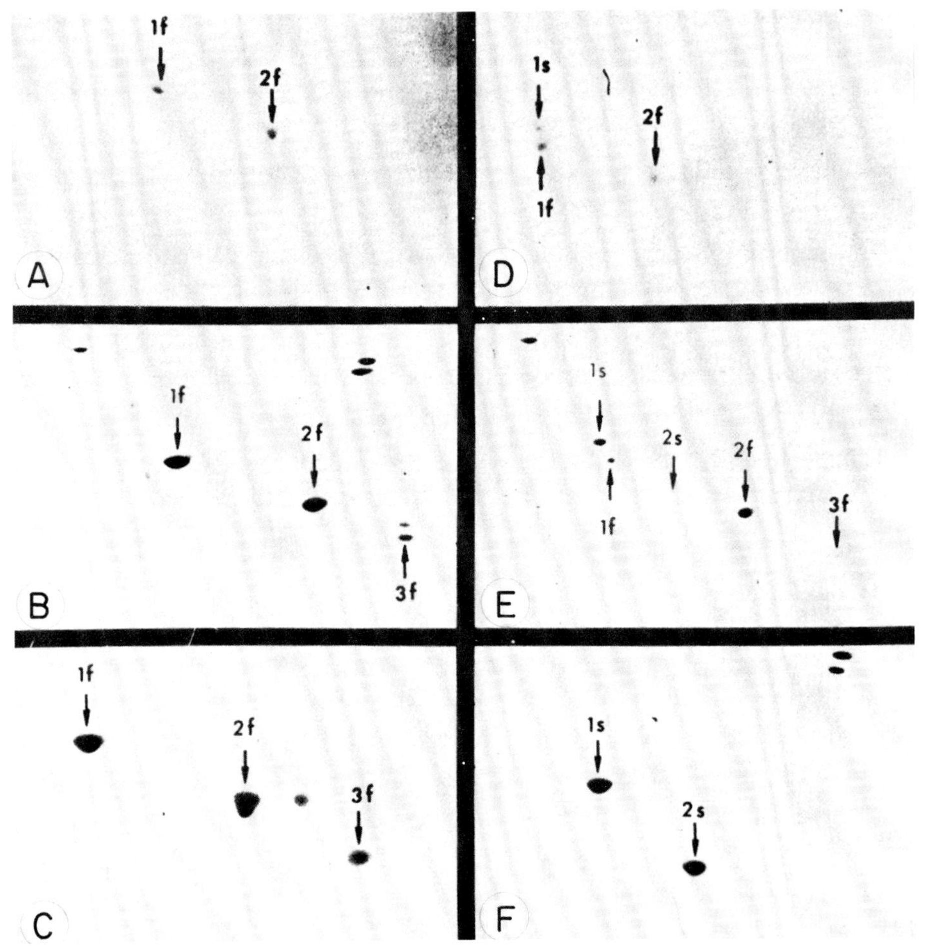

FIG. 21. Two-dimensional electrophoresis of EDL and soleus myosin light chains at different ages. *A–C*: EDL myosin light chains at 19 days in utero, 2 days postpartum, and adult age, respectively. *D–F*: soleus myosin light chains at 19 days in utero, 2 days postpartum, and adult age, respectively. Fast myosin light chains represented as follows: LC1F = 1f, LC2F = 2f, LC3F = 3f. Slow myosin light chains are LC1S = 1s, LC2S = 2s. [From Rubinstein and Kelly (152).]

light chains and there is a parallel increase in type II fibers (151). These observations have since been confirmed by Steinbach et al. (170), who observed a complete transformation from slow to fast in light chains of the soleus immobilized by cordotomy for over a year. Similarly, when the hindlimbs of neonatal kittens were rendered electrically silent by spinal cord transection coupled with section of the lumbar dorsal roots, Buller et al. (29) noted that the increase in speed of contraction of the developing fast-twitch muscles was very close to normal. Conversely the contraction time of the prospective slow-twitch muscle increased, and in a few weeks the speed of contraction of the soleus became nearly as fast as that of a normal fast muscle (Fig. 22). Gallego et al. (59) have since confirmed these early findings in the cat, and Danieli-Betto and Midrio (46) have described comparable electrophysiological changes in neonatally cordotomized rats. All of these studies suggest that slow muscle is uniquely dependent on tonic patterns of impulse activity from the motoneuron (157, 158), and if this is modified there is an inherent tendency to acquire some of the characteristics of fast-twitch muscle. Though the light chains in perturbed slow muscles may be identical to those of fast muscle, presently nothing is known of the heavy chains to which they are attached. Recent studies suggest that there is more heterogeneity among myosin heavy than light chains (190), and variations in the heavy chains may explain some of the confusing histochemical and physiological events (56, 66) occurring after denervation.

A series of studies by Hoh et al. (77) has demonstrated a great deal more of the complexity of these responses. These authors, by using pyrophosphate gel electrophoresis, examined the myosin isozymes in rat hindlimbs 8 wk after cordotomy. This technique affords the opportunity of examining myosin under nondenaturing conditions (75). The light-chain composition of each isozyme can be further analyzed by cutting the isozymes from pyrophosphate gels and subjecting the slices to conventional SDS gel electrophoresis.

In normal rat hindlimb muscles five isozymes can be resolved, isozyme 1 having the greatest electrophoretic mobility and isozyme 5 the least. The soleus is predominantly composed of isozyme 5 with small proportions of isozyme 4. The rat EDL has the fast isozymes 1, 2, 3, and 4 (Fig. 23) and in this respect is distinct from the rabbit and chicken, which have only isozymes 1, 2, and 3. When run on SDS gels, isozyme 5 from the soleus contains roughly equal proportions

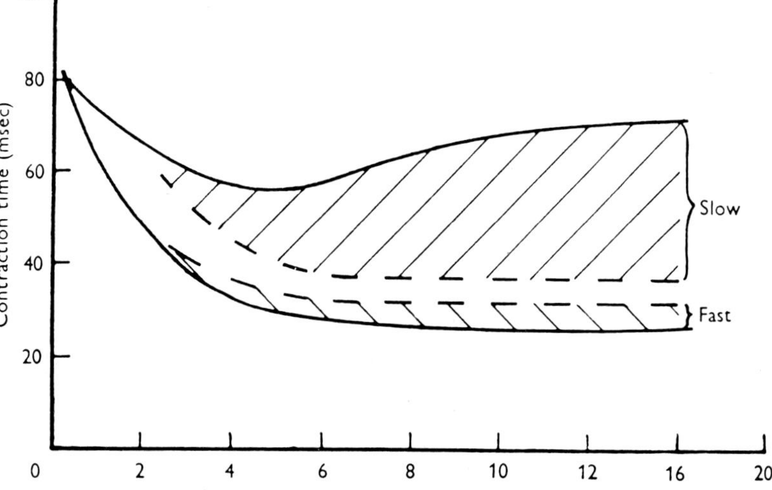

FIG. 22. *Solid lines,* standard developmental time courses (contraction time–age curves) for slow and fast muscles in the cat. *Broken lines,* postulated time course for these muscles in the absence of suprasegmental neural influences. [From Buller et al. (29).]

of LC1S and LC2S (Fig. 23). No details of the composition of isozyme 4 in the normal soleus are given here.

Although the profile of EDL was not significantly changed after cordotomy, which is consistent with previous studies, the soleus underwent a dramatic change (Fig. 24). Isozyme 5 was almost completely suppressed, and the profile was dominated by isozymes 3 and 4. Analysis of isozyme 4 revealed that it was composed of LC1S, LC1F, and LC2F in a ratio of 1:1:2. There was no LC2S. This unusual stoichiometry suggests the presence of a light-chain heterodimer LC1S-LC2F, LC1F-LC2F synthesized within individual cells. An isozyme with comparable light-chain mixture was also found in cross-innervation experiments by Hoh et al. (77). The heavy-chain composition of isozyme 4 is unclear, but they speculate that it may be a unique species.

These interesting results refine the understanding of nerve influences on muscle. Maintenance of isozyme 5 in the soleus appears to be critically dependent on normal, mature, motoneuron activity. If this activity is suppressed, as occurs after cordotomy, isozyme 5 is also suppressed. However, after 8 wk it is not replaced by an isozyme characteristic of mature fast muscle but by a new species with a unique, mixed or transitional, light-chain composition.

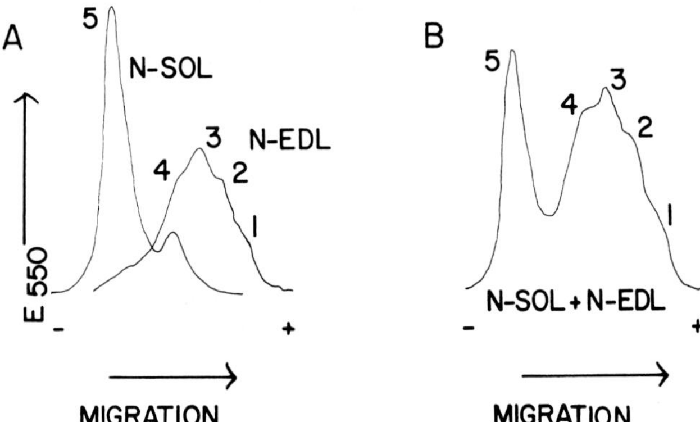

FIG. 23. Myosin isozyme profiles from normal slow-twitch soleus (N-SOL) and normal fast-twitch EDL (N-EDL) muscles of the rat. Electrophoresis with 4% polyacrylamide gels was performed for 9 h at 80 V and in 20 mM sodium pryophosphate buffer (pH 8.8, with 10% glycerol). Gels were stained in Coomassie blue and scanned at 550 nm. *A*: profile from each muscle superimposed. *B*: results of coelectrophoresis. Numbers indicate different types of myosin isozymes. [From Hoh et al. (77).]

DIFFERENTIATING MUSCLE HAS LIGHT CHAINS OF BOTH FAST AND SLOW MUSCLE. In contrast to the foregoing interpretation it has been proposed by other investigators that significant amounts of slow as well as fast isozymes of myosin coexist in the same fibers during early development (62). This interpretation, consistent with earlier and less critical analyses (113), is primarily based on work with developing rat muscle and involves immunocytochemical studies with a variety of highly specific antisera. Gauthier et al. (62) report that all fibers in 19-day fetal rat diaphragm and EDL muscles react strongly with both antifast and antislow sera.

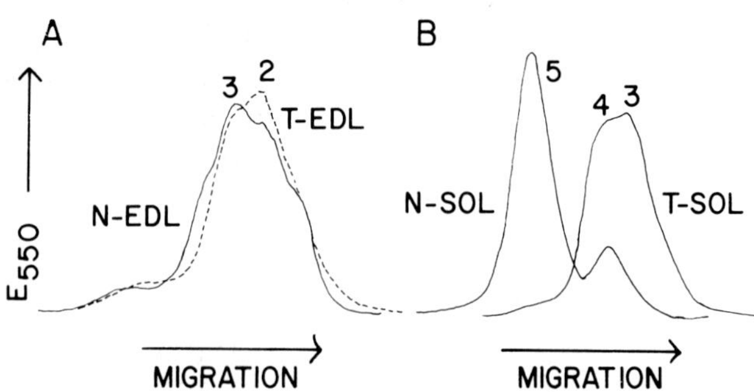

FIG. 24. Myosin isozyme profiles of EDL and soleus muscles of normal and cordotomized rat. *A*: superimposed myosin isozyme profiles for EDL from normal (N-EDL, *solid line*) and cordotomized (T-EDL, *broken line*) rats. *B*: superimposed myosin isozyme profiles for soleus from normal (N-SOL) and cordotomized (T-SOL) rats. Muscles from cordotomized rat, 8 wk postoperatively, and from normal rat of same age. [From Hoh et al. (77).]

The pattern of staining changed slowly postpartum, and it was not until after approximately 21 days that the adult pattern was fully established—with a majority of the fibers in the EDL staining with antifast myosin but not with antislow myosin. From these results it was concluded that synthesis of slow myosin or of an embryonic myosin with antigenic determinants common to slow myosin is switched off in most fast-twitch muscle fibers during the course of differentiation and that an alternate sequence of events occurred in differentiating slow muscle. The authors speculate that the presence of both fast and slow myosin within immature cells is correlated with the occurrence of polyneural innervation characteristic of early developing muscle (7, 15, 25, 47, 48, 142). Inappropriate myosins are tuned out in response to withdrawal of multiple innervation as the neuromuscular system matures. This idea introduced the concept that as evolution progresses, quantitative rather than qualitative differences emerge between muscle fibers. The continuous spectrum of metabolic enzyme concentrations found in various mature myofibers is consistent with this, as are recent biochemical studies of the forms of myosin in single fibers in both humans (17) and bovines (196). These fibers reveal a great deal more heterogeneity than is apparent from histochemical stains of muscle made by the myosin ATPase reaction.

Additional studies of the synthetic activity of cultured chick and quail muscle with [^{35}S]methionine and gel electrophoresis (94, 171, 172) are consistent with the interpretation of Gauthier et al. (62). The entire subset of five light chains can be recognized in autoradiograms prepared from two-dimensional gels, although they are inapparent in the same gels conventionally stained with Coomassie blue. The reason for the discrepancy lies in the observation by Keller and Emerson (94) that fast light chains in these cultured muscles are synthesized at 4–5 times the rate of slow light chains. Thus one effect of the nerve operating in vivo may be to selectively increase low rates of endogenous synthesis of slow myosin, and this acceleration proceeds at different rates in various motor units as a response to functional demand. Conversely, endocrine secretions such as thyroid hormone may selectively suppress synthesis of slow myosin or increase its rate of degradation in order to foster differentiation of fast fibers.

Although they are present in these cultured avian muscles, both sets of light chains have not yet been found in cultured mammalian muscle. Whalen and his colleagues (186), for example, used [^{35}S]methionine to investigate the light-chain complement of cultured muscle cells from rats and did not observe slow light chains in their two-dimensional gel autoradiograms.

DIFFERENTIATING MUSCLE HAS UNIQUE EMBRYONIC ISOZYMES. A third analysis of the myosin synthesized by developing muscle in vivo and in vitro has been advanced by Hoh and Yeoh (78), Rushbrook and Stracher (155), and Whalen and his colleagues (185–188, 190). Using two-dimensional gel electrophoresis, Whalen et al. (186) investigated the earliest forms of myosin produced by postfusion myotubes in culture and identified a polypeptide with a molecular weight similar to that of LC1F but with slightly more acidic charge properties. By rigorous criteria this was shown to be a myosin light chain that is not present in adult muscle. In primary rat cultures it is more abundantly synthesized than LC1F during the first several days after fusion, but this pattern of gene expression changes and by 6 days after fusion LC1F predominates. This prototype light chain is also present in small amounts in fetal and neonatal rat muscle but is not found after 12 days postpartum. This suggests that its synthesis is turned off as development proceeds (Fig. 25), and thus it was designated as an embryonic light chain. Further studies revealed embryonic light chains in fetal skeletal muscles of mice, rabbits, and calves, as well as in differentiating cardiac tissues (185, 189, 191). In fetal guinea pig skeletal muscle, Kelly and Rubinstein (unpublished observations) have identified an embryonic light chain that, consistent with the results of Whalen and Thornell (191), comigrates with the heaviest light chain of atrial myosin. In chick muscle, however, embryonic light chains have not yet been discovered.

In view of these results, as well as the previous observations of Huszar (81) and Sréter et al. (165), Whalen and his colleagues proceeded to investigate the heavy chains of differentiating muscle in vivo and in vitro by proteolytic cleavage of SDS-denatured myosin with either chymotrypsin or *Staphylococcus aureus* proteinase (182, 188, 190). By this technique large numbers of polypeptides are liberated, and they can then be analyzed by one- and two-dimensional gel electrophoresis. These peptide maps show that the heavy chains of slow and cardiac muscle are closely related and that there are differences between these and the degradation products of bulk, presumably fast muscle myosin. Myosins from in vivo embryonic tissues, primary cultures, and the myogenic cell line L6 also have analogous cleavage patterns. Although small amounts of fast myosin polypeptides are present, there are basic differences in these patterns compared with those of adult fast and slow muscles (Fig. 26). Again it was found that fast light chains may associate with these precursor forms of myosin as well as with the myosin of fully differentiated fast muscle.

Additional studies correlate with the analyses of Whalen and his colleagues. Hoh and Yeoh (78) have described the presence of a unique heavy chain in neonatal rabbit muscle. Rushbrook and Stracher (155) have demonstrated variations between the heavy chains of embryonic and adult fast and slow muscle in the chicken that probably represent different gene products. Rushbrook and Stracher also draw attention to the general similarity between the cleavage prod-

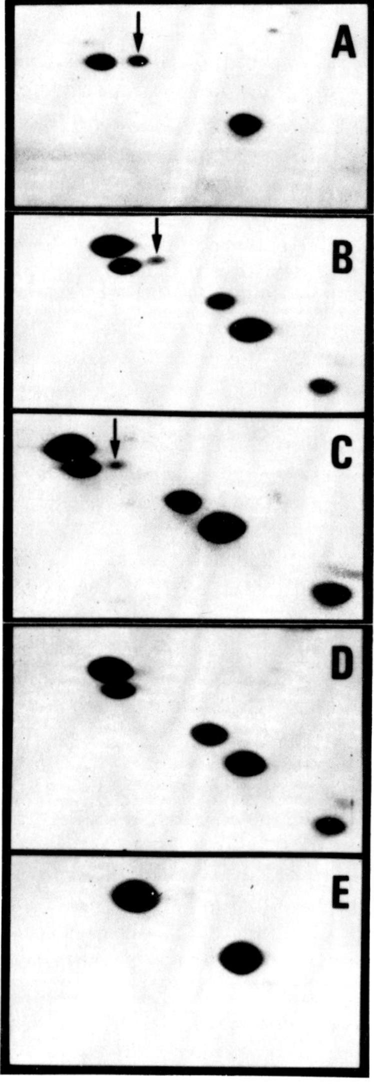

FIG. 25. Analysis of embryonic, newborn, and adult tissue myofibrils. Muscle tissue was dissected from 20-day-old rat embryos and was glycerinated. Soleus muscle was dissected from newborn rats of 3, 7, and 12 days as well as from an adult, and these were glycerinated. Crude myofibrils were analyzed by 2-dimensional gel electrophoresis. *A*: 20-day embryonic muscle (120 μl). *B*: 3-day soleus (100 μl). *C*: 7-day soleus (120 μl). *D*: 12-day soleus (100 μl). *E*: adult soleus (30 μl). *Vertical arrows*, embryonic light-chain LC1 protein. The 2 additional spots in *A* correspond to LC1F and LC2F. The 2 spots in *E* correspond to LC1S and LC2S. In *B–D* there are mixtures of fast and slow light chains. [From Whalen et al. (186).]

ucts from embryonic future fast white myosin and adult fast white myosin in the chicken. This may explain the cross-reactivity that has been observed between adult myosins and fetal myosins (62, 150).

More recently Whalen et al. (185, 190) have amplified their previous findings on the heavy chains of fetal rat muscle, and from results obtained by using a variety of approaches they have demonstrated the presence of an additional heavy chain in perinatal muscle that is distinct from both fetal and adult heavy chains. Whalen's analysis therefore reveals that myogenesis in the rat involves a series of transitions from fetal myosin (exclusively present at 18 days gestation) to neonatal myosin (20 days gestation to several days postpartum) to adult myosin (14 days after birth). The predominant form of myosin heavy chain in developing muscles is neither adult fast nor a mixture of fast and slow but a unique gene product that is synthesized prior to the evolution of adult patterns of neural activity. Thus variations between developing and mature muscle principally involve genes transcribing for heavy chains as opposed to those for light chains, which change comparatively little during myogenesis. These results compare with those of Hoh's (76) previous investigation of isozymes in chick muscle, which showed sequential additions of myosin isozymes during development.

The studies of Whalen et al. (190), though not specifically directed to unraveling the evolution of diversity, imply that the specialized forms of fast and slow myosin do not emerge until late in postpartum development, coincident with the development of mature patterns of innervation and locomotor activity. Hoh and Yeoh's (78) finding of embryonic isozymes common to future fast and slow muscles in the 2-day-old rabbit is consistent with this, but it is presently hard to reconcile these results with those of a variety of histochemical (24, 98) and immunochemical (62, 86, 97, 152, 153) studies in the same species of animal showing that fiber diversity evolves during the fetal or perinatal period. In fetal rats distinctions in the complement of light chains that portend the destiny of the soleus and EDL muscles have also been reported; the EDL contains the three fast light chains LC1F, LC2F, and LC3F; the soleus contains not only the fast light chains but also the two slow light chains LC1S and LC2S (152). Presently, little is known about the heavy chains to which the slow light chains are coupled in immature muscle. This question and the cues that direct fast- as well as slow-myosin maturation must be elucidated. Another area for research is understanding why developing animals need precursor forms of myosin.

Tropomyosin and Troponin

Tropomyosin and troponin are involved in regulation of the calcium-dependent interaction of actin and myosin. The two subunits of tropomyosin, α and β, have similar amino acid sequences and molecular weights; α is the smaller and faster migrating of the two. The proportions of the subunits vary in different types of mature muscle, and this has been correlated with speeds of contraction (43, 50). Slow muscles are usually described as having higher contents of the β-subunit, whereas most fast muscles contain more of the α-subunit. For example, the adult rat soleus almost exclusively contains the β-subunit, whereas in the EDL both α- and β-subunits are present in roughly equal proportions (37). However, this relationship is not straightforward; it varies by species and type of

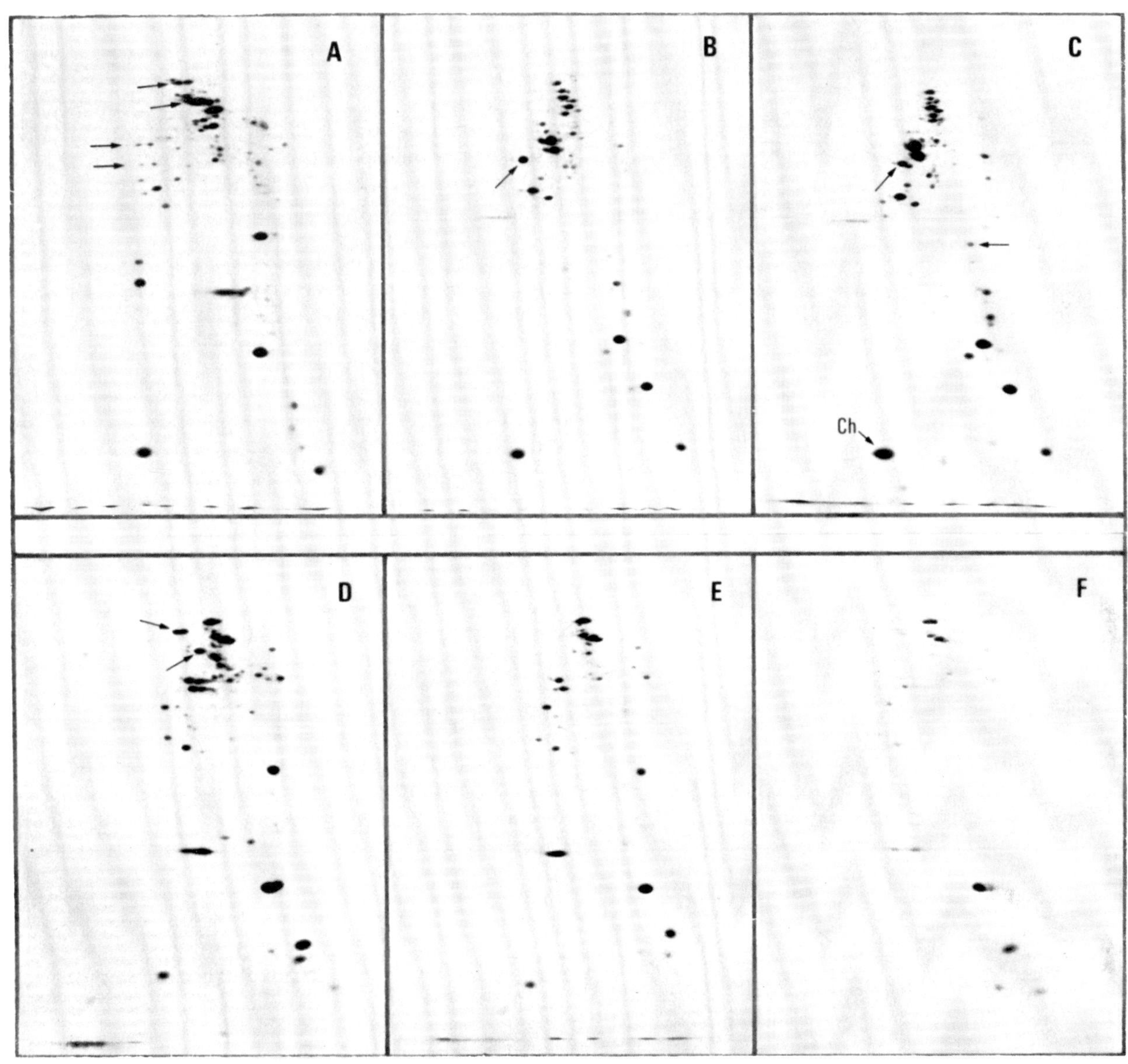

FIG. 26. Two-dimensional gel electrophoretic analysis of chymotryptic myosin cleavage products. Myosins from bulk tissue (*A*), soleus (*B*), cardiac tissue (*C*), 20-day embryonic bulk (*D*), L6 cultures (*E*), and primary cultures (*F*). Primary culture myosin degraded in the presence of nonradioactive L6 myosin. Approximately 15,000 count/min loaded in *F*. Gels are presented with samples in the basic pH range to the *left* and decreasing molecular weight from *top* to *bottom*. Excess chymotrypsin added to gel in *C*; its position is indicated (Ch). Corresponding Ch spot can be seen in all stained gels (*A–E*). This 2-dimensional analysis demonstrates that soleus and cardiac myosin degradation patterns are closely related but can be distinguished by some of the polypeptides present (see *arrows* in Figs. 3*B*, *C*). Myosin from embryonic tissue, primary cultures, and L6 cells have very similar cleavage patterns, but these patterns are different from those of adult myosins. [From Whalen et al. (188).]

muscle. In adult human muscle Billeter et al. (18) described α- and β-tropomyosin to be in roughly equal proportions within individual type I, IIA, IIB, and IIC fibers. Mikawa et al. (117) found that the α- and β-subunits in single fibers of the adult chicken are also in more or less equal proportions in the fast sartorius and slow soleus muscles of the limb. Among wing muscles, though, the fast pectoralis almost exclusively contained the α-subunit, and the slow anterior latissimus dorsi had a preponderance of the β-subunit. In cross-reinnervated rabbit soleus muscle the proportions of α- and β-tropomyosin are not significantly altered despite a twofold increase in the speed of muscle contraction (2). The lack of plasticity in this case is puzzling, since in transformation of rabbit muscle from fast to slow by chronic stimulation, Roy et al. (148) found that the subunit ratio was altered from 80:20 (the ratio of α to β characteristic of fast muscle) to 55:45 (the ratio characteristic of slow muscle). In these chronically stimulated muscles, tropomyosin transformation occurred after 3 wk; by contrast myosin light chains were not altered for 6 to 8 wk. Hence the syntheses of tropomyosin subunits and myosin light chains do not appear to be coordinately regulated (117, 148).

In the chicken, cow, and rabbit, both tropomyosin subunits are synthesized during development, but the β-subunit is the major species present [Fig. 27; (2, 45, 51, 114, 148, 149)]. This subunit constitutes approximately 70% of the tropomyosin in 20-day rabbit embryos. A unique embryonic form has not been identified. Studies by Roy et al. (148, 149) show that as the muscle develops, the β-subunit is progressively replaced by the α-subunit (Fig. 23), suggesting that there may be a relation between the species of tropomyosin present and the changes in speed of contraction of the developing muscle.

Using protease digestion and two-dimensional gel electrophoresis, Billeter et al. (18) have revealed differences in the cleavage patterns of α- and β-tropomyosins from isolated type I, IIA, and IIB fibers. This compares with the studies of Montarras et al. (121), who modified the conventional system of two-dimensional polyacrylamide gel electrophoresis and showed that it is possible to completely separate the α-subunit of chick fast and slow tropomyosins. These researchers also demonstrated that primary cultures of chick muscle synthesize a tropomyosin that is electrophoretically identical to the tropomyosin of fast muscle. Advances in technique such as these make it particularly interesting to learn more about the forms of tropomyosin in developing fast and slow muscle in vivo, as well as about the extent of their exchange in cross-innervated and chronically stimulated muscle.

Troponin and tropomyosin undergo an interesting maturational change in the chick pectoralis muscle. There is almost complete replacement of the β-subunit by the α-subunit. This is closely coordinated with alterations in troponin T, which in breast muscle has a significantly greater molecular weight than in leg muscle (133, 192). Matsuda et al. (114) showed that cultured muscle exclusively contained troponin T of the leg muscle variety, which is also present in leg muscles of the embryonic chick; like troponins I and C, it does not alter with development. Embryonic breast muscle, however, contains both the leg and breast muscle forms of troponin T in addition to troponins I and C. The I and C components do not change with development, although the leg muscle form of troponin T is progressively replaced by the breast muscle form and the latter predominates by 8 days after hatching. Since this unique exchange follows approximately the same time course as substitution of α- for β-tropomyosin, Matsuda et al. speculate that in contrast to other muscles the process may involve correlated control of gene expression between these two functionally related proteins.

Studies of troponin and myosin subunits in single fibers of the chick (117) show that the forms of troponin and myosin light chains are also consistently correlated, suggesting a similar coordinated regulation of the genetic expression of these subunits. As with tropomyosin, no evidence of a fetal form of troponin has been detected (51). Developmental aspects of the polymorphic forms of troponin have been described by Dhoot and Perry (50, 51), who used monospecific antibodies to adult troponins I, T, and C in their experiments. They found that all muscle cells in the

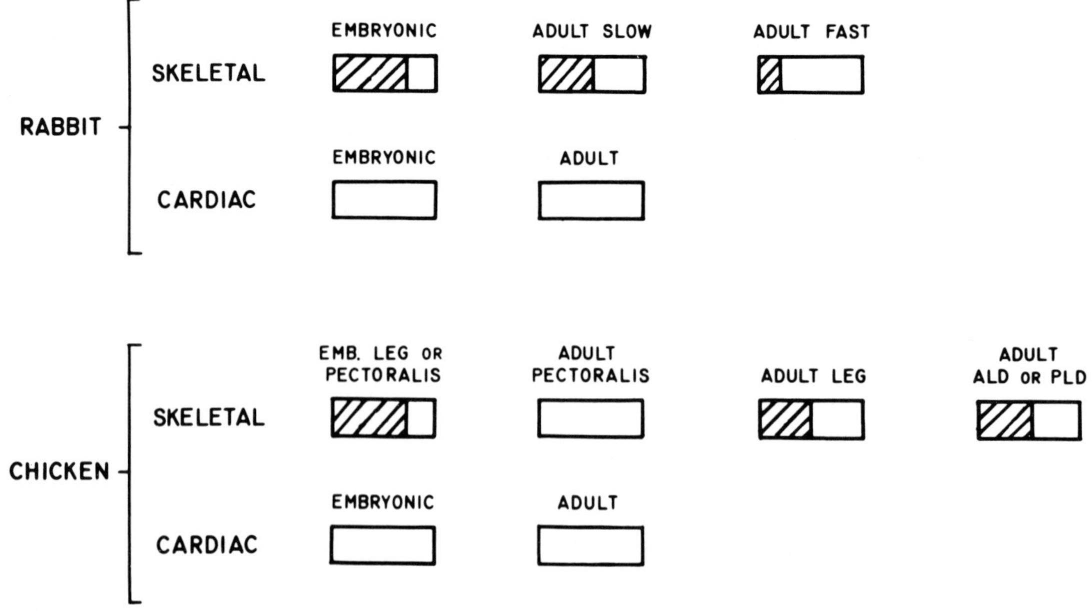

FIG. 27. Relative proportions of tropomyosin subunits α (*white area*) and β (*hatched area*) in various striated muscles of chicken and rabbit. ALD, anterior latissimus dorsi; PLD, posterior latissimus dorsi. [From Roy et al. (149).]

hindlimbs of 18-day fetal rats stained with fast skeletal muscle forms of troponins I, C, and T. A select population of cells, which had a characteristic distribution throughout the muscle, also stained with slow muscle forms of the three troponin components. Affinity for the fast components in these fibers progressively decreased and was no longer detected at 10 days postpartum. Reciprocally, affinity for the slow forms of troponin progressively increased in this select population. Since these fibers were far more numerous in the primordial soleus than in primordial fast muscles, they were identified as presumptive type I cells. The remainder of the cells, which stained exclusively for the fast components of troponin, were identified as presumptive type II cells. The pattern of antibody staining suggests that the fast forms of troponins I, T, and C predominate in early differentiating muscle—even in differentiating slow muscles.

These results correlate remarkably well with the staining pattern of fetal rat muscle described previously (97, 146, 152, 153) as well as with studies by Kerrick et al. (101), who demonstrated that embryonic rabbit fast and slow muscle fibers have the same sensitivity to calcium as do adult fast fibers. During development the calcium sensitivity of slow muscle changes but that of fast muscle remains constant.

This review presents a complex picture of contractile protein synthesis during development. There is a progressive evolution of myosin, particularly involving the heavy chains. At least three major species of contractile protein are sequentially synthesized in developing fast muscles: embryonic, neonatal, and adult. Embryonic and neonatal myosin have antigenic determinants in common with mature fast myosin. Differential patterns of myofiber staining with antibodies specific to slow myosin and the slow forms of troponin are evident early in ontogeny, and it is presently hard to correlate these observations with studies of the heavy chain and myosin isozymes.

Fiber populations change during ontogeny. Early in development primary-generation cells are produced, many of which are the forerunners of slow fibers (50, 51, 97, 153). Large numbers of secondary-generation cells follow, most of which develop into fast fibers. They have a different dependence on innervation than do primary cells (71), and as they are added to the contractile machinery they must progressively eclipse the properties of primary slow fibers, particularly in a differentiating fast muscle. It is still not known how these separate generations of cells relate to the presence of the fetal and neonatal forms of myosin or if there are precursor forms of slow as well as fast myosin. The present dichotomy between the biochemical and cytochemical studies cannot be adequately resolved until this point is clarified.

During myogenesis in the chicken, rabbit, and rat, myosin light chains, troponin, and tropomyosin (121) are very similar if not identical to those in mature fast muscle. However, these studies were performed on small laboratory animals that have high metabolic rates and the high circulating levels of thyroid hormone associated with these rates. The fiber composition in mature muscles of these species reflects this; for example, in the adult rat type II fibers usually outnumber slow fibers by ratios of at least 9 to 1. Ariano et al. (3) surveyed 27 muscles of the rat hindlimb; in 22 of them fast fibers represented over 90% of the total population and only in 2 muscles, the soleus and adductor longus, was there an excess of type I slow fibers. In many respects therefore the initial programs of contractile protein synthesis are conservative and anticipate adaptations of muscle in the mature animal. Whether the inaugural synthesis of contractile proteins is the same in all species has yet to be discovered; in larger animals with slower rates of metabolism slow fibers tend to be more numerous. For example, in the vastus lateralis muscle of the rat 2% are slow and 98% fast fibers (3), in humans 45% are slow and 55% fast fibers (161), and in the slow loris 63% are slow and 37% fast fibers. Thus to more completely understand the genetic controls over contractile protein synthesis it would be useful to investigate the initial patterns of myosin and regulatory protein synthesis in some of these larger species of animals.

REFERENCES

1. Allbrook, D. B., M. F. Ham, and A. E. Hellmuth. Population of muscle satellite cells in relation to age and mitotic activity. *Pathology* 3: 233–234, 1971.
2. Amphlett, G. W., S. V. Perry, H. Syska, H. Brown, and G. Vrbová. Cross innervation and the regulatory protein system of rabbit soleus muscle. *Nature London* 257: 602–604, 1975.
3. Ariano, M. A., R. B. Armstrong, and V. R. Ederton. Hindlimb muscle fiber populations of five mammals. *J. Histochem. Cytochem.* 21: 51–55, 1973.
4. Arndt, I., and F. A. Pepe. Antigenic specificity of red and white muscle myosin. *J. Histochem. Cytochem.* 23: 159–168, 1975.
5. Ashmore, C. R., P. B. Addis, and L. Doerr. Development of muscle fibers in the fetal pig. *J. Anim. Sci.* 36:1088, 1973.
6. Ashmore, C. R., D. W. Robinson, P. V. Rattray, and L. Doerr. Biphasic development of muscle fibers in the fetal lamb. *Exp. Neurol.* 37: 241, 1972.
7. Bagust, J., D. M. Lewis, and R. A. Westerman. Polyneural innervation of kitten skeletal muscle. *J. Physiol. London* 229: 241–255, 1973.
8. Bárány, M. ATPase activity of myosin correlated with speed of muscle shortening. *J. Gen. Physiol.* 50 (pt. 2): 197–218, 1967.
9. Bárány, M., and R. I. Close. The transformation of myosin in cross-innervated rat muscles. *J. Physiol. London* 213: 455–474, 1971.
10. Beermann, D. H., R. G. Cassens, and G. J. Hausman. A second look at fiber type differentiation in porcine skeletal muscle. *J. Anim. Sci.* 46: 125–132, 1978.
11. Bekoff, A. Ontogeny of leg motor output in the chick embryo: a neural analysis. *Brain Res.* 106: 271–291, 1976.
12. Benfield, P. A., S. Lowey, and D. D. LeBlanc. Fractionation and characterization of myosin from embryonic chicken pectoralis muscle. *Biophys. J.* 33: 243a, 1981.
13. Bennett, M. R., and A. Pettigrew. The formation of syn-

apses in striated muscle during development. *J. Physiol. London* 241: 515–545, 1974.

14. Benoit, P., and J. P. Changeux. Consequences of tenotomy on the evolution of multiinnervation in developing rat soleus muscle. *Brain Res.* 99: 354–358, 1975.
15. Betz, W. J., J. H. Caldwell, and R. R. Ribchester. The size of motor units during post-natal development of rat lumbrical muscle. *J. Physiol. London* 297: 463–478, 1979.
16. Betz, W. J., J. H. Caldwell, and R. R. Ribchester. The effect of partial denervation at birth on the development of muscle fibers and motor units in the rat lumbrical muscle. *J. Physiol. London* 303: 265–279, 1980.
17. Billeter, R., C. W. Heizmann, H. Howald, and E. Jenny. Analysis of myosin light and heavy chain types in single human skeletal muscle fibers. *Eur. J. Biochem.* 116: 389–395, 1981.
18. Billeter, R., C. W. Heizmann, U. Reist, H. Howald, and E. Jenny. α- and β-tropomyosin in typed single fibers of human skeletal muscle. *FEBS Lett.* 132: 133–136, 1981.
19. Bischoff, R. Myoblast fusion. In: *Membrane Fusion,* edited by G. Post and A. L. Nicolson. Amsterdam: Elsevier/North-Holland, 1978, p. 127–179.
20. Bischoff, R., and H. Holtzer. Mitosis and the process of differentiation of myogenic cells in vitro. *J. Cell Biol.* 41: 188–200, 1969.
21. Bixby, J. L., J. A. R. Maunsell, and D. C. Van Essen. Effects of motor unit size on innervation patterns in neonatal mammals. *Exp. Neurol.* 70: 516–524, 1980.
22. Blackshaw, S. E., and A. E. Warner. Low resistance junctions between mesoderm cells during development of trunk muscles. *J. Physiol. London* 255: 209–230, 1976.
23. Brooke, M. H., and K. K. Kaiser. Three "myosin adenosine triphosphatase" systems: the nature of their pH lability and sulfhydryl dependence. *J. Histochem. Cytochem.* 18: 670–680, 1970.
24. Brooke, M. H., E. Williamson, and K. K. Kaiser. The behavior of four fiber types in developing and reinnervated muscle. *Arch. Neurol. Chicago* 25: 360–366, 1971.
25. Brown, M. C., J. K. Jansen, and D. C. Van Essen. Polyneural innervation of skeletal muscle in newborn rats and its elimination during maturation. *J. Physiol. London* 261: 387–422, 1976.
26. Brown, M. D. Role of activity in the differentiation of slow and fast muscle. *Nature London* 244: 178–179, 1973.
27. Bucher, T., and D. Pette. In: *Verhandlungen der Deutschen Gesellschaft für innere Medizin,* edited by J. F. Bermann. Munich, West Germany: Bermann, 1965, p. 104–124.
28. Buchthal, F., and H. Schmalbruch. Motor unit of mammalian muscle. *Physiol. Rev.* 60: 90–142, 1980.
29. Buller, A. J., J. C. Eccles, and R. M. Eccles. Differentiation of fast and slow muscles in the cat hind limb. *J. Physiol. London* 150: 399–416, 1960.
30. Buller, A. J., and D. M. Lewis. Further observations on the differentiation of skeletal muscles in the kitten hind limb. *J. Physiol. London* 176: 335–370, 1965.
31. Buller, A. J., W. F. H. M. Mommaerts, and K. Seraydarian. Enzymic properties of myosin in fast and slow twitch muscles of the cat following cross-innervation. *J. Physiol. London* 205: 581–597, 1969.
32. Burke, R. E., D. W. Levine, P. Tsairis, and F. E. Zajae. Physiological types of histochemical profiles in motor units of the cat gastrocnemius. *J. Physiol. London* 234: 723–748, 1973.
33. Bursian, A. V., and G. E. Sviderskaya. Studies on the activity of motor units in newborn rats and kittens. *J. Evol. Biochem. Physiol. USSR* 7: 309–317, 1971.
34. Cardasis, C. A., and G. W. Cooper. An analysis of nuclear numbers in individual muscle fibers during differentiation and growth: a satellite cell-muscle fiber growth unit. *J. Exp. Zool.* 191: 347–358, 1975.
35. Carraro, U., C. Catani, D. Biral. Selective maintenance of neurotrophically regulated proteins in denervated rat diaphragm. *Exp. Neurol.* 63: 468–475, 1979.
36. Carraro, U., C. Catani, and L. Dalla Libera. Myosin light and heavy chains in rat gastrocnemius and diaphragm muscles after chronic denervation or reinnervation. *Exp. Neurol.* 72:401–412, 1981.
37. Carraro, U., C. Catani, L. Dalla Libera, M. Vascon, and G. Zanella. Differential distribution of tropomyosin subunits in fast and slow rat muscles and changes in long-term denervated hemidiaphragm. *FEBS Lett.* 128: 233–236, 1981.
38. Chi, J., N. Rubinstein, K. Strahs, and H. Holtzer. Synthesis of myosin heavy and light chains in muscle cultures. *J. Cell Biol.* 67: 523–537, 1975.
39. Church, J. Satellite cells and myogenesis: a study of the fruit bat. *J. Anat.* 105: 419–438, 1969.
40. Cihák, R., E. Gutmann, and V. Hanzliíková. Involution and hormone-induced persistence of the M. sphincter (levator) ani in female rats. *J. Anat.* 106: 93–110, 1970.
41. Close, R. I. Dynamic properties of fast and slow skeletal muscles of the rat during development. *J. Physiol. London* 173:74–95, 1964.
42. Close, R. I. Dynamic properties of mammalian skeletal muscles. *Physiol. Rev.* 52: 129–197, 1972.
43. Cummins, P., and S. V. Perry. Chemical and immunochemical characteristics of tropomyosins from striated and smooth muscle. *Biochem. J.* 141: 43–49, 1974.
44. Cuojunco, J. Development of the human motor end plate. *Contrib. Embryol.* 30: 129–142, 1942.
45. Dabrowska, R., J. Sosinski, and W. Drabikowski. Comparative studies of various kinds of tropomyosin. In: *Plasticity of Muscle,* edited by D. Pette. New York: de Gruyter, 1980, p. 225–240.
46. Danieli-Betto, D., and M. Midrio. Effect of the spinal section and of subsequent denervation on the mechanical properties of fast and slow muscle. *Experientia* 34: 55–56, 1978.
47. Dennis, M. J. Development of the neuromuscular junction: inductive interactions between cells. *Annu. Rev. Neurosci.* 4: 43–68, 1981.
48. Dennis, M. J., L. Ziskind-Conhaim, and A. J. Harris. Development of neuromuscular junctions in rat embryos. *Dev. Biol.* 81: 266–279, 1981.
49. Devlin, R. B., and C. P. Emerson. Coordinate regulation of contractile protein synthesis during myoblast differentiation. *Cell* 13: 599–611. 1978.
50. Dhoot, G. K., and S. V. Perry. Distribution of polymorphic forms of troponin components and tropomyosin in skeletal muscle. *Nature London* 278: 714–718, 1979.
51. Dhoot, G. K., and S. V. Perry. The components of the troponin complex and development of skeletal muscle. *Exp. Cell Res.* 127: 75–87, 1980.
52. Dow, J., and A. Stracher. Identification of the essential light chains of myosin. *Proc. Natl. Acad. Sci. USA* 68: 1107–1110, 1971.
53. Drachman, D. B., and D. M. Johnston. Development of a mammalian fast muscle: dynamic and biochemical properties correlated. *J. Physiol. London* 234: 29–42, 1973.
54. Drachman, D. B., and L. Sokoloff. The role of movement in embryonic joint development. *Dev. Biol.* 14: 401–420, 1966.
55. Dubowitz, V. Cross-innervated mammalian skeletal muscle: histochemical, physiological and biochemical observations. *J. Physiol. London* 193: 481–496, 1967.
56. Dubowitz, V., and J. Brooke. *Muscle Biopsy: A Modern Approach.* Philadelphia, PA: Saunders, 1973, p. 153–154.
57. Edström, L., and E. Kugelberg. Histochemical composition, distribution of fibres and fatigability of single motor units. Anterior tibial muscle of the rat. *J. Neurol. Neurosurg. Psychiatry* 31: 424–433, 1968.
58. Erulkar, S. D., D. B. Kelley, M. E. Jurman, F. P. Zemlan, G. T. Schneider, and N. R Krieger. *Proc. Natl. Acad. Sci. USA* 78: 5876–5880, 1981.
59. Gallego, R., P. Huizar, N. Kudo, and M. Kuno. Disparity of motoneurone and muscle differentiation following spinal transection in the kitten. *J. Physiol. London* 281: 253–265, 1978.
60. Gauthier, G. F., and S. Lowey. Polymorphism of myosin among skeletal muscle fiber types. *J. Cell Biol.* 74: 760–779, 1977.

61. GAUTHIER, G. F., AND S. LOWEY. Distribution of myosin isoenzymes among skeletal muscle fiber types. *J. Cell Biol.* 81: 10–25, 1979.
62. GAUTHIER, G. F., S. LOWEY, AND A. HOBBS. Fast and slow myosin in developing muscle fibres. *Nature London* 274: 27–29, 1978.
63. GORDON, T., AND G. VRBOVÁ. The influence of innervation on the differentiation of contractile speeds of developing chick muscle. *Pfluegers Arch.* 360: 199–218, 1975.
64. GOSPODAROWICZ, D., J. WESEMAN, J. S. MORAN, AND J. LONDSTROM. Effect of fibroblast growth factor on the division and fusion of bovine myoblasts. *J. Cell Biol.* 70: 395–402, 1976.
65. GUTH, L., P. K. WATSON, AND W. C. BROWN. Effects of cross-reinnervation on some chemical properties of red and white muscles of rat and cat. *Exp. Neurol.* 20: 52–69, 1968.
66. GUTMANN, E. Neurotrophic relations. *Annu. Rev. Physiol.* 38: 177-217, 1976.
67. GUTMANN, E., V. HANZLIKOVA, AND Z. LOJDA. Effect of androgens on histochemical fiber type. *Histochemie* 24: 287–291, 1970.
68. GUTMANN, E., J. MELCHNA, AND I. SYROVÝ. Developmental changes in contraction time, myosin properties and fibre pattern of fast and slow skeletal muscles. *Physiol. Bohemoslov.* 23: 19–27, 1974.
69. HAMBURGER, V. Changing concepts in developmental neurobiology. *Perspect. Biol. Med.* 18: 162–178, 1975.
70. HAMBURGER, V. The developmental history of the motor neuron. *Neurosci. Res. Program Bull. Suppl.* 15: iii–37, 1977.
71. HARRIS, A. J. Embryonic growth and innervation of rat skeletal muscles. Neural regulation of muscle fiber numbers. *Philos. Trans. R. Soc. London Ser. B.* 293: 258–275, 1981.
72. HARRIS, A. J. Embryonic growth and innervation of rat skeletal muscles. III. Neural regulation of junctional and extra junctional acetylcholine receptor clusters. *Philos. Trans. R. Soc. London Ser. B.* 293: 288–306, 1981.
73. HEILIG, A., AND D. PETTE. Changes induced in the enzyme activity pattern by electrical stimulation of fast-twitch muscle. In: *Plasticity of Muscle*, edited by D. Pette. New York: de Gruyter, 1980, p. 409–420.
74. HENNEMAN, E., G. SOMJEN, AND D. CARPENTER. Functional significance of cell size in spinal motoneurons. *J. Neurophysiol.* 28: 560–580, 1965.
75. HOH, J. F. Neural regulation of mammalian fast and slow muscle myosin: an electrophoretic analysis. *Biochemistry* 14: 742–747, 1975.
76. HOH, J. F. Developmental changes in chicken skeletal myosin isoenzymes. *FEBS Lett.* 98:267–270, 1979.
77. HOH, J. F., B. T. S. KWAN, C. DUNLOP, AND B. H. KIM. Effects of nerve cross-union and cordotomy on myosin isoenzymes in fast-twitch and slow-twitch muscles of the rat. In: *Plasticity of Muscle*, edited by D. Pette. New York: de Gruyter, 1980.
78. HOH, J. F., AND G. P. YEOH. Rabbit skeletal myosin isoenzymes from fetal fast-twitch and slow-twitch muscles. *Nature London* 280: 321–323, 1979.
79. HOLLYDAY, M. Motoneuron histogenesis and the development of limb innervation. In: *Current Topics in Developmental Biology: Emergence of Specificity in Neural Histogenesis*, edited by R. K. Hunt. New York: Academic, 1980, vol. 15, pt. I, p. 181–212.
80. HUIZAR, P., M. KUNO, AND Y. MIYATA. Differentiation of motoneurons and skeletal muscles in kittens. *J. Physiol. London* 252: 465–479, 1975.
81. HUSZAR, G. Developmental changes of the primary structure and histidine methylation in rabbit skeletal muscle myosin. *Nature London New Biol.* 240: 260–263, 1972.
82. IANUZZU, C. D., P. PATEL, V. CHEN, AND P. O'BRIEN. A possible thyroidal trophic influence on fast and slow skeletal muscle myosin. In: *Plasticity of Muscle*, edited by D. Pette. New York: de Gruyter, 1980, p. 593–606.
83. ISHIURA, S., A. TAKAGI, I. NONAKA, AND H. SUGITA. Effect of denervation of neonatal rat sciatic nerve on the differentiation of myosin in a single muscle fiber. *Exp. Neurol.* 73: 487–495, 1981.
84. ISHIURA, S., A. TAKAGI, I. NONAKA, AND H. SUGITA. Heterogeneous expression of myosin light chain 1 in a human slow twitch muscle fiber. *J. Biochem. Tokyo* 90: 279–282, 1981.
85. JANSEN, J. W., C. VAN HARDEVELD, AND A. A. H. KOSSENAAR. A methodological study in measuring T_3 and T_4 concentration in red and white skeletal muscle and plasma of euthyroid rats. *Acta Endocrinol. Copenhagen* 90: 81–89, 1979.
86. JENNY, E., H. WEBER, H. LUTZ, AND R. BILLETER. Fiber populations in rabbit skeletal muscles from birth to old age. In: *Plasticity of Muscle*, edited by D. Pette. New York: de Gruyter, 1980, p. 97–110.
87. JOHN, H. A. The myosin of developing and dystrophic skeletal muscle. *FEBS Lett.* 39: 278–282, 1974.
88. JOHNSON, M. A., F. L. MASTAGLIA, A. MONTGOMERY, B. POPE, AND A. G. WEEDS. A neurally mediated effect of thyroid hormone deficiency on slow-twitch skeletal muscle? In: *Plasticity of Muscle*, edited by D. Pette. New York: de Gruyter, 1980, p. 607–616.
89. JOLESZ, F., AND F. A. SRÉTER. Development, innervation and activity pattern induced changes in skeletal muscle. *Annu. Rev. Physiol.* 43: 531–552, 1981.
90. JULIAN, F. L., R. L. MOSS, AND G. S. WALLER. Mechanical properties and myosin light chain composition of skinned muscle fibres from adult and newborn rabbits. *J. Physiol. London* 311: 201–218, 1981.
91. KALDERON, H., M. L. EPSTEIN, AND N. GILULA. Cell-to-cell communication and myogenesis. *J. Cell Biol.* 75: 788–806, 1977.
92. KARPATI, G., AND W. K. ENGEL. Neuronal trophic function. *Arch. Neurol. Chicago* 17: 542–545, 1967.
93. KARPATI, G., AND W. K. ENGEL. Correlative histochemical study of skeletal muscle after suprasegmental denervation, peripheral nerve section and skeletal fixation. *Neurology* 18: 681–692, 1968.
94. KELLER, L. R., AND C. P. EMERSON. Synthesis of adult myosin light chains by embryonic muscle cultures. *Proc. Natl. Acad. Sci. USA* 77: 1020–1024, 1980.
95. KELLY, A. M. Satellite cells and myofiber growth in the rat soleus and extensor digitorum longus muscles. *Dev. Biol.* 65: 1–10, 1978.
96. KELLY, A. M., AND N. A. RUBINSTEIN. Patterns of myosin synthesis in regenerating normal and denervated muscles of the rat. In: *Plasticity of Muscle*, edited by D. Pette. New York: de Gruyter, 1980, p. 161–176.
97. KELLY, A. M., AND N. A. RUBINSTEIN. Why are fetal muscles slow? *Nature London* 288: 266–269, 1980.
98. KELLY, A. M., AND D. L. SCHOTLAND. The evolution of the 'checkerboard' in a rat muscle. In: *Research in Muscle Development and the Muscle Spindle*, edited by B. Q. Banker, R. J. Przybyliski, J. P. van der Meulen, and M. Victor. Amsterdam: Excerpta. Med., 1972, p. 32–49. (Int. Congr. Ser. 240.)
99. KELLY, A. M., AND S. I. ZACKS. The histogenesis of rat intercostal muscle. *J. Cell Biol.* 42: 135–153, 1969.
100. KELLY, A. M., AND S. I. ZACKS. The fine structure of motor end plate morphogenesis. *J. Cell Biol.* 42: 154–169, 1969.
101. KERRICK, W. G. L., D. SECRIST, R. COBY, AND S. LUCAS. Development of difference between red and white muscles in sensitivity to Ca^{2+} in the rabbit from embryo to adult. *Nature London* 260:440–441, 1976.
102. KOCHAKIAN, C. D. Body and organ weight and composition. III. Muscle. In: *Handbook of Experimental Pharmacology, Anabolic-Androgenic Steroids*, edited by C. D. Kochakian. Berlin: Springer-Verlag, 1976, vol. 43, p. 90–104.
103. KUGELBERG, E. Adaptive transformation of rat soleus motor units during growth. *J. Neurol. Sci.* 27: 269–289, 1976.
104. KULLBERG, R. W., T. LENTZ, AND M. W. COHEN. Development of the myotomal neuromuscular junction in *Xenopus laevis*: an electrophysiological and fine-structural study. *Dev. Biol.* 60: 101–129, 1977.
105. LANDMESSER, L. The distribution of motoneurones supplying chick hind limb muscles. *J. Physiol. London* 284: 371–389, 1978.
106. LANDMESSER, L. The development of motor projection patterns in the chick hind limb. *J. Physiol. London* 284: 391–414, 1978.

107. LANDMESSER. L. The generation of neuromuscular specificity. *Annu. Rev. Neurosci.* 3: 279–302, 1980.
108. LANDMESSER, L., AND D. G. MORRIS. The development of functional innervation in the hind limb of the chick embryo. *J. Physiol. London* 249: 301–326, 1975.
109. LETINSKY, M. S., AND K. MORRISON-GRAHAM. Structure of developing frog neuromuscular junctions. *J. Neurocytol.* 9: 321–342, 1980.
110. LØMO, T., R. H. WESTGAARD, AND L. ENGEBRETSEN. Different stimulation patterns affect contractile properties of denervated rat soleus muscles. In: *Plasticity of Muscle*, edited by D. Pette. New York: de Gruyter, 1980, p. 297–310.
111. LOWEY, S., AND D. RISBY. Light chains from fast and slow muscle myosins. *Nature London* 234: 81–85, 1971.
112. MARGRETH, A., V. CARRARO, AND G. SALVIATI. Effects of denervation on protein synthesis and on properties of myosin of fast and slow muscles. In: *Pathogenesis of Human Muscular Dystrophies*, edited by L. P. Rowland. Amsterdam: Excerpta Med., 1977, p. 161–167.
113. MASAKI, T., AND C. YOSHIZAKI. Differentiation of myosin in chick embryos. *J. Biochem. Tokyo* 76: 123–131, 1974.
114. MATSUDA, R., T. OBINATA, AND Y. SHIMADA. Types of troponin components during development of chicken skeletal muscle. *Dev. Biol.* 82: 11–19, 1981.
115. MAURO, A. Satellite cell of skeletal muscle fibers. *J. Biophys. Biochem. Cytol.* 9: 493–495, 1961.
116. MEVES, F. Über Neubildung quergestreifter Muskelfaser nach Beobachtungen am Hühnerembryo. *Anat. Anz.* 34: 161–183, 1909.
117. MIKAWA, T., S. TAKEDA, T. SHINIZU, AND T. KITAURA. Gene expression of myofibrillar proteins in single muscle fibers of adult chicken: micro two dimensional gel electrophoretic analysis. *J. Biochem. Tokyo* 89: 1951–1962, 1981.
118. MILBURN, A. The early development of muscle spindles in the rat. *J. Cell Sci.* 12: 175–195, 1973.
119. MIYATA, Y., AND K. YOSHIOKA. Selective elimination of motor nerve terminals in the rat soleus muscle during development. *J. Physiol. London* 309: 631–646, 1980.
120. MOMMAERTS, W. F., K. SERAYDARIAN, M. SUH, C. J. R. KEAN, AND A. J. BULLER. The conversion of some biochemical properties of mammalian skeletal muscles following cross-reinnervation. *Exp. Neurol.* 55: 637–653, 1977.
121. MONTARRAS, D., M. Y. FISZMAN, AND F. GROS. Characterization of the tropomyosin present in various chick embryo muscle types and in muscle cells differentiated in vitro. *J. Biol. Chem.* 256: 4081–4086, 1981.
122. MORPURGO, B. Über die postembryonale Entwicklung der quergestreiften Muskeln van weissen Ratten. *Anat. Anz.* 15: 200–262, 1898.
123. MULLER, G., M. ERMINI, AND E. JENNY. Studies on the differentiation of red and white skeletal muscle in the developing rabbit. *Experientia 31:* 723, 1975.
124. NARAYANAN, C. H., M. W. FOX, AND V. HAMBURGER. Prenatal development of spontaneous and evoked activity in the rat (*Rattus norvegicus albinus*). *Behaviour* 40: 100–134, 1971.
125. NAVARRETE, R., AND G. VRBOVÁ. Electromyographic activity of rat slow and fast muscles during postnatal development. *J. Physiol. London* 305: 33P–34P, 1980.
126. NEMETH, P. M., D. PETTE, AND G. VRBOVÁ. Malate dehydrogenase homogeneity of single fibers of the motor unit. In: *Plasticity of Muscle,* edited by D. Pette. New York: de Gruyter, 1980, p. 45–54.
127. OBINATA, T., T. MASAKI, AND H. TAKANO. Types of myosin light chains present during the development of fast skeletal muscle in chick embryo. *J. Biochem. Tokyo* 87: 81–88, 1980.
128. O'BRIEN, R., A. ÖSTBERG, AND G. VRBOVÁ. Observations on the elimination of polyneural innervation in developing muscle. *J. Physiol. London* 282: 571–582, 1978.
129. OH, T. H., AND G. J. MARKELONIS. Neurotrophic effects of a protein fraction isolated from peripheral nerves on skeletal muscle in culture. In: *Muscle Regeneration*, edited by A. Mauro. New York: Raven, 1980, p. 419–428.
130. ONTELL, M. Neonatal muscle: an electron microscopic study. *Anat. Rec.* 189: 669–690, 1977.
131. ONTELL, M. The source of "new" muscle fibers in neonatal muscle. In: *Muscle Regeneration*, edited by A. Mauro. New York: Raven, 1980, p. 137–146.
132. PELLONI-MÜLLER, G., M. ERMINI, AND E. JENNY. Myosin light chains of developing fast and slow rabbit skeletal muscle. *FEBS Lett.* 67: 68–74, 1976.
133. PERRY, S. V., AND H. A. COLE. Phosphorylation of troponin and the effects of interactions between the components of the complex. *Biochem. J.* 141: 733–743, 1974.
134. PERRY, S. V., AND G. K. DHOOT. Biochemical aspects of muscle development and differentiation. In: *Development and Specialization of Skeletal Muscle*, edited by D. Goldspink. Cambridge, UK: Cambridge Univ. Press, 1980, p. 51–64. (Soc. Exp. Biol. Semin. Ser. 7.)
135. PETTE, D., W. MULLER, E. LEISNER, AND G. VRBOVÁ. Time dependent effects on contractile properties, fibre population, myosin light chains and enzymes of energy metabolism in intermittently and continuously stimulated fast twitch muscles of the rabbit. *Pfluegers Arch.* 364: 103–112, 1976.
136. PETTE, D., AND U. SCHNEZ. Coexistence of fast and slow type myosin light chains in single muscle fibres during transformation as induced by long term stimulation. *FEBS Lett.* 83: 128–130, 1977.
137. PETTE, D., M. E. SMITH, H. W. STAUDTE, AND G. VRBOVÁ. Effect of long-term electrical stimulation on some contractile and metabolic characteristics of fast rabbit muscles. *Pfluegers Arch.* 338: 257–272, 1973.
138. PETTE, D., G. VRBOVÁ, AND R. C. WHALEN. Independent development of contractile properties and myosin light chains in embryonic chick fast and slow muscle. *Pfluegers Arch.* 178: 253–257, 1979.
139. PODLESKI, T. R., D. AXELROD, P. RAVDIN, I. GREENBERG, M. M. JOHNSON, AND M. M. SALPETER. Nerve extract induces increase and redistribution of acetylcholine receptors in cloned muscle cells. *Proc. Natl. Acad. Sci. USA* 75: 2035–2039, 1978.
140. RASH, J. E., AND D. FAMBROUGH. Ultrastructural and electrophysiological correlates of cell coupling and cytoplasmic fusion during myogenesis in vitro. *Dev. Biol.* 30: 168–186, 1973.
141. RASH, J. E., AND L. A. STAEHELIN. Freeze-cleave demonstration of gap junctions between skeletal myogenic cells in vivo. *Dev. Biol.* 36: 455–461, 1974.
142. REDFERN, P. Neuromuscular transmission in newborn rats. *J. Physiol. London* 209: 701–709, 1970.
143. RIDGE, R. M. The differentiation of conduction velocities of slow twitch and fast twitch muscle motor innervations in kittens and cats. *Q. J. Exp. Physiol.* 52: 293–304, 1967.
144. RILEY, D. A. Multiple axon branches innervating single endplates of kitten soleus myofibers. *Brain Res.* 110: 158–161, 1976.
145. RILEY, D. A. Multiple innervation of fiber types in the soleus muscles of postnatal rats. *Exp. Neurol.* 56: 400–409, 1977.
146. ROWLERSON, A. Histochemistry of developing muscle in rabbit and cat. *J. Physiol. London* 293: 18P, 1979.
147. ROWLERSON, A. Differentiation of muscle fibre types in fetal and young rats studied with a labelled antibody to slow myosin. *J. Physiol. London* 301: 19P, 1980.
148. ROY, R. K., F. A. SRÉTER, M. G. PLUSKAL, AND S. SARKAR. Tropomyosin transitions in avian and mammalian skeletal muscles. In: *Plasticity of Muscle*, edited by D. Pette. New York: de Gruyter, 1980, p. 241–254.
149. ROY, R. K., F. A. SRÉTER, AND S. SARKAR. Changes in tropomyosin subunits and myosin light chains during development of chicken and rabbit striated muscles. *Dev. Biol.* 69: 15–30, 1979.
150. RUBINSTEIN, N. A., AND H. HOLTZER. Fast and slow muscles in tissue culture synthesize only fast myosin. *Nature London* 280: 323–325, 1979.
151. RUBINSTEIN, N. A., AND A. M. KELLY. Myogenic and neurogenic contributions to the development of fast and slow twitch muscles in rat. *Dev. Biol.* 62: 473–483, 1978.
152. RUBINSTEIN, N. A., AND A. M. KELLY. The sequential appearance of fast and slow myosins during myogenesis. In: *Plasticity of Muscle*, edited by D. Pette. New York: de Gruyter, 1980, p. 147–160.

153. RUBINSTEIN, N. A., AND A. M. KELLY. Development of muscle fiber specialization in the rat hindlimb. *J. Cell Biol.* 90: 128–144, 1981.
154. RUBINSTEIN, N. A., F. A. PEPE, AND H. HOLTZER. Myosin types during the development of embryonic chicken fast and slow muscles. *Proc. Natl. Acad. Sci. USA* 74: 4524–4527, 1977.
155. RUSHBROOK, J. I., AND A. STRACHER. Comparison of adult, embryonic, and dystrophic myosin heavy chains from chicken muscle by sodium dodecyl sulfate/polyacrylamide gel electrophoresis and peptide mapping. *Proc. Natl. Acad. Sci. USA* 76: 4331–4334, 1979.
156. SALMONS, S., AND J. HENRICKSSON. The adaptive response of skeletal muscle to increased use. *Muscle Nerve* 4: 94–105, 1981.
157. SALMONS, S., AND F. A. SRÉTER. Significance of impulse activity in the transformation of skeletal muscle type. *Nature London* 263: 30–34, 1976.
158. SALMONS, S., AND G. VRBOVÁ. The influence of activity on some contractile characteristics of mammalian fast and slow muscles. *J. Physiol. London* 201: 533–549, 1969.
159. SARKAR, S., F. A. SRÉTER, AND J. GERGELY. Light chains of myosin from white, red and cardiac muscles. *Proc. Natl. Acad. Sci. USA* 68: 946–950, 1971.
160. SATO, N., N. MIZUNO, AND Z. KONISHI. Postnatal differentiation of cell body volumes of spinal motoneurons innervating slow-twich and fast-twitch muscles. *J. Comp. Neurol.* 175: 27–36, 1977.
161. SCHOTLAND, D., E. BONILLA, AND Y. WAKAYAMA. Freeze-fracture studies in human muscular dystrophy. In: *Disorders of the Motor Unit*, edited by D. Schotland. New York: Wiley, 1982, p. 475–487.
162. SCHULTZ, E. A quantitative study of the satellite cell population in post-natal mouse lumbrical muscle. *Anat. Rec.* 180: 589–599, 1974.
163. SINGER, M. Trophic Functions of the Neuron. VI. Other trophic systems. Neurotrophic control of limb regeneration in the newt. *Ann. NY Acad. Sci.* 228: 308–321, 1974.
164. SISTO-DANEO, L., AND G. FILOGAMO. Ultrastructure of early neuromuscular contacts in the chick embryo. *J. Submicrosc. Cytol.* 5: 219–229, 1973.
165. SRÉTER, F. A., M. BÁLINT, AND J. GERGELY. Structural and functional changes of myosin during development: comparison with adult fast, slow and cardiac myosin. *Dev. Biol.* 46: 317–325, 1975.
166. SRÉTER, F. A., J. GERGELY, AND A. L. LUFF. The effect of cross reinnervation on the synthesis of myosin light chains. *Biochem. Biophys. Res. Commun.* 56: 84–89, 1974.
167. SRÉTER, F. A., J. GERGELY, S. SALMONS, AND F. ROMANUL. Synthesis by fast muscle of myosin light chains characteristic of slow muscle in response to long-term stimulation. *Nature London New Biol.* 241: 17–19, 1973.
168. SRÉTER, F. A., S. HOLTZER, J. GERGELY, AND H. HOLTZER. Some properties of embryonic myosin. *J. Cell Biol.* 55: 586–594, 1972.
169. SRÉTER, F. A., J. C. SEIDEL, AND J. GERGELY. Studies on myosin from red and white muscles of rabbit. I. Adenosine triphosphatase activity. *J. Biol. Chem.* 241: 5772–5776, 1966.
170. STEINBACH, J. H., D. SCHUBERT, AND L. ELDRIDGE. Changes in cat muscle contractile proteins after prolonged muscle activity. *Exp. Neurol.* 67:655–669, 1980.
171. STOCKDALE, F. E., H. BADEN, AND N. RAMAN. Slow muscle myoblasts differentiating in vitro synthesize both slow and fast myosin light chains. *Dev. Biol.* 82: 168–171, 1981.
172. STOCKDALE, F. E., N. RAMAN, AND H. BADEN. Myosin light chains and developmental origin of fast muscle. *Proc. Natl. Acad. Sci. USA* 78: 931–935, 1981.
173. SYROVY, I. Changes in light chains of myosin during animal development. *Int. J. Biochem.* 10: 223–227, 1979.
174. SYROVY, I., AND E. GUTMANN. Differentiation of myosin in soleus and extensor digitorum longus muscles in different animal species during development. *Pfluegers Arch.* 369: 85–89, 1977.
175. TAKAHASI, M., AND Y. TONOMURA. Developmental changes in the structure and kinetic properties of myosin adenosinetriphosphatase of rabbit skeletal fast muscle. *J. Biochem. Tokyo* 78: 1123–1133, 1975.
176. THOMPSON, W., D. P. KUFFLER, AND J. K. JANSEN. The effect of prolonged, reversible block of nerve impulses on the elimination of polyneural innervation of new-born rat skeletal muscle fibers. *Neuroscience* 4: 271–278, 1979.
177. TRAYER, I. P., C. I. HARRIS, AND S. V. PERRY. 3-Methyl histidine and adult and foetal forms of skeletal muscle myosin. *Nature London* 217: 452–454, 1968.
178. VRBOVÁ, G. The effects of motoneurone activity on the contraction speed of striated muscle. *J. Physiol. London* 169: 513–526, 1963.
179. VRBOVÁ, G. Innervation and differentiation of muscle fibers. In: *Development and Specialization of Skeletal Muscle*, edited by D. Goldsink. Cambridge, UK: Cambridge Univ. Press, 1980, p. 37–50. (Soc. Exp. Biol. Semin. Ser. 7.)
180. WEEDS, A. G. Myosin: polymorphism and promiscuity. *Nature London* 274: 417–418, 1978.
181. WEEDS, A. G. Light chains from slow-twitch muscle myosin. *Eur. J. Biochem.* 66: 157–173, 1976.
182. WEEDS, A. G., AND S. LOWEY. Substructure of the myosin molecule. II. The light chains of myosin. *J. Mol. Biol.* 61: 701–725, 1971.
183. WEEDS, A. G., D. R. TRENTHAM, C. J. C. KEAN, AND A. J. BULLER. Myosin from cross-innervated cat muscles. *Nature London* 247: 135–139, 1974.
184. WEISS, P. Nerve patterns, the mechanisms of nerve growth. *Growth* 5: 16, 1941.
185. WHALEN, R. G. Contractile protein isozymes in muscle development: the embryonic phenotype. In: *Plasticity of Muscle*, edited by D. Pette. New York: de Gruyter, 1980, p. 177–192.
186. WHALEN, R. G., G. S. BUTLER-BROWNE, AND F. GROS. Identification of a novel form of myosin light chain present in embryonic muscle tissue and cultured muscle cells. *J. Mol. Biol.* 126: 415–431, 1978.
187. WHALEN, R. G., G. S. BUTLER-BROWNE, S. SELL, AND F. GROS. Transitions in contractile protein isozymes during muscle differentiation. *Biochimie* 61: 625–632, 1979.
188. WHALEN, R. G., K. SCHWARTZ, P. BOUVERET, S. M. SELL, AND F GROS. Contractile protein isozymes in muscle development: identification of an embryonic form of myosin heavy chain. *Proc. Natl. Acad. Sci. USA* 76: 5197–5201, 1979.
189. WHALEN, R. G., AND S. M. SELL. Myosin from fetal hearts contains the skeletal muscle embryonic light chain. *Nature London* 286: 731–733, 1980.
190. WHALEN, R. G., S. M. SELL, G. S. BUTLER-BROWNE, K. SCHWARTZ, P. BOUVERET, AND I. PINSET-HÄRSTRÖM. Three myosin heavy-chain isozymes appear sequentially in rat muscle development. *Nature London* 292: 805–809, 1981.
191. WHALEN, R. G., AND L.-E. THORNELL. Heart Purkinje fibers contain both atrial-embryonic and ventricular-type myosin light chains (Abstract). *Int. Cong. Cell Biol., 2nd, Berlin, 1980.* Stuttgart, West Germany: Wissenschaftliche Verlagsgesellschaft, 1980, p. 319.
192. WILKINSON, J. M. The components of troponin from chicken fast skeletal muscle. A comparison of troponin T and troponin I from breast and leg muscle. *Biochem. J.* 169: 229–238, 1978.
193. WILLSHAW, D. J. The establishment and the subsequent elimination of polyneural innervation of developing muscle: theoretical considerations. *Proc. R. Soc. London Ser. B.* 212: 233–252, 1981.
194. WINDER, W., R. FITTS, J. HOLLOSZY, K. KAISER, AND M. H. BROOK. Effects of thyroid hormones on different types of skeletal muscle. In: *Plasticity of Muscle*, edited by D. Pette. New York: de Gruyter, 1980, p. 581–592.
195. WIRSEN, C., AND K. S. LARSSON. Histochemical differention of skeletal muscle in foetal and newborn mice. *J. Embryol. Exp. Morphol.* 12: 759, 1964.
196. YOUNG, O. A., AND C. L. DAVEY. Electrophoretic analysis of proteins from single bovine muscle fibers. *Biochem. J.* 195: 317–327, 1981.

CHAPTER 18

Alterations in myofibril size and structure during growth, exercise, and changes in environmental temperature

GEOFFREY GOLDSPINK | *Muscle Research Unit, University of Hull, Hull, England*

CHAPTER CONTENTS

ONE OF THE FASCINATING ASPECTS of muscle is its inherent adaptability. Athletes who train by lifting heavy weights develop large and powerful muscles; athletes who train for long-duration events develop muscles that are resistant to fatigue. In addition to these more obvious examples, much adaptation takes place during the normal growth and development of the tissue. This chapter is devoted mainly to adaptation during growth and is almost entirely confined to alterations in the myofibrillar system. The myofibrils are the contractile elements and as such they determine much of the physiology of muscle tissue. Nevertheless reference is made to other ultrastructural alterations, for example, changes in the mitochondria and sarcoplasmic reticulum (SR), where these have a profound effect on the contractile response of the tissue. Although exercise changes are not dealt with in detail, the effects of exercise on size, number, and type of the myofibrils are covered because these changes are closely related to growth changes.

Knowledge of the diversity and mutability of muscle fiber types and hence the type of proteins they contain has changed in recent years. This is dealt with in the chapter by B. R. Eisenberg in this *Handbook*; however, some mention is made here of the changes at the myofibrillar level that are associated with artificial stimulation and cross innervation. Also described are some of the alterations that occur in response to changes in environmental temperatures in the myofibrillar system of certain species of fish. These illustrate the adaptability of the myofibrillar system as well as show how the locomotory requirements are met in poikilothermic (ectothermic) animals that experience a wide range of environmental temperatures.

CHANGES IN MYOFIBRILS DURING GROWTH

The length and girth of myofibrils in striated muscle are important in determining the amount and rate at which force is produced. The overall rate of force production depends on the intrinsic rate of shortening and the number of sarcomeres in series. Therefore the longer the fiber (myofibrils) the greater the overall rate of shortening. The force produced by the muscle is, however, proportional to the myofibrillar cross-sectional area. It is therefore important to know how myofibrils increase in length and girth during growth.

Increase in Length of Myofibrils

Measurements made on the number of sarcomeres and the length of the filaments (35) indicated that longitudinal growth of myofibrils is associated with an increase in the number of sarcomeres in series. The length of the sarcomeres may change from very short in the young animal to somewhat longer in the adult animal. In vertebrate muscle, however, this does not involve a change in the length of the filaments. The situation is rather different in some invertebrate muscle where the filaments are known to change length during growth (2, 4). The production of myofibrils with extra long sarcomeres is important because these myofibrils are able to develop more force by having more cross bridges per sarcomere. The extra length of these sarcomeres means, however, that there are fewer sarcomeres in series, therefore the overall rate of shortening of the myofibrils is less. In certain invertebrates this is one method by which muscle fibers are specialized for high production of force as opposed to a high rate of shortening.

The fact that the longitudinal growth of vertebrate muscle is associated with increases in the number of sarcomeres in series was established beyond doubt by Williams and Goldspink (114), who teased out whole fibers from muscles of animals at different ages and counted the number of sarcomeres along the length of these fibers (Fig. 1). In the mouse soleus the fibers increased during postnatal growth from about 700 to 2,200. The point or points at which the sarcomeres are added has been rather uncertain until recently. With radioactively labeled amino acids and radioactively labeled adenosine the site of longitudinal growth was shown to be at the ends of the myofibrils (46, 114). In this work the muscles removed from animals that had received injections of isotope were serially sectioned on a cryostat. The sections from the different regions of the muscle were then assayed for radioactivity by placing batches of them in scintillation-counter vials. Some sections were mounted on microscope slides so that the area of the muscle and hence the volume of tissue in the vials could be measured. As Figure 2 shows most of the radioactivity was incorporated into the end regions of the muscle fibers, which indicates that the new sarcomeres are added to the ends of the fibers. Alternatively the isotope was located by radioautography in mammalian muscle and tadpole muscle. The advantage of using tadpoles is that they can be raised in a solution of the isotope, so a high level of activity can be obtained. Figure 3 is a radioautograph of a tadpole tail. There is a very distinct band of labeling near the ends of the fiber, indicating the region of longitudinal growth of the myofibrils. Light microscopy did not show whether the radioactive label was in the muscle fibers or in the tendon, since there are many folds at the myotendon junction. Experiments in which the tadpoles were first placed in an isotope solution and then transferred to isotope-free water for several days still resulted in bands of labeling; however, these were nearer the middle of the fibers because additional sarcomeres that had a low level of labeling had been added. Examination of the myotendon junction in growing animals with the electron microscope reveals that there are quite large numbers of polysome assemblies and free filaments in this region, indicating again that the new sarcomeres are formed at the ends of the existing myofibrils.

In insect muscle longitudinal growth is rather different; recent evidence suggests that elongation of muscles during metamorphosis is associated with the vertical splitting of the Z disks and the insertion of new sarcomeres at points along the myofibrils. (D. F. Houlihan and J. R. L. Newton, personal communication). The process in insects should really be regarded as embryonic differentiation, and the vertical splitting of Z disks may possibly occur in vertebrate muscle during the very early stage of myofibrillogenesis. Indeed, a similar mechanism was proposed by Schmalbruck (92) for myofibril elongation during postnatal growth of vertebrate muscle; however, the suggestion cannot be reconciled with the evidence from radioisotope studies.

What regulates the length of the muscle fibers and the number of sarcomeres laid down in series is not fully understood. In growing animals the addition of sarcomeres can be suppressed by immobilizing the limb in a plaster cast (114). Under these conditions the length of the muscle plus tendon is the same as in the normal limb, but the muscle fibers are shorter and have fewer sarcomeres in series (103, 116). When the plaster casts are removed, however, the muscle fibers produce sarcomeres rapidly and acquire the correct length within a few days. This demonstrates that

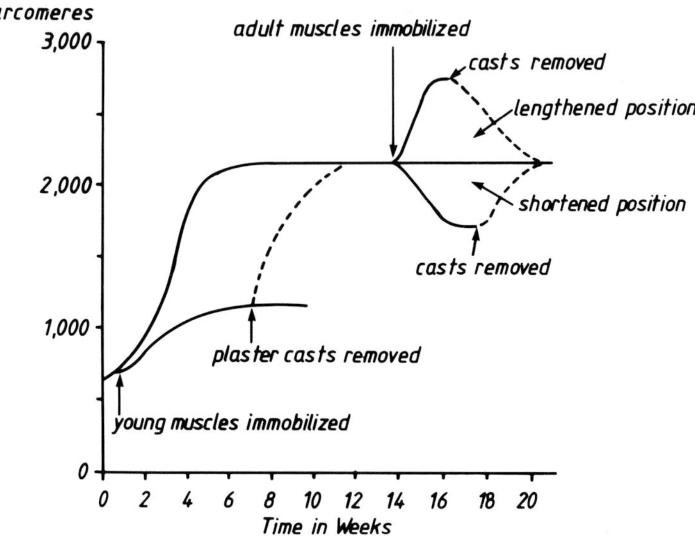

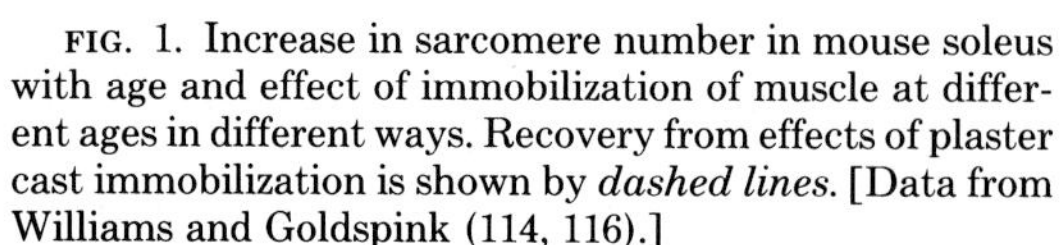

FIG. 1. Increase in sarcomere number in mouse soleus with age and effect of immobilization of muscle at different ages in different ways. Recovery from effects of plaster cast immobilization is shown by *dashed lines*. [Data from Williams and Goldspink (114, 116).]

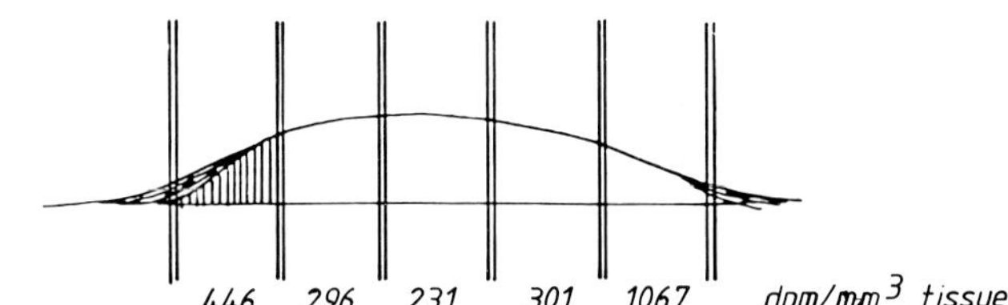

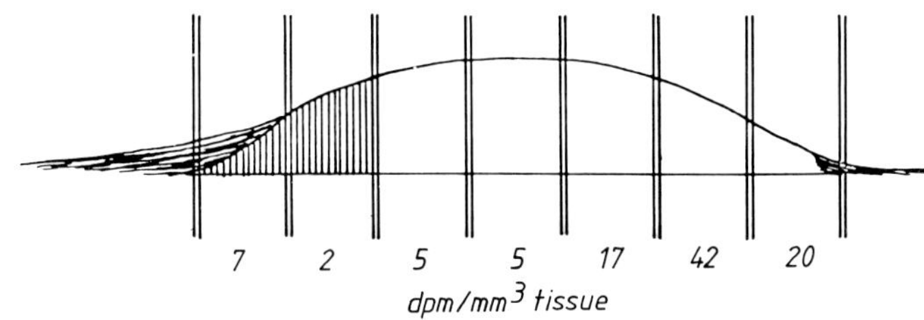

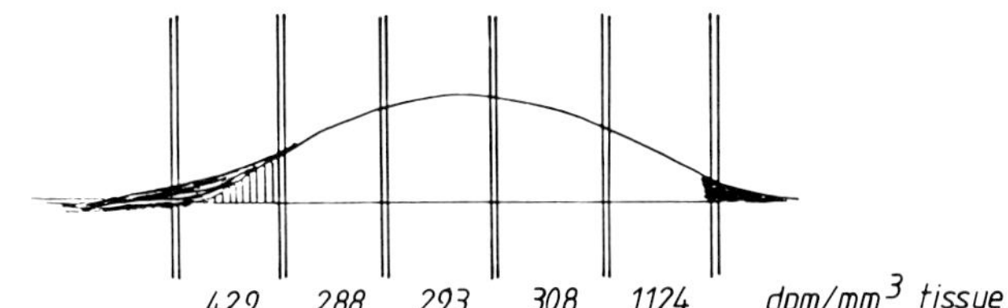

FIG. 2. Level of labeling in end and middle regions of young (*top*) and mature (*center*) muscles after a single injection of tritiated adenosine (adenosine is incorporated into structural ADP of actin monomers). *Bottom*: level of labeling for adult muscles recovering from immobilization in shortened position is also given. In *top* and *bottom*, end regions are more heavily labeled than middle ones, indicating that the site of longitudinal growth is at end regions.

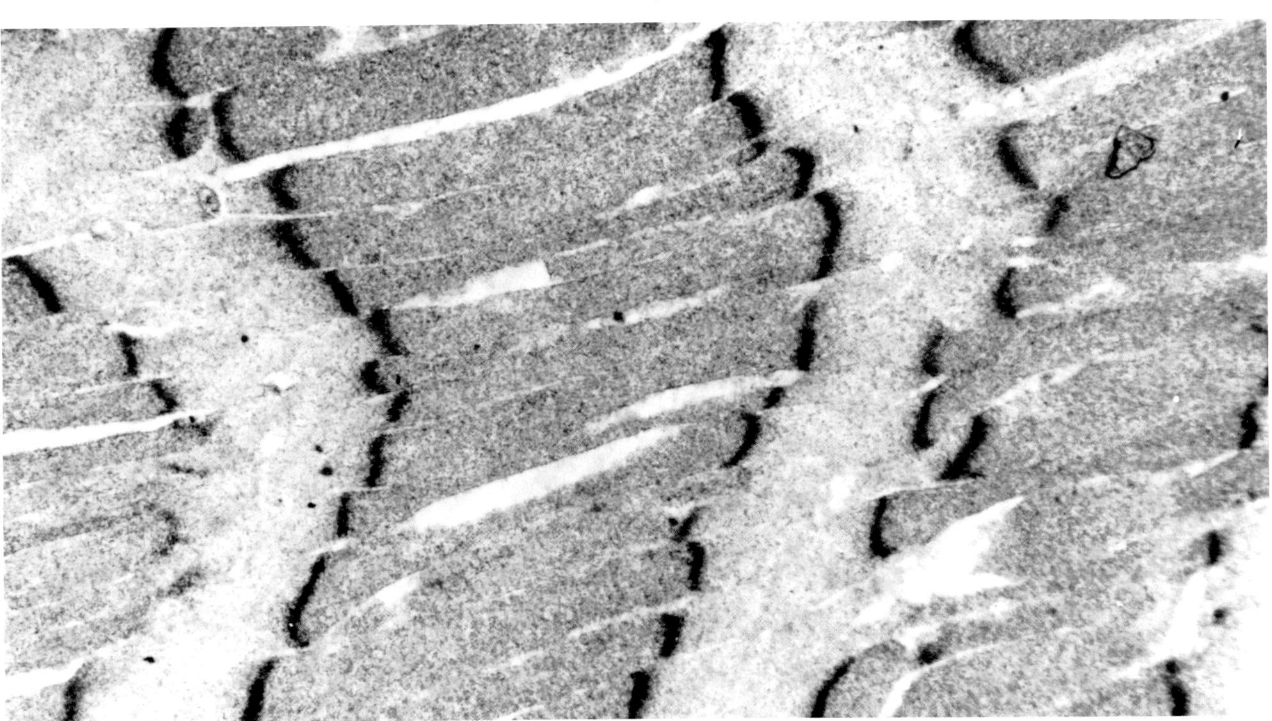

FIG. 3. Autoradiograph of tail muscle from *Xenopus* tadpole reared for a few days in a medium containing [^{3}H]leucine. Muscle fibers are arranged in myotomes and ends of fibers show bands of heavy labeling. This is further evidence that new sarcomeres are added serially to ends of existing myofibrils.

muscles in growing animals can adapt very quickly to changes in length.

More recently Tabary et al. (102), Williams and Goldspink (115), and Goldspink et al. (42) studied the cellular mechanisms involved in length adaptation. The muscles of adult animals were immobilized in different positions using plaster casts, and the muscle adapted in length to these positions. For example, when the soleus muscle of the mouse was immobilized in the lengthened position, it produced 20%–30% more sarcomeres in series. On the other hand when this muscle was immobilized in the shortened position, it lost 40% of its sarcomeres in series. When the plaster casts were removed from the immobilized muscles, however, the sarcomere numbers rapidly returned to normal, so the sarcomere number changes were in fact completely reversible. Rather surprisingly a muscle could adapt in this way even if its nerve supply was severed prior to the experiment. Thus it is assumed that the sensing mechanism for the adaptation must lie in each individual muscle fiber.

The adaptation in sarcomere numbers in growing and adult muscle is physiologically significant because the force that a muscle can develop depends on the degree of overlap of the thick and thin filaments (44, 45). The optimum sarcomere length is that which allows the maximum interaction of the myosin cross bridges with the actin filaments. The length of the thick and thin filaments is fixed, and therefore the only way in which the muscle fiber can adjust its sarcomere length is to adjust the number of sarcomeres along the length of the myofibrils. It seems that each muscle fiber can "sense" when its mechanical output is diminished and add or remove sarcomeres to regain the maximum functional overlap of the thick and thin filaments.

Increase in Myofibrillar Cross-Sectional Area

It is generally accepted that the number of muscle fibers does not change once embryonic differentiation of the tissue is complete (32, 66, 83, 101). The increase in girth of the muscle during growth and exercise is therefore the result of an increase in the diameter of the existing muscle fibers. In contrast the number of myofibrils within the fibers increases considerably. In the fibers of a mouse muscle, for example, the number of myofibrils increases from about 50 in the myotube or newly formed muscle fiber to over 1,000 in the fully mature fiber. This proliferation of myofibrils is accompanied by an increase in the SR and the transverse tubular system (T system), which are responsible for activation of the myofibrils and other organelles such as mitochondria, although not necessarily at the same rate. The increase in the number of myofibrils in the cross-sectional area and hence the size of the muscle fibers is functionally significant, because it enables the muscle to produce the additional force required when the animal becomes heavier and more active.

The mechanism of myofibril proliferation has been investigated (36, 37), and it appears that when myofibrils reach a certain critical size, they split longitudinally. Consequently the myofibrillar mass subdivides during growth, permitting the invasion of the mass by the developing SR and T system. Longitudinal splitting of myofibrils can often be seen in muscles of young animals and muscles of animals that have been exercised [Fig. 4; (36)]. Indeed the splitting of myofibrils was observed in trout muscle by Heidenhain as long ago as 1913 (51). Without the aid of the electron microscope, however, the mechanism could not be elucidated. Recent work has suggested that the longitudinal splitting of myofibrils results from a mismatch in the spacing of the thick-filament and thin-

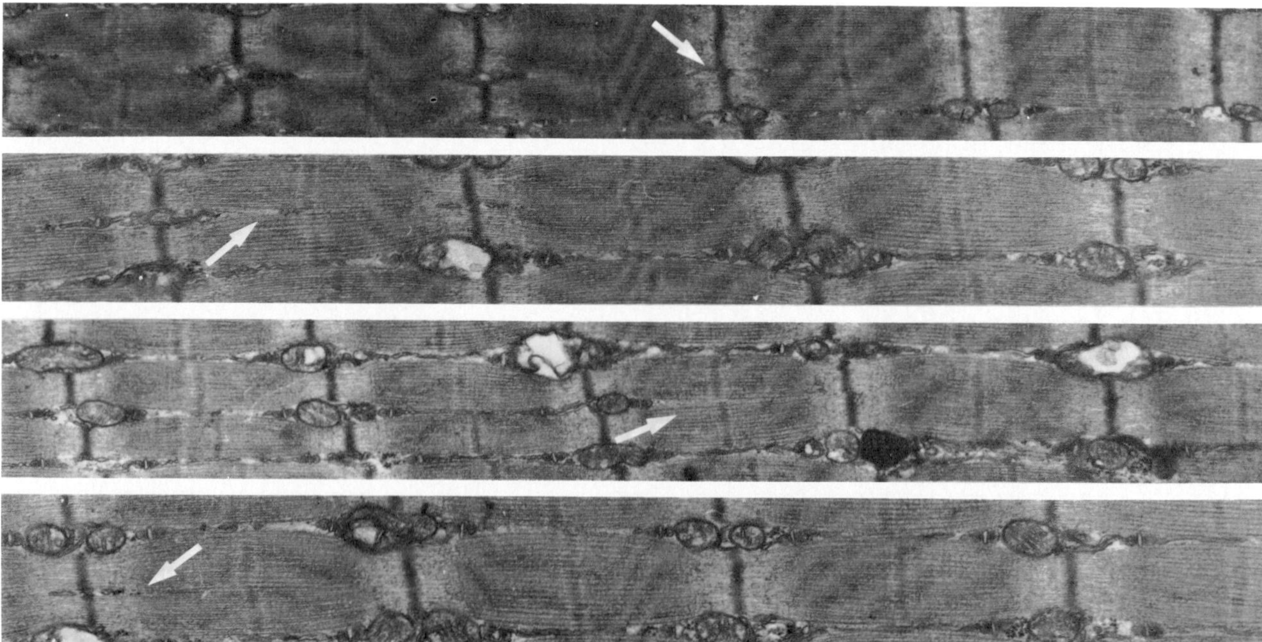

FIG. 4. Myofibrils in process of splitting longitudinally. Position of split is marked by *white arrow*. Some Z disks in myofibrils are still intact, whereas others have split, and there are already elements of the sarcoplasmic reticular system and some mitochondria in the fork of each split.

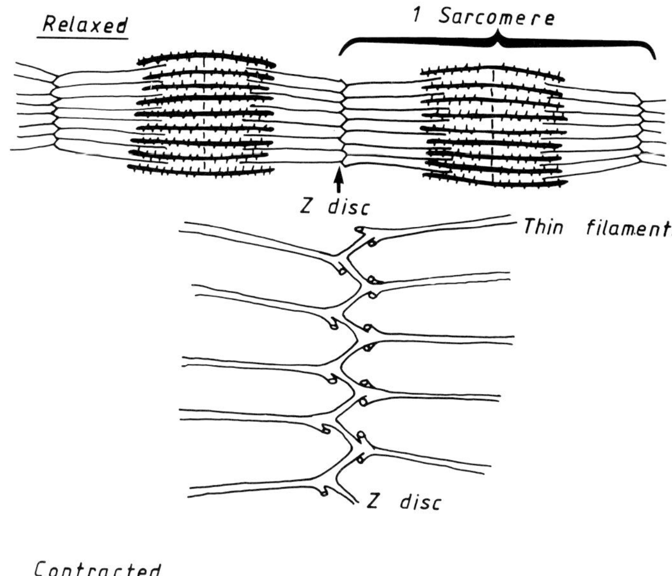

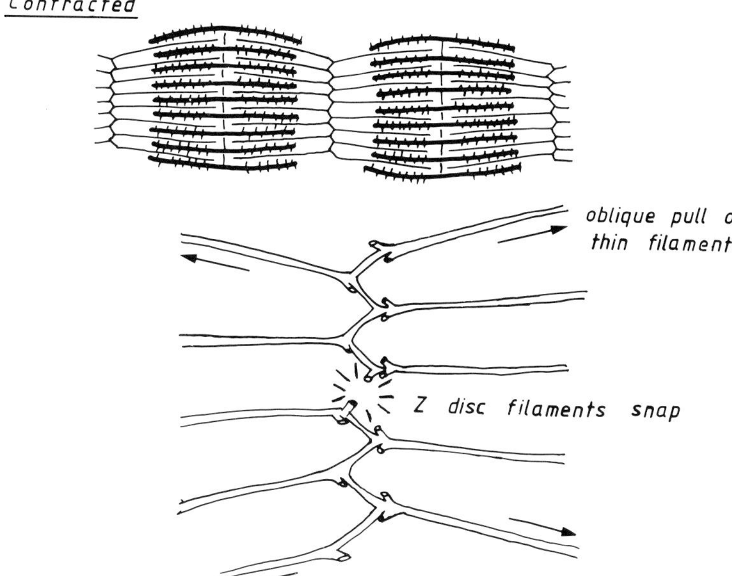

FIG. 5. Mechanism of myofibril splitting seems to depend on oblique pull of peripheral actin filaments. This oblique pull is due to mismatch in actin and myosin lattices. Obliqueness of actin filaments increases as myofibrils grow and also as sarcomeres shorten during contraction. When force is developed very rapidly, this oblique pull of actin filaments is believed to result in splitting of Z disks.

filament lattices. The thin filaments run from the Z disk, where the lattice is square or slightly rhombic, into the thick-filament lattice, where they take up a hexagonal configuration so that each thick filament is surrounded by six thin filaments. To achieve this transformation with a minimum displacement of thin filaments, the ratio of thin- to thick-filament lattice spacing has to be 1:1.5. When this ratio is achieved, the rhombic lattice can be transformed into a hexagonal one by displacing each thin filament by a small and equal amount. Measurements of myofibrils at all states of contraction and relaxation show that the ratio is always greater than this theoretical ratio. This means that the thin filaments are displaced more than they would be in the theoretical transition and the farther the thin filaments are from the center of the Z disk, the greater the displacement. This mismatch also means that as the myofibrils increase in size, the distance through which the peripheral thin filaments are displaced increases. When the sarcomere contracts, the oblique pull of the peripheral thin filaments results in a mechanical stress developing at the center of the Z disk (Fig. 5). If the force developed by the sarcomeres on each side of the Z disk is sufficient, then the Z disk will rip. The Z disk has a structure rather like a piece of cloth, and it is imagined that once a few of the central Z-disk filaments have been broken, then the rip will continue across the disk in the direction of the weave.

Another factor leading to myofibril splitting (in addition to their size) is the rate at which sarcomeres develop force. The most effective way of ripping a piece of cloth is to pull it very quickly. In fast-contracting muscles the myofibrils invariably appear to be more punctate and discrete, whereas in slow-contracting muscles the myofibrils appear to branch, presumably because the splitting is incomplete. It has been suggested (94) that this gives rise to the characteristic *Felderstruktur* and *Fibrillenstruktur* appearance of the myofibrils in slow- and fast-contracting muscle fibers, respectively. To demonstrate that development of force is important in the splitting of myofibrils, some muscles were stimulated electrically for periods of up to 30 min while the animals were anesthetized. After this short-term artificial exercise there was a considerable reduction in the numbers of large myofibrils in the experimental muscles as compared with unstimulated contralateral muscles. The longitudinal splitting of myofibrils may be important for two reasons. One is that it permits the extensive development of the SR and T system. The other is that it may expose new sites that may "seed" the polymerization of actin and myosin monomers and in this way encourage the formation of new thick and thin filaments. What is still unclear is how the myofibrils are built up in size and how the rate of synthesis of the contractile proteins in the muscle is controlled.

Synthesis and Assembly of Myofibrillar Proteins

The mechanism of differential gene expression in vertebrate cells is still very much a mystery. Certainly in muscle cells very little is known as yet about the control of transcription of DNA into messenger RNA (mRNA). Some information is available, however, about the translation of mRNA into protein. Using a cell-free system Heywood and Rich (55) showed that large polysomes of 50–60 ribosomes were capable of synthesizing myosin. In this work they used a radioactively labeled amino acid as the precursor, and the newly formed protein was identified using polyacrylamide gel electrophoresis. Similar studies have been carried out on polysomes of other sizes, showing that some of these synthesize the other contractile proteins such as actin and the light chains of myosin, the size of the polysome cluster corresponding to the molecular weight of the protein (91). These findings indicate that the different contractile proteins are synthesized independently and not produced from the one polycistronic strand of mRNA. This in turn means that the rate of synthesis of the different proteins may be independent of one another and therefore may be controlled by separate mechanisms. Heywood and Nwagwu (54) were able to isolate the mRNA of myosin from the large polysome clusters and have shown that the size of the mRNA corresponds to the large subunit of the myosin molecule, which has a molecular weight of about 200,000.

Although it is relatively easy to measure the rate of accumulation of the different contractile proteins during growth, it is much more difficult to estimate their rates of synthesis and turnover. There are several problems associated with the measurement of the rates of synthesis (108). In such studies it is desirable to choose a radioactive form of an amino acid that is neither synthesized nor degraded by the tissue concerned, e.g., tyrosine or phenylalanine for skeletal muscle. Perhaps the greatest problem in measuring protein synthesis lies in identifying and measuring the specific activity of the precursor amino acid pool(s). The specific activity of the one or more pools is influenced in time by several parameters, including the transport of the amino acid into and out of the cell and the intracellular rate of protein breakdown. Some of the latter factors are, in turn, influenced by the blood supply, which varies between different individual muscles and to the same muscle as a function of the age of the animal.

In spite of the difficulties experienced in studying the factors that influence the ratio of protein synthesis in vivo, some information has been obtained about protein synthesis in muscle during growth (31, 108). Several workers have noted that the total RNA and the ribosomal RNA per unit weight of muscle decreased during postnatal growth (26, 31). Besides the decrease in the total ribosomal content, the percentage of the ribosomes in polyribosome clusters also decreases during growth (7, 100). Polysome aggregates are certainly much more frequently observed with the electron microscope in embryonic or neonatal muscles than in adult tissue. Often they are seen in helical configurations around individual myosin filaments (63, 114).

Breuer and Florini (7) found that the ability of the cell-free systems to synthesize proteins was related to their polysome content; in other words, their mRNA content. The polysome content of the total ribosomal fraction was found to be 83% in the muscle of young rats and 72% in the muscle of older rats. Similar results have also been obtained for chick muscle. Although the concentration of ribosomes decreases with age, it seems that the production of mRNA becomes the limiting factor in myofibrillar production because the decrease in the percentage of ribosomes in polysomes that occurs during growth is probably a reflection of the reduction in mRNA synthesis. This has been verified by Srivastava (100), who demonstrated that synthetic mRNA could stimulate protein synthesis of muscle ribosome preparations and that the extent to which they were stimulated depended on the age of the muscle.

The accumulation of muscle mass during growth is the result of the balance between the synthetic and the degradative processes. Although the rate of synthesis of muscle protein can be estimated from the rate of incorporation of labeled amino acids, it is considerably more difficult to estimate the rate of degradation (29, 108)—particularly for specific proteins such as myosin. Estimates of turnover rates for myosin range from a few days to a few weeks; however, most of these studies measure incorporation over too long a time and do not account for the reutilization of the radioactive amino acids (108). Certainly there seems to be considerable turnover in the myofibrils both during growth and in adult muscle. How the contractile proteins are broken down is not known. This may involve the lysis of complete myofibrils, complete filaments, or parts of filaments, or it may involve the removal of individual protein monomers. In the latter case it is difficult to see how, for instance, an actin monomer could be removed without the actin filament breaking. The mechanism of turnover is not yet known, but what has emerged is that degradation may be as important as synthesis and that it does not necessarily take place at a constant rate (29). Goldspink (30) has shown that in muscles immobilized in the lengthened position there is an elevation of the rates of synthesis and degradation; however, synthesis is predominant and therefore there is accumulation of muscle mass, which includes the formation of extra sarcomeres in series.

It is not always appreciated that muscle represents a large reserve of protein. It has been estimated that about 12% of muscle protein is broken down each day (69), and as the musculature constitutes almost 45% of the body weight, this represents a lot of protein. In cases of emergency, for example, starvation and disease, some of this protein becomes available for purposes of energy production. Starvation has been shown to result in a reduction in the number of myofibrils and in the size of muscle fibers (34, 81). However, during short-term starvation myofibrillar proteins tend to be spared, and it is sarcoplasmic proteins that are used (17, 50, 71). More prolonged malnutrition does cause myofibrillar breakdown with the result that the ratio of myofibrillar to sarcoplasmic proteins becomes the same as in normal animals (109). Roy et al. (85) found the myofibrils in protein-deficient monkeys to be much thinner than in control animals, and they observed a loss of myofilaments from the periphery of the myofibrils.

The way in which myofibrils are assembled is rather a mystery. There are probably two mechanisms involved, one being the de novo assembly of myofibrils that takes place during embryonic development and the other being the building up of existing myofibrils that occurs in adult muscle after longitudinal splitting has taken place. Fischman suggested (25) that the construction of myofibrils may involve completed A and I filaments being assembled by the interaction of the myosin cross bridges with the actin filaments. This may be one reason why the sarcomeres in postnatal animals may not involve any de novo process as such but merely the adding of filaments to existing myofibrils. Certainly labeling studies have indicated that the newly formed proteins tend to be found around the periphery of existing myofibrils (72). Labeling studies on fish muscle (76) also confirmed this view. It was found that the outermost myofibrils (within the muscle fibers) tended to be the ones that were more heavily labeled. Etlinger et al. (24) were able to isolate some myosin filaments with a high specific activity after injections of [^{3}H]leucine into rats. They suggested that these represent the newly synthesized myosin filaments, which are probably relatively easily detached from the periphery of the myofibrils. Therefore it seems that myofibril assembly during postnatal growth involves the building up of existing myofibrils; however, the details of the process are not known.

Changes in Myofibrillar Proteins During Differentiation

Most muscles in adult animals are heterogeneous in that they were made up of different types of muscle fibers, some slow contracting and some fast contracting. The physiological properties of the fibers and of the muscles as a whole are to a large extent a reflection of the types of myofibrillar proteins they contain. Since the cross bridges (the force generators) belong to the myosin filaments, one might expect differences between the myosins of fast- and slow-contracting fibers. Indeed, the myosin of fast-contracting fibers is known to have the ability to hydrolyse adenosine 5′-triphosphate (ATP) much more rapidly than that from slow fibers. There are also differences in some of the other proteins, for example, the troponins, which are involved in the activation of the thin filaments. Recent evidence suggests that individual muscle fibers possess different kinds of myosin, although of course a fast-contracting fiber would be expected to have more fast myosin (65). There is some controversy, however, about fetal muscle. Some authors consider fetal myosin to be identical to adult fast-twitch myosin. Others suggest that it is a mixture of fast- and slow-twitch myosins. A third group of workers maintain that a distinct fetal form of myosin differs in primary structure from all adult myosin.

Although neonatal muscle is physiologically slow contracting (11, 12), when stained for myofibrillar ATPase using alkaline preincubation it stains in a way similar to adult fast-contracting muscle. (47). The ability of this histochemical method to distinguish between fast and slow myosin depends on the susceptibility of the different myosins to denaturation at alkaline and acid pH values rather than on their ATPase activity at physiological pH; therefore it may be that fetal and adult fast myosins are alike only in the ability to withstand denaturation at alkaline pH.

Rubinstein and Holtzer (86), using affinity-purified antibodies to adult chicken fast and slow myosin on cultures of embryonic pectoralis (presumptive fast) and embryonic anterior latissimus dorsi (presumptive slow), found that the fibers from both of these embryonic muscles would react only with the anti–fast myosin antibody. Other workers have claimed that antibodies to fast and slow myosins would react with chicken fast and slow myosins (67). Rubinstein and Holtzer (86) comment, however, that the antigens used by some workers are too impure. Other workers counter by stating that muscle cells do not differentiate normally in tissue culture. Nevertheless some biochemists, including Hoh and Yeoh (56) and Whalen et al. (112, 113), claim that fetal myosin has a distinct identity, because the separation of myosin light chains with two-dimensional electrophoresis is different for fetal muscle compared to adult muscle. Very recently Rowlerson (84) has been successful in distinguishing different fibers in fetal rat muscle (5 days before birth) by using antibodies developed to cat soleus muscle myosin, although all the fibers did react to some extent. The nature of fetal myosin therefore remains unclear. Although the basic molecule (heavy chains) exhibits properties of fast myosin in that it stains in a similar way for the myofibrillar ATPase method and it reacts with anti-fast myosin antibodies, the light chains seem somewhat different. Another confusing aspect of this type of work is that some workers use proteins from avian slow tonic muscles to generate antibodies and regard these as being equivalent to those prepared from the slow-twitch muscles of mammals. However, results from recent work indicate that these two types of muscle are quite different. Also the immunochemical approach is beset with difficulties, because it is almost certain that the antibody does not correspond to the active site of the myosin molecule and there are problems about the purity of the original antigen. The other main method for characterizing two-dimensional electrophoresis is a very complex technique, and the interpretation of the different patterns that are obtained can lead to differences of interpretation. The question of whether fetal myosin is different from adult myosin will no doubt be answered with improvements in technique.

MUSCLE FIBER TYPES IN ADULT MUSCLE

As stated, the contractile proteins of the myofibrils in young muscle fibers and adult muscle fibers may differ. Similarly most adult muscles are composed of different kinds of fibers that may be fast contracting or slow contracting. There are two main types of striated muscle fibers: tonic and phasic. The phasic fibers are diverse, and unfortunately the various methods of classification can be confusing. The classification used below is one of the simplest and most convenient.

Tonic Muscle Fibers

These fibers are very slow contracting and do not usually show a propagated muscle action potential; hence when stimulated with a single stimulus, they do not produce a significant response. They are multiply innervated (en grappe motor end plates) and have a graded response to stimulation of different frequencies. Tonic fibers usually have a very low specific myosin ATPase activity, and this is no doubt why they are capable of developing and maintaining isometric tension very economically (38, 68). A good example of this type of muscle is the anterior latissimus dorsi muscle in the bird, which holds the wings against the body. The fibers of this muscle, like other tonic fibers, are able to remain contracted for long periods of time with very little utilization of energy.

Phasic Muscle Fibers

SLOW-TWITCH, PHASIC FIBERS. These slow-twitch, phasic fibers are also called SO or type I. They are slow contracting but they are not usually as slow as the tonic muscle fibers. They have a propagated action potential and are hence referred to as twitch fibers. Slow-twitch, phasic fibers are responsible for both maintaining posture and carrying out slow repetitive movements and are economical and efficient in carrying out these functions (38). Since they usually contain many mitochondria and since their myofibrils hydrolyze ATP only very slowly, this type of fiber is very fatigue resistant.

FAST-TWITCH, PHASIC, GLYCOLYTIC FIBERS. These fast-twitch, phasic, glycolytic fibers are also known as FG, FF, or type IIB. These fibers are adapted for a high-power output and have a reasonable thermodynamic efficiency for producing work. They have a high or very high intrinsic speed of shortening and hence a high myosin ATPase specific activity. Fast-twitch, phasic fibers are usually used only when very rapid movement is required. They usually possess very few mitochondria because they cannot possibly replenish ATP as fast as it is used. They therefore fatigue very rapidly and their energy supplies are replenished while the fibers are inactive. During contraction the energy that is supplied comes mainly from glycolysis and the immediate energy stores (ATP and phosphocreatine).

FAST-TWITCH, PHASIC, OXIDATIVE FIBERS. These fast-twitch, phasic, oxidative fibers are also called FOG, FR, or type IIA. These fibers are essentially the same as the fast glycolytic fibers except that they contain more mitochondria. In some cases they may have a slightly lower intrinsic rate of shortening than the fast-twitch glycolytic fibers. Fast-twitch oxidative fibers are apparently adapted for fast movements of a repetitive nature and are probably recruited next after the slow-twitch fibers. Because of the larger numbers of mitochondria, they are less subject to fatigue and are able to recover relatively quickly after exercise.

Structural Differences Between Myofibrils of Different Fiber Types

The usual way of distinguishing between different fiber types is based on their histochemical staining for myofibrillar (myosin) ATPase, after preincubation at acid or alkaline pH. The fibers are distinguished by their susceptibility to pH denaturation and not on true myofibrillar activity at physiological pH. Therefore there has been some criticism of this method. There is now good reason to believe that this approach is valid, however, because myosin extracted from physiologically fast and slow muscles has been shown to have different specific activities, pH sensitivities, and isoenzymic forms (90, 99). Also Essen et al. (23), using homogenates and extracts of single fibers identified by their acid and alkali-stable myofibrillar ATPase, were able to confirm the histochemical observations of relative oxidative, glycolytic, and myofibrillar activity. It therefore appears that the myofibrillar ATPase method is in general valid, although there are still pitfalls, particularly in the identification of the subtypes of fast fibers. In human muscle the fast fibers may be divided into three types: IIA, IIB, and IIC on the basis of acid sensitivity (8, 9). This is possible with some animal muscle; however, care must be exercised in identifying the subtypes because sometimes the pH sensitivities of the fast-twitch, oxidative fibers and the fast-twitch, glycolytic fibers are reversed. For instance, the FOGs in mouse muscle are more alkali stable than the FGs, although in hamster muscle it is the FGs that are more alkali stable (43). For this reason most workers still combine the myofibrillar ATPase stain with histochemical staining for oxidative enzymes, for example, succinic dehydrogenase (75) and NADH-tetrazolium reductase (19, 74), as shown in Figure 6. Recently Spurway (97), using a microphotometer, measured the intensity of staining individual fibers with different staining methods on serial sections. He found that four different fiber types could be identified: FG, FOG, FO, and SO, although this distinction cannot apparently be achieved with oxidative enzymes alone.

An alternative approach to making measurements on individual fibers in sections is to carry out microbiochemical analysis on the myofibrils of isolated fibers (23, 79, 110). This has been very useful in some studies, although it is not yet clear just how many fiber types can be identified by this method because

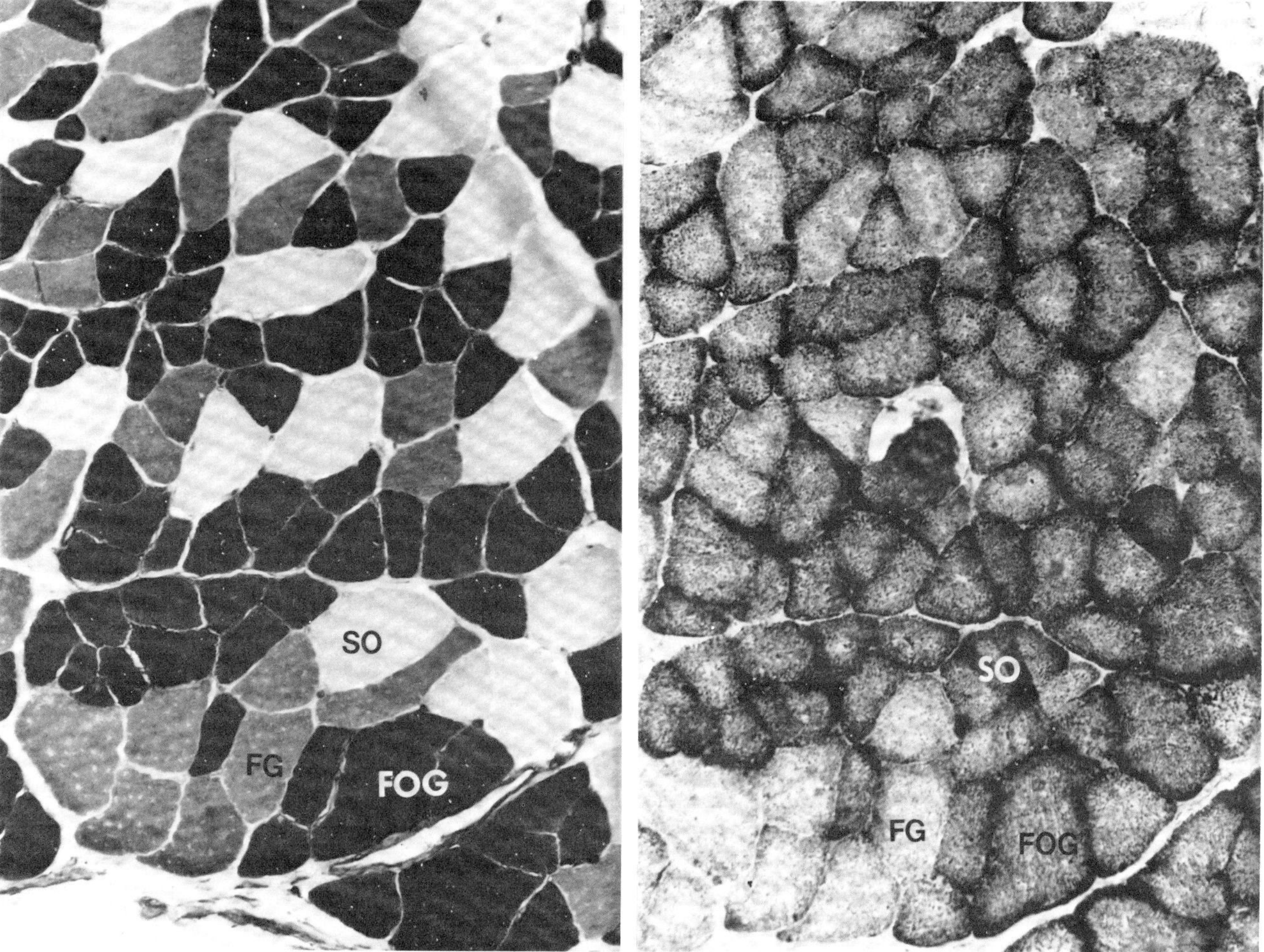

FIG. 6. Method of distinguishing different fiber types with myofibrillar ATPase stain (*left*) and oxidative enzymes such as succinic dehydrogenase (*right*). With these methods, at least 3 fiber types can be distinguished in most mammalian muscles. The ATPase method includes preincubation at pH 9.4, and therefore alkaline-resistant fibers stain more darkly. Three fiber types—slow twitch, oxidative (SO), fast twitch, glycolytic (FG), and fast twitch, oxidative, glycolytic (FOG)—are indicated. (Photomicrographs by P. Watt of Muscle Research Unit, University of Hull, England.)

of the problems of sampling the less common fiber types.

One other source of information concerning fiber types has been electrophysiological studies in motor units (16, 20, 61). These methods involve either splitting the ventral root and stimulating a single motor axon or stimulating a simple motoneuron by impaling the nerve cell body in the spinal cord with a microelectrode. In brief, these studies indicate three types of fibers: FF, FR, and S (15). There is often some overlap, however, in the physiological properties of these motor units, and there is again a sampling problem for the less common fiber types, particularly the IIC.

Ultrastructural differences among the fiber types have been investigated by several workers, including Eisenberg, Kuda, and Peter (22), Eisenberg and Kuda (21), Gauthier (27), and Sjöstrom et al. (96). These include differences in M-line structure as well as Z-line thickness. In addition to differences in myofibril structure there are also differences between the form and number of other organelles in the fiber types. These include the mitochondrial content (27), the myofibrillar content (57), the SR and T system (22, 77), and the plasma membrane (93). The slow-twitch fibers tend to have wider Z lines, a higher mitochondrial content, and smaller area of T and SR tubules than the fast-twitch fibers. Eisenberg and Kuda (21) found that if all three parameters were considered, there was a 90% certainty of identifying the fibers as fast or slow twitch, and they found Z-line thickness to be the single best parameter.

CHANGES IN MUSCLE FIBER TYPES DURING GROWTH

Several workers have investigated the change in proportion of fiber types during growth. Kugelberg (62) reported that there is an increase in the number of fibers low in ATPase in the soleus muscle of the rat with growth, whereas Tomanek (104) reported a decrease in the number of fibers high in ATPase in the soleus muscle of the cat with growth. Recently Goldspink and Ward (43) made measurements of the number and sizes of the major fiber types in hamster muscle with age (Fig 7). They found that in the hamster biceps brachii, which is predominantly composed of fibers high in ATPase, there was a decrease in the number of fibers low in ATPase. In the soleus muscle, which is predominantly composed of fibers low in ATPase, there was a decrease in the fibers high in ATPase with age. Although there was a change in the proportion of fiber types, there was no change in the total number of fibers within the muscle. It was therefore suggested that some reinnervation may take place during growth and that this is why the less predominant fiber type tends to decrease in number. Certainly the mechanism of conversion may involve alterations in the innervation of the muscle fibers, because it is

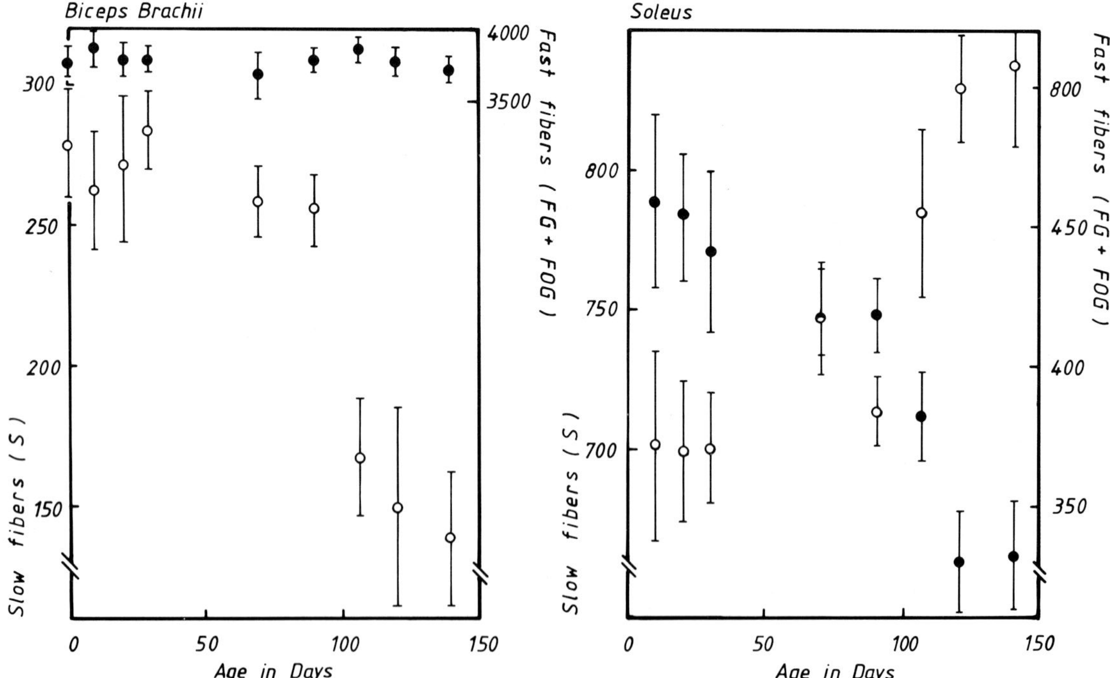

FIG. 7. Change in number of fast (●) and slow (○) fibers in mouse biceps brachii and soleus muscles during growth. Because total number of fibers does not change, change in number of different types means that there is some interconversion of types. Predominant fiber type is the one that tends to increase, and this may be the result of some reinnervation. [From Goldspink and Ward (43).]

known from cross-innervation experiments (11, 12) that the nerve supply of the muscle is one of the most important factors determining muscle fiber type. Alterations in the motor input of skeletal muscles may increase with age, and this may involve a turnover of the neuromuscular connections themselves (6, 105) or in the pattern of neuromuscular transmission (49). Therefore the change in the percentage of fiber types may involve one or both of these factors.

EFFECT OF EXERCISE AND INACTIVITY ON MYOFIBRILLAR CONTENT OF MUSCLE FIBERS

Hypertrophy of muscle fibers in response to exercise training was noted many years ago by Morpurgo (73). Although Morpurgo attributed hypertrophy to an increase in the sarcoplasm rather than in the myofibrils, it is now known from biochemical studies (53) and cytological studies (33, 36) that work-induced hypertrophy is usually associated with a large increase in the myofibrillar material of the fibers. The number of myofibrils increases (40), and this is almost certainly due to the longitudinal splitting of existing myofibrils rather than de novo assembly. An increase in the myofibrillar content of muscle fibers makes physiological sense, because this is the means for increasing the contractile force of the muscle. As stated, most mammalian muscles are composed of fast- and slow-twitch fibers, and one kind of fiber may be converted into another in a manner similar to what apparently takes place during growth. There seems to be no convincing evidence, however, for any change in the proportions of fiber types in adult muscle as a result of exercise. Indeed there is a reasonable amount of evidence to the contrary. Walsh and colleagues (107) studied the physiological properties of individual motor units in soleus muscles that had undergone compensatory hypertrophy after excision or denervation of the gastrocnemius muscle. Although they found a large increase in mean tetanic tension, they found no change in the twitch contraction times or fatigue resistance of any of the types of motor unit. Others indicated that although hypertrophy had taken place, this was not associated with qualitative changes in the myofibrils. Also, Burke et al. (14) had found that inactivity induced by chronic immobilization produced no change in the proportions of fiber types, although there was selective atrophy, with the fast-twitch, oxidative, glycolytic (fatigue-resistant) motor units affected more severely.

Goldspink and Ward (43) studied the effects of weight-lifting exercise on the size and proportion of fiber types in certain rodent muscles. They found no change in the proportion of fiber types or total number of fibers within the muscles. There was selective hypertrophy of some fiber types, however, depending on the nature of the exercise and the location of the muscle. The fast-twitch, glycolytic fibers usually hypertrophied more than the fast-twitch, oxidative, glycolytic fibers or the slow-twitch fibers. Thus it seems that exercise produces hypertrophy of one or more fiber types in the muscle and that this is associated with a quantitative rather than a qualitative change in the myofibrillar content of the muscle fibers. Although the proportions of the fiber types are apparently unchanged by activity or inactivity, the total cross-sectional area of the fast myofibrils or the slow myofibrils is very much affected by the differential hypertrophy or atrophy of the different fiber types, and therefore the physiological characteristics of the muscle as a whole will change. This may not be the end of the story, because it may be possible to convert fast-twitch fibers into slow-twitch fibers if the recruitment pattern of the fibers can be substantially altered by the exercise. This can be achieved by artificial stimulation, as described next.

ULTRASTRUCTURAL CHANGES ASSOCIATED WITH CROSS INNERVATION AND ARTIFICIAL STIMULATION

The speed of contraction of fast muscles and slow muscles can be reversed by crossing their nerve supplies (11, 12). Therefore the nerve supply apparently is very important in determining what type of myofibrils are produced by the individual muscle fibers. This is a fascinating problem because it implies that the motoneurons, by some means, can selectively activate the genes for the synthesis of either fast-contracting myofibrils or slow-contracting myofibrils. The motoneurons might act via some chemotrophic substance or by the impulse pattern; it is known, for instance, that "slow" motoneurons have a sustained low-frequency pattern, whereas "fast" motoneurons tend to deliver impulses intermittently at a high frequency.

Changes in contractile speed have been shown to be accompanied by changes in myosin ATPase (5, 13) and changes in the types of myofibrillar protein subunits (80, 88, 98, 111). Therefore the transformation of contractile speeds undoubtedly involves alterations in the myofibrils. The changes are not confined to the myofibrils, however: the activity of the SR changes (70) and the metabolic enzyme levels also change (19, 48, 82). Changes in the ultrastructure of myofibrils as a result of a changed impulse pattern have clearly been shown for the Z band (87, 22a), the M line (95), and the SR (52, 22a).

The question as to whether it is a chemotrophic effect or impulse activity seems to have been answered to some extent by the experiments of Salmons and Vrbova (89), Al-Amood et al. (1), and Lømo et al. (64), who showed that contraction speeds could be changed by imposing the opposite type of impulse pattern using implanted electrodes and electrical stimulation. More recently Salmons and Sréter (88), using stimulation in conjunction with cross innervation, were able to prevent the transformation from fast to slow contraction by supplying the appropriate stimulation pattern. This again tends to mitigate against a chemotrophic effect, although possibly there are two effects and under these circumstances the impulse pattern is the most important. Nevertheless there is some sort of trophic effect of the motoneurons, because if the muscle is denervated, the fibers degenerate. In hemiplegia or cordotomy the fibers of the affected muscles are not functional, although the motoneuron-muscle connections are still intact. Under these circumstances the muscle fibers atrophy but do not degenerate, and the ratio of fiber types on a given muscle is unaltered. Therefore there is a trophic effect. There is no good evidence, however, that it is involved in the determination of fiber type. Indeed the stimulation experiments strongly suggest that activity is the important determinant of the type of myofibrils produced within an individual fiber.

Changing the nerve supply to the muscle or superimposing a different activity pattern by artificial stimulation may not be the only means of altering the synthesis of specific myofibrillar proteins, since recent work has shown that there may be some hormonal control. Vaughan et al. (106) showed that the ratio of fiber types is different in male and female mice and that castration of the males changes the ratio, making it similar to that of the female animal. This suggests that androgens can influence the type of myofibrils produced. Also recent work has shown that the fiber-type ratio may be radically altered in hypo- and hyperthyroidism (3, 10, 58).

TEMPERATURE ADAPTATION IN MYOFIBRILS OF ECTOTHERMIC ANIMALS

Muscles in endothermic animals work over a restricted temperature range, but those in some ectothermic animals have to work at more extreme temperatures. Antarctic fish, for example, experience environmental temperatures of −1°C–4°C; at the other end of the scale, fish in the hot springs of the Rift Valley in East Africa live at temperatures of 35°C–38°C. Assuming the same basic force-producing mechanism of the myofibrils, how can antarctic fish move about at these low temperatures? Recent work has shown that the contractile apparatus of antarctic fish differs from that of fish living in warm water or moderate-temperature water in that it hydrolyzes ATP more rapidly at low temperature [Goldspink et al. (60)]. The increased specific activity of the myofibrillar ATPase seems to be associated with a difference in the tertiary structure of the proteins, because the myofibrils are very susceptible to heat denaturation (Fig. 8). At higher environmental temperatures fish

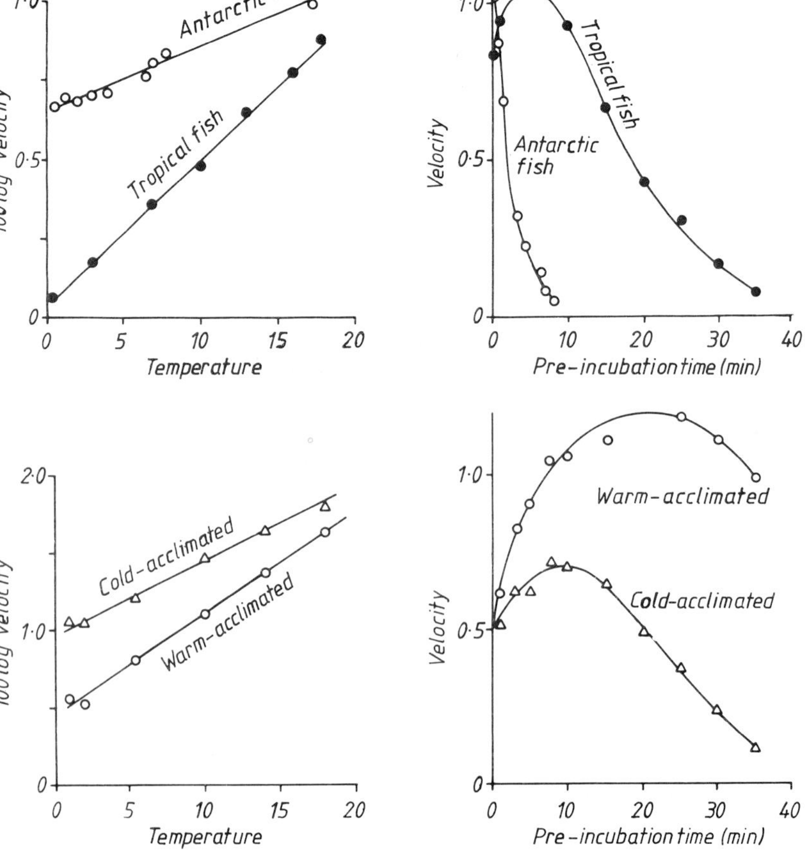

FIG. 8. Plots of ATPase activity (mol $P_i \cdot mg^{-1} \cdot min^{-1}$) and rate of temperature denaturation for myofibrils of antarctic and tropical fish (*top*) and warm- and cold-acclimated carp (*bottom*). Plots on *left* show specific ATPase activity of myofibrils at different temperatures; those on the *right* show residual ATPase activity after preincubation for different periods of time at 37°C. Production of different kinds of myofibril according to environmental temperature is seen from results of warm- and cold-adapted fish. [From Johnston, Goldspink, et al. (60).]

require a fairly heat-stable contractile system; therefore these fish have evolved myofibrillar proteins with a more rigid molecular structure.

Many species of fish live within a very restricted temperature range, and hence they have evolved a myofibrillar system that is adapted for this range. A few species, however, can adapt to a wide range of temperatures; the carp family provides several examples of fish with this ability. For instance, the common goldfish can survive and move around reasonably well at temperatures of about +1°C in an ice-bound garden pool, and yet it can live quite happily in an ornamental pool in the tropics. The carp family can acclimate to these temperatures because they have the ability to alter the characteristics of the contractile proteins. During acclimation to a low environmental temperature they produce myofibrils with an ATPase that is active at the lower end of the temperature scale but that is more readily denaturated by heat. Fish acclimated to a high environmental temperature have a myosin ATPase that is only active at the higher temperatures but that is relatively heat stable [Fig. 8; (69)].

Alterations in the rate of muscular contraction during temperature acclimation may involve changes in the rate at which the cross bridges work (myosin ATPase activity), but they may also involve the rate at which the active sites become available on the actin filaments. Work by I. A. Johnston at the University of St. Andrews and in our own laboratory (59) has indicated that the troponin complex changes during temperature acclimation. Indeed if the troponin is removed from myofibrils prepared from warm- and cold-adapted fish, the myofibrils no longer show the elevated ATPase activity at low temperatures. The difference is again obtained when the troponins are replaced (59). This may not mean that the troponins are directly involved in this adaptation but merely that the myofibrillar complex must be intact to show differences between warm- and cold-adapted fish.

Excitation-activation coupling has also been studied in fish acclimated to high and low temperatures. Penney and Goldspink (78) were unable to find any change in the composition and Ca^{2+}-binding properties of the SR. The SR was more extensive and the myofibrils were smaller, however, in the cold-adapted fish, so both the relaxation and the activation processes are more rapid than they would otherwise be at the low temperatures. Adaptation to low environmental temperature therefore involves morphological changes in the myofibrils as well as in types of protein they contain.

CONCLUSION

The sliding-filament mechanism occurs throughout the animal kingdom, undoubtedly because it is adaptable and very effective in producing force. I have attempted to show how the mechanism is altered during growth, exercise, and changes in environmental temperature to meet the locomotory requirements of particular animals. There are still many gaps in our understanding of how the myofibrillar system is altered, because mechanisms at the molecular level are involved; however, our knowledge undoubtedly will increase in the next 10 or 20 years. Certainly the study of adaptation at the cellular and molecular level is very exciting, and muscle, perhaps more than any other tissue, is a good example of this type of adaptation.

REFERENCES

1. AL-AMOOD, W., A. J. BULLER, AND R. POPE. Long-term stimulation of cat fast-twitch skeletal muscle. *Nature London* 244: 225–227, 1973.
2. ARONSON, J. Sarcomere size in developing muscles of a tarsonemidmite. *J. Biophys. Biochem. Cytol.* 11: 147–156, 1961.
3. ASHTON, J. A., A. G. MONTGOMERY, AND S. N. WEBB. Motor unit characteristics of hypothyroid slow-twitch rat muscle. *J. Physiol. London* 310: 54P, 1980.
4. AUBER, J. L'accroissement en longueur des myofibrilles et la formation de nouveaux sarcomeres au cours du developpement des muscles du vol chez *Calliphora erythrocephala* (Mg). *C. R. Acad. Sci.* 261: 4845–4848, 1965.
5. BÁRÁNY, M., AND R. I. CLOSE. The transformation of myosin in cross-innervated rat muscles. *J. Physiol. London* 213: 455–474, 1971.
6. BARKER, D., AND M. C. IP. The probable existence of motor end-plate replacement. *J. Physiol. London* 176: 11P–12P, 1965.
7. BREUER, C. B., AND J. R. FLORINI. Amino acid incorporation into protein by cell-free preparations from rat skeletal muscle. IV. Effects of age, androgens and anabolic agents on activity of muscle ribosomes. *Biochemistry* 4: 1544–1549, 1965.
8. BROOKE, M. H., AND K. K. KAISER. Muscle fiber types: how many and what kind? *Arch. Neurol. Chicago* 23: 369–379, 1970.
9. BROOKE, M. H., AND K. K. KAISER. The use and abuse of muscle histochemistry in the trophic functions of the neuron. *Ann. NY Acad. Sci.* 228: 121–144, 1974.
10. BRUCE, D. S., AND C. J. M. NICOL. Contractile and fibre population changes induced by hyperthyroidism in rat skeletal muscle. *J. Physiol. London* 310: 57P–58P, 1980.
11. BULLER, A. J., J. C. ECCLES, AND R. M. ECCLES. Differentiation of fast and slow muscles in the cat hindlimb. *J. Physiol. London* 150: 399–416, 1960.
12. BULLER, A. J., J. C. ECCLES, AND R. M. ECCLES. Interactions between motorneurons and muscles in respect of the characteristic speed of their responses. *J. Physiol. London* 150: 417–439, 1960.
13. BULLER, A. J., W. H. F. M. MOMMAERTS, AND K. SERAYDARIAN. Enzymatic properties of myosin in fast and slow-twitch muscles of the cat following cross-innervation. *J. Physiol. London* 205: 581–597, 1969.
14. BURKE, R. E., K. KANDA, AND R. F. MAYER. The effect of c' ronic immobilization on defined types of motor units in cat medial gastrocnemius. *Soc. Neurosci. Abstr.* 1: 1174, 1975.
15. BURKE, R. E., D. N. LEVINE, F. E. ZAJAC, P. TSAIRIS, AND W. K. ENGEL. Mammalian motor units: physiological-histochemical correlation in three types of cat gastrocnemius. *Science* 174: 709–712, 1971.
16. BURKE, R. E., AND P. TSAIRIS. The correlation of physiological properties with histochemical characteristics in single motor units. *Ann. NY Acad. Sci.* 228: 145–159, 1974.
17. DICKENSON, J. W. T., AND R. A. MCCANCE. The early effects of rehabilitation on the chemical structure of the organs and

whole bodies of undernourished pigs and cockerels. *Clin. Sci.* 27: 123–136, 1964.

18. DUBOWITZ, V. Cross-innervated mammalian skeletal muscle: histochemical, physiological and biochemical observations. *J. Physiol. London* 193: 481–496, 1967.
19. DUBOWITZ, V., AND M. H. BROOKE. *Major Problems in Neurology. Muscle Biopsy: a Modern Approach.* Philadelphia, PA: Saunders, 1973, vol. 2.
20. EDSTROM, L., AND E. KUGELBERG. Histochemical mapping of motor units in experimentally reinnervated skeletal muscle. *Experientia* 25: 1044–1045, 1969.
21. EISENBERG, B. R., AND A. M. KUDA. Discrimination between fibre populations in mammalian skeletal muscle by using ultrastructural parameters. *J. Ultrastruct. Res.* 54: 76–88, 1976.
22. EISENBERG, B. R., A. M. KUDA, AND J. B. PETER. Stereological analysis of mammalian skeletal muscle. I. Soleus muscle of the guinea pig. *J. Cell Biol.* 60: 732–754, 1974.

22a. EISENBERG, B. R., AND S. SALMONS. The reorganization of subcellular structure in muscle undergoing fast to slow type transformation: a stereological study. *Cell Tissue Res.* In press.

23. ESSEN, B., E. JANSSON, J. HENRIKSSON, A. W. TAYLOR, AND B. SALTIN. Metabolic characteristics of fibre types in human skeletal muscles. *Acta Physiol. Scand.* 95: 153–165, 1975.
24. ETLINGER, J. D., R. ZAK, D. A. FISCHMAN, AND M. RABINOWITZ. Isolation of newly synthesized myosin filaments from skeletal muscle homogenates and myofibrils. *Nature London* 255: 259–261, 1975.
25. FISCHMAN, D. A. An electron microscope study of myofibril formation in embryonic chick skeletal muscle. *J. Cell Biol.* 32: 557–575, 1967.
26. FLORINI, J. R., AND C. B. BREUER. Amino acid incorporation into protein by cell-free preparations from rat skeletal muscle. III. Comparison of muscle and liver ribosomes. *Biochemistry* 4: 253–257, 1965.
27. GAUTHIER, G. F. Some ultrastructural and cytochemical features of fibre populations in the soleus muscle. *Anat. Rec.* 180: 551–552, 1975.
28. GAUTHIER, G. F. Ultrastructural identification of muscle fibre types by immunocytochemistry. *J. Cell Biol.* 82: 391–401, 1979.
29. GOLDBERG, A. L., AND J. F. DICE. Intracellular protein degradation in mammalian and bacterial cells. *Annu. Rev. Biochem.* 43: 835–869, 1974.
30. GOLDSPINK, D. F. The influence of immobilization and stretch on protein turnover of rat skeletal muscle. *J. Physiol. London* 264: 267–282, 1977.
31. GOLDSPINK, D. F., AND G. GOLDSPINK. Age-related changes in protein turnover and ribonucleic acid of the diaphragm muscle of normal and dystrophic hamsters. *Biochem. J.* 162: 191–194, 1977.
32. GOLDSPINK, G. Fixation of muscle. *Nature London* 192: 1305–1306, 1961.
33. GOLDSPINK, G. The combined effects of exercise and reduced food intake on skeletal muscle fibres. *J. Cell. Comp. Physiol.* 63: 209–216, 1964.
34. GOLDSPINK, G. Cytological basis of decrease in muscle strength during starvation. *Am. J. Physiol.* 209: 100–104, 1965.
35. GOLDSPINK, G. Sarcomere length during the post-natal growth of mammalian muscle fibre. *J. Cell Sci.* 3: 539–548, 1968.
36. GOLDSPINK, G. The proliferation of myofibrils during muscle fibre growth. *J. Cell Sci.* 6: 593–603, 1970.
37. GOLDSPINK, G. Ultrastructure changes in striated muscle fibres during contraction and growth with particular reference to the mechanism of myofibril splitting. *J. Cell Sci.* 9: 123–138, 1971.
38. GOLDSPINK, G. Biochemical energetics for fast and slow muscles. In: *Comparative Physiology: Functional Aspects of Structural Materials,* edited by L. Bolis, S. H. P. Maddrell, and K. Schmidt-Nielsen. Amsterdam: Elsevier, 1975. (Proc. Int. Conf., Ascona, 1974.)
39. GOLDSPINK, G., A. HAYAT, AND P. E. WILLIAMS. The relationship between the activity pattern of a muscle and the synthesis of fast and slow contractile proteins (Abstract). *Proc. Int. Congr. Physiol. Sci., 28th, Budapest, 1980,* vol. 14, p. 124.
40. GOLDSPINK, G., AND K. HOWELLS. Work-induced hypertrophy in exercised normal muscles of different ages and the reversibility of hypertrophy after cessation of exercise. *J. Physiol. London* 239: 179–193, 1974.
41. GOLDSPINK, G., R. E. LARSON, AND R. E. DAVIES. Thermodynamic efficiency and physiological characteristics of the chick anterior latissimus dorsi muscle. *Z. Vgl. Physiol.* 66: 379–388, 1970.
42. GOLDSPINK, G., J. C. TABARY, C. TABARY, C. TARDIEU, AND G. TARDIEU. Effect of denervation on the adaptation of sarcomere number and muscle extensibility to the functional length of the muscle. *J. Physiol. London* 236: 733–742, 1974.
43. GOLDSPINK, G., AND P. S. WARD. Changes in rodent muscle fibre types during post-natal growth, undernutrition and exercise. *J. Physiol. London* 296: 453–469, 1979.
44. GORDON, A. M., A. F. HUXLEY, AND F. J. JULIAN. Tension development in highly stretched vertebrate muscle fibres. *J. Physiol. London* 184: 170–192, 1966.
45. GORDON, A. M., A. F. HUXLEY, AND F. J. JULIAN. The variation in isometric tension with sarcomere length in vertebrate muscle fibres. *J. Physiol. London* 184: 143–169, 1966.
46. GRIFFIN, G., G. GOLDSPINK, AND P. E. WILLIAMS. Region of longitudinal growth in striated muscle fibres. *Nature London New Biol.* 232: 28–29, 1971.
47. GUTH, L., AND F. J. SAMAHA. Erroneous interpretations which may result from the application of the "myofibrillar ATPase" histochemical procedure to developing muscle. *Exp. Neurol.* 34: 465–475, 1972.
48. GUTH, L., P. K. WATSON, AND W. C. BROWN. Effects of cross-reinnervation on some chemical properties of red and white muscles in the rat and cat. *Exp. Neurol.* 20: 52–69, 1968.
49. GUTTMAN, E. Age changes in the neuromusclar system and aspects of rehabilitation medicine. In: *Neurophysiological Aspects of Rehabilitation Medicine,* edited by A. A. Buerger and J. S. Jobsis. Springfield, IL: Thomas, 1976, p. 42–61.
50. HAGAN, S. N., AND R. O. SCOW. Effect of fasting on muscle proteins and fat in young rats of different ages. *Am. J. Physiol.* 188: 91–94, 1957.
51. HEIDENHEIN, M. Über die Entstelung der quergestreiften Muskelsubstanz. *Arch. Mikroskop. Anat. Entwicklungsmech.* 83: 427–653, 1913.
52. HEILMAN, C., AND D. PETTE. Molecular transformations in sarcoplasmic reticulum of fast-twitch muscle by electro-stimulation. *Eur. J. Biochem.* 93: 437–446, 1979.
53. HELANDER, E. A. S. Influence of exercise and restricted activity on the protein composition of skeletal muscle. *Biochem. J.* 78: 478–482, 1961.
54. HEYWOOD, S. M., AND M. NWAGWU. Partial characterization of presumptive myosin messenger ribonucleic acid. *Biochemistry* 8: 3839–3845, 1969.
55. HEYWOOD, S. M., AND A. RICH. *In vitro* synthesis of native actin tropomyosin from embryonic chick polyribosomes. *Proc. Natl. Acad. Sci. USA* 57: 1002–1004, 1968.
56. HOH, J. F. Y., AND G. P. S. YEOH. Rabbit skeletal myosin insoenzymes from foetal, fast-twitch and slow-twitch muscles. *Nature London* 280: 321–323, 1979.
57. HOWELLS, K. F., T. C. JORDAN, AND J. D. HOWELLS. Myofibril content of histochemical fibre types in rat skeletal muscle. *Acta Histochem.* 63: 177–182, 1978.
58. IANUZZO D., P. PATEL, B. CHEN, P. O'BRIAN, AND C. WILLIAMS. Thyroidal trophic influence on skeletal muscle myosin. *Nature London* 270: 74–76, 1977.
59. JOHNSTON, I. A. Calcium regulatory proteins and temperature acclimation of actomyosin ATPase, from a eurythermal teleost, *Carassius auratus,* L. *J. Comp. Physiol.* 129: 163–167, 1979.
60. JOHNSTON, I. A., N. J. WALESBY, W. DAVISON, AND G. GOLDSPINK. Temperature adaptation in myosin of Antarctic fish. *Nature London* 254: 74–75, 1975.
61. KUGELBERG, E. Properties of the hind-limb motor units. In: *New Developments in Electromyography and Clinical Neurophysiology,* edited by J. E. Desmedt. Basel: Karger, 1973, vol. I.

62. Kugelberg, E. Adaptive transformation of rat soleus motor units during growth. *J. Neurol. Sci.* 22: 269–289, 1976.
63. Larson, P. F., P. Hudgson, and J. N. Walton. Morphological relationship of polyribosomes and myosin filaments in developing and regenerating skeletal muscle. *Nature London* 222: 1169–1170, 1969.
64. Lømo, T., R. H. Westgaard, and A. H. Dahl. Contractile properties of muscle: control by pattern of muscle activity in the rat. *Proc. R. Soc. London Ser. B* 187: 99–103, 1974.
65. Lutz, H., H. Weber, R. Billeter, and E. Jenny. Fast and slow myosin within skeletal muscle fibres of adult rabbits. *Nature London* 281: 142–144, 1979.
66. MacCallum, J. B. Histogenesis of the striated muscle fibre and the growth of the human sartorius. *Johns Hopkins Hosp. Bull.* 9: 208–212, 1898.
67. Masaka, T., and C. Yoshizaki. Differentiation of myosin in chick embryos. *J. Biochem.* 76: 123–131, 1974.
68. Matsumoto, Y. T., T. Hoekman, and B. C. Abbott. Heat measurements associated with isometric contraction in fast and slow muscles of the chicken. *Comp. Biochem. Physiol. A* 46: 785–797, 1973.
69. Millward, D. J. Protein turnover in skeletal muscle. 1. The measurement of rates of synthesis and catabolism of skeletal muscle protein using [^{14}C] Na^2CO_3 to label protein. *Clin. Sci.* 39: 577–590, 1970.
70. Mommaerts, W. F. H. M., A. J. Buller, and K. Seraydarian. The modification of some biochemical properties of muscle by cross-innervation. *Proc. Natl. Acad. Sci. USA* 64: 128–133, 1969.
71. Montgomery, R. D., J. W. T. Dickerson, and R. A. McCance. Severe undernutrition in growing and adult animals. 13. The morphology and chemistry of development and undernutrition in the sartorius muscle of the fowl. *Br. J. Nutr.* 18: 587–593, 1964.
72. Morkin, E. Postnatal muscle fiber assembly: localization of newly synthesised myofibrillar proteins. *Science* 167: 1499–1501, 1970.
73. Morpurgo, B. On the nature of functional hypertrophy of voluntary muscle. *Arch. Sci. Med.* 19: 327–336, 1897.
74. Novikoff, A. B., W. Shin, and J. Drucker. Mitochondrial localization of oxidative enzymes. Staining results with two tetrazolium salts. *J. Biophys. Biochem. Cytol.* 9: 47–54, 1961.
75. Padykula, H. A. The localization of succinic dehydrogenase in tissue sections of the rat. *Am. J. Anat.* 91: 107–132, 1952.
76. Paterson, S., and G. Goldspink. Fibre growth and myofibril proliferation in red and white fish muscle. *J. Cell Sci.* 22: 607–616, 1976.
77. Peachey, L. D. The sarcoplasmic reticulum and transverse tubules of the frog's sartorius. *J. Cell Biol.* 25: 209–231, 1965.
78. Penney, R. K., and G. Goldspink. Temperature adaptation of sarcoplasmic reticulum of fish muscle. *J. Therm. Biol.* 5: 63–68, 1980.
79. Pette, D., J. Henriksson, and M. Emmerich. Myofibrillar protein patterns of single fibres from human muscle. *FEBS Lett.* 103: 152–155, 1979.
80. Pette, D., W. Müller, E. Leisner, and G. Vrbová. Time-dependent effects on contractile properties, fibre population, myosin light chains and enzymes of energy metabolism in intermittently and continuously stimulated fast twitch muscles of the rabbit. *Pfluegers Arch.* 364: 103–112, 1976.
81. Raccla, A. S., H. J. Grady, J. Higginson, and D. J. Svobava. Protein deficiency in rhesus monkeys. *Am. J. Pathol.* 49: 419–443, 1966.
82. Romanul, F. C. A., and J. P. Van der Meulen. Slow and fast muscles after cross-reinnervation. Enzymatic and physiological changes. *Arch. Neurol. Chicago* 17: 387–402, 1967.
83. Rowe, R. W. D., and G. Goldspink. Studies on post-embryonic growth and development of skeletal muscle. II. Physiological changes associated with the growth of the rat biceps brachii. *Proc. R. Ir. Acad. Sect. B* 66: 85–89, 1969.
84. Rowlerson, A. Differentiation of muscle fibre types in fetal and young rats studied with a labelled antibody to slow myosin. *J. Physiol. London* 301: 19P, 1980.
85. Roy, S., N. Singh, M. G. Deo, and V. Ramalingaswami. Ultrastructure of skeletal muscle and peripheral nerve in experimental protein deficiency and its correlation with nerve conduction studies. *J. Neurol. Sci.* 17: 399–409, 1972.
86. Rubinstein, N. A., and H. Holtzer. Fast and slow muscles in tissue culture synthesize only fast myosin. *Nature London* 208: 323–325, 1979.
87. Salmons, S., D. R. Gale, and F. A. Sreter. Ultrastructural aspects of the transformation of muscle fibre type by long term stimulation: changes in Z discs and mitochondria. *J. Anat.* 127: 17–31, 1978.
88. Salmons, S., and F. A. Sreter. Significance of impulse activity in the transformation of skeletal muscle type. *Nature London* 263: 30–34, 1976.
89. Salmons, S., and G. Vrbova. The influence of activity on some contractile characteristics of mammalian fast and slow muscles. *J. Physiol. London* 210: 535–549, 1969.
90. Samaha, F. J., L. Guth, and W. R. Albers. The neural regulation of gene expression in the muscle cell. *Exp. Neurol.* 27: 276–282, 1970.
91. Sarkar, S., and P. H. Cooke. In vitro synthesis of light and heavy polypeptide chains of myosin. *Biochem. Biophys. Res. Commun.* 41: 918–925, 1970.
92. Schmalbruck, H. Z. Noniusperioden und Langenwachstum der quergestreiften Muskelfaster. *Z. Mikrosk. Anat. Forsch.* 79: 493–507, 1968.
93. Schmalbruck, H. Z. "Square arrays" in the sarcolemma of human skeletal muscle fibres. *Nature London* 281: 145–146, 1979.
94. Shear, C. R., and G. Goldspink. Structural and physiological changes associated with the growth of avian fast and slow muscle. *J. Morphol.* 135: 351–372, 1971.
95. Sjöström, M., A. C. Edman, and S. Salmons. Changes in M-Band structure accompanying the transformation of rat fast muscle by long-term stimulation. *Muscle Nerve Abstr.* 3: 277, 1980.
96. Sjöström, M., S. Kidman, K. Larsén, and K. Ängqvist. Sarcomeric appearance in different histochemically defined types of human skeletal muscle fibre. *Muscle Nerve Abstr.* 3: 265–266, 1980.
97. Spurway, N. C. Histochemical typing of muscle fibres by microphotometry. In: *Plasticity of Muscle*, edited by D. Pette. New York: de Gruyter, 1979.
98. Sréter, F. A., J. Gergely, and A. L. Luff. The effect of cross reinnervation on the synthesis of myosin light chains. *Biochem. Biophys. Res. Commun.* 56: 84–89, 1974.
99. Sréter, F. A., J. C. Seidel, and J. Gergely. Studies on myosin from red and white skeletal muscles of the rabbit. 1. Adenosine triphosphatase activity. *J. Biol. Chem.* 241: 5772–5776, 1966.
100. Srivastava, U. Polyribosome concentration of mouse skeletal muscle as a function of age. *Arch. Biochem. Biophys.* 130: 129–139, 1969.
101. Stickland, N. C., and G. Goldspink. A possible indicator muscle for the fibre content and growth characteristics of porcine muscle. *Anim. Prod.* 16: 135–146, 1973.
102. Tabary, J. C., C. Tabary, C. Tardieu, G. Tardieu, and G. Goldspink. Physiological and structural changes in the cat's soleus muscle due to immobilization at different lengths by plaster cast. *J. Physiol. London* 224: 231–244, 1972.
103. Tardieu, C., J. C. Tabary, C. Tabary, and E. H. De La Tour. Is sarcomere number adaptation different in young and in grown up animals. *Proc. Int. Congr. Physiol. Sci., 27th, Paris, 1977*, vol. 13.
104. Tomanek, R. J. A histochemical study of postnatal differentiation of skeletal muscle with reference to functional overload. *Dev. Biol.* 42: 305–314, 1975.
105. Tuffrey, A. R. Growth and degeneration of motor end-plates in normal cat hind limb muscles. *J. Anat.* 110: 221–247, 1971.
106. Vaughan, H. S., Aziz-Ullah, G. Goldspink, and N. W. Nowell. Sex and stock differences in the histochemical myo-

fibrillar ATPase reaction in the soleus muscle of the mouse. *J. Histochem. Cytochem.* 22: 155–159, 1974.

107. WALSH, J. V., JR., R. E. BURKE, W. Z. RYMER, AND P. TSAIRIS. Effect of compensatory hypertrophy studied in individual motor units in medial gastrocnemius muscle of the cat. *J. Neurophysiol.* 41: 496–508, 1978.

108. WATERLOW, J. C., P. J. GARLICK, AND D. J. MILLWARD (editors). *Protein Turnover in Mammalian Tissues and in the Whole Body.* Amsterdam: Elsevier, 1978.

109. WATERLOW, J. C., AND J. M. L. STEPHEN. Adaptation of the rat to a low-protein diet: the effect of a reduced protein intake on the pattern of incorporation of L-$^{(14C)}$ lysine. *Br. J. Nutr.* 20: 461–484, 1966.

110. WEEDS, A. G., R. HALL, AND N. C. S. SPURWAY. Characterization of myosin light chains from histochemically identified fibres of rabbit psoas muscle. *FEBS Lett.* 49: 320–342, 1975.

111. WEEDS, A. G., D. R. TRENTHAM, C. J. KEAN, AND A. J. BULLER. Myosin from cross-reinnervated cat muscles. *Nature London* 247: 135–139, 1974.

112. WHALEN, R. G., G. S. BUTLER-BROWNE, AND F. GROS. Identification of a novel form of myosin light chain present in embryonic muscle tissue and cultured muscle cells. *J. Mol. Biol.* 126: 415–431, 1978.

113. WHALEN, R. G., K. SCHWARTZ, P. BOUVERET, S. M. SELL, AND F. GROS. Contractile protein isozymes in muscle development: identification of an embryonic form of myosin heavy chain. *Proc. Natl. Acad. Sci. USA* 76: 5197–5201, 1979.

114. WILLIAMS, P., AND G. GOLDSPINK. Longitudinal growth of striated muscle fibres. *J. Cell Sci.* 9: 751–767, 1971.

115. WILLIAMS, P., AND G. GOLDSPINK. The effect of immobilization on the longitudinal growth of striated muscle. *J. Anat.* 116: 45–55, 1973.

116. WILLIAMS, P., AND G. GOLDSPINK. Changes in sarcomere length and physiological properties in immobilized muscle. *J. Anat.* 127: 459–468, 1978.

CHAPTER 19

Skeletal muscle adaptability: significance for metabolism and performance

BENGT SALTIN | *August Krogh Institute, University of Copenhagen, Copenhagen, Denmark*

PHILIP D. GOLLNICK | *Department of Physical Education for Men, Washington State University, Pullman, Washington*

CHAPTER CONTENTS

Living systems are worn out by inactivity
and developed by use.
A. Szent-Györgyi

SKELETAL MUSCLES ARE AGGREGATES of muscle fibers that can be controlled individually or collectively. The multiplicity of movement patterns produced by man in daily life testifies to the intricate control that the nervous system has over the muscles and indicates the diverse characteristics of the muscle fibers. The same muscle or muscle group can respond and adapt to the need for either fine control, short intense effort, or prolonged activity, which reveals the plastic nature of this tissue.

The individual motor units that unite to form an entire muscle have different characteristics. The adaptive responses seen in muscle may therefore depend on a combination of the types of motor units contained in the muscle and the pattern or patterns of activity that they engage in. This chapter begins with a brief description of the motor unit and the basis for classification by fiber type that is used throughout to enable the reader to understand our approach to the subject of adaptations to use or disuse. The topic of motor unit properties has been reviewed in depth by Close (122) and by Buchthal and Schmalbruch (91).

MOTOR UNIT

The awareness that skeletal muscle is composed of different fiber types is not new. Although it is difficult to establish the first systematic description of these differences, it is frequently attributed to Ranvier (569).

Major advances in identifying the properties and organization of motor units within muscles came from the histochemical staining for glycogen in cross sections of muscle combined with isolating and stimulating individual motoneurons repetitively (176). A loss of glycogen identified those fibers (motor units) that had been active. A number of characteristics of the active fibers could then be identified from serial cross sections stained by histochemical methods. The initial studies were done with rats (176, 437, 439, 440), after which similar data were added from cat hindlimb muscle (97, 99, 101, 102). Because of their invasive nature, these methods cannot be applied directly to the study of motor unit properties in human skeletal muscle.

However, some motor-unit mapping of human skeletal muscle has been done with electrophysiological methods (237, 485, 486). Such studies have demonstrated a remarkable degree of similarity in the organizational pattern from human and animal muscle. The general characteristics of the motor unit are enumerated. *1*) All fibers in a single motor unit are homogeneous with regard to histochemically identifiable contractile and metabolic properties (237, 437, 441). *2*) The fibers in a motor unit are distributed in a fairly large part of the cross-sectional area of the muscle (10%–30% for the rat tibialis anterior muscle) (183). *3*) Fibers belonging to a single motor unit are rarely positioned immediately proximal to each other. *4*) A central locus for a motor unit exists with the density of fibers in the unit declining as a function of the distance from the center (176, 440). In the cat gastrocnemius muscle, fibers belonging to 40 or 50 motor units may be found in the same region (mm^2) of the muscle (101). In man, there appear to be only 15–30 motor units contained in a 5- to 10-mm^2 cross-sectional area (86–88). Motor units found in a given area can belong to all of the types represented in the muscle.

Fibers per Motor Unit

Data are available on the number of fibers per motor unit for a few muscles of several animals including man. For some animal studies the glycogen-depletion method was used to make these estimates. In others the number of motoneurons entering the muscle along with estimates of the total fiber number were used to calculate this ratio. In the rat soleus, containing a total of about 2,500 fibers, there are approximately 35 motor units (297). The range of fibers per motor unit in the rat is from 50 to 178 with a mean of 125 (176, 438). The tibialis anterior muscle of the cat has been reported to contain 56,000 fibers (156). The range for the slow-twitch (ST) motor units has been reported to be from 469 to 1,323 fibers per motor unit with the average being 775. For the fast-twitch (FT) motor units the average was 169 fibers per motor unit with a range of from 43 to 382 (156). In the studies of cat skeletal muscle only a small percent of the total number of motor units was examined.

Data from man are quite difficult to obtain. The most reliable estimates have come from counting the total number of motor nerves and muscle fibers (115, 121, 216). Estimates based on electrophysiological (485) measurements are less reliable. The range of fibers per motor unit is from 110 for the lumbricalis to 1,720 for the gastrocnemius medius muscles (216). At present there are no exact determinations of the number of fibers in the different types of motor units found in human skeletal muscle.

Contractile Properties

The basic feature that differentiates motor units into types is their contractile properties. These are identified from the time to peak tension in a twitch and the closely related one-half relaxation time. Two general classes of motor units and in some cases of complete muscles can be identified from these contractile properties. One group of motor units possesses a relatively long time to peak tension (a slow twitch) and the other a short time to peak tension (a fast twitch). Available data on the contractile properties of various motor units or muscle fibers within a single muscle illustrate the existence of a clear dichotomy of contractile speeds between fiber types (98–102, 223, 437, 438, 540). A discrete dichotomy does not extend, however, to the individual motor units, where there is a wide range of contractile speeds in spite of similar histochemical characteristics.

Biochemical Basis for Differences in Twitch Properties

A prime determinant of the twitch property of muscle is the rate at which myosin splits adenosine 5′-triphosphate (ATP), that is, its ATPase activity (31, 32, 606, 656). This is best illustrated when pure myosin is activated by actin. With such an assay system the specific activity of the pure protein is obtained without the dilution effect produced by the presence of other contaminating proteins. The relationship between the specific ATPase activity of myosin and contractile speed for a variety of muscles with varying twitch times is presented in Figure 1.

The differences in the specific ATPase activity of myosin are attributable to the existence of multimolecular forms of the protein (76–78, 240, 242, 243, 351, 352, 466, 533). These polymorphic forms of myosin can be identified and differentiated from a number of physicochemical characteristics. The simplest method for identifying the myosin isozymes is based on their susceptibility to loss of ATPase activity in response to changes in pH (77, 78). Myosin from FT muscles is alkaline stable but acid labile (Fig. 2). The opposite is true for myosin from ST muscles.

The multimolecular nature of myosin becomes a feature of all of the components that are assembled to form the functional protein complex (64a). This complex is composed of both a heavy- and a light-chain portion (463, 467, 655, 717). The heavy-chain portion can be divided into the structural subunits of the rod and the head. The ATPase activity is localized in the head subunit of myosin. Proteins of low molecular

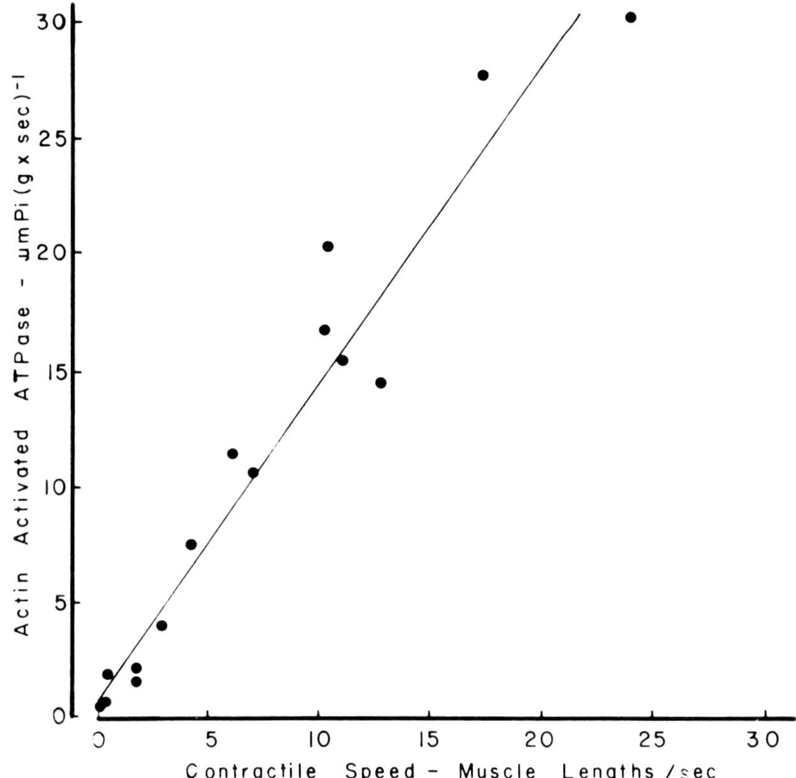

FIG. 1. Relationship between maximal speed of shortening and actin-activated ATPase of myosin from a variety of animal species. Equation from the regression line is $y = 0.34 + 1.37\ x$, and for the 2 variables, $r = 0.97$. [Plotted from original data published by Bárány (31).]

weight, the myosin light chains, are associated with the head portion of the heavy myosin. Identification of the components of myosin can be made through the use of immunological methods used in conjunction with histochemistry (Fig. 3). With these methods specific antibodies have been prepared against all subunits of the heavy chain and the individual light chains. Two classes of slow and three classes of fast ATP-splitting myosin have been identified with these techniques (595, 596). In general each muscle fiber contains only one class of myosin (that is slow or fast) but the relative proportion of the different isozymes in this class can vary. There are, however, instances in which fibers may contain a mixture of classes of myosin (421, 552, 715). These immunological methods hold great promise for positively establishing the existence of a specific type of myosin in a given fiber and the possible interconversion of fiber types in response to experimental perturbations such as chronic use or disuse.

Electrophoretic methods have also demonstrated the existence of different types of myosin in skeletal muscle (351, 352, 552, 715). With these methods five myosin isozymes have been identified in rat muscle, which is like the findings with immunological methods. These isozymes result from varying combinations of the light chains associated with the heavy chains. Of the five isozymes of myosin, the FT extensor digitorum longus muscle of the rat contains principally the first four with only trace amounts of the fifth. In contrast the ST soleus muscle contains only the fourth and fifth isozymes. In addition to isozymes of myosin, it has also been demonstrated that other proteins of the myofibrillar complex exist in polymorphic forms (148–151, 669). Table 1 summarizes the variations in the proteins found in the contractile apparatus of skeletal muscle. In summary there are major differences between the proteins of the myofibrils of the FT and the ST muscles. On the basis of these differences the fibers can be most reliably typed.

The present data suggest that under normal conditions the assembly of the individual units of the myofibrillar proteins occurs in such a manner that a complete randomization of the subunits does not or only rarely takes place. Thus it is unlikely that the light chains associated with the fast-type heavy myosin will be assembled with the slow-type myosin. The general observation that only one class of contractile protein is found in a single muscle fiber does not preclude the existence of minor components of other types of proteins. Examples of this can be found in fetal and neonatal stages (240, 476, 595, 716, 718), during chronic electrical stimulation (437, 438, 552, 596, 715), and after cross innervation and reinnervation (33, 421, 475). The presence of more than one form of myosin in fetal and neonatal muscle is probably due to the existence of polyinnervation, which disappears with maturation (81, 82, 525–527). Fast-twitch muscle fibers also possess a greater concentration of sarcoplasmic reticulum (218), and it changes with development

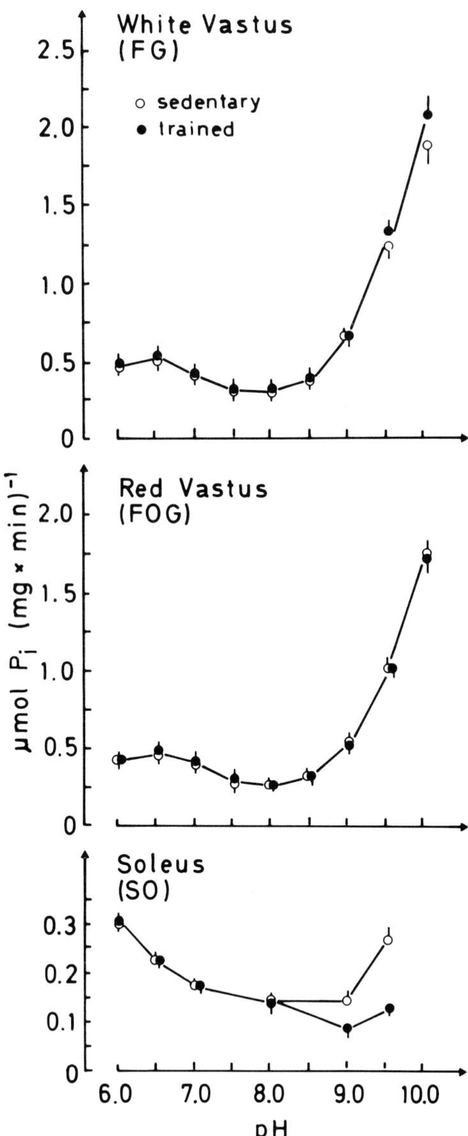

FIG. 2. Influence of pH on Ca^{2+}-activated ATPase activites of myosin from white [fast-twitch, glycolytic (FG)] and red [fast-twitch, oxidative, glycolytic (FOG)] portions of the vastus muscle and soleus [slow-twitch, oxidative (SO)] muscle of the sedentary (○) and endurance-trained (●) rats. ATPase activities were determined at 25°C. [From Watrus (713).]

(152), electrical stimulation (323, 325), and cross innervation (157, 654).

Histochemical Differentiation of Muscle Fibers

The difference in the sensitivity of myosin for retaining or losing ATPase activity after exposure to either high or low pH is a reliable method for the histochemical classification of muscle fibers (192, 533). It is a simple, rapid, and inexpensive method for determining the fiber composition of whole muscle or portions of muscles. This histochemical method for fiber identification is based on the ATPase activity remaining in myofibrils after preincubation of serial sections at pH 4.3, 4.6, and 10.3 (77). Preincubation of muscle sections at pH 10.3 results in a loss of the histochemically demonstrable stain for myofibrillar ATPase in fibers that have a low specific ATPase activity of purified myosin. These fibers have ST contractile properties. Conversely all classes of FT fibers stain intensely after alkaline preincubation. Preincubation of muscle sections at pH 4.3 results in a loss of ATPase staining in a majority of the FT fibers, whereas the ST fibers stain intensely. A preincubation of the sections at pH 4.6 produces a subdivision of the FT fibers. After such preincubation a population of FT fibers, as identified by staining after treatment at pH 10.3, exists that retains some ATPase staining. Immunological methods have demonstrated that these histochemical staining patterns produced by manipulation of the preincubation pH are the result of the presence of different myosin isozymes (239, 240, 242). This finding extends to the different classes of FT fibers, including those with either high or low oxidative capacities present in the limb muscle of most animals (240). The staining pattern that exists in most mammalian muscles in response to variation in the pH of the preincubation is presented in Figure 3.

Engel (192, 193) proposed that the fibers be identified as type I and type II. Brooke and Kaiser (76–79) have proposed a scheme for classifying fibers in skeletal muscle based on the different sensitivities of the myofibrillar ATPase toward acid and alkaline inactivation. Based on the differential staining pattern as illustrated in Figure 4, the fibers have been designated as type I or type II. The type I fibers are acid stable and alkaline labile, whereas the converse is true for the type II fibers. Type I fibers are found in ST muscle and type II in FT muscle. The type II fibers are further subdivided into IIA, IIB, and IIC based on their resistance to loss of histochemically demonstrable myofibrillar ATPase at the low pH values.

In this chapter classification of skeletal muscle fibers is based on the histochemical differentiation of myofibrillar ATPase (602, 642). The assumption being made is that the acid stable and the alkaline stable myofibrillar ATPase correspond to slow and fast contractile characteristics, respectively. Justification for using the myofibrillar ATPase staining pattern after acid or alkaline preincubation as an indication for the contractile properties of the fibers comes from the finding that the ATPase activity of myosin purified from either FT or ST muscle behaves similarly when exposed to acid or alkaline preincubation (33). Moreover a homology exists for the reaction of antibodies prepared from purified myosin or its subunits (including rod, head, or light chains), with the FT or ST fibers as identified from the histochemical methods depending on the source of the original protein used in antibody production (240). Hence the basic designation of the fibers is ST or FT. The FT fibers are further subdivided into FT_a, FT_b, and FT_c on the basis of differences in myofibrillar ATPase stability to low pH (see Fig. 4). The choice of the ST and FT desig-

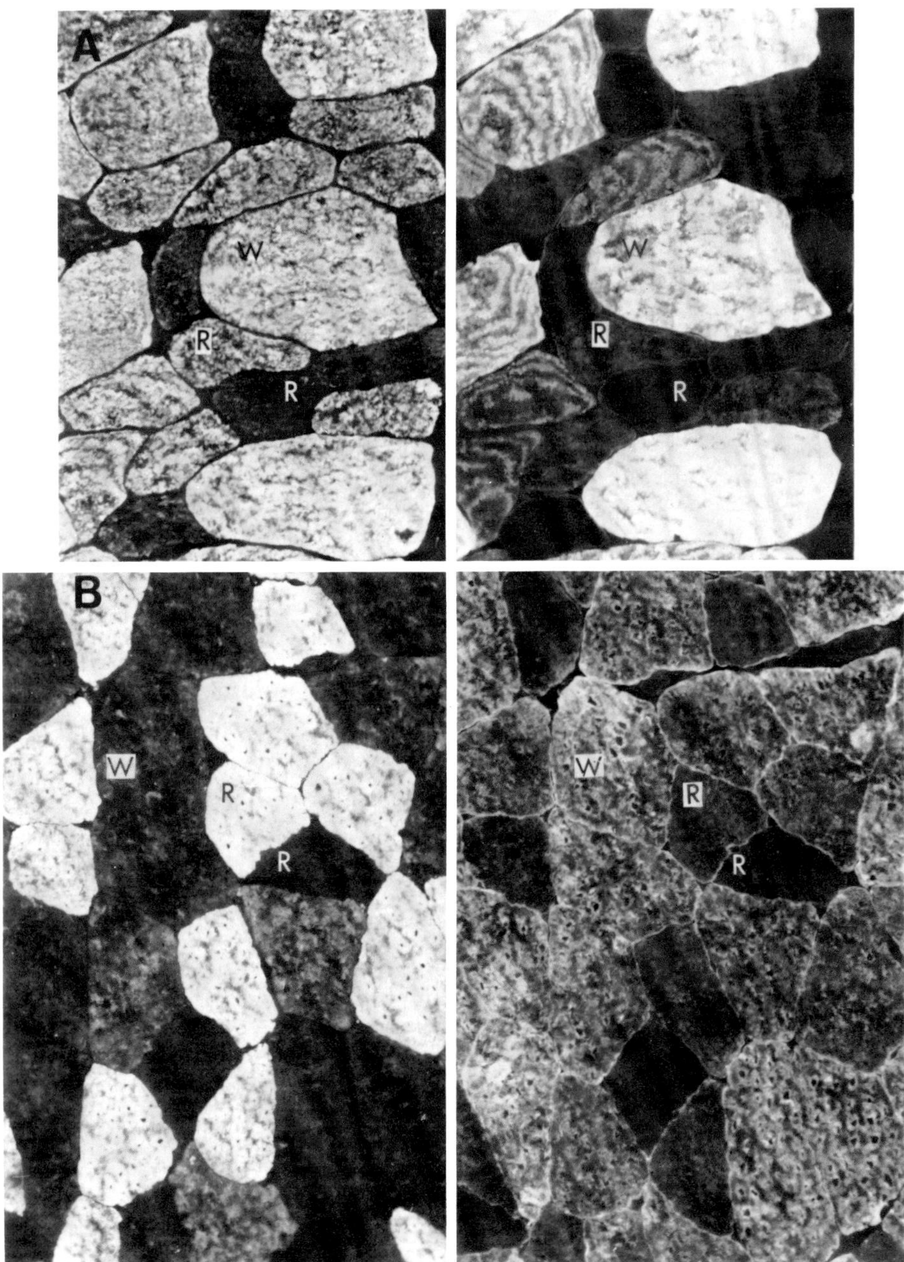

FIG. 3. *A*: rat diaphragm, serial transverse sections. *Left* stained with antibody specific for alkali 1 light chain (anti-Δ1); *right* stained with antibody for alkali 2 light chain (anti-Δ2). Both antibodies react with same fibers (*W, I, black R*) that react with antibodies against whole white myosin. However, level of response to anti-Δ2 is lower in fast-twitch red fibers (*black R*) than in other fast-twitch fibers (*W, I*). *B*: cat flexor digitorum longus, serial sections. *Left*, anti-Δ1; *right*, anti-Δ2. Response of most fast-twitch fibers (*W*) is weak; compare with unreactive fibers (*white R*). However, level of response to anti-Δ1 (*left*) is more intense in one type of red fibers (*black R*) than in other fast-twitch fibers. Response to anti-Δ2 is less intense in this fiber (*black R*) than in other fast-twitch fibers. [From Gauthier (240).]

nation is not the result of any objection to the type I and II designation. It is merely an attempt to give the classification more physiological meaning.

This nomenclature is similar to that proposed by Peter et al. (540) from the histochemical study of guinea pig limb muscle. In this and most other animal species the subgroups of FT fibers are easily discernible on the basis of large differences in metabolic profiles. This is most marked for the mitochondrial enzymes where one of the subgroups of FT fibers has a high or higher oxidative potential than the ST fibers, whereas another is very low in oxidative enzymes. The FT fiber types were therefore designated fast-twitch, oxidative, glycolytic (FOG) or fast-twitch, glycolytic (FG). Also the designation into the basic subgroups of FT fibers or ST fibers was based on a standard ATPase stain (pH 10.3 preincubation) and a staining for oxidative and glycolytic enzymes, and not on the basis of ATPase staining after a combination of alkaline and acid preincubations. In the skeletal muscle of sedentary man, differences in metabolic potential can be identified from both histochemical (Fig. 4) and biochemical (see Tables 2 and 4) techniques when comparing subgroups of FT fibers, but these are small and an overlap is present. When subgrouping of the fiber types in human skeletal muscle is based on ATPase stains after both alkaline and acid preincubations rather than stains for oxidative or glycolytic enzymes, rather large differences are obtained in which fibers can readily be assigned to the various groups (74–77).

TABLE 1. *Distribution of Multimolecular Forms of Myofibrillar Proteins in Type I and Type II Fibers of Mammalian Skeletal Muscle*

Protein	Type I Fiber	Type II Fiber*
Myosin	Slow A1 homodimer Slow A1 A2 heterodimer Slow A2 homodimer	Fast A1 homodimer Fast A1 A2 heterodimer Fast A2 homodimer
Actin	α	α
Tropomyosin	β	β
Troponin C	Slow	Fast
Troponin T	Slow	Fast
Troponin I	Slow	Fast

* Note that data of Gauthier and Lowey (242) suggest that differences exist in distribution of isomeric form of myofibrillar proteins, which could account for the presence of subpopulations of type II fibers. [Adapted from Dhoot and Perry (151).]

Moreover this system eliminates the uncertainty that arises when changes in the oxidative potential occur in response to altered patterns of chronic physical activity. Thus with extensive endurance training all fiber types in the trained muscle may stain similarly for oxidative capacity, thereby making identification of fiber types based on this characteristic difficult if not impossible. Therefore it may be wrong to include abbreviations for the metabolic profile in the names to identify fibers as these, at least for man, can be misleading. The subscripts a, b, and c that we prefer to use indicate that there are certain differences in the populations of FT fibers. Whether they are related to differences in the myosin isozymes, energy metabolism, or other features of the muscle fiber cannot presently be evaluated. The studies of Gauthier and Lowey (240, 242, 243) do suggest that differences in the isozymes of the contractile proteins exist for the FT muscle of the rat.

Ultrastructural Basis for Skeletal Muscle Fiber Typing

Attempts have been made to identify the fiber types in skeletal muscle by ultrastructural features detectable by electron microscopy (238, 241, 538, 696). The width of the Z band has been reported to vary in a systematic manner in the different fibers of some animals (238, 241, 696). In early studies with the rat a fairly consistent pattern exists of a wider Z band in the ST fibers (238, 241). In more recent studies this relationship is less clear (239). A similar pattern has not been demonstrated in human skeletal muscle, however, nor has it been possible to identify the subtypes of FT muscle based on this criterion. Sjöström and co-workers (643) have examined the ultrastructural features of the Z and M bands of human skeletal muscle (Fig. 5). The fibers were identified by histochemical staining for myofibrillar ATPase prior to electron microscopy. The ST fibers had wide Z and M bands with five strong (high-density) M-bridge lines. The FT_a fibers had Z bands of intermediate width and three strong and two weak (low-density) M-bridge lines. The FT_b fibers had narrow Z bands and three strong and two very weak M-bridge lines. A higher degree of accuracy for fiber identification existed from examination of the M rather than the Z band (95% vs. 70%). The identification of ultrastructural differences in skeletal muscle fibers supports the concept that the basic constitution of a fiber lies in the contractile proteins.

Other features commonly examined with electron microscopy are the size, shape, and concentration of the mitochondria. Examination of mitochondria is based on the assumption that ST muscle possesses higher oxidative capacity and therefore a higher concentration of mitochondria than FT muscle. This relationship between mitochondrial concentration and contractile characteristics is not valid for FT muscles that possess high mitochondrial concentrations (240, 540, 696). Moreover the mitochondrial content of skeletal muscle is markedly influenced by the amount and type of activity of that muscle. Thus an examination of mitochondrial features holds little promise as a reliable method for fiber identification.

Maximal Contractile Force

Considerable interest exists in identifying the factor or factors that contribute to the capacity of skeletal muscle to develop tension. A plethora of reports describe muscular strength increases in response to heavy-resistance exercise and decreases after inactivity. An interesting aspect of this topic is the question of whether any changes occur in the contractile properties of the fibers themselves in response to different patterns of physical activity. The central issue is whether changes occur at the level of the individual fiber. The capacity of a muscle or fiber to develop force is best related to the tension produced per unit of cross-sectional area (427). The isometric tension developed by single, skinned, human muscle fibers in response to ionized Ca^{2+} has been reported to be about 15 N/cm^2 (726). Ikai and Fukunaga (381, 382) examined this relationship in man by determining both the maximal voluntary contractile strength (MVC) and the cross-sectional area of the arm flexor muscle in children and adults. Cross-sectional area of the muscles was estimated from ultrasound echoes; MVC was estimated to be 6.4 kg/cm^2 (64 N/cm^2) with no differences between male and female subjects.

The maximal voluntary force as reported by Ikai and Fukunaga (381, 382) is an overestimate of the true capacity of human skeletal muscle. The total muscle mass involved in elbow flexion includes the pronator teres, extensor carpi radialis longus, and brachioradialis muscles (66, 69). Moreover the placement of the origin and insertion of the biceps brachii muscle on the skeleton is such that in the position of elbow flexion used by Ikai and Fukunaga there is a 1:4.9

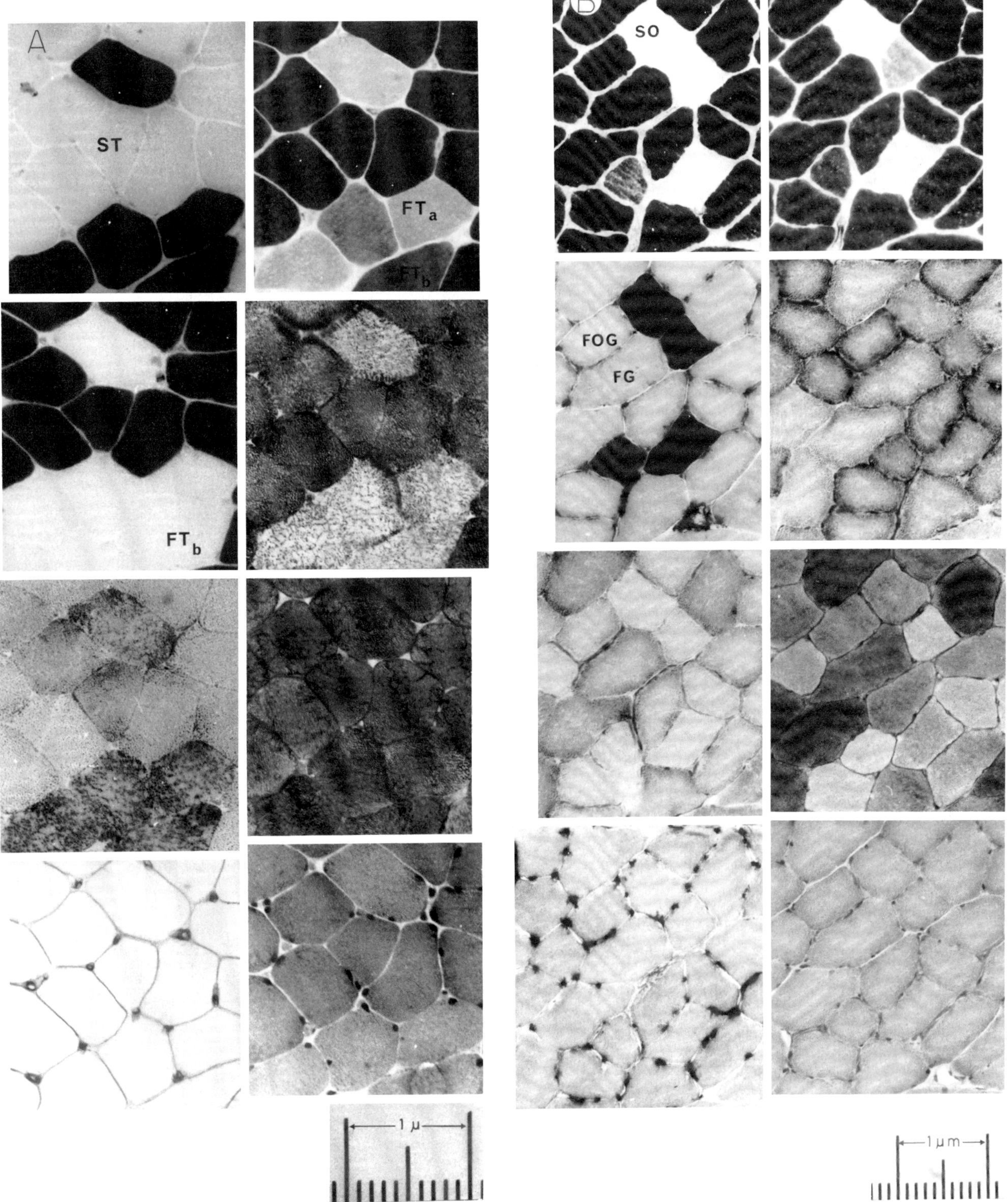

FIG. 4. Serial transverse-sectioned frozen skeletal muscle from the lateral head of the gastrocnemius muscle of man (*A*) and the same muscle from rat (*B*). From *top* to *bottom* are the following stains (myofibrillar ATPase stained at pH 9.4 and preincubated at pH 10.3, 4.6, 4.3): nicotinamide adenine dinucleotide, reduced-tetrazolium reductase (NADH); α-GPDH, glycogen (periodic acid-Schiff, PAS); capillaries (man = amylase-treated sections stained with PAS; rat = alkaline phosphatase); and hematoxylin-eosin.

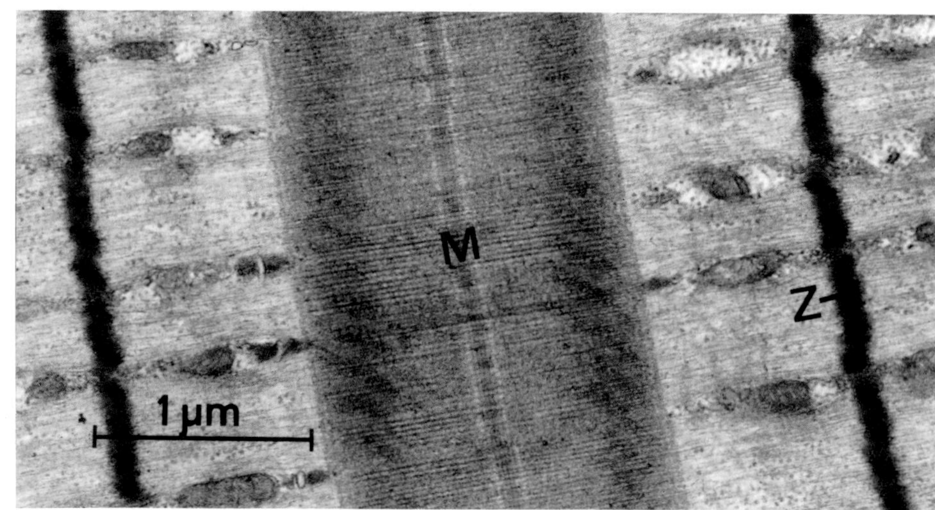

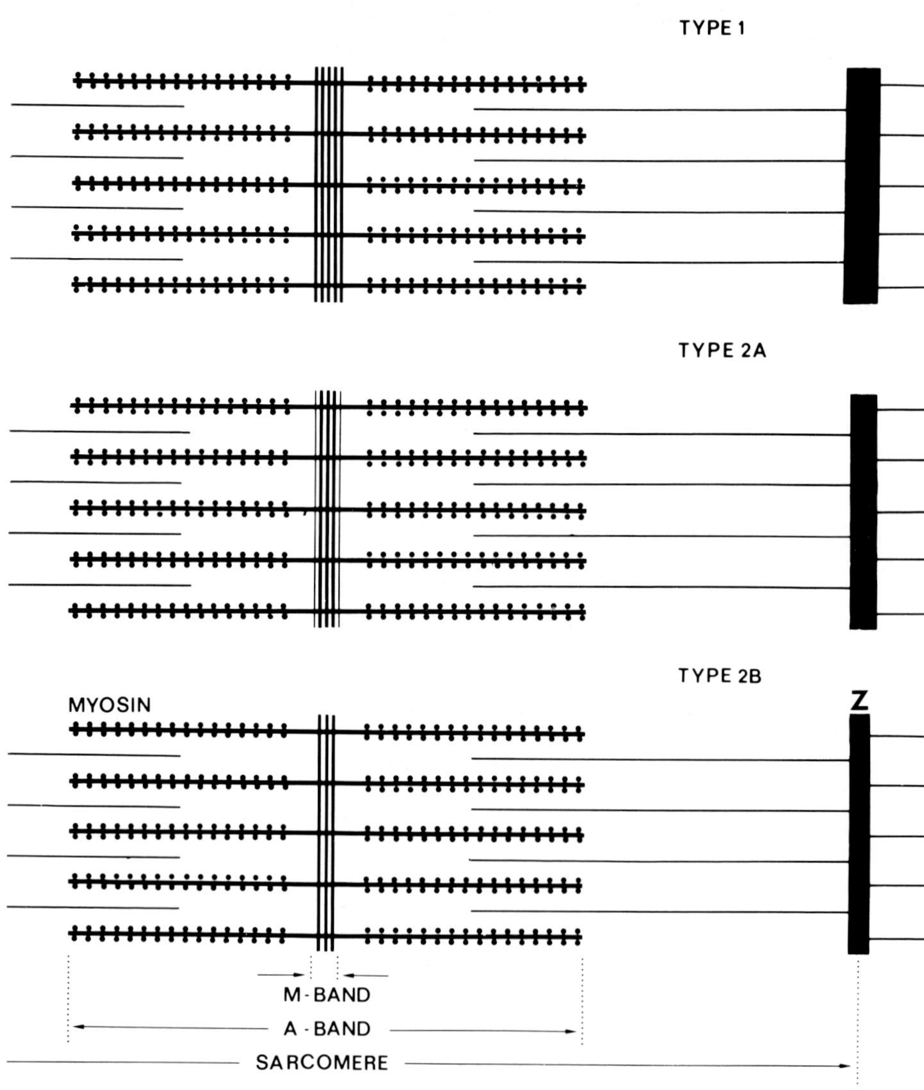

FIG. 5. Part of a sarcomere from slow-twitch, ST (*micrograph* and *top panel*), fast-twitch, subtype a, FT_a (*middle panel*), and fast-twitch, subtype b, FT_b (*bottom panel*) fibers in combination with a schematic drawing of the respective fiber types. [From Ängquist (9).]

mechanical advantage (309, 721). On the basis of these factors the value given by Ikai and Fukunaga can be calculated to be about 47 N/cm^2. This is similar to a value of 40 N/cm^2 reported for the biceps brachii by Nygaard (520) and 39 N/cm^2 as determined for the calf muscles by Haxton (314).

The cross-sectional area of the upper arm flexors and knee extensors of man has also been estimated from X-ray computerized tomography (100, 384, 578). In two of these studies (100, 578) the fiber composition of the muscles was estimated from biopsy samples. This revealed that the maximal voluntary strength of human skeletal muscle is related to fiber composition in only a minor way. Instead total cross-sectional area appeared to be the decisive factor.

The ability of the different types of muscle and motor units to produce maximal tetanic tension has been examined in the mouse, rat, and cat. Maximal tensions ranging from 15.7 to 21.5 N/cm^2 have been reported for the soleus muscle of the mouse (592). For the rat soleus and extensor digitorum longus muscles maximal tetanic tensions ranged from 19 to 21 and from 20 to 30 N/cm^2, respectively (33, 119, 120, 122, 124). Sexton and co-workers (626, 627) reported that there was no difference in force development between ST and FT muscles in maximally activated, glycerol-extracted fibers. Independent measurements of the maximal tetanic force developed by the cat soleus and extensor digitorum longus (215) muscles support the concept that the intrinsic capacity of the contractile elements to develop tension is similar for ST and FT muscle. Burke and co-workers (97, 101), however, reported the maximal tetanic tension of FT motor units in cat muscle to be between 15 and 29 N/cm^2 as compared to 6 N/cm^2 for ST motor units. This difference could be due to the technical difficulties in accurately assessing the cross-sectional area of the motor units that were stimulated. If such large differences in force-developing capacity do exist between ST and FT motor units, its molecular basis is obscure. Differences could exist in excitation-contraction coupling, which ultimately involves the control of free calcium by the sarcoplasmic reticulum. Further studies into this problem are needed. One preparation that may prove useful for studies is the skinned muscle fiber. With this preparation activation of the contractile process can be initiated without involvement of the sarcolemma or sarcoplasmic reticulum. Moreover exact assessments of the cross-sectional area of the individual fibers can be made so that force development per square centimeter is accurately determined. These data, combined with assessments of the isozyme composition of the fibers being tested, should clarify the issue of whether or not intrinsic differences in the capacity to develop tension exist between the types of muscle and whether this is related to the polymorphic forms of myosin or the other proteins in the contractile elements. Data from these methods do not appear to support the existence of a difference in force-generating capacity of ST and FT fibers (155).

Speed of Contraction

The speed of contraction, that is, the time to peak isometric tension, of individual motor units has been studied most extensively in cat and rat skeletal muscle (33, 35, 84, 98–101, 120, 121, 217, 223, 437, 438, 489). For the rat the mean time to peak isometric tension is 13 ms and 38 ms for the FT and ST motor units, respectively (33, 120, 121, 217, 437, 438). In the cat the values for FT units in the gastrocnemius muscle range from 32 to 43 ms (99–101). The ST motor units in the cat soleus muscle range from 77 to 97 ms (98). In the guinea pig these values are 82 ms for ST muscle and 21 ms for FT muscle (35).

As described earlier, a close relationship exists between the contractile speed of a muscle and the specific activity of its myosin. There is, however, considerable variation around the mean value for the contractile times of motor units, more than that which could be expected from differences in the staining intensity for myofibrillar ATPase. Differences in the isozyme composition of myosin do exist in the different motor units, such as between the different types of FT fibers (239, 240, 242, 243), however, and these may contribute to the variation in contractile speeds.

Other elements in the excitation-contraction coupling system may also exert a regulatory influence on maximal speed of contraction of the individual motor units. Included are properties of the nerve and motor end plate, interneuronal modulations, characteristics of the sarcolemma and transverse-tubular system for transmission of the neural impulse, the sarcoplasmic reticulum and its abilty to release and sequester calcium, and finally, the role of the isozymes of troponin and tropomyosin in binding calcium and initiating contraction. Very little is known regarding these other regulatory factors.

Studies with man have lacked the precision for establishing contractile properties of the individual muscle or motor units of those from animals. In situ stimulation of motor units has demonstrated the existence of FT and ST motor units (85, 89, 90, 94, 143–147, 237, 293, 294, 485, 600). Thus in the biceps muscle, bimodal distributions of contraction times with maximal values of 36 ms and 90 ms were observed, whereas in the medial head of the gastrocnemius muscle the respective peak times were slightly longer. This does not necessarily signify that differences exist in contraction times between similar fiber types of these two muscles since the methods for recording tensions were different in the two studies. The longer contraction times were observed in experiments where the torque of the whole ankle joint was measured, probably causing an elongation of the real time to peak isometric tension due to the inertia in the system.

In both studies the variation around the mean values for time to peak tension was large, especially for the faster contraction times. There are also reports of contractile properties of biopsy samples of human skeletal muscle (162, 163, 181, 504). These support the existence of FT and ST motor units. The exact times for attainment of peak tension as reported in such studies, although they do not differ markedly from the values cited above, are open to question since the fibers had been cut and the integrity of the excitation-contraction coupling system compromised. However, membrane potential was maintained at near normal levels in these cut but ligated muscle bundles. In these preparations one-half relaxation times were also established and found to be approximately four times shorter in FT than in ST fibers (179, 504, 720). When measurements were performed in intact man, assuming a selective recruitment of ST fibers at low static contraction and that all fibers engaged in maximal contractions only twice as fast, a relaxation rate was estimated for the ST as compared to the FT fibers (504).

Fatigue Characteristics

Burke and co-workers (96, 98–100, 102) have examined the response of individual motor units of cat muscle to contractile activity (Fig. 6). In these studies individual motor units were stimulated through the motoneuron and the tension development and fatigue characteristics determined. Three types of fast motor units were discernible in the medial gastrocnemius muscle and one slow unit in the soleus muscle of the cat. All fast-twitch units produced high tetanic tension. One type of these fast-twitch units fatigued rapidly and was designated as fast twitch, easily fatigued (FF). A second type was fatigue resistant (FR), and a third was intermediate to the FF and FR and was identified as F(int). All motor units of the soleus muscle produced low tension and were resistant to fatigue. They were designated simply as slow twitch (S). Histochemical examination of the muscle revealed that the FT and ST motor units show patterns of staining for myofibrillar ATPase typical for the respective muscles.

It has been suggested that the fast-twitch motor unit with intermediate fatigue characteristics, F(int), is the result of differences in the activity level of the cats. Thus cats that were allowed freedom to exercise had higher percentages of such motor units than cats maintained in cages. Considerable variation existed in fatigue properties (within each group of fibers). This continuum of resistance to fatigue was probably associated with the normal state of fiber use in these cats during daily life. Resistance to fatigue was closely related to the activities of the oxidative enzymes as demonstrated by the staining intensity for succinate dehydrogenase. This is similar to the findings in the rat (176, 437, 441).

A similar classification of human skeletal muscle motor units has been made (237). In these experiments a total of 57 single motor units of the medial gastrocnemius muscle were activated with a bipolar stimulating electrode (Fig. 7). An electromyogram (EMG) of a single motor unit was recorded, and tension produced by activation of a motor unit was estimated from the torque produced in the ankle joint. As was true for cat muscle, some motor units were more resistant to fatigue than others. The slowest contracting motor units demonstrated a small decline (2%–20%) in twitch tension from the initial level after 3,000 stimuli delivered over a 50-min period. Two groups of FT fibers were discernible. One had fatigue-resistance properties similar to the ST fibers, and the other had a reduction in tension from 50% to 75% during the same experiment period.

Metabolic Characteristics

SUBSTRATES. Human skeletal muscle contains stores of glycogen and lipids in addition to the more immediate energy sources of ATP and creatine phosphate (CP). A summary giving the average values for these stores as compiled from several studies where they were estimated from biopsy samples (see ref. 49) of the extremity muscles is presented in Table 2.

Triglyceride content. The triglyceride content of human skeletal muscle varies between 5 and 15 mmol/kg wet wt (197, 198, 200, 203, 233, 234). Although these values are from measurements made on samples of mixed-fiber muscle freed from visible fat, the possibility remains that part of this fat is localized in the extrafiber space. However, since bundles of fibers, carefully liberated from freeze-dried muscle samples, contain similar amounts of triglyceride as those given in Table 2, the extrafiber lipid store does not appear to have been appreciable.

The magnitude of the variation in the triglyceride stores between various muscles of the body is unknown. Measurements made on biopsy samples of muscles from the leg and arm suggest that the variation is small. The localization of fat within the muscle appears to be heterogeneous. When determinations were made on small samples (5–10 mg wet wt) the high values were three- to five-fold higher than the lowest value found in 30- to 50-mg pieces of the same muscle. Ultrastructural evaluations support the concept that fat is localized in small droplets at varying intervals in a fiber. An additional factor contributing to the variation of the triglyceride content in skeletal muscle is the distinct difference in the lipid content of the individual fibers with the ST fibers containing three to five times higher levels than the FT fibers (202). Therefore differences in the lipid content must be expected when variation exists in the fiber composition of the tissue samples being analyzed.

Differences in the lipid content of the fiber types can be demonstrated when sections are stained with either Sudan black or oil red O (454). With these treatments the ST fibers stain more intensely than the FT fibers (89, 90). Since mitochondrial membrane contains large amounts of lipid, which is also stained

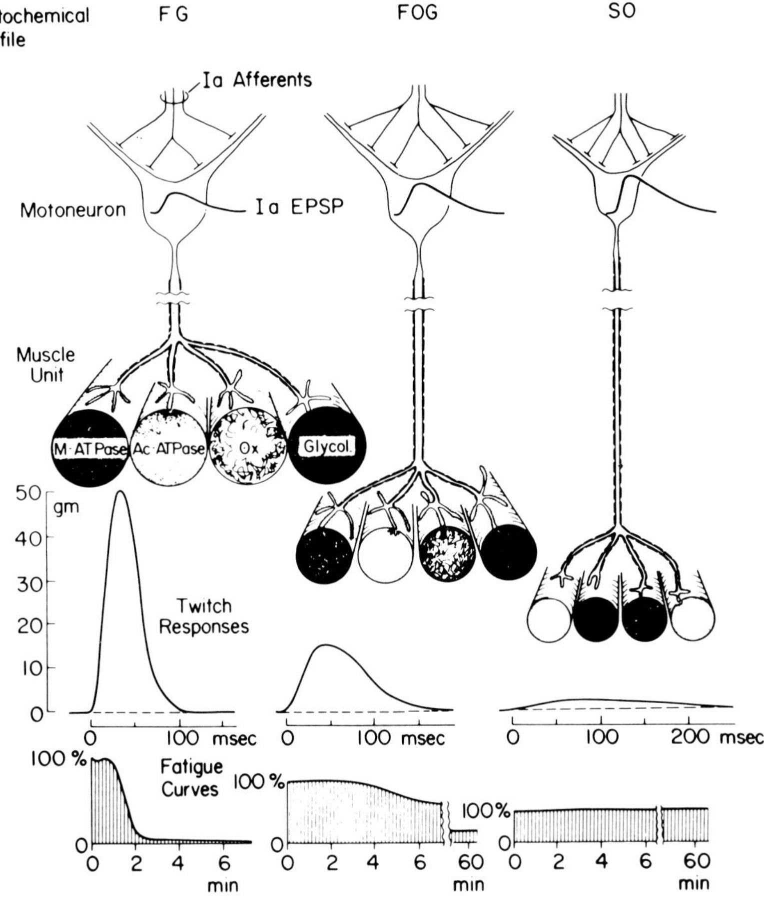

FIG. 6. Important features of organization of motor units in medial gastrocnemius muscle of cat. Diameters of muscle fibers and unit mechanical responses are scaled appropriately for respective groups, representing typical observations. Shading in muscle fiber outlines denotes relative staining intensities found for each histochemical reaction (identified in the FF unit fibers). Note differences in pattern as well as intensity of staining in the oxidative enzyme reaction (3rd fiber from *left* in each unit sequence). Note also the somewhat smaller motoneuron innervating type S unit and relation between number of group Ia synapses and cell size; a low density of terminals (as in the FF unit) produces a relatively small Ia excitatory postsynaptic potential (EPSP), whereas increasing densities (in the FR and higher still in the type S unit) produce larger EPSPs. Motor unit type nomenclature: FF, fast twitch, fatiguable; FR, fast twitch, fatigue resistant; S, slow twitch. Histochemical profiles: FG, fast twitch, glycolytic; FOG, fast twitch, oxidative, glycolytic; SO, slow twitch, oxidative. These 2 systems are essentially interchangeable. [From Burke and Edgerton (97).]

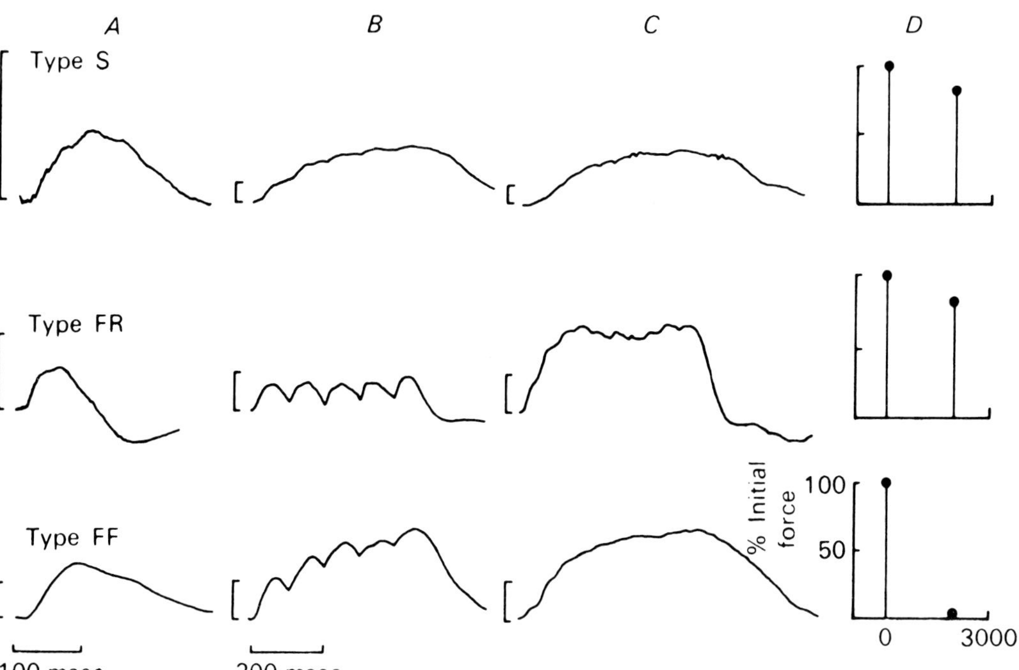

FIG. 7. Examples of the 3 motor unit types found in human medial gastrocnemius. *A*, isometric twitch; *B*, isometric tetanus 10 pulses/s; *C*, isometric tetanus 20 pulses/s; and *D*, fatigue test, control and after 3,000 stimuli, expressed as a percentage of initial isometric tension. [From Garnett et al. (237).]

TABLE 2. *Human Skeletal Muscle Substrate in Vastus Lateralis Muscle*

Substrate	Mixed Muscle, μmol/g wet wt	Fiber Types, μmol/g wet wt			
		ST	FT	FT_a	FT_b
Triglyceride	9.9 ± 0.6	7.1 ± 1.7	4.2 ± 1.2		
Glycogen (glucose units)	83.8 ± 18	77.8 ± 18	84.7 ± 19	83.1 ± 18	89.2 ± 21
ATP	5.0 ± 0.2	4.9 ± 0.1	5.1 ± 0.2	5.3 ± 0.2	4.9 ± 0.1
CP	10.7 ± 0.6	12.6 ± 0.2	14.7 ± 1.4	14.5 ± 1.1	14.8 ± 1.6

ST, slow twitch; FT, fast twitch; FT_a, fast twitch, a type; FT_b, fast twitch, b type; ATP, adenosine triphosphate; CP, creatine phosphate. Values are means ± 1 SD and are given for triglycerides in mixed muscles from refs. 197, 198, 200, 269, 396; glycogen from refs. 197, 198, 262, 263, 267, 341, 373; ATP and CP from refs. 374, 415, 418, 428. Corresponding values on fiber types are from refs. 202 (triglycerides); 199, 201–203 (glycogen); 312, 375 (ATP and CP).

by Sudan black or oil red O, caution must be exercised in the interpretation of the histochemical staining method to estimate the triglyceride stores of the individual fibers. Consequently this method seems to hold little promise for evaluating differences in lipid stores of the different fiber types or in estimating changes induced by either exercise, diet, or training.

Glycogen content. The average glycogen content (Table 2) of human extremity muscle lies in the range of from 50 to 90 mmol/kg wet wt. (All glycogen concentrations given as millimoles of glycosyl units.) Part of this rather wide variation appears to be related to the diet and state of physical activity of the subject (51, 271, 373). Overall the glycogen granules are homogeneously distributed throughout the muscle fibers with only small differences existing in the glycogen content of ST and FT fibers or in the subgroups of FT fibers of man (191, 201–203). Moreover only minor variation in muscle glycogen is found when determinations are made on multiple samples from the same muscle or when assays performed on small samples are compared with those made on larger samples from the same muscle (373).

The glycogen content of the gastrocnemius, the quadriceps femoris, the triceps brachii, and the biceps brachii muscles of man all lie within the range of 50–90 mmol/kg wet wt (373, 641). Quantitative determinations of the glycogen content of the individual fiber types present in the vastus lateralis of the quadriceps muscle have revealed that at a glycogen concentration of about 75 mmol/kg wet wt (≈300 mmol/kg dry wt) there is a 10–15 mmol/kg wet wt mean difference between the ST and FT fibers with the latter fibers having the higher glycogen content (201–203). It appears that for the subgroups of the FT fibers, the FT_b fibers may contain more glycogen than the FT_a fibers. These differences in glycogen content of the muscle fibers can be detected with periodic acid–Schiff (PAS) stain, but at a glycogen content of 80–100 mmol/kg wet wt or above, the staining intensity is homogeneous and neither subjective ratings nor spectrophotometric methods can detect differences between fibers or fiber types (171, 559). The variation in the glycogen content within a single fiber type has been reported to be from about 50 to 650 mmol/kg dry wt for both the ST and FT fiber types (199, 201–203). The reason for this variation is unknown, but it may be due in part to the technical difficulties of separating the fiber from the support tissue and of accurately weighing the small tissue fragments. Thus although a close relationship has been demonstrated between the histochemical evaluation of the glycogen content of muscle and the value determined biochemically, it is surprising that these differences are not more evident in tissue stained by standard histochemical methods.

Phosphagen. The phosphagen stores of skeletal muscle constitute 23–25 mmol/kg wet wt with the CP concentration being 18–20 and the ATP 4–5 mmol/kg wet wt [Table 2; (374, 418, 428)]. Variations between muscles are small. The magnitude of the variation of these stores in the major fiber types of human muscle has been examined (312, 375). This has demonstrated a slightly higher ATP and CP concentration in ST fibers. These differences, however, are so small, 0.05 mmol/kg wet wt for ATP and 1–3 mmol/kg wet wt for CP, as to be physiologically unimportant. Measurements performed on samples with large differences in fiber composition also have failed to demonstrate any major differences in the concentrations of the high-energy phosphates (375).

The ATP and CP concentrations in mixed-fiber muscle of nonhuman species (primarily the rat) are similar to those observed in human skeletal muscle (Table 3). In spite of this, significant differences do exist in the concentrations of ATP and CP in the slow- and fast-twitch muscles, with the ATP content of FT muscle being about 60% higher than that of the ST fibers and the CP content being from 70% to 100% higher (375).

The glycogen and triglyceride (Table 3) stores of rat muscle and other species are generally present at lower concentrations than that obtained in mixed muscle of man. Thus the triglyceride and glycogen concentrations of rat skeletal muscle are only 25%–33% and 33%–50%, respectively, of that found in human skeletal muscle. For glycogen, a similar pattern of distribution between fiber types appears to exist in most species, with the lowest concentrations being found in the ST muscle and only minor differences existing between the different types of FT muscles. In contrast, the red portion of the vastus muscle in the rat, an FT muscle, contains the higher triglyceride content, with similar amounts being found in the ST soleus and FT white portion of the vastus muscle. In the guinea pig the triglyceride content is highest in the ST soleus, lowest in the FT oxidative red vastus, and intermediate in the FT glycolytic white vastus (219).

ENZYME ACTIVITIES. The content and/or activities of enzymes for contraction and energy metabolism differ in the various fiber types of skeletal muscle. This can be demonstrated in a variety of nonhuman species when quantitative biochemical assays are performed on portions of muscles or whole muscles that contain only one fiber type (15). For man, in whom most muscles are homogeneous mixtures of the different types, quantitative data are more difficult to obtain, and results at the individual fiber level are scarce. It has been possible, with the method developed by Essén, Saltin, et al. (203), to tease apart fragments of single fibers from freeze-dried muscle samples and to histochemically identify them according to type. The remaining portion is then weighed on a quartz balance and microchemical methods are applied.

The Ca^{2+}-activated myosin ATPase determined on pooled samples of a single fiber type was 2.5-fold higher in the FT than ST fibers (203). The absolute values in these studies were somewhat low due to a loss of activity that occurred during the process of freeze-drying and isolating the individual fibers. To estimate the absolute values, samples containing 100% ST fibers were obtained from soleus muscle and from other muscles that contained increasing percentages of FT fibers. The myosin ATPase activity of the ST fibers averaged 0.16 μmol $P_i \cdot mg^{-1} \cdot min^{-1}$, and the value obtained by extrapolating the FT fiber content to 100% was 0.48 μmol $P_i \cdot mg^{-1} \cdot min^{-1}$ (203). This value is only slightly less than the 0.59 μmol $P_i \cdot mg^{-1} \cdot min^{-1}$ reported by Bárány (31) for the biceps brachii muscle, a mixed-fiber muscle. The differences between the activities reported in these studies appear to be the result of a better purification of the protein by Bárány (31) made possible by the availability of a larger tissue sample.

Some representative data about the ATPase activity of myosin prepared from both ST and FT rat skeletal muscle are presented in Figure 8. The ATPase activities were activated by Ca^{2+}, K^+, or actin. Of these activators, actin clearly is better for differentiating the myosin from ST as compared to FT muscle. The approximately threefold difference in the actin-activated ATPase that exists between the myosin prepared from the soleus or from white portion of the gastrocnemius or vastus muscles corresponds closely to the differences in the time to peak isometric tension that have been reported for ST and FT muscle of the rat (713). Estimations of the Michaelis constants (K_m) for the different types of myosin demonstrated that the affinity of myosin for actin was only about one-fourth as great for myosin from slow-twitch as compared to that from fast-twitch muscles (Fig. 9).

Creatine kinase. Major differences in creatine kinase activity of the fiber types appear to exist in all skeletal muscle. For example, in human muscle the average creatine kinase activity has been reported to be about 222 and 333 $\mu mol \cdot mg^{-1} \cdot min^{-1}$ for the ST and FT fibers, respectively (686, 689, 690). When the FT fibers are further identified as either FT_a or FT_b, the FT_b fibers appear to have slightly higher activities than the FT_a fibers. In the rat the creatine kinase activity for the FT rectus femoris muscle has been reported to be 424 $\mu mol \cdot mg^{-1} \cdot min^{-1}$ as compared to

TABLE 3. *Summary of Substrate Level in Rat Heart and Various Fiber Types in Rat Muscles*

Substrate	Heart, μmol/g wet wt	Fiber Type, μmol/g wet wt		
		SO	FOG	FG
Triglyceride				
Mean	1.35	2.13	2.45	1.95
Range	0.53–1.79	1.35–3.10	2.02–3.08	1.52–2.45
	(231, 282, 576)		(230–232, 235, 282, 576)	
Glycogen (glucose units)				
Mean	27.5	30.3	40.8	42.6
Range	24.4–31.2	20.7–37.8	21.7–58.2	24.8–56.1
	(27, 282, 469, 576, 679)		(25, 27, 36, 126, 282, 346, 469, 488, 572, 576, 577, 581, 608, 625, 676, 679)	
ATP				
Mean	4.03	4.54	6.20	6.28
Range	3.6–4.31	3.9–5.8	5.8–6.5	6.1–6.4
	(375, 576)*		(375, 576)*	
Creatine phosphate				
Mean	4.6	11.65	16.8	18.14
Range	4.1–4.9	9.1–12.4	13.4–18.2	16.8–20.4
	(375, 576)*		(375, 576)*	

SO, slow-twitch, oxidative type from soleus; FOG, fast-twitch, oxidative, glycolytic type from red vastus lateralis; FG, fast-twitch, glycolytic type from white vastus lateralis or psoas. Numbers in parentheses are references. * Unpublished data by P. D. Gollnick, G. A. Klug, and L.-J. Cartier are also included.

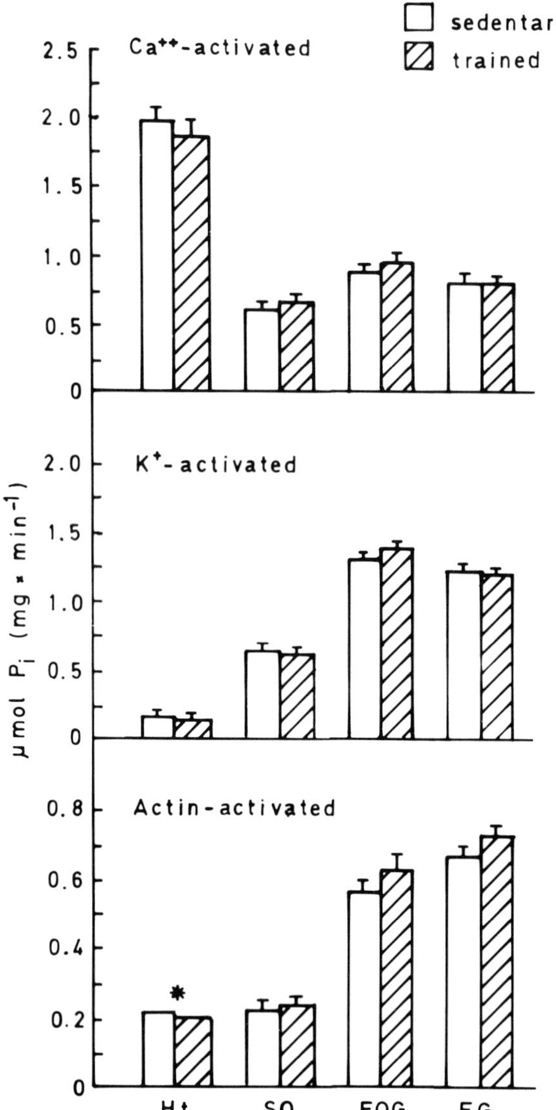

FIG. 8. Ca^{2+}-activated, K^+-activated, and actin-activated ATPase activities of myosin from heart, soleus, red vastus, and white vastus muscles of sedentary and trained rats. Temperature, 37°C; pH 7.4. Vertical lines, SEM. * Sedentary vs. trained, $P < 0.05$. Ht, heart; SO, slow-twitch, oxidative type from soleus; FOG, fast-twitch, oxidative, glycolytic type from red vastus lateralis; FG, fast-twitch, glycolytic type from white vastus lateralis. [Adapted from Watrus (713).]

114 μmol·mg^{-1}·min^{-1} for the ST soleus muscle (659).

Histochemical staining of human skeletal muscle has demonstrated the existence of major differences in the metabolic profiles of the ST and FT fibers (see Fig. 2). The general pattern is for the ST fibers to be well endowed with enzymes for end-terminal oxidation and a low anaerobic potential, with the reverse being true for the FT fibers. There is not, however, a discrete relationship, and enzyme activities vary considerably within each of the fiber types. Some insight into this diversity within a given fiber type can be achieved from the varying staining intensities of the fibers. It has been further quantified from biochemical studies where enzyme activities for carbohydrate and fat metabolism were determined at the level of the individual muscle fiber (198, 203, 347, 468, 515, 554). In some cases the fiber types were not histochemically identifed. Instead, the activities of several enzymes were measured on each fiber and of these, lactate dehydrogenase (LDH) activity was used to type the fibers (347, 468, 469). The results of these studies are summarized together with values for mixed-fiber muscles in Table 4. Glycolytic and mitochondrial enzymes are quite consistent, that is, mitochondrial enzymes are higher in ST than in FT fibers, and the reverse is true for the glycolytic enzymes. An overlap is almost nonexistent. For all four glycolytic enzyme studies there is a twofold-higher mean value in the FT than in ST fibers. The subgroups of FT fibers also differ, with activities being 20%–50% higher in the FT_b than in FT_a fibers.

The activities of 3-hydroxyacyl-CoA dehydrogenase (HAD), succinate dehydrogenase (SDH), and citrate synthase (CS) are 30% to 50% higher in the ST than in the FT fiber groups. When comparisons are made between FT_a and ST fibers of the vastus lateralis muscle, however, the difference for CS is small or nonexistent. In contrast, HAD and SDH activities are 20% and 30% lower in the FT_a than in ST fibers. In the study by Lowry et al. (468) of the biceps brachii muscle, CS activity was about 20% lower in the FT_a than in ST fibers. The activity of these enzymes in the FT_a fibers was approximately 50% of that found in the ST fibers and 50%–67% that of the activity in FT_b fibers. Unfortunately no data are available for human skeletal muscle for the activities of any respiratory chain enzymes at the individual fiber level.

In samples of muscle containing a mixture of fiber types the activity of the mitochondrial enzymes appears to be about 6–10 μmol·mg^{-1}·min^{-1}. In this case little difference exists between activities for the three major oxidative pathways (fatty acid oxidation, citric acid cycle, or electron-transport system). A constant porportionality exists among mitochondrial enzymes (549).

The activities of the glycolytic enzymes are generally higher than those for the end-terminal oxidation. In this pathway the enzymes also appear to be present in a constant proportion to one another (543, 546–548). No obvious deviation from this rule appears to exist when comparisons are made at the individual fiber level.

Data recording the activities of a wide array of enzymes in the metabolic pathways of skeletal muscle from several nonhuman species are shown in Table 5. Only those for the laboratory rat are discussed because this is perhaps the most studied of the nonhuman animals with regard to adaptive responses to varying patterns of physical activity. The general picture that emerges for rat tissue is that ST muscle, such as the soleus muscle, possesses a low potential for glycolytic

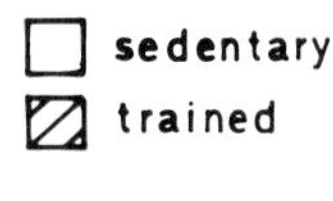

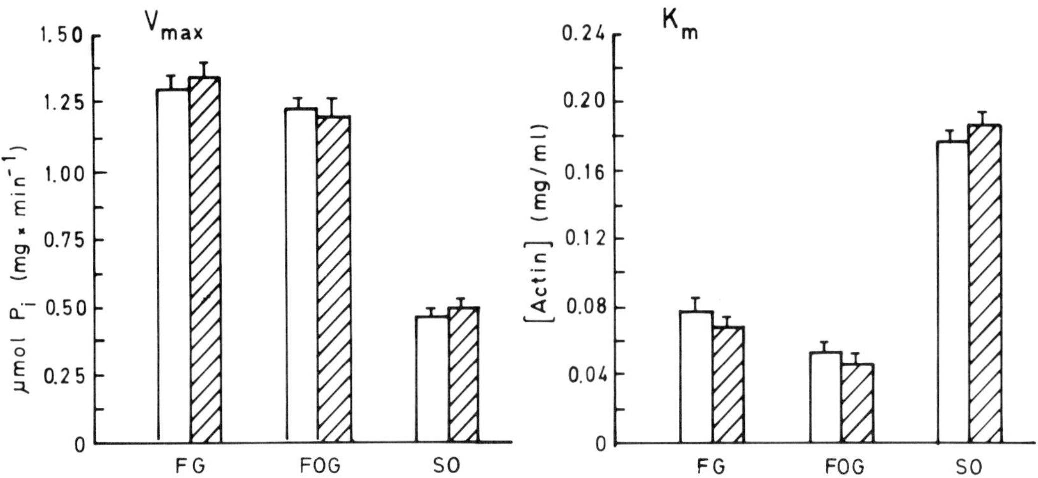

FIG. 9. Predicted V_{max} and apparent K_m of actin-activated ATPase activity of myosin from white vastus, red vastus, and soleus muscles of sedentary and trained rats. Vertical lines, SEM. FG, fast-twitch, glycolytic type from white vastus; FOG, fast-twitch, oxidative, glycolytic from red vastus; SO, slow-twitch, oxidative type from soleus. [Adapted from Watrus (713).]

TABLE 4. *Enzyme Activities in Human Skeletal Muscle (Vastus Lateralis) for Carbohydrate and Fat Metabolism Determined on Whole Muscle and on Fiber Types*

Enzyme	Mixed Muscle, $\mu mol \cdot g^{-1} \cdot min^{-1}$	Fiber Types, $\mu mol \cdot g^{-1} \cdot min^{-1}$				Ref.
		ST	FT	FT_a	FT_b	
Phosphorylase	6–7	2.8	7.3	5.8	8.8	202
Phosphofructokinase	20–25	7.5	15.4	13.7	17.5	203
		6.2	11.9			202
Lactate dehydrogenase	107–210	59	257	221	293	202
		94 ± 16	195 ±12	179 ± 18	211 ± 3	347, 468, 469
Triosephosphate-dehydrogenase	134±10	92 ± 3	175 ± 19	158 ± 9	191 ± 29	347, 468, 469
3-Hydroxyacyl-CoA dehydrogenase	6.2–12.0	14.8	9.3	11.6	7.1	202
		6.2 ± 0.2	3.4 ± 0.4	3.7 ± 0.2	3.1 ± 0.6	347, 468, 469
Succinate dehydrogenase	5.6–8.0	7.1	4.6	4.8	2.5	202, 203
Citrate synthase	6.0–11.5	10.8	7.5	8.6	6.5	202, 203

Activities are measured at 25°C.

TABLE 5. *Enzyme Activities for Fat and Carbohydrate Metabolism in Rat Skeletal Muscle*

Enzyme	SO	FOG	FG	Ref.
	$\mu mol \cdot g^{-1} \cdot min^{-1}$			
Phosphorylase	14	115	171	24, 608
Phosphofructokinase	21	69	100	24, 29, 608
Pyruvate kinase	64	493	696	24, 608
Lactate dehydrogenase	205	486	773	24, 659
Glycogen synthase	6	10	5	679
α-Glycerophosphate dehydrogenase	5	26	57	24
Triosephosphate dehydrogenase	175	432	607	24
Hexokinase	2	2	0.8	24, 659, 679
Succinate dehydrogenase	7	9	5	608
Citrate synthase	23	41	9	29, 723

Mean activities measured at 25°C. SO, slow twitch, oxidative; FOG, fast twitch, oxidative, glycolytic; FG, fast twitch, glycolytic.

activity as indicated by the low activities of the key enzymes of phosphorylase (PHOS) and phosphofructokinase (PFK). Conversely this type of muscle (SO fibers) contains a rich supply of oxidative enzymes. Two classes of FT muscle are identifiable in rat skeletal muscle. In the sedentary animal one type (FG) is white to the eye, whereas the other is deeply red (FOG). Fibers from FG muscle have high activities of enzymes of the Embden-Meyerhof pathway but low activities of the enzymes for end-terminal oxidation. This high anaerobic capacity is characterized by activities of PHOS and PFK that are 5–10 times higher than those of the ST muscle. This metabolic profile suggests a primary reliance on the anaerobic breakdown of glycogen. The FOG portion of the FT muscle possesses high activities for both glycolytic and oxidative enzymes. This tissue can have higher activities for end-terminal oxidation than SO fibers. This situation is distinctly different from that of man where ST fibers have the higher oxidative potential. Note that all of the different types of fibers found in rat skeletal muscle can be identified on the basis of differences in the contractile proteins.

An important result from single fiber analysis is the finding of a wide variation in the content of enzymes for ATP production when comparing fibers of the same type from a single muscle (347, 468, 554, 651–653). Both SDH and PFK activities varied up to 50% in ST fibers in the muscle from one subject (202, 203). Part of this variation can probably be attributed to the 5%–10% variability in the precision of weighing the fragments of fibers on the quartz balance. Furthermore the amount of extramuscular material remaining on the fibers may vary from fiber to fiber. These two factors could account for 5%–15% of the observed variability in enzyme activities, but they cannot detract from the very large differences that exist in the enzyme content of fibers of the same type. This observation has been substantiated by quantitative histochemical studies where variations in staining intensity were shown to exist for fibers in different motor units (555–557). This variability does not exist for fibers belonging to the same motor unit (511–513). Quantitative histochemical studies revealed that the variation in enzyme content along the length of a fiber is small (558). This can account for the relative consistency of enzyme activities when muscle biopsy samples are divided by cutting across the longitudinal axis of the fibers. The uniformity of structural characteristics along the length of a skeletal muscle fiber supports these findings (212).

TABLE 6. *Water Spaces and Electrolytes in Predominantly Red (SO) and White (FG and FOG) Muscles*

	Predominantly Red (SO)	Predominantly White (FG and FOG)	Species	Ref.
Total H_2O, ml/100 g dry wt	344	310	Rat	158
	325	308	Rat	657
	350	339	Rat	116
	324	329	Guinea pig	109
H_2O extracellular, ml/100 g dry wt	72	46	Rat	158*
	53	33	Rat	657*
	39	35	Guinea pig	109†
H_2O intracellular, ml/100 g dry wt	272	264	Rat	158
	272	275	Rat	657
	285	294	Guinea pig	109
Na in muscle, mmol/100 g dry wt	15	11	Rat	158
	14	9	Rat	657
	14	8	Rat	116
$[Na]_i$, mM	13	10	Rat	158
	23	13	Rat	657
	28	19	Rat	109
	44	50	Guinea pig	109
K in muscle, mM/100 g dry wt	38	45	Rat	158
	42	47	Rat	657
	44	51	Rat	116
$[K]_i$, mM	141	179	Rat	158
	154	169	Rat	657
	138	172	Guinea pig	109
Mg in muscle, mM/100 g dry wt	4.6	5.5	Rat	116

Values are means. * Inulin space. † Chloride space.

Ionic Composition of Skeletal Muscle

The various fiber types also contain different amounts of intracellular ions (Tables 6 and 7). Sodium is low in all fibers but the FT fibers contain only about 50% of that found in ST fibers. This is true for rat muscle but species differences may exist. Campion (109) has reported slightly higher values in guinea pig muscle with no difference between ST and FT fibers (Tables 6 and 7). In humans, the sodium content of the muscle fiber appears to be quite low with no difference between fiber types. Species differences may also be present for intramuscular potassium concentrations. Rat and guinea pig muscle fiber types are different: the concentration of K^+ of ST fibers being 140–150 mM whereas the FT fibers have a K^+ concentration of 170–180 mM. In man no differences can be detected when comparing the different fiber types, the mean value for both ST and FT fibers being approximately 160 mM. Recently electron probe analysis has been used to study electrolyte concentration and intracellular distribution. In addition to confirming that K^+ is of similar concentration in the ST and FT fibers in human skeletal muscle, with this method no differences between fiber types have been found for chlorine, sulfur, or phosphorus (478, 727). Magnesium, on the other hand, appeared to be slightly higher in the FT than in ST fibers. These ions may not be evenly distributed within the muscle fiber (478, 727).

In this context we add that the rather large variation in intracellular space of a muscle that exists in the rat may be related to the percent fiber composition. The higher the percentage of ST fibers, the larger the extracellular space of the muscle (443, 657). In human skeletal muscle such a relationship has not been observed (641). There is also some variation between human skeletal muscles (33–53 ml/g dry wt), but there is no explanation for this rather large variation.

Summary

Some of the major similarities and dissimilarities in the properties of the fiber types in the skeletal muscle from various mammalian species may be summarized. The first distinguishing feature is clearly the time to peak isometric tension. On this basis FT and ST motor units can be identified. This feature is most easily demonstrated for the limb muscles of animals. From such studies clearly the time to peak isometric tension and one-half relaxation time for the FT and ST units

TABLE 7. *Muscle Electrolytes in Healthy Subjects*

Muscle	Na_m	K_m	Mg_m	Ref.
	mmol/100 g FFW			
Vastus lateralis	11.6 (2.7)	44.7 (2.0)		49
Vastus lateralis	15.9 (2.9)	43.1 (4.1)		284
Different*	12.1 (2.0)	43.3 (2.5)	3.73 (0.58)	700
Vastus lateralis	9.3 (1.5)	46.7 (0.9)	4.48 (0.08)	50
	mmol/100 g dry wt†			
Triceps brachii	12.7 (5.0)	45.0 (2.0)	3.86 (0.33)	641
Vastus lateralis	8.9 (2.5)	44.9 (5.4)	4.12 (0.18)	641
Soleus	12.5 (3.3)	43.3 (4.7)	4.07 (0.45)	641
Triceps brachii				
ST fibers	13.0	44.0	3.98	
FT fibers	11.6	46.2	4.15	641
Homogenate	11.7	44.5	3.79	
Vastus lateralis				
ST fibers	8.0	42.6	4.58	
FT fibers	8.9	43.0	4.76	641
Homogenate	8.3	44.2	4.12	
Soleus				
ST fibers	9.6	42.6	4.36	
FT fibers	9.6	43.2	4.52	641
Homogenate	10.7	41.8	4.09	

Values are means with 1 SD in parentheses. FFW, fat-free weight; ST, slow twitch; FT, fast twitch. * In 6 subjects from sartorius or pectineus muscles and in 6 subjects from the internal oblique muscle. † Fat content averaged 8% (5%–14%) of dry weight. If expressed per 100 g FFW, value should be increased by this amount.

vary not only among species but also between muscles of the same animal. For human skeletal muscle few precise data are available, but indications are that the time to peak isometric tension is about 40 ms for FT units and 80–100 ms for ST units. It is unknown whether differences exist between the subgroups of FT units or what variation exists for the ST and FT units of different muscles.

The ability of FT and ST units to develop force per unit transectional area of muscle is a matter of controversy. There are reports of major differences in the tension produced per square centimeter by the ST and FT units of the cat. In the rat, evidence seems to suggest that the force-developing capacity is similar for both FT and ST motor units. The force developed per square centimeter for mixed-fiber skeletal muscle of man appears to be greater than the values reported for either cat or rat skeletal muscle. Although direct measurements of the force per unit area of ST or FT motor units are not available for human muscle, they appear to be similar.

Some similarities exist in the fatigue characteristics of the motor units in cat and human skeletal muscle. On the other hand there are also major differences. In the cat the tension developed by ST units remains rather constant over a 60-min period of stimulation, whereas in human skeletal muscle there is an approximately 25% decline in the force developed during a similar period and type of stimulation. The differences are more pronounced when comparisons are made between the FF units of cats and the FT_b fibers of man. The force of FF units falls to near zero after 1 min of stimulation. In contrast the FT_b fibers in human skeletal muscle retain up to 40% of the initial force developed after 50 min of stimulation and 3,000 contractions. The FT_a fibers of man are more fatigue resistant than the FR units of the cat. In man the ST and FT_a units have similar fatigue patterns, whereas in the cat the FR units lose about 50% of their initial force-developing capacity within 5 min of stimulation.

The metabolic potential of the fiber types differs in various species. The most obvious difference is between the FT_a fibers in human skeletal muscle and FOG fibers found in many other species. The FT_a fiber has a rather low triglyceride content and a low concentration of enzymes for β-oxidation. The enzymes for the citric acid cycle and electron-transport chain are usually present at lower concentrations than those found in the ST fibers in the muscle of sedentary man. This is in sharp contrast to the FOG fiber in the cat, where the oxidative system is equal to or higher than that found in the SO fibers. Briefly, we feel that striking differences exist in the characteristics of fibers found in human skeletal muscles as compared with those of other species. These differences are exemplified most dramatically by comparisons of the FT_a and the FOG fibers. A major difference is in the significantly greater resistance of the FT_a and FT_b motor units of man to fatigue as compared to all FT motor units of the cat.

MUSCLE FIBER COMPOSITION IN HUMAN SKELETAL MUSCLE

There is considerable interest in the percent composition and the size of the different fiber types in the skeletal muscle of normal humans and of athletes. Table 8 is a compilation of such data for normal sedentary subjects as reported by a number of laboratories. Table 9 is a summary of the fiber composition and fiber area for several muscles from subjects who were either elite athletes or who had undergone specific training programs. In addition to the data compiled in Tables 8 and 9, other studies containing more information on this subject can be found in references 47, 118, 136, 288, 289, 300, 315, 405, 430, 574, 579, 598, 673. These data are mostly from studies where the muscle samples were obtained by the biopsy (either the needle or open) method. Data are also available from entire muscles obtained at autopsy. Values for fiber composition and fiber size from such studies can be found in references 173, 401–403, 406, 407, 520, 562. Comparisons have also been made between the open and needle biopsy methods (160).

Perhaps the most extensively studied human muscle

TABLE 8. *Summary of Some Published Values for Percent Distribution and Size of Fibers in Limb Muscles of Humans as Estimated From Biopsy Samples*

Sex	Muscle	No.	Mean	Range	Slow-Twitch Fibers				Fast-Twitch Fibers			Ref.
					%	Range	X Area, $\mu m^2 \times 10^2$	Range	%	X Area, $\mu m^2 \times 10^2$	Range	
	VM	11			42	26–63			58			174
	BB	7			49	39–61			51			174
M, F	VL	6			57	50–71	45.6	29.7–60.3	43	48.9	33.1–63.9	177
M, F	BB	7			48	37–61	40.6	27.2–54.3	52	61.4	34.2–87.1	177
M	G	2			64	55–69	33.7	33.0–34.4	36	46.0	39.8–50.2	177
M	S	2			72	65–78	53.3	47.8–58.7	28	94.3	71.1–117.5	177
M	VL	26	34	24–52	36	13–73	40.2	11.4–98.4	64	52.2	17.4–94.7	261
M	D	26	34	24–52	46	14–60			54			261
M	VL	8		23–32	48	29–65	45.6	33.0–60.3	52	50.7	37.0–71.7	175
M	VL	6		28–37	32	18–41	55.0	30.6–92.0	38	66.4	43.1–75.9	260
M	VL	4		16–18	41		50.6		59	55.0		687, 688
M	G	19	27		58		54.6		42	49.5		132
M	G	11	27	17–42	53	38–73	57.0	34.0–87.2	47	49.7	38.8–68.6	130
F	G	10	22	20–30	51	27–72	38.8	25.5–50.4	49	41.9	25.7–61.6	130
M	VL	4			36	20–48	33.0	22.6–41.8	64	37.6	22.3–51.9	565
F	VL	5			36	27–42	27.8	20.5–35.8	64	29.1	17.1–41.6	566
M	VL	19	27		58		54.6		42	49.5		96
M	VL	69		16–18	54		48.4		32[a]	52.7		398
									13[b]			
									1[c]			
M, F	VL	5		24–41	51	47–67			49			272
M, F	S	11		24–41	80	64–100			20			272
M, F	G	6		24–41	60	45–82			40			272
M	G	4	24	20–26	51	37–66	43.1	31.6–51.0	49	47.3	35.0–69.3	8
M	S	4	24	20–26	71	53–88	75.2	49.5–90.0	29	110.6	81.1–147.3	8
M	VL	8	24	20–31	53	45–62			47			681
M	VL	9	23		49	26–60	52.9		37[a]	55.7		289
									18[b]	51.5		
M	VL	5	24		47		55.9		29[a]	68.0		129
									24[b]	62.7		
M	G	19	32		53				23[a]			131
									24[b]			
F	VL	24	24		51				49			108
M	VL	6	6		43	42–72			57			45
F	VL	6	7		56	41–68			44			45
M	VL	11	26	20–29	60		29.4		40	36.6		445
M	VL	10	35	30–39	63		28.5		337	35.1		445
M	VL	8	43	40–49	52		31.3		48	33.6		445
M	VL	12	55	50–59			28.8		52	28.0		445
M	VL	10	62	60–69	45		22.6		55	21.2		445
M, F			59	21–83								173
					Autopsy Material							
	S	20			70	12–95			30			
	Med. gast.	24			50	14–84			50			
	Lat. bast.	9			48	37–62			52			
	Whole gast.	33			50	33–63			50			
	Vast. int.	14			47	30–71			53			
	VL deep	10			35	22–50			65			
	VL superf.	15			30	11–53			70			
	VL whole	25			32	19–48			68			
	BB autopsy			17–30	42	34–51			58			408
	D				53	43–63			47			408
	VL				38	27–48			62			408

M, male; F, female; G, gastrocnemius; S, soleus; BB, biceps brachialis; D, deltoid; VL, vastus lateralis; VM, vastus medialis; X, cross-sectional area. [a] Fast twitch, a type. [b] Fast twitch, b type. [c] Fast twitch, c type.

is the lateral portion of the quadriceps femoris (vastus lateralis). In an early study biopsy samples were obtained from 74 male subjects from 17 to 58 yr of age, including sedentary men and highly trained athletes (261). For this group the average fiber composition was 52.2% ST with a range from 13% to 98% ST fibers. In an attempt to provide further information concerning the normal fiber composition of this muscle, 69 males and 48 females (Fig. 10), all 16 yr old and representing a random sample for this age group, were studied (602). The mean fiber composition of the vastus lateralis muscle for this group was 54% and 52%

ST fibers for the males and females, respectively. Within the FT fibers the FT_a fibers were approximately twice as common as the FT_b fibers. Similar mean values for the percentages of ST, FT_a, and FT_b fibers were observed in studies of 26 men and 25 women around 25 yr of age (521). Thus ample evidence is available to suggest that in the vastus lateralis muscle the ST and FT fibers are about equally common, and no differences exist between the sexes.

In the studies cited above, the relative percentage of fibers was estimated from small muscle samples obtained with the needle biopsy (49) technique where fragments of 200–1,000 fibers are contained in each sample. The large variation observed in these samples could be a reflection of a heterogeneous mixture of fibers in the cross section of the vastus lateralis muscle. The variability of the relative frequency and of the size of the various fiber types has been examined in whole cross sections of muscles obtained at autopsy (173, 186, 402, 403).

A variation in the relative occurrence of the fiber types in a muscle does not exist but it does exceed 5%–15% when calculated for adjacent regions of the muscle. A tendency for ST fibers to comprise a higher percent of the total in the deeper parts of the muscle is sometimes found, but this is limited and does not exceed 5%–10%. Fiber size varies slightly in different parts of the muscle with the ratio between ST and FT fibers being relatively constant throughout the entire muscle. Another approach to the study of the variation in fiber composition and size is to take multiple biopsy samples from the same muscle. When this was done in the vastus lateralis muscle the coefficient of variation for the relative occurrence of a fiber type was 5%–15% and for the size of the corresponding type it was 5% (261, 302, 686). A similar pattern of variation was also found when data from 36 human muscles were analyzed (406, 407). Other studies of the vastus lateralis muscle and the biceps brachii confirm these findings (520).

The large range of the percentages of ST and FT fibers observed in the population in these studies implies that for a certain percent of the population of males and females, their muscles are predominantly of one or the other fiber type. This interindividual variation appears to be genetically determined because studies with mono- and dizygotic twins have shown almost identical fiber composition of the vastus lateralis muscle in the monozygotic but not in the dizygotic twins [Fig. 11; (431)].

The various muscles of the human body differ in fiber composition. The extent of this variation is illustrated by data from an autopsy study where the same muscles from several subjects were analyzed (173, 402, 403, 406, 407, 667). The results from six men and three women, who died suddenly without having a known muscle disease, are given in Figure 12*B*. It is apparent that some similarities exist among muscles from the same person. It is also apparent that although most muscles have a mean fiber composition of about 50% ST fibers, some muscles, like the soleus and triceps brachii, have a predominance of either ST or FT fibers. In man the respiratory and trunk muscles have mixed ST and FT fibers. The diaphragm and intercostal muscles of man contain approximately equal percentages of ST and FT fibers (311). Muscles around the spine appear to contain nearly 50% ST fibers but a fairly wide interindividual variation as is seen in the muscles of the extremities. In addition to the results from autopsy studies, data are available from studies where several muscles in the same subjects were biopsied and the fiber composition estimated (Fig. 12*A*). In all important aspects these findings are analogous to the autopsy study.

An important question is whether small muscle samples from a human muscle, such as those obtained with a biopsy technique (49), will give acceptable information about the fiber composition, fiber size, or chemical composition of the entire muscle (160, 180, 181, 520, 563). Repeated sampling from the same muscles gives a coefficient of variation of 5%–10% for fiber composition and size (SD in percent of the mean fiber size or fiber composition). Large samples do not reduce this variation substantially nor does an open versus needle biopsy produce a significant difference (186, 261). The problem of a differential distribution of fibers in the central as compared to the superficial part of a muscle can be accommodated by a greater precision in the sampling site (186). We may justifiably conclude that for most cases the mean value for a group of subjects closely reflects the true value for a given muscle. However, there are instances where considerable deviation from the mean value may occur (186, 644); for these more reliable informaton can be obtained from multiple biopsies taken from different sites. This is especially true for the assessment of the percent fiber composition.

Similar problems may also be encountered in the determination of substrate concentrations and enzyme activities where these are distinctly different for the different fiber types. This problem can only be adequately resolved by analysis of individual fibers. This problem also extends to the analysis of substrate changes in muscle where only select motor units have been active. Under these conditions analysis of whole muscle samples will seriously underestimate a change such as the depletion of glycogen or an increase in a metabolite.

Human beings, in contrast to other species, have a more homogeneous mixture of fibers in nearly all muscles. Thus the higher degree of specialization, with the result that a single fiber type is seen in a muscle or large area in some animals, rarely occurs in man.

MOTOR-UNIT RECRUITMENT

The contractile and metabolic properties that combine to produce the physiological characteristics of the individual motor units in skeletal muscle enable them

TABLE 9. *Summary of Some Published Values for Percent Distribution and Size of Fibers in Limb Muscles of Humans in Training as Estimated From Biopsy Samples*

Sex	Muscle	No.	Age		Slow-Twitch Fibers				Fast-Twitch Fibers			Experiment	Ref.
			Mean	Range	%	Range	X Area, $\mu m^2 \times 10^2$	Range	%	X Area, $\mu m^2 \times 10^2$	Range		
M	VL	6	33	29–40	32[a]	18–41	55.0	30.6–92.0	68	66.4	36.8–95.8	Endurance training on cycle ergometer, 6 mo	688
					36[b]	27–42	67.8	55.5–89.0	64	61.4	43.1–76.0		
M	VL	4	24	18–33	61	48–73	86.5[c]	58.0–127.6	39	99.5	75.4–147.9	Elite bicyclists	261
	D				51	40–64	54.7[c]	40.6–72.5	49	73.4	46.4–92.8		
M	VL	4	26	25–27	61	45–72	64.4[c]	36.6–91.4	39	51.0	36.6–65.8	Elite canoeists	261
	D				58	48–66	82.4[c]	58.5–131.6	42	83.9	54.8–109.8		
M	VL	4	25	23–29	46	25–60	60.4[c]	17.4–101.5	54	95.6	58.0–145.0	Weight lifters	261
	D				53	43–67	55.5[c]	29.0–75.4	47	89.2	43.5–145.0		
M	VL	8	23	19–33	59	53–70			41			Distance runners	261
M	VL	11	52	47–58	69	47–96			31			Orienteers	261
	D				63	31–98			37				
F	G	2	20	18–21	27	27–28	37.5	35.4–39.4	73	39.3	33.7–45.0	Trained sprinters	130
M	G	2	20	17–22	24	21–27	58.8	39.8–77.8	76	60.3	58.8–61.9	Trained sprinters	130
F	G	7	20	16–25	61	44–73	60.7	30.8–99.5	39	56.4	40.1–75.0	Trained middle-distance runners	130
M	G	7	23	19–32	52	41–69	61.0	45.5–84.5	48	71.2	48.9–92.1	Trained middle-distance runners	130
M	G	5	24	20–32	69	63–74	66.1	36.4–101.1	31	76.3	47.3–113.3	Trained distance runners	130
F	G	3	22	21–23	49	37–61	41.6	35.0–50.8	51	51.1	43.5–66.2	Long and high jumpers	130
M	G	2	29	26–32	47	44–49	47.2	44.8–49.6	53	65.2	63.0–67.5	Long and high jumpers	130
F	G	3	21	17–26	42	41–42	48.6	42.6–54.6	58	45.7	42.7–48.7	Javelin throwers	130
M	G	3	25	23–30	50	46–56	55.9	25.7–82.5	50	57.7	42.1–76.1	Javelin throwers	130
F	G	2	24	21–26	51	48–54	51.9	32.9–70.9	49	58.5	47.7–69.4	Shot and discus throwers	130
M	G	4	27	21–32	38	13–52	77.0	50.4–103.5	62	94.8	91.3–97.2	Shot and discus throwers	130
M	VL	4	21	17–28	69	60–83			20[d]		14–30	Distance runners after 18 wk aerobic training	399
									10[e]		1–20		
									1[f]		0–1		
M	VL	4	21	17–28	52	34–77			18[d]		7–28	Distance runners after 11 wk anaerobic training	399
									18[e]		4–29		
									12[f]		7–15		
M	G	13	35		55				43[d]			Trained distance runners	131
									2[e]				
		12	23		23				47[d]				
									2[e]				
F	G			18–26	39		32.5		61	35.0		Sprinters	290
F	G			18–26	54		37.5		46	30.0		Pentathletes	290
F	G			18–26	63		32.5		37	27.5		Middle-distance runners	290
F	G			18–26	73		36.0		27	21.0		Distance runners	290
M	G	26			56		54.3		44	54.2		Well-trained distance runners	227
M	VL	8			68				24[d]			Elite orienteers	398
									3[e]				
									4[f]				
M	G	7			67				29[d]			Elite orienteers	398
									2[e]				
									2[f]				

TABLE 9—*Continued*

Sex	Muscle	No.	Age		Slow-Twitch Fibers				Fast-Twitch Fibers			Experiment	Ref.
			Mean	Range	%	Range	X Area, $\mu m^2 \times 10^2$	Range	%	X Area, $\mu m^2 \times 10^2$	Range		
M	D	4			68				14[d] 17[e] 0[f]			Elite orienteers	398
M	VL	3	21	20–22	60	51–70			40			Elite skiers	681
M	VL	11	25		57		63.3		43	61.2		Elite cyclists	96
M	VL	11	25		53		60.6		47	57.6		Well-trained cyclists	96
F	VL	7	20		51		54.9		49	52.2		Well-trained cyclists	96
F	VL	5	23	20–32	48	24–82	43.1	31.1–71.7	52	38.2	15.2–76.9	Field hockey players	566
M	VL	3			45	30–60	44.3	31.6–58.9	55	67.7	58.1–76.6	Weight lifters	565
M	VL	3			44	29–54	46.1	33.9–69.0	56	43.1	25.1–69.0	Distance runners	565
M	VL	5	24		45		61.1		30[d] 25[e]	73.7 67.7		Leg 1 control	129
M	VL	5	24		42		58.9		35[d] 23[e]	73.8 71.2		Leg 1 after 7 wk of training 6 s, 4 times per wk	129
M	VL	5	24		48		48.7		28[d] 23[e]	62.3 57.7		Leg 2 control	129
M	VL	5	24		47		49.6		32[d] 21[e]	75.9 56.3		Leg 2 after 7 wk of training 30 s, 4 times per wk	129
M	D	6	23	18–28	53	41–74			47			Elite canoeists	682
M	G	14	26	21–32	79	50–98	83.42	48.5–151.4	21	64.9	31.8–115.2	Elite distance runners	132
M	VL	19	22		50	20–71	50.9		38[d] 12[e]	58.7 53.6		Elite ice hockey players	289
M	VL	8	20	16–29	44	24–55	45.5	35.7–65.8	56	74.3	59.5–92.4	Weight lifters	175
M	VL	4		16–18	41[a] 44[b]		50.6 51.9		59 56		55.0 57.4	Sprint training	687

M, male; F, female; VL, vastus lateralis; D, deltoid; G, gastrocnemius. [a] Before training. [b] After training. [c] Samples for single representative subjects. [d] Fast twitch, a type. [e] Fast twitch, b type. [f] Fast twitch, c type.

to engage in a wide variety of activities. The ST motor units, in all species, are well designed for prolonged activity, where ATP can be produced by directing substrate flux through the oxidative pathways of the mitochondria. In animals other than man the FT motor units in red muscle rely primarily on either the terminal-oxidative process or the glycolytic pathway (or both) for ATP production. These motor units appear uniquely suited for joining the ST units during prolonged activity when the intensity is relatively high. The FT motor units in white skeletal muscle (FT$_b$) appear best suited for high-intensity short-duration activity, where a glycolytic degradation of glycogen to lactate is the primary method for ATP production.

Some differences exist in the properties of FT motor units contained in human skeletal muscle as compared with those of other animals, which may result in slightly different patterns of use for these motor units during locomotion. First, the capacity of the ST fibers to develop force per unit of cross-sectional area does not appear to be significantly different from that of FT fibers. This would reduce the need for an early recruitment of the FT motor units when additional tension development is required. Second, the oxidative potential of the FT$_a$ fibers is considerably lower than that of the ST fibers in the muscle of sedentary man. For most other animals the mitochondrial density of the FT$_a$ fibers may be equal to or in some cases higher than that of ST fibers.

The systematic use of the different motor units in response to distinct physiological demands depends on the existence of an orderly procedure for their recruitment by the central nervous system. This system is based on the existence of motoneurons of varying size, threshold for activation, and conduction velocity. These properties of nerves were identified by Hursh (377) and Rushton (597). Their importance in the control of motor recruitment was elaborated by Henneman and co-workers (327–331). In this scheme,

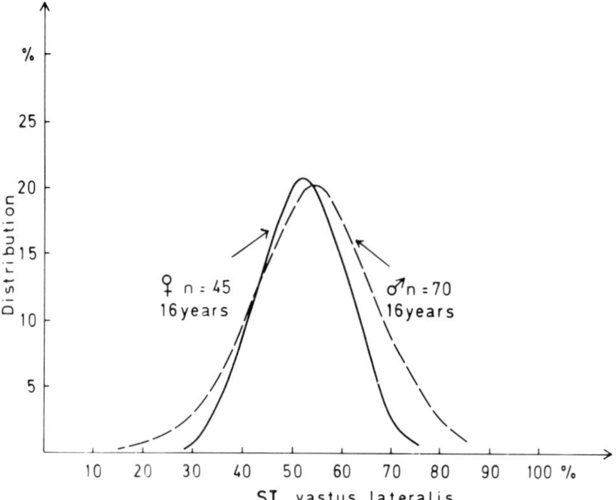

FIG. 10. The distribution of relative occurrence of ST fibers in vastus lateralis in young men and women. [Adapted from a study by Hedberg and Jansson (319); some results are presented in Saltin et al. (602).]

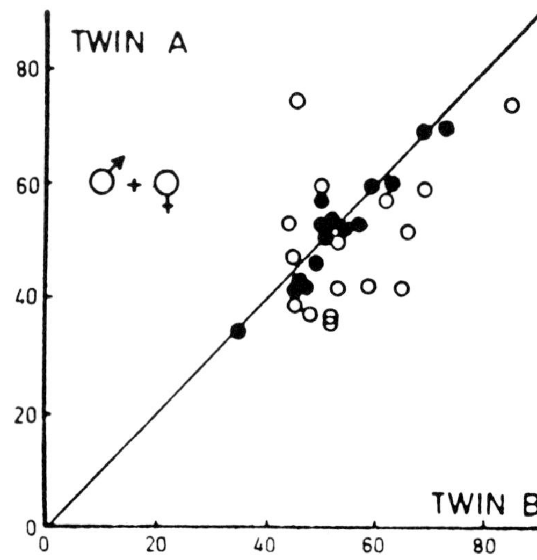

FIG. 11. Intrapair comparison of slow-twitch fiber distribution of m. vastus lateralis in monozygous (●) and dizygous (○) twins. [From Komi et al. (431).]

now commonly referred to as the size principle, ST motor units are innervated by small, low-threshold, slowly conducting motor nerves; FT motor units are innervated by large, higher threshold, fast-conducting motor nerves. Rather than discrete differences in motoneurons it appears that a continuum of thresholds for activation exists. In this manner a systematic procedure for mobilizing motor units exists whereby the tension requirements for a specific muscular contraction pattern can be initiated by the central nervous system.

Evidence for an orderly recruitment of motor units in man during a variety of physical activities has come from both histochemical (133, 237, 262, 263, 267, 270, 271, 286, 287, 522) (based on the depletion of glycogen from the fibers in biopsy samples) and electrophysiological data (143–147, 293, 294, 299, 308, 493, 494). The method of biopsy and glycogen depletion is limited to exercise of sufficient duration and intensity to produce a discernible loss of PAS stain in the fibers. In some instances the metabolic profile of the fibers results in underestimating the involvement of ST units. Thus during high-intensity exercise the loss of glycogen from FT_b units would be greater than from ST units simply because the ST units would also consume large amounts of oxygen, free fatty acids (FFA), and glucose, resulting in a smaller degradation of glycogen. Electrophysiological methods lack a definitive proof of the type of motor unit from which the electrical potential is recorded.

Histochemical studies (Fig. 13) have verified a primary involvement of ST motor units during low-intensity exercise in man (262, 270). When such activity is prolonged or when its intensity is above a certain level, there is a progressive involvement of FT motor units, with the FT_a units being involved first, until, if the exercise extends to exhaustion, all motor units will have been involved (263). With high-intensity dynamic exercise, that is, above maximal oxygen uptake ($\dot{V}O_{2\,max}$) capacity, all types of motor units may be activated (263, 270). For some individuals exhaustion does not result in a complete depletion of glycogen from all FT fibers regardless of whether the exercise has been of a moderate or high intensity (262, 270).

The exercise intensity required to activate FT motor units is debated. It has been suggested that this may occur at intensities as low as 60%–70% of the $\dot{V}O_{2\,max}$ and that this may be responsible for the elevation of lactate in the blood at these exercise intensities (392, 598). Definite proof for this concept is lacking in the published literature, and data are available to suggest that it is unlikely. The increase in the lactate concentration of blood that occurs during prolonged, moderately severe (60%–70% $\dot{V}O_{2\,max}$) exercise usually peaks at about 10–20 min and then declines toward rest values as the exercise continues (270, 341, 418). If the lactate production is a result of FT fiber use, its decline could be explained either as a fatigue and inactivation of these fibers or by assuming that they have switched to terminal oxidation to support their energy requirements. If the FT fibers were exhausted they could be expected to be depleted of glycogen as occurs during short, heavy exercise (263). This is not the case. Since the power output is constant during such exercise a loss of some motor units would necessitate the addition of others. Based on the concept of ST recruitment before FT units, this would imply addition of more FT units (143–145), but this would produce more lactate rather than less. If the FT fibers had converted to oxidative metabolism, the total oxygen uptake would increase. This does not occur (262, 270). As the exercise continues, however, and ST fibers become glycogen depleted, there is evidence of a use of FT units (262, 270). This occurs without any rise in the lactate con-

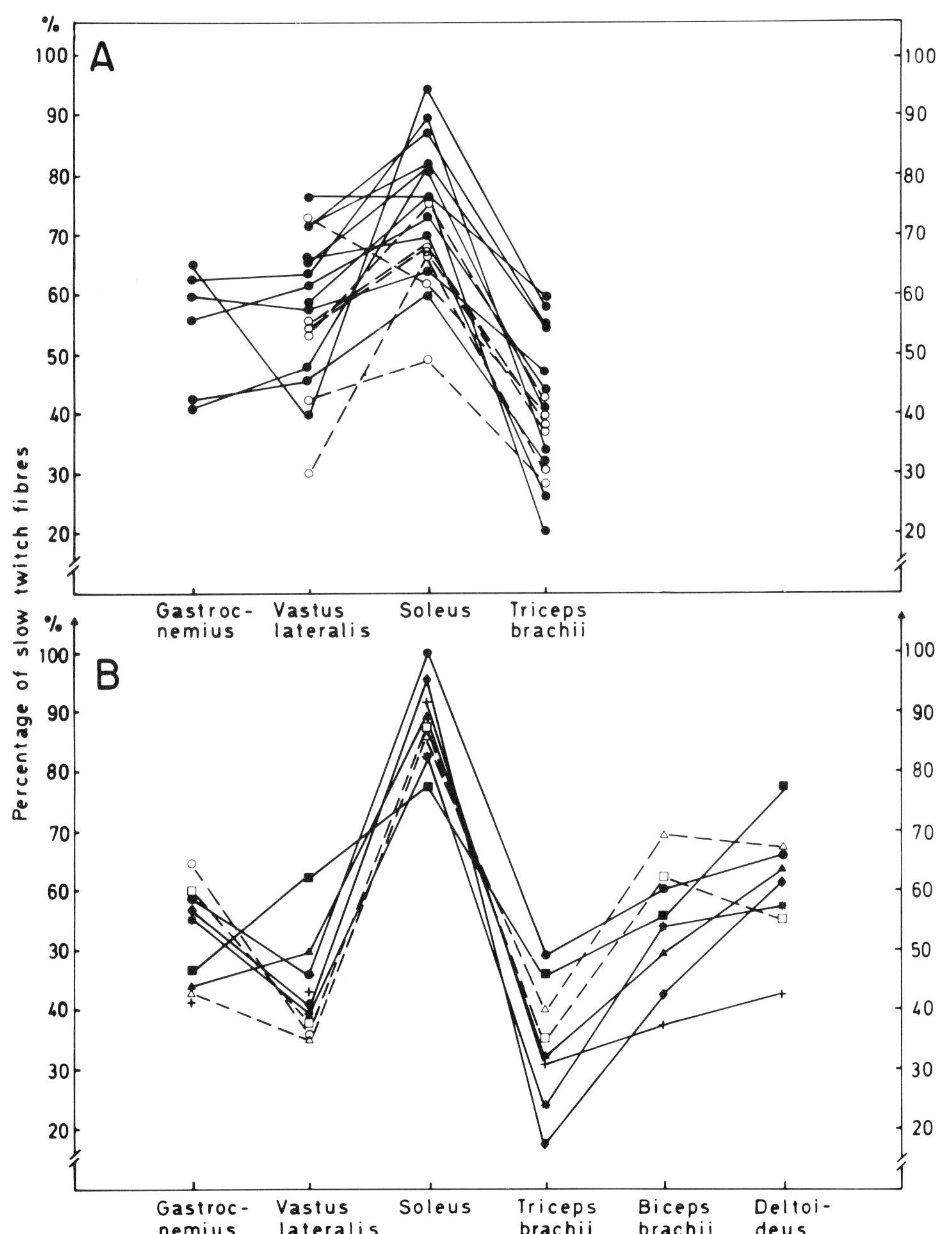

FIG. 12. Relative occurrence of ST fibers in some muscles of the body. *A*: muscle samples are obtained by multiple needle biopsy samples or (*B*) postmortem within 24 h after death. [*A* from Sjøgaard (641) and G. Sjøgaard, unpublished material. *B* from Johnson et al. (406).]

centrations of the blood or in total-body oxygen uptake (270). The latter circumstances suggest either that the FT fibers possess adequate mitochondrial enzymes and receive sufficient blood flow to support the terminal oxidation required for the levels of tension they produce during such exercise or that the lactate produced is taken up and oxidized by other muscles. Such lactate could also be cleared by the liver.

Some of the discrepancies that exist in the literature concerning the fiber type involvement at different exercise intensities may be attributable to the use of different modes of exercise. For example, cycle ergometers that are mechanically braked and have light flywheels often possess little inertial momentum. Thus for each pedal thrust a brisk contraction may be needed to keep a steady pace. From EMG studies it is known that the threshold for activation of a motor unit is reduced during brisk or ballistic-type contractions (143, 146). This situation basically applies to dynamic exercise performed by man. Motor unit involvement in various gaits has been studied, e.g., in the rat, lion, and horse (17, 19, 21, 457, 663). It is apparent from these studies that during walking and trotting at rather low intensities both ST motor units

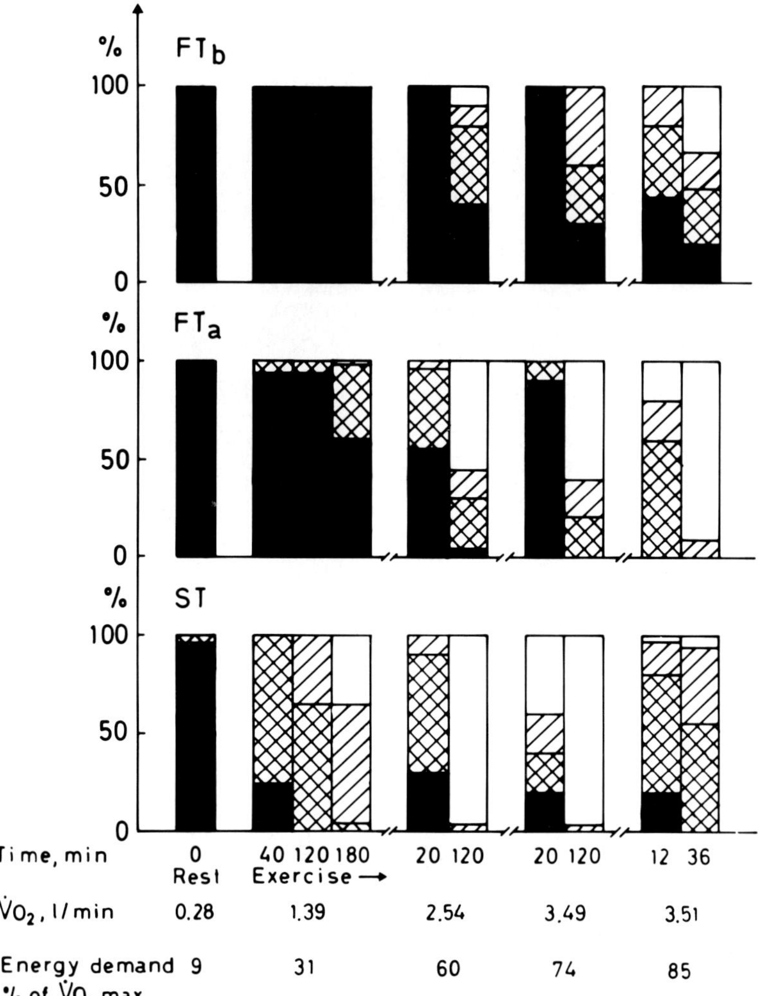

FIG. 13. Schematic illustration of intensity of periodic acid–Schiff (PAS) stain (glycogen) in human skeletal muscle fibers at rest and after various times during prolonged exercise at relative work intensities ranging from 31% to 85% of the subject's maximal oxygen uptake. Graph is a summary of several studies. Findings at 74% $\dot{V}O_{2\,max}$ show the PAS stain evaluated by microphotometry, whereas in the other studies results are based on a subjective rating (dark = *filled;* and white = *unfilled,* with various levels between as *crosshatched* and *hatched*). [Data from Gollnick, Saltin, et al. (262, 263, 270, 271). Findings at 74% $\dot{V}O_{2\,max}$ from K. Vøllestad, unpublished material.]

and FT motor units of oxidative type (FOG) become depleted of glycogen early in the exercise. In contrast, the FG motor units do not become depleted of glycogen in these gaits even at high speeds but only during galloping. This is additional evidence for a basic difference between the FT motor units of man and other animals that have been studied.

These findings do not detract from the concept of an orderly recruitment of motor units but point to species differences in the programming of the recruitment of the fiber types. This has implications for how they are used in various activities.

Clearly recruitment order in man may be related either to the requirement for tension development or to the availability of oxygen or to both. To obtain some perspective of what fraction of the voluntary contractile strength is used in dynamic exercise, peak force for a pedal thrust during cycle ergometer exercise was measured (267, 269, 349, 640). Less than 10% of the MVC was used at power productions demanding less than the subjects' $\dot{V}O_{2\,max}$. At exercise intensities eliciting $\dot{V}O_{2\,max}$, the corresponding value ranged from 10% to 15% of MVC. These measurements take into consideration the knee angle at which the peak force was developed but not the speed of contraction. When the speed of contraction was also considered, the relative values ranged from 20% to 40% of the MVC that could be produced at the speed of contraction obtained at 60 rpm. Thus even at exercise intensities that produce exhaustion in 4 min, less than one-half of the strength of the muscle was utilized.

In experiments where static contractions were held with the knee extensors at tensions representing from 10%–20% of the MVC, only ST units became glycogen depleted (270). At higher tensions FT units also became depleted of glycogen. This suggests that with this type of muscular activity the availability of oxygen and the development of force influenced recruitment of FT units since blood flow in the knee extensor group is restricted during sustained contraction above about 20% MVC (58, 59, 376).

The EMG recordings from single fibers support the concept of an orderly recruitment of motor units in a progression from ST to FT units (143–147, 279, 493, 494, 539). The observation that the individual motor unit is activated at specific levels of tension and ceases discharging when the tension falls below this set level points to the level of tension development as the primary factor in controlling motor unit recruitment (53–55). Though there is evidence for an activation of FT motor units before or without ST units during high-intensity exercise (293, 294, 661), the data in support of this concept are equivocal.

There are reports using either histochemical or electrophysiological techniques indicating exceptions to the orderly treatment of motor units as described above (294, 295, 661). The histochemical studies are difficult to evaluate since there is a lack of definite proof as to the ST fiber involvement. In such studies the reduction in glycogen was too small to be evident from histochemical staining procedures. The EMG recordings from single ST and FT fibers in brisk contractions or at contractions close to MVC demonstrate that FT units may be electrically active before ST units, but the ST fibers are not silent (143). In voluntary efforts with simultaneous, preprogrammed activation of neurons in the motor cortex (40, 147), it could be anticipated that FT units of muscle would display electrical activity prior to ST units simply because of a difference in the conduction velocity of the motoneurons and the number of interconnecting neurons. The recruitment pattern might also differ in reflex activation of motor units by input from sensory receptors in the skin.

The specific mechanism or sensing system to which the central nervous system responds with varying patterns of motor unit recruitment is unknown. It is easy to envisage a system centered around the stretch receptors in muscle spindles or golgi organs. Information from these receptors could signal the need for adding or subtracting motor units from the contraction. During prolonged submaximal exercise, where it appears that a progressive recruitment of motor units occurs starting with ST and finally using all units including FT units, this could occur as a result of failure of the ST units to produce the needed tension as their glycogen stores are depleted and their ability to produce the ATP needed to support contraction is diminished.

ADAPTIVE RESPONSE IN SKELETAL MUSCLE

Different types of motor units exist in skeletal muscles, and they are endowed with properties that uniquely qualify them for specific types of activity. In addition to the differences between major types of motor units there are also differences between motor units that are histologically similar. Thus there is a broad array of contractile speeds, fiber numbers, and metabolic potentials for the motor units in a single muscle. This section considers what effects growth and patterns of use (either overload or inactivity) have in establishing, maintaining, or changing the characteristics of skeletal muscle. Since activation of skeletal muscle by electrical stimulation or by voluntary means can produce very different mechanical and metabolic demands on the muscle, depending on which fibers are engaged in generating the force, this must be considered when discussing muscle adaptation. To evaluate whether the mode of usage may elicit different adaptive responses, exercise is categorized as: *1*) high-resistance, few-repetition exercise (strength training); *2*) low-resistance, high-repetition exercise (endurance training); or *3*) varying intermediate combinations (for example, sprint training).

Clearly the changes in skeletal muscle that accompany either use or disuse as described in this chapter involve alterations in either the rate of protein synthesis or degradation. Recently attempts have been made to investigate these changes and to determine the mechanisms by which they are induced and controlled (60, 62, 244–246, 313, 332, 339, 350, 393, 414, 610, 618, 620, 677). This is an area for future investigation.

Muscle Size

In terms of its ability to adjust its size to physiological demands, skeletal muscle is a very plastic tissue. This is illustrated by the changes in weight that occur during normal growth and development and in the adult or growing animal in response to alterations in activity patterns. Since skeletal muscle consists of about 85% (by weight) fibers and 15% extrafiber material (224, 348, 429, 447, 458), a change in total weight is a simple, yet reliable, method for estimating changes in the fiber component of muscle. Exceptions to this are instances where experimental perturbations or pathological changes produce modifications in the water and collagen content of muscle (16, 378). The growth potential of skeletal muscle can be illustrated in inbred animal strains such as the rat or chicken. For the rat, the limb muscles increase about 28-fold from fetal stage to 80 days (190) and 9- to 21-fold in weight from the 16th to the 86th day after birth (191). For the chicken, the weights of the gastrocnemius and pectoralis muscle increase 40- to 90- and 300- to 600-fold, respectively, from hatching to 266 days of age (502). From hatching to 10 wk of age the sartorius muscle of the chicken increased from 0.129 to 4.930 g (745). Human skeletal muscles possess a growth characteristic similar to that of other animals. This is illustrated by the increase in weight of the biceps brachii from about 2.0 g at birth to 110–150 g in the adult (B. Saltin, E. Nygaard, and A.-S. Colling-Saltin, unpublished observations). In addition to illustrating the great growth potential for skeletal muscle, these data also demonstrate that the absolute increase in the size of muscle depends on its function as determined by its location on the skeleton.

With changes in muscle size as a result of growth and maturity there are also changes in the chemical composition of muscle of the fetus as compared to that of the adult. Fetal skeletal muscle is about 90% water

(123–125, 153). At 4–7 mo of age this value is about 78.5% water with only minor changes occurring thereafter until attaining the adult value of about 76% water. There are also major changes in the protein fractions of muscle (Fig. 14). This is exemplified by a 2.8-fold increase in total protein from the 14th wk of gestation to the adult human being. Of the various protein fractions, the biggest increase occurs in the fibrillar fraction, which increases 3.5-fold. There are also changes in the intracellular ion concentration from fetal life to maturity (Fig. 15).

POSTNATAL DEVELOPMENT. *Nonhuman species.* There has been considerable interest in the question of the relative importance of changes in the size (cross-sectional area or diameter) and number of fibers in animal muscle. This has been an active area of research for those interested in meat production. As a result, data are available on the size and in some cases the number of fibers in the muscle of the chicken, pig, sheep, rabbit, and steer (114, 219, 343, 410, 487, 490, 564, 585, 645, 660). The general conclusion from these studies is that there is a large increase in fiber size during normal growth and development. An example of such data is the report that the fiber diameter of the pig increased from an average of about 7 μm at birth to over 70 μm in the adult (660). This 10-fold change in diameter would be equal to about a 100-fold increase in cross-sectional area if one were to assume that the fiber areas were geometrically similar (which they are not). Other factors that influenced the magnitude of the fiber enlargement were the strain of the animals and their state of nutrition. The lack of any change in fiber number extended to instances where the total muscle weight had increased more than 600 times during the growth period (507).

The number of fibers in the limb muscles of the rat has been reported to be essentially unchanged over the period from 4–6 days postpartum to 300 days (190, 191). The average fiber weight in the neonatal rat has been estimated to be slightly over 2 μg as compared to 22.4 μg/fiber in the biceps brachii and 63.1 μg/fiber in the gastrocnemius muscle in the adult animal (191). The relative increase in weight per fiber exceeds that

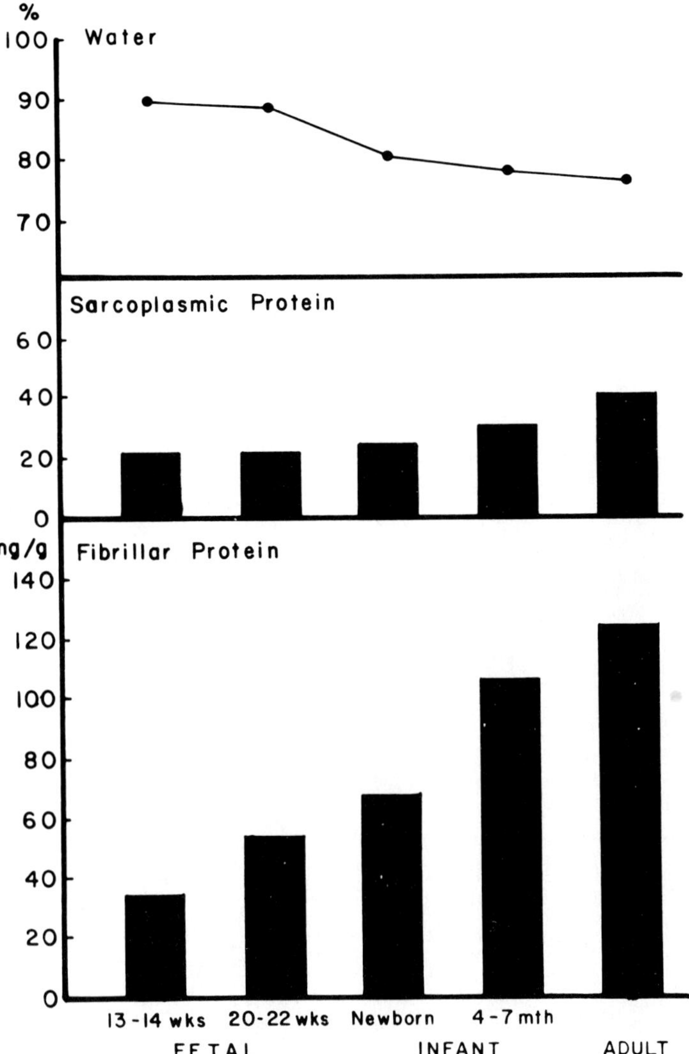

FIG. 14. Changes in the percent water and concentration of protein in the sarcoplasmic and fibrillar fractions of human skeletal muscle as a result of growth and development. [Adapted from Dickerson and Widdowson (153).]

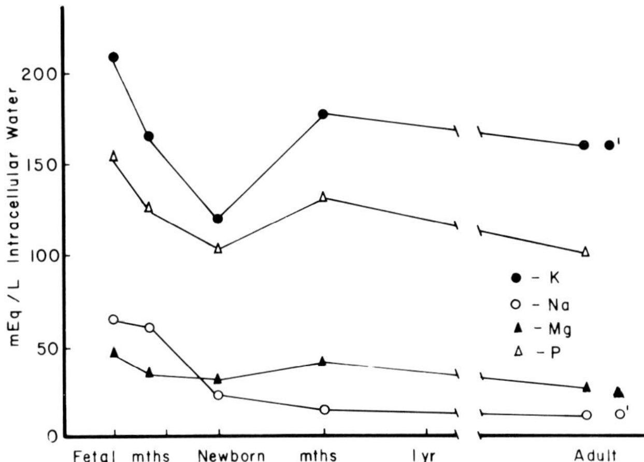

FIG. 15. Intracellular ion concentrations for human skeletal muscle from fetal life to adulthood. The data points marked (′) are averages of samples collected from the triceps brachii, vastus lateralis, and soleus of 6 male and 6 female adults. [Data from Dickerson and Widdowson (153), except those marked (′) from Sjøgaard (641).]

of the overall gain in weight during postnatal skeletal muscle growth.

In contrast to the above, there are reports of increases in the number of fibers in skeletal muscle of the rat during the period from birth to 3 wk of age (72, 114, 571) and in the muscles of an Australian marsupial (71). Conversely, decreases in the fiber number of the dog, guinea pig, and rat have been reported with age (213, 214, 380, 571).

Man. Aherne et al. (2) examined changes in the fibers of the deltoid, biceps brachii, rectus femoris, and gastrocnemius muscle of man in the age range of from 37 wk of gestation to 18 yr of age. This material was from 22 individuals, 14 males. Only rarely was there more than one sample for a given age and not all years were represented. In this sample the fibers in the muscles at 37 wk of gestation ranged from 36.5 to 48.2 μm^2 with the smallest fibers in the rectus femoris and the largest in the gastrocnemius muscles. Over the entire age range examined, there was a nearly linear increase in the cross-sectional area of the muscle fibers as a function of body dimension (Fig. 16*A*, *B*). Unfortunately, the fibers were not subdivided into the different types. In mature individuals, the average fiber areas were approximately 2,000 μm^2 with those in the leg muscles being larger than those of the arm muscles. Nevertheless during skeletal growth the longitudinal growth of the muscle fibers is such that the average sarcomere length in the mature muscle fibers is not markedly different from that of the young animal (122, 252).

Colling-Saltin (123–125, 697) has examined muscular growth in the lateral portion of the quadriceps, rectus abdominis, deltoid, biceps brachii, soleus, and gastrocnemius muscle of 86 fetuses and 50 infants and children to age 7. The fetal samples included material from as early as 12–14 wk of gestation. The majority of the samples were from males. The samples were fresh frozen and stained with histochemical methods to identify the different fiber types. These data illustrated that early in fetal life the muscle fibers had not developed to a stage where they could be typed. For animals also, it is difficult to identify fiber types in fetal life (157, 159, 240, 404, 475, 595). Some differentiation of fibers into types appeared at about the 21st wk of gestation and thereafter continued with differentiation being nearly complete at approximately 1 yr of age (Fig. 17). These studies revealed that at about 12 wk of gestation the average cross-sectional area was 36.3 μm^2. This remained relatively constant until about 21 wk of gestation when ST fibers with an average area of about 128 μm^2 appeared in cross sections. These ST fibers constituted about 3% of the total fiber population with the remainder still being small, undifferentiated fibers. During the subsequent period of gestation the percent of fibers that could be identified as a specific type increased as did the average cross-sectional area of the fibers. At the time interval of 38 to 42 wk of fetal life, approximately 80% of the fibers could be typed. These fibers averaged about 200 μm^2 in cross-sectional area. At the age of 1 yr the cross-sectional area of the fibers ranged from 500 to 600 μm^2. The cross-sectional areas reported by Colling-Saltin are larger than those observed by Aherne et al. (2). This difference can probably be attributed to the different methods used to prepare the tissue.

Aherne et al. (2) used paraffin embedding as contrasted to the fresh-frozen tissue technique used by Colling-Saltin (123–125). Paraffin embedding produces a significant shrinkage of the tissue during the dehydration procedure. Normally this amounts to about a 20% reduction in area. However, since the water content of fetal muscle is considerably greater (e.g., see *Muscle Size*, p. 579) than that of postnatal muscle, this could also contribute to the variability between the fetal and mature muscles. Cross-sectional areas ranging from about 2,500 to 10,000 μm^2 have been observed in cryostat sections of fresh-frozen adult human limb skeletal muscle (see Table 9). There are a number of other studies where fiber size was determined in muscle of children and adults (67, 74, 75).

In addition to problems associated with methods of fixation, paraffin versus fresh frozen, there are a number of difficulties associated with the assessment of the cross-sectional area of skeletal muscle fibers (183, 326, 637, 662). First is that once removed from the intact muscle there is usually a shortening of the fibers (363). In fresh-frozen sections, sarcomere length averages 2.0 μm (range 1.8–2.2 μm) (320, 520). This contrasts with 2.8 μm in the stretched state (520). Similarly, Holly et al. (359) observed a 25% reduction in the length of a muscle after removal from its skeletal attachments. This results in an overestimate of 33% in the fiber area. Moreover several methods can be applied in the actual determination of the area, which can also influence the results. The method used is

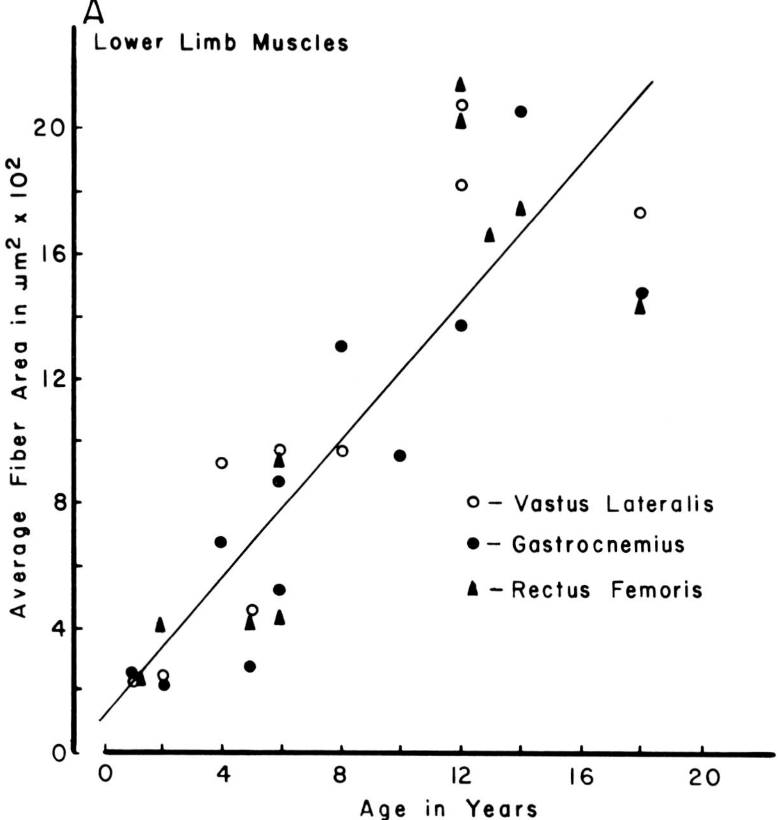

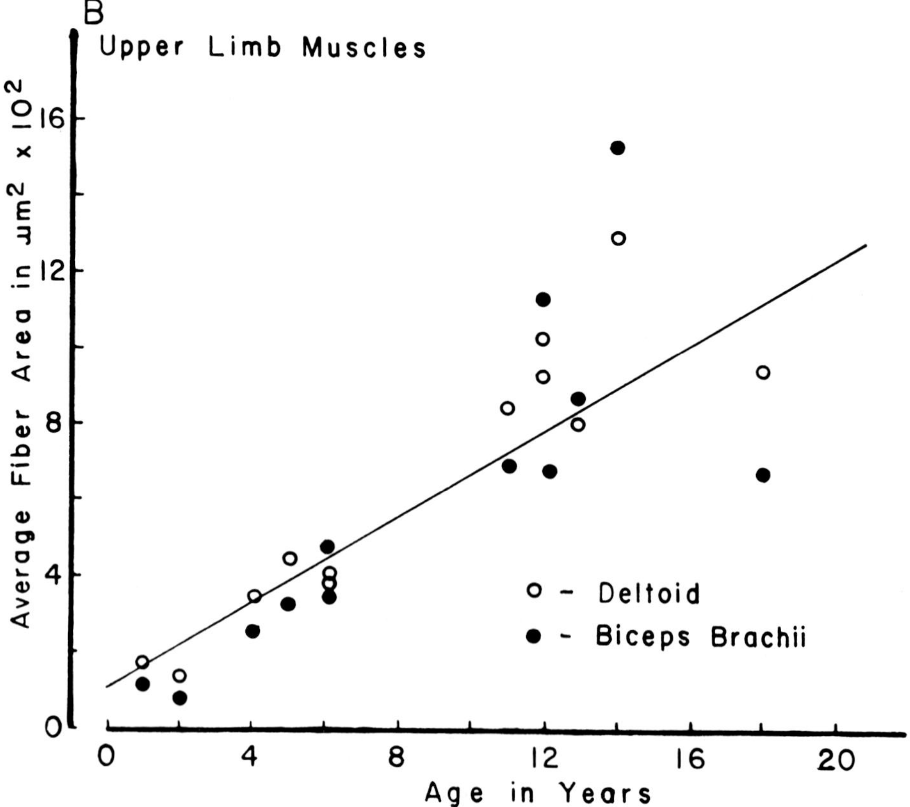

FIG. 16. Data are for muscle from human subjects ranging in age from 2 mo to 18 yr. Fiber areas for infants less than 1 yr are not plotted. *A*: relationship between age and muscle fiber cross-sectional area in the lower limb muscles of humans. Equation of the regression line $y = 115 + 111x$. Between age and fiber area $r = 0.92$; between age and body height $r = 0.98$. *B*: relationship between age and muscle fiber cross-sectional area in the upper limb muscles of humans. Equation of the regression line is $y = 112 + 56x$. Between age and fiber area $r = 0.85$ [Data from Aherne et al. (2).]

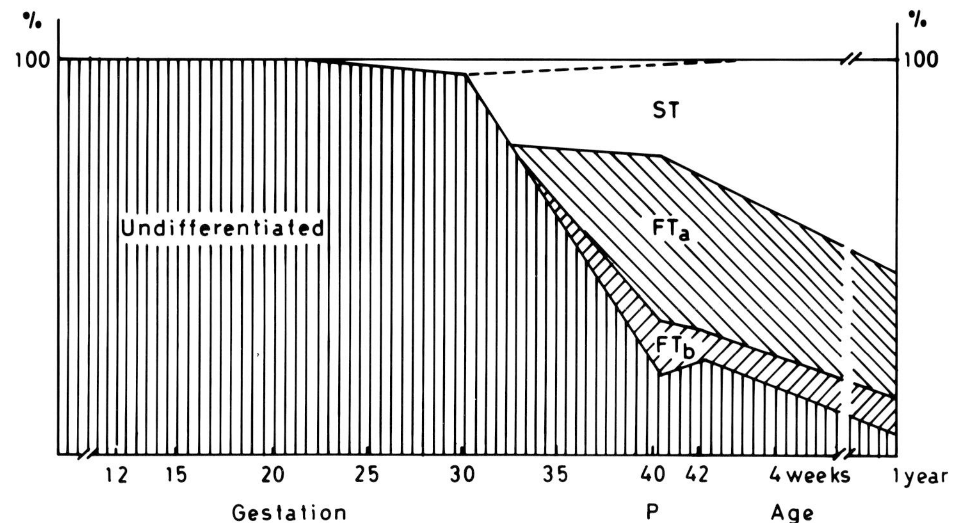

FIG. 17. A summary description of the relative occurrence of various fiber types in human skeletal muscle during gestation and 1st year of life. The slow-twitch (ST) fibers are divided by size with the small fraction of Wohlfart's B fiber above the *dashed line* (725). [Data from Colling-Saltin (123, 125).]

usually one of the following: *1)* direct measurement by planimetry, *2)* analysis by a grid technique (or particle size analysis), and *3)* assessment of the shortest diameter and estimation of cross-sectional area from the assumption that the fibers are circular. The validity of these methods has been discussed by Edström and Torlegård (178), Aniansson et al. (11), and Song et al. (649). Because of its ease of application one of the most frequently used methods for estimating the cross-sectional area of the fibers is measuring the least diameter. The method is valid if the fiber area is circular, which appears to be the case in fetal and infant skeletal muscle. However, with increasing age the fiber areas become less round and the result is a consistent underestimate of the fiber area. This situation is illustrated in Figure 18, where it is evident that as the fibers become larger there is a progressive deviation from the line of identity. This method can be used if an appropriate correction factor is employed.

Postnatal increases in muscle size are closely associated with hypertrophy of the preexisting fibers (e.g., see POSTNATAL DEVELOPMENT, p. 580). Data on the number of fibers in human skeletal muscle come primarily from studies of the sartorius muscle as reported by MacCallum (470) and Montgomery (496). MacCallum made fiber counts from cross sections of five fetuses and one full-term infant and concluded that fiber number was established before birth. Montgomery employed similar methods to estimate the total number of fibers in the sartorius muscle from samples including three stillborn (two fetal and one full-term) infants, two well-nourished infants (4 and 13 mo old), and two adults (64 and 74 yr old) of unspecified sex. The number of fibers appearing in the cross section of the 4-mo-old infant was about twice that observed for the 32-wk-old fetus. There were no major differences in total fiber number with advanced age. Histological examination of the muscle sections in the late stages of fetal life did not reveal any evidence of mitotic activity or of fibers undergoing "longitudinal splitting." On this basis Montgomery concluded that the apparent increase in fiber number of the sartorius muscle of man during later fetal and early postnatal life was the result of a longitudinal fiber growth such that more fibers appeared in the histological cross section. The mechanisms for such a longitudinal and circumferential growth through the addition of sarcomeres on the distal ends of the fibers and myofibrils has been discussed in the chapter by Goldspink in this *Handbook*. The lack of increase in fiber number in the sartorius muscle is in agreement with the observation that there is no evidence of fiber division in the biceps brachialis muscle of man after midgestation. Moreover no myoblasts have been observed in the muscle of human beings after birth, and the number of fibers in the biceps of infants is similar to that of adults (115, 344, 520).

USE AND DISUSE. *Muscular strength.* Heavy-resistance exercise results in increases in muscle bulk in excess of that which occurs during normal growth and development. This is exemplified by the conspicuous musculature of persons who engage in heavy physical labor or in athletic events where heavy-resistance exercise is practiced (body building). The importance of the increase in size in response to functional overloads lies in the fact that the strength of a muscle is closely related to its cross-sectional area (381, 382, 520). This principle is based on the concept that all motor units are maximally activated during MVC (181, 643). Moreover there was little difference in the strength per square centimeter among boys, sedentary males, and highly trained judo athletes (381, 382). This supports the general contention that the capacity of

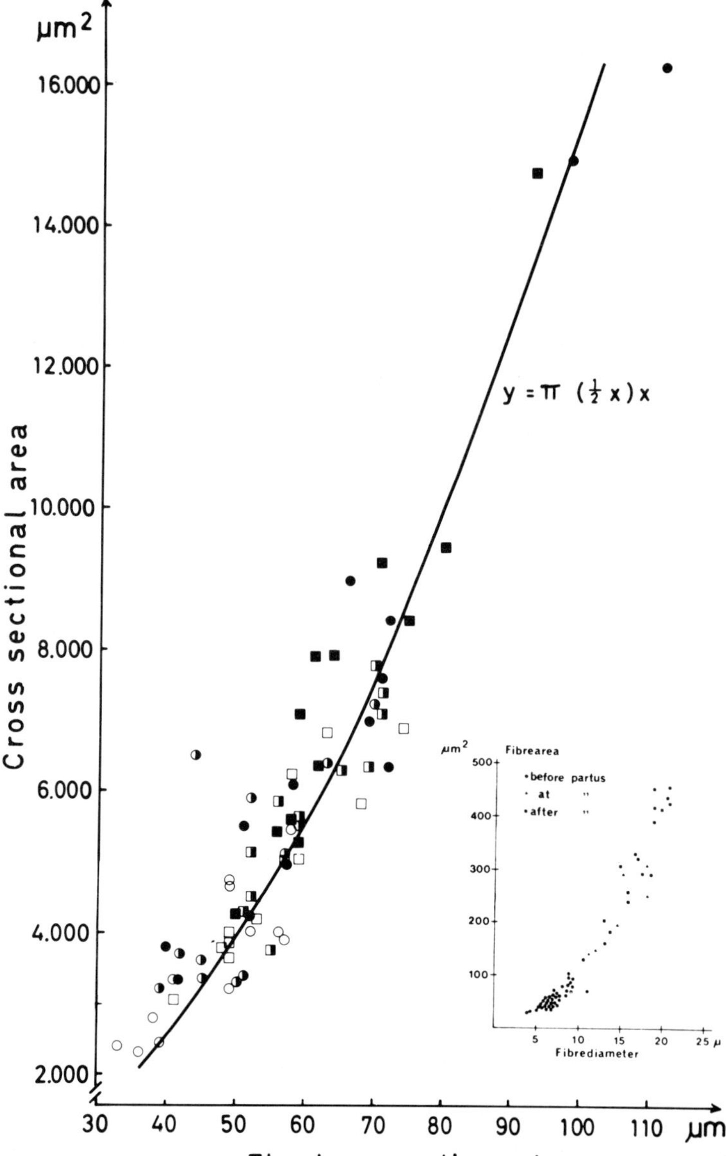

FIG. 18. Relationship between cross-sectional fiber area and lesser diameter in human skeletal muscle during gestation and 1st years of life (*small graph*), and adults (*large graph*). [*Small graph* from Colling-Saltin (123); *large graph* from Sjøgaard (641).]

muscle to develop force per unit of cross-sectional area is constant. If one accepts the concept that all individuals can maximally activate all motor units in a muscle (55), it is difficult to explain the increases in force-developing capacity that occur in the nontrained limbs of individuals who train a contralateral limb or in instances where the training does not produce increases in the cross-sectional area of a muscle (443, 689). Such changes in the force-developing capacity may be a function of the central nervous system rather than of the muscle (493). Moreover isometric training consisting of three maximal contractions sustained for 10 s and separated by 1 min of rest continued for 100 days has been reported to produce a near doubling of the volitional strength of the forearm flexor muscles (399). This increase occurs with only a 23% increase in the cross-sectional area of the muscles. The non-trained arms of these subjects increased in strength by 30% without any change in cross-sectional area of the muscles.

Fiber cross-sectional area. There are several reports in which the cross-sectional area of the fibers in skeletal muscle of weight lifters or those who have engaged in a variety of sports events have been examined (see Table 9). The general conclusion from such studies has been that weight lifters generally have larger fiber areas than sedentary individuals or those who engage in endurance-type activities (261). Edström and Ekblom (175), Costill et al. (129), and MacDougall and co-workers (471, 472) have reported that a period of strength training results in increases in the cross-sectional area of the FT fibers. Thorstensson et al. (689), however, did not observe a similar finding in subjects who had participated in 8 wk of strength training. In the latter study this was true in spite of an increased muscle mass and total body potassium. Muscle mass increased by only 1 kg (2.5%), however, which is probably too little to detect in fiber size if the increase is not confined to only a few muscle groups. Gollnick, Saltin, et al. (260) did observe a selective enlargement of ST fibers after a 6-mo endurance-training program. MacDougall et al. (471, 472) have also examined the effect of weight-lifting activities on the cross-sectional area of the fibers in the triceps muscle of man and found muscle-fiber hypertrophy.

Forced inactivity, for example, after injury, reduces the cross-sectional area of the fibers in skeletal muscle (301, 471, 578). Subjects whose legs are immobilized in fixed casts as a result of radical knee surgery readily demonstrate this phenomenon (299). In these subjects the cross-sectional area of the fibers was similar in the normal and the injured leg prior to surgery. After a 5-wk immobilization there was a 27% decline in the cross-sectional area of the ST fibers of the vastus lateralis muscle. There was, however, no change in the area of FT fibers. Data are also available from subjects whose one leg had been immobilized for 15 wk as a result of fracture (607). Such immobilizations did not alter the composition of the muscle in terms of the percentages of the different fiber types. However, the cross-sectional area of both ST and FT fibers was lower by an average of 47% and 38%, respectively. The reduced FT fiber area after a 15-wk immobilization as opposed to no change after a 5-wk immobilization is probably attributable to the fact that in the latter study the patients were encouraged to perform intensive isometric contractions of the thigh. With such contractions FT fibers are recruited, and this may be an adequate stimulus for maintaining normal size of the FT fibers. This was evident from the relatively large FT fibers in these patients. When such exercise is not performed, the FT fibers also become smaller after a 4- to 6-wk period of inactivity induced by putting a cast on the leg (299).

The effect of physical conditioning on the fiber size of a normal leg and a leg after 6–8 wk of immobilization has also been examined (301). In these experiments computerized tomography was used to establish the total cross section of the thigh muscles. These experiments have firmly established an atrophy of the thigh muscles as a result of chronic immobilization. This atrophy was almost exclusively restricted to the knee extensors, whereas the hamstring muscles were almost unchanged (301). Moreover the relative changes in the knee extensor cross section and fiber size were closely correlated. A similar conclusion was reached by Renström in his study of the knee extensors in below-the-knee amputees (578). In these investigations the total cross-sectional area was reduced by 30% and that of the fibers by 26%.

In animals there is also an increase in fiber area of muscle exposed to overloads (248, 254, 255). With a return to normal physical activity there is a return of fiber size to normal (255).

The nutritional status of the animal can also influence the rate and magnitude of the growth of muscle fibers (250, 251, 309, 321, 424). In one case it was reported that a short period of complete starvation of young (weanling) rats resulted in an approximately 20% loss of fiber number in the skeletal muscles. In starved and refed rats the number of fibers was normal (321). These data are questionable, however, since the changes reported in muscle weight, fiber diameter, and fiber number are such that to accommodate the overall changes there would have had to have been an elongation of the fibers during starvation and a subsequent shortening with refeeding. These data appear to be limited by an accurate determination of total fiber number.

HYPERTROPHY VERSUS HYPERPLASIA. There has been considerable interest over the years in the mechanism(s) by which skeletal muscles increase in size in response to heavy-resistance exercise. The early studies of Morpurgo (500, 501) where increases in muscle weight produced by training did not alter the number of fibers contained in the cross section of the sartorius muscle of the dog (one muscle having been removed before and the other after training) have been the cornerstone of evidence that muscular growth in response to functional overloads occurs by hypertrophy of the fibers and not by hyperplasia. Subsequent studies (624, 655, 685) supported this general concept. There is also general agreement with the concept that normal growth of muscle occurs by hypertrophy of the fibers present in the muscle at birth.

The concept of a postnatal growth of muscle occurring by a combination of longitudinal and circumferential hypertrophy of the preexisting fibers has recently been challenged by reports of larger numbers of fibers in enlarged muscle as compared to control muscle (276, 280, 379, 593, 609, 610, 612, 648, 704, 731). In some cases the suggestion has been made that the increase in fiber number was the result of new fibers formed by a longitudinal division of preexisting fibers (168, 303–305, 573, 593, 612, 648, 668, 701, 704, 731). This suggestion is based in part on the observation that fibers with points of branching or with central cleavages exist in skeletal muscle (172, 280, 390, 573, 612, 614, 622, 668). It should be pointed out that the existence of such fibers in skeletal muscle was reported in 1866 by Eulenberg and Cohnheim (207) and in 1891 by Erb (194). The major impetus for espousing the concept that increases in fiber number occur as a result of fiber division (a so-called fiber splitting) during muscular enlargement produced by functional overload came from the studies of Van Linge (701) and Reitsma (573). These investigators produced muscular enlargement in the hindlimb muscles of the rat by either denervation or surgical ablation of synergistic muscles. In some cases exercise was used in combination with inactivation of a synergist to produce further muscular enlargement. Van Linge (701) observed what were considered to be new fibers in histological sections of the overloaded, enlarged muscles. These "new fibers" were described as small fibers interspersed among normal-sized fibers. It was suggested that these represented "young muscle fibers, the growth of which was stimulated by strenuous training." Technical difficulties were cited by Van Linge as making it impossible to count all of the fibers in the muscle from histological cross sections. Subsequently Reitsma (573) reported the existence of similar small fibers in histological cross section of experimentally enlarged muscle. Moreover when enlarged muscles were digested in nitric acid and fibers teased free, some fibers with branches and appendages of varying length were isolated. The presence of such fibers was interpreted as evidence that a longitudinal splitting of the fibers was occurring. Unfortunately the total number of fibers in the muscles was not determined nor was the frequency of the branched fibers established.

Little is known about the number of fibers in human skeletal muscle. Etemadi and Hosseini (205) reported that the number of fibers in the human biceps brachii muscle was larger in an athletic subject (316,243 fibers) as compared to two sedentary individuals (227,233 and 199,240 fibers). Of these subjects, the one with well-developed musculature also had the greater fiber diameter (45.25 μm as compared to about 23 μm for the sedentary individuals). The difference in fiber size is similar between large and small breeds of dogs (413).

The total number of fibers in the human biceps has been estimated from measurements of the total cross-sectional area of the muscle determined by computerized tomography and the area of the individual fibers determined from biopsy samples (519, 521), assuming that the majority of the fibers extend through the whole muscle (623). In sedentary male and female subjects the cross-sectional area of the muscle averaged 11.6 cm^2 (range: 9.8–16.1) and 8.7 cm^2 (6.8–10.6), respectively. These values were 12.3 cm^2 (11.9–12.9) and 9.0 cm^2 (7.7–9.7) for trained male and female swimmers. The total number of fibers in the biceps averaged 280,000 (280,000–290,000) and 420,000 (340,000–500,000) for the sedentary female and male subjects as compared to 320,000 (240,000–380,000) and 350,000 (280,000–400,000) for the trained female and male subjects. These data demonstrate the existence of considerable variation between the fiber number of subjects and considerable overlap between the sexes and the sedentary and trained groups. There is no evidence of a systematic difference between the sedentary and the trained groups, the greater total cross-sectional area of the muscle being attributable to the larger cross-sectional area of the individual fibers.

A greater number of fibers in the cross section of the anterior latissimus dorsi muscle has also been reported for chicken where enlargement was produced by hanging a weight on one wing (648). However, in another study the increased cross-sectional area of the fibers in the enlarged muscles of the shoulder of chicken, where growth was induced by a chronic stretch, could account for the observed greater muscle weight (359).

Schiaffino et al. (612) surgically removed the tibialis anterior muscle of 1- to 65-day-old rats. At time intervals ranging from 4 to 76 wk postsurgery, the remaining extensor digitorum longus muscles were on an average 32% heavier, and cross sections contained 25% more fibers than the contralateral control muscles. The presence of fibers with branches in those teased from nitric acid–treated muscles was used as evidence for proliferation of fibers via splitting.

Ianuzzo, Gollnick, et al. (379) reported the existence of 30% more fibers in the cross sections of the plantaris muscle of rats where a doubling of its weight was induced by the surgical removal of the gastrocnemius muscle. The cross-sectional areas of the major fiber types in the muscles had increased from 30% to 60%. In this study there was no change in the fiber number in the soleus muscle in spite of a 45% increase in its weight. No evidence of fiber branching was observed from the histological observation of the sections used to determine fiber numbers.

Gonyea and associates (276, 279, 280) trained cats to perform a weight-lifting type of activity to produce muscular enlargement. This experimental procedure was claimed to be a more physiological method for producing muscular growth than the denervation or surgical removal of synergistic muscle. Differences in weight of from 6% to 16% between the flexor carpi radialis muscles of the control and experimental legs were produced by this procedure. The enlarged muscles were reported to contain an average of up to 20% more muscle fibers, and the average fiber diameters were 9%–15% larger than those of the contralateral control muscles. Fiber number was assessed from a histological cross section made at the point of greatest girth of muscle belly. The identification of fibers in serial sections with branch points was cited as evidence of fiber splitting. However, there was no evidence of the frequency of this phenomenon. To produce a 20% increase it would have had to occur in every fifth fiber. Even if one accounts for the time it takes to induce the change, split fibers would have to occur at a very high rate.

The number of fibers in the plantaris muscle has been reported to decline between the ages of 6 and 45 wk in sedentary but not in trained guinea pigs (213, 214). Termination of training resulted in a progressive loss of fibers. This suggested that a normal attrition of fibers occurs, which could be prevented by physical activity. In a subsequent paper (481), however, a mathematical model, based on changes in fiber angles with growth, was described to demonstrate that the determination of fiber number from counts made of histological cross sections was invalid for penniform muscles. On this basis it was suggested that the earlier data were in error.

The tedious nature of isolating all of the fibers of a muscle has deterred the application of this method to the study of normal growth and development and of hypertrophy versus hyperplasia during work-induced muscular enlargement. Gollnick and co-workers (275) dissected, counted, and examined each fiber over its entire length for bifurcations. In these studies there was no change in fiber number in enlarged as compared to control skeletal muscle in the rat. Muscular enlargement ranging from 10% to 115% was induced in the penniform plantaris and extensor digitorum longus and in the parallel-fibered soleus muscle by surgical ablation of a synergist and treadmill exercise. Muscles were examined from 4 to 40 wk after the ablation of the synergistic muscle. Treadmill running was for 6–8 wk and was initiated at least 4 wk (18, 378) after the surgical removal of the synergistic muscle. Although considerable variation in the number of fibers per muscle existed among animals, the total fiber number in the same muscle from the right and left leg was similar regardless of whether it was normal or enlarged (Fig. 19). It should be pointed out that considerable variation exists among animals for the total number of fibers for the same muscle (Fig. 20). The differences in dry weight of individual fibers of the enlarged muscle as compared to those from the normal muscle demonstrated that the increase in weight was the result of hypertrophy and not hyperplasia. The incidence of branched fibers was similar for normal and enlarged muscles. However, the observation that points of branching can occur anywhere along the length of the fiber illustrates the technical difficulty of using histological cross sections to evaluate its frequency (275, 303–305, 573, 612). The appearance of branched fibers in all muscles was interpreted as an indication that these abnormal fibers are normally present in small percentages and do not represent an active process of a longitudinal division of fibers.

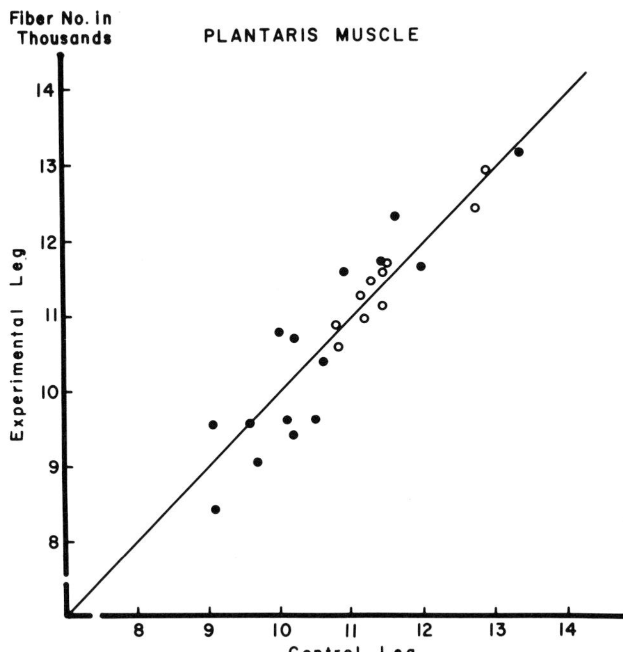

FIG. 19. Comparison of the number of fibers in a control and enlarged plantaris muscle of the rat. Muscular enlargement was induced either by ablation of the gastrocnemius muscle (●) or a combination of ablation of the gastrocnemius muscle and treadmill exercise (○). [From Gollnick et al. (275).]

The finding of Gollnick et al. (275) supports the older concept that the number of fibers in skeletal muscle is established early in life (188, 470, 496, 624, 712) and that the exceptional enlargement that occurs in response to a variety of overloads is a true hypertrophy. This supports the conclusion of Hall-Craggs and co-workers (303–305) and of James (394) that if a splitting of fibers in skeletal muscle does occur during enlargement, it is of minimal importance in the overall increase in muscular size. Moreover James concluded from the changes in fiber cross-sectional area during hypertrophy of the mouse extensor digitorum longus muscle that a hypoplasia of fibers must have occurred (395).

There are reports of increases in the DNA content of skeletal muscle during normal growth and work-induced hypertrophy (307, 368, 499). This could be interpreted as an indication of the addition of new fibers. However, the bulk of the increase in DNA arises from the addition of connective tissue to support enlarged fibers (18, 393). Part of the increase in DNA is associated with a proliferation of the satellite cells of muscle (3, 502, 503, 610, 611, 615, 616, 628). Some of these are apparently incorporated into the existing muscle fibers. This has been proposed as a mechanism whereby the ratio of nuclear material to other cellular components is maintained at a constant level within the cell. Of some interest is the observation that blocking DNA synthesis does not stop the hypertrophy of muscle fibers in the rat soleus muscle after tenotomy of the synergists (225). This did completely inhibit connective tissue proliferation: an almost complete lack of new nuclei was observed in histological sections.

Since there has been a rather wide acceptance of the concept that the total number of fibers in skeletal muscle can increase with work-induced growth, it seems appropriate to comment on the methodology that was used to arrive at this conclusion. Basically there are three methods that are used to determine total fiber number in skeletal muscle. These are: *1*) counting all fibers that appear in a cross-sectional cut of the muscle; *2*) counting the fibers in a given cross-sectional area cut and then estimating total fiber number by an extrapolation to the total area of the section; and *3*) making a cross-sectional cut, dispersing the fibers in saline, and counting the fragments with an electronic device (684). All methods appear valid for estimating the total number of fibers in the cross

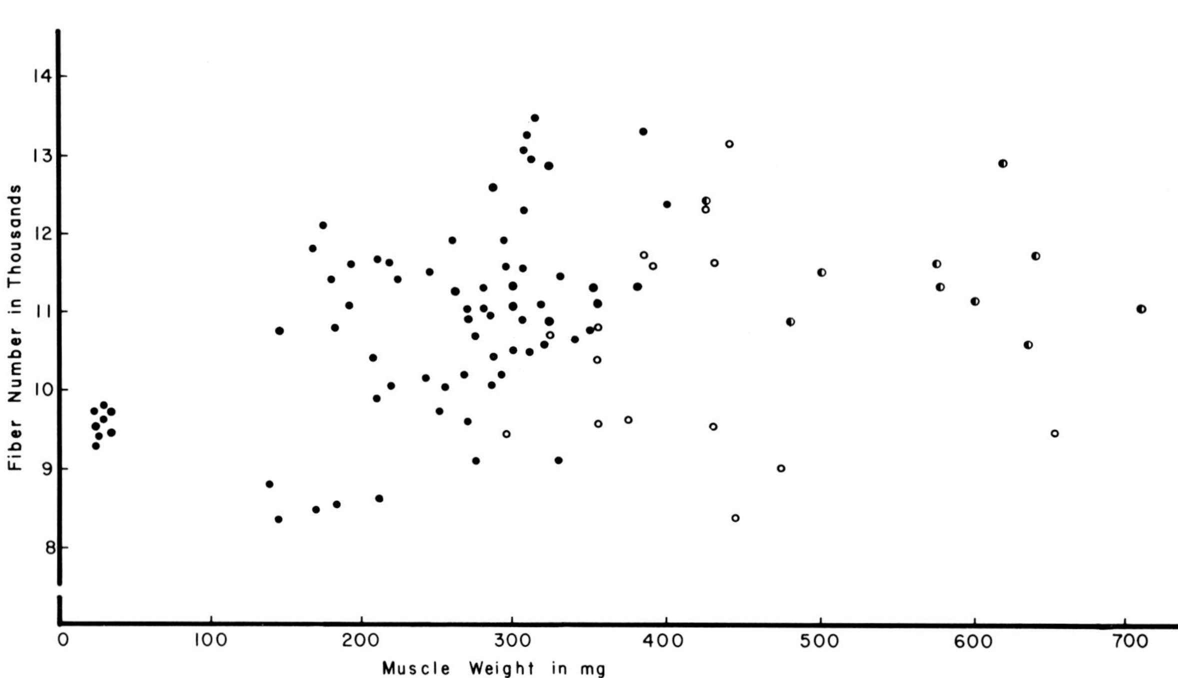

FIG. 20. A plot of the number of fibers vs. total wet weight for the plantaris muscles. ●, Control muscles (including normal weanling, sham-operated, thyroidectomized, and control muscles from experimental animals); ○, muscles enlarged by ablation of the gastrocnemius muscle; and ◐, muscles enlarged by ablation of the gastrocnemius muscle and exercise. The smallest muscle weighed 25 mg and the heaviest 712 mg. [From Gollnick et al. (275).]

section of muscle. However, these methods assume that all of the fibers in a muscle are either contained in the cross section or that changes in the number of fibers contained in the single section are representative of any change in the entire muscle. These assumptions appear to be tenable only when the fibers lie parallel to the long axis of the muscle and traverse the point where the cross section is made. This, however, is not the case for muscles where the fiber arrangement is penniform. The problem with determining the total fiber number in muscles with pennate fiber arrangement has been discussed by Clark (117) and alluded to by others (478, 490, 571, 704). In muscles with a single pennate fiber arrangement all fibers could be included in carefully spaced, multiple cross-sectional cuts. With multipennate fiber arrangements the problem is greatly compounded. It cannot be assumed that a cross-sectional cut made through the same point of the muscle, for example, the point of greatest girth, includes the same number of fibers of a normal versus an enlarged muscle since this depends on the angle that the fibers form with the longitudinal axis of the muscle (275). This fiber angle is known to change during muscular enlargement (57, 309, 490). A change in fiber angle in the mature animal is necessary to accommodate the larger fiber diameter without any change in the total length of the muscle. Since increases in fiber number with work-induced growth have been reported primarily for muscle with penniform fiber arrangements where fiber number was determined from histological cross sections, these data are open to doubt. Also the estimation of the size of the fibers depends on the ability to section the muscle perpendicular to the long axis of the fibers. When the cuts are made at a tangent to the long axis of the fiber the area and diameter will be overestimated.

The difficulty in determining the fiber number in a muscle with a multipennate fiber arrangement is illustrated from the studies of Gollnick and associates (275) and of Gonyea et al. (276, 280). Gonyea et al. reported that the flexor carpi radialis muscle of the cat contained about 7,500 fibers as estimated from a cross section made at the point of greatest girth. When this muscle was treated in a manner that permitted isolation of each fiber it was found to contain about 28,000 fibers (275). Similarly, Schiaffino et al. (612) estimated the number of fibers from cross sections of the extensor digitorum longus to be about 3,400. When counted directly this muscle, with a single pennate fiber arrangement, was found to contain about 5,200 fibers.

SUMMARY. From birth to full maturity there is an increase in muscle weight of from 100- to 200-fold in the skeletal muscle of most mammals. This increased muscle size is the result of a longitudinal growth produced by the addition of sarcomeres to the ends of the existing muscle fibers and by circumferential growth produced by the addition of myofibrils. During the growth process the total number of nuclei increases such that the ratio between cellular material and nuclei remains rather constant. With added physical demands, such as heavy manual labor or weight lifting, there is an additional increase in muscle mass. This increased muscle mass is produced by further increases in total cross-sectional area of the individual fibers and not by the addition of more muscle fibers. With disuse or with inadequate nutrition there is a loss of muscle mass as a result of a decrease in cross-sectional area.

Metabolic Capacity

POSTNATAL DEVELOPMENT. The skeletal muscle of the newborn contains substrate concentrations and enzyme activities that are only slightly below those found in later life when these are expressed per unit dry weight (124). This could be interpreted as indicating that parallel increases occur in all muscular components with postnatal maturation. However, with growth there is a continued differentiation of the fiber types that necessitates a preferential synthesis of either mitochondrial, cytoplasmic, or myofibrillar proteins depending on the type of fiber that develops. This is illustrated by the observation that at birth histochemical staining for NADH-tetrazolium reductase and α-glycerophosphate dehydrogenase (αGPDH) does not discriminate between fiber types (714). In the skeletal muscle of adults these histochemical procedures identify major differences in the metabolic profiles of the fibers (35, 540). Based on dry weight measure the increase in end-terminal oxidation enzymes of the mitochondria does not parallel that of the contractile proteins in all fibers (627). This has been illustrated in mixed-fiber skeletal muscle where the checkerboard appearance of the muscle only appears with maturation (249, 253, 524, 695). The loss of mitochondrial density in the FT_b fibers appears to be a function of a preferential production of myofibrillar proteins. This growth effect can be modified by endurance training (4).

How this differential growth is regulated is unknown. Since it is the rule rather than the exception, different stimuli and regulatory mechanisms must be present for the increases in contractile proteins and metabolic enzymes. Evidence suggests that this is regulated, at least in part, by the motor nerve (83, 323, 334, 371, 465, 525–527, 544, 551, 567).

USE AND DISUSE. *Phosphagen stores.* There are reports of increases and of no change in the ATP and CP concentrations of human skeletal muscle with either endurance or strength training (195, 415, 418, 472). Increases in both ATP and CP concentrations have been reported in the limb muscles of adolescent (195) and adult (415, 418) males after programs of endurance training. However, when the training was extended from 3 to 6 mo in the adult group, the ATP and CP concentrations returned to the pretraining level. Only a few studies are available dealing with the effects of immobilization or termination of training on the phosphagen stores of muscle. Studies with animals suggest that although there may be increases in the phosphagen stores after training (228, 534), these modifications are small and probably biologically unimportant. Further proof that changes in the immediately available energy stores of ATP and CP are not important features of adaptation to training comes from observations of elite athletes. In these individuals, whether they have trained for strength development or for endurance, the ATP and CP concentrations in the muscles do not differ more than a few moles per kilogram wet weight (~10%) from that of sedentary individuals. Attempts have been made to determine whether differences exist between the ST and FT fibers (375). In these studies the ATP and CP concentrations were found to be slightly higher in the ST as compared to FT fibers in the muscle of female athletes competing in endurance events (312).

Glycogen. In the first studies on the glycogen stores of human skeletal muscle where the influence of exercise was examined, it was noted that higher values existed in trained than in sedentary individuals (341). Thereafter several studies, both longitudinal and cross-sectional, demonstrated that subjects undergoing strength-, sprint-, or endurance-training programs possessed larger muscle glycogen stores (260, 373, 418, 472), although in some instances the difference between the trained and sedentary state was small. Conversely immobilization or detraining results in a reduction in the glycogen concentration of skeletal muscle (299). The changes observed with activity and inactivity are, however, well within the more dramatic variation in the glycogen concentration of skeletal muscle that can be induced with dietary manipulations with or without exercise (51, 271, 396, 397, 560). The one-leg model, that is where one leg is trained and the other left untrained, has been useful to assess objectively the quantitative effect of exercise, divorced from either dietary or hormonal influences, on muscle glycogen stores. At least three (333, 559, 603) such studies are available where the vastus lateralis muscle of a control and an endurance-trained leg was examined. In these studies the glycogen concentration of the trained leg was from 6 to 60 mmol/kg wet wt higher than that of the untrained leg. An alternative approach to this problem has been to examine the glycogen content in the arm and leg muscles of individuals whose training is primarily with either the arms or the legs, for example, bicyclists, canoeists, and swimmers. Such studies have revealed that the muscle glycogen content is higher in the trained than in the control muscles with differences varying from 20 to 101 mmol/kg wet wt. Training increases glycogen synthase activity (95, 365, 366, 497, 559, 624, 675, 682). When activities of hexokinase and glycogen synthase were also compared in the two legs where only one leg was trained (559), both enzymes were found to be increased in the trained leg with the relative increments being about 30%–50%. The muscle glycogen concentrations in these studies were also increased from 38 to 50 mmol/kg wet wt. These differences represented relative increases of 47%–100%.

Although results vary, endurance training appears to increase the glycogen stores of rat skeletal muscle (25, 268, 273, 672). The magnitude of the increases varies from about 25% to 70%. There are, however, reports of no difference in the glycogen concentration of skeletal muscle of trained as compared with sedentary rats (674). Moreover this increase in glycogen appears to be localized, occurring in some muscles but not others after endurance training (25, 268, 672). This cannot be attributed to a specific use of the gastrocnemius muscle since swimming results in a large reduction in the glycogen content of all hindlimb muscles (572, 679). Sprint training has no effect on the glycogen concentration of any of the fiber types found in rat hindlimb muscle (608).

Triglyceride stores. Few studies have measured the triglyceride concentration in human skeletal muscle, and of these, only three were longitudinal with measurements made on the same subjects before and after training (104, 333, 498). Quantitative morphometric techniques applied to electron micrographs have demonstrated that the lipid content in muscles of sedentary man varies between 0.1 and 0.6 vol% depending on the muscle examined (364, 422, 423). In muscle from trained subjects the range for the same muscles was from 0.2–0.8 vol%. Strength and endurance training altered the triglyceride content of muscle. Morgan et al. (497, 498) and Bylund-Fellenius et al. (104) observed elevation in the triglyceride content of the quadriceps muscle after endurance training. The increase was about 50% from an initial value of approximately 10 μmol/g wet wt. Of special interest, however, are results from a study where subjects trained only one leg thereby permitting comparison with the nontrained leg to obviate the effects of diet. In this instance there was no difference in triglyceride content of the muscles of the two legs (333). Variations in the percent of lipid in the diet is a major factor contributing to the fluctuation in the triglyceride stores of skeletal muscle (396). Jansson and Sylvén (396, 400) found that after 5 days of consuming a fat-enriched diet (70% fat, 5% protein, 8 mJ/day), the triglyceride content of the quadriceps was 22 μmol/g wet wt, and the same after consumption of a low-fat diet (10% fat, 20% protein, 8 mJ/day). The problem of whether physical training has a significant effect on the muscle triglyceride content can also be examined from cross-sectional studies. When data from several studies in which the same methods were used are pooled, there is a slight tendency for higher muscle triglyceride stores in the most highly trained individuals (B. Essén, personal communication). The variation is, however, large. Thus factors other than physical activity may dominate in determining the triglyceride content of skeletal muscle. There are reports of a decline in the triglyceride content of skeletal muscle of man with exercise (234).

The triglyceride content of both the red and white portion of the gastrocnemius muscle of the rat has been reported to be reduced by training (232, 235). Data are also available, however, suggesting that endurance exercise does (231, 232, 282, 572, 658) and does not alter (27, 282, 658) the triglyceride stores in the different skeletal muscle fiber types in the rat.

Glycolytic enzymes. The number of longitudinal training studies focusing on changes in the activities of glycolytic enzymes in human skeletal muscle is limited. When these studies are divided into reports concentrating on improving strength, speed (sprinting), or endurance capacity, only one, or at the most two, reports are available in each area. Although this is the case, the adaptive response of the glycolytic enzymes in skeletal muscle to varying patterns of increased use is rather clear. Training regimens designed to increase maximal strength have not produced alterations in the activities of PHOS, PFK, or LDH (129, 443). This is true both for dynamic and static exercise. The response of muscle appears to be related to the total duration of the exercise. Thus no changes were noted in muscle when the resistance was so high that the total number of repetitions to exhaustion was completed in 6 s (129). When the resistance was lowered and the exercise extended to 30 s, however, there was a 10%–20% elevation in PHOS and PFK activities but LDH was unchanged. A high-intensity endurance training did produce an increase in PFK activity (195, 260). Hexokinase also has been reported to be elevated with training (497).

Further information concerning the adaptive response of the glycolytic system comes from cross-sectional studies of athletes competing in typical strength and sprint-type events. Shot-putters, weight lifters, and discus throwers have PHOS, PFK, and LDH activities well within the range of sedentary subjects (130, 261), whereas sprinters, jumpers, and runners (400–800 m) usually have elevated levels of these enzymes (130).

The influence of sprint and endurance training on total LDH activity and on the isozymes of LDH has been examined (638, 639). Cross-sectional comparisons were also made between weight lifters and endurance athletes (419, 638, 683, 688, 689). Total LDH activity was not altered by sprint training. These results and also the report of high values in the muscles of weight lifters (419, 638) contrast to some mentioned above. It has been found that the muscle of sprint-trained individuals contains a relatively high percent of LDH_{4-5}, whereas muscle from endurance-trained individuals is especially high in LDH_{1-2} (638). Part of the explanation for the differences between athletic groups may lie in the fiber composition of the muscle. Thus it is known that ST fibers show not only lower LDH activities but also have high percentages of LDH_{1-2} (638,

683). The type and cellular location of the LDH is also different for the fiber types and could be an important factor in their function (210, 211, 259, 416, 542, 702). Clearly in future studies where adaptations of LDH are investigated, close attention must be given to the nature of the muscle sample that is analyzed.

How varying types and intensities of physical activity influence the activities of enzymes of the Embden-Meyerhof pathway in rat skeletal muscle has been described in numerous reports (see ref. 265). There appear to be two major problems with many of these investigations: *1*) the exercise used for training was often of insufficient intensity to place significant demands on this system, and *2*) in many cases the enzymes assayed were not those generally considered to be rate limiting or regulatory. The earliest of these used rather short periods of swimming as the mode of exercise. The general finding was that this mild exercise stress did not elicit any change in the activities of PHOS, LDH, or aldolase (ALD) in the rat hindlimb muscles (264, 279, 283, 316, 318, 357). An exception was the early report of an increased LDH activity in rat muscle after a program of swimming 1 min the first day and increasing the duration of the swim 1 min per day for 30 days (729, 730).

More strenuous programs of treadmill running (up to 2 h) have been used to train rats. These have used speeds up to 31 m/min and in some cases have included periodic sprints at 42 m/min (353). Increases in PFK, pyruvate kinase (PK), triosephosphatase dehydrogenase (TPDH), and αGPDH of the soleus muscle and decreases in these enzymes as well as PHOS have been reported in the red portion of the quadriceps muscle after such training programs (29). The activities of these enzymes were unchanged in the white portion of the quadriceps. In the soleus, LDH activity was unchanged, but it was lower in both the red and white portions of the quadriceps muscle. The effect of sprint training on the activities of select glycolytic enzymes has been reported (345, 608, 659). These studies employed treadmill running with speeds up to 99 m/min. In one study (659) the exercise was 45-s bouts of running—two bouts in the morning and two in the afternoon. At the end of a 3-wk training program the running speed was 80 m/min. With the exception of an increase in TPDH in the soleus muscle, there were no differences in PHOS, TPDH, and LDH activities in the soleus and rectus femoris muscles 24 h after the final exercise session. In a second experiment, training consisted of 18 alternate periods of 30 s of exercise and 30 s of rest (608). The training program covered 11 wk with the final running speed of 80 m/min attained during the 11th week. Activities of PHOS, PFK, and PK were unchanged in fast-twitch muscle (both red and white), whereas for the slow-twitch soleus PHOS and PK activities were higher by 70% and 35%, respectively.

An exercise program of 10 s of running (speeds up to 99 m/min) with 45 s of rest between bouts has also been used to study high-intensity training (345). One bout consisted of six sprints, which were repeated eight times with 2.5-min rest periods between bouts. An endurance program of running 12.5 min at 35 m/min was also studied. Activities of phosphoglucomutase (PGM), LDH, and phosphoglucoisomerase (PGI) were determined in the soleus, plantaris, and white portion of the gastrocnemius muscle after 8–16 wk of training. Small but statistically significant reductions in the LDH activities of the soleus and white portion of the gastrocnemius muscles were reported after 8 wk of sprint training. The activity of PGI was higher in the plantaris but lower in the white gastrocnemius muscles, whereas LDH and PGM were both lower in the soleus muscle after endurance training. After 16 wk of training, LDH activity was lower in the soleus and white portion of the gastrocnemius muscle of the endurance-trained group, whereas PGM was lower in all muscles. In the soleus muscle of sprint-trained animals, PGM activity was lower. Overall the magnitude of these changes was small but statistically significant.

Of the enzymes normally considered glycolytic, hexokinase activity increases with endurance and sprint training, as observed in rats (29, 659) and guinea pigs (38, 541). This increased activity appears to be related to changes in oxidative capacity of the muscle (29, 41, 137). Even in sedentary animals the highest activities are found in the most oxidative enzymes. Hexokinase activity is also many times lower than that of other enzymes in the Embden-Meyerhof pathway. It responds rapidly, increasing shortly after the onset of training and decreasing as quickly after termination of a training program (38). Since hexokinase is more involved with glucose transport across the cell membrane than in glycolysis, it cannot be considered to be a glycolytic enzyme in the traditional sense. Modifications in its activity appear to facilitate the uptake and oxidation of glucose from the blood.

Two points should be considered when evaluating the results of the experiments with rats. First, was the exercise severe enough to stress the glycolytic pathway? Second, were the results influenced by the time at which the tissue samples were obtained after the final training session? In the early experiments rats were exercised by swimming. The oxygen uptake of the rat during swimming is about 4.6 $ml \cdot 100\ g^{-1} \cdot min^{-1}$ (19, 23, 484). This corresponds to less than 50% of $\dot{V}O_{2\,max}$ for the rat (44, 78, 142, 629). This is below the exercise intensity that usually elicits an increase in the lactate concentration in the blood of man. The lack of an increase in blood lactate of swimming rats supports the contention that this is a mild metabolic stress (257, 274). The rate of glycogen depletion and the increase in blood lactate that occur in the rat are functions of exercise intensity (19, 288). At running speeds below 22 m/min the lactate concentration of the blood is about 3 mM and glycogen breakdown averages about 1.5 $mmol \cdot kg^{-1} \cdot min^{-1}$. At running speeds above about 25 m/min there is a sharp rise in the lactate in the blood with a maximum of about 20 mM having been observed at running speeds of about 70 m/min. At this point the rate of glycogen depletion was 20 $mmol \cdot kg^{-1} \cdot min^{-1}$. These data support the contention that for the high-intensity exercise used in the sprint studies there is a significant substrate flux via the glycolytic pathway. With regard to the time of obtaining the tissue samples after the final exercise session, this varies from 1 to 3 days. This is an important consideration since the turnover rate of the glycolytic enzymes lies between about one-half hour and a few days (154, 383, 544). An example of the importance of this is illustrated by the observation that a period of prolonged exercise can increase the PFK activity of rat skeletal muscle (61). Since rats have usually been studied from 1 to 3 days after the last exercise session, it is possible that the training effect may have been totally or partially missed. Moreover athletes are not usually studied at the point of peak performance, and in training studies with man the muscle samples may be obtained one to several days after completion of the exercise. Because of these differing experimental protocols, the true extent of the adaptability of these enzymes in response to physical activity may not be fully understood.

Immobilization of the leg for from 1 to 6 wk did not produce any change in PFK activity (299). A similar lack of change was observed with detraining (367). In the latter study PFK activity was similar to that of sedentary subjects in the control phase for these groups. Inactivity produced by denervation of rat skeletal muscle results in a decline in the PK, ALD, and LDH activities of the gastrocnemius muscle (316, 350) that is evident as early as 7 days after nerve section. Thereafter a progressive decline in enzyme activities occurred until 8 wk after denervation if activities were only 25%–38% of those of the control animals (350). There were, however, no changes in the activities of PK and ALD of the soleus muscle over the same period of time, whereas LDH had declined by 57%. There were also major histochemical changes (589). These data support the concept that a differential response to forced inactivity exists for the different fiber types.

At first inspection there are conflicting reports of the adaptive response of the glycolytic capacity of skeletal muscle to endurance training. Several reports show no effect, whereas others observed substantial increases. This apparent disparity may be due, at least in part, to variations in the training protocols employed. In studies where elevations in $\dot{V}O_{2\,max}$ were induced by continuous strenuous but not maximal exercise, glycolytic enzyme activities were unaltered (337). In contrast, in those experiments (196, 260) where 50%–115% increases in PFK activities were observed, the exercise was performed at or very close to $\dot{V}O_{2\,max}$. This probably resulted in a high demand for pyruvate formation throughout the exercise. Likewise for sprint exercise an increased demand on glycolysis appears to cause adaptive changes in the glycolytic pathways. In the study where the largest increase in PFK was observed after endurance training, histochemical staining of tissue samples for αGPDH demonstrated an increased staining intensity of the FT fibers with no apparent change in the ST fibers (260). Chronic electrical stimulation of animal muscle via the nerve has also been shown to alter the glycolytic capacity of skeletal muscle (323, 550, 553). In contrast, quantitative biochemical methods have failed to reveal any differences in the total PFK activity or in that of the individual muscle fiber types after endurance training in the rat (29, 337). Clearly further investigations regarding the adaptability of the glycolytic pathway to varying types of training are needed.

Mitochondrial enzymes. Though it has been known for a long time that the capacity of muscle to consume oxygen was related to the level of activity of the citric acid cycle and electron-transport system, studies of adaptations in the mitochondrial enzymes of human skeletal muscle were not undertaken until the late 1960s and early 1970s. At that time results over a period of time from cross-sectional studies of men and women performing physical activity of an endurance type were published (6, 7, 10, 48, 103, 104, 130, 132, 175, 195, 260, 261, 360, 364, 389, 398, 419, 422, 423, 529–531, 559, 565, 566, 602–604, 639, 664, 703, 705). Cytochrome oxidase (CYTOX) and SDH activities were found to be elevated in the trained skeletal muscle.

Exercise designed to develop strength does not alter the activities of the mitochondrial enzymes (129, 261, 471). When this type of exercise is practiced over a long time, it leads to a disproportionate proliferation of the contractile proteins, resulting in a dilution of the mitochondrial concentration in the muscle fiber, and the activities of the enzymes expressed per unit of muscle become lower than those of muscle from sedentary individuals (261, 471). This situation is analogous to the growth dilution that occurs during the early development in animals (249, 253).

Sprint training, in contrast to high-resistance training, causes a definite adaptive response with significant elevation of the mitochondrial enzymes (603). When performed intermittently, thereby placing a severe stress on oxygen utilization, isometric strength training also induces increases in mitochondrial enzymes (291). Thus it appears that the concentration of mitochondrial enzymes is increased whenever there is a chronic demand for a high-oxygen consumption by the muscle. In line with this is the finding that the largest increases in these enzymes occur after typical endurance-training programs (260, 603). It appears to make little difference whether the exercise is performed intermittently or continuously, although changes at the level of the individual fiber may be affected (337). Other evidence for differences in the concentration of oxidative enzymes based on the relative use of a muscle can be obtained from sedentary individuals where the activities of the oxidative enzymes for end-terminal oxidation are higher in the leg than the arm muscles in spite of a similar fiber-type distribution (261). The muscles of the legs are presumably used more in endurance activity than those of the arms.

The time course for the change in oxidative enzyme activities and the concomitant change in whole-body $\dot{V}O_{2\,max}$ (Fig. 21) suggests that there is a close relationship of these variables over the first 3–4 wk of training (6). Thereafter the increase in $\dot{V}O_{2\,max}$ levels off, but the activity of the mitochondrial enzymes continues to rise. This disparity in the response of the $\dot{V}O_{2\,max}$ and mitochondrial enzyme activities is further illustrated by comparisons of endurance athletes and sedentary individuals. The $\dot{V}O_{2\,max}$ of the athletes may be twice that of the control subjects, whereas the activity of the mitochondrial enzymes of the muscle is 3- to 4-fold higher than those of the sedentary individuals (605). As pointed out earlier, the adaptive response in enzyme activity is local in nature. Competitive cyclists and endurance runners have higher activity levels for the mitochondrial enzymes in their legs than sedentary individuals. Canoeists resemble sedentary people in their leg muscles but have elevated enzyme concentrations in arm muscles (261). Moreover training one limb induces changes in the muscle of that limb but not in the muscle of the contralateral untrained limb (Fig. 22).

The enzymes in the various metabolic pathways of the muscle cell are found in a rather constant ratio one to another (543, 546–549). The question arises as to whether this constant proportionality is retained when adaptations occur in response to increased muscular usage. This relationship does not appear to be disturbed in rabbit skeletal muscle in response to either normal physical activity, inactivity, or to chronic electrical stimulation (551, 553). Comparisons of enzyme activities for terminal oxidation in the hindlimb muscles of sedentary and trained rats also support this concept (142). Note, however, the finding of a slightly smaller increase in mitochondrial protein than that observed for the citric acid cycle or respiratory-chain enzymes (353–355, 495, 532). This may be due to the fact that some mitochondrial enzymes are unchanged with muscular usage, for example, creatine kinase, adenylate kinase, and αGPDH (355, 532). An alternate explanation might be that the enlargement of the mitochondria that occurs with endurance training (268) alters the surface-to-volume ratio with

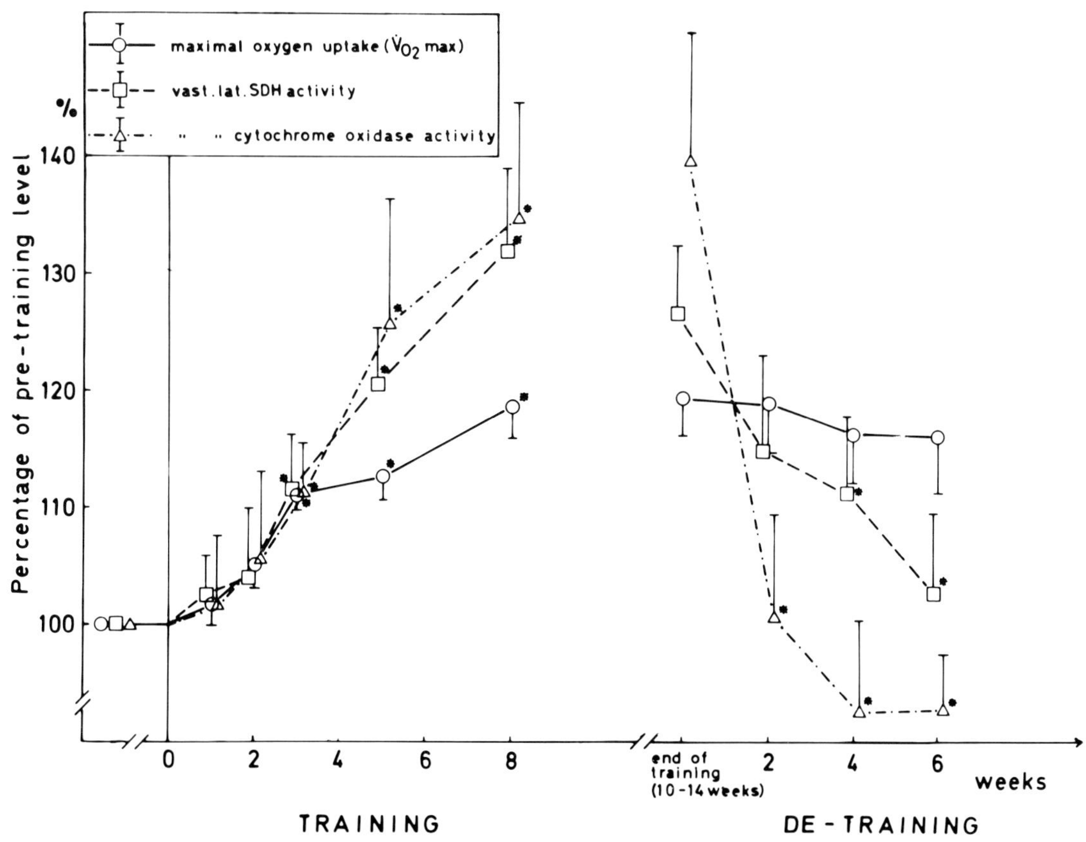

FIG. 21. Time courses for changes in 2 mitochondrial enzymes and $\dot{V}_{O_2\,max}$ during physical conditioning and deconditioning. *Significant changes in time (paired *t* test) for the selected variables. [Adapted from Henriksson and Reitman (338).]

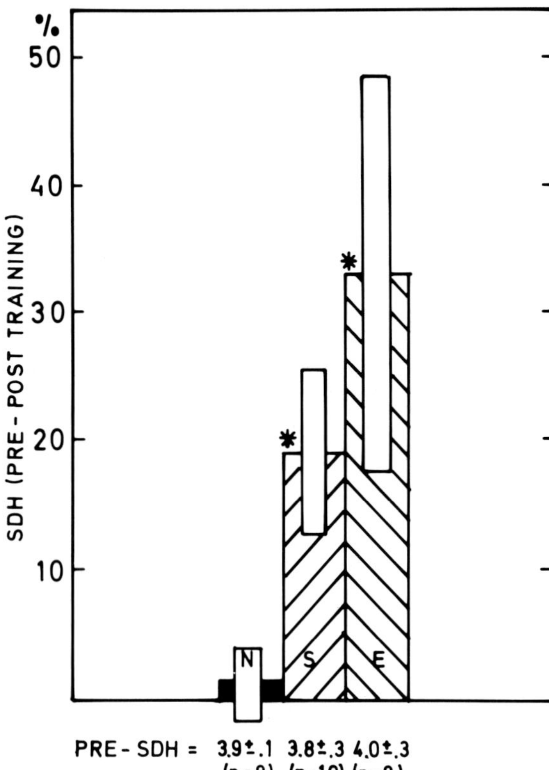

FIG. 22. Mean change in percent of succinate dehydrogenase (SDH) activity of vastus lateralis with different training procedures. Note that the mean values ± SD for the absolute activities are similar before the training started. N, no training; S, sprint; E, endurance trained; *, significant difference, $P < 0.05$. [Adapted from Saltin, Gollnick, et al. (603).]

smaller amounts of surface protein needed to support the cristae. Other studies (142, 422, 423) do not support this contention.

For human skeletal muscle almost all existing data support the concept of a constant proportionality of enzymes. Thus increases in SDH and CYTOX activities occur in concert (322, 338). Thus the capacities of the citric acid cycle and the electron-transport chain change in parallel. Whether enzymes in the β-oxidation pathway adapt in similar proportion is unknown. In one of the few studies where marker enzymes for all of the major mitochondrial pathways were followed, CS and CYTOX increased similarly though with a slightly different time course, but HAD was unchanged (104). In fact a small decline was noted after 6 mo of training. These data are in contrast to those from a study with middle-aged men where a similar type of training (jogging, playing basketball, etc.) produced parallel increases in SDH, CS, and HAD activities (43). The activity of HAD was observed to be present in a constant proportion to either SDH, CS, or CYTOX in cross-sectional studies of endurance-trained subjects with the ratio being close to 1.0 (0.8–1.4) (364, 398). It is, however, conceivable that training could produce differential responses in enzymes of β-oxidation as compared to the citric acid cycle or the electron-transport chain as a function of the type or intensity of the exercise regimen. With intense interval training, which is as effective in producing increases in $\dot{V}O_{2\,max}$ as continuous exercise, FFA utilization may be less and thereby fail to elicit any adaptive response in the enzymes of the β-oxidation pathway. An indication of this possibility is found in a study of eight long-distance runners all having $\dot{V}O_{2\,max}$ above 70 $ml \cdot kg^{-1} \cdot min^{-1}$ (398). Those who trained with continuous exercise possessed higher HAD activities in the leg muscles than those who trained with intermittent exercise, despite the fact that SDH activities were identical. Additional support for this possibility comes from sprint-training studies where CS, SDH, and CYTOX were elevated but HAD was unchanged (104). In concert with this are the results from a study of sedentary subjects and individuals involved in a variety of sport activities (43). Those persons who participated in game-type activities had lower HAD/CS ratios than the sedentary or endurance-trained individuals.

Histochemical staining for NADH-nitrotetrazolium reductase or SDH clearly demonstrates that the elevation of oxidative enzymes can occur in all fiber types. Morphometric studies have demonstrated that mitochondrial volumes increase in FT_b and FT_c as well as ST fibers with physical conditioning (9, 104). These findings are consistent with quantitative biochemical assessments of the SDH activity of ST and FT fibers after interval and continuous training that elicited elevations in both the total body $\dot{V}O_{2\,max}$ and the SDH activity of mixed-fiber muscle preparation of the two groups (337, 338). The largest increases in SDH activities of pooled samples of the ST and FT fibers occurred after continuous or interval training, respectively. Cross-sectional studies have demonstrated that SDH activities of FT_a and FT_b fibers can reach values as high as those of ST fibers with extensive training (398). In such instances the SDH activities of FT_a and FT_b fibers were 4-fold higher than those of sedentary subjects, whereas the activity of the ST fibers was only 2.5-fold above that in the sedentary individuals (Table 10).

TABLE 10. *Succinate Dehydrogenase Activity of Thigh Muscle Fiber Types in Response to Conditioning and Deconditioning*

Condition	Range for Maximal Oxygen Uptake	Muscle Fiber Types			Mixed Muscle
		ST	FT_a	FT_b	
	$ml \cdot kg^{-1} \cdot min^{-1}$	$\mu mol \cdot g \cdot min^{-1}$			
Deconditioning	30–40	5.0	4.0	3.5	4.0
Sedentary	40–50	9.2	5.8	4.9	7.0
Conditioning (months)	45–55	12.1	10.2	5.5	11.0
Endurance athletes	>70	23.2	22.1	22.0	22.5

ST, slow twitch. FT_a, FT_b, fast-twitch fibers of the thigh muscles. Approximate values for maximal oxygen uptake are included. (Adapted from data in refs. 299, 337, 398, 602.)

Immobilization or inactivity causes SDH activity to fall. This is true for sedentary and well-trained subjects. In sedentary subjects the largest reductions occur in the ST fibers such that the difference in SDH activity of the various fiber types in deconditioned muscle is small (299). This is somewhat in contrast to the findings for the glycolytic enzymes and indicates that physical activity regulates the level of the mitochondrial more than the glycolytic enzymes.

An important aspect of the detraining studies is that rate constants for the turnover of the enzymes can be estimated from them. Thus it has been estimated that the half-life of cytochrome oxidase is about 8 days in rat skeletal muscle (62, 677). Data on this subject for man are incomplete, and an exact evaluation of the regulation of enzyme levels is currently not available. A single exercise bout has been shown to produce an increase in the synthesis of components of cytochrome *c* (358). Some evidence suggests that the turnover rates are similar for the muscle of man and rat. In studies with man, comparisons can also be made between the rate of change in $\dot{V}O_{2\,max}$ and the aerobic capacity of the limb muscles (Fig. 21). From such studies it is apparent that the enzyme activities decline faster than the $\dot{V}O_{2\,max}$ (7, 425), the former approaching pretraining values in 2–3 wk. At this time $\dot{V}O_{2\,max}$ was still 10% higher than the pretraining value.

Lipoprotein lipase is an enzyme located on the intraluminal surface of the capillaries, and it has a key position in the utilization of plasma triglycerides by the tissues. The enzyme is synthesized by skeletal muscle cells and found in skeletal muscle of man (459, 460). Lipoprotein lipase activity is related to the degree of capillarization of the skeletal muscle (461), and it could therefore be expected that it would become elevated when capillary density is increased with physical training. No studies are yet available on this subject in man. It is demonstrated, however, that prolonged exercise causes an acute pronounced enhancement of the lipoprotein lipase activity (462). Variations due to the previous 24-h physical activity level may mask any changes due to a more permanent elevation of the physical activity level. On the other hand it could be anticipated that along with more capillaries there would be more binding sites for the lipoprotein enzyme, and this would provide an explanation for higher lipoprotein lipase activity after prolonged exercise in the trained stage.

The effect of physical activity on the oxidative capacity of skeletal muscles of animals has been extensively and intensively investigated. The models used for increasing activity have included electrical stimulation (either direct or via the motor nerve), varying durations of swimming, endurance running, sprint running, and isometric contractions. Inactivity has been imposed on the muscles by denervation and by limb immobilization either by the application of restrictive casts or joint immobilization.

One of the earliest indications of an adaptive response of the oxidative systems of skeletal muscle to physical activity was the report of 50%–100% increases in SDH activity in the hindlimb muscles of the rabbit after 20–30 min/day of direct electrical stimulation for 15 days (113). Subsequent studies where rats were exercised with programs of swimming did not confirm the existence of high activities for SDH or malic dehydrogenase (283, 317, 353).

The application of methods where rats were forced to run either on treadmills or in exercise wheels for prolonged periods of time (up to 2 h) at speeds between 27 and 32 m/min firmly established the fact that endurance training increases the capacity of the citric acid cycle, fat oxidation, and the electron-transport system (26, 46, 62, 142, 328, 345, 353, 354, 357, 434, 495, 678, 723, 732). When the exercise is sufficiently intense, the increases in mitochondrial enzymes occur somewhat in parallel in all fiber types present in the muscles (678). The effect is a result of an increase in mitochondria (39, 266, 268, 353, 422, 505). Histochemical staining of muscles from sedentary and trained animals for oxidative enzymes results in an increased staining intensity. As the staining intensity of the fibers that are normally low in mitochondrial enzymes (FT fibers) increases, it becomes increasingly difficult to discriminate between these and the normally oxidative fibers (ST). This has lead some investigators to conclude that endurance training produces a conversion of one fiber type to another (39, 172, 213, 214, 497). But since the oxidative capacity of all fiber types increases with the relative ratio between fiber types remaining rather constant, this does not constitute a change in the basic phenotype of the fibers.

Since all components of the oxidative system appear to respond in parallel to endurance training, the result is that the skeletal muscles of endurance-trained animals possess greater capacities for the oxidation of pyruvate, fatty acid, and ketone bodies. Although the majority of the work in describing the adaptive response of skeletal muscle to endurance training has used the rat as an experimental subject, similar responses have been reported for the guinea pig, bushbaby, and horse (36, 39, 169, 646, 692). Similar changes have also been observed in the rat diaphragm when airway resistance was increased by an experimentally imposed stenosis of the trachea (420). It should also be noted that the metabolic potential of the neuromuscular junction also adapts to endurance training (138).

Short, high-intensity exercise such as sprinting produces smaller augmentations of the oxidative pathways (608). Thus 11 wk of training rats with a sprint program of alternate periods of 30 s of running and 30 s of rest with the final running speed being 80 m/min did not alter SDH activity in any of the fiber types (608). A sprint program with fewer repetitions has been reported to increase the CS and hexokinase activities in the rectus femoris and soleus muscles of the rat (659). Creatine kinase was unchanged in the rectus femoris and increased in the soleus muscle in this experiment. Similarly 16 wk of sprint training was reported to increase the fumarase activity for the soleus, the white portion of the gastrocnemius, and the plantaris muscles of the rat (345). A training program of isometric contractions had no effect on the oxidative potential of rat skeletal muscle (208). Chronic electrical stimulation of skeletal muscle via the motor nerve produces an overall increase in the activity of the oxidative enzymes (323, 371).

Inactivity by various experimental procedures causes a precipitous fall in the oxidative capacity of skeletal muscle (316, 350, 670, 671). This has been reported to be about 70% for succinate–cytochrome *c* reductase, and about 50% for CYTOX of the rat gastrocnemius in 21 days. Malate dehydrogenase was 40% and 70% lower in the gastrocnemius and soleus muscles, respectively, of the rat after denervation. The overall picture for inactivity produced by denervation is for a major reduction in the oxidative capacity of all types of skeletal muscle.

Immobilization of limbs has also been reported to result in decreases in the oxidative capacity of animal muscle (60, 64, 439, 474, 479, 582). This effect, however, is less dramatic than that occurring with denervation and may be minimal when the enzyme activities are expressed per unit of muscle (170). There are, however, reports of changes in the mitochondria with reduced capacities to oxidize glucose, pyruvate, palmitate, and β-hydroxybutyrate (583). The changes are more rapid in ST than FT muscle (64). These data suggest that qualitative and quantitative changes had occurred in the mitochondria with immobilization.

Studies conducted with man closely parallel those with animals for changes in the mitochondrial enzymes. This includes the methods for tissue analysis and many procedures for producing increases and decreases of physical activity. Interestingly most of the enzyme assays were first developed with animal models and then applied to man. Overall the responses observed in skeletal muscle to altered physical activity are similar for animals and man. In each group of subjects there are certain advantages and disadvantages for their use. It has been possible to use some experimental perturbations with animals that are not possible with man, for example, the experiments with chronic electrical stimulation of the muscle via the motor nerve. There is some activity in the area of direct electrical stimulation of muscle of man via the nerves at motor points. Such studies may apply to rehabilitation medicine and also to athletes during periods of injury. Conversely there are advantages in the study of man. Foremost among these is the ability to use specific experimental protocols that require the cooperation of the subjects, such as the one-leg model, and a wide variety of individuals are available who naturally engage in physical activity or who are sedentary.

Contractile properties and fiber conversion. One important question concerning the adaptability of skeletal muscle to varying types of overload is whether there is a change in the fiber types. As stated initially in this chapter, skeletal muscle fibers are classified only on the basis of their contractile properties as can be identified from histochemical, immunological, electrophoretic, or biochemical characterization of myofibrillar proteins. Thus a true interconversion of a fiber is characterized by changes in contractile properties and in the manner that a fiber is utilized during exercise.

There is no question that under appropriate conditions muscle fibers are mutable. Perhaps the first of these situations occurs during maturation after birth. At birth many of the skeletal muscles of the limbs of mammals possess contractile properties similar to the ST muscle of the adult (92). During the early postnatal period some of these muscles undergo changes in their biochemical composition such that their speed of contraction attains that of the adult FT muscle (157). During this process the myosin in fetal muscle, which is initially undifferentiated, takes on the characteristics associated with the myosin of mature FT muscle (157, 718). The relative speed with which this conversion occurs is a function of the initial size of the newborn and the rate at which a given species matures (92, 93, 119, 122). For example, for the rat the extensor digitorum longus attains a contractile speed similar to that of the mature animal by 21 days of age (157). During this period the ATPase of actomyosin increases in parallel with the time to peak tension. Conversely the one-half relaxation time changes in concert with the development of the Ca^{2+}-sequestering capacity of the sarcoplasmic reticulum (157).

It is also a consistent observation that the reinnervation of a denervated muscle with a motoneuron that normally innervates a muscle with dissimilar contractile properties (i.e., an ST muscle with a nerve normally innervating an FT muscle or vice versa) results in the muscle taking on the contractile and biochemical properties associated with the new nerve (33, 121, 122, 151, 351, 421). The experimental basis of this cross innervation came from the observation of Eccles and co-workers (165–167) that the contractile properties of a muscle were associated with the characteristic pattern of the neural impulses delivered to the muscle. For the adult cat, ST muscle is innervated by motoneurons that discharge tonically at low frequencies, whereas FT muscles receive chronic impulses in a phasic manner at higher rates (167). These data suggested that the stimulation frequency of the nerve or the release of some neurotrophic substance associated with the pattern of nervous discharge was responsible for determining the contractile properties of the muscle or of the individual motor units. The cross-innervation studies support such a contention. Chronic electrical stimulation produced by electrodes implanted on the motor nerves and applying stimulation frequencies mimicking those of the opposite nerve produces a similar conversion of the contractile and chemical properties of the muscles (323–325, 371, 551–553, 568, 599, 600). These data conclusively demonstrated that all muscle cells retain a "genetic memory" for the synthesis of all kinds of proteins associated with the regulation of the contractile properties.

Whether the conversion of a muscle from an ST to an FT or the reverse depends exclusively on the frequency of the stimulation or on a neurotrophic substance released from the nerve independently of the impulse frequency has been questioned. Two experimental approaches have been taken to this problem. In the first study the soleus muscle of the rat was denervated and electrodes implanted in it. Low-frequency impulses delivered at a mean of either 1 or 9 Hz did not alter the time to peak tension but at a mean of 9 Hz the one-half relaxation time was prolonged (465, 488). Both the time to peak tension and one-half relaxation times were reduced when the stimulation was 100 Hz for 0.01 or 1 s. At a mean stimulation rate of 1 Hz, endurance was reduced. Reinnervation of the denervated muscle by nerves normally innervating ST muscle resulted in the appearance of the ST contractile characteristics in spite of a continued direct electrical stimulation (469). These data demonstrate that although direct stimulation can have a regulatory role in the contractile properties of muscle, ultimately the motor nerve is dominant. These data do not, however, answer the question of whether this neural dominance is due to the natural impulse traffic mediated by acetylcholine or to neurotrophic substances. Chordotomy, which produces electrical silence of the nerves, may give some insight into this question. When the spinal cord is sectioned, there is a conversion of ST to FT muscles (187). This change is rather slow and occurs in concert with a shift of the myosin isozymes to those of the FT muscle. When considered in light of the results from electrical stimulation applied directly to denervated muscle, these data suggest that the prime determinant of the contractile properties of muscle fibers is the electrical activity rather than a neurotrophic factor. These studies do not rule out the existence of neurotrophic regulators, only that without normal electrical traffic over the end-plate region they are not effective, or that electrical traffic in the nerve is required for a normal transport of these substances from the nerve or across the motor end plate. The observation that there is a conversion of ST to FT fibers after chordotomy suggests that the maintenance of ST properties depends on chronic electrical activity.

Experimental chordotomy is like spinal cord section in man resulting from accidents. In such patients all fibers in the paralyzed muscle stain histochemically as FT fibers (292). Also, in hemiplegic patients there is an increase in percentage of FT fibers in the muscles of the affected side (444). These data illustrate the mutability of human skeletal muscle. This is consistent with the conversion of ST to FT fibers in the muscles where the nerve is intact but electrically silent. These data suggest that for the maintenance of slow-twitch properties the nerve must be chronically active.

Although interesting and important the above experimental approaches do not answer the question of whether or not the fiber distribution of skeletal muscle can be altered by an interconversion of one type to the other as a result of some form of "normal" physical activity. The logical conversion would be for an increase in the ST fibers in response to endurance type activity and the appearance of a greater percentage of FT fibers for those activities where short explosive contractions are required. In most of the early studies with animal species other than man the fibers were identified simply as red or white on the basis of staining intensities for oxidative enzymes. With such methods it was reported by a number of investigators that there was a higher percentage of red than white fibers in the muscles of endurance-trained animals (39, 172, 213, 214). Termination of the training program resulted in a return to the control situation. By some this has been interpreted as a conversion of white to red fibers. A similar report also exists in a longitudinal study of the effect of training on human skeletal muscle (497). Such an alteration in the staining intensity for mitochondrial enzymes is consistent with biochemical studies demonstrating that endurance training induces increases in mitochondrial protein concentrations and in the activities of the oxidative enzymes associated with the mitochondria. As seen in Table 10 this increase in oxidative potential of the muscle can occur in all types of fibers if the intensity and duration are adequate to produce recruitment of all motor units in the muscle. On the other hand the short, heavy-resistance exercise of weight lifting results in a decrease in the oxidative potential of skeletal muscle. This could be viewed as an increase in the white fibers. The criterion that has been established to identify fiber type is a difference in the myofibrillar proteins. On this basis changes in oxidative potential do not represent a change in fiber type.

A significant amount of data are available on the fiber composition of muscles of athletes. The majority of these data have come from studies that determined the fiber composition in biopsy samples. As a result, there is appreciable descriptive information on the fiber distribution of several muscles from athletes specializing in a variety of athletic events (see Table 8). In most of these studies the fiber composition has been assessed from the histochemical identification of fibers on the basis of the histochemical demonstration of myofibrillar ATPase. In some instances this has been combined with procedures that illustrate the metabolic profiles of the fibers from histochemical staining procedures. From cross sections the fiber composition of athletes has been found to fall within the range for normal subjects (602). Since the range encompassed by normal subjects is rather large, this is not surprising.

In spite of the fact that most athletic subgroups have fiber distributions in their muscles that are within the range of normal subjects, there are some indications of selective fiber distributions in certain athletic groups. Most notably, individuals who excel in events requiring great endurance usually possess a predominance of ST fibers in their muscles. Conversely there is a tendency for a person with sprint abilities to have slightly higher percentages of FT fibers. In the latter case, however, the situation is less dramatic than for endurance athletes. On this basis it has been tempting for some to speculate that prolonged exposure to a given type of muscular activity can induce a conversion of one fiber type to another. There are, however, few longitudinal studies to substantiate this supposition. Gollnick, Saltin, and coworkers (260) examined the fiber composition of biopsy samples from the vastus lateralis muscle of six subjects before and after a 6-mo training program consisting of bicycle exercise. Since this type of exercise depends to a large extent on the quadriceps muscle group, this muscle should have undergone extensive use. The oxidative potential of the muscle was doubled at the completion of the training period, which supports this contention. The fiber composition, as determined by staining procedures to identify fibers only as FT or ST, was not altered by the training. Since the FT fibers were not further differentiated into the FT_a, FT_b, and FT_c, there was no indication of shifts in the distribution within this fiber group. However, if a major shift in the fibers in the two major types did occur, it should have been detectable with the methods that were used. Jansson et al. (399) have examined the fiber composition in samples from the vastus lateralis muscles of four subjects after 18 wk of endurance training and again after an additional 11 wk of training that included exercise at high relative oxygen consumption. During the period of endurance training the subjects ran an average of 110 km/wk. The second training program included some high-intensity exercise (at 90%–100% of the $\dot{V}O_{2\,max}$) in conjunction with endurance running. The average distance run per week was 71 km. Since samples were not taken before initiation of training, no comparisons could be made between the sedentary and endurance-trained state. After the second training period there was a 17% reduction in ST fibers. This was accomodated by an increase in the FT_c (type IIC) fibers. The suggestion was made from these data that a major conversion of fiber types could occur as a result of training. These authors also referred to data where the percent of ST fibers decreased from 81% to 57% in the muscle of a well-trained cross-country skier after a 6-wk period of limb immobilization due to an injury. This conversion of the ST fibers to a class of FT fibers as a result of high-intensity exercise is not in agreement with the data of Saltin, Gollnick, et al. (603) comparing the fiber composition of legs of subjects studied in combinations of no training, endurance-training, and sprint-training practices with one leg. Henriksson et al. (335) examined the effect of a 50-day program of endurance training (skiing 18 mi/day) on the fiber composition of the human triceps brachii muscle. There was no difference in the percent of ST fibers before and after the training. However, there was a reduction of about 11% in the total population of FT_a and FT_b fiber. This was in part compensated for by a 5% increase in the FT_c fiber population. Six months after termination of the training there were no differences in fiber distribution as compared to that at the end of the training period.

Pette et al. (545) have observed a similar pattern of myofibrillar proteins when comparing FT_a and FT_b fibers. There is also a lack of definitive proof that normal physical activity produces a change from a fast- to a slow-type fiber or the reverse in animals. Bagby, Gollnick, et al. (22) did not observe any change in the percent distribution of the fibers of the gastrocnemius muscle after either an endurance- or sprint-training program. Chronic overload, however, produced by inactivation or ablation of a synergistic muscle or by chronic stretch produces an increase in the percentage of ST fibers in rat (296, 379) and chicken (359) skeletal muscle. Thus the potential for an interconversion of fibers does exist when the stimulus is appropriate.

In summary, it appears that training does not produce any major shifts in the population of ST and FT fibers in skeletal muscle. Unfortunately there is currently a lack of longitudinal studies that have encompassed a large enough sample and included all of the techniques that can be used to identify fiber-type interconversion to settle this issue. The current data suggest that it may be possible to induce some shifts in distribution of the subgroups of the FT fibers.

Mechanical properties. There are few reports that examined the contractile properties of enlarged skeletal muscle. Some of the early experiments in this field produced a muscular enlargement by elimination of the synergistic muscle via tenotomy. With this model a slowing of the normally ST soleus muscle was observed in both the cat (709) and rat (451). There was also a decrement in the maximal tetanic tension per square centimeter 6 days after the onset of the overload. There was no change in the contractile properties of the FT plantaris muscle of the rat after enlargement produced by denervation of the soleus and gastrocnemius muscles or by the combination of denervation of the synergistic muscle and treadmill exercise (56, 57). In the latter experiments the time span between imposition of the overload and assessment of the contractile properties of the enlarged muscles was 10 wk. The muscular enlargement averaged about 35% and was similar whether the rats were exercised or not. The major differences between these experiments were the choice of muscle studied (an ST vs. an FT muscle) and the time span between the imposition of the overload and assessment of the contractile properties. The latter difference may be significant since it has been demonstrated that there is a major increase in the water content of the overloaded muscle after tenotomy or ablation of the synergistic muscles (378). Thus even if the contractile properties are corrected for such differences and expressed on a dry weight basis, this does not preclude the possibility that in the intact cell normal contractile activity was disrupted as a result of the superhydrated state. After 4 wk this situation no longer exists, and the protein content and activities of the glycolytic and oxidative pathways are normal (18, 378).

Only a few reports are available that examined the contractile properties of skeletal muscle fibers after physical training. A program of sprint training was reported to shorten the time to peak tension of the rat soleus muscle by 14% (659). However, this program did not alter the contractile properties of the FT rectus femoris muscle. This could be interpreted as a specific change to enhance running speed. In cats a weight-lifting program that lasted from 10 to 61 wk was reported to increase the time to peak tension for the flexor carpi radialis and palmaris longus muscles (both normally FT muscles) (277, 278). In neither of the aforementioned experiments were measurements made of the ATPase activity of myosin. In the latter experiments there was no evidence of a change in fiber type as demonstrated from the histochemical staining for myofibrillar ATPase. In contrast to these observations, Buchthal and Schmalbruch (89, 90) did not observe any differences in the contractile properties of the biceps brachii and triceps muscle of weight lifters. Endurance training did not alter the contractile properties of the plantaris muscle of the *Galago senegalensis* [lesser bushbaby; (169)] or of the gastrocnemius-plantaris muscle group of the guinea pig (37). An exception to this general pattern of a lack of a major change in the contractile characteristics of muscle after training is the report of a 14% decrease in the time to peak tension of the rat soleus after treadmill exercise (223). An increase in myofibrillar ATPase activity has also been reported after endurance training (28), and a decrease with overload produced by surgical ablation of a synergistic muscle (67). The latter change is consistent with the greater percentage of ST fibers as identified by the histochemical method in the enlarged plantaris after ablation of the gastrocnemius muscle (378).

Forced inactivity such as occurs after immobilization of a limb has been studied from the standpoint of its effect on the contractile properties of skeletal muscle. Immobilization of the hindlimb of the *Galago senegalensis* for 5 to 6 mo did not alter the contractility of the FT plantaris muscle (170). In contrast an elongation in the contraction times for both the ST and FT muscles of the cat hindlimb was noted after 22 wk of immobilization (127).

The general consensus from the literature appears to be that there are no major changes in the contractile characteristics in response to varying types of physical training or inactivity. In cases where changes have been reported there is a lack of an unequivocal demonstration that there has been a change in the basic type of fibers of the muscles.

REGULATION. Clearly the adaptive response of substrate levels and enzyme activities that occurs in skeletal muscle varies as a function of the type, duration, and frequency of the exercise stimulus. This suggests that specific stimuli are generated by different patterns of use and that these are somehow sensed and translated into adaptations in the muscle. Presently very little is known concerning the nature of the stimuli or the manner in which they are translated into a genetic expression.

The increased tension associated with high-intensity muscular contractions may be responsible for increases in muscle mass. Such increases in muscle size can be demonstrated with chronic stretch of either normal or denervated muscle (206, 427, 648). This stretching of muscle can also prevent the atrophy associated with limb immobilization (64). The unanswered question is how stretch stimulus is communicated as a specific chemical signal to the genes to induce the synthesis of proteins specific for muscular enlargement. A commonly suggested chemical messenger is the level of free calcium (206). The idea is attractive, but it has not been demonstrated that the elevation of free calcium associated with muscular contractions induces adaptations in these systems. Furthermore it is difficult to imagine this applying to growth and development as influenced by physical activity or to weight-lifting activities as practiced by humans. In the latter instances the actual time of the physical activity when the muscle experiences high tensions may be extremely brief. Under these conditions it would be expected that the level of free calcium would return to normal as it would after all types of motor activity. Direct electrical stimulation of skeletal muscle cell has also been reported to increase the synthesis of myosin (70).

It has been suggested that the level of free creatine could induce protein synthesis, based on early experiments measuring the rate of actin and myosin synthesis in muscle cultures from the chicken embryo (388, 389). More rigorous tests of this possibility have failed to reproduce the initial observation (236). Since CP is reduced in the muscle during submaximal and heavy exercise, the release of free creatine should occur under both conditions. But since there is no increase in total muscle bulk with the submaximal exercise, it seems unlikely that creatine could be a major factor controlling the synthesis of myofibrillar protein. Another possibility would be that an intracellular elevation either of specific or general amino acids induces protein synthesis. This hypothesis is related to the fact that after exercise there is an increased entrance of amino acids into the muscle cell (245–247). Animal studies have also indicated that overloads produce increases in ribonucleic acid (RNA) and RNA polymerase in skeletal muscle (307, 586, 647). Similar measurements on denervated muscle also support this notion (426).

The situation regarding the control mechanism for the increases in energy-releasing enzymes is equally unclear. Several hypotheses have been proposed. Because the activities of the enzymes for end-terminal oxidation respond most dramatically to prolonged activity, it has been suggested that this is a response to hypoxia. This assumes that the total muscle or parts of the muscle become hypoxic during exercise. This may be false. Low oxygen tension has been measured in skeletal muscle at rest when the number of perfused capillaries is lower than during activity (361, 362, 648). In fact with exercise the variation in intracellular muscle fiber oxygen tension is reduced and fibers with very low values are not observed at higher exercise rates than in resting muscle (361, 362). Moreover hypoxia during exercise could be assumed to be accompanied by elevations in the lactate concentration of both muscle and blood. Mitochondrial enzymes increase in muscle in response to training regimens where no appreciable elevation in lactate occurs in either blood or muscle. Some support for the lack-of-oxygen hypothesis as a stimulus for inducing increases in oxidative enzymes comes from studies on patients with intermittent claudication and on high-altitude natives (9, 42, 105, 140, 580). Mitochondrial enzyme levels, as well as mitochondrial volumes, have been reported to be higher in the most severely affected leg of such patients (9, 105). These values were higher than those of control subjects. However, examination of the rare patients with unilateral stenosis of the arteries to the leg has failed to verify the existence of a different level of SDH or CYTOX activities between the normal and the affected leg (336).

The notion that high-altitude residents have higher oxidative enzyme activities in their muscles is based on measurements from permanent residents of the Andes (580). When these measurements were repeated and the work capacity of the subjects taken into account, it was found that men native to an altitude of 3,700 m had oxidative enzyme levels similar to sea-level residents with comparable patterns of physical activity (604). Conversely sea-level natives who sojourn at high altitude do not have an increase in the activities of oxidative enzymes in the skeletal muscles (Fig. 23). In fact if anything, there is a slight decrease. The latter finding may be due to a reduction in activity associated with living at high altitude. Thus the strength of the arguments for tissue hypoxia as the major stimulus for the adaptive response of the oxidative enzymes of the mitochondria appears to be limited. The observation that the greatest increases in the oxidative enzymes occur with endurance-type training, as compared to sprint and weight-lifting activities during which hypoxia would be greatest, is also indirect evidence against tissue hypoxia as the specific inducer of protein synthesis. Moreover it would appear that the FT_b fibers of man and the FG fibers of animals would function most often under conditions of low oxygen tension either because they have a poor capillary supply or because they are recruited during periods of high-intensity exercise. If hypoxia were a stimulus for inducing the synthesis of oxidative enzymes, these fibers could be expected to show very high activities, which they clearly do not.

Stimulation of the β-receptors of the skeletal muscle has also been suggested as a mechanism for inducing alterations with training (313, 314). When this hypothesis was tested in rats through a chronic β-blockade and sympathectomy, CS, CYTOX, and SDH increased equally in the treated and untreated animals with endurance training (339).

In the vast number of experiments varying the electrical stimulation pattern to a muscle, distinct adaptations are obtained related to the type of stimulation. Tonic, slow-impulse traffic generates an enhancement of the oxidative enzymes, whereas high-frequency, phasic stimulation does not (465). The adaptations occur whether the stimulation is via the nerve or directly to the denervated muscle (465). This suggests that it is the pattern of muscular usage produced by the electrical activity that is the controlling factor.

The findings described above lead to the general conclusion that the stimulus for adaptive changes in the muscle fiber is related directly to the actual use of the fiber. This suggests that the inducers of these modifications are local in nature and depend on the internal conditions within the muscle fibers. Since similar adaptations can be induced by continuous or interval exercise, there are obviously many methods for inducing these local changes. Presently there is no indication as to the nature of the inducer for the synthesis-specific proteins or how it is related to physical activity. The adaptations preclude the existence of a general inducing factor such as a change in the level of an unknown factor in the blood.

A number of reports have appeared in which elimination of the major hormones known to be regulators of protein synthesis and body growth has not blocked the adaptation in mitochondrial enzymes to chronic exercise (266, 680, 694) or in muscle mass in response to acute overloads (52, 244, 693). Furthermore increases in RNA, amino acid uptake, and protein synthesis occur in the isolated, overloaded heart (618–622) where there is no hormonal control. Thus nonhormonal factors must be given close examination. It is known that synthesis of enzymes can be induced by elevation in substrate concentrations (221). There are a number of substrates that become elevated during exercise including citrate, lactate, malate, and glucose 6-PO_4 (198, 200, 269). None of these has been demonstrated to be an inducer for the synthesis of components of the metabolic pathways. The fact that all components of the oxidative system increase in concert appears to suggest that the general flux of substrates through the system may be the inducer. Fitch and Chaikoff (221) suggested the involvement of a concept of "throughput" since the enzyme content of tissue appears to be directly related to the amount of substrate conversion occurring in a given tissue. With the elevated metabolic rates associated with exercise, and the total substrate conversion during prolonged endurance-type exercise, it is entirely possible that a

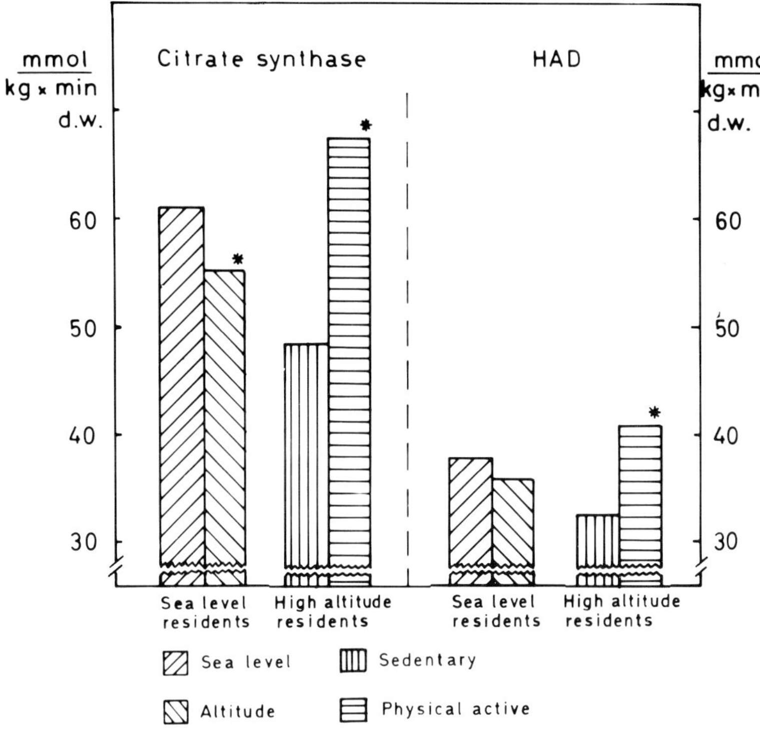

FIG. 23. Mean values for 2 mitochondrial enzymes [citrate synthase and 3-hydroxyacyl-CoA dehydrogenase (HAD)] determined from muscle samples from vastus lateralis in 9 sea-level residents at sea level and after an average 32-wk stay (6–52 wk) at elevation 3,700 m and 16 men born and permanently living at this altitude. Note that high-altitude residents are divided into 2 groups, those who were physically inactive (job and leisure time) and those who were active. Maximal oxygen uptake (ml · kg^{-1} · min^{-1}) for the sea-level residents was 39 ml and 36 ml · kg^{-1} · min^{-1} at sea level and high altitude, respectively; inactive high-altitude residents had 28 ml and active 46 ml · kg^{-1} · min^{-1}. [Adapted from Saltin et al. (604).]

substrate flux through the system could be involved in the induction of the increased oxidative capacities of the different fiber types. This may be important from the standpoint of the stability of enzymes. Enzymes are known to be more stable in the presence of their substrates (128).

In recent years a great deal of information has been generated concerning the adaptability of skeletal muscle to a variety of patterns of use and disuse. It would appear that there is little need for further experiments to explore additional types and intensities of exercise that can influence some of these well-documented changes. Therefore more attention should be directed toward furthering the understanding of the processes that induce the specific synthesis of proteins and control the genetic apparatus of the cells involved.

CONNECTIVE TISSUE

The influence of altered states of physical activity on the strength of ligaments, or in most cases the force required to separate the bone from ligament, has been studied in a number of species including the rat, dog, rabbit, and primate (518, 691, 692, 706–708). The general conclusion from these investigations is that the fluctuations in the strength of the bone-ligament junction parallels the state of physical activity. Moreover early mobility promotes a more rapid return of ligament strength after surgical repair. It has also been shown that normal ligament strength did not exist 12 wk after surgical repair when 6 wk was immobilization and 6 wk was exercise training (691). In primates ligament strength was below normal 20 wk after resumption of activity after a period of immobilization from wearing a cast (518).

The differences in ligament strength appear to be a function of the total amount of ligament present, that is, the total cross-sectional area of the ligament. This is analogous to skeletal muscle in which strength is a function of the cross-sectional area of the muscle with strength per unit area of muscle being rather constant.

Limited data are available that show the effects of training on the connective tissue of skeletal muscle and of differences between the types of skeletal muscle. However, it has been demonstrated that with a work-induced growth of muscle there is an increased synthesis of both deoxyribonucleic acid (DNA) and RNA in skeletal muscle (225, 393) and in the myocardium (491, 498). The bulk of this DNA has been shown to be localized in the connective tissue (225, 393, 491). When DNA synthesis was inhibited, chronic overload still produced an increase in the cross-sectional area of the muscle fibers but without a concomitant proliferation of the interfiber support structures (225). Similarly the induction of muscular growth in the rat plantaris muscle by sectioning of the tendon to the gastrocnemius muscle has been reported to increase the activity of protocollagen proline hydroxylase activity, thereby suggesting an increased synthesis of connective tissue (698). Endurance training of mice (treadmill running) has also been reported to stimulate connective tissue synthesis in the skeletal muscle and tendons of mice (666) and to increase the activities of some of the enzyme for energy metabolism (322). The effects of an endurance-training program on the connective tissue of the rat has produced less conclusive data. Overall this resulted in little or no change in the total collagen or the chemical composition of the collagen (433). The training was rather short, however, and did not induce the usual increase in activity of mitochondrial enzymes. Interestingly, a greater collagen content was reported in ST as compared to FT muscle for the chicken and rat (433, 446). There was an increase in the concentration of collagen in muscle of chicken during stretch-induced hypertrophy (446). Only limited data are available that concern the effect of training on the connective tissue of human skeletal muscle. In one study (665) it was reported that an 8-wk training program increased the activity of propyl hydroxylase in the vastus lateralis muscle of 69-yr-old female but not male subjects. In a population of men ranging in age from 33 to 70 yr Suominen and Heikkinen (664) observed higher activities of propyl hydroxylase in the vastus lateralis muscle of those who were habitually active as compared to the sedentary individuals. Clearly this is an area where additional data are needed.

CAPILLARIES

The capillary is the interface between the skeletal muscle and the vascular supply that makes the exchange of blood-borne materials possible. Many of the features of this exchange were described by Krogh (435, 436) in his now-classic studies. Since these pioneering studies there has been considerable effort directed towards furthering the understanding of this system. Since the functioning of skeletal muscle during exercise depends to a large extent on the perfusion of the muscle with blood, attention is focused here on some of the factors that contribute to this process. This includes a description of the number, length, and diameter of the capillaries as they are related to and surround the muscle fibers. Although such measures do not give any indication of the number of open capillaries, of blood flow either at rest or during exercise, or of the permeability characteristics for the exchange process, all of which are essential in determining the transport rate for specific substances, they do give estimates of the upper capacity for blood flow in the muscle. This situation is similar to the use of maximal activity (V_{max}) for enzymes as an indicator of the potential substrate flux through a specific metabolic pathway.

There has been some attention paid to the effect of varying patterns of physical activity on the capillary supply to muscles and of the differences in capillary supply that may exist among the different types of muscle fibers. Since the results of such studies may depend on the methodology used, a brief discussion of some of the problems associated with each method is given. Further, a short description of the present understanding of capillary architecture is included.

Methodology

There are basically three methods that have been used to visualize capillaries in skeletal muscle: *1*) injection of a dye into the capillary lumen, *2*) staining the capillary wall, and *3*) vital microscopy. There are problems associated with all three methods. Spalteholz (650) pioneered this work with injection of a dye into the vascular tree. This method can give good estimates both of number and length of capillaries. In addition the anatomy, i.e., the structural relationship between capillaries and muscle fibers, is seen. The drawbacks are that not all capillaries may be filled and that in the preparation for microscopy a profound shrinkage occurs. The latter problem can in part be accounted for by determination of a shrinkage factor, but it does not account for possible distortion in the preparative work. Various techniques have been used to overcome the nonhomogeneous filling, but at the present time this problem appears to be unsolved and an underestimation in the total number of capillaries can be the result. In preparing the tissue to identify the muscle cells, a hematoxylin-eosin stain has been used. In doing so the nuclei of the cell are stained quite dark. It is possible that some of the peripherally located nuclei have been misinterpreted as capillaries stained with dye, resulting in an erroneously high capillary count. This could be a likely explanation for the extremely high capillary densities found in some earlier studies, as first pointed out by Pappenheimer (535).

Techniques to stain the capillaries, either the basal membrane or the endothelial cells, have not been used as extensively as the injection methods. These techniques have the advantage that they can be combined with staining of cross sections of the muscle so that the fibers in the section can be identified with regard to contractile and metabolic characteristics. Further, these stains can be used on sections of frozen samples, which minimize shrinkage, and the distortion may also be at an acceptable level. The major drawback is that only the number of capillaries in cross sections can be counted. Further, there is a risk that not all capillaries are stained. Alkaline phosphatase appears to be the safest stain for capillaries, but myofibrillar ATPase after acid preincubation also functions in many species. However, neither of these reactions stain capillaries in human skeletal muscle well (5, 6). The reason for this is obscure. The PAS reaction stains the basal membrane of the capillaries in human muscle. If the sections are pretreated with amylase, the capillaries can easily be identified [Fig. 4; (5)]. The PAS stain or electron-microscopic technique for identifying capillaries in human skeletal muscle gives the same number of capillaries per fiber (520).

The vital microscopy technique gives detailed information about the number of capillaries and their length and diameter. The flow rate can also be estimated in the various capillaries. The problem with the technique is that only a few muscles are suitable for use. Moreover the surgical procedure and the light to visualize the structures can offset the normal state. This is probably not a major problem when counting the capillaries but the diameter of the capillary and the flow may be affected (196, 281, 477, 483, 509).

Anatomy

The arrangement of the capillaries in skeletal muscle was the focus of many of the early studies [(477, 570, 650); for further references, see ref. 370]. In sum, in white muscle the majority of capillaries run parallel with the muscle fibers, but there are also capillaries that encircle the fibers. In red muscle the capillaries have a more tortuous arrangement. They also seem to form parallel loops. In addition several studies point to definite widening of some capillaries in the venous end where capillaries join the venules (for references, see ref. 369).

In more recent studies, Eriksson and Myrhage have worked out some of the details of the configuration of the microvascular supply in the thin and flat tenuissimus muscle of the rabbit [(196); Fig. 24]. In many essential parts their results confirm the earlier observations. Running parallel to the muscle and along its side are the main feeding artery and a vein. From these vessels transverse arterioles and venules branch off at angles of 45°–90°. From such a transverse arteriole and vein there is a mean of 10–15 branches. After a distance of 1–2 mm the smallest arterioles subdivide into capillaries. These run essentially parallel to the muscle fibers. Two capillaries may join in one small venule or end at an almost right angle in a larger venule. The capillaries are joined at regular distances by anastomoses. The average length of the capillary in this muscle is 1,000 μm with a large variation around this mean. The average diameter is slightly smaller than the diameter of the red blood cell of the rabbit (5.7 vs. 5.5 μm) and somewhat wider in the venular than the arterial side. In spite of large differences in the size of the muscle fibers, an almost identical number of capillaries was found around each of three fiber types (3.5 capillaries per fiber) with a mean of one capillary per fiber giving a sharing factor of 3. With the same technique other muscles and other species have been studied and the same general arrangements of the vessels have been found although the values for number and length of the capillaries vary (477, 507, 509).

Hammersen (306) has presented evidence that the very regular pattern for the microvascular tree observed in these thin muscles studied by vital microscopy may not apply to all muscles. In his own studies using an injection technique to visualize the capillaries in various rat and rabbit muscles, the arrangement was more complex. He found ramification to adjacent capillary beds to be much more frequent. Further, close to the venous end of the capillary the number of interconnections rose considerably. Several of the capillaries unite to form small venous stems. In addition, unramified capillaries were found that ran along the external surface of the fiber bundle, sometimes joining

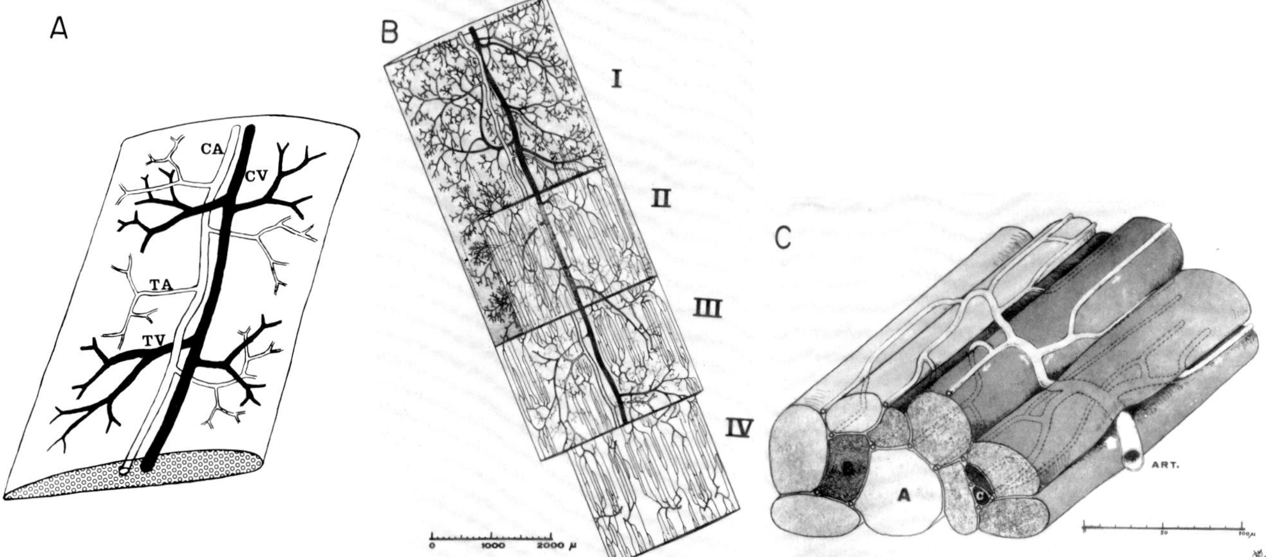

FIG. 24. *A*: schematic representation of the vascular arrangement in the tenuissimus muscle. CA, central artery; CV, central vein; TA, transverse arteriole; TV, transverse venule. *B*: detailed schematic representation of the vascular architecture of the tenuissimus muscle. Arterial vessels, open; venous vessels, filled. Sections of different depth are made into the muscle at *II*, *III*, and *IV*. At *I* a projection of the pre- and postcapillary vessels is shown. The section at *II* shows the vessels above, at *III* at the same, and *IV* under the level of the central vessels. *C*: graphic representation of a small arteriole (ART) subdividing into capillaries. Capillaries then run parallel to the muscle fibers. [*A* adapted from Eriksson and Myrhage (196).]

a distant capillary bed. Hammersen's conclusion is that the concept for a "terminal vascular unit" does not fit for skeletal muscle tissues. Basically, Myrhage and Eriksson (507) reached the same conclusion when extending their studies to cat gastrocnemius muscle and with an injection technique. These more recent studies have also brought new evidence on controversial topics such as arteriovenous anastomoses and capillary sphincters (161, 196, 361, 362, 477). In none of the studies with vital microscopy could the presence of arteriovenous anastomoses be verified. Besides, the ultralong unramified capillaries described by Hammersen did not function as an arteriovenous anastomosis (306). The explanation offered for regulation of flow in various capillaries is that smooth muscle cells in the wall of the terminal arteriole surround the capillary at the branching point and function as "sphincters," because no precapillary sphincters can be detected with a vital microscopy technique. However, Hammersen has pointed out that these can be difficult to visualize with this technique (306), and the existence of capillary sphincters remains to be proved.

Capillary Density

From the very first studies of skeletal muscle capillaries, the number per fiber or unit area has been estimated. Rather complete lists can be found in reviews by Hudlická (369, 370). The significance of an estimate of the number of capillaries in a muscle is limited as long as length and diameter of the vessel are unknown. However, capillary number in a cross section of a muscle fiber bundle can give information on several subjects of importance for the understanding of skeletal muscle capillary physiology.

GROWTH AND DEVELOPMENT. Postnatal growth of skeletal muscle is due to enlargement in both diameter and length of existing muscle fibers. This means that the capillaries surrounding the fibers are pushed apart, and the number of capillaries per square millimeter (density) decreases. The most detailed studies have been in growing rats, where capillary density and muscle fiber size in various muscles have been examined in rats weighing from 90 to over 600 g. Over this range of weights, the number of capillaries per square millimeter was lowered from 1,300 to 400–500 in the gastrocnemius and soleus muscles (584, 633, 634). A similar trend was found for the tibialis anterior muscle, but the absolute values were higher. The number of capillaries surrounding the fibers increases with enlarged muscle fiber size, with a concomitant increase in sharing factor. The reduction in capillary density is less, however, and the increase in capillaries surrounding the fibers is larger than could be anticipated from the growth of fiber size. This is due then to an increase in capillaries per fiber found with development. In the aforementioned muscles of the rat the number of capillaries per fiber increased from 1 to 2 (gastrocnemius) and 1 to 3 (soleus) (633, 634). Similar results are available for the chicken, where the number of capillaries per fiber is approximately 0.5 at birth and increases to 1–1.5 in the adult muscle (65).

In growing rats a very close relationship exists between body weight and muscle fiber size [r = 0.98 (633)]. Thus with enlargement of the body and a smaller metabolic rate per weight of the animal, skeletal muscle capillarization also goes down. This is in line with the old observations [for references, see Hudlická (369)] that small animals have a higher capillary count than larger species. A good illustration of this is found in the work by Schmidt-Neilsen and Pennycuik (617). They studied the masseter muscle from 10 species varying in weight from 9 g (bat) to 200–450 kg (pig, cattle). The number of capillaries per fiber was surprisingly similar (1–2.5) but the number of muscle fibers per square millimeter was around 2,000 in the bat and 500–1,000 in pigs and cattle, resulting in over 3,000 capillaries/mm^2 in the bat and fewer than 500 in the pig.

MUSCLE FIBER TYPES AND POTENTIAL FOR OXIDATIVE METABOLISM. Ranvier was the first to demonstrate a difference in red and white muscles in degree of capillarization (570). Since then quite a few studies have presented evidence in support of this early finding, but systematic studies on the subject are scarce. The explanation is that with injection techniques it is difficult to identify fiber types and their metabolic potential. Romanul (588), combining a stain for alkaline phosphatase to visualize capillaries in muscles from the rat, rabbit, and man with stains for mitochondrial enzymes, has made a plea for a very close coupling between the oxidative metabolic capacity of a fiber and the number of capillaries surrounding the fiber. Further, in studies with cross innervation of muscles the capillary count did change in relation to alteration in the oxidative capacity of the muscle fibers (590). He supports his contention with excellent micrographs, but no detailed mathematical treatment of the results is presented. Ample evidence is available, however, demonstrating differences in capillaries of ST and FT fibers (cf. Fig. 4). This appears to be true for both human and nonhuman species. In the medial gastrocnemius muscle of the guinea pig and the rabbit, the difference is not pronounced (473), but in the lateral head of the gastrocnemius muscle and tibialis anterior muscles of the rabbit, the difference is more substantial (633). This is not directly apparent from values of capillaries per square millimeter or per fiber. The size of the various fiber types also has to be taken into account, as ST fibers usually are smaller than FT fibers.

Gray and Renkin (285) found in their detailed study of muscles of the rabbit that the average capillary density was twice as high for ST as for FT fibers. On this particular topic a considerable amount of information is available on human muscle, as so many of the studies of capillaries in human muscle have utilized serial frozen sections where staining of the capillary basement membranes was done concurrently with evaluation of metabolic profile and muscle fiber type (5, 8, 11, 313, 326, 520, 523, 602). In mixed muscles such as the gastrocnemius, the number of capillaries surrounding a specific fiber type is between 3–4 for ST fibers and 2.5–3 for FT_a and 2–3 for FT_b fibers. Not until the fiber size is taken into account can a significant difference in capillarization of the various fiber types be established. In the untrained muscles studied the average area a capillary supplies is 20%–30% more for FT_b and 10%–20% more for FT_a than for ST fibers. The absolute values may vary markedly between individuals and also between muscles but the overall pattern is remarkably stable. What contributes to this rather small difference is the fact that in large parts of mixed muscle, FT fibers share capillaries with adjacent ST fibers. In locally homogeneous areas of mixed muscle where an individual muscle fiber is surrounded only by those of similar type, it was found that there are 1–4 capillaries per FT fiber but 4–11 capillaries per ST fiber (G. Sjøgaard, personal communication). Accounting for differences in fiber size, the ratio for the fiber-type area each capillary had to supply could be estimated to be in the order of 3:1 for ST and FT fibers, respectively. The value found in human muscle is not much different from similar calculations made by Renkin and co-workers (285, 575) on rabbit muscle. It must be reiterated, however, that such extreme differences are rarely seen in human muscles since especially FT (FT_b) fibers are seldom surrounded only by fibers of the same type.

The concept of a coupling between aerobic potential of the muscle and its capillary supply has been challenged by Maxwell and colleagues (482). They studied fiber composition, oxidative potential of whole muscle, and degree of capillarization of various skeletal muscles from five species and found no significant relation among any of the variables. This conflicts with a large number of other reports, but it must be pointed out that Maxwell et al. did find significant correlations among several of these variables within a species (482). The metabolic potential of a given muscle fiber type may vary considerably between species, and indeed may vary within a given animal. Thus the approach taken by Maxwell et al. may not be the most fruitful to elucidate the problem of a coupling between aerobic potential of a fiber and its capillary supply (482).

From among variables used to quantitate capillarization, the question of which serves as the best indicator of diffusing conditions is still unsettled. Based on a comparative study of various species, Plyley and Groom (561) have come to the conclusion that the number of capillaries per fiber is an appropriate measure, whereas others favor Krogh's concept of a capillary and its "diffusing" cylinder (6, 226, 295). Although it appears essential to include an estimate of diffusing distance, it is not immediately apparent whether the critical distance is to the center of the muscle fiber or to the most distant point between capillaries along the periphery of a fiber in cross section; the point being that mitochondrial density is largest underneath the sarcolemma with fewer mitochondria found centrally (364, 422). What adds to the importance of this question is that although it is commonly believed that the diffusion of oxygen is the key factor, there may be situations during exercise where substrate uptake, release of a metabolite, or heat dissipation is just as essential.

Capillary Length and Diameter

There are few detailed studies on capillary length and diameter for most species, and for man they are nonexistent. Thus available information on capillary surface area and volume in skeletal muscles is limited. In the early studies the capillaries were estimated to account for 10% or more of total muscle volume, which was much too high a value as could be deduced from measurements of total vascular volume (535). Pappenheimer et al. (536) estimated the values to be approximately 0.1 of those previously reported; i.e., capillary surface area was estimated to be 0.7 m^2/100 g muscle tissue and the volume 1.6%. Later studies have all given estimates of the same order of magnitude although there appears to be some variation related to species and muscles studied (111, 285, 492, 728).

The most direct measurements are obtained with vital microscopy. In the rabbit's tenuissimus muscle the diameter averages 5.4 μm and is slightly narrower at the arteriolar end of the capillary [4.7 μm (196)]. Cat tenuissimus muscle capillaries have the same diameter, whereas those of the dog gastrocnemius (4.2 μm) and rat extensor hallucis proprius (4.8 μm) are slightly smaller (477, 507). Length of muscle capillaries varies markedly in the same capillary bed, and by comparing various muscles and muscles in various species figures between 100 μm and 2,000 μm have been reported (196, 507, 509). Assuming a length of 1,000 μm for mean capillary length in human muscle and a mean diameter of 6 μm (slightly less than the mean diameter of a red blood cell), this will give a capillary surface area of 0.62 cm^2/cm^2 muscle in a muscle with 330 capillaries/mm^2. In muscles with predominantly FT fibers this value may be slightly less and in muscle with many ST fibers somewhat higher. Based on the same assumptions capillary volume in human skeletal muscle is around 1%.

In these estimations of capillary surface area and volume it is usually assumed that the capillaries are straight, as the most precise numbers for length and diameter of the capillaries are obtained on thin and flat muscles. The capillaries may have a rather tortuous arrangment, especially in muscles with many ST fibers. Thus an underestimation of the true surface area and volume of the capillaries is likely in these muscles. All of these estimates concern the total number of capillaries in a muscle, only a small fraction of which may be exposed to circulating blood at any given time.

Use and Disuse

CAPILLARY DENSITY. Long before systematic studies of the effect of training on skeletal muscle capillarization were performed, it was noted that the domesticated animal held in sheds or cages had fewer skeletal muscle capillaries than its counterpart living in the wild (65, 710). Early training studies on rats also revealed a pronounced increase in the number of skeletal muscle capillaries, although the significance of some of these early reports can be questioned as exceptionally high capillary counts were observed. No doubt exists, however, that there is a true proliferation of capillaries associated with an enhanced physical activity level in these nonhuman species (for references, see ref. 370). Further, the adaptation is a local response, i.e., it occurs in the exercised muscle and only around those muscle fibers that are recruited in the training schedule.

For a long time comparable data were not available in man. In the first systematic study, cross-sectional material of sedentary men and endurance athletes was examined, and the same number of capillaries per fiber was observed in both groups (342). Further, in a study where the physical activity level was varied, no significant changes in any of the variables to stimulate capillarization could be detected (601). In both of these studies electron microscopy was used to identify the capillaries. Judged by the low numbers of capillaries per fiber reported by these investigators, all capillaries may not have been identified.

More recent studies using both electron microscopy and histochemistry have demonstrated that human skeletal muscle adapts to use by increasing the number of capillaries (6, 73, 385, 387, 402, 521, 523). In fact all variables (capillaries per fiber, capillaries per square millimeter, and number of capillaries found around a fiber) are increased. As the latter two variables also are a function of muscle fiber size, the variable most frequently used is capillaries per fiber. This indicator of capillarization is in trained muscle closely linked to whole-body maximal oxygen uptake of a subject (Fig. 25), and alteration in activity level causing a change in maximal oxygen uptake results in a parallel change in the number of capillaries per fiber. From such plots it is apparent that the percentage changes of these two variables are comparable. A doubling of maximal oxygen uptake corresponds approximately to a doubling of the number of capillaries per fiber. Including the size of the fibers in the evaluation of diffusing conditions of skeletal muscle with training makes the picture somewhat more complex but also gives a deeper insight into the problems. In most training studies of the endurance type, skeletal muscle fibers are slightly enlarged. If in the exercise all fiber types are involved, both the number of capillaries around the various fiber types and the size of the fibers are increased (6, 402, 523). However, the increase in capillaries is larger than the increase in fiber size resulting in a definite reduction in the fiber-type area each capillary has to supply (Fig. 26). The present reduction in diffusing area is found to be largest for FT (FT_b) fibers. This is quite similar to the observation for the activity of mitochondrial enzymes. In untrained muscles FT (FT_b) fibers have the largest fiber area per capillary and the lowest level of oxidative capacity, but with use these fibers adapt and become almost indistinguishable from ST fibers for these variables. This supports the concept of Romanul and others (569, 588, 590) that there is a close coupling between the number of capillaries and the capacity for oxidative metabolism of the fibers they supply. Further, in experiments where the time course for changes has been followed in rat and rabbit muscle during chronic stimulation, it appears as if the capillaries begin to proliferate before changes can be noted in the oxidative enzymes. Just as importantly, it proves that the FT fibers have the ability to adapt to aerobic metabolism, which is similar to the metabolism of ST fibers.

In the experiments with chronic stimulation of a muscle it was found that along with enhanced aerobic potential of the muscle fibers and increased number of capillaries adjacent to a fiber, the fibers also became slightly smaller, thereby contributing to the shortening of diffusing distances in the muscle (134, 135). Also, with endurance-type training in animals as in standard-bred horses and rats, the mean muscle fiber area is reduced in trained muscles [(110, 204); unpublished observations by P. Henckel on horses]. This reduction is mainly a function of smaller FT (FG and FOG) fibers. Similar findings from man are available. In well-trained endurance swimmers, mean muscle fiber area was the smallest in the most trained muscles (523), and in marathon runners the areas of muscle fibers in the gastrocnemius muscle were also small (367). Further, 2 wk of no training caused the muscle fibers of the gastrocnemius to become slightly larger (367). These findings may support the notion that the distance to the center of the muscle cell is a critical factor. Whether it is the transport of gas or substrate that is crucial is, however, still obscure. Because myoglobin markedly enhances the oxygen transport within the cell (724) and is elevated with enhanced oxidative capacity, the reduction in diffusing distances of substrates other than oxygen may be the crucial limiting factor.

The effect of inactivity on muscle capillarization is less well studied in man (Fig. 26). The picture that emerges from available detraining studies or studies where a limb is placed in a cast is that the number of capillaries per fiber is reduced. Notably it appears as if early in the time course the reduction in the number of capillaries is slightly slower than a possible change in fiber size, resulting in slightly shorter diffusing distances the 1st wk of inactivity (605). After some

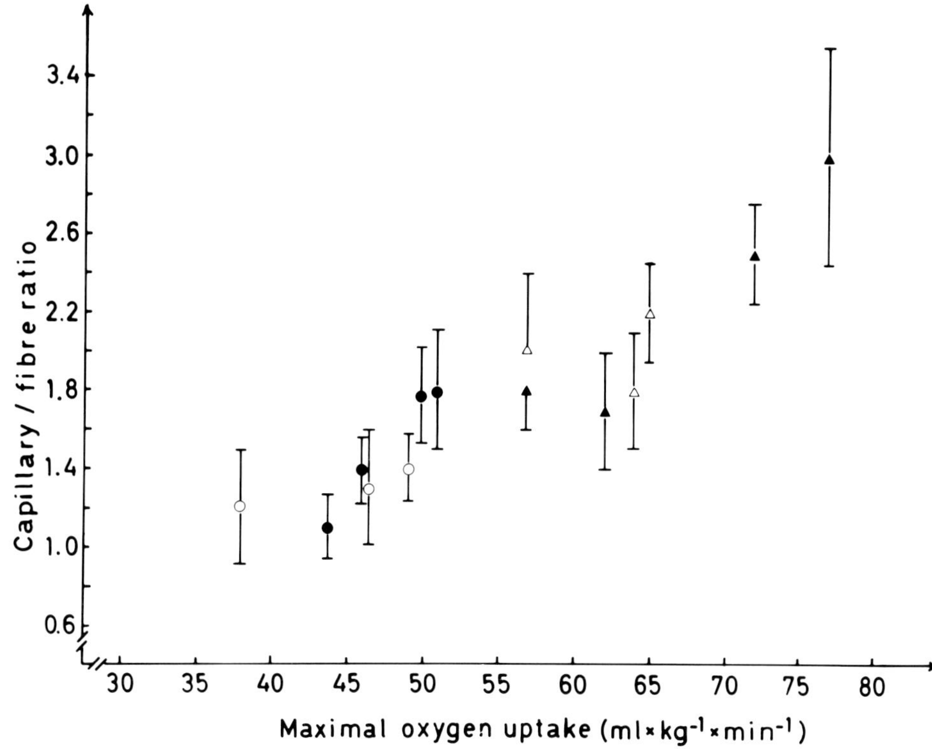

FIG. 25. Capillaries per muscle fiber related to maximal oxygen uptake. Diagram includes mean values obtained from the following: PAS method, light microscopy (PAS + LM) studies, *open symbols* (5, 6, 521, 523), and electron microscopy (EM) studies, *closed symbols* (73, 385–387). *Circles*, females; *triangles*, males. $P = 0.001$; $r = 0.917$. [From E. Nygard and H. Schmalbruch, unpublished observations.]

weeks both variables approach a new level of adaptation (425). With tenotomy, reduction in capillary density has also been observed (411, 412).

CAPILLARY LENGTH AND DIAMETER. The only exact data available are from studies on rats and rabbits, where muscles have been chronically stimulated and evaluated with vital microscopy (509). Along with a quite rapid proliferation of capillaries, which is noticeable within days, there is a reduction in mean capillary length. The increase in number of capillaries is larger than the decrease in length. The capillary surface area and volume do enlarge with increased use of the muscle. Further, the diameter of the capillaries is increased and may amount to 1 μm in the arteriolar end and 2.3 μm in the venular end of the capillary.

In addition to increased branching, as a result of more muscle activity the capillaries may become more tortuous (13). Precise data on this point are not available, however.

MYOGLOBIN. The redness of a muscle fiber depends on its myoglobin content, and for a long time this has been the basis for classifying muscle fibers. The oxidative capacity of the muscle fiber and its myoglobin content are closely coupled in a large range of animal species (448–450). With physical training in rats myoglobin content is increased parallel to the enhancement of the aerobic enzymes (537). Further, an increase is only observed in muscles engaged in the training program. Studies on human muscles are scarce. In preliminary reports by Jansson and Sylvén (400) a clear-cut difference was observed when ST and FT fibers were compared, with the mean value for ST fibers being 60% higher than for the FT fibers. So far, however, they have been unable to detect a training effect, i.e., when examining cross-sectional material of trained bicyclists with sedentary people, the same myoglobin content is noted in the leg muscles although a difference in mitochondrial enzyme is noted (E. Jansson, personal communication).

Regulation

Little is known about the factors involved in capillary proliferation. Myrhage and Hudlická (509) cite Ashton (20) saying that "endothelial cells themselves are in some way directly sensitive to oxygen—multiplying at low O_2 levels, resting at normal O_2 levels, and dying at high O_2 concentrations." They base this belief in tissue partial pressure of O_2 (P_{O_2}) being the crucial variable on the same reports of high capillary counts in skeletal muscle of animals living at or exposed to high altitude (14, 112, 699). Other studies have revealed that it is questionable whether any new capil-

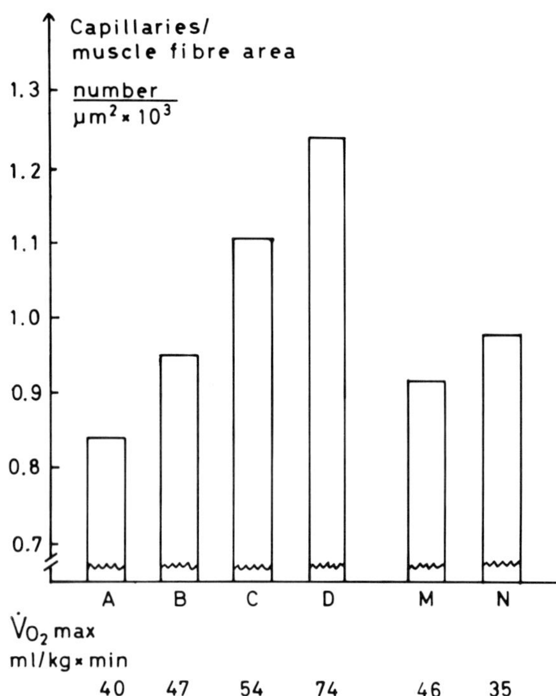

FIG. 26. Mean values for number of capillaries per 1,000 μm^2 of muscle fiber area. *Bar A* shows results from a group of sedentary subjects (602). *Bars B* and *C* show values before and after 8 wk of conditioning (6, 425). *Bar D* shows values from well-trained men (367, 398, 523, 602). *Bars M* and *N* are values from subjects deconditioned for 7–14 days (ref. 425; B. Saltin, unpublished observations). $\dot{V}O_{2\,max}$ below *bars M* and *N* was estimated from heart rate response to submaximal exercise (subjects were recovering from minor knee injury).

laries are formed when exposed to low oxygen pressure in inspired air. Systematic studies in various species by Banchero and associates (30, 164, 631, 632, 635) clearly demonstrate that the larger number of capillaries per square millimeter is due to the decrease in the cross-sectional size of the muscle fibers. The number of capillaries per fiber is unchanged in their studies. The same appears to be true for human muscle (604). When sea-level residents stay at high altitude (elevation 3,700 m) for months, the muscle fibers become slightly smaller but the number of capillaries per fiber is unchanged (Fig. 27). Further, permanent residents at this altitude do not have a high number of capillaries per fiber, but they have small muscle fibers resulting in high values for capillaries per square millimeter. When the high-altitude residents are divided into physically inactive and physically active, the latter group has the higher number of capillaries per fiber, similar to the results found in sea-level residents. Thus it appears likely that tissue oxygen tension is not the key factor for capillary proliferation.

Unfortunately no other obvious alternative for a stimulus and regulatory factor has been suggested. In tissue injury some substance is thought to be released, serving as a stimulus for capillary proliferation (68); but with increased use of a muscle, no signs of tissue damage or inflammation are observed (509). Because sprouting capillaries are most frequently found branching off where the capillary is bent and its diameter widens (509), the pressure in the capillaries both at arteriolar and venular ends may serve as stimulus for proliferation. This hypothesis is, however, not experimentally tested.

SIGNIFICANCE OF ADAPTATION

In this section we analyze what the specific role may be for the adaptations that occur in skeletal muscle as a result of changes in patterns of use and disuse. More specifically the focus is on how these may alter metabolism and performance. A schematic overview of the varying systems and the interaction between them is given in Figure 28. We briefly sum up the possibilities that exist for each of the essential adaptations under study and discuss their contribution to a change in the metabolic response to exercise. Further, we evaluate whether such a change would aid in explaining a change in performance capacity. Finally, we feel that it is equally important to discuss why certain adaptations do not occur in spite of the fact that at first glance they would appear likely and beneficial.

Muscular Size

The capacity of skeletal muscle to develop tension per unit of cross-sectional area is not altered by training. At the molecular level this implies that the tension developed per cross-bridge interaction is constant. This is what could be anticipated. A large variation does exist in the number of fibers contained in the same muscle of man and rat. This is probably a function of genetic endowment and a likely factor in limiting the maximal growth potential of a muscle. As fiber number is uninfluenced by the activity level, the only resource available for increasing total muscular strength is for the muscles to increase in cross-sectional area (427). This is accomplished by a hypertrophy of the existing muscle fibers. It may appear that it would be just as logical to have mechanisms for increasing the number of fibers in a muscle rather than restricting the number of those present either at or shortly after birth. There are, however, a number of arguments against the efficacy of adding fibers to preexisting muscles. First, this could disturb the existing architecture in the muscle by having to provide for new attachments on the bone or tendons that serve as origin and insertions. If the fibers arose within the muscle without appropriate attachments they would be ineffective (506). Second, and perhaps of greater importance, is the problem of how they would be innervated and incorporated into preexisting motor units. A lateral sprouting of the existing motor units might also result in reducing the capacity for neuromuscular coordination.

Although the capacity for skeletal muscle to enlarge appears to be great, there may not always be a direct

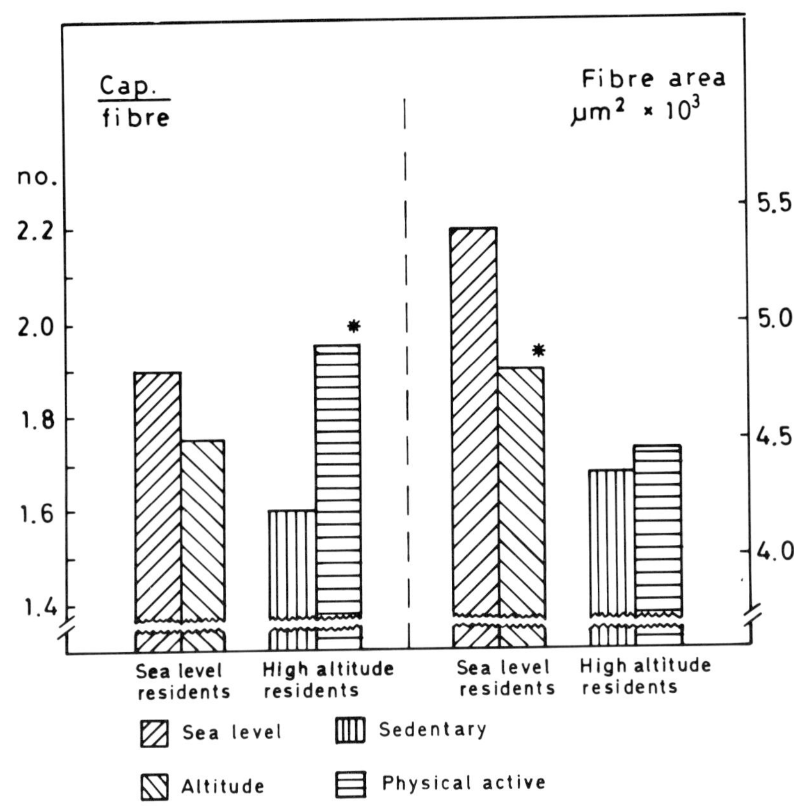

FIG. 27. Capillaries per fiber and fiber area in sea-level residents at sea level and after an average 32 wk (6–52 wk) at elevation 3,500 m and in high-altitude residents. For further details see Fig. 23. [Adapted from Saltin et al. (604).]

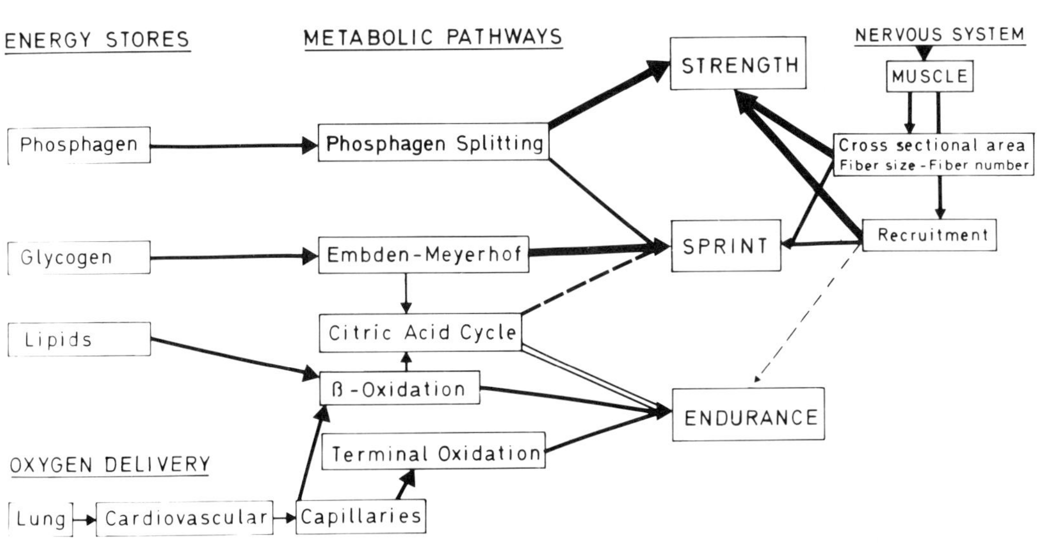

FIG. 28. A schematic summary with indication of relative importance of various energy stores and metabolic pathways for performance in strength, sprint, and endurance events. Included in the scheme are also indications of how oxygen delivery and the nervous system are interacting.

relationship between the degree of enlargement and the torque that a muscle can develop around a joint. This is because for muscles with pennate fiber arrangements the angle of attachment to the tendon becomes greater as they are enlarged (57, 490). Since the force developed along the long axis of the muscle depends on the angle of attachment, this change in angle will result in a diminution in the tension transferred to the tendon. A mathematical model illustrating this principle was published by Lindhard (456). Although increases in strength can be closely related to changes in the total cross-sectional area of a muscle, there are many reports of increases in muscular strength without changes in muscle bulk. This can be explained on the basis of an increased capacity for motor unit recruitment and activation.

Substrate Stores

The resting levels of ATP and CP in skeletal muscle of man are in the range of 5 and 20 mol/kg wet wt, respectively, and these stores are influenced by the state of training only to a very minor extent. The amount of energy contained in the phosphagen stores is very small and would only support 3–4 s of maximal contractile activity. With a few exceptions even a doubling of these stores would have little physiological meaning. Instead it would be more judicious to enlarge the capacity for resynthesizing ATP through an increased capacity for energy release via end-terminal oxidation and/or glycolysis.

That the energy per unit of weight in ATP and CP is quite small supports such a conclusion. Further, by keeping the ATP-ADP-AMP pool low in muscle, any changes among these components result in a large change in their ratio, which is important in view of the regulatory function this ADP/ATP ratio has on the metabolic reactions both in the cytosol and in the mitochondria.

The glycogen stores of the muscle are only slightly elevated as a result of changed activity level. Any specific role of this increase for brief exhaustive exercise, where muscle lactate reaches levels of 20–25 mmol/kg wet wt, can hardly be anticipated, as muscle of sedentary man already contains approximately 80 mmol/kg wet wt of glycogen. In repeated efforts a high initial glycogen storage may be of some importance.

The question can then be asked, how important are changes in the intramuscular energy stores in terms of the capacity for aerobic energy production? This can be considered from two standpoints. First, how would an augmentation of the local energy reserves relate to the maximal work capacity of a muscle if this were the only source of substrate? The aerobic capacity of skeletal muscle is a function of the maximal flux of substrates through the oxidative systems of the mitochondria and the supply of oxygen. The maximal substrate flux through the metabolic pathways can be estimated from the V_{max} of selected enzymes (see Table 1). From such data it can be estimated that the maximal substrate flux through the oxidative enzymes would require an oxygen uptake of about 850 $ml \cdot kg^{-1} \cdot min^{-1}$ and a blood flow of about 5 $liter \cdot kg^{-1} \cdot min^{-1}$ (based on an oxygen extraction of 170 ml/liter of blood). If this oxygen uptake can be attained by man it is only with exercise of a small muscle group (1). With exercise (such as walking, running, or cycling) that is sustainable for 8–10 min, the oxygen consumption may average about 150 ml/kg of active muscle per minute. When the exercise intensity is about one-half that sustainable for 8–10 min, it can be performed for many hours. If fully oxidized, the glycogen and triglyceride stores of human muscle are equal to about 200 and 80 kJ/kg wet wt, respectively. At the maximal rate of oxidation with a small muscle group, the local energy stores would last 17–18 min. Such efforts, however, cannot be sustained for this period of time, and factors other than the local availability of substrate must be limiting. Thus it would appear that augmenting the local energy stores, whether this be as glycogen or triglyceride, would be of little importance for maximal efforts. With short, intense exercise there is a rapid depletion of glycogen from the FT fibers in skeletal muscle. A failure to sustain multiple bouts of such exercise may be related to an exhaustion of the local glycogen in the FT fibers. An elevation in the glycogen stores could forestall exhaustion in such activities.

A second aspect of the importance of changes in intramuscular energy stores relates to submaximal exercise. As indicated, the exercise capacity of man at power outputs of about 50% of maximal is several hours. The immediate energy stores of muscle are sufficient for up to 200 min of such exercise. Thus it is obvious that extramuscular substrates also are important. This has been demonstrated in experiments where mobilization of fats has been inhibited. At exhaustion the carbohydrate stores of the body are nearly depleted (341), and the importance of this energy store as a determinant of exercise capacity has been demonstrated (51, 222, 260, 577, 725). Consumption of a fat and protein diet decreases exercise tolerance by about 25%, whereas exercise capacity was doubled following consumption of a high-carbohydrate diet (51, 271). Subsequent experiments have established that these dietary manipulations alter the glycogen store of the muscle and that a linear relationship existed between exercise capacity and the muscle glycogen concentration (51). The role of stored triglyceride is unknown. It is, however, well known that increases in the local glycogen store can increase exercise capacity. This is even more important when coupled with the increased oxidation of fat that occurs with training.

Enzyme Activities

ANAEROBIC METABOLISM. There are reports of increases in the activities of some enzymes in the glycolytic pathway. In some instances these changes are small and appear to exist in only select enzymes of the system. Moreover in some cases the enzymes that have been reported to increase are not those whose activity is known to be regulated (PHOS, PFK) and which thus exert control over the flux of substrate through the system. Overall the data available concerning adaptations in the glycolytic system are less certain than those for the enzymes for end-terminal oxidation.

An increase in the enzymes for glycolysis has an unknown role in the overall economy of the metabolic response to exercise. All fiber types are very well endowed with such enzymes. For example, the PFK activity of the ST and FT fibers of human muscle has been reported to be 25 and 50 $mmol \cdot kg^{-1} \cdot min^{-1}$ (203).

This enzyme usually has an activity similar to that of PHOS. Both enzymes are regulated and are generally believed to regulate the flow of substrate through the glycolytic pathway. If fully activated this would result in the production of 50 and 100 mmol lactate·kg^{-1}·min^{-1} for the ST and FT fiber, respectively. These values far exceed those that have been observed during maximal voluntary muscular activity. It has been estimated that a 5% activation of PHOS could account for the maximal lactate production in skeletal muscle if glycolysis depended on PHOS (220). Further augmentation of this system would not seem useful. Moreover it does not appear that increasing the total amount of enzyme available would increase the precision for regulating substrate flux through the system.

As pointed out, the concentration (activities) of the enzymes of the Embden-Meyerhof pathway is very high in most skeletal muscle, particularly in the FT fibers. This activity would appear to be greater than that which would ever be required for the degradation of glycogen. This brings up the question of why these enzymes are maintained at such high levels. This metabolic pathway would be most important during periods of short, intense muscular activity where a major part of the ATP production was derived from the degradation of glycogen to lactate. During such activity lactate concentrations in muscle and blood in excess of 20 mM are frequently attained (265). It has been suggested that such high lactate concentrations would interfere with subsequent efforts, either by lowered pH or by end-product inhibition of enzymes (417). The low pH could affect the oxidative system and the glycolytic pathway. If so, attempts at repeating high-intensity efforts would be characterized by a reduced exercise tolerance, a decrease in the $\dot{V}o_{2\,max}$, and a decline in total lactate production. With such repeated efforts $\dot{V}o_{2\,max}$ is reached earlier, however, and there is a continued elevation in the blood lactate. This suggests that lactate per se is not responsible for terminating the exercise, nor are the enzymes for metabolism significantly inhibited.

The question of whether the lactate levels as seen in the blood and muscle of man after short, high-intensity exercise could inhibit a further degradation of glycogen can also be asked. Some information relating to this possibility may come from studies of diving mammals. The glycolytic enzyme levels in these animals are not conspicuously different from those of man (432). When these animals dive there is an almost complete shunting of the blood from the peripheral muscles to the heart, lung, and brain circuit. The exercising muscles may be nearly ischemic. Muscular activity can continue for rather long periods of time under these conditions. After such exercise the muscle lactate may exceed 50 mmol/kg. This suggests that an end-product inhibition of the glycolytic pathway probably does not occur or is of only minor importance in those animals.

The question remains as to why the very high concentrations of enzymes exist in the glycolytic pathway. These levels are obviously higher than would be required to produce the substrate flux that occurs through this pathway. It would appear that the answer lies in the overall regulation of this system. There are rate-limiting enzymes in this pathway. However, most of the enzymes are of the equilibrium type and obey Michaelis-Menten kinetics and thus are substrate controlled (Fig. 29). With such enzymes the higher the enzyme concentration the greater will be the activity at very low substrate concentrations. This allows for a better control over the system. For example, with an enzyme such as pyruvate kinase the activity of which is about 400 μmol of substrate converted per gram per minute, it is highly unlikely that a substrate concentration could ever be reached to produce V_{max}. However, a low substrate concentration, for example, 10% of the K_m, would induce an activity of about 40 μmol of substrate split per minute per gram. This activity is higher than that required for the maximal rates of lactate production that occur during heavy exercise. With high enzyme levels it is possible to attain high rates of substrate fluxes at low substrate concentrations. Since there are a number of enzymes involved in the pathways for ATP production, the induction of high activities via elevations in substrate levels would

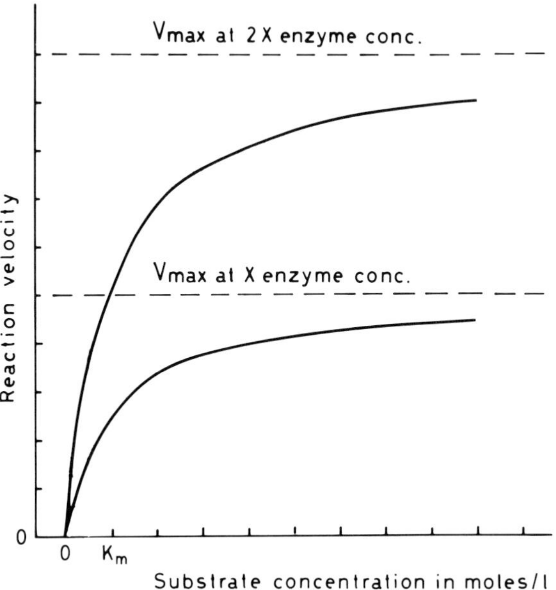

FIG. 29. A representation of the influence of changing the total enzyme concentration on the specific activity based on the rate (V_r). The velocity and any substrate concentration [S] can be estimated from the Michaelis constant (K_m) and the maximal velocity (V_{max}) for the equation $V_r = \frac{[S]}{K_m + [S]} \cdot V_{max}$. With a doubling of enzyme concentration, velocity of the reaction will be doubled at any substrate concentration. This relationship would be most important at low substrate concentrations where substrate could thereby be more efficiently directed into end-terminal oxidative pathways. Conversely with a reduction in enzyme concentration such control would be lost. [From Gollnick and Saltin (256).]

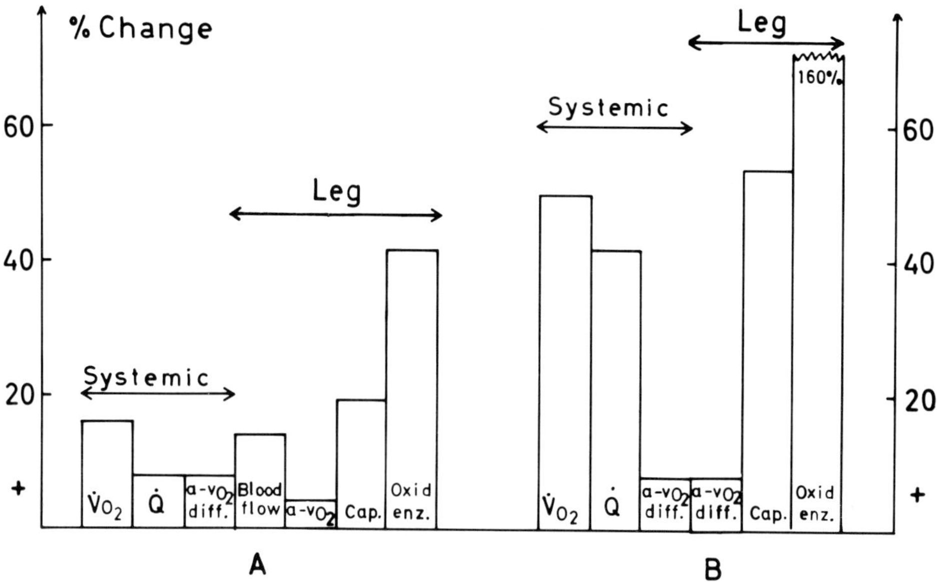

FIG. 30. Summary of changes associated with a moderate (*panel A*) and a large (*panel B*) increase in $\dot{V}O_{2\,max}$ in response to physical conditioning. *A*: from longitudinal studies in which sedentary subjects were conditioned for 2–3 mo. *B*: (also longitudinal studies) subjects participated either in a conditioning program for 2–3 yr starting from a sedentary level [$\dot{V}O_{2\,max}$ 45 ml·kg^{-1}·min^{-1} (184)] or in an intense conditioning program for some months starting from very low $\dot{V}O_{2\,max}$ [34 ml O_2·kg^{-1}·min^{-1} (601)]. [*A*: circulatory data: (184, 594, 601). Leg blood flow and arteriovenous O_2 differences are collected from several studies: (408, 603, 711) and B. Saltin, unpublished observations. Muscle data: (338) for enzymes, (8) for capillaries. *B*: central circulatory data: (184, 601). Leg arteriovenous O_2 differences: (601); muscle capillarization and enzyme data are from unpublished studies by B. Saltin, J. Halkjær-Kristensen, and T. Ingemann-Hansen.]

increase the particle level to a point where the osmotic pressure within the cell would be unacceptable.

AEROBIC METABOLISM. In addition to substrate levels and mitochondrial enzymes, the role of oxygen delivery is important for a discussion of the aerobic energy yield in muscle. To thoroughly discuss this subject we need to summarize some of the adaptations that occur within the cardiovascular system as a response to varied levels of physical activity. From the results in Figure 30 it is apparent that at maximal exercise (running or bicycling) that elicits maximal oxygen uptake both systemic cardiac output and a widening of the arteriovenous difference contribute to the improved maximal oxygen uptake. After a short period of adaptation to endurance training these two factors increase to the same extent. After a longer period of training, enlargement of the cardiac output contributes the most to the increased maximal oxygen uptake. Muscle capillary density and mitochondrial enzyme activities are enhanced both after shorter and longer periods of adaptation. The percentage increase in capillarization occurs in parallel with maximal oxygen uptake, whereas the increase in mitochondrial enzyme potential is far in excess. The question then is whether these changes in the muscle are necessary to increase maximal oxygen uptake. Since close relationships exist among the degrees of capillarization, the activity of a marker enzyme for oxidative capacity, and maximal oxygen uptake in experimental material with large variations in training studies, many researchers use it as a criterion to illustrate the importance of these variables in attaining maximal oxygen uptake.

It is true that many links in the transport of oxygen to the tissues are closely related, but this does not mean that they are limiting (63, 636). Exercise with a single muscle group, such as the knee extensor muscles, illustrates this problem. In a sedentary person blood flow to these muscles at maximal exercise may average 2,000–3,000 ml·kg^{-1} of muscle·min^{-1}, $\dot{V}O_2$ may attain values of 400–500 ml O_2·kg^{-1} of muscle·min^{-1}, while the arterial-femoral venous oxygen difference is maintained at around 160–180 ml/liter (1). Thus when the capacity of the cardiovascular system can be diverted to a small, maximally activated muscle mass, considerably larger blood flow and oxygen uptake (milliliter per kilogram of active muscle) are observed than in ordinary whole-body exercise when systemic cardiac output is shared by a much larger muscle mass. Although blood flow through the knee extensors is tremendous, an extremely wide arterial-femoral venous oxygen difference is maintained. Taken in total, we conclude from these results that neither the capillarization of the muscle nor the concentration of mitochondrial enzymes are limiting to whole-body aerobic power in healthy man.

If we cannot ascribe any significant role to the adaptation in capillarization or mitochondrial enzyme concentrations for attainment of maximal oxygen uptake, why do these variables change so dramatically in response to physical training? An obvious effect of increasing the number of capillaries, and also the observed small decrease in the size of the muscle fibers with extreme endurance training, would be to reduce the diffusion distances within the muscle. This may be crucial for gas and substrate transport, especially FFA, from the blood to the muscle cell.

In the trained state the number and volume of mitochondria increase, which increases the surface area for the exchange of metabolites, cofactors, and end products between the cytosol and the mitochondrial matrix. Of particular interest here might be an increased capacity for the transport of fatty acids into the mitochondria and the ATP out into the cytosol. This could in part be responsible for the increased use of FFA, the decreased rate of glycogen depletion, and the lower lactate levels that occur in response to a standard exercise test after training. These differences occur despite lack of change in oxygen uptake and cardiac output at standard work loads before and after training.

A possible effect of increasing the activities of oxidative enzyme in muscle would be to elevate the capacity for the low oxidative fibers for terminal oxidation. Thus the FT fibers, and particularly the FT_b fibers, could more effectively utilize the intracellular glycogen stores and perhaps rely to a greater extent on the oxidation of FFA during prolonged exercise. This would be important where such fibers ultimately are recruited during prolonged exercise, and during more intense exercise, where there may be engagement of these motor units from onset of exercise.

Although the above considerations might be important for the understanding of the overall metabolism of skeletal muscle during exercise, they fail to adequately explain why there is such a large increase in the oxidative capacity. The answer to this question could be related to how enzyme concentration influences the sensitivity of enzyme regulation. Thus with higher enzyme concentrations it would be easier to regulate the oxidative system on the basis of a substrate and cofactor regulation of the enzymes. This effect would be important for both the nonrate-limiting and the rate-limiting enzyme reactions. The underlying principle is that most enzyme reactions appear to obey Michaelis-Menten kinetics (256). Under these conditions increases in substrate exert profound control over the reaction rate at the lower levels of substrate (Fig. 29). The substrate concentration that produces 50% of the V_{max} is the well-known Michaelis constant (K_m). This figure illustrates that by doubling the enzyme concentration the reaction velocity at K_m will also be doubled. This is true since K_m is independent of enzyme concentration. Further, at very low substrate levels large differences in the reaction rate in response to a given substrate concentration would be realized by increases in total enzyme content. Since the substrate levels needed to attain V_{max} for a given enzyme are probably never attained in vivo, the absolute V_{max} for a given enzyme is probably of minor importance, and most enzymes function at most at about 50% of the V_{max} or near the K_m in the intact system. Another illustration of this concept is that to elicit an increase in the enzyme velocity from 10% to 90% of the V_{max} requires an 81-fold increase in substrate concentration. Such a flooding of the tissue with any metabolite is extremely unlikely. However, an elevation in the total enzyme concentration would increase the sensitivity for control at low substrate levels and also increase total activity. This could result in a more efficient use of the substrate stores by directing them through the oxidative pathways with the result being to maintain a constant ADP/ATP ratio in the cytoplasm thereby inhibiting anaerobic glycolysis at the level of PFK. Such a fine tuning of the control of oxidative metabolism could be responsible for the lower respiratory exchange ratio and lactate levels in muscle and blood that occur during exercise after training. Conversely a decrease in physical activity with a resultant loss of oxidative capacity would have an opposite effect on metabolic control.

Could the increase in the enzymes for oxidation be operative in controlling the entry of substrates into the citric acid cycle? The key enzyme for such substrate entry is thought to be citrate synthase (722). The activity of this enzyme increases with endurance training; it is also regulated by the levels of both acetyl-CoA and oxaloacetate (722). This is not to imply that substrate flux through the citric acid cycle is under such simplistic control but only to point out that an increased enzyme concentration would facilitate this control. It is known, for example, that the flux of substrate through the citric acid cycle is a function of the coordinated control of citrate synthase, isocitrate dehydrogenase, and α-ketoglutarate dehydrogenase (722). These activities are linked not only to oxaloacetate and acetyl-CoA concentrations, but also to the NAD/NADH ratio and citrate levels. When the NADH level in the mitochondria is high, due either to a lack of oxygen or to ADP, isocitrate dehydrogenase is inhibited and citrate accumulates. Such an elevation of citrate concentration results in an increase in the K_m of citrate synthase. With the oxidation of NADH the citrate level will fall and the K_m of citrate synthase will be lowered. The increased enzyme concentration would aid in the directing of acetyl-CoA units derived either from decarboxylation of pyruvate or β-oxidation into the citric acid cycle. Since most of the enzymes of the citric acid cycle have been shown to increase in skeletal muscle in response to training, the overall effect would be to increase the response of this system to lower substrate levels.

The question can be asked, why would an organism adapt to an increased metabolic demand by increasing the level of proteins that would require energy for synthesis and maintenance rather than by simply storing more intramuscular substrates? In the latter instance it might be possible to raise the metabolite levels during periods of maximal activity to attain close to V_{max} of the enzymes. Part of this answer lies in the fact that the substrate levels needed to attain V_{max} of the enzymes are unreasonably high and might cause an increase in osmolality. In such a case this could be complicated because the intramitochondrial and cytoplasmic metabolic reactions may occur at different rates. Just as important is the possibility that glycogen, although it contains rather large amounts of energy per unit weight, will create a weight disturbance because it is stored with 2–3 g of water per gram of glycogen. Migrating birds and insects have a metabolism almost completely geared to fat metabolism (719). It is likely that in terrestrial animals the overall economy of movement calls for limitation in the storage of glycogen.

The stores of lipids in human skeletal muscle are rather small and no changes due to increased physical activity levels are apparent. Why this energy source is kept so low in the muscles of man and rodents is presently unknown. Instead, especially in man the extramuscular lipid stores are high and would, in individuals of normal body weight, support many hours, in fact days, of submaximal exercise.

In contrast, glycogen is stored only in small amounts outside the skeletal muscles, the total in the liver being only 40–70 g (373). The primary purpose of this glycogen store is to maintain blood glucose concentration as a continuous supply to the nervous system. Its role for muscle is limited. In fact at least two regulatory mechanisms are brought into play during exercise to minimize its uptake by skeletal muscle. These are a reduction in plasma insulin levels and an elevation in the intracellular concentration of glucose 6-PO_4, which inhibits hexokinase and the phosphorylation of glucose needed for its transport across the cell membrane.

Summary

The stage is then set. In submaximal exercise with limited amounts of glycogen (also after dietary manipulation) and with the predominant fraction of the lipids stored outside the muscle cell, the ultimate factor that determines the intensity and duration of work is the body's capacity to utilize extramuscular fat stores. There are at least five steps required for the transport of FFA from the adipocytes to the skeletal muscles, where the lipids are being finally oxidized in the mitochondria. These are *1)* the release from the fat cell, *2)* transport to the muscle via the blood, *3)* transport from the capillary across the interstitial space to the muscle cell, *4)* transport into the muscle and mitochondria, and *5)* oxidation by the mitochondria. Both in the untrained and in the trained state the mobilization of lipids appears to be sufficient, and the exercising muscles are offered ample amounts of FFA. Only a very small percentage (3%–5%) of the FFA that is offered by the blood is taken up by the muscle (258, 269). This is also true in situations lacking all other substrates, indicating that the limitations in the utilization of FFA lie either within the muscle or in the transport of the FFA from the blood into the muscle cell (510, 591). There may be a larger FFA uptake by trained muscle but if this is so, it is within the methodological variation and thus has not been substantiated (332, 333). It is not known which of the three remaining possibilities for limiting the uptake of FFA by skeletal muscle is the most important. Presently, it appears that the transport of FFA through the interstitial space with its low protein concentration may constitute the major hindrance. For obvious reasons (colloid osmotic pressure and hydrostatic pressure balance over the capillary wall) interstitial protein concentration cannot be elevated. With training, adaptations take place on both sides of this hindrance, by increasing the number of capillaries and by elevations in mitochondrial volume and the capacity for β-oxidation. The importance of these adaptations is illustrated in Figure 31, which shows that when subjects who have trained one leg exercise using both, the

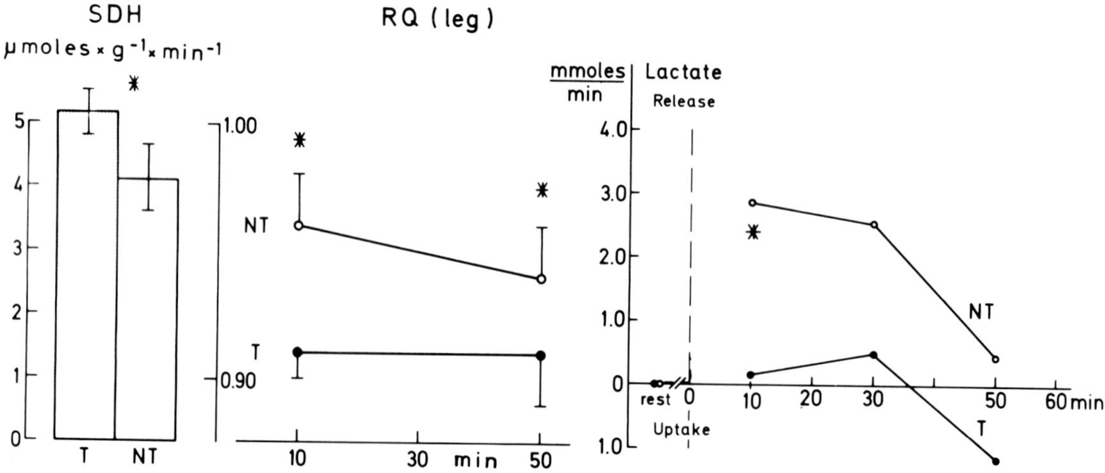

FIG. 31. Succinate dehydrogenase activity (μmol·g^{-1} wet wt·min^{-1}) in trained (T) and nontrained (NT) leg (*left*), respiratory quotient (RQ) values (*middle*), and release/uptake of lactate (*right*) for both legs during a posttraining metabolic study. Means ± SE are given. * Significant difference between trained and nontrained leg ($P < 0.05$). [Adapted from Henriksson (332).]

utilization of FFA is greater and the production of lactate less by the trained leg in spite of the fact that both legs were offered similar amounts of oxygen and FFA. Of note is that the increase in mitochondrial protein is maintained as long as the training stimulus persists. After termination of training the "excessive" metabolic apparatus is rapidly disassembled and the muscle returns to the nontrained state.

Part of the answer to why increases occur in total oxidative capacity rather than in substrate storage with training may lie in the fact that the total protein needed to produce a doubling of mitochondria and the oxidative enzymes is relatively small, amounting to only a few milligrams per gram fresh weight. Such an increase appears to add very little to the overall bulk of the muscle and to produce no measurable disturbance of the ionic and osmotic balance.

REFERENCES

1. ADAMS, R. P., P. ANDERSEN, G. SJØGAARD, A. THORBOE, AND B. SALTIN. Knee-extension as a model for the study of isolated exercising muscle in man (Abstract). *Med. Sci. Sports Exerc.* 13: 99, 1981.
2. AHERNE, W., D. R. AYYAR, P. A. CLARKE, AND J. N. WALTON. Muscle fibre size in normal infants, children and adolescents. *J. Neurol. Sci.* 14: 171–182, 1971.
3. ALLBROOK, D. B., M. F. HAN, AND A. E. HELLMUTH. Population of muscle satellite cells in relation to age and mitotic activity. *Pathology* 3: 233–243, 1971.
4. ALLEN, G. D. The influence of endurance training upon the fiber composition of rat skeletal muscle. Pullman: Washington State Univ., 1975. PhD thesis.
5. ANDERSEN, P. Capillary density in skeletal muscle of man. *Acta Physiol. Scand.* 95: 203–205, 1975.
6. ANDERSEN, P., AND J. HENRIKSSON. Capillary supply of the quadriceps femoris muscle of man: adaptive response to exercise. *J. Physiol. London* 270: 677–690, 1977.
7. ANDERSEN, P., AND J. HENRIKSSON. Training induced changes in the subgroups of human type II skeletal muscle fibres. *Acta Physiol. Scand.* 99: 123–125, 1977.
8. ANDERSEN, P., AND A. J. KROESE. Capillary supply in soleus and gastrocnemius muscles of man. *Pfluegers Arch.* 375: 245–249, 1978.
9. ÄNGQUIST, K. A. Human skeletal muscle fibre structure. Effects of physical training and arterial insufficiency. Umeå, Sweden: Umeå Univ. Medical Dissertations, 1978. New Series, No. 39.
10. ÄNGQUIST, K. A., A. C. BYLUND, T. BJURÖ, G. CEDERBLAD, J. HOLM, K. LUNDHOLM, T. SCHERSTÉN, AND M. SJÖSTRÖM. Physical training in man. Skeletal muscle metabolism in relation to muscle morphology and running ability. *Eur. J. Appl. Physiol. Occup. Physiol.* 36: 151–169, 1977.
11. ANIANSSON, A., G. GRIMBY, M. HEDBERG, AND M. KROTKIEWSKI. Muscle morphology, enzyme activity and muscle strength in elderly men and women. *Clin. Physiol.* 1: 73–86, 1981.
12. ANIANSSON, A., G. GRIMBY, E. NYGAARD, AND B. SALTIN. Muscle fiber composition and fiber area in various age groups. *Muscle Nerve* 3: 271–272, 1980.
13. APPELL, H.-J. Zur Faserzusammensetzung und Kapillarversorgung besonders beanspruchter Muskeln. Untersuchungen am "roten" M. semitendinosus des Kaninchens (*Lepus cuniculus*) sowie dem M. gastrocnemius und M. tibialis ant. der japanischen Tanzmaus (*Mus wagneri rotans*). Cologne, W. Germany: Deutschen Sportshochschule Köln, 1977. Dissertation.
14. APPELL, H.-J. Morphological studies on skeletal muscle capillaries under conditions of high-altitude training. *Int. J. Sport Med.* 1: 103–109, 1980.
15. ARIANO, M. A., R. B. ARMSTRONG, AND V. R. EDGERTON. Hindlimb muscle fiber populations of five mammals. *J. Histochem. Cytochem.* 21: 51–55, 1973.
16. ARMSTRONG, R. B., P. D. GOLLNICK, AND C. D. IANUZZO. Histochemical properties of skeletal muscle fibers in streptozotocin-diabetic rats. *Cell Tissue Res.* 162: 387–394, 1975.
17. ARMSTRONG, R. B., P. MARUM, C. W. SAUBERT IV, H. J. SEEHERMAN, AND C. R. TAYLOR. Muscle fiber activity as a function of speed and gait. *J. Appl. Physiol.: Respirat. Environ. Exercise Physiol.* 43: 672–677, 1977.
18. ARMSTRONG, R. B., P. MARUM, P. TULLSON, AND C. W. SAUBERT IV. Acute hypertrophic response of skeletal muscle to removal of synergists. *J. Appl. Physiol.: Respirat. Environ. Exercise Physiol.* 46: 835–842, 1979.
19. ARMSTRONG, R. B., C. W. SAUBERT IV, W. L. SEMBROWICH, R. E. SHEPHERD, AND P. D. GOLLNICK. Glycogen depletion in rat skeletal muscle fibers at different intensities and durations of exercise. *Pfluegers Arch.* 352: 243–256, 1974.
20. ASHTON, W. Neovascularization in ocular disease. *Trans. Ophthalmol. Soc. U.K.* 81: 145–161, 1961.
21. BAGBY, G. J., H. J. GREEN, S. KATSUTA, AND P. D. GOLLNICK. Glycogen depletion in exercising rats infused with glucose, lactate, or pyruvate. *J. Appl. Physiol.: Respirat. Environ. Exercise Physiol.* 45: 425–429, 1978.
22. BAGBY, G. J., W. L. SEMBROWICH, AND P. D. GOLLNICK. Myosin ATPase and fiber composition from trained and untrained rat skeletal muscle. *Am. J. Physiol.* 223: 1415–1417, 1972.
23. BAKER, M. A., AND S. M. HORVATH. Influence of water temperature on oxygen uptake by swimming rats. *J. Appl. Physiol.* 19: 1215–1218, 1964.
24. BALDWIN, K. M., W. G. CHEADLE, O. M. MARTINEZ, AND D. A. COOKE. Effect of functional overload on enzyme levels in different types of skeletal muscle. *J. Appl. Physiol.: Respirat. Environ. Exercise Physiol.* 42: 312–317, 1977.
25. BALDWIN, K. M., R. H. FITTS, F. W. BOOTH, W. W. WINDER, AND J. O. HOLLOSZY. Depletion of muscle and liver glycogen during exercise: protective effect of training. *Pfluegers Arch.* 354: 203–212, 1975.
26. BALDWIN, K. M., G. H. KLINKERFUSS, R. L. TERJUNG, P. A. MOLÉ, AND J. O. HOLLOSZY. Respiratory capacity of white, red, and intermediate muscle: adaptative response to exercise. *Am. J. Physiol.* 222: 373–378, 1972.
27. BALDWIN, K. M., J. S. REITMAN, R. L. TERJUNG, W. W. WINDER, AND J. O. HOLLOSZY. Substrate depletion in different types of muscle and in liver during prolonged running. *Am. J. Physiol.* 225: 1045–1050, 1973.
28. BALDWIN, K. M., W. W. WINDER, AND J. O. HOLLOSZY. Adaptation of actomyosin ATPase in different types of muscle to endurance exercise. *Am. J. Physiol.* 229: 422–426, 1975.
29. BALDWIN, K. M., W. W. WINDER, R. L. TERJUNG, AND J. O. HOLLOSZY. Glycolytic enzymes in different types of skeletal muscle: adaptation to exercise. *Am. J. Physiol.* 225: 962–966, 1973.
30. BANCHERO, N. Capillary density of skeletal muscle in dogs exposed to simulated altitude. *Proc. Soc. Exp. Biol. Med.* 148: 435–439, 1975.
31. BÁRÁNY, M. ATPase activity of myosin correlated with speed of muscle shortening. *J. Gen. Physiol.* 50, Suppl., pt. 2: 197–218, 1967.
32. BÁRÁNY, M., K. BÁRÁNY, T. RECKARD, AND A. VOLPE. Myosin of fast and slow muscles of the rabbit. *Arch. Biochem. Biophys.* 109: 185–191, 1965.
33. BÁRÁNY, M., AND R. I. CLOSE. The transformation of myosin in cross-innervated rat muscles. *J. Physiol. London* 213: 455–474, 1971.
34. BARCROFT, H., AND J. L. E. MILLEN. The blood flow through muscle during sustained contractions. *J. Physiol. London* 97: 17–31, 1939.

35. BARNARD, R. J., V. R. EDGERTON, T. FURUKAWA, AND J. B. PETER. Histochemical, biochemical, and contractile properties of red, white, and intermediate fibers. *Am. J. Physiol.* 220: 410–414, 1971.
36. BARNARD, R. J., V. R. EDGERTON, AND J. B. PETER. Effect of exercise on skeletal muscle. I. Biochemical and histochemical properties. *J. Appl. Physiol.* 28: 762–766, 1970.
37. BARNARD, R. J., V. R. EDGERTON, AND J. B. PETER. Effect of exercise on skeletal muscle. II. Contractile properties. *J. Appl. Physiol.* 28: 767–770, 1970.
38. BARNARD, R. J., AND J. B. PETER. Effect of training and exhaustion on hexokinase activity of skeletal muscle. *J. Appl. Physiol.* 27: 691–695, 1969.
39. BARNARD, R. J., AND J. B. PETER. Effect of exercise on skeletal muscle. III. Cytochrome changes. *J. Appl. Physiol.* 31: 904–908, 1971.
40. BASMAJIAN, J. V., M. BAEZA, AND C. FABRIGAR. Conscious control and training of individual spinal motor neurons in normal human subjects. *J. New Drugs* 5: 78–85, 1965.
41. BASS, A., D. BRIDCZKA, P. EYER, S. HOFFER, AND D. PETTE. Metabolic differentiation of distinct muscle types at the level of enzymatic organization. *Eur. J. Biochem.* 10: 198–206, 1969.
42. BASS, A., E. GUTMANN, V. HANZLIKOVÁ, AND J. TEISINGER. Effects of ischaemia on enzyme-activities in the soleus muscle of the rat. *Pfluegers Arch.* 379: 203–208, 1979.
43. BASS, A., K. VONDRA, R. RATH, AND V. VÍTEK. M. quadriceps femoris of man, a muscle with an unusual enzyme activity pattern of energy supplying metabolism in mammals. *Pfluegers Arch.* 354: 249–255, 1975.
44. BEDFORD, T. G., C. M. TIPTON, N. C. WILSON, R. A. OPPLIGER, AND C. V. GISOLFI. Maximum oxygen consumption of rats and its changes with various experimental procedures. *J. Appl. Physiol.: Respirat. Environ. Exercise Physiol.* 47: 1278–1283, 1979.
45. BELL, R. D., J. D. MACDOUGAL, R. BILLETER, AND H. HOWALD. Muscle fiber types and morphometric analysis of skeletal muscle in six-year-old children. *Med. Sci. Sports Exerc.* 12: 28–31, 1980.
46. BENZI, G., P. PANCERI, M. DE BERNARDI, R. VILLA, E. ARCELLI, L. D'ANGELO, E. ARRIGONI, AND F. BERTÈ. Mitochondrial enzymatic adaptation of skeletal muscle to endurance training. *J. Appl. Physiol.* 38: 565–569, 1975.
47. BERGH, U., A. THORSTENSSON, B. SJÖDIN, B. HULTÉN, K. PIEHL, AND J. KARLSSON. Maximal oxygen uptake and muscle fiber types in trained and untrained humans. *Med. Sci. Sports Exerc.* 10: 151–154, 1978.
48. BERGMAN, H., P. BJÖRNTORP, T.-B. CONRADSON, M. FAHLÉN, J. STENBERG, AND E. VARNAUSKAS. Enzymatic and circulatory adjustments to physical training in middle-aged men. *Eur. J. Clin. Invest.* 3: 414–418, 1973.
49. BERGSTRÖM, J. Muscle electrolytes in man. *Scand. J. Clin. Lab. Invest. Suppl.* 68: 1–110, 1962.
50. BERGSTRÖM, J., A. ALVESTRAND, P. FÜRST, E. HULTMAN, K. SAHLIN, E. WINNARS, AND A. WIDSTRÖM. Influence of severe potassium depletion and subsequent repletion with potassium on muscle electrolytes, metabolites, and amino acids in man. *Clin. Sci. Mol. Med.* 51: 589–599, 1976.
51. BERGSTRÖM, J., L. HERMANSEN, E. HULTMAN, AND B. SALTIN. Diet, muscle glycogen, and physical performance. *Acta Physiol. Scand.* 71: 140–150, 1967.
52. BEZNAK, M. The effect of different degrees of subdiaphragmatic aortic constriction on heart weight and blood pressure of normal and hypophysectomized rats. *Can. J. Biochem. Physiol.* 33: 985–994, 1955.
53. BIGLAND-RITCHIE, B. EMG and fatigue of human voluntary and stimulated contractions. In: *Human Muscle Fatigue: Physiological Mechanisms.* London: Pitman Medical, 1981, p. 130–156. (Ciba Found. Symp. 82.)
54. BIGLAND, B., AND O. C. J. LIPPOLD. The relation between force, velocity, and integrated electrical activity in human muscles. *J. Physiol. London* 123: 214–224, 1954.
55. BIGLAND, B., AND O. C. J. LIPPOLD. Motor unit activity in the voluntary contraction of human muscle. *J. Physiol. London* 125: 322–335, 1954.
56. BINKHORST, R. A. The effect of training on some isometric contraction characteristics of a fast muscle. *Pfluegers Arch.* 309: 193–202, 1969.
57. BINKHORST, R. A., AND M. A. VAN'T HOF. Force-velocity relationship and contraction time of the rat fast plantaris muscle due to compensatory hypertrophy. *Pfluegers Arch.* 342: 145–158, 1973.
58. BONDE-PETERSEN, F., H. GRADUAL, J. W. HANSEN, AND H. HVID. The effect of varying the number of muscle contractions on dynamic muscle training. *Int. Z. Angew. Physiol. Einschl. Arbeitsphysiol.* 18: 268–273, 1961.
59. BONDE-PETERSEN, F., A.-L. MØRK, AND E. NIELSEN. Local muscle blood flow and sustained contractions of human arms and back muscle. *Eur. J. Appl. Physiol.* 34: 43–50, 1975.
60. BOOTH, F. W. Time course of muscular atrophy during immobilization of hindlimbs in rats. *J. Appl. Physiol: Respirat. Environ. Exercise Physiol.* 43: 656–661, 1977.
61. BOOTH, F. W., AND E. W. GOULD. Effects of training and disuse on connective tissue. In: *Exercise and Sports Sciences Reviews*, edited by J. H. Wilmore and J. F. Keogh. New York: Academic, 1975, p. 83–112.
62. BOOTH, F. W., AND J. O. HOLLOSZY. Cytochrome *c* turnover in rat skeletal muscle. *J. Biol. Chem.* 252: 416–419, 1977.
63. BOOTH, F. W., AND K. A. NARAHARA. Vastus lateralis cytochrome oxidase activity and its relationship to maximal oxygen consumption in man. *Pfluegers Arch.* 349: 319–324, 1975.
64. BOOTH, F. W., AND M. J. SEIDER. Effects of disuse by limb immobilization on different muscle fiber types. In: *Plasticity of Muscle*, edited by D. Pette. New York: de Gruyter, 1980, p. 374–383.
64a. BORMIOLI, S. P., S. SARTORE, M. VITADELLO, AND S. SCHIAFFINO. "Slow" myosins in vertebrate skeletal muscle. An immunofluorescence study. *J. Cell Biol.* 85: 672–681, 1980.
65. BÖSIGER, E. Vergleichende Untersuchungen über die Brust-Muskulatur von Huhn, Wachtel und Star. *Acta Anat.* 10: 385–429, 1950.
66. BOUISSET, S., F. LESTIENNE, AND B. MATON. Relative work of main agonists in elbow flexion. *Biomechanics*, edited by P. V. Komi. Baltimore, MD: University Park, 1969, vol. A, p. 272–279. (Int. Ser. Biomech. vol. 1a)
67. BOWDEN, D. H., AND R. A. GOYER. The size of muscle fibres in infants and children. *Arch. Pathol.* 69: 188–189, 1960.
68. BRÅNEMARK, P.-I. Capillary form and function.—The microcirculation of granulation tissue. *Bibl. Anat.* 7: 9–28, 1965.
69. BRAUNE, W., AND O. FISCHER. Die Rotationsmomente der Beugemuskeln am Ellbogengelenk des Menschen. *Abh. Saechs. Ges. (Akad.) Wiss.* 15: 243–310, 1890.
70. BREVET, A., E. PINTO, J. PEACOCK, AND F. E. STOCKDALE. Myosin synthesis increased by electrical stimulation of skeletal muscle cell culture. *Science* 193: 1152–1154, 1976.
71. BRIDGE, D. T., AND D. ALLBROOK. Growth of striated muscle in an Australian marsupial (*Setonix brachyurus*). *J. Anat.* 106: 285–295, 1970.
72. BRISKEY, E. J. Muscle. In: *Animal Growth and Nutrition*, edited by E. S. E. Hafez and I. A. Dyer. Philadelphia, PA: Lea & Febiger, 1969, chapt. 11, p. 193–216.
73. BRODAL, P., F. INGJER, AND L. HERMANSEN. Capillary supply of skeletal muscle fibers in untrained and endurance-trained men. *Am. J. Physiol.* 232 (*Heart Circ. Physiol.* 1): H705–H712, 1977.
74. BROOKE, M. H., AND W. K. ENGEL. The histographic analysis of human muscle biopsies with regard to fiber types. 1. Adult male and female. *Neurology* 19: 221–223, 1969.
75. BROOKE, M. H., AND W. K. ENGEL. The histographic analysis of human muscle biopsies with regard to fiber types. 4. Children's biopsies. *Neurology* 19: 591–605, 1969.
76. BROOKE, M. H., AND K. KAISER. Muscle fiber types: how many and what kind? *Arch. Neurol.* 23: 369–379, 1970.
77. BROOKE, M. H., AND K. K. KAISER. Three "myosin adenosine triphosphatase" systems: the nature of their pH lability and

sulfhydryl dependence. *J. Histochem. Cytochem.* 18: 670–672, 1970.

78. BROOKE, M. H., AND K. K. KAISER. The use and abuse of muscle histochemistry. *Ann. NY Acad. Sci.* 228: 121–144, 1974.
79. BROOKE, M. H., E. WILLIAMSON, AND K. K. KAISER. The behavior of four fiber types in developing and reinnervated muscle. *Arch. Neurol.* 25: 360–366, 1971.
80. BROOKS, G. A., AND T. P. WHITE. Determination of metabolic and heart rate responses of rats to treadmill exercise. *J. Appl. Physiol.: Respirat. Environ. Exercise Physiol.* 45: 1009–1015, 1978.
81. BROWN, M. C., J. K. S. JANSEN, AND D. VAN ESSEN. Polyneuronal innervation of skeletal muscle in new-born rats and its elimination during maturation. *J. Physiol. London* 261: 387–422, 1976.
82. BROWN, M. D. Role of activity in the differentiation of slow and fast muscle. *Nature London* 244: 178–179, 1973.
83. BROWN, M. D., M. A. COTTER, O. HUDLICKÁ, AND G. VRBOVÁ. The effects of different patterns of muscle activity on capillary density, mechanical properties and structure of slow and fast rabbit muscles. *Pfluegers Arch.* 361: 241–250, 1976.
84. BRUST, M., AND H. W. COSLA. Contractility of isolated abdominal skeletal muscle. *Arch. Phys. Med. Rehabil.* 48: 543–555, 1967.
85. BUCHTHAL, F., K. DAHL, AND P. ROSENFALCK. Rise time of the spike potential in fast and slowly contracting muscle of man. *Acta Physiol. Scand.* 79: 435–452, 1970.
86. BUCHTHAL, F., F. ERMINO, AND P. ROSENFALCK. Motor unit territory in different human muscles. *Acta Physiol. Scand.* 45: 72–87, 1959.
87. BUCHTHAL, F., C. GULD, AND P. ROSENFALCK. Multielectrode study of the territory of a motor unit. *Acta Physiol. Scand.* 39: 83–104, 1957.
88. BUCHTHAL, F., Z. KAMIENIECKA, AND H. SCHMALBRUCH. Fibre types in normal and diseased human muscles and their physiological correlates. In: *Exploratory Concepts in Muscular Dystrophy II.* Amsterdam: Excerpta Med., 1974, p. 526–551. (Int. Congr. Ser. 333.)
89. BUCHTHAL, F., AND H. SCHMALBRUCH. Spectrum of contraction times of different fibre bundles in the brachial biceps and triceps muscles of man. *Nature London* 22: 89, 1969.
90. BUCHTHAL, F., AND H. SCHMALBRUCH. Contraction times and fibre types in intact human muscle. *Acta Physiol. Scand.* 79: 435–452, 1970.
91. BUCHTHAL, F., AND H. SCHMALBRUCH. Motor unit of mammalian muscle. *Physiol. Rev.* 60: 90–142, 1980.
92. BULLER, A. J., J. C. ECCLES, AND R. M. ECCLES. Differentiation of fast and slow muscles in the cat hind limb. *J. Physiol. London* 150: 399–416, 1960.
93. BULLER, A. J., AND D. M. LEWIS. Further observations on the differentiation of skeletal muscles in the kitten hind limb. *J. Physiol. London* 176: 355–370, 1965.
94. BULLER, N. P., H. M. ISMAIL, AND K. W. RANATUNGA. Recording of isometric contractions of human biceps brachii muscle (proceedings). *J. Physiol. London* 277: 11P–12P, 1978.
95. BURKE, E. R., F. CERNY, D. COSTILL, AND W. FINK. Characteristics of skeletal muscle in competitive cyclists. *Med. Sci. Sports* 9: 109–112, 1977.
96. BURKE, R. E. Motor unit types of cat triceps surae muscle. *J. Physiol. London* 193: 141–160, 1967.
97. BURKE, R. E., AND V. R. EDGERTON. Motor unit properties and selective involvement in movement. *Exercise Sport Sci. Rev.* 3: 31–81, 1975.
98. BURKE, R. E., D. N. LEVINE, M. SALCMAN, AND P. TSAIRIS. Motor units in cat soleus muscle: physiological, histochemical and morphological characteristics. *J. Physiol. London* 238: 503–514, 1974.
99. BURKE, R. E., D. N. LEVINE, P. TSAIRIS, AND F. E. ZAJAC III. Physiological types and histochemical profiles in motor units of the cat gastrocnemius. *J. Physiol. London* 234: 723–748, 1973.
100. BURKE, R. E., D. N. LEVINE, F. E. ZAJAC III, P. TSAIRIS, AND W. K. ENGEL. Mammalian motor units: physiological-histological correlation in three types in cat gastrocnemius. *Science* 174: 709–712, 1971.
101. BURKE, R. E., AND P. TSAIRIS. Anatomy and innervation ratios in motor units of cat gastrocnemius. *J. Physiol. London* 234: 749–765, 1973.
102. BURKE, R. E., AND P. TSAIRIS. The correlation of physiological properties with histochemical characteristics in single muscle units. *Ann. NY Acad. Sci.* 301: 144–159, 1977.
103. BYLUND, A. C. Skeletal muscle metabolism in man. Studies with special reference to methodology and effects of physical training. Göteborg, Sweden: Univ. of Göteborg, 1977. Thesis.
104. BYLUND-FELLENIUS, A. C., T. BJURÖ, G. CEDERBLAD, J. HOLM, K. LUNDHOLM, M. SJÖSTRÖM, K.-A. ÄNGQVIST, AND T. SCHERSTÉN. Physical training in man. Skeletal muscle metabolism in relation to muscle morphology and running ability. *Eur. J. Appl. Physiol. Occup. Physiol.* 36: 151–169, 1977.
105. BYLUND-FELLENIUS, A. C., J. HAMMARSTEN, J. HOLM, AND T. SCHERSTÉN. Enzyme activities in skeletal muscles from patients with peripheral arterial insufficiency. *Eur. J. Clin. Invest.* 6: 425–429, 1976.
106. BYLUND, A. C., J. HOLM, K. LUNDHOLM, AND T. SCHERSTÉN. Incorporation rate of glucose carbon, palmitate carbon and leucine carbon into metabolites in relation to enzyme activities and RNA levels in human skeletal muscles. *Enzyme* 21: 39–52, 1976.
107. BYLUND, A. C., J. HOLM, AND T. SCHERSTÉN. Oxidation of palmitate by human skeletal muscles in vitro. Method and normal values. *Scand. J. Clin. Lab. Invest.* 35: 413–418, 1975.
108. CAMPBELL, C. J., A. BONEN, R. L. KIRBY, AND A. N. BELCASTRO. Muscle fiber composition and performance capacities of women. *Med. Sci. Sports* 11: 260–265, 1979.
109. CAMPION, D. S. Resting membrane potential and ionic distribution in fast- and slow-twitch mammalian muscle. *J. Clin. Invest.* 54: 514–518, 1974.
110. CARROW, R. E., R. E. BROWN, AND W. D. VAN HUSS. Fiber sizes and capillary to fiber ratios in skeletal muscle of exercised rats. *Anat. Rec.* 159: 33–40, 1967.
111. CASLEY-SMITH, J. R., H. S. GREEN, J. L. HARRIS, AND P. J. WADEY. The quantitative morphology of skeletal muscle capillaries in relation to permeability. *Microvasc. Res.* 10: 43–64, 1975.
112. CASSIN, S., R. D. GILBERT, C. E. BUNNELL, AND E. M. JOHNSON. Capillary development during exposure to chronic hypoxia. *Am. J. Physiol.* 220: 448–451, 1971.
113. CHEPENOGA, O. P. Muscle tissue dehydrogenase in training and fatigue. *Ukr. Biokhim. Zh.* 14: 5–12, 1939.
114. CHIAKULUS, J. J., AND J. E. PAULY. A study of postnatal growth of skeletal muscle in the rat. *Anat. Rec.* 152: 55–62, 1965.
115. CHRISTENSEN, E. Topography of terminal motor innervation in striated muscles from stillborn infants. *Am. J. Phys. Med.* 38: 65–78, 1959.
116. CHUTKOV, J. G. Magnesium, potassium and sodium in "red" and "white" muscle in the rat. *Proc. Soc. Exp. Biol. Med.* 143: 430–443, 1973.
117. CLARK, D. A. Muscle counts of motor units: a study in innervation ratios. *Am. J. Physiol.* 96: 296–304, 1931.
118. CLARKSON, P. M., W. KROLL, AND T. C. MCBRIDE. Plantar flexion fatigue and muscle fiber type in power and endurance athletes. *Med. Sci. Sports Exercise* 12: 262–267, 1980.
119. CLOSE, R. Dynamic properties of fast and slow skeletal muscles of the rat during development. *J. Physiol. London* 173: 74–95, 1964.
120. CLOSE, R. Properties of motor units in fast and slow skeletal muscles of the rat. *J. Physiol. London* 193: 45–55, 1967.
121. CLOSE, R. I. Dynamic properties of fast and slow skeletal muscle of the rat after nerve cross-union. *J. Physiol. London* 204: 331–346, 1969.
122. CLOSE, R. I. Dynamic properties of mammalian skeletal muscles. *Physiol. Rev.* 52: 129–197, 1972.
123. COLLING-SALTIN, A.-S. Enzyme histochemistry on skeletal

muscle of the human foetus. *J. Neurol. Sci.* 39: 169–185, 1978.

124. COLLING-SALTIN, A.-S. Some quantitative biochemical evaluations of developing skeletal muscles in the human foetus. *J. Neurol. Sci.* 39: 187–198, 1978.

125. COLLING-SALTIN, A.-S. Skeletal muscle development in the human foetus and during childhood. In: *Children and Exercise IX*, edited by K. Berg and B. Eriksson. Baltimore, MD: University Park, 1980, p. 193–207.

126. CONLEE, R. K., R. C. HICKSON, W. W. WINDER, J. M. HAGBERG, AND J. O. HOLLOSZY. Regulation of glycogen resynthesis in muscles of rats following exercise. *Am. J. Physiol.* 235 (*Regulatory Integrative Comp. Physiol.* 4): 145–150, 1978.

127. COOPER, R. R. Alterations during immobilization and regeneration of skeletal muscle in cats. *J. Bone Jt. Surg.* 45: 919–953, 1972.

128. COOPERSTEIN, S. J., A. LAZAROW, AND N. J. KURFESS. A microspectrophotometric method for the determination of succinic dehydrogenase. *J. Biol. Chem.* 186: 129–139, 1950.

129. COSTILL, D. L., E. F. COYLE, W. F. FINK, G. R. LESMES, AND F. A. WITZMANN. Adaptations in skeletal muscle following strength training. *J. Appl. Physiol.: Respirat. Environ. Exercise Physiol.* 46: 96–99, 1979.

130. COSTILL, D. L., J. DANIELS, W. EVANS, W. FINK, G. KRAHENBUHL, AND B. SALTIN. Skeletal muscle enzymes and fiber composition in male and female track athletes. *J. Appl. Physiol.* 40: 149–154, 1976.

131. COSTILL, D. L., W. J. FINK, L. H. GETCHELL, J. L. IVY, AND F. A. WITZMANN. Lipid metabolism in skeletal muscle of endurance-trained males and females. *J. Appl. Physiol.: Respirat. Environ. Exercise Physiol.* 47: 787–791, 1979.

132. COSTILL, D. L., W. J. FINK, AND M. L. POLLOCK. Muscle fiber composition and enzyme activities of elite distance runners. *Med. Sci. Sports* 8: 96–100, 1976.

133. COSTILL, D. L., P. D. GOLLNICK, E. J. JANSSON, B. SALTIN, AND E. M. STEIN. Glycogen depletion patterns in human muscle fibres during distance running. *Acta Physiol. Scand.* 89: 374–383, 1973.

134. COTTER, M., O. HUDLICKÁ, D. PETTE, H. STAUDTE, AND G. VRBOVÁ. Changes of capillary density and enzyme patterns in fast rabbit muscles during long term stimulation. *J. Physiol. London* 230: 34P–35P, 1973.

135. COTTER, M., O. HUDLICKÁ, AND G. VRBOVÁ. Growth of capillaries during long-term activity in skeletal muscle. *Bibl. Anat.* 11: 395–398, 1973.

136. COYLE, E. F., D. L. COSTILL, AND G. R. LESMES. Leg extension power and muscle fiber composition. *Med. Sci. Sports* 11: 12–15, 1979.

137. CRABTREE, B., AND E. A. NEWSHOLME. The activities of phosphophorylase, hexokinase, phosphofructokinase, lactate dehydrogenase, and the glycerol-3-phosphate dehydrogenase in muscle from vertebrates and invertebrates. *Biochem. J.* 126: 49–58, 1972.

138. CROCKETT, J. L., V. R. EDGERTON, S. R. MAX, AND R. J. BARNARD. The neuromuscular junction in response to endurance training. *Exp. Neurol.* 51: 207–215, 1976.

139. CURLESS, R. G., AND M. B. NELSON. Needle biopsies of muscle in infants for diagnosis research. *Dev. Med. Child Neurol.* 17: 592–601, 1975.

140. DAHLLÖF, A.-G., P. BJÖRNTORP, J. HOLM, AND T. SCHERSTÉN. Metabolic activity of skeletal muscle in patients with peripheral arterial insufficiency. *Eur. J. Clin. Invest.* 4: 9–15, 1974.

141. DATTA, A. K., AND J. A. STEPHENS. Differences in reflex effect of digital nerve stimulation on the firing of low and high threshold motor units in human first dorsal interosseous muscle. *Soc. Neurol. Sci.* 9: 367, 1979.

142. DAVIES, K. J. A., L. PACKER, AND G. A. BROOKS. Biochemical adaptation of mitochondria, muscle, and whole-animal respiration to endurance training. *Arch. Biochem. Biophys.* 209: 538–553, 1981.

143. DESMEDT, J. E., AND E. GODAUX. Ballistic contractions in man: characteristic recruitment pattern of single motor units of the tibialis anterior muscle. *J. Physiol. London* 264: 673–693, 1977.

144. DESMEDT, J. E., AND E. GODAUX. Fast motor units are not preferentially activated in rapid voluntary contractions in man. *Nature London* 267: 717–719, 1977.

145. DESMEDT, J. E., AND E. GODAUX. Mechanism of the vibration paradox: excitatory and inhibitory effects of tendon vibration on single soleus muscle motor units in man. *J. Physiol. London* 285: 197–207, 1978.

146. DESMEDT, J. E. AND E. GODAUX. Recruitment patterns of single motor units in the human masseter muscle during brisk jaw clenching. *Arch. Oral. Biol.* 24: 171–178, 1979.

147. DESMEDT, J. E., AND E. GODAUX. Voluntary motor commands in human ballistic movements. *Ann. Neurol.* 5: 415–421, 1979.

148. DHOOT, G., N. FREARSON, AND S. V. PERRY. Polymorphic forms of troponin T and tropinin C and their localization in striated muscle cell types. *Exp. Cell Res.* 122: 339–350, 1979.

149. DHOOT, G. K., P. G. H. GELL, AND S. V. PERRY. The localization of the different forms of troponin I in skeletal and cardiac muscle cells. *Exp. Cell Res.* 117: 357–370, 1978.

150. DHOOT, G. K., AND S. V. PERRY. Distribution of polymorphic forms of troponin components and tropomyosin in skeletal muscle. *Nature London* 278: 714–718, 1979.

151. DHOOT, G. K., AND S. V. PERRY. Factors determining the expression of the genes controlling the synthesis of the regulatory proteins in striated muscle. In: *Plasticity of Muscle*, edited by D. Pette. New York: de Gruyter, 1980, p. 256–267.

152. DICKERSON, J. W. T., AND P. A. MCANULTY. The response of hindlimb muscles of the weanling rat to undernutrition and subsequent rehabilitation. *Br. J. Nutr.* 33: 171–180, 1975.

153. DICKERSON, J. W. T., AND E. M. WIDDOWSON. Chemical changes in skeletal muscle during development. *Biochem. J.* 74: 247–257, 1960.

154. DÖLKEN, G., AND D. PETTE. Turnover of several glycolytic enzymes in rabbit heart, soleus muscle and liver. *Hoppe-Seyler's Z. Physiol. Chem.* 355: 289–299, 1974.

155. DONALDSON, S., S. K. BOLITHO, AND L. HERMANSEN. Differential, direct effects of H^+ on Ca^{2+} activated force of skinned fibres from soleus, cardiac and adductor magnus muscles of rabbits. *Pfluegers Arch.* 376: 55–65, 1978.

156. DOYLE, A. M., AND R. F. MAYER. Studies of the motor unit in the cat. *Bull. Sch. Med., Univ. MD* 54: 11–17, 1969.

157. DRACHMAN, D. B., AND D. M. JOHNSTON. Development of mammalian fast muscle: dynamic and biochemical properties correlated. *J. Physiol. London* 234: 29–42, 1973.

158. DRAHOTA, Z. Ionic composition of various types of muscle in relation to their functional activity. In: *Membrane Transport and Metabolism*, edited by A. Kleinzeller and A. Kotyk. New York: Academic, 1961, p. 571–578.

159. DUBOWITZ, V. Enzyme histochemistry of skeletal muscle. *J. Neurol. Neurosurg. Psychiatry* 28: 516–524, 1965.

160. DUBOWITZ, V. Contribution of histochemistry to the diagnosis of muscle pathology. *Isr. J. Med. Sci.* 13: 126–130, 1977.

161. DULING, B. R., AND E. STAPLES. Microvascular effects of hypertonic solutions in the hamster. *Microvasc. Res.* 11: 51–56, 1976.

162. EBERSTEIN, A., AND J. GOODGOLD. The use of biopsies in the study of human skeletal muscle. *Life Sci.* 6: 655–661, 1967.

163. EBERSTEIN, A., AND J. GOODGOLD. Slow and fast twitch fibers in human skeletal muscle. *Am. J. Physiol.* 215: 535–541, 1968.

164. EBY, S. H., AND N. BANCHERO. Capillary density of skeletal muscle in Andean dogs. *Proc. Soc. Exp. Biol. Med.* 151: 795–798, 1976.

165. ECCLES, J. C. The effect of nerve cross-union on muscle contraction. In: *Explanatory Concepts in Muscular Dystrophy and Related Disorders*, edited by A. T. Milhorat. Amsterdam: Excerpta Med., 1967, p. 151–160.

166. ECCLES, J. C., R. M. ECCLES, AND W. KOZAK. Further investigations on the influence of motoneurones on the speed of muscle contraction. *J. Physiol. London* 163: 324–339, 1962.

167. ECCLES, J. C., R. M. ECCLES, AND A. LUNDBERG. The action potentials of the alpha motoneurones supplying fast and slow muscles. *J. Physiol. London* 142: 275–291, 1958.

168. EDGERTON, V. R. Morphology and histochemistry of the soleus

muscle from normal and exercised rats. *Am. J. Anat.* 127: 81–88, 1970.

169. EDGERTON, V. R., R. J. BARNARD, J. B. PETER, C. A. GILLESPIE, AND D. R. SIMPSON. Overloaded skeletal muscle of a nonhuman primate (*Galago senegalensis*). *Exp. Neurol.* 37: 322–339, 1972.
170. EDGERTON, V. R., R. J. BARNARD, J. B. PETER, A. MAIER, AND D. R. SIMPSON. Properties of immobilized hind-limb muscles of the *Galago senegalensis. Exp. Neurol.* 46: 115–131, 1975.
171. EDGERTON, V. R., B. ESSÉN, B. SALTIN, AND D. R. SIMPSON. Glycogen depletion in specific types of human skeletal muscle fibers in intermittent and continuous exercise. In: *Metabolic Adaptation to Prolonged Physical Exercise*, edited by H. Howald and J. R. Poortmans. Basel: Birkhäuser, 1975, p. 402–416.
172. EDGERTON, V. R., L. GERCHMAN, AND R. CARROW. Histochemical changes in rat skeletal muscle after exercise. *Exp. Neurol.* 24: 110–123, 1969.
173. EDGERTON, V. R., J. L. SMITH, AND D. R. SIMPSON. Muscle fibre type populations of human leg muscles. *Histochem. J.* 7: 259–266, 1975.
174. EDSTRÖM, L. Histochemical changes in upper motor lesions, parkinsonism and disuse. Differential effect on white and red muscle fibers. *Experientia* 24: 916–918, 1968.
175. EDSTRÖM, L., AND B. EKBLOM. Differences in sizes of red and white muscle fibres in vastus lateralis of musculus quadriceps femoris of normal individuals and athletes. Relation to physical performance. *Scand. J. Clin. Lab. Invest.* 30: 175–181, 1972.
176. EDSTRÖM, L., AND E. KUGELBERG. Histochemical composition, distribution of fibres and fatiguability of single motor units. *J. Neurol. Neurosurg. Psychiatry* 31: 424–433, 1968.
177. EDSTRÖM, L., AND B. NYSTRÖM. Histochemical types and sizes of fibres in normal human muscles. *Acta Neurol. Scand.* 45: 257–269, 1969.
178. EDSTRÖM, L., AND K. TORLEGÅRD. Area estimation of transversely sectioned muscle fibres. *Z. Wiss. Mikr.* 69: 166–178, 1969.
179. EDWARDS, R. H. T. Physiological analysis of skeletal muscle weakness and fatigue. *Clin. Sci. Mol. Med.* 54: 463–470, 1978.
180. EDWARDS, R. H. T., C. MAUNDER, D. A. JONES, AND G. J. BATRA. Needle biopsy for muscle chemistry. *Lancet* 1: 736–740, 1975.
181. EDWARDS, R. H. T., A. YOUNG, G. P. HOSKING, AND D. A. JONES. Human skeletal muscle function: description of tests and normal values. *Clin. Sci. Mol. Med.* 52: 283–290, 1977.
182. EDWARDS, R. H. T., A. YOUNG, AND M. WILES. Needle biopsy of skeletal muscle in the diagnosis of myopathy and the clinical study of muscle function and repair. *N. Engl. J. Med.* 302: 261–271, 1980.
183. EISEN, A., G. KARPATI, S. CARPENTER, AND J. DANTON. The motor unit profile of the rat soleus in experimental myopathy and reinnervation. *Neurology* 24: 878–884, 1974.
184. EKBLOM, B. The effect of physical training on oxygen transport system in man. *Acta Physiol. Scand. Suppl.* 328: 1–45, 1969.
185. EKBLOM, B., P.-O. ÅSTRAND, B. SALTIN, J. STENBERG, AND B. WALLSTRÖM. Effect of training on the circulatory response to exercise. *J. Appl. Physiol.* 24: 518–528, 1968.
186. ELDER, G. C. B., J. FENSE, D. SALE, AND J. R. SUTTON. Relationship between the fatigue index of the quadriceps and the %FT distribution of the vastus lateralis (Abstract). *Med. Sci. Sports Exercise* 12: 143, 1980.
187. ELDRIGE, L., AND W. MOMMAERTS. Ability of electrically silent nerves to specify fast and slow muscle characteristics. In: *Plasticity of Muscle*, edited by D. Pette. New York: de Gruyter, 1980, p. 325–338.
188. ELIOT, T. S., R. C. WIGGINTON, AND K. B. CORBIN. The number and size of muscle fibres in the rat soleus in relation to age, sex, and exercise. *Anat. Rec.* 85: 307–308, 1943.
189. ELLIOTT, G. F., J. LOWY, AND C. R. WORTHINGTON. An X-ray and light-diffraction study of the filament lattice of striated muscle in the living state and in rigor. *J. Mol. Biol.* 6: 295–305, 1963.
190. ENESCO, M., AND C. P. LEBLOND. Increase in cell number as a factor in the growth of the organs and tissues of the young male rat. *J. Embryol. Exp. Morphol.* 10: 530–562, 1962.
191. ENESCO, M., AND D. PUDDY. Increase in the number of nuclei and weight in skeletal muscle of rats of various ages. *Am. J. Anat.* 111: 235–244, 1964.
192. ENGEL, W. K. The essentiality of histo- and cytochemical studies of skeletal muscle in the investigation of neuromuscular disease. *Neurology* 12: 778–794, 1962.
193. ENGEL, W. K. Fiber-type nomenclature of human skeletal muscle for histochemical purposes. *Neurology* 24: 344–348, 1974.
194. ERB, W. H. Dystrophia muscularis progressiva. Klinische und pathologische Studien. *Dtsch. Z. Nervenheilk.* 1: 173–261, 1891.
195. ERIKSSON, B. O., P. D. GOLLNICK, AND B. SALTIN. Muscle metabolism and enzyme activities after training in boys 11–13 years old. *Acta Physiol. Scand.* 87: 485–497, 1973.
196. ERIKSSON, E., AND R. MYRHAGE. Microvascular dimensions of blood flow in skeletal muscle. *Acta Physiol. Scand.* 86: 211–222, 1972.
197. ESSÉN, B. Intramuscular substrate utilization during prolonged exercise. *Ann. NY Acad. Sci.* 301: 30–44, 1977.
198. ESSÉN, B. Studies on the regulation of metabolism in human skeletal muscle using intermittent exercise as an experimental model. *Acta Physiol. Scand. Suppl.* 454, 1978.
199. ESSÉN, B. Glycogen depletion of different fibre types in human skeletal muscle during intermittent and continuous exercise. *Acta Physiol. Scand.* 103: 446–455, 1978.
200. ESSÉN, B., L. HAGENFELDT, AND L. KAIJSER. Utilization of blood-borne and intramuscular substrates during continuous and intermittent exercise in man. *J. Physiol. London* 265: 489–506, 1977.
201. ESSÉN, B., AND J. HENRIKSON. Glycogen content of individual muscle fibres in man. *Acta Physiol. Scand.* 90: 645–647, 1974.
202. ESSÉN, B., AND J. HENRIKSON. Metabolic characteristics of human type 2 skeletal muscle fibers (Abstract). *Muscle Nerve* 3: 263, 1980.
203. ESSÉN, B., E. JANSSON, J. HENRIKSON, A. W. TAYLOR, AND B. SALTIN. Metabolic characteristics of fibre types in human skeletal muscle. *Acta Physiol. Scand.* 95: 153–165, 1975.
204. ESSÉN, B., A. LINDHOLM, AND J. THORNTON. Histochemical properties of muscle fibre types and enzyme activities in skeletal muscles of standard bred trotters of different ages. *Equine Vet. J.* 12: 175–180, 1980.
205. ETEMADI, A. A., AND F. HOSSEINI. Frequency and size of muscle fibers in athletic body build. *Anat. Rec.* 162: 269–274, 1968.
206. ETLINGER, J. D., T. KAMEYAMA, K. TONER, D. VAN DER WESTHUYZEN, AND K. MATSUMOTO. Calcium and stretch-dependent regulation of protein turnover and myofibrillar disassembly in muscle. In: *Plasticity of Muscle*, edited by D. Pette. New York: de Gruyter, 1980, p. 541–557.
207. EULENBERG, A. VON, AND R. COHNHEIM. Ergebnisse der anatomischen Untersuchung eines Falles von sogenannter Muskelhypertrophie. *Verh. Ber. Med. Ges.* 1: 191–210, 1866.
208. EXNER, G. U., H. W. STAUDTE, AND D. PETTE. Isometric training of rats—effects upon fast and slow muscle and modification by an anabolic hormone (nandrolone decanoate). *Pfluegers Arch.* 345: 1–14, 1973.
209. EZEKWO, M. O., AND R. J. MARTIN. Cellular characteristics of skeletal muscle in selected strains of pigs and mice and the unselected controls. *Growth* 39: 95–106, 1975.
210. FAHIMI, H. D., AND C. R. AMARASINGHAM. Cytochemical localization of lactic dehydrogenase in white skeletal muscle. *J. Cell Biol.* 22: 29–48, 1964.
211. FAHIMI, H. D., AND M. J. KARNOVSKY. Cytochemical localization of two glycolytic dehydrogenases in white skeletal muscle. *J. Cell Biol.* 29: 113–128, 1966.
212. FARRELL, P. R., AND M. R. FEDDE. Uniformity of structural characteristics throughout the length of skeletal muscle fibers. *Anat. Rec.* 164: 219–230, 1969.
213. FAULKNER, J. A., L. C. MAXWELL, D. A. BROOK, AND D. A.

LIEBERMAN. Adaptation of guinea pig plantaris muscle fibers to endurance training. *Am. J. Physiol.* 221: 291-297, 1971.

214. FAULKNER, J. A., L. C. MAXWELL, AND D. A. LIEBERMAN. Histochemical characteristics of muscle fibers from trained and detrained guinea pigs. *Am. J. Physiol.* 222: 836-840, 1972.

215. FAULKNER, J. A., J. H. NIEMEYER, L. C. MAXWELL, AND T. P. WHITE. Contractile properties of transplanted extensor digitorum longus muscles of cats. *Am. J. Physiol.* 238 (*Cell Physiol.* 7): C120-C126, 1980.

216. FEINSTEIN, B., B. LINDEGÅRD, E. NYMAN, AND G. WOHLFART. Morphologic studies of motor units in normal human muscles. *Acta Anat.* 23: 127-142, 1955.

217. FIDLER, M. W., R. L. JOWETT, AND J. D. G. TROUP. Myosin ATPase activity in multifidus muscle from cases of lumbar spinal derangment. *J. Bone Jt. Surg.* 57: 220-227, 1975.

218. FIEHN, W., AND J. B. PETER. Properties of the fragmented sarcoplasmic reticulum from fast twitch and slow twitch muscles. *J. Clin. Invest.* 50: 570-573, 1971.

219. FIEHN, W., AND J. B. PETER. Lipid composition of muscles of nearly homogenous fiber type. *Exp. Neurol.* 39: 372-380, 1973.

220. FISCHER, E. H., L. M. G. HEILMEYER, JR., AND R. H. HASCHKE. Phosphorylase and the control of glycogen degradation. *Curr. Top. Cell Regul.* 3: 211-251, 1971.

221. FITCH, W. M., AND I. L. CHAIKOFF. Extent and patterns of adaptation of enzyme activities in livers of normal rats fed diets high in glucose and fructose. *J. Biol. Chem.* 235: 554-562, 1960.

222. FITTS, R. H., F. W. BOOTH, W. W. WINDER, AND J. O. HOLLOSZY. Skeletal muscle respiratory capacity, endurance, and glycogen utilization. *Am. J. Physiol.* 228: 1029-1033, 1975.

223. FITTS, R. H., AND J. O. HOLLOSZY. Contractile properties of rat soleus muscle: effects of training and fatigue. *Am. J. Physiol.* 233 (*Cell Physiol.* 2): C86-C91, 1977.

224. FLEAR, C. T. G., R. F. CRAMPTON, AND D. M. MATTHEWS. An in vitro method for the determination of the inulin space of skeletal muscle with observations on the composition of human muscle. *Clin. Sci.* 19: 483-493, 1960.

225. FLECKMAN, P., R. S. BAILYN, AND S. KAUFMAN. Effects of the inhibition of DNA synthesis on hypertrophying skeletal muscle. *J. Biol. Chem.* 253: 3320-3327, 1978.

226. FLETCHER, J. E. Mathematical modeling of the microcirculation. *Math. Biosci.* 38: 159-202, 1978.

227. FOSTER, C., D. L. COSTILL, J. T. DANIELS, AND W. J. FINK. Skeletal muscle enzyme activity, fiber composition and V_{O_2} max in relation to distance running performance. *Eur. J. Appl. Physiol.* 39(2): 73-80, 1978.

228. FREDMAN, D., AND O. FEINSCHMIDT. Über Einfluss des Trainierens des Muskels auf seinen Gehalt and Phosphorverbindungen. *Hoppe-Seyler's Z. Physiol. Chem.* 183: 216-268, 1929.

229. FREUND, H.-J., H. J. BUEDINGEN, AND V. DIETZ. Activity of single motor units from human forearm muscles during voluntary isometric contractions. *J. Neurophysiol.* 38: 933-946, 1975.

230. FRÖBERG, S. O. Determination of muscle lipids. *Biochim. Biophys. Acta* 144: 83-93, 1967.

231. FRÖBERG, S. O. Effect of acute exercise on tissue lipids in rats. *Metabolism* 20: 714-720, 1971.

232. FRÖBERG, S. O. Effects of training and of acute exercise in trained rats. *Metabolism* 20: 1044-1051, 1971.

233. FRÖBERG, S. O., E. HULTMAN, AND L. H. NILSSON. Effect of noradrenaline on triglyceride and glycogen concentrations in liver and muscle from man. *Metabolism* 24: 119-126, 1975.

234. FRÖBERG, S. O., AND F. MOSSFELDT. Effect of prolonged strenuous exercise on the concentration of triglycerides, phospholipids and glycogen in muscle of man. *Acta Physiol. Scand.* 82: 167-171, 1971.

235. FRÖBERG, S. O., I. ÖSTMAN, AND N. O. SJÖSTRAND. Effect of training on esterified fatty acids and carnitine in muscle and on lipolysis in adipose tissue in vitro. *Acta Physiol. Scand.* 86: 166-174, 1972.

236. FRY, M. D., AND M. F. MORALES. A reexamination of the effects of creatine on muscle protein synthesis in tissue culture. *J. Cell Biol.* 84: 294-297, 1980.

237. GARNETT, R. A. F., M. J. O'DONOVAN, J. A. STEPHENS, AND A. TAYLOR. Motor unit organization of human medical gastrocnemius. *J. Physiol. London* 287: 33-43, 1978.

238. GAUTHIER, G. F. On the relationship of ultrastructural and cytochemical features to color in mammalian skeletal muscle. *Z. Zellforsch. Mikroskop. Anat.* 96: 462-482, 1969.

239. GAUTHIER, G. F. Ultrastructural identification of muscle fiber types by immunochemistry. *J. Cell Biol.* 82: 391-400, 1979.

240. GAUTHIER, G. F. Distribution of myosin isoenzymes in adult and developing muscle fibers. In: *Plasticity of Muscle*, edited by D. Pette. New York: de Gruyter, 1980, p. 83-96.

241. GAUTHIER, G. F., AND R. A. DUNN. Ultrastructural and cytochemical features of mammalian skeletal muscle fibres following denervation. *J. Cell Sci.* 12: 525-547, 1973.

242. GAUTHIER, G. F., AND S. LOWEY. Polymorphism of myosin among skeletal muscle fiber types. *J. Cell Biol.* 74: 760-779, 1977.

243. GAUTHIER, G. F., AND S. LOWEY. Distribution of myosin isoenzymes among skeletal muscle fiber types. *J. Cell Biol.* 81: 10-25, 1979.

244. GOLDBERG, A. L. Work-induced growth of skeletal muscle in normal and hypophysectomized rats. *Am. J. Physiol.* 213: 1193-1198, 1967.

245. GOLDBERG, A. L., AND H. M. GOODMAN. Amino acid transport during work-induced growth of skeletal muscle. *Am. J. Physiol.* 216: 1111-1115, 1969.

246. GOLDBERG, A. L., AND H. M. GOODMAN. Effects of disuse and denervation on amino acid transport by skeletal muscle. *Am. J. Physiol.* 216: 1116-1119, 1969.

247. GOLDBERG, A. L., C. JABLECKI, AND J. B. LI. Effects of use and disuse on amino acid transport and protein turnover in muscle. *Ann. NY Acad. Sci.* 228: 190-201, 1974.

248. GOLDSPINK, D. F. The influence of activity on muscle size and protein turnover. *J. Physiol. London* 264: 283-296, 1977.

249. GOLDSPINK, G. Biochemical and physiological changes associated with the postnatal development on the biceps brachii. *Comp. Biochem. Physiol.* 7: 157-168, 1962.

250. GOLDSPINK, G. The combined effects of exercise and reduced food intake on skeletal muscle fibers. *J. Cell. Comp. Physiol.* 63: 209-216, 1964.

251. GOLDSPINK, G. Cytological basis of decrease in muscle strength during starvation. *Am. J. Physiol.* 209: 100-104, 1965.

252. GOLDSPINK, G. Sarcomere length during post-natal growth of mammalian muscle fibres. *J. Cell Sci.* 3: 539-548, 1968.

253. GOLDSPINK, G. Succinic dehydrogenase content of individual muscle fibers at different ages and stages of growth. *Life Sci.* 8: 791-808, 1969.

254. GOLDSPINK, G. The proliferation of myofibrils during muscle fibre growth. *J. Cell Sci.* 6: 593-604, 1970.

255. GOLDSPINK, G., AND K. F. HOWELLS. Work-induced hypertrophy in normal muscles of different ages and the reversibility of hypertrophy after cessation of exercise. *J. Physiol. London* 239: 179-193, 1974.

256. GOLLNICK, P. D., AND B. SALTIN. Significance of skeletal oxidative enzyme enhancement with endurance training. *Clin. Physiol.* 2: 1-12, 1982.

257. GOLLNICK, P. D. Exercise, adrenergic blockage, and free fatty acid mobilization. *Am. J. Physiol.* 213: 734-738, 1967.

258. GOLLNICK, P. D. Free fatty acid turnover and the availability of substrates as a limiting factor in prolonged exercise. *Ann. NY Acad. Sci.* 301: 64-71, 1977.

259. GOLLNICK, P. D., AND R. B. ARMSTRONG. Histochemical localization of lactate dehydrogenase isozymes in human skeletal muscle fibers. *Life Sci.* 18: 27-32, 1976.

260. GOLLNICK, P. D., R. B. ARMSTRONG, B. SALTIN, C. W. SAUBERT IV, W. L. SEMBROWICH, AND R. E. SHEPHERD. Effect of training on enzyme activity and fiber composition of human skeletal muscle. *J. Appl. Physiol.* 34: 107-111, 1973.

261. GOLLNICK, P. D., R. B. ARMSTRONG, C. W. SAUBERT IV, K. PIEHL, AND B. SALTIN. Enzyme activity and fiber composition in skeletal muscle of untrained and trained men. *J. Appl.*

Physiol. 33: 312–319, 1972.
262. GOLLNICK, P. D., R. B. ARMSTRONG, C. W. SAUBERT IV, W. L. SEMBROWICH, R. E. SHEPHERD, AND B. SALTIN. Glycogen depletion patterns in human skeletal muscle fibers during prolonged work. *Pfluegers Arch.* 344: 1–12, 1973.
263. GOLLNICK, P. D., R. B. ARMSTRONG, W. L. SEMBROWICH, R. E. SHEPHERD, AND B. SALTIN. Glycogen depletion pattern in human muscle fibers after heavy exercise. *J. Appl. Physiol.* 34: 615–618, 1973.
264. GOLLNICK, P. D., AND G. R. HEARN. Lactic dehydrogenase activities of heart and skeletal muscle of exercised rats. *Am. J. Physiol.* 201: 694–696, 1961.
265. GOLLNICK, P. D., AND L. HERMANSEN. Biochemical adaptations to exercise: anaerobic metabolism. In: *Exercise and Sport Sciences Reviews*, edited by J. H. Wilmore. New York: Academic, 1973, p. 1–43.
266. GOLLNICK, P. D., AND C. D. IANUZZO. Hormonal deficiencies and the metabolic adaptations of rats to training. *Am. J. Physiol.* 223: 278–282, 1972.
267. GOLLNICK, P. D., J. KARLSSON, K. PIEHL, AND B. SALTIN. Selective glycogen depletion in skeletal muscle fibres of man following sustained contractions. *J. Physiol. London* 241: 59–67, 1974.
268. GOLLNICK, P. D., AND D. W. KING. Effect of exercise and training on mitochondria of rat skeletal muscle. *Am. J. Physiol.* 216: 1502–1509, 1969.
269. GOLLNICK, P. D., B. PERNOW, B. ESSÉN, E. JANSSON, AND B. SALTIN. Availability of glycogen and plasma FFA for substrate utilization in leg muscle of man during exercise. *Clin. Physiol.* 1: 27–42, 1981.
270. GOLLNICK, P. D., K. PIEHL, AND B. SALTIN. Selective glycogen depletion pattern in human muscle fibers after exercise of varying intensity and at varying pedalling rates. *J. Physiol. London* 241: 45–57, 1974.
271. GOLLNICK, P. D., K. PIEHL, C. W. SAUBERT IV, R. B. ARMSTRONG, AND B. SALTIN. Diet, exercise, and glycogen changes in human muscle fibers. *J. Appl. Physiol.* 33: 421–425, 1972.
272. GOLLNICK, P. D., B. SJÖDIN, J. KARLSSON, E. JANSSON, AND B. SALTIN. Human soleus muscle: a comparison of fiber composition and enzyme activities with other leg muscles. *Pfluegers Arch.* 348: 247–255, 1974.
273. GOLLNICK, P. D., R. G. SOULE, A. W. TAYLOR, C. WILLIAMS, AND C. D. IANUZZO. Exercise-induced glycogenolysis and lipolysis in the rat: hormonal influence. *Am. J. Physiol.* 219: 729–733, 1970.
274. GOLLNICK, P. D., P. J. STRUCK, AND T. P. BOGYO. Lactic dehydrogenase activities of heart and skeletal muscle after exercise and training. *J. Appl. Physiol.* 22: 623–627, 1967.
275. GOLLNICK, P. D., B. F. TIMSON, R. L. MOORE, AND M. RIEDY. Muscular enlargement and the number of fibers in the skeletal muscles of rats. *J. Appl. Physiol: Respirat. Environ. Exercise Physiol.* 50: 936–943, 1981.
276. GONYEA, W. J. Role of exercise in inducing increases in skeletal muscle fiber number. *J. Appl. Physiol.: Respirat. Environ. Exercise Physiol.* 48: 421–426, 1980.
277. GONYEA, W., AND F. BONDE-PETERSEN. Contraction properties and fiber types of some forelimb and hind limb muscles in the cat. *Exp. Neurol.* 57: 637–644, 1977.
278. GONYEA, W., AND F. BONDE-PETERSEN. Alterations in muscle contractile properties and fiber composition after weight-lifting exercise in cats. *Exp. Neurol.* 59: 75–84, 1978.
279. GONYEA, W. J., AND G. C. ERICSON. An experimental model for the study of exercise-induced skeletal muscle hypertrophy. *J. Appl. Physiol.* 40: 630–633, 1976.
280. GONYEA, W., G. C. ERICSON, AND F. BONDE-PETERSEN. Skeletal muscle fiber splitting induced by weight-lifting exercise in cats. *Acta Physiol. Scand.* 99: 105–109, 1977.
281. GORCZYNSKI, R. J., AND B. R. DULING. Role of oxygen in arteriolar functional vasodilation in hamster striated muscle. *Am. J. Physiol.* 235 (*Heart Circ. Physiol.* 4): H505–H515, 1978.
282. GORSKI, J., AND T. KIRYLUK. The post-exercise recovery of triglycerides in rat tissues. *Eur. J. Appl. Physiol. Occup. Physiol.* 45: 33–41, 1980.
283. GOULD, M. K., AND W. A. RAWLINSON. Biochemical adaptation as a response to exercise. I. Effect of swimming on the levels of lactic dehydrogenase, malic dehydrogenase, and phosphorylase in muscles of 8-, 11-, and 15-week-old rats. *Biochem. J.* 73: 41–44, 1959.
284. GRAHAM, J. A., J. F. LAMB, AND A. L. LINTON. Measurements of body water and intracellular electrolytes by means of muscle biopsy. *Lancet* 2: 1172–1176, 1967.
285. GRAY, S. D., AND E. M. RENKIN. Microvascular supply in relation to fiber metabolic type in mixed skeletal muscles of rabbits. *Microvasc. Res.* 16: 404–425, 1978.
286. GREEN, H. J. Glycogen depletion patterns during continuous and intermittent ice skating. *Med. Sci. Sports Exercise* 10: 183–187, 1978.
287. GREEN, H. J., B. D. DAUB, D. C. PAINTER, AND J. A. THOMSON. Glycogen depletion patterns during ice hockey performance. *Med. Sci. Sports Exercise* 10: 289–293, 1978.
288. GREEN, H. J., AND M. E. HOUSTON. Blood lactate response to continuous and intermittent running in the rat. *Pfluegers Arch.* 360: 283–286, 1975.
289. GREEN, H. J., J. A. THOMSON, W. D. DAUB, M. E. HOUSTON, AND D. A. RANNEY. Fiber composition, fiber size and enzyme activities in vastus lateralis of elite athletes involved in high intensity exercise. *Eur. J. Appl. Physiol. Occup. Physiol.* 41: 109–117, 1979.
290. GREGOR, R. J., V. R. EDGERTON, J. J. PERRINE, D. S. CAMPION, AND C. DEBUS. Torque-velocity relationships and muscle fiber composition in elite female athletes. *J. Appl. Physiol.: Respirat. Environ. Exercise Physiol.* 47: 388–392, 1979.
291. GRIMBY, G., P. BJÖRNTORP, M. FAHLÉN, T. A. HOSKINS, O. HÖÖK, H. OXHÖJ, AND B. SALTIN. Metabolic effects of isometric training. *Scand. J. Clin. Lab. Invest.* 31: 301–305, 1973.
292. GRIMBY, G., C. BROBERT, I. KROTKIEWSKA, AND M. KROTKIEWSKI. Muscle fiber composition in patients with traumatic cord lesion. *Scand. J. Rehabil. Med.* 8: 37–42, 1976.
293. GRIMBY, L., AND J. HANNERZ. Recruitment order of motor units on voluntary contraction: changes induced by proprioceptive afferent activity. *J. Neurol. Neurosurg. Psychiatry* 31: 565–573, 1968.
294. GRIMBY, L., AND J. HANNERZ. Firing rate and recruitment order of toe extensor motor units in different modes of voluntary contraction. *J. Physiol. London* 264: 865–879, 1977.
295. GRUNEWALD, W. The influence of the three-dimensional capillary pattern on the intercapillary oxygen diffusion—a new composed model for comparison of calculated and measured oxygen distribution. In: *Oxygen Transport in Blood and Tissue*, edited by D. W. Lübbers, V. C. Luft, G. Thews, and E. Witzleb. Stuttgart, West Germany: Thieme, 1968, p. 5–17.
296. GUTH, L., AND H. YELLIN. The dynamic nature of the so-called "fiber types" of mammalian skeletal muscle. *Exp. Neurol.* 31: 277–300, 1971.
297. GUTMANN, E., AND V. HANZLIKOVÁ. Motor unit in old age. *Nature London* 209: 921–922, 1966.
298. GYDIKOV, A., AND D. KOSAROV. Some features of different motor units in human biceps brachii. *Pfluegers Arch.* 347: 75–88, 1974.
299. HÄGGMARK, T. A study of morphologic and enzymatic properties of the skeletal muscles after injuries and immobilization in man. Stockholm: Karolinska Institute, 1978. Thesis.
300. HÄGGMARK, T., AND A. THORSTENSSON. Fibre types in human abdominal muscles. *Acta Physiol. Scand.* 107: 319–325, 1979.
301. HALKJAER-KRISTENSEN, J., T. INGEMANN-HANSEN, AND B. SALTIN. Cross-sectional and fiber size changes in the quadriceps muscle of man with immobilization and physical training (Abstract). *Muscle Nerve* 3: 275, 1980.
302. HALKJAER-KRISTENSEN, J., AND T. INGEMANN-HANSEN. Variations in single fibre areas and in fiber composition in needle biopsies from the quadriceps muscle in man. *Scand. J. Clin. Lab. Invest.* 41: 391–396, 1981.
303. HALL-CRAGGS, E. C. B. The longitudinal division of fibres in overloaded rat skeletal muscle. *J. Anat.* 107: 459–470, 1970.

304. Hall-Craggs, E. C. B. The significance of longitudinal fibre division in skeletal muscle. *J. Neurol. Sci.* 15: 27–33, 1972.
305. Hall-Craggs, E. C. B., and C. A. Lawrence. Longitudinal fibre division in skeletal muscle: a light- and electronmicroscopic study. *Z. Zellforsch. Mikrosk. Anat.* 109: 481–494, 1970.
306. Hammersen, F. The pattern of the terminal vascular bed and the ultrastructure of capillaries in skeletal muscle. In: *Oxygen Transport in Blood and Tissue*, edited by D. W. Lübbers, V. C. Luft, G. Thews, and E. Witzleb. Stuttgart, West Germany: Thieme, 1968, p. 184–197.
307. Hamosh, M., M. Lesch, J. Baron, and S. Kaufman. Enhanced protein synthesis in a cell-free system from hypertrophied skeletal muscle. *Science* 157: 935–937, 1967.
308. Hannerz, J. Discharge properties of motor units in relation to recruitment order in voluntary contraction. *Acta Physiol. Scand.* 91: 374–384, 1974.
309. Hansen, T. E., and J. Lindhard. On the maximum work of human muscles especially the flexors of the elbow. *J. Physiol. London* 57: 287–300, 1923.
310. Hansen-Smith, F. M., D. Picou, and M. H. Golden. Growth of muscle fibres during recovery from severe malnutrition in Jamaican infants. *Br. J. Nutr.* 41: 275–282, 1979.
311. Hanson, J. Effects of repetitive stimulation on membrane potentials and muscle contraction. In vitro studies of muscle fibres from frog, rat and man. Stockholm: Karolinska Institute, 1974. Thesis.
312. Härkönen, M., S. Rehunen, H. Näveri, and K. Kuoppasalmi. High-energy phosphate compounds in human slow-twitch muscle fibers: methodological and functional aspects (Abstract). *Muscle Nerve* 3: 264, 1980.
313. Harri, M. N. E. Effect of prolonged beta-blockade on energy metabolism and adrenergic responses in the rat. *Med. Biol.* 55: 268–276, 1977.
314. Haxton, H. A. Absolute muscle force in the ankle flexors of man. *J. Physiol. London* 103: 267–273, 1944.
315. Havu, M., H. Rusko, P. V. Komi, J. Vos, and V. Vihko. Muscle fiber composition, work performance capacity and training in Finnish skiers. *Int. Res. Commun. System/Hum. Biol.* (73-10)5-7-8, 1973.
316. Hearn, G. R. Succinate-cytochrome c reductase, cytochrome oxidase, and aldolase activities of denervated rat skeletal muscle. *Am. J. Physiol.* 196: 465–466, 1959.
317. Hearn, G. R., and W. W. Wainio. Succinic dehydrogenase activity of the heart and skeletal muscle of exercise rats. *Am. J. Physiol.* 185: 348–350, 1956.
318. Hearn, G. R., and W. W. Wainio. Aldolase activity of the heart and skeletal muscle of exercised rats. *Am. J. Physiol.* 190: 206–208, 1957.
319. Hedberg, G., and E. Jansson. Skelettmuskelfiberkomposition. Kapacitet och intresse för olika fysiska aktiviteter bland elever i gymnasieskolan. Umeå, Sweden: Pedagogiska Inst., 1976. (Rep. 54.)
320. Hegarty, P. V. J., and A. C. Hooper. Sarcomere length and fibre diameter distributions in four different mouse skeletal muscles. *J. Anat.* 110: 249–257, 1971.
321. Hegarty, P. V. J., and K. O. Kim. Changes in skeletal muscle cellularity in starved and refed young rats. *Br. J. Nutr.* 44: 123–127, 1980.
322. Heikkinen, E., H. Suominen, M. Vihersaari, I. Vuori, and A. Kiiskinen. Effect of physical training on enzyme activities of bones, tendons, and skeletal muscle in mice. In: *Metabolic Adaptation to Prolonged Physical Exercise*, edited by H. Howald and J. R. Poortmans. Basel: Birkhäuser, 1973, p. 448–450.
323. Heilig, A., and D. Pette. Changes induced in the enzyme activity pattern by electrical stimulation of fast-twitch muscle. In: *Plasticity of Muscle*, edited by D. Pette. New York: de Gruyter, 1980, p. 409–420.
324. Heilmann, C., and D. Pette. Molecular transformation in sarcoplasmic reticulum of fast-twitch muscle by electrostimulation. *Eur. J. Biochem.* 93: 437–446, 1979.
325. Heilmann, C., and D. Pette. Molecular transformations of sarcoplasmic reticulum in chronically stimulated fast-twitch muscle. In: *Plasticity of Muscle*, edited by D. Pette. New York: de Gruyter, 1980, p. 421–440.
326. Henderson, D. W., D. E. Goll, and M. E. Stromer. A comparison of shortening and Z-line degradation in post-mortem bovine, porcine, and rabbit muscle. *Am. J. Anat.* 128: 117–136, 1970.
327. Henneman, E. Relation between size of neurons and their susceptibility to discharge. *Science* 126: 1345–1347, 1957.
328. Henneman, E., H. P. Clamann, J. D. Gillies, and R. D. Skinner. Rank order of motoneurons within a pool: law of combination. *J. Neurophysiol.* 37: 1338–1349, 1974.
329. Henneman, E., and C. B. Olson. Relations between structure and function in the design of skeletal muscles. *J. Neurophysiol.* 28: 581–598, 1965.
330. Henneman, E., G. Somjen, and D. O. Carpenter. Functional significance of cell size in spinal motoneurons. *J. Neurophysiol.* 28: 560–580, 1965.
331. Henneman, E., G. Somjen, and D. O. Carpenter. Excitability and inhibitability of motoneurons of different sizes. *J. Neurophysiol.* 28: 599–620, 1965.
332. Henriksson, J. Human skeletal muscle adaptation to physical activity. Copenhagen: Univ. of Copenhagen, 1976. PhD thesis.
333. Henriksson, J. Training-induced adaptation of skeletal muscle and metabolism during submaximal exercise. *J. Physiol. London* 270: 677–690, 1977.
334. Henriksson, J., H. Galbo, and E. Blomstrand. The importance of the motor nerve for the stimulation-induced oxidative enzymatic adaptation in cat skeletal muscle (Abstract). *Muscle Nerve* 3: 274, 1980.
335. Henriksson, J., E. Jansson, and P. Schantz. Increase in myofibrillar ATPase intermediate skeletal muscle fibers with endurance training of extreme duration in man (Abstract). *Muscle Nerve* 3: 274, 1980.
336. Henriksson, J., E. Nygaard, J. Andersson, and B. Eklöf. Enzyme activities, fibre types and capillarization in calf muscles of patients with intermittent claudication. *Scand. J. Clin. Lab. Invest.* 40: 361–369, 1980.
337. Henriksson, J., and J. S. Reitman. Quantitative measures of enzyme activities in type I and type II muscle fibres of man after training. *Acta Physiol. Scand.* 97: 392–397, 1976.
338. Henriksson, J., and J. S. Reitman. Time course of changes in human skeletal muscle succinate dehydrogenase and cytochrome oxidase activities and maximal oxygen uptake with physical activity and inactivity. *Acta Physiol. Scand.* 99: 91–97, 1977.
339. Henriksson, J., J. Svedenhag, E. A. Richter, and H. Galbo. Significance of the sympathetic-adrenal system for the exercise-induced enzymatic adaptation of skeletal muscle (Abstract). *Muscle Nerve* 3: 277, 1980.
340. Hermann, L. Zur Messung der Muskelkraft am Menschen. *Pfluegers Arch. Gesamte Physiol. Menschen Tiere* 73: 429–437, 1898.
341. Hermansen, L., E. Hultman, and B. Saltin. Muscle glycogen during prolonged severe exercise. *Acta Physiol. Scand.* 71: 129–139, 1967.
342. Hermansen, L., and M. Wachtlova. Capillary density of skeletal muscle in well-trained and untrained men. *J. Appl. Physiol.* 30: 860–863, 1971.
343. Herring, H. K., R. G. Cassens, and E. J. Briskey. Sarcomere length of free and restrained muscle at low temperature as related to tenderness. *J. Sci. Food Agr.* 16: 379–384, 1965.
344. Hewer, E. E. The development of muscle in the human foetus. *J. Anat.* 62: 72–78, 1927/28.
345. Hickson, R. C., W. W. Heusner, and W. D. Van Huss. Skeletal muscle enzyme alterations after sprint and endurance training. *J. Appl. Physiol.* 40: 868–872, 1975.
346. Hickson, R. C., M. J. Rennie, R. K. Conlee, W. W. Winder, and J. O. Holloszy. Effects of increased plasma fatty acids on glycogen utilization and endurance. *J. Appl. Physiol.: Respirat. Environ. Exercise Physiol.* 43: 829–833, 1977.

347. HINTZ, C. S., C. V. LOWRY, K. K. KAISER, D. MCKEE, AND O. H. LOWRY. Enzyme levels in individual rat muscle fibers. *Am. J. Physiol.* 239 (*Cell Physiol.* 8): C58–C65, 1980.

348. HOCHREIN, H., M. REINERT, AND B. KRIEGSMANN. Der Extracellulärraum des Herz- und Skelettmuskels. *Z. Gesamte Exp. Med.* 139: 79–93, 1965.

349. HOES, M. J. A. J. M., R. A. BINKHORST, A. E. M. C. SMEEKES-KUYL, AND A. C. A. VISSERS. Measurements of forces exerted on pedal and crank during work on a bicycle ergometer at different loads. *Int. Z. Angew. Physiol. Einschl. Arbeitsphysiol.* 26: 33–42, 1968.

350. HOGAN, E. L., D. M. DAWSON, AND F. C. A. ROMANUL. Enzymatic changes in denervated muscle. *Arch. Neurol.* 13: 274–282, 1965.

351. HOH, J. F. Y. Neural regulation of mammalian fast and slow muscle myosins: an electrophoretic analysis. *Biochemistry* 14: 742–747, 1975.

352. HOH, J. F. Y., P. A. MCGRATH, AND R. I. WHITE. Electrophoretic analysis of multiple forms of myosin in fast-twitch and slow-twitch muscles of the chick. *Biochem. J.* 157: 87–95, 1976.

353. HOLLOSZY, J. O. Biochemical adaptations in muscle. Effects of exercise on mitochondrial oxygen uptake and respiratory enzyme activity in skeletal muscle. *J. Biol. Chem.* 242: 2278–2282, 1967.

354. HOLLOSZY, J. O., AND F. W. BOOTH. Biochemical adaptations to endurance exercise in muscle. *Annu. Rev. Physiol.* 38: 273–291, 1976.

355. HOLLOSZY, J. O., AND L. B. OSCAI. Effect of exercise on α-glycerophosphate dehydrogenase activity in skeletal muscle. *Arch. Biochem.* 130: 653–656, 1969.

356. HOLLOSZY, J. O., L. B. OSCAI, I. J. DON, AND P. A. MOLÉ. Mitochondrial citric acid cycle and related enzymes: adaptive response to exercise. *Biochem. Biophys. Res. Commun.* 40: 1368–1373, 1970.

357. HOLLOSZY, J. O., L. B. OSCAI, P. A. MOLÉ, AND I. J. DON. Biochemical adaptations to endurance exercise in skeletal muscle. In: *Muscle Metabolism During Exercise*, edited by B. Pernow and B. Saltin. New York: Plenum, 1977, p. 51–61.

358. HOLLOSZY, J. O., AND W. W. WINDER. Induction of δ-aminolevulinic acid synthetase in muscle by exercise or thyroxine. *Am. J. Physiol.* 236 (*Regulatory Integrative Comp. Physiol.* 5): R180–R183, 1979.

359. HOLLY, R. G., J. G. BARNETT, C. R. ASHMORE, R. G. TAYLOR, AND P. A. MOLÉ. Stretch-induced growth in chicken wing muscles: a new model of stretch hypertrophy. *Am. J. Physiol.* 238 (*Cell Physiol.* 7): C62–C71, 1980.

360. HOLM, J., P. BJÖRNTORP, AND T. SCHERSTÉN. Metabolic activity in human skeletal muscle. *Eur. J. Clin. Invest.* 2: 321–325, 1972.

361. HONIG, C. R. Contributions of nerves and metabolites to exercise vasodilation: a unifying hypothesis. *Am. J. Physiol.* 236 (*Heart Circ. Physiol.* 5): H705–H719, 1979.

362. HONIG, C. R., AND T. E. J. GAYESKI. Capillary recruitment in exercise; relation to control mechanisms and tissue Po_2 (Abstract). *Proc. Int. Congr. Physiol. Sci. 28th, Budapest, 1980.* vol. 14, p. 23.

363. HOOPER, A. C., AND J. P. HANRAHAN. The diameter and mean sarcomere length of individual muscle fibres. *Life Sci.* 16: 775–778, 1975.

364. HOPPELER, H., P. LÜTHI, H. CLAASSEN, E. R. WEIBEL, AND H. HOWALD. The ultrastructure of the normal human skeletal muscle: a morphometric analysis on untrained men, women, and well-trained orienteers. *Pfluegers Arch.* 344: 217–232, 1973.

365. HOUSTON, M. E. The use of histochemistry in muscle adaptation: a critical assessment. *Can. J. Appl. Sport Sci.* 3: 109–118, 1978.

366. HOUSTON, M. E. Metabolic responses to exercise, with special reference to training and competition in swimming. In: *Swimming Medicine IV*, edited by B. Eriksson and B. Furberg. Baltimore, MD: University Park, 1978, p. 207–232.

367. HOUSTON, M. E., H. BENTZEN, AND H. LARSEN. Interrelationships between skeletal muscle adaptations and performance as studied by detraining and retraining. *Acta Physiol. Scand.* 105: 163–170, 1979.

368. HUBBARD, R. W., C. D. IANUZZO, W. T. MATTHEW, AND J. D. LINDUSKA. Compensatory adaptation of skeletal muscle composition to a long-term functional overload. *Growth* 39: 85–93, 1975.

369. HUDLICKÁ, O. *Muscle Blood Flow. Its Relation to Muscle Metabolism and Function.* Amsterdam: Swetz & Zeitlinger, 1973.

370. HUDLICKÁ, O. Effect of training on macro- and microcirculatory changes in exercise. *Exercise Sport Sci. Rev.* 6: 181–230, 1980.

371. HUDLICKA, Ó., M. BROWN, M. COTTER, M. SMITH, AND G. VRBOVÁ. The effect of long-term stimulation of fast muscles on their blood flow, metabolism, and ability to withstand fatigue. *Pfluegers Arch.* 369: 141–149, 1977.

372. HULTÉN, B., A. THORSTENSSON, B. SJÖDIN, AND J. KARLSSON. Relationship between isometric endurance and fibre types in human leg muscles. *Acta Physiol. Scand.* 93: 135–138, 1975.

373. HULTMAN, E. Studies on muscle metabolism of glycogen and active phosphate in man with special reference to exercise and diet. *Scand. J. Clin. Lab. Invest.* 19, Suppl. 94: 1–63, 1967.

374. HULTMAN, E., J. BERGSTRÖM, AND N. MCLENNAN ANDERSSON. Breakdown and resynthesis of phosphorylcreatine and adenosine triphosphate in connection with muscular work in man. *Scand. J. Clin. Lab. Invest.* 19: 56–66, 1967.

375. HULTMAN, E., H. SJÖHOLM, K. SAHLIN, AND L. EDSTRÖM. The contents of adenine nucleotides and phosphagens in fast-twitch and slow-twitch muscles of rats and human (Abstract). *Muscle Nerve* 3: 264, 1980.

376. HUMPHREYS, P. W., AND R. A. LIND. The blood flow through active and inactive muscles of the forearm during sustained hand-grip contractions. *J. Physiol. London* 166: 120–135, 1963.

377. HURSH, J. B. Conduction velocity and diameter of nerve fibers. *Am. J. Physiol.* 127: 131–139, 1939.

378. IANUZZO, C. D., AND V. CHEN. Metabolic character of hypertrophied rat muscle. *J. Appl. Physiol.: Respirat. Environ. Exercise Physiol.* 46: 738–742, 1979.

379. IANUZZO, C. D., P. D. GOLLINICK, AND R. B. ARMSTRONG. Compensatory adaptations of skeletal muscle fibre types to a long-term functional overload. *Life Sci.* 19: 1517–1524, 1976.

380. IHEMELANDU, E. C. Decrease in fibre numbers of dog pectineus muscle with age. *J. Anat.* 130: 69–73, 1980.

381. IKAI, M., AND T. FUKUNAGA. Calculation of muscle strength per unit cross-sectional area of human muscle by means of ultrasonic measurement. *Int. Z. Angew. Physiol. Einschl. Arbeitsphysiol.* 26: 26–32, 1968.

382. IKAI, M., AND T. FUKUNAGA. A study on training effect on strength per unit cross-sectional area of muscle by means of ultrasonic measurement. *Int. Z. Angew. Physiol. Einschl. Arbeitsphysiol.* 28: 173–180, 1970.

383. ILLG, D., AND D. PETTE. Turnover rates of hexokinase I, phosphofructokinase, pyruvate kinase, and creatinine kinase in slow-twitch soleus muscle and heart of the rabbit. *Eur. J. Biochem.* 97: 267–273, 1979.

384. INGEMANN-HANSEN, T., AND J. HALKJAER-KRISTENSEN. Computerized tomographic determinations of human thigh components. *Scand. J. Rehabil. Med.* 12: 27–31, 1980.

385. INGJER, F. Maximal aerobic power related to the capillary supply of the quadriceps femoris muscle in man. *Acta Physiol. Scand.* 104: 238–240, 1978.

386. INGJER, F. Effects of endurance training on muscle fibre ATP-ase activity, capillary supply, and mitochondrial content in man. *J. Physiol. London* 294: 419–422, 1979.

387. INGJER, F., AND P. BRODAL. Capillary supply of skeletal muscle fibers in untrained and endurance-trained women. *Eur. J. Appl. Physiol. Occup. Physiol.* 38: 291–299, 1978.

388. INGWALL, J. S., M. F. MORALES, AND F. E. STOCKDALE. Creatine and the control of myosin synthesis in differentiating skeletal muscle. *Proc. Natl. Acad. Sci. USA* 69: 2250–2253, 1972.

389. INGWALL, J. S., C. D. WEINER, M. F. MORALES, E. S. DAVIS,

AND F. E. STOCKDALE. Specificity of creatine in the control of protein synthesis. *J. Cell Biol.* 63: 145–151, 1974.

390. ISAACS, E. R., W. G. BRADLEY, AND G. HENDERSON. Longitudinal fibre splitting in muscular dystrophy: a serial cinematographic study. *J. Neurol. Neurosurg. Psychiatry* 36: 813–819, 1973.
391. ISMAIL, H. M., AND K. W. RANATUNGA. Isometric tension development in a human skeletal muscle in relation to its working range of movement: the length-tension relation of biceps brachii muscle. *Exp. Neurol.* 62: 595–604, 1978.
392. IVY, J. L., R. T. WITHERS, P. J. VAN HANDEL, D. H. ELGER, AND D. L. COSTILL. Muscle respiratory capacity and fiber type as determinants of the lactate threshold. *J. Appl. Physiol.: Respirat. Environ. Exercise Physiol.* 48: 523–527, 1980.
393. JABLECKI, C. K., J. E. HEUSER, AND S. KAUFMAN. Autoradiographic localization of new RNA synthesis in hypertrophying skeletal muscle. *J. Cell Biol.* 57: 743–759, 1973.
394. JAMES, N. T. Compensatory hypertrophy in the extensor digitorum longus muscle of the rat. *J. Anat.* 116: 57–65, 1973.
395. JAMES, N.T. Compensatory muscular hypertrophy in the extensor digitorum longus muscle of the mouse. *J. Anat.* 122: 121–131, 1976.
396. JANSSON, E. Diet and muscle metabolism in man. *Acta Physiol. Scand. Suppl.* 487: 1980.
397. JANSSON, E. Acid soluble and insoluble glycogen in human skeletal muscle. *Acta Physiol. Scand.* 113: 337–340, 1981.
398. JANSSON, E., AND L. KAIJSER. Muscle adaptation to extreme endurance training in man. *Acta Physiol. Scand.* 100: 315–324, 1977.
399. JANSSON, E., B. SJÖDIN, AND P. TESCH. Changes in muscle fibre type distribution in man after physical training. *Acta Physiol. Scand.* 104: 235–237, 1978.
400. JANSSON, E., AND C. SYLVÉN. Myoglobin and fibre types in human skeletal muscle. *Acta Physiol. Scand.* 112: 12A, 1981.
401. JENNEKENS, F. G. I., B. E. TOMLINSON, AND J. N. WALTON. The sizes of the two main histochemical fiber types in five limb muscles in man. *J. Neurol. Sci.* 13: 281–292, 1971.
402. JENNEKENS, F. G. I., B. E. TOMLINSON, AND J. N. WALTON. Data on the distribution of fibre type in five human limb muscles. *J. Neurol. Sci.* 14: 245–257, 1971.
403. JENNEKENS, F. G. I., B. E. TOMLINSON, AND J. N. WALTON. Histochemical aspects of five limb muscles in old age. *J. Neurol. Sci.* 14: 259–276, 1971.
404. JENNY, E., H. WEBER, H. LUTZ, AND R. BILLETER. Fibre populations in rabbit skeletal muscles from birth to old age. In: *Plasticity of Muscle*, edited by D. Pette. New York: de Gruyter, 1980, p. 97–109.
405. JERUSALEM, F., A. G. ENGEL, AND H. A. PETERSON. Human muscle fiber fine structure: morphometric data on controls. *Neurology* 25: 127–134, 1975.
406. JOHNSON, M. A., J. POLGAR, D. WEIGHTMAN, AND D. APPLETON. Data on the distribution of fiber types in thirty-six human muscles. *J. Neurol. Sci.* 18: 111–129, 1973.
407. JOHNSON, M. A., G. SIDERI, D. WEIGHTMAN, AND D. APPLETON. A comparison of fibre size, fibre type constitution and spatial fibre type distribution in normal human muscle and in muscle from cases of spinal muscular atrophy and from other neuromuscular disorders. *J. Neurol. Sci.* 20: 345–361, 1973.
408. JORFELDT, L., AND J. WAHREN. Leg blood flow during exercise in man. *Clin Sci. Mol. Med.* 41: 459–473, 1971.
409. JØRGENSEN, K., AND S. BANKOV. Maximum strength of elbow flexors with pronated and supinated forearm. *Med. Sports Basel* 6: 174–180, 1971.
410. JOUBERT, D. M. A study of pre-natal growth and development in the sheep. *J. Agric. Sci.* 47: 382–388, 1956.
411. JÓZSA, L., J. BÁLINT, A. RÉFFY, M. JÄRVINEN, AND M. KVIST. Capillary density of tenotomized skeletal muscles. II. Observations on human muscles after spontaneous rupture of the tendon. *Eur. J. Appl. Physiol. Occup. Physiol.* 44: 183–188, 1980.
412. JÓZSA, L., M. JÄRVINEN, M. KVIST, M. LEHTO, AND A. MIKOLA. Capillary density of tenotomized skeletal muscles. I. Experimental study in the rat. *Eur. J. Appl. Physiol. Occup. Physiol.* 44: 175–181, 1980.
413. JULIAN, L. M., AND G. H. CARDINET III. Fiber sizes of the biceps brachii muscle of dogs which differ greatly in body size. *Anat. Rec.* 139: 243, 1961.
414. KAMEYAMA, T., AND J. D. ELTINLEG. Calcium-dependent regulation of protein synthesis and degradation in muscle. *Nature London* 279: 344–346, 1979.
415. KARLSSON, J., B. DIAMANT, AND B. SALTIN. Muscle metabolites during submaximal and maximal exercise in man. *Scand. J. Clin. Lab. Invest.* 26: 358–394, 1971.
416. KARLSSON, J., K. FRITH, B. SJÖDIN, P. D. GOLLNICK, AND B. SALTIN. Distribution of LDH isozymes in human skeletal muscle. *Scand. J. Clin. Lab. Invest.* 33: 307–312, 1974.
417. KARLSSON, J., B. HULTÉN, AND B. SJÖDIN. Substrate activation and product inhibition of LDH activity in human skeletal muscle. *Acta Physiol. Scand.* 92: 21–26, 1974.
418. KARLSSON, J., L.-O NORDESJÖ, L. JORFELDT, AND B. SALTIN. Muscle lactate, ATP, and CP levels during exercise after physical training in man. *J. Appl. Physiol.* 33: 199–203, 1972.
419. KARLSSON, J., B. SJÖDIN, A. THORSTENSSON, B. HULTÉN, AND K. FRITH. LDH isoenzymes in skeletal muscles of endurance and strength trained athletes. *Acta Physiol. Scand.* 93: 150–156, 1975.
420. KEENS, T. G., V. CHEN, P. PATEL, P. O'BRIEN, H. LEVISON, AND C. D. IANUZZO. Cellular adaptations of the ventilatory muscles to a chronic increased respiratory load. *J. Appl. Physiol.: Respirat. Environ. Exercise Physiol.* 44: 905–908, 1978.
421. KELLY, A. M., AND N. A. RUBINSTEIN. Patterns of myosin synthesis in regenerating normal and denervated muscles of the rat. In: *Plasticity of Muscle*, edited by D. Pette. New York: de Gruyter, 1980, p. 161–175.
422. KIESSLING, K.-H., L. PILSTRÖM, A.-C. BYLUND, B. SALTIN, AND K. PIEHL. Enzyme activities and morphometry in skeletal muscle of middle-aged men after training. *Scand. J. Clin. Lab. Invest.* 33: 63–69, 1974.
423. KIESSLING, K.-H., L. PILSTRÖM, A.-C. BYLUND, B. SALTIN, AND K. PIEHL. Morphometry and enzyme activities in skeletal muscle from middle-aged men after training and from alcoholics. In: *Metabolic Adaptation to Prolonged Physical Exercise*, edited by H. Howald and J. R. Poortmans. Basel: Birkhäuser, 1975, p. 384–389.
424. KIM, K. O., AND P. V. J. HEGARTY. Effect of total starvation on the number and size of fibres in different muscles from the young of four species. *Proc. Nutr. Soc.* 37: 114A, 1978.
425. KLAUSEN, K., L. B. ANDERSEN, AND I. PELLE. Adaptive changes in work capacity, skeletal capillarization and enzyme levels during training and detraining. *Acta Physiol. Scand.* 113: 9–16, 1981.
426. KLEMPERER, H. G. Lowered proportion of polysomes and increased amino acid incorporation by ribosomes from denervated muscle. *FEBS Lett.* 28: 169–172, 1972.
427. KNOWLTON, G. C., AND H. M. HINES. The effects of growth and atrophy upon the strength of skeletal muscle. *Am. J. Physiol.* 128: 521–525, 1939/40.
428. KNUTTGEN, H. G., AND B. SALTIN. Muscle metabolites and oxygen uptake in short-term submaximal exercise in man. *J. Appl. Physiol.* 32: 690–694, 1972.
429. KOBAYASHI, N., AND Y. YONEMURA. The extracellular space in red and white muscle of the rat. *Jpn. J. Physiol.* 17: 698–707, 1967.
430. KOMI, P. V., AND J. KARLSSON. Skeletal muscle fibre types, enzyme activities and physical performance in young males and females. *Acta Physiol. Scand.* 103: 210–218, 1978.
431. KOMI, P. V., J. H. T. VIITASALO, M. HAVU, A. THORSTENSSON, B. SJÖDIN, AND J. KARLSSON. Skeletal muscle fibres and muscle enzyme activities in monozygous and dizygous twins of both sexes. *Acta Physiol. Scand.* 100: 385–392, 1977.
432. KOOYMAN, G. L., M. A. CASTELLINI, AND R. W. DAVIS. Physiology of diving in marine mammals. *Annu. Rev. Physiol.* 43: 343–356, 1981.
433. KOVANEN, V., H. SUOMINEN, AND E. HEIKKINEN. Connective

tissue of "fast" and "slow" skeletal muscle in rats—effects of endurance training. *Acta Physiol. Scand.* 108: 173–180, 1980.

434. KRAUS, H., AND R. KIRSTEN. Die Wirkung von Schwimm- und Lauftraining auf die celluläre Funktion und Struktur des Muskels. *Pfluegers Arch.* 308: 57–79, 1969.

435. KROGH, A. The number and distribution of capillaries in muscles with calculations in the oxygen pressure head necessary for supplying the tissue. *J. Physiol. London* 52: 405–415, 1919.

436. KROGH, A. The supply of oxygen to the tissues and the regulation of the capillary circulation. *J. Physiol. London* 52: 457–474, 1919.

437. KUGELBERG, E. Histochemical composition, contraction speed, and fatiguability of rat soleus motor units. *J. Neurol. Sci.* 20: 177–198, 1973.

438. KUGELBERG, E. Adaptive transformation of rat soleus motor units during growth. Histochemistry and contraction speed. *J. Neurol. Sci.* 27: 269–289, 1976.

439. KUGELBERG, E., AND L. EDSTRÖM. Differential histochemical effects of muscle contractions on phosphorylase and glycogen in various types of fibers: relation to fatigue. *J. Neurol. Neurosurg. Psychiatry* 31: 415–423, 1968.

440. KUGELBERG, E., L. EDSTRÖM, AND M. ABRUZZESE. Mapping of motor units in experimentally reinnervated rat muscle. *J. Neurol. Neurosurg. Psychiatry* 33: 319–329, 1970.

441. KUGELBERG, E., AND B. LINDEGREN. Transmission and contraction fatigue of rat motor units in relation to succinate dehydrogenase activity of motor unit fibres. *J. Physiol. London* 288: 285–300, 1979.

442. LAMB, D. R., J. B. PETER, R. N. JEFFRESS, AND H. A. WALLACE. Glycogen, hexokinase, and glycogen synthetase adaptations to exercise. *Am. J. Physiol.* 217: 1628–1632, 1969.

443. LANDIN, S., L. HAGENFELDT, B. SALTIN, AND J. WAHREN. Muscle metabolism during exercise in patients with Parkinson's disease. *Clin. Sci. Mol. Med.* 47: 493–506, 1974.

444. LARSSON, M. Studies on the extracellular fluid volume in the rat. Stockholm: Karolinska Institute, 1980. Thesis.

445. LARSSON, L., G. GRIMBY, AND J. KARLSSON. Muscle strength and speed of movement in relation to age and muscle morphology. *J. Appl. Physiol.: Respirat. Environ. Exercise Physiol.* 46: 451–456, 1979.

446. LAURENT, G. J., M. P. SPARROW, P. C. BATES, AND D. J. MILLWARD. Turnover of muscle protein in the fowl. Collagen content and turnover in cardiac and skeletal muscles of the adult fowl and the changes during stretch-induced growth. *Biochem. J.* 176: 419–427, 1978.

447. LAW, R. O., AND C. F. PHELPS. The size of the sucrose, raffinose, and inulin spaces in the gastrocnemius muscle of the rat. *J. Physiol. London* 186: 547–557, 1966.

448. LAWRIE, R. A. The activity of the cytochrome system in muscle and its relation to myoglobin. *Biochem. J.* 55: 298–305, 1953.

449. LAWRIE, R. A. The relation of energy-rich phosphate in muscle to myoglobin and to cytochrome oxidase activity. *Biochem. J.* 55: 305–309, 1953.

450. LAWRIE, R. A. Effect of enforced exercise on myoglobin concentration in muscle. *Nature London* 171: 1069–1070, 1953.

451. LESCH, M., W. W. PARMLEY, M. HAMOSH, S. KAUFMAN, AND E. H. SONNENBLICK. Effects of acute hypertrophy on the contractile properties of skeletal muscle. *Am. J. Physiol.* 214: 685–690, 1968.

452. LEWIS, S., E. NYGAARD, AND B. SALTIN. Circulatory control during isometric exercise studied by one-legged strength training and autonomic blockade (Abstract). *Med. Sci. Sports Exercise* 12: 139, 1980.

453. LIEB, F. J., AND J. PERRY. Quadriceps function. An anatomical and mechanical study using amputated limbs. *J. Bone Jt. Surg.* 50A: 1535–1548, 1968.

454. LILLIE, R. D. Various oil soluble dyes as fat stains in the supersaturated isopropanol technic. *Stain Technol.* 19: 55–58, 1944.

455. LIN, E. C. C. Glycerol utilization and its regulation in mammals. *Annu. Rev. Biochem.* 46: 765–796, 1977.

456. LINDHARD, J. Der Skeletmuskel und seine Funktion. *Ergeb. Physiol.* 33: 337–557, 1931.

457. LINDHOLM, A., H. BJERNELD, AND B. SALTIN. Glycogen depletion pattern in muscle fibres of trotting horses. *Acta Physiol. Scand.* 90: 475–484, 1974.

458. LING, G. N., AND M. H. KROMASH. The extracellular space of voluntary muscle tissue. *J. Gen. Physiol.* 50: 677–694, 1967.

459. LITHELL, H. Lipoprotein-lipase activity in human skeletal muscle and adipose tissue. *Acta Universitatis Upsaliensis*, 272. Uppsala, Sweden: 1977. Thesis.

460. LITHELL, H., AND J. BOBERG. Determination of lipoprotein-lipase activity in human skeletal muscle tissue. *Biochim. Biophys. Acta* 528: 58–68, 1978.

461. LITHELL, H., F. LINDGÄRDE, E. NYGAARD, AND B. SALTIN. Capillary supply and lipoprotein-lipase activity in skeletal muscle in man. *Acta Physiol. Scand.* 111: 383–384, 1981.

462. LITHELL, H., J. ÖRLANDER, R. SCHELE, B. SJÖDIN, AND J. KARLSSON. Changes in lipoprotein-lipase activity and lipid stores in human skeletal muscle with prolonged heavy exercise. *Acta Physiol. Scand.* 107: 257–261, 1979.

463. LOCKER, R. H., AND C. J. HAGYARD. The myosin of rabbit red muscles. *Arch. Biochem. Biophys.* 127: 370–375, 1968.

464. LØMO, T., AND J. ROSENTHAL. Control of ACh sensitivity by muscle activity in the rat. *J. Physiol. London* 221: 493–513, 1972.

465. LØMO, T., R. H. WESTGAARD, AND L. ENGEBRETSEN. Different stimulation patterns affect contractile properties of denervated rat soleus muscle. In: *Plasticity of Muscle*, edited by D. Pette. New York: de Gruyter, 1980, p. 297–309.

466. LOWEY, S. An immunological approach to the isolation of myosin isoenzymes. In: *Plasticity of Muscle*, edited by D. Pette. New York: de Gruyter, 1980, p. 69–81.

467. LOWEY, S., AND D. RISBY. Light chains from fast and slow muscle myosin. *Nature London* 234: 81–85, 1971.

468. LOWRY, C. V., J. S. KIMMEY, S. FELDER, M. M.-Y. CHI, K. K. KAISER, P. N. PASSONNEAU, K. A. KIRK, AND O. H. LOWRY. Enzyme patterns in single human muscle fibers. *J. Biol. Chem.* 253: 8269–8277, 1978.

469. LOWRY, O. H., C. V. LOWRY, M. M.-Y. CHI, C. S. HINTZ, AND S. FELDER. Enzymological heterogeneity of human muscle fibers. In: *Plasticity of Muscle*, edited by D. Pette. New York: de Gruyter, 1980, p. 3–18.

470. MACCALLUM, J. B. On the histogenesis of the striated muscle fiber, and the growth of the human sartorius muscle. *Johns Hopkins Hosp. Bull.* 9: 208–215, 1898.

471. MACDOUGALL, J. D., D. G. SALE, J. R. MOROZ, G. C. B. ELDER, J. R. SUTTON, AND H. HOWALD. Mitochondrial volume density in human skeletal muscle following heavy resistance training. *Med. Sci. Sports Exercise* 11: 164–166, 1979.

472. MACDOUGALL, J. D., G. R. WARD, D. G. SALE, AND J. R. SUTTON. Biochemical adaptation of human skeletal muscle to heavy resistance training and immobilization. *J. Appl. Physiol.: Respirat. Environ. Exercise Physiol.* 43: 700–703, 1977.

473. MAI, J. V., V. R. EDGERTON, AND R. J. BARNARD. Capillary of red, white and intermediate muscle fibers in trained and untrained guinea-pigs. *Experientia* 26: 1222–1223, 1970.

474. MANN, W. S., AND B. SALAFSKY. Enzyme and physiological studies of normal and disused developing fast and slow cat muscles. *J. Physiol. London* 208: 33–47, 1970.

475. MARGRETH, A., L. D. LIBERA, AND G. SALVIATI. Postnatal changes in myosin composition of slow muscle in relation to the differentiation of the motoneurons (Abstract). *Muscle Nerve* 3: 273, 1980.

476. MARGRETH, A., G. SALVIATI, L. D. LIBERA, R. BETTO, D. BIRAL, AND S. SALVATORI. Transition in membrane macromolecular composition and in myosin isozymes during development of fast-twitch and slow-twitch muscles. In: *Plasticity of Muscle*, edited by D. Pette. New York: de Gruyter, 1980, p. 193–208.

477. MARTIN, E. G., E. C. WOOLLEY, AND M. MILLER. Capillary counts in resting and active muscle. *Am. J. Physiol.* 100: 407–416, 1932.

478. MAUNDER, C. A., R. YAROM, AND V. DUBOWITZ. Electron-

microscopic X-ray microanalysis of normal and diseased human muscle. *J. Neurol. Sci.* 33: 323–334, 1977.

479. MAX, S. R. Disuse atrophy of skeletal muscle: loss of functional activity of mitochondria. *Biochem. Biophys. Res. Commun.* 46: 1394–1398, 1972.

480. MAXWELL, L. C., J. K. BARCLAY, D. E. MOHRMAN, AND J. A. FAULKNER. Physiological characteristics of skeletal muscles of dogs and cats. *Am. J. Physiol.* 233: (*Cell Physiol.* 2): C14–C18, 1977.

481. MAXWELL, L. C., J. A. FAULKNER, AND G. J. HYATT. Estimation of number of fibers in guinea pig skeletal muscles. *J. Appl. Physiol.* 37: 259–264, 1974.

482. MAXWELL, L. C., T. P. WHITE, AND J. A. FAULKNER. Oxidative capacity, blood flow, and capillarity of skeletal muscles. *J. Appl. Physiol.: Respirat. Environ. Exercise Physiol.* 49: 627–633, 1980.

483. MAYROVITZ, H. N., M. P. WIEDEMAN, AND A. NOORDEGRAAF. Microvascular hemodynamic variations accompanying microvessel dimensional changes. *Microvasc. Res.* 10: 322–339, 1975.

484. MCARDLE, W. D. Metabolic stress of endurance swimming in the laboratory rat. *J. Appl. Physiol.* 22: 50–54, 1967.

485. MCCOMAS, A. J., P. R. W. FAWCETT, M. J. CAMPBELL, AND R. E. P. SICA. Electrophysiological estimation of the number of motor units within human muscle. *J. Neurol. Neurosurg. Psychiatry* 34: 121–131, 1971.

486. MCCOMAS, A. J., AND H. C. THOMAS. Fast and slow twitch muscles in man. *J. Neurol. Sci.* 7: 301–307, 1968.

487. MCKEEN, C. P. Growth and development in the pig, with special reference to carcass quality characters. *J. Agric. Sci.* 30: 276, 1940.

488. MCLANE, J. A., AND J. O. HOLLOSZY. Glycogen synthesis from lactate in the three types of skeletal muscle. *J. Biol. Chem.* 254: 6548–6553, 1979.

489. MCPHEDRAN, A. M., R. B. WUERKER, AND E. HENNEMAN. Properties of motor units in a homogeneous red muscle (soleus) of the cat. *J. Neurophysiol.* 28: 71–84, 1965.

490. MEARA, P. J. Post-natal growth and development of muscle, as exemplified by the gastrocnemius and psoas muscles of the rabbit. *Onderstepoort J. Vet. Sci. Anim. Ind.* 21: 329–482, 1947.

491. MEERSON, F. Z. The myocardium in hyperfunction and heart failure. *Circ. Res.* 25, Suppl. 2: 1–163, 1969.

492. MELLANDER, S. Differentiation of fiber composition, circulation, and metabolism in limb muscles of dog, cat, and man. In: *Mechanisms of Vasodilatation*, edited by P.M. Vanhoutte and I. Leusen. New York: Raven, 1981, p. 243–254.

493. MILNER-BROWN, H. S., R. B. STEIN, AND R. G. LEE. Synchronization of human motor units: possible roles of exercise and suprasinal reflexes. *Electroencephalogr. Clin. Neurophysiol.* 38: 245–254, 1975.

494. MILNER-BROWN, H. S., R. B. STEIN, AND R. YEMM. The orderly recruitment of human motor units during voluntary isometric contractions. *J. Physiol. London* 230: 359–370, 1973.

495. MOLÉ, P. A., L. B. OSCAI, AND J. O. HOLLOSZY. Adaptation of muscle to exercise. Increase in levels of palmityl CoA synthetase, carnitine palmityltransferase, and palmityl CoA dehydrogenase, and in the capacity to oxidize fatty acids. *J. Clin. Invest.* 50: 2323–2330, 1971.

496. MONTGOMERY, R. D. Growth of human striated muscle. *Nature London* 195: 194–195, 1962.

497. MORGAN, T. E., L. A. COBB, F. A. SHORT, R. ROSS, AND D. R. GUNN. Effects of long-term exercise on human muscle mitochondria. In: *Muscle Metabolism During Exercise*, edited by B. Pernow and B. Saltin. New York: Plenum, 1971, p. 87–95.

498. MORGAN, T. E., F. A. SHORT, AND L. A. COBB. Effect of long-term exercise on skeletal muscle lipid composition. *Am. J. Physiol.* 216: 82–86, 1969.

499. MORKIN, E., AND T. P. ASHFORD. Myocardial DNA synthesis in experimental cardiac hypertrophy. *Am. J. Physiol.* 215: 1409–1413, 1968.

500. MORPURGO, B. Über Aktivitäts-Hypertrophie der willkürlichen Muskeln. *Virchows Arch. Pathol. Anat. Physiol.* 150: 522–554, 1897.

501. MORPURGO, B. Über die postembryonale Entwickelung der quergestreiften Muskeln von weissen Ratten. *Anat. Anz.* 15: 200–206, 1898.

502. MOSS, F. P. The relationship between the dimensions of the fibers and the number of nuclei during normal growth of skeletal muscle in the domestic fowl. *Am. J. Anat.* 122: 555–564, 1968.

503. MOSS, F. P., AND C. P. LEBLOND. Nature of dividing nuclei in skeletal muscle of growing rats. *J. Cell. Biol.* 44: 459–462, 1970.

504. MOULDS, R. F. W., A. YOUNG, D. A. JONES, AND R. H. T. EDWARDS. A study of the contractility, biochemistry, and morphology of an isolated preparation of human skeletal muscle. *Clin. Sci. Mol. Med.* 52: 291–297, 1977.

505. MÜLLER, W. Temporal progress of muscle adaptation to endurance training in hind limb muscles of young rats. *Cell Tissue Res.* 156: 61–87, 1975.

506. Muscle fibre splitting—a reappraisal. *Lancet* 1: 646, 1978.

507. MYRHAGE, R., AND E. ERIKSSON. Vascular arrangements in hind limb muscles of the cat. *J. Anat.* 131: 1–17, 1980.

508. MYRHAGE, R., AND O. HUDLICKÁ. The microvascular bed and capillary surface area in rat extensor hallucis proprius muscle (EHP). *Microvasc. Res.* 11: 315–323, 1976.

509. MYRHAGE, R., AND O. HUDLICKÁ. Capillary growth in chronically stimulated adult skeletal muscle. As studied by intravital microscopy and histological methods in rabbit and rat. *Microvasc. Res.* 12: 218–225, 1977.

510. NEELY, J. R., M. J. ROVETTO, AND J. F. ORAM. Myocardial utilization of carbohydrates and lipids. *Progr. Cardiovasc. Dis.* 15: 389–396, 1972.

511. NEMETH, P., H.-W. HOFER, AND D. PETTE. Metabolic heterogeneity of muscle fibers classified by myosin ATPase. *Histochemistry* 63: 191–201, 1979.

512. NEMETH, P., D. PETTE, AND G. VRBOVÁ. Malate dehydrogenase activity indicating metabolic homogeneity of single fibres of the motor unit. *J. Physiol. London* 301: 73P–74P, 1979.

513. NEMETH, P., D. PETTE, AND G. VRBOVÁ. Malate dehydrogenase homogeneity of single fibers of the motor unit. In: *Plasticity of Muscle*, edited by D. Pette. New York: de Gruyter, 1980, p. 45–54.

514. NIKKILÄ, E., M.-R. TASKINEN, S. REHUNEN, AND M. HÄRKÖNEN. Lipoprotein lipase activity in adipose tissue and skeletal muscle of runners: relation to serum lipoproteins. *Metabolism* 27: 1661–1671, 1978.

515. NOLTE, J., AND D. PETTE. Microphotometric determination of enzyme activity in single cells in cryostat sections. II. Succinate dehydrogenase, lactate dehydrogenase and triosephosphate dehydrogenase activities in red, intermediate and white fibers of soleus and rectus femoris muscles of rat. *J. Histochem. Cytochem.* 20: 577–582, 1972.

516. NORRIS, F. N., AND E. L. GASTEIGER. Action potential of single motor units in normal tissue. *Electroencephalogr. Clin. Neurophysiol.* 7: 115–126, 1955.

517. NOVIKOFF, A. B., W.-Y. SHIN, AND J. DRUCKER. Mitochondrial localization of oxidative enzymes: staining results with two tetrazolium salts. *J. Biophys. Biochem. Cytol.* 9: 47–61, 1961.

518. NOYES, F. R., P. J. TORVIK, W. B. HYDE, AND J. L. DELUCAS. Biomechanics of ligament failure. II. An analysis of immobilization, exercise, and reconditioning effects in primates. *J. Bone Jt. Surg.* 56A: 1406–1418, 1974.

519. NYGAARD, E. Number of fibers in skeletal muscle of man (Abstract). *Muscle Nerve* 3: 268, 1980.

520. NYGAARD, E. Morfologi og funktion i m. biceps brachii. Copenhagen: Univ. of Copenhagen, 1981. Thesis.

521. NYGAARD, E. Skeletal msucle fibre characteristics in young women. *Acta Physiol. Scand.* 112: 299–304, 1982.

522. NYGAARD, E., P. ANDERSEN, P. NILSSON, E. ERIKSSON, T. KJESSEL, AND B. SALTIN. Glycogen depletion pattern and lactate accumulation in leg muscles during recreation downhill skiiing. *Eur. J. Appl. Physiol. Occup. Physiol.* 39: 261–269, 1978.

523. NYGAARD, E., AND E. NIELSEN. Skeletal muscle fiber capillarization with extreme endurance training in man. In: *Swimming*

Medicine IV, edited by B. Eriksson and B. Furberg. Baltimore, MD: University Park, 1978, p. 282–293.

524. NYSTRÖM, B. Succinic dehydrogenase in developing cat leg muscles. *Nature London* 212: 954–955, 1966.
525. O'BRIEN, R. A. D., A. J. C. ÖSTERBERG, AND G. VRBOVÁ. Observations on the elimination of polyneuronal innervation in developing mammalian skeletal muscle. *J. Physiol. London* 282: 571–582, 1978.
526. O'BRIEN, R. A. D., R. D. PURVES, AND G. VRBOVÁ. Effect of activity on the elimination of multiple innervation in soleus muscles of rats (Abstract). *J. Physiol. London* 271: 54P, 1977.
527. O'BRIEN, R. A. D., AND G. VRBOVÁ. Nerve muscle interactions during early development. In: *Plasticity of Muscle*, edited by D. Pette. New York: de Gruyter, 1980, p. 271–281.
528. OLSON, C. B., AND C. P. SWETT. A functional and histochemical characterization of motor units in a heterogeneous muscle (flexor digitorum longus) of the cat. *J. Comp. Neurol.* 128: 475–498, 1966.
529. ÖRLANDER, J., AND A. ANIANSSON. Effects of physical training on skeletal muscle metabolism and ultrastructure in 70 to 75-year-old men. *Acta Physiol. Scand.* 109: 149–154, 1980.
530. ÖRLANDER, J., K.-H. KIESSLING, AND B. EKBLOM. Time course of adaptation to low intensity training in sedentary men: dissociation of central and local effects. *Acta Physiol. Scand.* 108: 85–90, 1980.
531. ÖRLANDER, J., K.-H. KIESSLING, J. KARLSSON, AND B. EKBLOM. Low intensity training, inactivity and resumed training in sedentary men. *Acta Physiol. Scand.* 101: 351–362, 1977.
532. OSCAI, L. B., AND J. O. HOLLOSZY. Biochemical adaptations in muscle. II. Response of mitochondrial adenosine triphosphatase, creatinine phosphokinase, and adenylate kinase activities in skeletal muscle to exercise. *J. Biol. Chem.* 246: 6968–6972, 1971.
533. PADYKULA, H. A., AND E. HERMAN. The specificity of the histochemical method for adenosine triphosphatase. *J. Histochem. Cytochem.* 3: 170–183, 1955.
534. PALLADIN, A., AND D. FERDMANN. Über den Einfluss der Trainings der Muskeln auf ihren Kreatingehalt. *Hoppe-Seyler's. Z. Physiol. Chem.* 174: 284–294, 1928.
535. PAPPENHEIMER, J. R. Passage of molecules through capillary walls. *Physiol. Rev.* 33: 387–423, 1953.
536. PAPPENHEIMER, J. R., E. M. RENKIN, AND L. M. BORRERO. Filtration, diffusion and molecular sieving through peripheral capillary membranes. A contribution to the pore theory of capillary permeability. *Am. J. Physiol.* 167: 13–46, 1951.
537. PATTENGALE, P. K., AND J. O. HOLLOSZY. Augmentation of skeletal muscle myoglobin by a program of treadmill running. *Am. J. Physiol.* 213: 783–785, 1967.
538. PAYNE, C. M., L. Z. STERN, R. G. CURLESS, AND L. K. HANNAPEL. Ultrastructural fiber typing in normal and diseased human muscle. *J. Neurol. Sci.* 25: 99–108, 1975.
539. PERSON, R. S., AND L. P. KUDINA. Discharge frequency and discharge pattern of human motor units during voluntary contraction of muscle. *Electroencephalogr. Clin. Neurophysiol.* 32: 471–483, 1972.
540. PETER, J. B., R. J. BARNARD, V. R. EDGERTON, C. A. GILLESPIE, AND K. E. STEMPEL. Metabolic profiles of three fiber types of skeletal muscle in guinea pigs and rabbits. *Biochemistry* 11: 2627–2633, 1972.
541. PETER, J. B., R. N. JEFFRESS, AND D. A. LAMB. Exercise: effects of hexokinase activity in red and white skeletal muscle. *Science* 160: 200–201, 1968.
542. PETER, J. B., S. SAWAKI, R. J. BARNARD, V. R. EDGERTON, AND C. A. GILLESPIE. Lactate dehydrogenase isoenzymes: distribution in fast-twitch red, fast-twitch white, and slow-twitch intermediate fibers of guinea pig skeletal muscle. *Arch. Biochem. Biophys.* 144: 304–307, 1971.
543. PETTE, D., AND T. BÜCHER. Proportionskonstante Gruppen in Beziehung zu Differenzierung der Enzymaktivitätsmuster von Skelettmuskeln des Kaninchen. *Hoppe-Seyler's Z. Physiol. Chem.* 331: 180–195, 1963.
544. PETTE, D., AND G. DÖLKEN. Some aspects of regulation of enzyme levels in muscle energy-supplying metabolism. *Adv. Enzyme Regul.* 13: 355–377, 1975.
545. PETTE, D., J. HENRIKSSON, AND M. EMMERICH. Myofibrillar protein patterns of single fibers from human muscle (Abstract). *Muscle Nerve* 3: 264, 1980.
546. PETTE, D., AND H. W. HOFER. The constant proportion enzyme group concept in the selection of reference enzymes in metabolism. *Trends in Enzyme Histochemistry and Cytochemistry.* Amsterdam: Excerpta Med., 1980, vol. 73, p. 231–244. (Ciba Found. Symp.)
547. PETTE, D., AND W. LUH. Constant-proportion groups of multilocated enzymes. *Biochem. Biophys. Res. Commun.* 8: 283–287, 1962.
548. PETTE, D., W. LUH, AND T. BÜCHER. A constant-proportion in the enzyme activity pattern of the Embden-Meyerhof chain. *Biochem. Biophys. Res. Commun.* 7: 419–424, 1962.
549. PETTE, D., W. LUH, M. KLINGENBERG, AND T. BÜCHER. Comparable and specific proportions in the mitochondrial enzyme activity pattern. *Biochem. Biophys. Res. Commun.* 7: 425–429, 1962.
550. PETTE, D., W. MÜLLER, E. LEISNER, AND G. VRBOVÁ. Time dependent effect on contractile properties, fibre population, myosin light chains and enzymes of energy metabolism in intermittently and continuously stimulated fast-twitch muscles of the rabbit. *Pfluegers Arch.* 364: 103–112, 1976.
551. PETTE, D., B. A. RAMIREZ, W. MÜLLER, R. SIMON, G. U. EXNER, AND R. HILDEBRAND. Influence of intermittent long-term stimulation of contractile, histochemical, and metabolic properties of fibre populations in fast and slow rabbit muscles. *Pfluegers Arch.* 361: 1–7, 1975.
552. PETTE, D., AND U. SCHNEZ. Coexistence of fast and slow type myosin light chains in single muscle fibers during transformation as induced by long term stimulation. *FEBS Lett.* 83: 128–130, 1977.
553. PETTE, D., M. E. SMITH, H. W. STAUDTE, AND G. VRBOVÁ. Effects of long-term electrical stimulation on some contractile and metabolic characteristics of fast rabbit muscles. *Pfluegers Arch.* 338: 257–272, 1973.
554. PETTE, D., AND C. SPAMER. Metabolic subpopulations of muscle fibers. *Diabetes* 28, Suppl. 1: 25–29, 1979.
555. PETTE, D., H. WASMUND, AND M. WIMMER. Principle and method of kinetic microphotometric enzyme activity determination in situ. *Histochemistry* 64: 1–10, 1979.
556. PETTE, D., AND M. WIMMER. Kinetic microphotometric activity determination in enzyme containing gels and model studies with tissue secretions. *Histochemistry* 64: 11–22, 1979.
557. PETTE, D., AND M. WIMMER. Microphotometric determination of enzyme activities in cryostat sections by the gel film technique. *Trends in Enzyme Histochemistry and Cytochemistry.* Amsterdam: Excerpta Med., 1980, vol. 73, p. 121–134. (Ciba Found. Symp.)
558. PETTE, D., M. WIMMER, AND P. NEMETH. Do enzyme activities vary along muscle fibres? *Histochemistry* 67: 225–231, 1980.
559. PIEHL, K., S. ADOLFSSON, AND K. NAZAR. Glycogen storage and glycogen synthetase activity in trained and untrained muscle of man. *Acta Physiol. Scand.* 90: 779–788, 1974.
560. PIEHL, K. Time course for refilling of glycogen stores in human fibres following exercise-induced glycogen depletion. *Acta Physiol. Scand.* 90: 297–302, 1974.
561. PLYLEY, M. J., AND A. C. GROOM. Geometrical distribution of capillaries in mammalian striated muscle. *Am. J. Physiol.* 228: 1376–1383, 1975.
562. POLGAR, J., M. A. JOHNSON, D. WEIGHTMAN, AND D. APPLETON. Data on fibre size in thirty-six human muscles. *J. Neurol. Sci.* 19: 307–318, 1973.
563. PORRO, R. S., H. DE F. WEBSTER, AND W. TOBIN. Needle biopsy of skeletal muscle: a phase and electron microscopic evaluation of its usefulness in study of muscle disease. *J. Neuropathol. Exp. Neurol.* 28: 229–242, 1969.
564. POWELL, S. E., AND E. D. ABERLE. Cellular growth of skeletal muscle in swine differing in muscularity. *J. Anim. Sci.* 40: 476–485, 1975.

565. PRINCE, F. P., R. S. HIKIDA, AND F. C. HAGERMAN. Human muscle fiber types in power lifters, distance runners and untrained subjects. *Pfluegers Arch.* 363: 19–26, 1976.

566. PRINCE, F. P., R. S. HIKIDA, AND F. C. HAGERMAN. Muscle fiber types in women athletes and non-athletes. *Pfluegers Arch.* 371: 161–165, 1977.

567. PURVES, D. Long-term regulation in the vertebrate peripheral nervous system. In: *Neurophysiology II*, edited by R. Porter. Baltimore, MD: University Park, 1976, vol. 10, p. 125–177. (Int. Rev. Physiol. Ser.)

568. RAMIREZ, B. U., AND D. PETTE. Effects of long-term electrical stimulation on sarcoplasmic reticulum of fast rabbit muscle. *FEBS Lett.* 49: 188–190, 1974.

569. RANVIER, L. Propriétés et structures différentes des muscles rouges et des muscles blancs chez les lapins et chez les raies. *C. R. Acad. Bulg. Sci.* 77: 1030–1034, 1873.

570. RANVIER, L. Note sur les vaisseaux sanguine et la circulation dans muscles rouges. *C. R. Hebd. Seances Mem. Soc. Biol.* 26: 28–31, 1874.

571. RAYNE, J., AND G. N. C. CRAWFORD. Increase in fiber number of the rat pterygoid muscles during post-natal growth. *J. Anat.* 119: 347–357, 1975.

572. REITMAN, J., K. M. BALDWIN, AND J. O. HOLLOSZY. Intramuscular triglyceride utilization by red, white, and intermediate skeletal muscle and heart during exhausting exercise. *Proc. Soc. Exp. Biol. Med.* 142: 628–631, 1973.

573. REITSMA, W. Skeletal muscle hypertrophy after heavy exercise in rats with surgically reduced muscle function. *Am. J. Phys. Med.* 48: 237–258, 1969.

574. RENIERS, J., L. MARTIN, AND C. JORIS. Histochemical and quantitative analysis of muscle biopsies. *J. Neurol. Sci.* 10: 349–367, 1970.

575. RENKIN, E. M., S. D. GRAY, L. R. DODD, AND B. D. LIA. Heterogeneity of capillary distribution and capillary circulation in mammalian skeletal muscles. Symposium on O_2 transport. *Underwater Physiology. Proc. 7th Symp.*, edited by A. J. Bachrach and M. Matzen. Bethesda, MD: Undersea Med. Soc., 1981, p. 465–474.

576. RENNIE, M. J., AND J. O. HOLLOSZY. Inhibition of glucose uptake and glycogenolysis by availability of oleate in well-oxygenated perfused skeletal muscle. *Biochem. J.* 168: 161–170, 1977.

577. RENNIE, M. J., W. W. WINDER, AND J. O. HOLLOSZY. A sparing effect of increased plasma fatty acids on muscle and liver glycogen content in the exercising rat. *Biochem. J.* 156: 647–655, 1976.

578. RENSTRÖM, P. The below-knee amputee. Thigh muscle atrophy in below-knee amputees. Göteborg, Sweden: Univ. of Göteborg, 1981, p. 72–83. Thesis.

579. RESKE-NIELSEN, E., C. COËRS, AND A. HARMSEN. Qualitative and quantitative histological study of neuromuscular biopsies from healthy young men. *J. Neurol. Sci.* 10: 369–384, 1970.

580. REYNAFARJE, B. *Myoglobin content and enzymatic activity of human skeletal muscle. Their relation with the process of adaptation to high altitude.* San Antonio, TX: U.S. Air Force Sch. Med., Aerosp. Med. Div., 1962. (Rep. 62:89, 1:8)

581. RICHTER, E. A., H. GALBO, AND N. J. CHRISTENSEN. Control of exercise-induced muscular glycogenolysis by adrenal medullary hormones in rats. *J. Appl. Physiol.: Respirat. Environ. Exercise Physiol.* 50: 21–26, 1981.

582. RIFENBERICK, D. H., J. G. GAMBLE, AND S. R. MAX. Response of mitochondrial enzymes to decreased muscular activity. *Am. J. Physiol.* 225: 1295–1299, 1973.

583. RIFENBERICK, D. H., AND S. R. MAX. Substrate utilization by disused rat skeletal muscles. *Am. J. Physiol.* 226: 295–297, 1974.

584. RIPOLL, E., A. H. SILLAU, AND N. BANCHERO. Changes in the capillarity of skeletal muscle in the growing rat. *Pfluegers Arch.* 380: 153–158, 1979.

585. ROBINSON, D. W. The cellular response of porcine skeletal muscle to prenatal and neonatal nutritional stress. *Growth* 33: 231–240, 1969.

586. ROGOZKIN, V., AND B. FELDKOREN. The effect of retabolil and training on activity of RNA polymerase in skeletal muscle. *Med. Sci. Sports Exercise* 11: 345–347, 1979.

587. ROMANUL, F. C. A. Enzymes in muscle. I. Histochemical studies of enzymes in individual muscle fibers. *Arch. Neurol.* 11: 355–368, 1964.

588. ROMANUL, F. C. A. Capillary supply and metabolism of muscle fibers. *Arch. Neurol.* 12: 497–509, 1965.

589. ROMANUL, F. C. A., AND E. L. HOGAN. Enzymatic changes in denervated muscle. I. Histochemical studies. *Arch. Neurol.* 13: 263–273, 1965.

590. ROMANUL, F. C. A., AND M. POLLOCK. The parallelism of changes in oxidative metabolism and capillary supply of skeletal muscle fibers. In: *Modern Neurology*, edited by S. Locke. Boston, MA: Little, Brown, 1969, p. 203–214.

591. ROSE, C. P., AND C. A. GORESKY. Constraints on the uptake of labeled palmitate by the heart. *Circ. Res.* 41: 534–545, 1977.

592. ROWE, R. W. D. The effect of hypertrophy on the properties of skeletal muscle. *Comp. Biochem. Physiol.* 28: 1449–1453, 1969.

593. ROWE, R. W. D., AND G. GOLDSPINK. Surgically induced hypertrophy in skeletal muscles of the laboratory mouse. *Anat. Rec.* 161: 69–75, 1968.

594. ROWELL, L. B. Factors affecting the prediction of the maximal oxygen intake from measurements made during submaximal work with observations related to factors which may limit maximal oxygen intake. Minneapolis: Univ. of Minnesota, 1962. Thesis.

595. RUBINSTEIN, N. A., AND A. M. KELLY. The sequential appearance of fast and slow myosins during myogenesis. In: *Plasticity of Muscle*, edited by D. Pette. New York: de Gruyter, 1980, p. 147–159.

596. RUBINSTEIN, N., K. MABUCHI, F. PEPE, S. SALMONS, J. GERGELY, AND F. SRETÉR. Use of type-specific antimyosins to demonstrate the transformation of individual fibers in chronically stimulated rabbit fast muscles. *J. Cell Biol.* 79: 252–261, 1978.

597. RUSHTON, W. A. H. A theory of the effects of fibre size in medullated nerve. *J. Physiol. London* 115: 101–122, 1951.

598. RUSKO, H., P. RAHKILA, AND E. KÄRVINEN. Anaerobic threshold, skeletal muscle enzymes and fiber composition in young female cross-country skiers. *Acta Physiol. Scand.* 108: 263–268, 1980.

599. SALMONS, S., AND F. A. SRÉTER. Significance of impulse activity in the transformation of skeletal muscle type. *Nature London* 263: 30–34, 1976.

600. SALMONS, S., AND G. VRBOVÁ. The influence of activity on some contractile characteristics of mammalian fast and slow muscles. *J. Physiol. London* 20: 535–549, 1969.

601. SALTIN, B., G. BLOMQVIST, J. H. MITCHELL, R. L. JOHNSON, JR., K. WILDENTHAL, AND C. B. CHAPMANN. Response to exercise after bed rest and after training. *Circulation* 38, Suppl. 7: 1–78, 1968.

602. SALTIN, B., J. HENRIKSSON, E. NYGAARD, E. JANSSON, AND P. ANDERSEN. Fiber types and metabolic potentials of skeletal muscles in sedentary man and endurance runners. *Ann. NY Acad. Sci.* 301: 3–29, 1977.

603. SALTIN, B., K. NAZAR, D. L. COSTILL, E. STEIN, E. JANSSON, B. ESSÉN, AND P. GOLLNICK. The nature of the training response; peripheral and central adaptations to one-legged exercise. *Acta Physiol. Scand.* 96: 289–305, 1976.

604. SALTIN, B., E. NYGAARD, AND B. RASMUSSEN. Skeletal muscle adaptation in man following prolonged exposure to high altitude (Abstract). *Acta Physiol. Scand.* 109: 31A, 1980.

605. SALTIN, B., AND L. B. ROWELL. Functional adaptations to physical activity and inactivity. *Federation Proc.* 39: 1506–1513, 1980.

606. SAMAHA, F. J., L. GUTH, AND R. W. ALBERS. Differences between slow and fast muscle myosin. Adenosine triphosphatase activity and release of associated proteins by *p*-chloromercuriphenylsulfonate. *J. Biol. Chem.* 245: 219–224, 1970.

607. SARGEANT, A. J., A. YOUNG, C. T. M. DAVIES, C. MAUNDER,

AND R. H. T. EDWARDS. Functional and structural changes following disuse of human muscle. *Clin. Sci. Mol. Med.* 52: 337–342, 1977.

608. SAUBERT, C. W., IV, R. B. ARMSTRONG, R. E. SHEPHERD, AND P. D. GOLLNICK. Anaerobic enzyme adaptations to sprint training in rats. *Pfluegers Arch.* 341: 305–312, 1973.
609. SCHIAFFINO, S. Hypertrophy of skeletal muscle induced by tendon shortening. *Experientia* 30: 1163–1164, 1974.
610. SCHIAFFINO, S., S. P. BORMIOLI, AND M. ALOISI. Cell proliferation in rat skeletal muscle during early stages of compensatory hypertrophy. *Virchows Arch. B* 11: 268–273, 1972.
611. SCHIAFFINO, S., S. P. BORMIOLI, AND M. ALOISI. The fate of newly formed satellite cells during compensatory muscle hypertrophy. *Virchows Arch. B* 21: 113–118, 1976.
612. SCHIAFFINO, S., S. P. BORMIOLI, AND M. ALOISI. Fiber branching and formation of new fibers during compensatory muscle hypertrophy. In: *Muscle Regeneration*, edited by A. Mauro. New York: Raven, 1979, p. 177–188.
613. SCHMALBRUCH, H. The morphology of regeneration of skeletal muscles in the rat. *Tissue Cell* 8: 673–692, 1976.
614. SCHMALBRUCH, H. Muscle fibre splitting and regeneration in diseased human muscle. *Neuropathol. Appl. Neurobiol.* 2: 3–19, 1976.
615. SCHMALBRUCH, H. Satellite cells of rat muscles as studied by freeze-fracturing. *Anat. Rec.* 191: 371–376, 1978.
616. SCHMALBRUCH, H., AND H. HELLHAMMER. The number of satellite cells in normal human muscle. *Anat. Rec.* 185: 279–282, 1976.
617. SCHMIDT-NIELSEN, K., AND P. PENNYCUIK. Capillary density in mammals in relation to body size and oxygen consumption. *Am. J. Physiol.* 200: 746–750, 1961.
618. SCHREIBER, S. S., M. ORATZ, C. D. EVANS, I. GUEYIKIAN, AND M. A. ROTHSCHILD. Myosin, myoglobin, and collagen synthesis in acute cardiac overload. *Am. J. Physiol.* 219: 481–486, 1970.
619. SCHREIBER, S. S., M. ORATZ, C. EVANS, E. SILVER, AND M. A. ROTHSCHILD. Effect of acute overload on cardiac muscle mRNA. *Am. J. Physiol.* 215: 1250–1259, 1968.
620. SCHREIBER, S. S., M. ORATZ, AND M. A. ROTHSCHILD. Effect of acute overload on protein synthesis in cardiac muscle microsomes. *Am. J. Physiol.* 213: 1552–1555, 1967.
621. SCHREIBER, S. S., M. ORATZ, AND M. A. ROTHSCHILD. Nuclear RNA polymerase activity in acute hemodynamic overload in the perfused heart. *Am. J. Physiol.* 217: 1305–1309, 1969.
622. SCHWARTZ, M. S., M. SARGEANT, AND M. SWASH. Longitudinal fibre splitting in neurogenic muscular disorders—its relation to the pathogenesis of "myopathic" change. *Brain* 99: 617–636, 1976.
623. SCHWARZACHER, H. G. Über die Länge und Anordnung der Muskelfasern in menschlichen Skelettmuskeln. *Acta Anat.* 37: 217–231, 1959.
624. SEIBERT, W. W. Untersuchungen über Hypertrophie des Skelettmuskels. *Z. Klin. Med.* 109: 350–360, 1928.
625. SEMBROWICH, W. L., C. D. IANUZZO, C. W. SAUBERT IV, R. E. SHEPHERD, AND P. D. GOLLNICK. Substrate mobilization during prolonged exercise in 6-hydroxydopamine treated rats. *Pfluegers Arch.* 349: 57–62, 1974.
626. SEXTON, A. W. Isometric tension of glycerinated muscle fibers following adrenalectomy. *Am. J. Physiol.* 212: 313–316, 1967.
627. SEXTON, A. W., AND J. W. GERSTEN. Isometric tension differences in fibers of red and white muscles. *Science* 157: 199, 1967.
628. SHAFIQ, S. A., M. A. GORYCKI, AND A. MAURO. Mitosis during postnatal growth in skeletal and cardiac muscle of the rat. *J. Anat.* 103: 135–141, 1968.
629. SHEPHERD, R. E., AND P. D. GOLLNICK. Oxygen uptake of rats at different work intensities. *Pfluegers Arch.* 362: 219–222, 1976.
630. SICA, R. E. P., AND A. J. MCCOMAS. Fast and slow twitch units in a human muscle. *J. Neurol. Neurosurg. Psychiatry* 34: 113–120, 1971.
631. SILLAU, A. H., L. AQUIN, M. V. BUI, AND N. BANCHERO. Chronic hypoxia does not affect guinea pig skeletal muscle capillarity. *Pfluegers Arch.* 386: 39–45, 1980.
632. SILLAU, A. H., AND N. BANCHERO. Effects of hypoxia on capillary density and fiber composition in rat skeletal muscle. *Pfluegers Arch.* 370: 227–232, 1977.
633. SILLAU, A. H., AND N. BANCHERO. Effect of maturation on capillary density, fiber size and composition in rat skeletal muscle. *Proc. Soc. Exp. Biol. Med.* 154: 461–466, 1977.
634. SILLAU, A. H., AND N. BANCHERO. Skeletal muscle fiber size and capillarity. *Proc. Soc. Exp. Biol. Med.* 158: 288–291, 1978.
635. SILLAU, A. H., AND N. BANCHERO. Effect of hypoxia on the capillarity of guinea pig skeletal muscle. *Proc. Soc. Exp. Biol. Med.* 160: 368–373, 1979.
636. SIMON, L. M., AND E. D. ROBIN. Relationship of cytochrome oxidase activity to vertebrate total and organ oxygen consumption. *Int. J. Biochem.* 2: 569–573, 1971.
637. SINK, J. D., R. G. CASSENS, W. G. HOEKSTRA, AND E. J. BRISKEY. Rigor mortis pattern of skeletal muscle and sarcomere length of the myofibril. *Biochim. Biophys. Acta* 102: 309–311, 1965.
638. SJÖDIN, B. Lactate dehydrogenase in human skeletal muscle. *Acta Physiol. Scand. Suppl.* 436: 5–32, 1976.
639. SJÖDIN, B., A. THORSTENSSON, K. FRITH, AND J. KARLSSON. Effect of physical training on LDH activity and LDH isozyme pattern in human skeletal muscle. *Acta Physiol. Scand.* 97: 150–157, 1976.
640. SJØGAARD, G. Force-velocity curve for bicycle work. In: *Biomechanics VI A*, edited by E. Asmussen and K. Jørgensen. Baltimore, MD: University Park, 1978, p. 93–99.
641. SJØGAARD, G. Water spaces and electrolyte concentrations in human skeletal muscle. Copenhagen: Univ. of Copenhagen, 1979. Thesis.
642. SJØGAARD, G., M. E. HOUSTON, E. NYGAARD, AND B. SALTIN. Subgrouping of fast twitch fibres in skeletal muscles of man. *Histochemistry* 58: 79–87, 1978.
643. SJÖSTRÖM, M., S. KIDMAN, K. LARSEN-HENRIKSSON, AND K. A. ÄNGQUIST. Z- and M-band appearance in different histochemically defined types of human skeletal muscle fibers. *J. Histochem. Cytochem.* 30: 1–11, 1982.
644. SJÖSTRÖM, M., J. LEXELL, AND K. LARSEN-HENRIKSSON. Distribution of different fibres in m. vastus lateralis. *Panamerican Congress and Int. Course on Sports Medicine and Exercise Science.* Abstracts. May, 1981, Miami, p. 12.
645. SMITH, J. H. Relation of body size to muscle cell size and number in the chicken. *Poult. Sci.* 12: 283–290, 1963.
646. SNOW, D. H., AND P. S. GUY. The effect of training and detraining on several enzymes in horse skeletal muscle. *Arch. Int. Physiol. Biochim.* 87: 87–93, 1979.
647. SOBEL, B. E., AND S. KAUFMAN. Enhanced RNA polymerase activity in skeletal muscle undergoing hypertrophy. *Arch. Biochem. Biophys.* 137: 469–476, 1970.
648. SOLA, O. M., D. L. CHRISTENSEN, AND A. W. MARTIN. Hypertrophy and hyperplasia of adult chicken anterior latissimus dorsi muscles following stretch with and without denervation. *Exp. Neurol.* 41: 76–100, 1973.
649. SONG, S. K., N. SHIMADA, AND P. J. ANDERSON. Orthogonal diameters in the analysis of muscle fibre size and form. *Nature London* 200: 1220–1221, 1963.
650. SPALTEHOLZ, W. Die Vertheilung der Blutgefässe im Muskel. *Abh. Math.-Phys. K. Königl. Saechs. Ges. Wiss.* 14: 509–528, 1888.
651. SPAMER, C., AND D. PETTE. Activity patterns of phosphofructokinase, glyceraldehydephosphate dehydrogenase, lactate dehydrogenase, and malate dehydrogenase in microdissected fast and slow fibers from rabbit psoas and soleus muscle. *Histochemistry* 52: 201–216, 1977.
652. SPAMER, C., AND D. PETTE. Activities of malate dehydrogenase, 3-hydroxyacyl-CoA dehydrogenase and fructose-1,6-diphosphatase with regard to metabolic subpopulations of fast- and slow-twitch fibers in rabbit muscles. *Histochemistry* 60: 9–19, 1979.
653. SPAMER, C., AND D. PETTE. Metabolic subpopulations of rabbit skeletal muscle fibres. In: *Plasticity of Muscle*, edited by D. Pette. New York: de Gruyter, 1980, p. 19–30.

654. SRÉTER, F. A., A. R. LUFT, AND J. GERGELY. Effect of cross-reinnervation on physiological parameters and on properties of myosin and sarcoplasmic reticulum of fast and slow muscles of the rabbit. *J. Gen. Physiol.* 66: 811–821, 1975.
655. SRÉTER, F. A., S. SARKAR, AND J. GERGELY. Myosin light chains of slow twitch muscle. *Nature London* 239: 124–125, 1972.
656. SRÉTER, F. A., J. C. SEIDEL, AND J. GERGELY. Studies on myosin from red and white skeletal muscles of the rabbit. I. Adenosine triphosphatase activity. *J. Biol. Chem.* 241: 5772–5776, 1966.
657. SRÉTER, F. A., AND G. WOO. Cell water, sodium, and potassium in red and white mammalian muscle. *Am. J. Physiol.* 205: 1290–1294, 1963.
658. STANKIEWICZ-CHOROSZUCHA, B., AND J. GORSKI. Effect of beta-adrenergic blockade on intramuscular triglyceride mobilization during exercise. *Experientia* 34: 357–358, 1978.
659. STAUDTE, H. W., G. U. EXNER, AND D. PETTE. Effects of short-term, high intensity (sprint) training on some contractile and metabolic characteristics of fast and slow muscle of the rat. *Pfluegers Arch.* 344: 159–168, 1973.
660. STAUN, H. Various factors affecting number and size of muscle fibers in the pig. *Acta Agric. Scand.* 13: 293–322, 1963.
661. STEPHENS, J. A., AND T. P. USHERWOOD. The mechanical properties of human motor units with special reference to their fatigability and recruitment threshold. *Brain Res.* 125: 91–97, 1977.
662. STROMER, M. H., AND D. E. GOLL. Molecular properties of post-mortem muscle. *J. Food Sci.* 32: 386–389, 1967.
663. SULLIVAN, T. E., AND R. B. ARMSTRONG. Rat locomotory muscle fiber activity during trotting and galloping. *J. Appl. Physiol.: Respirat. Environ. Exercise Physiol.* 44: 358–363, 1978.
664. SUOMINEN, H., AND E. HEIKKINEN. Enzyme activities in muscle and connective tissue of m. vastus lateralis in habitually training and sedentary 33- to 70-year-old men. *Eur. J. Appl. Physiol. Occup. Physiol.* 34: 249–254, 1975.
665. SUOMINEN, H., E. HEIKKINEN, AND T. PARKATTI. Effect of eight weeks' physical training on muscle and connective tissue of the m. vastus lateralis in 69-year-old men and women. *J. Gerontol.* 32: 33–37, 1977.
666. SUOMINEN, H., A. KIISKINEN, AND E. HEIKKINEN. Effects of physical training on metabolism of connective tissues in young mice. *Acta Physiol. Scand.* 108: 17–22, 1980.
667. SUSHEELA, A. K., AND J. N. WALTON. Note on the distribution of histochemical fibre types in some normal human muscles. *J. Neurol. Sci.* 8: 201–207, 1969.
668. SWASH, M., AND M. S. SCHWARTZ. Implications of longitudinal muscle fibre splitting in neurogenic and myopathic disorders. *J. Neurol. Neurosurg. Psychiatry* 40: 1152–1159, 1977.
668a. SYROVY, I., E. GUTMANN, AND J. MELICHNA. Effect of exercise on skeletal muscle myosin ATPase activity. *Physiol. Bohemoslov.* 21: 633–638, 1972.
669. SYSKA, H., S. V. PERRY, AND I. P. TRAYER. A new method for preparation of troponin I (inhibitory protein) using affinity chromatography. Evidence for three different forms of troponin I in striated muscle. *FEBS Lett.* 40: 253–257, 1974.
670. TAKÁCS, Ö., I. SOHÁR, T. PELLE, F. GUBA, AND T. SZILÁGYI. Experimental investigations on hypokinesis of skeletal muscles with different functions. III. Changes in protein fractions of subcellular components. *Acta Biol. Acad. Sci. Hung.* 28: 213–219, 1977.
671. TAKÁCS, Ö., I. SOHÁR, T. SZILÁGYI, AND F. GUBA. Experimental investigations on hypokinesis of skeletal muscles with different function. IV. Changes in the sarcoplasmic proteins. *Acta Biol. Acad. Sci. Hung.* 28: 221–230, 1977.
672. TAYLOR, A. W., S. CARY, M. MCNULTY, J. GARROD, AND D. C. SECORD. Effects of food restriction and exercise upon the disposition and mobilization of energy stores in the rat. *J. Nutr.* 104: 218–222, 1974.
673. TAYLOR, A. W., S. LAVOIE, G. LEMIEUX, C. DUFRESNE, J. S. SKINNER, AND J. VALLÉE. Effects of endurance training on the fiber area and enzyme activities of skeletal muscle of French-Canadians. In: *Biochemistry of Exercise*, edited by F. Landey and W. A. R. Orban. Miami, FL: Symposia Specialists, 1978, p. 267–278.
674. TAYLOR, A. W., D. C. SECORD, P. MURRAY, AND G. BAILEY. The effect of castration and repositol testosterone treatment on exercise-induced glycogen and free fatty acid mobilization. *Endokrinologie* 61: 13–20, 1973.
675. TAYLOR, A. W., R. THAYER, AND S. RAO. Human skeletal muscle glycogen synthase activities with exercise and training. *Can. J. Physiol. Pharmacol.* 50: 411–415, 1972.
676. TERBLANCHE, S. E., R. D. FELL, A. C. JUHLIN-DANNFELT, B. W. CRAIG, AND J. O. HOLLOSZY. Effects of glycerol feeding before and after exhausting exercise in rats. *J. Appl. Physiol.: Respirat. Environ. Exercise Physiol.* 50: 94–101, 1981.
677. TERJUNG, R. L., Cytochrome c turnover in skeletal muscle. *Biochem. Biophys. Res. Commun.* 66: 173–178, 1975.
678. TERJUNG, R. L. Muscle fiber involvement during training of different intensities and durations. *Am. J. Physiol.* 230: 946–950, 1976.
679. TERJUNG, R. L., K. M. BALDWIN, W. W. WINDER, AND J. O. HOLLOSZY. Glycogen repletion in different types of muscle and in liver after exhausting exercise. *Am. J. Physiol.* 226: 1387–1391, 1974.
680. TERJUNG, R. L., AND J. E. KOERNER. Biochemical adaptations in skeletal muscle of trained thyroidectomized rats. *Am. J. Physiol.* 230: 1194–1197, 1976.
681. TESCH, P., L. LARSSON, A. ERIKSSON, AND J. KARLSSON. Muscle glycogen depletion and lactate concentration during downhill skiing. *Med. Sci. Sports Exerc.* 10: 85–90, 1978.
682. TESCH, P., K. PIEHL, G. WILSON, AND J. KARLSSON. Physiological investigations of Swedish elite canoe competitors. *Med. Sci. Sports* 8: 214–218, 1976.
683. TESCH, P., B. SJÖDIN, AND J. KARLSSON. Relationship between lactate accumulation, LDH activity, LDH isozyme and fibre type distribution in human skeletal muscle. *Acta Physiol. Scand.* 103: 40–46, 1978.
684. THOMPSON, E. H., A. S. LEVINE, P. V. J. HEGARTY, AND C. E. ALLEN. An automated technique for simultaneous determinations of muscle fiber number and diameter. *J. Anim. Sci.* 48: 328–337, 1979.
685. THORNER, S. H. Trainierungsversuche an Hunde. 3. Histologische Beobachtungen an Herz und Skelettmuskel. *Arbeitsphysiologie* 8: 359–370, 1935.
686. THORSTENSSON, A. Muscle strength, fibre types and enzyme activities in man. *Acta Physiol. Scand. Suppl.* 443: 1976.
687. THORSTENSSON, A., L. LARSSON, P. TESCH, AND J. KARLSSON. Muscle strength and fiber composition in athletes and sedentary men. *Med. Sci. Sports* 9: 26–30, 1977.
688. THORSTENSSON, A., B. SJÖDIN, AND J. KARLSSON. Enzyme activities and muscle strength after "sprint training" in man. *Acta Physiol. Scand.* 94: 313–318, 1975.
689. THORSTENSSON, A., B. SJÖDIN, AND J. KARLSSON. Separation of isozymes of creatine phosphokinase and lactate dehydrogenase in human heart muscle by isoelectric focusing. In: *Progress sin Isoelectric Focusing and Isotachophoresis*, edited by P. G. Righetti. Amsterdam: North-Holland, 1975, p. 213–222.
690. THORSTENSSON, A., B. SJÖDIN, P. TESCH, AND J. KARLSSON. Actomyosin ATPase, myokinase, CPK and LDH in human fast and slow twitch muscle fibres. *Acta Physiol. Scand.* 99: 225–229, 1977.
691. TIPTON, C. M., R. D. MATTHES, J. A. MAYNARD, AND R. A. CAREY. The influence of physical activity on ligaments and tendons. *Med. Sci. Sports* 7: 165–175, 1975.
692. TIPTON, C. M., R. D. MATTHES, A. C. VAILAS, AND C. L. SCHONEBELEN. The response of the *Galago senegalensis* to physical training. *Comp. Biochem. Physiol.* 63A: 29–36, 1979.
693. TIPTON, C. M., AND T. K. TCHEN. Influence of physical training, aortic constriction and exogenous anterior pituitary hormones on the weights of hypophysectomized rats. *Pfluegers Arch.* 325: 103–112, 1971.
694. TIPTON, C. M., R. L. TERJUNG, AND R. J. BARNARD. Response

of thyroidectomized rats to training. *Am. J. Physiol.* 215: 1137–1142, 1968.

695. TOMANEK, R. J. A histochemical study of postnatal differentiation of skeletal muscle with reference to functional overload. *Dev. Biol.* 42: 305–314, 1975.

696. TOMANEK, R. J. Ultrastructural differentiation of skeletal muscle fibers and their diversity. *J. Ultrastruct. Res.* 55: 212–227, 1976.

697. TOMANEK, J., AND A. S. COLLING-SALTIN. Cytological differentiation of human fetal skeletal muscle. *Am. J. Anat.* 149: 227–246, 1977.

698. TURTO, H., S. LINDY, AND J. HALME. Protocollagen proline hydroxylase activity in work-induced hypertrophy of rat muscle. *Am. J. Physiol.* 226: 63–65, 1974.

699. VALDIVA, E. Total capillary bed in striated muscle of guinea pigs native to the Peruvian mountains. *Am. J. Physiol.* 194: 585–589, 1958.

700. VALENTIN, N., AND K. H. OLESEN. Measurements of muscle tissue water and electrolytes. *Scand. J. Clin. Lab. Invest.* 32: 155–160, 1973.

701. VAN LINGE, B. The response of muscle to strenuous exercise. *J. Bone Jt. Surg.* 44B: 711–721, 1962.

702. VAN WIJHE, M., M. C. BLANCHAER, AND S. ST. GEORGE-STUBBS. The distribution of lactate dehydrogenase isozymes in human skeletal muscle fibres. *J. Histochem. Cytochem.* 12: 608–614, 1964.

703. VARNAUSKAS, E., P. BJÖRNTORP, M. FAHLÉN, I. PREROVSKY, AND J. STENBERG. Effects of physical training on exercise blood flow and enzymatic activity in skeletal muscle. *Cardiovasc. Res.* 4: 418–422, 1970.

704. VAUGHAN, H. S., AND G. GOLDSPINK. Fibre number in a surgically overloaded muscle. *J. Anat.* 129: 293–303, 1979.

705. VIHKO, V., Y. HIRSIMAKI, H. RUSKO, M. HAVU, P. V. KOMI, AND A. U. ARSTILLA. Adaptation of skeletal muscle to endurance training: succinate dehydrogenase activities in highly trained skiers. *Int. Res. Commun. System* 2: 1033, 1974.

706. VIIDIK, A. The effect of training on the tensile strength of isolated rabbit tendons. *Scand. J. Plast. Reconstr. Surg.* 1: 141–147, 1967.

707. VIIDIK, A. Elasticity and tensile strength of the anterior cruciate ligaments in rabbits as influenced by training. *Acta Physiol. Scand.* 74: 372–380, 1969.

708. VIIDIK, A. Tensile strength properties of achilles tendon systems in trained and untrained rabbits. *Acta Orthop. Scand.* 40: 261–272, 1969.

709. VRBOVÁ, G. The effect of motoneurone activity on the speed of contraction of striated muscle. *J. Physiol. London* 169: 513–526, 1963.

710. WACHTLOVÁ, M., AND J. PARÍZKOVÁ. Comparison of capillary density in skeletal muscles of animals suffering in respect of their physical activity—the hare (*Lepus europaeus*), the domestic rabbit (*Oryctolagus domesticus*), the brown rat (*Rattus norvegicus*), and the trained and untrained rat. *Physiol. Bohemoslov.* 21: 489–495, 1972.

711. WAHREN, J., B. SALTIN, L. JORFELDT, AND B. PERNOW. Influence of age on the local circulatory adaptation to leg exercise. *Scand. J. Clin. Lab. Invest.* 33: 79–86, 1974.

712. WALKER, M. G. The effect of exercise on skeletal muscle fibres. *Comp. Biochem. Physiol.* 19: 791–797, 1966.

713. WATRUS, J. M. Influence of chronic exercise on myosin from cardiac and skeletal muscles of hamster and rats. Pullman: Washington State University, 1980. PhD thesis.

714. WATTENBERG, L. W., AND J. L. LEONG. Effects of coenzyme Q_{10} and menadione on succinic dehydrogenase activity as measured by tetrazolium salt reduction. *J. Histochem. Cytochem.* 8: 296–303, 1960.

715. WEEDS, A. Myosin: polymorphism and promiscuity. *Nature London* 274: 417–418, 1978.

716. WEEDS, A. Myosin light chains, polymorphism and fibre types in skeletal muscles. In: *Plasticity of Muscle*, edited by D. Pette. New York: de Gruyter, 1980, p. 55–68.

717. WEEDS, A. G., AND B. POPE. Chemical studies on light chains from cardiac and skeletal muscle. *Nature London* 234: 85–88, 1971.

718. WHALEN, R. G. Contractile protein isozymes in muscle development: the embryonic phenotype. In: *Plasticity of Muscle*, edited by D. Pette. New York: de Gruyter, 1980, p. 177–191.

719. WIGGLESWORTH, V. B. The utilization of reserve substances in *Drosophila* during flight. *J. Exp. Biol.* 26: 150–163, 1949.

720. WILES, C. M., A. YOUNG, D. A. JONES, AND R. H. T. EDWARDS. Relaxation rate of constituent muscle-fibre types in human quadriceps. *Clin. Sci.* 56: 47–52, 1979.

721. WILKIE, D. R. The relation between force and velocity in human muscle. *J. Physiol. London* 110: 249–280, 1950.

722. WILLIAMSON, J. R., AND R. H. COOPER. Regulation of the citric acid cycle in mammalian systems. *FEBS Lett.* 117, Suppl.: K73–K85, 1980.

723. WINDER, W. W., K. W. BALDWIN, AND J. O. HOLLOSZY. Enzymes involved in ketone utilization in different types of muscle: adaptation to exercise. *Eur. J. Biochem.* 47: 461–467, 1974.

724. WITTENBERG, B., AND J. B. WITTENBERG. Role of myoglobin in the oxygen supply to red skeletal muscle. *J. Biol. Chem.* 250: 9038–9043, 1975.

725. WOHLFART, G. Über das Vorkommen verscheidener Arten von Muskelfasern in der Skelettmuskulatur des Menschen und einiger Säugetiere. *Acta Psychiatr. Neurol. Scand. Suppl.* 12: 1–119, 1937.

726. WOOD, D. S., J. ZOLLMAN, J. P. REUBEN, AND P. W. BRANDT. Human skeletal muscle: properties of the "chemically skinned" fiber. *Science* 187: 1075–1076, 1975.

727. WROBLEWSKI, R., G. M. ROOMANS, E. JANSSON, AND L. EDSTRÖM. Electron probe X-ray microanalysis of human muscle biopsies. *Histochemistry* 55: 281–292, 1978.

728. YAMAKI, T., S. BAEZ, AND L. R. ORKIN. Microvasculature in open cremaster muscle of mouse. *Microcirculation 1*, edited by J. Grayson and W. Zingg. New York: Plenum, 1976, p. 402–403.

729. YAMAMOTO, Y. Comparison of histochemical and physiological characteristics. of *m. digastricus* and *m. semitendinosus* of the guinea pig. *Jpn. J. Physiol.* 23: 509–528, 1973.

730. YAMPOLSKAYA, L. I. Biochemical changes in the muscle of trained and untrained animals under the influence of small loads (English translation). *Sechenov Physiol. J. USSR* 39: 91–99, 1952.

731. YELLIN, H. Changes in fibre types of the hypertrophying denervated hemidiaphragm. *Exp. Neurol.* 42: 412–428, 1974.

732. ZÍKA, K., Z. LOJDA, AND M. KUCERA. Activities of some oxidative and hydrolytic enzymes in musculus biceps brachii of rats after tonic stress. *Histochemie* 35: 153–164, 1973.

CHAPTER 20

Diseases of skeletal muscle

R. H. T. EDWARDS
D. A. JONES | *Department of Medicine, Faculty of Clinical Science, University College London, London, England*

CHAPTER CONTENTS

AN INTEREST IN NORMAL muscle physiology, a compassionate response to suffering, and a fascination with physical fitness and athletic performance are motives for research leading to our present understanding of muscle disease. How muscle diseases present to the clinician, the ways in which muscle disease can be examined, and the specific disorders as they have been investigated comprise this chapter. The field is large so only an introduction and guide to the relevant literature are given. We concentrate on muscle disorders that are thought to originate in the muscle itself and do not discuss those that are a consequence of degeneration of motoneurons or nerves. The latter diseases are fully discussed by Bradley (33), Bradley and Thomas (36), and Liversedge and Campbell (249).

HISTORY

Although normal muscle physiology was of interest to Galvani and other scientists in the eighteenth century [for review see Needham (293)], it was not until the latter part of the nineteenth century that descriptions of human muscle diseases were recorded. Some of the first accounts were those of Meryon (269, 270),

Duchenne (115, 116), Gowers (166), and Landouzy and Déjèrine (232). These authors described the pseudohypertrophic and the facioscapulohumeral types of muscular dystrophy and recognized their intractable nature.

Since the 1950s many advances in the study of muscle disease have been made in the field of biochemical pathways. The genetic disorders of glycogen metabolism in other tissues were described over 50 years ago in patients in whom there was an excessive accumulation of glycogen in tissues [reviewed by DiMauro (98)]. The physiological implications of glycogen storage in muscle and the occurrence of abnormalities in this system were highlighted by McArdle's (259) elegant demonstration of a failure in lactate production during ischemic forearm exercise in a patient with muscle cramps after exercise. The enzyme defect (absence of myophosphorylase) responsible for this was demonstrated simultaneously by two groups only a few years later (277, 335). The subsequent discovery of a defect in acid maltase activity heralded the recognition of a succession of inherited disorders of lysosomal metabolism (e.g., see GLYCOLYTIC DISORDERS, p. 652).

Since the 1950s our knowledge of the number and diversity of muscle diseases has increased rapidly, largely through the development of sensitive electromyographic methods and the use of histochemical techniques to examine the fine structure of diseased muscle.

The cross-innervation experiments of Buller et al. (54), which demonstrated the importance of the nerve supply in determining the functional characteristics of the muscle, were the first of the observations that led to the proposal of the neurogenic theory of muscular dystrophy (264). This theory suggests that the primary defect may be in the nerve supply to the muscle rather than in the muscle itself. Other theories have also been considered, such as the possibility that muscle degeneration could be due to defects of the microcirculation (91) or to an abnormal response to serotonin (for review see ref. 143).

In recent years investigators have argued that there may be membrane defects in the muscle and other tissues of dystrophic patients; the "leaky" cell membrane allows the accumulation of intracellular calcium, which leads to cellular damage. Calcium appears to play an important role not only in the control of contractile activity but also in many other cellular metabolic processes.

Much of the progress is the result of support by the Muscular Dystrophy Group of Great Britain, the Muscular Dystrophy Association of America, and similar organizations throughout the world.

CLINICAL PRESENTATION OF MUSCLE DISEASE

Muscle diseases are expressed in many different ways. The most obvious manifestation of muscle involvement is when a patient can be shown to be objectively weak, that is, unable to produce the force expected of a person of his or her stature, age, or sex. A child may fail to achieve the motor milestones such as sitting and walking, whereas an adult may not be able to rise from a chair, climb stairs, or sit up in bed. In general these patients do not complain of the sensation of weakness, but rather of its consequences, the failure to perform everyday tasks. Such patients are weak even when rested, in contrast to a second group who are of normal strength at rest but in whom only a small amount of exercise leads to premature or excessive fatigue. A third category is patients who are not necessarily weak or especially fatigable but have some disturbance of function such as spasticity, inability to relax the muscle after contraction (myotonia), or abnormally severe cramps or episodes of weakness. Patients who are difficult to categorize are those whose various muscle aches and pains have not been diagnosed. These patients tend to be labeled hysterical, but in many cases this merely hides our considerable ignorance of the origins of pain in muscle. If any objective evidence of abnormality (either of function, structure, or chemistry) can be found, it is often a great relief to these patients, who are reassured to know that their problem has some organic basis.

The most common characteristics of muscle diseases are briefly described here and discussed at greater length with the diseases that may be responsible.

Weakness

The force generated by any muscle is proportional to the cross-sectional area of the contractile proteins; consequently hypertrophy or atrophy of the muscle fibers results in an increase or decrease in force, whereas growth in length does not change the isometric force generated.

Except for a few rare muscle diseases, muscle weakness is almost always due to loss of contractile tissue. This may occur in two ways: muscle fibers may be damaged and destroyed (destructive myopathies) or the fibers may shrink and atrophy but not disappear altogether (atrophic myopathies). In both cases the cross-sectional area of contractile tissue is decreased. In the destructive myopathies the replacement of muscle fibers with fat and connective tissue may sometimes mask the loss of muscle bulk (pseudohypertrophy), but in the atrophic myopathies the weakness is associated with thin and wasted muscles.

Fatigue

The physiological basis of human muscle fatigue was the subject of a recent Ciba Foundation symposium (383). Fatigue can be defined as the failure to achieve or maintain an expected force or power output. A person with reduced muscle bulk, if asked to maintain the same absolute force as a normal subject, will inevitably tire more rapidly. There are patients, however, who have apparently normal amounts of muscle but still fatigue rapidly. These patients fall into two main categories: those with myasthenic symptoms in whom a defect of the neuromuscular junction leads to neuromuscular block during an attempted sustained contraction and those with some defect of muscle energy metabolism leading to unduly rapid depletion of muscle energy stores and fatigue. Interestingly abnormal muscle metabolism does not always result in more rapid fatigue: patients with hypothyroidism, in whom there is a decrease in muscle adenosine 5′-triphosphate (ATP) turnover, can sustain isometric contractions for appreciably longer periods than normal subjects (384).

Myoglobinuria

The appearance of myoglobin in the urine is a serious matter because it indicates the destruction of muscle and may also lead to renal damage. It can occur as a consequence of physical damage to the muscle, such as crush injuries, but it is more often seen in clinical practice as a result of rhabdomyolysis or active myositis or more rarely as a symptom of some metabolic muscle disease such as carnitine palmitoyltransferase or a myophosphorylase deficiency.

Unusual Function

Spasticity and myotonia are the most common forms of disordered function. Spasticity originates in the central nervous system and therefore is not considered here. Myotonia, or the inability to fully relax the muscle following contraction, may be a symptom of such diseases as myotonia congenita and myotonic dystrophy and probably has a different physiological basis in each instance.

Table 1 gives a brief guide to the various types of neuromuscular disease, the presenting symptoms, and the subsequent time course of the various disorders.

INVESTIGATION OF PATIENTS WITH MUSCLE DISEASE

Current procedures used for patients referred to the Charles Dent Metabolic Unit, University College Hospital, are similar to the practice of many other centers, although the procedures described for muscle function testing may be more extensive than usual.

Clinical History and Examination

Clinical investigation has two main parts. First there is the routine history-taking and description of symptoms of the patient and family from which may emerge details suggesting a genetic basis for the complaint. [Good recent accounts of this procedure include those of Brooke (42) and Dubowitz (111).] The physical examination afterward is intended to demonstrate any defects in performance due to weakness of particular muscle groups. Posture is checked because alteration in the shape of the spine is often a consequence of weakness of the proximal muscles. Such weakness can also result in a characteristic waddling gait, which is a form of postural adaptation (343).

Blood Biochemistry

Investigation of patients with myopathy includes evaluation of plasma electrolytes, thyroid hormones and thyroid-stimulating hormone, full blood count and erythrocyte sedimentation rate, plasma proteins and immunoglobulins, and serum creatine kinase (CK). If there is any history of pigmenturia, myoglobin is measured in the urine, although a more sensitive test would be to measure it in serum because this gives positive results in a variety of conditions, including muscular dystrophy, even in the absence of myoglobinuria (216, 217). Hypo- and hyperkalemia are associated with episodes of flaccid paralysis (see *Periodic Paralysis*, p. 655), and altered thyroid function can result in considerable changes in muscle function (384).

Normal calcium chemistry helps to eliminate bone disease (e.g., osteomalacia) as a cause of muscle weakness, and a raised erythrocyte sedimentation rate points to the presence of inflammatory disease. Plasma proteins and immunoglobulins are important in the diagnosis of autoimmune states, some of which may include muscle symptoms. The most widely used test for these is the plasma CK activity. This enzyme is released from muscle cells in a wide variety of conditions, and increased activity is an indicator of active disease (306). In severe destructive muscle disease the CK activity may be raised by 2–3 orders of magnitude. Marginally raised values may occur because of exercise, local damage to the muscle after an intramuscular injection, or other reasons. For the diagnosis of putative carriers of Duchenne muscular dystrophy, CK activities have often been used, but marginally raised levels must be interpreted with care.

Electromyography

Clinical electromyography (EMG) is a valuable tool for differentiating diseases that are primarily myopathic from those that are neuropathic in origin (261). In myopathic disorders the characteristic EMG features include an increased number of small polyphasic action potentials that can be distinguished from the "giant" action potentials seen when collateral sprouting of nerves, leading to fiber grouping, has occurred in neurogenic atrophy with reinnervation. In denervated muscle, fibrillation and sharp waves can be detected (163). Myotonic discharges are easily recognized if the signal is played through a loudspeaker. The sound has been variously described as like a motorcycle or dive bomber.

Although valuable in the hands of an experienced clinician, EMG changes are difficult to quantify; nev-

TABLE 1. *Summary of Major Neuromuscular Diseases in Humans*

	Clinical Onset	Initial Symptoms	Progression
		Primary Myopathies (Muscular Dystrophy)	
Major types			
Pseudohypertrophic Duchenne	Early childhood.	Swayback, a waddling gait, and difficulty in rising from the floor and climbing stairs, due to pelvic girdle muscle weakness. Fat deposits replace wasting muscle tissue in the calves.	Rapid, ultimately involving all voluntary muscles. Death usually occurs within 10–15 yr of clinical onset.
Becker		Similar but less severe.	Slower progress.
Facioscapulohumeral Landouzy-Déjèrine	Early adolescence, occasionally in the 20's.	Lack of facial mobility, difficulty in raising arms over head, forward slope of shoulders, due to initial weakness of face and shoulder gridle muscles.	Very slow, often with intervals in which the disease marks time. Average life-span rarely shortened, despite considerable disability.
Limb girdle Includes juvenile dystrophy of Erb	Any time from 1st to 3rd decade of life.	Usually weakness of proximal muscles of both the pelvic and shoulder girdles.	Variable, sometimes slow and sometimes fairly rapid. Disability may remain slight and some patients live to old age.
Less common types			
Congenital dystrophy	Manifest at birth, indicating that the disease runs its course prenatally.	Small, weak muscles, sometimes multiple contractures.	Rapid, leading to the infant's early death.
Ophthalmoplegic dystrophy	Adulthood usually.	Weakness of extraocular muscles, causing drooping upper eyelids. Gradually spreads to pharyngeal muscles with resultant difficulty in swallowing and speaking.	Slow but inexorable.
Distal dystrophy	Middle age (40–60 yr).	Weakness in small muscles of hands and feet.	Slow and relatively benign.
		Neurogenic Atrophies (Noninfectious)	
Infantile spinal muscular atrophy Werdnig-Hoffman disease	Prenatal, at birth, or in 1st few months of life.	Symmetrical weakness of proximal muscles and "double joints." Infant can hardly crawl and is never able to walk.	The earlier the onset, the more rapid the course. Respiratory failure and/or infection usually cause death.
Benign congenital hypotonia Oppenheim's disease, amyotonia congenita	At birth or in 1st few months of life.	Similar to above, but milder and not so crippling. Child can walk.	None.
Juvenile spinal muscular atrophy Kugelberg-Welander disease	Late childhood or early adolescence as a rule.	Proximal muscle weakness similar to that in limb-girdle muscular dystrophy, with difficulty in rising from floor and climbing stairs.	Variable but usually very slow. Most patients live to old age.
Spinal muscular atrophy of adults Aran-Duchenne type	4th or 5th decade of life.	Distal muscles, especially fine hand muscles, are first affected, often with twitching of hand and arm muscles.	Variable. Some patients remain active for years.
Amyotrophic lateral sclerosis	Varying, from 20 to 60 yr of age.	Usually spastic irritability and weakness of leg muscles, later of pharyngeal muscles with difficulty in chewing, swallowing, and speaking. Sometimes it begins and progresses in reverse order.	Rapid, leading to death usually within 3–5 yr.
Peroneal muscular atrophy Charcot-Marie-Tooth disease	Between 5 and 50 yr of age.	Muscle weakness in feet and legs, spreading to hands and forearms, but sparing proximal muscles as a rule. Often inability to move big toe and tendency to walk on outer sides of feet are first signs.	Slow, leading to deformities of hands and feet, but rarely to death.
		Neuromuscular Junction Disease	
Myasthenia gravis	Any time of life, but commonly in 2nd decade in women, 4th to 6th decade in men.	Ptosis (eyelid drop) in some cases, difficulty in swallowing or speaking in others, often weakness in leg or arm muscles, especially after activity.	Some cases progress slowly, others improve or remain stationary. There may be occasional spontaneous remissions and exacerbations.
Myotonias			
Myotonia congenita Thomsen's disease	Early childhood.	Difficulty in relaxing muscles after contracting them, aggravated by cold.	None. Mild, lifelong disability.
Myotonic dystrophy Steinert's disease	Young adulthood, occasionally as early as puberty.	Weakening of hand and forearm muscles, with myotonic stiffness and inability to relax handgrip. Eye and tongue muscles often affected. Sometimes cataracts.	Variable but reaches severe disability 15–20 yr after onset. Patients rarely attain a normal life span.
Myositis			
Polymyositis	Any time of life.	Proximal muscle weakness not connected with any identifiable systemic disorder.	Variable, may be mild and chronic, severe and chronic, or rapidly fatal. Occasional periods of remission.
Dermatomyositis	Any time of life.	Similar to polymyositis symptoms, with a reddish skin eruption on face and upper trunk.	Similar to polymyositis.
		Congenital Myopathies (Rare, Sometimes Classed as Dystrophies)	
Central core disease Nemaline myopathy Mitochondrial disease Myotubular myopathy Idiopathic myopathy	Manifest at birth.	Hypotonic muscles and slowness in learning to walk. Later diffuse, mainly proximal, weakness.	Very slow, except in central core disease, which is nonprogressive.

ertheless in recent years some progress has been made by the measurement of "turns" and the mean amplitude between turns (189, 190). Another measurement that could have an application in clinical practice is power-spectrum analysis. This gives quantitative information about interference patterns but so far has been used mainly in the study of muscle fatigue (174, 215, 218).

Nerve stimulation in conjunction with EMG recording is used in the diagnosis of myasthenia, where abnormal decremental responses can be restored to normal by the administration of cholinesterase inhibitors (see ELECTROPHYSIOLOGICAL STUDIES, p. 653). More specialized techniques involve the recording of single-fiber activity (134). Recording from two muscle fibers of the same motor unit permits the measurement of the delay in firing between the first and second fibers. Variations in this time give rise to the phenomenon of "jitter." Excessive jitter and the occasional failure of the second fiber to fire at all are indications of neuromuscular block. Measurements of jitter have been useful in the diagnosis of myasthenia (350), and abnormalities have also been reported in muscular dystrophy (351).

Muscle Biopsy

Study of the muscle biopsy and the clinical examination are the most important investigations leading to a diagnosis. The biopsy specimen is also the raw material for much of the clinical research into muscle disease. Duchenne used a device, his "harpoon," very similar to a modern biopsy needle, to obtain samples that revealed the "living pathological anatomy" of diseased muscle (70).

Muscle biopsy has been of prime importance since the development in the late 1950s of histochemical techniques for the examination of muscle composition (114). Muscle samples are usually taken from the larger proximal muscle groups, either quadriceps or deltoid muscles, and can be obtained either by an open biopsy through an incision in the skin (3–5 cm long) or, as is becoming increasingly common in Europe, with a percutaneous needle biopsy method. The latter technique was reintroduced for the study of tissue electrolytes (20), tissue metabolites (200), and for clinical diagnosis (129).

The various biopsy techniques have their own advantages and disadvantages; the choice of method depends on many factors, including the types of tests to be carried out on the material obtained. One major advantage of the needle biopsy method is that it is possible to do repeated biopsies either to investigate metabolite changes during exercise or to follow the patient's progress in treatment over a longer period (133).

Histochemical (112) and biochemical (127, 130) techniques have been developed that allow many different determinations to be made on small samples of muscle, 50–100 mg being sufficient for most purposes. In clinical use the priorities of investigation are usually histochemical and electron-microscope examination, followed by specific enzyme measurements of both glycolytic and oxidative pathways, and then measurements of metabolites and electrolytes. Of the histological stains, hematoxylin-eosin is most commonly used to give an overall impression of the muscle fiber architecture and to show damage and inflammatory responses. From the histochemical studies the first task is to identify the different fiber types to determine whether there is any preferential involvement of one type or another. For this the myosin ATPase and oxidative enzyme stains are the most useful. Specific enzyme defects can be demonstrated by histochemical stains (e.g., myophosphorylase deficiency in McArdle's disease), and these can be a valuable screening procedure.

The needle biopsy technique and its clinical application for pathological and biochemical diagnosis have been reviewed recently (133).

Nuclear Magnetic Resonance

In the last few years the noninvasive technique of nuclear magnetic resonance (NMR) has been used to study chemical changes in intact muscles (85). Unusual phosphodiesters have been found in dystrophic muscle (69). With the development of new and larger magnets it is now becoming possible to use topical NMR to make measurements of human muscle constituents in situ (77, 131a). Further development of this technique may improve the study of chemical composition and metabolism of both normal and diseased human muscle. It may also provide a much-needed means of measuring muscle metabolism on repeated occasions during drug trials.

Measurement of Muscle Cross-Sectional Area

The force-generating capacity of a muscle depends on the cross-sectional area and the intrinsic strength of the contractile elements. Absolute measurements of force in human muscle are difficult to make because the lever systems through which the force is measured are not well defined, but in any one patient they remain constant and serial measurements can be valuable. Cross-sectional area is also difficult to measure in a limb that contains other muscles, fat, and bone. Total thigh volume can be calculated on the assumption that the form of the thigh can be represented by a series of truncated cones (212), and volume has been shown to correlate well with serial measurements of quadriceps muscle force made on a patient recovering from polymyositis (131).

ULTRASOUND. Ultrasound has been used to determine the cross-sectional area of muscles and to measure changes produced by programs of strength-training exercises (105, 202, 203). The principle underlying the imaging of muscle by ultrasound is that there is a reflection of sound waves at tissue interfaces. Although a clear distinction can be made between muscle and subcutaneous fat at the interface represented by the fascia covering the muscle and between muscle and the underlying bone, it is not reliable when there is replacement of muscle with fat and connective tissue, as in the dystrophies. In these circumstances there is a loss of reflection from the femur due to abnormal attenuation of the sound waves (191). Ultrasound can be a valuable guide to the treatment of wasting resulting from fracture of the lower limb when muscle is wasted without replacement with fat (393).

COMPUTERIZED TOMOGRAPHY. Although recently developed and used to visualize the cross-sectional area of the muscle, computerized tomography also gives information about the composition of the tissue. The method can be used to distinguish differences in density between muscle tissue and fat that may be occupying space within the fascial envelope [Fig. 1; (53, 124)]. Computerized tomography has also been used in the diagnosis of a unilateral swelling of the calf muscle, which was eventually found to be caused by an infiltrating lipoma (148).

Tests of Muscle Function

In his book on the physiology of motion, Duchenne (116) explored the function of most human muscles. With faradic stimulation, he studied the action of muscles in the living body and in freshly amputated limbs. Subsequent work on the response to electrical stimulation in human muscle has largely been carried out with small peripheral muscles with accessible motor nerves. Muscles studied in this way include the extensor digitorum brevis (263), the abductor digiti minimi (57), the adductor pollicis (268), and the first dorsal interosseus muscle of the hand (352).

Small distal muscles have been useful in the investigation of neuromuscular function in a number of conditions, including myasthenia (96), myotonia (382), and Duchenne muscular dystrophy (96a). Disadvantages of distal muscles are: *1*) the muscle temperature must be carefully controlled or it may fall below that of other muscle groups, creating the appearance of abnormal behavior; and *2*) most muscle disorders are proximal, with distal muscles being relatively spared until late in the course of the disease.

There are a number of factors that particularly recommend the quadriceps muscle for investigation: *1*) it is a proximal muscle group often severely affected in muscle disease, *2*) the group is load bearing and is therefore important to a patient for the maintenance of mobility, and *3*) it is also relatively free of major blood vessels and nerves so that a biopsy can be safely taken. Studies of function, structure, and chemistry can therefore be carried out on the same muscle. In the objective assessment of muscle strength the first measurement to be made is the force of a maximum voluntary contraction (MVC) of a well-defined muscle group. Isometric contractions of the quadriceps can be conveniently measured with a muscle-testing chair (360). For isokinetic contractions the commercial Cybex machine has been effectively used for determining the relation between the force-velocity characteristics

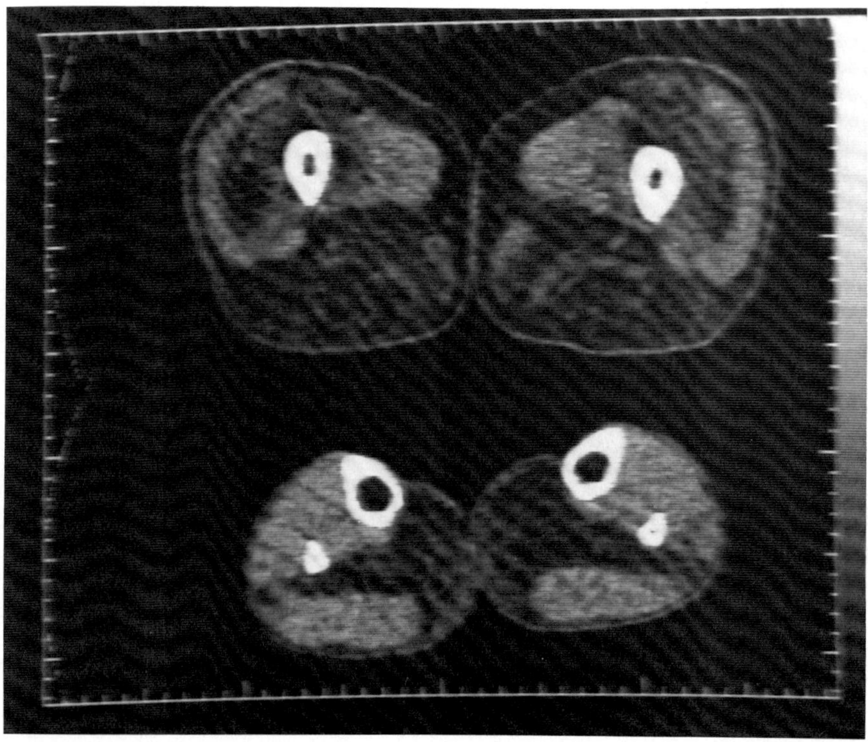

FIG. 1. Computerized tomography in a male West Indian (age 44 yr) with limb-girdle dystrophy. *Top*: cross sections in midthigh region. There is partial replacement of quadriceps muscle and almost complete replacement of posterior thigh (hamstring) muscles with fat. *Bottom*: cross sections in region of maximum calf circumference. There is hypertrophy of anterior tibial muscles, preservation of gastrocnemius, and replacement of soleus muscle by fat.

of the quadriceps muscle and its fiber-type composition (359).

Training, activity, occupation, age, sex, and build all influence muscle strength. As a practical guide for assessing a patient's weakness it has been found that for a wide range of body sizes the maximum quadriceps strength is linearly related to the body weight (132). In normal subjects the force (kg force) generated at the ankle during a maximum isometric contraction is approximately 75% of the body weight (in kg) with a lower limit of normal (3rd percentile) at about 50% of the body weight. Patients who generate less than this begin to experience difficulty performing everyday movements such as rising from a chair or walking up stairs. Walking on the level, however, requires only a low force to be generated in the quadriceps and is continued, often in the presence of very severe muscle wasting.

A number of muscles can be made to contract by electrical stimulation of the motor nerve, and this technique has been applied to the adductor pollicis stimulated via the ulnar nerve (132). The quadriceps has been maximally stimulated via the femoral nerve (22), and although in normal subjects this procedure is not without risk, it has been used with care in the study of selected patients (197).

For practical clinical purposes, however, reproducible stimulated contractions of the quadriceps can be easily elicited by percutaneous stimulation of the nerve terminals in the motor end-plate region. This is accomplished with large pad electrodes that activate 30%–50% of the whole muscle. Unstimulated parts of the muscle, in parallel with contracting portions, do not influence the contractile properties, such as relaxation rate. The procedure of percutaneous electrical stimulation is acceptable to the subject in terms of discomfort, is almost entirely free of risk, yields useful information, and has been used in the investigation of both adults (132) and children (197).

Percutaneous stimulation of motor nerve branches has been used to study the sternomastoid muscle as an indicator of respiratory muscle function (288), and stimulation of the phrenic nerve has been used to assess diaphragm function by measuring the transdiaphragmatic pressure produced (287).

In each of these studies stimulation of the muscle has been indirect, via the motor nerve. Human muscle has been intentionally stimulated directly in vivo only when massive discharges (1,000–1,500 V) were applied to the adductor pollicis (193). In these studies direct stimulation was adduced from the fact that the time from the stimulus to the latency relaxation was shorter with direct stimulation than when the muscle was stimulated with more usual voltages via the motor nerve branches.

Electrical stimulation gives an objective measurement of muscle function uncomplicated by the patient's emotional or psychological problems. It is also a valuable tool for studying the causes of muscle fatigue.

Isolated Human Muscle Preparations

The only practical in vitro human muscle preparation with intact cells is that from intercostal muscle (176). This preparation has been used to investigate the properties of muscle fiber membranes in periodic paralysis (319), and a preparation with an intact nerve supply has been used in the study of myasthenia gravis (79).

More accessible preparations employ fiber bundles with cut but ligatured ends (286). These can be made from samples of human muscle taken during routine surgery and remain viable for several hours. The contractile properties measured in vitro generally agree well with measurements of quadriceps and adductor pollicis function in vivo. This isolated preparation was originally developed to screen patients with suspected malignant hyperpyrexia. Abnormally large contractures were seen with preparations from susceptible patients when halothane was added to the bathing fluid (284, 285).

Mechanically skinned rabbit muscle fibers have been used to study the differential effects of H^+ on calcium-activated force generation (104). Chemically skinned muscle fibers have been used to investigate the relationship between possible defects in calcium activation and those of the contractile mechanism itself (390). The advantage of this preparation is that calcium and substrates can be independently varied. The force per unit cross-sectional area generated by this preparation agreed well with those for normal muscle with intact cell membranes, whereas somewhat lower values were observed in muscle from patients with Duchenne muscular dystrophy (391).

Exercise and Fasting as Provocation Tests

Exercise testing is a well-established technique in the assessment and diagnosis of patients with cardiac or pulmonary disorders. The same techniques [summarized by Jones et al. (211)] can be applied to the study of patients with metabolic myopathies. Exercise alone was used by Brooke and co-workers (43, 67) to distinguish three categories of patients: *1*) those with psychogenic symptoms and relatively normal responses to exercise; *2*) those with metabolic myopathies who showed signs of abnormal muscle damage as a consequence of exercise, namely, a raised CK; and *3*) those with mitochondrial abnormalities, who showed abnormally high levels of lactate after exercise. Results from a patient with a mitochondrial abnormality, an inability to oxidize pyruvate in the muscle, are shown in Figure 2. Not only was there a very large rise in plasma lactate for a relatively small amount of work, but the levels were also very slow to return to normal.

Although the exercise tests can provide an aid to diagnosis, the various factors that affect performance and the way in which muscle diseases influence these are still unclear so that the exercise test remains essentially a research tool.

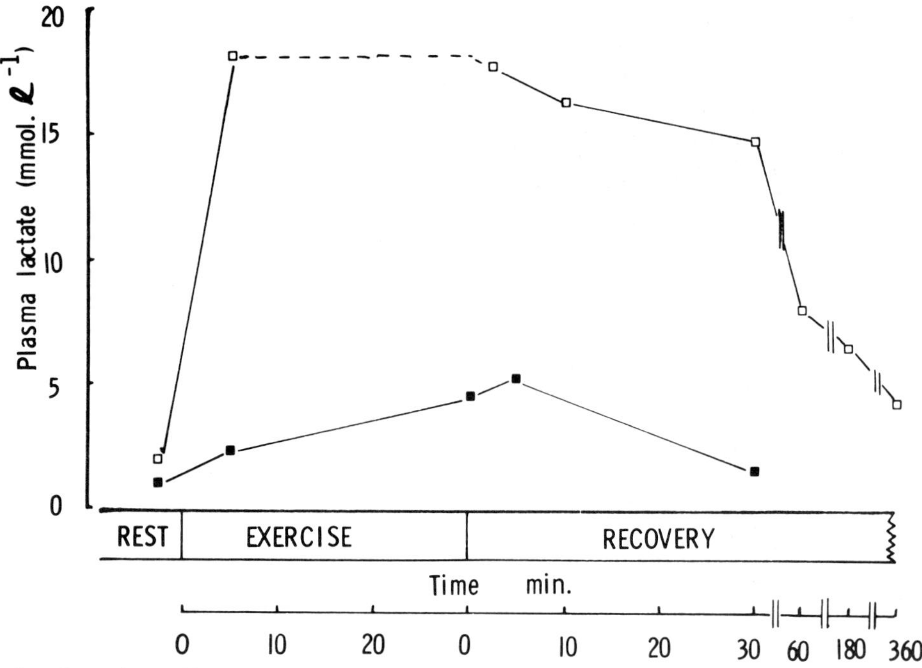

FIG. 2. Abnormal response to exercise of a patient with defect of mitochondrial metabolism. ■, Normal subject; work done = 196 W (70% max). □, Patient with a defect in mitochondrial pyruvate metabolism; work done = 65 W (59% max). Note that despite doing less absolute and relative work, patient had a much greater rise in plasma lactate, which was slow to recover. [From Edwards et al. (130)]

Fasting alone or in conjunction with exercise may provide an additional stress that reveals underlying metabolic abnormalities. In general those patients with defects in fatty acid metabolism are more severely affected by fasting, because during this period the body comes to rely on fat and ketone bodies as the major substrate. Patients with defective glycolytic pathways are less affected and may even show some improvement in their exercise performance during fasting (66).

Studies of Protein Turnover

In assessing turnover of total-body protein, the nitrogen balance can be used to study the course of a myopathy and its treatment. Changes in nitrogen balance have been shown to mirror quadriceps strength during deterioration and subsequent recovery in a patient with polymyositis (131).

Muscle bulk can be determined from the daily excretion of creatinine. Approximately 1 g of creatinine is formed per 20 kg of muscle by the degradation of creatine and is quantitatively excreted in the urine (169). The administration of [^{15}N]creatine by mouth and the measurement of its dilution in muscle biopsy samples have been used in children to measure muscle bulk (315). The determination of whole-body potassium gives a less specific indication of muscle bulk but could well be used to monitor loss of muscle (310).

Myofibrillar catabolism can be estimated by measuring the urinary excretion of 3-methylhistidine, which is derived from muscle actin and myosin and is excreted without further metabolism in humans. To measure the catabolic rate, 3-methylhistidine excretion is related to total muscle mass, most conveniently by expressing the results as the ratio of urinary 3-methylhistidine to creatinine.

The intracellular free 3-methylhistidine content of muscle appears to correlate with the rate of muscle breakdown as measured by its urinary excretion (317). Although 3-methylhistidine is predominantly derived from skeletal muscles, smooth muscle in the gut and skin also make a contribution to urinary excretion (275). In cases where the skeletal muscles are wasted, the smooth muscle contribution may be disproportionately large, making changes in the observed excretion difficult to interpret; the precise contributions from the different sources remain to be determined. Rates of protein synthesis in muscle have been determined in normal subjects by infusing labeled lysine (182). Techniques for measuring protein turnover in humans have recently been reviewed in detail (377).

ANALYSIS OF MUSCLE WEAKNESS

Muscle weakness is by far the most common clinical observation in patients with muscle diseases. Muscle strength is directly proportional to the cross-sectional area of the contractile material, and in the majority of cases weakness is due to muscle wasting and loss of contractile material.

Dystrophies

The term *dystrophy* includes all those hereditary progressive disorders of muscle that generally result in cell destruction and replacement of the muscle with fat and fibrous tissue. Several dystrophies can be distinguished clinically by their progress, the muscles affected, the pattern of inheritance, and the microscopic appearance of the affected muscles. In most dystrophies light microscopy reveals the presence of internal cell nuclei (as opposed to peripheral nuclei in normal fibers), with a wide variation in fiber size (see Fig. 3). Increased lysosomal enzyme activity is seen in fibers stained for acid phosphatase. In addition to these destructive changes, numerous large round hypertrophied fibers and small basophilic fibers are seen (80); the latter are thought to be regenerating cells. As the condition progresses the muscle is replaced with fat and connective tissue until there is virtually no contractile tissue left.

The most serious, though not the most common, type is Duchenne muscular dystrophy (pseudohypertrophic muscular dystrophy), which has a sex-linked recessive mode of inheritance. This form of dystrophy is receiving the most attention because it leads to progressive disability and death in the second or third decade (157). A slightly less severe form is Becker dystrophy, which also has a sex-linked mode of inheritance. It usually appears in the teens (282). There are a few clinical differences between these two severe forms of muscular dystrophy, but the essential pathological features are the same and the course is progressive in both.

Another form of dystrophy is limb-girdle (scapulohumeral) muscular dystrophy, which usually has a recessive form of inheritance although in rare instances there are families in which the inheritance is dominant (374). This type of dystrophy has a more benign course than Becker or Duchenne dystrophies, and sufferers may survive late into adult life but often with considerable disability due to profound limb-girdle weakness. The histopathological appearances are

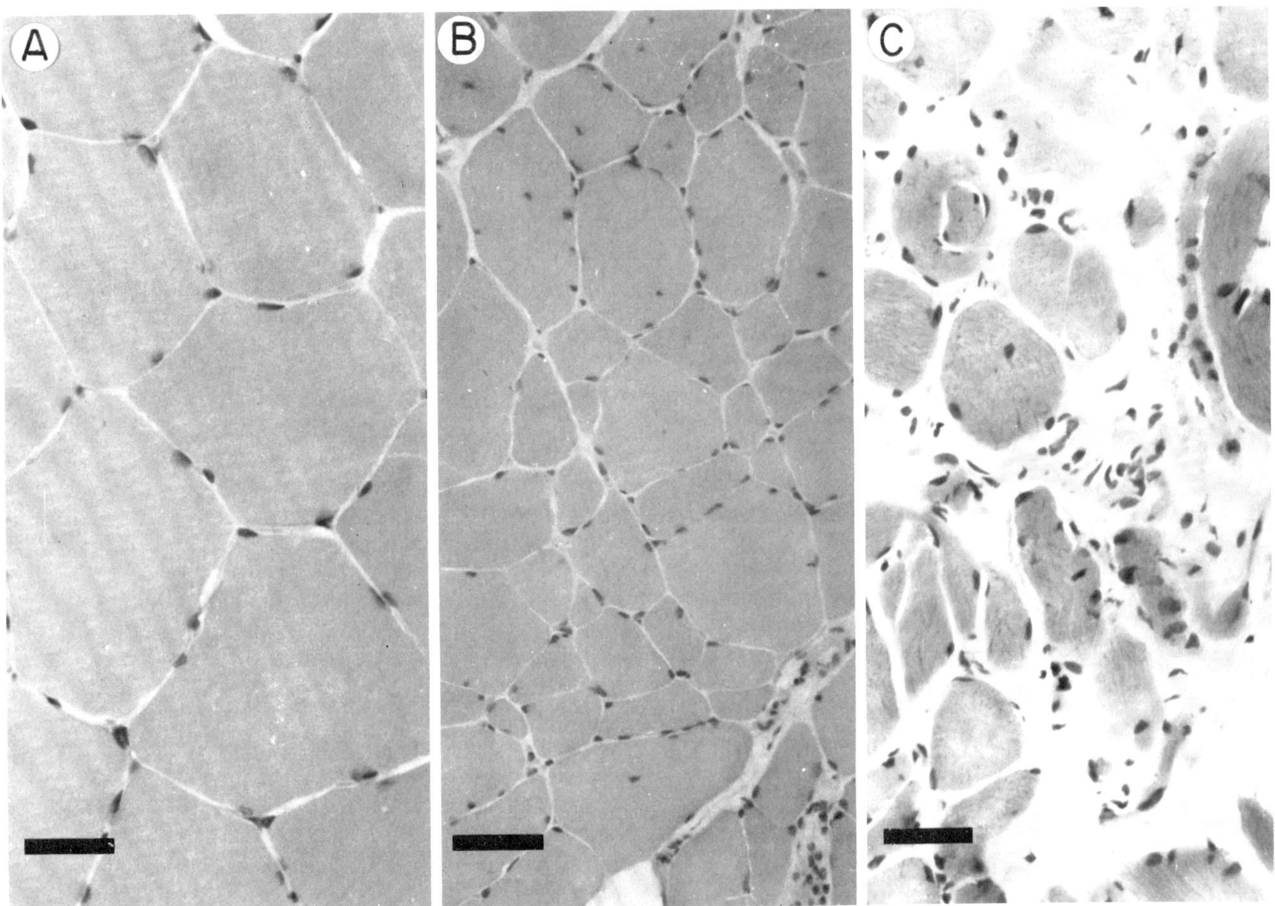

FIG. 3. Dystrophic changes in muscle: cross sections of quadriceps muscle stained with hematoxylin-eosin. *A*: normal (male, 22 yr). *B*: early dystrophy (male, 9 yr); note internal nuclei and variations in fiber size. The overall difference in fiber size between *A* and *B* reflects age difference between the 2 subjects and is not abnormal. *C*: advanced dystrophy (male, 17 yr); note loss of contractile material, which is replaced by fat and fibrous tissue. Scale bar = 50 μm.

similar to those in Duchenne dystrophy. It is almost certain that this diagnostic category includes a number of different diseases. The same clinical picture can be produced by a disorder of the central nervous system, the Kugelberg-Welander disease, a mild form of spinal muscular atrophy (348). Although the weakness is very similar to that in limb-girdle muscular dystrophy, the pathological and electromyographic features are quite different, showing evidence of group fiber atrophy and enlargement of motor units due to collateral reinnervation. Hypertrophy may also be a feature in this condition (29, 175, 365).

A well-recognized type of muscular dystrophy first described in the nineteenth century is facioscapulohumeral dystrophy (232). Here the inheritance is dominant; there is a wide variation of gene expression within a family, and patients usually have a normal life span. As its name implies, the distribution of the weakness is predominantly in the upper limb girdle, but later in the disease the lower limbs may be affected.

In general clinical practice the type of muscular dystrophy most likely to be seen in adults is myotonic dystrophy. This is dominantly inherited, but gene penetration varies considerably. The patients usually survive well into adult life, although severe forms may appear in childhood or adult life with progression and ensuing disability. This condition differs from most other diseases involving muscle; weakness starts peripherally and only later involves proximal muscle groups. Myotonia of the hands is often the initial symptom. Myotonic dystrophy is a multisystem disease involving the membranes of many tissues, including blood cells, brain, heart, endocrine system, skin, and eyes (184). There is evidence of impaired insulin sensitivity in patients with myotonic dystrophy that is out of proportion to the degree of muscle wasting (289). It is thought to be peripheral, involving several organs including the liver, and the excessive cell response to glucagon, fructose, and galactose is thought to be secondary to reduced affinity of insulin receptors (356).

There are a number of rare variants of these main forms of dystrophy, including the X-linked scapuloperoneal dystrophy, which may be considered a variant of limb-girdle muscular dystrophy (323, 358). An interesting variant is the dominantly inherited oculopharyngeal type (368) in which abnormalities in mitochondrial structure and function have been found (214, 281) as well as alterations in immune tolerance. There are some congenital dystrophies, disorders of muscle occurring in utero. At birth the child presents with muscular weakness, joint dislocation, or the features of arthrogryposis multiplex. A feature distinguishing this disease from the true dystrophies is that the muscle disorder progresses little after birth. Autosomal recessive inheritance seems likely, but acquired intrauterine disease is a possible cause in some cases (157). The importance for normal muscle development of intrauterine movement has not been explained but may be a factor in the etiology of these conditions. Depressed ventilatory response to exercise has been reported in oculocraniosomatic neuromuscular disease (Kearns-Sayer syndrome; ref. 67).

Apart from the dystrophies there are a few so-called congenital myopathies. These may be manifested as a failure in the development of one particular fiber type (42) or the presence of rodlike bodies (nemaline myopathy) or cores (central core disease). Diseases due to abnormalities of mitochondrial structure or chemistry are also often included in the category of congenital myopathy. The pathological and clinical features of myopathies are well described elsewhere (42, 111, 112).

Inflammatory Myopathies

Polymyositis and dermatomyositis are the most commonly seen types of acute muscle disease. The loss of muscle tissue may sometimes be severe enough to cause myoglobinuria (228) and consequent renal failure. The loss of muscle leads to weakening and immobilization of the patient, and if the respiratory muscles are involved, there is then the risk of a life-threatening respiratory failure.

The disease is characterized by weakness and less often tender or wasted muscles. A biopsy in the early stages shows marked variation in fiber size, infiltrations of macrophages into the muscle tissue, and increased lysosomal activity [Fig. 4; (340)]. In the advanced stages the destruction may be severe enough to resemble that in dystrophic muscle.

Several classifications have been proposed, and it seems likely that polymyositis is a heterogeneous group of conditions, whereas dermatomyositis is homogeneous (326). Both are almost certainly the result of autoimmune reactions against the muscle, which are probably cell mediated (304, 322). Several studies showed that lymphocytes from animals and human patients with polymyositis are cytotoxic toward muscle cells grown in culture (209).

The factors responsible for initiating the autoimmune response are not known but probably include virus infections, drugs, and neoplasia. The primary treatment is with immunosuppressive drugs and high doses of corticosteroids. This may lead to complications, however, because high doses of steroids can themselves cause muscle wasting. It is therefore important during treatment to balance the beneficial and harmful effects of the steroids (131). In doing this, quantitative information about muscle strength and the course of the disease is clearly essential in making a therapeutically useful distinction between residual weakness due to continuing disease and that from therapy with corticosteroids.

Atrophy and Hypertrophy

It is well known that immobilization and inactivity result in muscle atrophy and that increased activity,

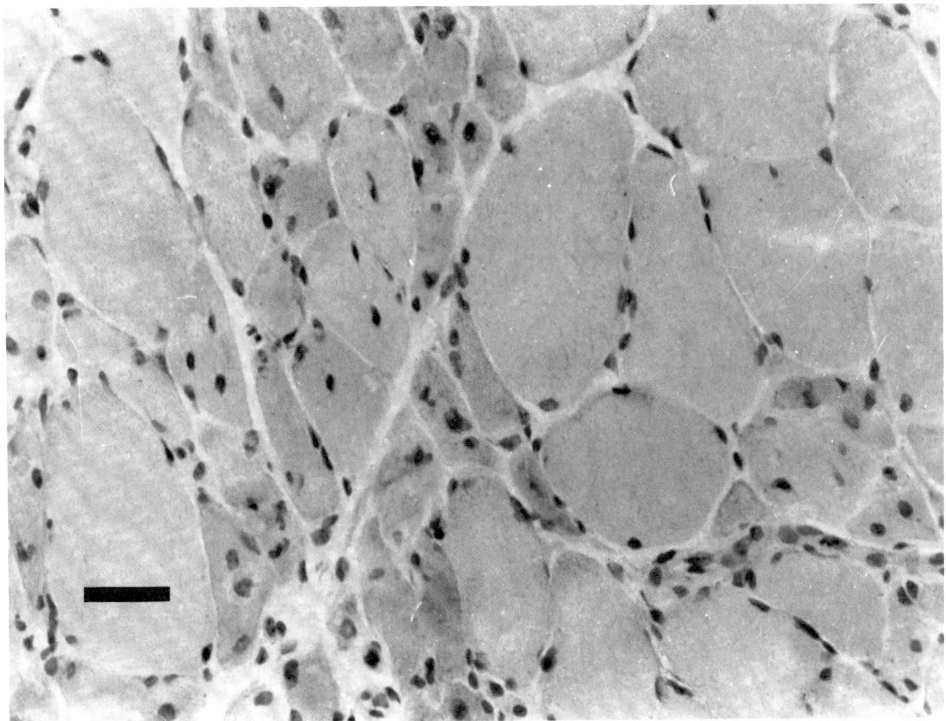

FIG. 4. Cross section of quadriceps muscle in patient with polymyositis (female, 48 yr); note marked differences in fiber size, internal nuclei, and infiltration with macrophages. Scale bar = 50 μm.

particularly when associated with strength-training exercise, results in hypertrophy.

The effect of prolonged submaximal activity is to improve the oxidative capacity of the muscle with the induction of mitochondrial oxidative enzymes (192) but with little or no increase in myofibrillar mass and consequently little or no increase in strength (75, 122, 161). Resistive exercises are capable of increasing both muscle strength and muscle mass. Both fiber types increase in size but changes are more noticeable in the type II fibers (105, 332).

Two mechanisms could lead to an overall growth of a muscle. The individual cells may increase in size (hypertrophy) or increase in number (hyperplasia). Evidence suggests that human muscle changes are the result of an increased or decreased cell size rather than a changed number because there is a good correlation between cell size and overall muscle cross-sectional area determined by computerized tomography (179) or ultrasonography (393). Although muscle fiber splitting is often seen in the destructive myopathies (354), demonstrating the possibility of hyperplasia, it is probably not a major mechanism for muscle growth in normal subjects, being in all probability a response to damage.

ATROPHIC MYOPATHIES. In the atrophic myopathies there is typically a reduction in the cross-sectional area of the individual muscle fibers, which often affects one type more than another, the effect on the whole muscle being the loss of a proportion of the contractile material. Most frequently it is the type II fibers that show the greatest atrophy (Fig. 5), a common observation in muscle biopsy samples regarded as a nonspecific finding of little diagnostic significance. Type II fiber atrophy is commonly seen in hypothyroidism (266, 394), osteomalacia (82, 392), and in a number of other conditions including chronic alcoholism, prolonged steroid therapy, rheumatoid arthritis, and wasting occurring as the result of carcinoma and malnutrition (112, 123).

Atrophic fibers become small and angular in appearance, but there is usually no evidence of abnormal lysosomal or inflammatory responses. Preferential atrophy of type I fibers is far less common. It has been reported in myotonic dystrophy (144, 184) and in some childhood myopathies (112).

Type II atrophy is believed to be the result of inactivity imposed on the patient by illness. We have also observed such atrophy in specimens of gluteus and quadriceps muscle obtained during the course of surgery for total hip replacement as have others (346) in patients who had been immobile for some time. Surprisingly, patients with immobilized limbs after knee injury or lower-limb fracture have the opposite: type I atrophy in the affected quadriceps (121, 178, 333). A striking absence of type I fibers in the quadriceps has been reported in patients after traumatic cervical cord transection (172).

If the underlying disorder (e.g., osteomalacia) is successfully treated, muscle strength recovers in parallel with the growth of the previously atrophied fibers (392).

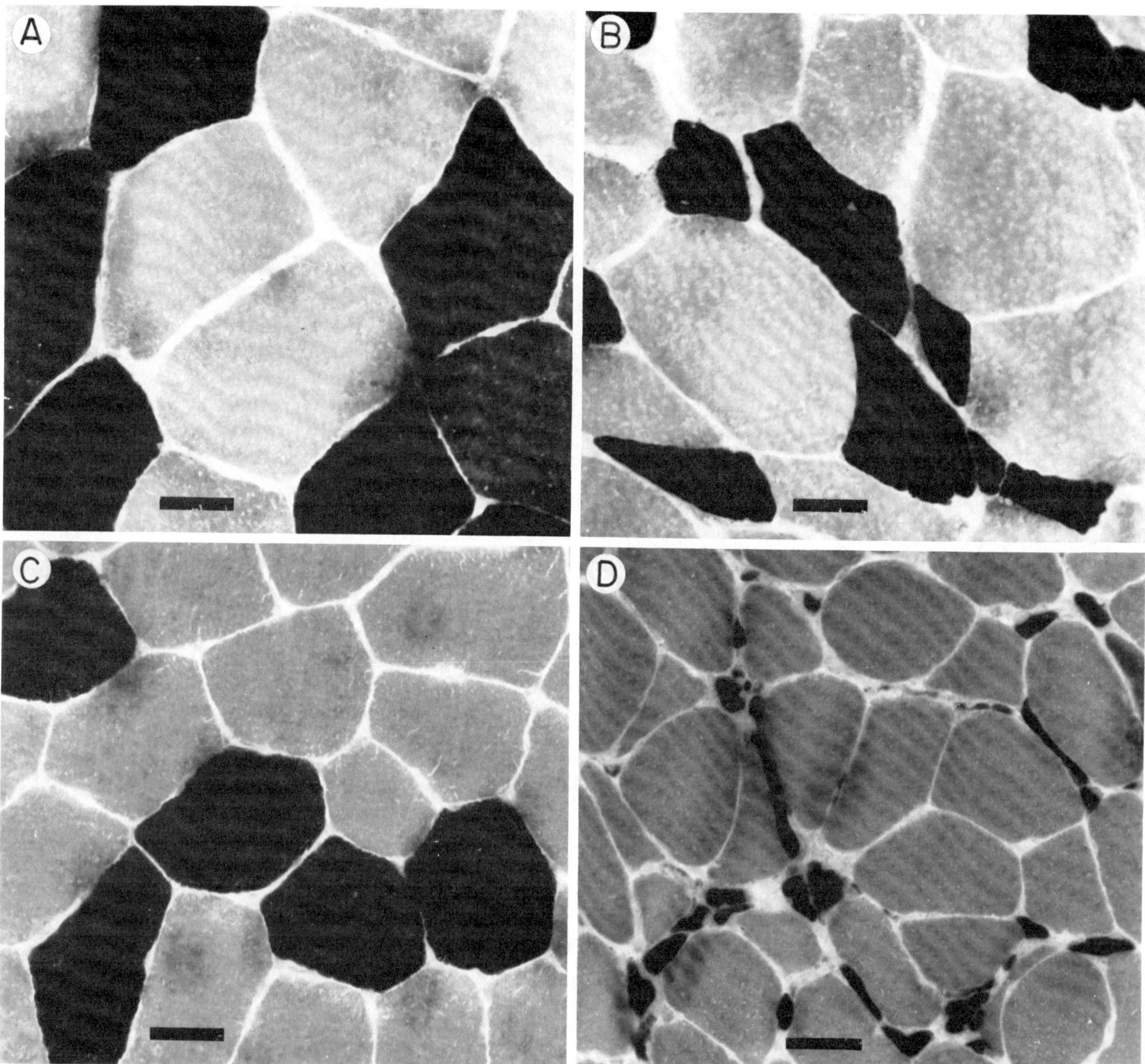

FIG. 5. Atrophic changes. Cross sections of quadriceps muscle stained for myosin ATPase at pH 9.4. Type I fibers, light staining; type II fibers, dark staining. *A*: normal male. *B*: male patient showing type II fiber atrophy after steroid therapy. *C*: normal female. *D*: female with Cushing's syndrome showing severe type II fiber atrophy. Scale bar = 50 μm.

Factors Affecting Protein Turnover in Muscle

Any attempt to explain the causes of hypertrophy and atrophy requires a consideration of the factors that control the normal growth and maintenance of cellular proteins (273, 274, 377, 394).

The protein content of the fiber is determined by the balance between synthesis and breakdown. Thus overall atrophy or hypertrophy of the whole muscle can be accomplished by either increased or decreased rates of protein degradation, provided that the corresponding synthesis rates are appropriately changed. There can be situations where a net increase in muscle protein is accompanied by an increased rate of protein degradation; this is the case during periods of rapid growth where overall weight gain, with a very rapid rate of protein synthesis, is also accompanied by a very rapid degradation (257). In regenerating adult muscle a similar situation may occur. Measurements of urinary 3-methylhistidine in a patient with polymyositis taken during both the active and the recovery phases showed that the excretion remained high even when there was a net protein synthesis and increase in muscle bulk (317). Increased 3-methylhistidine excretion has also been seen in children suffering from Duchenne muscular dystrophy (16, 265). In this case it is debatable whether the increased 3-methylhistidine excretion was caused by destruction of the muscle or was a consequence of increased protein turnover in regenerating fibers. This uncertainty raises an important question concerning the putative treatment of destructive myopathies. It has been suggested that the destructive process might be arrested by inhibitors of protein degradation (160, 353), but it could be that much of the increased protein degradation is an essential part of the regenerative activity of the remaining muscle fibers (316a). Inhibiting this process might therefore have undesirable consequences. Furthermore it now seems likely that the abnormality in Duchenne dystrophy is not so much an increased protein breakdown as a decreased synthetic rate (316b).

When atrophy is present in muscle it is most often seen in the type II, faster-contracting fibers. Animal studies have shown differences in protein-turnover rates between the two muscle fiber types. In the rat the slower-contracting muscles have an actomyosin-turnover rate that is approximately twice that seen in the faster-contracting muscles. For the anterior and posterior latissimus dorsi muscles in the chicken the difference is threefold (ref. 377, p. 504). The explanation for the different turnover rates in normal muscle fibers and why one fiber type should be more susceptible to atrophy than another are quite unknown, but it seems logical to imagine that there might be some link between these two questions, which are currently being researched.

The actions of insulin, thyroid hormones, and corticosteroids on muscle growth have been extensively studied in animal models. Thyroid hormones help to maintain normal protein-turnover rates in healthy animals. After thyroidectomy both synthesis and degradation rates are reduced. Thyroid replacement therapy restores turnover rates to normal (274). The influence of insulin on muscle protein is well documented (256). Stimulation of protein synthesis has been seen in vitro and also in whole animals by Hay and Waterlow [(188); see also ref. 378, p. 668].

In diabetic animals the fractional synthesis rate of skeletal muscle protein has been found to be between one-half and one-third normal and was accompanied by a marked decrease in the RNA content. Administration of insulin reversed these changes. Insulin causes the increased transport of amino acids into muscle, and there is debate as to whether the increase in protein synthesis is a consequence of this or is due to some other action of insulin within the cell; the evidence [reviewed by Waterlow et al. (377)] suggests that insulin may have a direct effect on intracellular protein synthetic mechanisms acting through an as yet unspecified "second messenger."

Glucocorticoids and insulin have opposing effects on protein turnover in muscle, and muscle growth may be predicted by the ratio of these two substances (377). The mechanism of action of corticosteroids is not clearly understood, but they may bind to receptor proteins and influence gene expression (258). It has also been suggested that they act by inhibiting glucose uptake by the muscle fiber (290). In the physiological range glucocorticoids probably induce muscle wasting by suppressing protein synthesis with little effect on protein breakdown. At high doses, such as those used during treatment, there is some evidence of an increased rate of protein degradation (317).

Growth hormone probably exerts an effect on muscle growth, but it is difficult to separate its action from that of insulin and changes in food intake because hypophysectomized rats show marked changes in both these variables (194, 364). The action of growth hormone on protein synthesis in muscle is probably mediated via the somatomedins. Purified somatomedin A stimulated amino acid incorporation into isolated diaphragm preparations without the lag period observed with growth hormone (367). It is possible that somatomedins and insulin may exert their influence on protein turnover at the same or similar receptor sites (181).

Neuropathies

Muscle requires an intact, healthy, and active nerve supply for its development and normal function. Damage to or dysfunction of either central motoneurons or peripheral motor axons leads to pathological changes in the muscle (261). Loss of an individual axon or motoneuron results in the atrophy of all the fibers of that motor unit that are of the same fiber type. Later there may be reinnervation of denervated muscle fibers by collateral sprouting of nearby motor axons. This gives rise to the predominance of a single fiber type in certain areas of the muscle, evident when the muscle is examined histochemically (Fig. 6), and the resultant large motor units are the reason for the EMG finding of giant action potentials (261).

ANALYSIS OF ABNORMAL FATIGABILITY

Everyone experiences muscular fatigue at one time or another, but in some individuals these symptoms can be profound enough to limit their activity and daily life. The assessment of these patients is complicated because the limiting factor may be the intensity with which these symptoms are perceived, rather than the objective changes in muscle function. Fatigue may be due to one or more changes in the central nervous system, the neuromuscular junction, or within the muscle itself. To identify abnormalities that lead to excessive fatigue in patients, we consider first the mechanisms leading to fatigue in normal subjects.

Muscle Fatigue in Normal Subjects

Several characteristics of muscle mechanics including fatigue were demonstrated in frog muscle by Fick (149), and Kennelly (227) described a "law of fatigue" in which there was a mathematical relationship be-

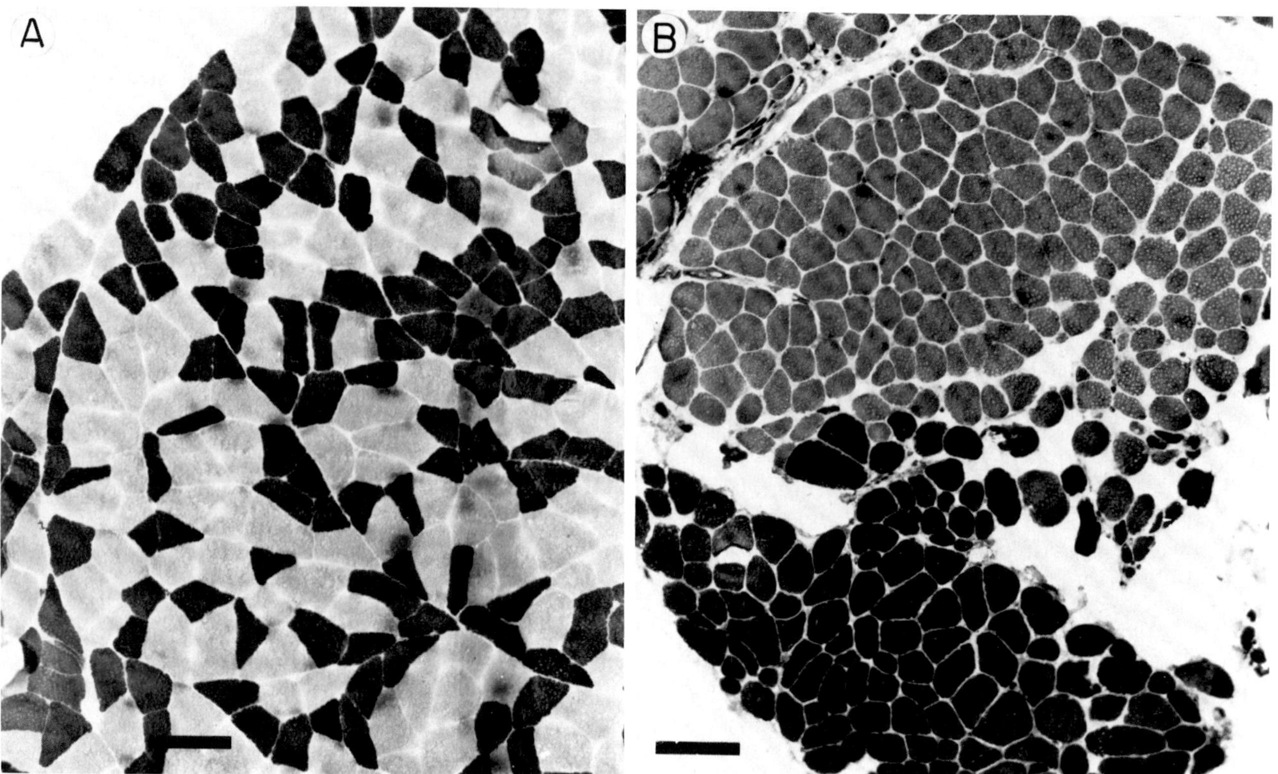

FIG. 6. Consequences of muscle denervation. Low-power views of cross sections of quadriceps muscle, stained for myosin ATPase at pH 9.4. *A*: normal muscle; note the even distribution of type I and II fibers. *B*: muscle from a patient with a neuropathy. A number of small atrophied fibers can be seen; these are a consequence of denervation. Main feature is pronounced fiber grouping, which is due to reinnervation of fibers by sprouting of nearby surviving motor nerve axons. Scale bar = 500 μm.

tween power output in running and endurance time for exercise in many different species. In his book on muscle fatigue in humans, Mosso (283) described studies of the finger flexors. With an ergograph, he investigated the effects of altitude, exercise, and emotional stress on the capacity to generate force in a series of brief contractions. He concluded that fatigue was central in origin; that is, the central nervous system was liable to reduce its motor drive before there was any evidence of failure in the contractile processes of muscle. That fatigue in voluntary contractions was central in origin had also been the conclusion of a long and reasoned argument by Waller (373). This became fully accepted when Reid (316) showed that in a series of fatiguing contractions the force of electrically stimulated contractions was retained when there was failure of voluntary contractions. This view was unchallanged until 1954, when Merton (268) showed in his studies of fatigue in the adductor pollicis muscle that there was evidence of failure in the muscle itself. The other main site where fatigue may occur is the neuromuscular junction; the work of Naess and Storm-Mathison (292) and more recently that of Stephens and Taylor (352) has shown that failure here may be a component of force loss in both stimulated and voluntary contractions. Abnormalities of neuromuscular transmission are an important cause of fatigue in some patients and this is discussed in *Myasthenia Gravis*, p. 647. Failure of action potential propagation along the surface membranes of the muscle has been suggested as another source of fatigue (23, 210).

One of the consequences of continued activity is slowing of muscle relaxation; this has been recognized for many years in animal muscle (147, 283) and more recently in human muscle (126). Edwards, Hill, and Jones (127) suggested that relaxation might reflect the rate of cross-bridge turnover and considered that the slowing of ATP turnover found in slowly relaxing muscle supports this idea. With phosphorous NMR, Dawson et al. (85), did not find any change in ATP turnover in frog muscle and favored a decreased rate of calcium reuptake by the sarcoplasmic reticulum as the explanation. There is, however, general agreement that the slowing is associated with a reduced muscle phosphagen level (ATP + phosphocreatine). Relaxation rate recovers with a time course similar to that of phosphocreatine resynthesis (186, 381).

After periods of heavy or ischemic exercise there are changes in the shape of the force/frequency curve; the force generated at the lower frequencies of stimulation is depressed relative to the force at higher frequencies (Fig. 7). It may take several hours to fully recover, and in some cases it has been observed as long as 24 h after exercise (128). This phenomenon has been called "low-

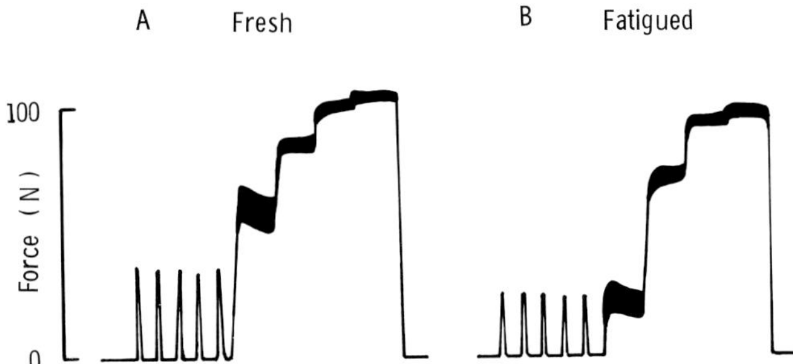

FIG. 7. Force generated by percutaneous stimulation of quadriceps muscle at different frequencies. Muscle was stimulated with 5 impulses at 1 Hz and then for 2 s successively at 10, 20, 50, and 100 Hz. *A*: fresh, rested muscle. *B*: same muscle tested after 10-min rest after a 20-min step test. Note that although maximum tetanic force is nearly fully recovered, force generated at low frequencies is much reduced.

frequency" fatigue and may be the result of damage to cell membranes that require de novo protein synthesis for their repair.

The perception of effort is an important factor influencing central fatigue; if a given task is perceived as requiring greater effort, it will become more difficult to complete. The study of such fatigue is fraught with difficulties. Where the sensation of effort arises is debated: it is not known whether it is contributed to by the perception of efferent motor drive to the muscle (155, 156) or by the various types of sensory information returning to the brain from the muscles, tendons, and joints involved in the contractions (60).

Change in perception of effort as a cause of unusual fatigability is not discussed at length, but it is important that this possible cause be recognized; it can be evaluated by comparing voluntary and electrically stimulated contractions. For large muscle groups, such as the quadriceps muscle, central fatigue is often a significant cause of force loss in normal subjects during the later stages of prolonged maximal voluntary contractions (22).

Myasthenia Gravis

The symptoms of myasthenia are well known and have been documented over the years (61, 94, 261, 344, 345, 369).

The onset of the weakness and fatigability, which can be rapid or insidious, may occur at any age but is most common in the second decade of life. The incidence is between 1:10,000 and 1:50,000 of the population, with twice as many females affected as males (261).

All muscles of the body may be involved, but weakness of the facial muscles with drooping eyelids often gives the patient a characteristic appearance. There may be difficulty with speech and swallowing, and involvement of the respiratory muscles may prove fatal. After a period of rest, muscles can have normal strength but weakness develops after brief activity. Diagnostic features are the characteristic EMG behavior, a rapid and sometimes dramatic improvement in muscle strength after injection of a cholinesterase inhibitor (edrophonium chloride, the Tensilon test), and an increased sensitivity to curare, although the last is infrequently used for diagnosis.

ELECTROMYOGRAPHY CHANGES IN MYASTHENIA. The characteristic behavior of myasthenic muscle is to show abnormal decrements of both force and action potential amplitude during repetitive nerve stimulation (96). This is seen at 20 or 30 Hz, when normal muscle would be expected to maintain force and action potential amplitude for at least 30 s. This stimulation may be a little unpleasant for patients, so the possibility of movement artifact could complicate the assessment. Desmedt (94) has described a test in which the response of the muscle to brief stimulation at 3 Hz is measured in a train of six impulses; the size of the fifth action potential is compared with that of the first and the decrement recorded. In normal subjects there is no such decrement. In myasthenic patients neuromuscular transmission appears to be improved by cooling (28).

SITE OF MUSCLE LESION. Normal nerve conduction and the beneficial effects of cholinesterase inhibitors (371, 372) pointed to a defect of the neuromuscular junction. The debate in recent years has been whether the lesion is pre- or postsynaptic.

Elmqvist et al. (139) made the observation that miniature end-plate potentials (MEPPs) in myasthenic muscles are decreased in amplitude. It was subsequently found that they are of normal frequency and increase in frequency (as would be expected) with the application of potassium (138). The reduced MEPPs could occur for two reasons: either the acetylcholine quanta are reduced in size or the receptor sites are reduced in number. The results of Dahlback et al. (81) and Elmqvist et al. (139) suggested that the sensitivity of the postsynaptic membrane to acetylcholine and cholinergic analogues is normal, indicating that the abnormality is a reduced quantity of acetylcholine released at the presynatptic membrane. On the basis of these arguments and his EMG observations showing posttetanic depression, Desmedt (95) has argued against the idea of myasthenic symptoms being due to curarelike substances, causing postsynaptic block. Despite these objections there remained sufficient similarities between myasthenia and partial curarization (the decremental EMG response, the action of anticholinesterases) to stimulate speculation that blood-borne curarelike substances cause myasthenic symptoms. This was reinforced by the existence of the neonatal form of myasthenia, which clearly suggested a blood-borne factor passing across the placenta (344).

In 1959 and 1960 a number of independent workers suggested that myasthenia gravis might have an autoimmune origin. These suggestions originated from observations of the frequent involvement of the thymus in myasthenia and the similarities between the presentation of myasthenia and other autoimmune diseases such as systemic lupus erythematosus. It was widely thought that either myasthenia gravis was due to an inflammatory reaction of the thymus (thymitis), which caused the release of a substance toxic to the neuromuscular junction, or that the thymus was the site of antibody production against the neuromuscular junction (for reviews see refs. 344 and 345). Acceptance of this theory, however, had to wait until the development of sensitive radioimmune assays for antibodies and techniques for measuring cholinergic binding sites, both based on the specific binding of snake venom toxins. As with other muscle diseases much of the impetus for research has come from the use of experimental animal models.

Patrick and Lindstrom (301) inoculated rabbits with electric eel acetycholine receptors (AChR) and demonstrated simultaneous muscle weakness and decremental EMG responses to repetitive stimulation in the presence of circulating antieel AChR antibodies. In the same year Fambrough et al. (146) demonstrated reduced numbers of acetylcholine-binding sites in human myasthenic muscle with a bungarotoxin-binding technique. Since then there has been a rapid advance in understanding both the immunological background and the nature of the damage to the receptors at the neuromuscular junction in myasthenia gravis.

Circulating AChR antibodies have been demonstrated in myasthenic patients with titers that are roughly proportional to the severity of the symptoms (243). It has also been shown that myasthenic immunoglobulin G (IgG) fractions can induce myasthenic symptoms when injected into mice (362, 363).

In contrast to the original findings of Elmqvist and co-workers it has now been shown that the myasthenic end plate does have a reduced acetylcholine sensitivity, the size of the MEPPs is related to the number of AChR sites (6, 146, 206) and inversely proportional to the amount of damage caused to the postsynaptic membrane (141a, 141b).

Although the action of the AChR antibody results in decreased MEPPs and decremental EMG response, characteristic postactivation exhaustion (94) has received little attention, and it is not clear whether the autoimmune mechanism can also account for this myasthenic property. The possibility that postactivation exhaustion may arise as a side effect of neuromuscular block is briefly mentioned by Satyamurti et al. (334) who found a form of posttetanic exhaustion in rat muscles that had been poisoned with cobra toxin, which specifically binds to receptor sites.

Changes in the postsynaptic receptor sites appear to occur for two reasons: *1)* the curarelike action of the antibodies blocks existing binding sites, and *2)* there is a reduction in the total number of sites. In studies of AChR turnover, Drachman et al. (106, 107) demonstrated an increased degradation of AChR when coupled to antibodies although synthesis was unaffected. The increased turnover appears to be caused by the antibodies' cross-linking adjacent receptor sites.

ETIOLOGY OF MYASTHENIA GRAVIS. The factors that may precipitate myasthenia are as elusive and problematic as they are in other autoimmune diseases; virus infections and emotional stress often appear to be precipitating factors. Apart from a very few cases there is little family history of myasthenia. Jacob et al. (207) found no secondary cases of myasthenia in 488 relatives of 70 patients. More recently, however, there have been reports of myasthenia associated with the human histocompatability antigen HLA-8 (344), suggesting that there may be predisposing factors that put certain people at risk of autoimmune complications after virus infection.

TREATMENT. Anticholinesterase inhibitors effectively relieve myasthenic symptoms; the object of treatment is to find the best long-lasting preparation, one that gives relief during periods of activity but avoids toxic side effects. Thymectomy is often helpful if carried out early in the course of the disease at a stage when the T cells are involved in antibody production. Later the production of antibody moves to extrathymic sites and thymectomy is ineffective. Plasmapheresis can give temporary relief by removing circulating antibodies (296), but its value as a routine form of treatment is still unproven despite claims that have been made for its usefulness (83).

Further developments in the treatment of myasthenia depend on advances in understanding and controlling the underlying autoimmune disease rather than treating the altered muscle function.

Disorders of Energy Metabolism

There are a number of genetically determined defects of muscle energy metabolism. These include defects in the glycolytic pathway, mitochondrial enzymes of both pyruvate and fatty acid metabolism, and the cytochrome components of the electron-transport chain. All are part of the pathways involved with the secondary supply of energy as the primary reserve, phosphocreatine, becomes depleted. As yet there have been no descriptions of defects in the actomyosin ATPase or the muscle creatine kinase reaction, perhaps because such defects might be lethal in utero.

In general, patients with metabolic defects are of normal or near normal strength when rested but are limited in their exercise endurance. When the defect is in the glycolytic pathway, the exercised muscle tends to go into a painful contracture (an electrically silent contraction). This is in contrast to those patients with mitochondrial disorders in whom a limited exercise capacity is associated with high blood lactate concentrations as if their muscles were partially ischemic.

GLYCOLYTIC DISORDERS. The present interest and research into the metabolic disorders of muscle began with the discovery of a myopathy with a defect in glycolysis (McArdle's disease) (259). The recognition of the enzyme defect (277, 355) and studies of whole-body exercise with substrate administration (308) have greatly stimulated interest in the physiological implications of specific enzyme defects in muscle. Since the discovery of myophosphorylase deficiency (type 5 glycogenosis) several other types have been discovered. Type 7 glycogenosis (355) is due to lack of phosphofructokinase (PFK). This has several features in common with McArdle's disease because the muscle is unable to produce lactate during anaerobic glycolysis. A number of other glycogen storage diseases may affect muscle (for reviews see refs. 101 and 255). The disorders affecting muscle are summarized in Table 2.

In these glycogen storage diseases the cause of weakness is not clear but is probably the result of mechanical damage to the contractile mechanism resulting from the accumulations of abnormal and less soluble forms of glycogen.

Type 2 glycogenosis (Pompe's disease); acid maltase deficiency. Type 2 glycogenesis is due to a deficiency of the lysosomal enzyme α-1,4-glucosidase and usually presents at birth as severe muscle hypotonia with respiratory failure. Apart from the specific enzyme deficiency the condition is characterized by large accumulations of glycogen in the muscle. The disease is usually fatal in early life (255) although there are now reports of adult patients presenting with similar symptoms (11, 102).

Type 3 glycogenosis; debrancher deficiency. Lack of debrancher enzyme leads to an accumulation of large amounts of structurally abnormal glycogen in the muscle. In the absence of this enzyme, myophosphorylase removes glycosyl units attached by a 1,4 linkage until a branch point is reached; the remaining glycogen molecule, called a limit dextrin, can be identified by the red color produced by its reaction with iodine. The clinical symptoms are diverse, ranging from severe muscle weakness in childhood to an asymptomatic form in the adult.

Type 4 glycogenosis (Andersen's disease); brancher enzyme deficiency. Type 4 glycogenosis is the result of a deficiency of brancher enzyme in which large amounts of abnormal glycogen are stored. It is a rapidly progressive childhood disease in which cirrhosis is a prominent feature (10).

Type 5 glycogenosis (McArdle's disease); myophosphorylase deficiency. McArdle's disease is caused by a specific lack of the adult form of myophosphorylase. Patients have normal strength at rest, but pain is experienced in the muscles during exercise. If the exercise is continued at a high level this leads to very painful contractures; these may occlude the local muscle circulation and lead to severe ischemic damage with the release of myoglobin into the circulation and the consequent risk of renal damage (18). If the exercise is continued at a lower level, the patients experience a "second wind," the pain diminishes, and they are able to continue with the exercise. The absence of myophosphorylase and the resultant inability to use stored glycogen severely limit the ability of the muscle to function under anaerobic conditions. During a prolonged voluntary contraction of normal muscle, approximately one-half of the total ATP turnover is derived from glycolysis; the total ATP flux available to the McArdle's patient is therefore reduced. When stimulated electrically the muscle loses force more rapidly than normal, and this is associated with a failure of the muscle action potential. This would suggest that one of the consequences of impaired ATP supply is altering the excitability of the muscle membranes (130, 383). The contractures that develop after a fatiguing contraction are electrically silent. They may be analogous to the contractures of rigor mortis, but measurements of the ATP content of the muscle

TABLE 2. *Enzyme Defects of Carbohydrate Metabolism*

Disease	Enzyme Deficiency	Tissues Affected	Clinical Features
Type 1: Von Gierke's disease	Glucose-6-phosphatase	Liver, kidney, skeletal muscle	Hepatomegaly, growth retardation, hypoglycemia ketosis, hyperlipemia, lactic acidosis
Type 2: Pompe's disease			
In infancy	Acid (lysosomal) α-1,4- and α-1,6-glucosidase	All tissues	Cardiomegaly, extreme weakness, death within 1st year of life
In adults		Skeletal muscle and liver	Proximal myopathy of variable severity, respiratory failure
Type 3: Cori-Forbes disease	Debrancher system results in abnormal glycogen (phosphorylase—limit dextrin)	Liver muscle, red blood cells, fibroblasts	Hepatosplenomegaly, fasting hypoglycemia, weakness
Type 4: Andersen's disease, amylopectinosis	Branching system results in abnormal glycogen—longer peripheral chains, fewer branching points	Liver, kidney, white blood cells, muscle, central nervous system, spleen	Hepatosplenomegaly, cirrhosis of liver
Type 5: McArdle's disease, myophosphorylase deficiency	Glycogen phosphorylase	Skeletal muscle	Cramps after exertion, myoglobinuria
Type 6: Hers' disease	Glycogen phosphorylase	Liver, white blood cells; skeletal muscle normal	Hepatomegaly, hypoglycemia, lactic acidosis
Type 7: Tarui's disease	Phosphofructokinase	Skeletal muscle, red but not white blood cells	Cramps after exertion, myoglobinuria

Data from Edwards et al. (125).

in contracture have not shown very large changes (325). This may mean that there are localized depletions of ATP within individual fibers or that some fibers may be more affected than others.

The second-wind phenomenon is a result of the utilization of blood-borne substrates, such as glucose and fatty acids, by the muscle as an alternative to the unavailable muscle glycogen (308, 312). The second wind is impaired if nicotinic acid is given to inhibit fatty acid metabolism (308). Patients can be helped by eating carbohydrates to raise the blood glucose just before exercise.

Although McArdle's disease is caused by a genetically determined enzyme defect, phosphorylase activity can be demonstrated in regenerating and cultured muscle cells from these patients (321). This is probably a fetal form of the enzyme lost during childhood (99).

Type 7 glycogenosis; phosphofructokinase deficiency. The clinical symptoms of PFK deficiency are very similar to those of McArdle's disease (355). After heavy exercise patients develop painful contractures of the muscles. During light exercise they show the second-wind phenomenon, but the improvement is not due to the utilization of blood glucose because their enzyme defect precludes the utilization of both glycogen and pentose sugars. The patients are therefore dependent on free fatty acids in the blood as a source of energy. Ketogenic diets may benefit these patients (101). One characteristic distinguishing this condition from McArdle's disease is that the defect is also seen in the red blood cells, giving rise to a hemolytic anemia often detectable by a raised reticulocyte count (234).

ACQUIRED DEFECTS OF GLYCOLYSIS. Disorders of carbohydrate metabolism that are associated with acquired disorders of muscle function have also been described. The striking reduction in glycolysis that may be seen in alcoholic muscle disease has been well documented (27, 307). Histochemical studies showing a reduced phosphorylase content of muscle from hypothyroid patients suggest that there may be impaired glycolysis in these cases (266). In part this may have been a reflection of the type I fiber predominance often seen in hypothyroidism. A direct demonstration of impaired muscle glycolysis was obtained by serial needle biopsies during sustained isometric contractions of the quadriceps (384). This reduction in the contribution of anarobic glycolysis to overall energy exchange during such (ischemic) contractions was reversed after several months of thyroid treatment. A paradoxical finding is a disproportionate increase in lactate concentrations during dynamic exercise of patients with hypothyroidism, which may occur because of the reduced circulating oxygen supply to working muscle as a result of reduced cardiac output (56). Another disorder of carbohydrate metabolism in hypothyroid muscle is a deficiency of acid maltase. After some months of treatment with thyroid replacement the enzyme activity was found to have returned to normal (201).

Reduction in the activity of a number of glycolytic enzymes has been reported in steroid myopathy (341). However, the interpretation is not straightforward because this condition is often associated with atrophy of the type II (glycolytic) fibers.

Impaired lactate response to ischemic forearm exercise has been described not only in the inherited glycogenoses but also in alcoholic myopathy, myasthenia gravis, steroid myopathy, polymyositis, and spinomuscular atrophy (74, 204).

Disorders of Mitochondrial Oxidative Metabolism

The first reported abnormality of human mitochondrial function was the description by Luft et al. (252) of a young Swedish woman who was hypermetabolic but euthyroid. The principal abnormality found in the muscle biopsy was abnormal mitochondrial ultrastructure and evidence of partially uncoupled mitochondrial metabolism. This condition appears to be very rare; there is only one other confirmed case (339). Abnormalities of mitochondrial structure are not uncommon, but as yet there is no known pattern relating structure to abnormal mitochondrial function. Microscopic examination of muscle stained with trichrome from patients with mitochondrial myopathies shows characteristic ragged red fibers. The abnormal staining is due to subsarcolemmal aggregations of mitochondria around the periphery of the cells and is commonly associated with profound muscle weakness in childhood and with other specific muscle diseases such as oculopharangeal muscular dystrophy and facioscapulohumeral dystrophy (112).

Morgan-Hughes et al. (280) described a case of muscle cytochrome *b* deficiency; the principal clinical signs were exercise intolerance and persistent lactic acidosis. Land and Clark (231) have reviewed a number of cases of cytochrome and mitochondrial enzyme deficiencies. One problem in assessing mitochondrial function in muscle is that training, bed rest, and habitual activity all influence the mitochondrial content of the fibers; it is therefore difficult to define normal levels against which to judge patients. It is possible that a reduction in the number of mitochondria in muscle is produced by habitual inactivity, and this may give rise to pain in chronically inactive subjects during exercise. More easily defined are cases where there is a specific deficiency of either an enzyme or cytochrome in the electron-transport chain, as in the case described by Morgan-Hughes et al. (280). A specific decrease in cytochrome *c* was reported by Willems et al. (385). A similar specific deficiency has also been seen in a young man with exercise intolerance as well as a much more severe and fatal case in a baby (159).

A mitochondrial defect that has been extensively studied in brain and in fibroblasts is pyruvate dehydrogenase (PDH) deficiency (24). Patients with a PDH deficiency present with ataxia and have a tendency to lacticacidemia, which may be reduced somewhat by the administration of a high-fat diet. It is not clear, however, to what extent the PDH deficiency described in nervous tissue and fibroblasts may also be expressed in other tissues such as muscle. We have studied a young man with severe exercise intolerance and a maximum oxygen uptake of less than 1 l/min. When exercised he produced a massive lacticacidemia, from which he was slow to recover. Measurements of muscle mitochondrial function showed that they were unable to utilize pyruvate, and a defect of either the PDH complex or pyruvate transport into the mitochondria was diagnosed (130).

Defects in mitochondrial function have been produced in animals by the use of uncoupling agents and chloramphenicol, which inhibits mitochondrial protein synthesis (330). Changes in mitochondrial structure have been seen after ischemia (302).

Disorders of Fat Metabolism

Disorders of fat metabolism have only recently been described (for review see ref. 103). The symptoms are weakness, exercise intolerance, muscle stiffness, and pain (sometimes accompanied by myoglobinuria). Symptoms are most evident at times when free fatty acids are the main substrates for energy metabolism such as during prolonged submaximal exercise, particularly in the fasting state.

The existence of lipid-metabolism disorders was first suggested by the observation of excessive accumulations of lipid in some muscle biopsy specimens (34, 35, 142, 145) and by the results of metabolic studies on human muscle (145). Fat accumulation around muscle fibers is also seen in cases of Duchenne muscular dystrophy, but a specific accumulation of fat droplets uniformly distributed within the fibers is peculiar to disorders of fat metabolism. In 1973 two specific disorders were described: carnitine deficiency (140) and carnitine palmitoyltransferase deficiency (100).

The β-oxidation of fatty acids depends on the transfer of free fatty acids into the mitochondria by a shuttle mechanism involving carnitine and the carnitine palmitoyltransferase (CPT) enzymes. It is believed that there are two transferases situated on the inner mitochondrial membrane, CPT I on the outer surface and CPT II on the inner surface of the membrane. The two transferases are very similar, but it is not known whether they are the same enzyme (38).

CARNITINE DEFICIENCY. Carnitine is synthesized in the liver and transported in the bloodstream to other tissues (76), and there is evidence for an active uptake of carnitine into the muscle (387). Disorders of fat metabolism associated with carnitine deficiency may occur for two reasons. There may be a failure of synthesis in the liver or of carnitine uptake by the muscle. Both of these problems have been described in humans, and although they exhibit similar clinical symptoms, they may be distinguished by measuring serum and muscle carnitine levels. Normal serum carnitine was reported by Angelini et al. (12) in a number of patients, which suggests normal hepatic synthesis but failure of muscle uptake, whereas Karpati et al. (226) reported a patient with both reduced serum and liver carnitine levels.

Where there is evidence of carnitine deficiency the first priority is to try to raise concentrations with oral carnitine. This treatment has improved exercise tolerance in patients who have evidence of hepatic involvement (12, 198). Even in those patients who appeared to have the defect in muscle transport, this therapy has resulted in some clinical improvement, although muscle carnitine concentration did not increase (12, 140, 226).

ACQUIRED PARTIAL CARNITINE DEFICIENCY. Marked carnitine deficiency in muscle has been described in patients with renal failure receiving regular dialysis (26). In humans, sepsis has also been reported to cause low serum carnitine (27). Malnutrition associated with liver disease (especially if the diet is deficient in lysine or methionine) may also give rise to carnitine deficiency (329). The "fatty degeneration" of the myocardium that occurs as a result of diphtheria toxin in guinea pigs (39) and in humans (376) is also thought to involve a local deficiency of carnitine. The normal metabolism of carnitine and the factors that affect it are not yet fully understood. According to Carrier and Berthillier (63) there are changes in the urinary excretion of carnitine during growth and development; excretion is low at birth, rises in the first few weeks of life, falls during the next three years, and subsequently rises to reach adult levels by about 10 yr of age. These authors also distinguish between soluble muscle carnitine and intramitochondrial carnitine, raising the possibility that there may be abnormalities of distribution within the cell. They also found low levels of muscle carnitine in patients with Duchenne muscular dystrophy but raised levels in patients with neurogenic atrophy.

Patients with carnitine deficiency have a tendency to lacticacidosis, which may reflect an increased glycolytic flux to compensate for impaired oxidation of fats.

CARNITINE PALMITOYLTRANSFERASE DEFICIENCY. To date 22 patients with CPT deficiency have been identified, of which only 2 have been female. The features differ from those of carnitine deficiency in that the dominant characteristic is recurrent pain and myoglobinuria, which is frequently precipitated by fasting or prolonged exercise. The onset of these symptoms is usually preceded by a rise in plasma CK activity, indicating damage to muscle. Weakness is not a feature except when associated with the pain and myoglobinuria. The accumulation of lipid in the muscle is not so marked as in carnitine deficiency. The muscle carnitine content may be raised (140, 145).

Because there are possibly two transferase enzymes,

attempts have been made to identify which is deficient in individual patients by comparing the mitochondrial oxidation of palmitate with that of palmitoylcarnitine. Oxidation of palmitate requires both the transferase enzymes (CPT I and CPT II), whereas oxidation of palmitoylcarnitine requires only the enzymes on the inner surface of the membrane (CPT II). The patient of DiMauro and DiMauro (100) showed an oxidation of palmitate that was more severely affected than that of palmitoylcarnitine, indicating a preferential loss of CPT I activity. Another patient, reported by Pathen et al. (300), showed a similar defect in both substrates, suggesting that CPT II was at least equally affected. The deficiency in CPT is also evident in leukocytes (101, 234), platelets (235), and cultured fibroblasts (97). Evidence that the liver may also be affected is suggested from the effects of fasting, because patients with CPT deficiency tend to have a delayed or absent rise in ketones compared with normal subjects (64). The requirement for carnitine and CPT in the translocation of long-chain fatty acids into mitochondria may be overcome by treating patients with medium-chain triglycerides. A high-carbohydrate–low-fat diet is usually sufficient, however, to give appreciable improvement and to reduce the incidence of myoglobinuria.

SUMMARY. Disorders of fat metabolism have a wide spectrum of symptoms, but it is possible to make a broad distinction between those with carnitine deficiency and those lacking CPT. The former are weak, whereas the latter are of fairly normal strength at rest but after fasting or exercise tend to show evidence of muscle destruction such as raised plasma CK and myoglobinuria. It is not at all clear why there should be a difference between these two patient groups because it is assumed that the metabolic pathway affected is the same. It is no surprise therefore to find that we have investigated a patient with carnitine deficiency who also exhibited recurrent myoglobinuria. The storage and utilization of lipid by muscle and the possible damaging effects of free fatty acids remains an important and challenging field of research.

Changes in Muscle Function

GLYCOLYTIC DISORDERS. In patients with myophosphorylase or PFK deficiency, ischemic isometric contractions (either stimulated or voluntary) lead to a premature loss of force. A notable finding reported by Dyken et al. (118) and Brandt et al. (37) is that the muscle action potential amplitude decreases with a similar time course to the loss of force, implying that this may be the cause of force fatigue (383). During repeated contractions at low forces with the circulation to the muscle intact, myophosphorylase-deficient patients suffer transient discomfort but no low-frequency fatigue. There is little evidence of changes in conduction in the axonal branches, or of changes in transmission across the neuromuscular junction, although these have not been exhaustively investigated.

Differences in response to objective function testing between normal subjects and patients with glycolytic disorders only become apparent during high-force contractions or when the circulation has been occluded. The loss of force that occurs appears to be due to the failure of the muscle action potential, which is only restored when the muscle returns to aerobic conditions. Relaxation rate becomes slow earlier in these patients, and this also fails to recover until the circulation, and therefore aerobic metabolism, is restored.

MITOCHONDRIAL ABNORMALITIES. Oxidative metabolism is restricted in patients with a defect in the electron-transport chain. This may have two consequences: *1*) there will be a reduction in the rate of ATP synthesis and *2*) there will be an accumulation of pyruvate and lactate leading to metabolic acidosis. During muscle function testing, isometric contractions under ischemic conditions are comparable to those of normal subjects. With the circulation intact, repeated low-force contractions result in a progressive increase in muscular pain and discomfort with an eventual loss of force. The muscles in these patients are continually working under partially anaerobic conditions even when the circulation is intact.

These two groups of patients contrast because those with glycolytic defects cannot sustain high-force contractions, whereas those with defects of oxidative metabolism cannot keep up repeated low-force contractions.

DISORDERED FUNCTION

Myotonic Syndromes

Myotonia is the slow or delayed relaxation of muscle after contraction. It differs from the slow relaxation seen in conditions such as hypothyroidism or in fatigued muscle in that it is accompanied by continuing electrical activity.

Myotonia occurs in a number of muscle disorders; it can be produced experimentally and the various forms almost certainly have different causes (327). Of the human conditions myotonia congenita is the best understood.

Myotonia congenita (Thomsen's disease) is usually described as an autosomal dominant condition although there may be a more severe recessive variant. Unlike most other muscle diseases a characteristic feature is true muscle hypertrophy (as opposed to pseudohypertrophy where there is replacement of muscle with fat). The myotonic stiffness affects the limb muscles and a common complaint is that patients have difficulty in releasing their grip on hand tools. It is a common feature of myotonic conditions that they tend to be aggravated by the cold. (One of our patients found he had difficulty riding his bicycle in cold weather because he could not release the brakes once he had used them.) A useful diagnostic feature is that myotonic contractions may be produced by direct percussion of the muscle; the thenar muscle or the tongue are often used to demonstrate this sign. There is no evidence of persistent weakness although there may be a tendency to undue fatigue during tetanic contractions. During EMG examination characteristic dive-bomber discharges are heard when signals are played over a loudspeaker. These appear to be bursts of repetitive firing in response to mechanical disturbance by movement of the needle electrode.

Research into the nature of myotonia has been stimulated by and largely dependent on investigations of a type of myotonia seen in a strain of American goat. Myotonic goats develop muscle stiffness and rigidity after sudden movements, so that if startled they assume bizarre postures and may fall over. The strain of goat was first noticed in the latter part of the nineteenth century in the southern United States and has been perpetuated partly out of curiosity but possibly because the goats are disinclined to make sudden efforts such as jumping even low fences, which may have a distinct advantage for the poorer farmers of the area (48). The goats exhibit symptoms that appear very similar to those of human myotonia congenita; the myotonia is produced by percussion, worked off by repeated contractions, and aggravated by the cold. A common symptom, which remains unexplained in humans and goats, is that the myotonia is relieved by dehydration.

Before the development of suitable EMG-recording techniques there was doubt as to whether the myotonic contractions were electrically active or silent contractures. Brown and Harvey (45) clearly demonstrated that the slow relaxation in the goat was associated with continuing electrical activity, and they showed that the myotonia produced by percussion was still seen after nerve section and curarization. The myotonic muscles were also shown to be abnormally sensitive to close arterial injection of acetylcholine and KCl. Their findings clearly showed that myotonia is a disorder of the muscle itself rather than originating centrally. Experiments with nerve block in humans have led to similar conclusions (151, 230).

It is now generally believed that contractions in myotonia congenita are due to a disorder of the muscle itself, but Denny-Brown and Nevin (93) and more recently McComas (261) have pointed out that the myotonic discharge may contain motor unit potentials, implying an involvement of the motoneuron. Most of these observations were on patients with dystrophia myotonica or dystrophic mice so it is still not clear whether there is a central component to myotonia congenita. Spindles of affected muscle may also show myotonic activity, which would tend to augment any peripheral myotonic activity.

ELECTROPHYSIOLOGICAL STUDIES. The first important observation in understanding the goat myotonia was that the myotonic fibers have a higher-than-normal membrane resistance. With normal goat muscle, replacement of the external chloride with an impermeable anion both raises the membrane resistance and induces myotonic behavior. Various monocarboxylic aromatic amino acids also reduce the g_{Cl^-} and provoke myotonia (46, 47, 51, 245). The primary, or at least the major change, in goat myotonia appears to be an increased membrane resistance as a consequence of a decreased g_{Cl^-}.

Observation of human intercostal muscle preparations shows similar changes in myotonia congenita. Lipicky et al. (246) found an increased membrane resistance in myotonic fibers although it was notable that normal human fibers had a slightly higher resistance than normal goat fibers. Separation of the total membrane conductance into its component of Cl^- and K^+ conductances has shown that the g_{Cl^-} may be as low as 5% of the normal value but that the g_{K^+} is also reduced to about 50% (244). In this last respect the human condition differs from the goat myotonia where g_K is slightly raised.

SIGNIFICANCE OF REDUCED CHLORIDE CONDUCTANCE. Predictions about the form of the action potential in skeletal muscle are complicated by the presence of the complex system of the transverse tubules (T tubules) conducting the action potential radially to the center of the fiber.

Because the action potential takes a finite time to travel from the surface to the center of the fiber the compound action potential is prolonged (afterpotential). If the T tubules are disrupted by osmotic shock, the afterpotential disappears (152). A model illustrating the effect of the tubular conduction on the form of the action potential has been produced by Adrian and Peachey (4). One consequence of this is that at a time when the surface membrane has repolarized, the inner tubular membranes will be still relatively depolarized, establishing a voltage gradient between the inner and outer membranes. This effect of geometry will be accentuated by the tendency of K^+ to accumulate in the T tubules. The surface area of the T tubules is very large compared to the volume, and the diffusion path to the exterior is long and tortuous. Adrian and Peachey (4) calculated that for every action potential the Na^+ concentration might fall by 0.5 mM and the K^+ increase by 0.28 mM. Adrian and Bryant (2) calculated that this would result in a depolarization of 1.7 mV per impulse. The persistent afterdepolarization could be sufficient to open the surface Na^+-conductance channels, initiate a new action potential, and start repetitive firing. The fact that this does not happen in normal skeletal muscle is due to the presence of a large chloride leak conductance. As the membrane goes positive so Cl^- moves through the membrane, delaying the upstroke of the action potential and speeding the repolarization.

In muscle fibers with reduced g_{Cl^-} each action potential is followed by a significant afterpotential, which is cumulative during a train of impulses and amounts to approximately 1 mV per impulse (2), a figure close to the calculated 1.7 mV. With myotonic fibers, detubulation abolishes both the afterpotential and the myotonic behavior.

Adrian and Marshall (3), in a theoretical treatment, have shown that reducing the g_{Cl^-} by a factor of 10 should induce repetitive firing. Interestingly although repetitive firing was found to be enhanced by K^+ accumulation in the T tubules, it was not a prerequisite. This implies that the delayed repolarization due to the geometry of the T tubules is sufficient to induce repetitive firing in the absence of a large leak conductance. The authors also found that myotonic behavior was dependent on the g_{Na^+} not returning to normal too quickly, suggesting that in myotonic muscle there could be changes other than that of g_{Cl^-}.

EXPERIMENTAL MYOTONIAS. Substances that interfere with cholesterol synthesis have been found to produce myotonia in experimental animals. Winer et al. (388a) were the first to use 20,25-diazacholesterol in rats, and they found that myotonia was associated with an accumulation of desmosterol in the muscle membranes. Rüdel and Senges (328) showed that affected muscles had a decreased g_{Cl^-}, and it is presumed that the myotonia has the same ionic basis as the goat myotonia and human myotonia congenita. In the rat, different muscle types have different susceptibilities, the fast-twitch muscles develop myotonia, whereas the slow-twitch muscles are relatively resistant (162). Peter and Campion (309) have examined this further and have shown that in the fast-twitch muscles, in addition to a change in the g_{Cl^-}, there was also a decrease in the intracellular Na^+. This gave a higher E_{Na} and a larger overshoot potential. In the soleus muscle there was no significant difference in the Na^+ contents of the treated and untreated muscle.

Not all inhibitors of cholesterol synthesis produce myotonia. Peter and Campion (309) have observed that both 20,25-diazacholesterol and triparanol, which lead to desmosterol accumulation, result in myotonia, but AY-9944, which inhibits synthesis earlier in the pathway, does not produce myotonic symptoms. The authors estimate that replacement of one molecule in ten of cholesterol by desmosterol is sufficient to distort the lipid structure of the membrane and to change the g_{Cl^-}.

A number of aromatic monocarboxylic acids produce myotonic symptoms when injected into live animals and with isolated preparations (51). They appear to act by binding to or blocking the Cl^--conductance channels. The g_{K^+} is raised in treated normal goat fibers, a feature common to the naturally occurring myotonic goat muscle fibers, but differing from human myotonia congenita. Whether the g_{K^+} changes are significant in the development of myotonia in the goat is not known.

Veratrinic agents also produce a form of myotonia (137, 150, 366), but the mechanism appears to be quite different from that of the naturally occurring goat or human myotonias. Chloride conductance is not affected and membrane resistance tends to be reduced. The myotonia may thus be the result of partial depolarization of the membrane, bringing the resting potential nearer to the threshold for electrical excitation.

ETIOLOGY OF MYOTONIA. The following explanations of myotonia congenita and the goat myotonia have been suggested.

1. Circulating myotonic factor. Because the aromatic monocarboxylic acids produce a myotonia in animals so similar to the human condition, it has been suggested that the naturally occurring conditions may be the result of a circulating aromatic carboxylic acid metabolite (51). Bryant (49), however, found that monocarboxylic acids lowered the mechanical threshold of normal goat fibers in contrast to the naturally occurring myotonia in which the threshold is increased. Although this does not rule out other types of circulating factors, it makes the hypothesis less attractive. There have been no convincing reports of myotonia being transferred to experimental animals by transfusion of blood fractions either from patients with myotonia congenita or from myotonic goats.

2. Abnormal cholesterol synthesis. Although the accumulation of desmosterol in animals produces myotonia that is very similar to the human condition, Peter and Campion (309) report that they were unable to detect any abnormal accumulation of desmosterol in myotonic goats or patients with myotonia congenita or myotonia dystrophia.

3. Trophic factors. It is known that denervation leads to (among other things) an increase in the membrane resistance in the muscle (7). More recently it has been shown with rat fast-twitch muscle that the increased membrane resistance is largely due to a reduced g_{Cl^-} (59) and similarly in the goat gastrocnemius (50). Any changes occurring as the result of denervation could be due either to a lack of trophic factor from the nerve or lack of activity of the muscle itself. Camerino and Bryant (59) and DeCoursey et al. (88) attempted to resolve this question by poisoning the peroneal nerve with colchicine, which blocks axonal transport along the microtubular system but does not prevent conduction of action potentials. It was found that the muscles from the treated animals had a reduced g_{Cl^-}, indicating that this was dependent on a trophic substance derived from the innervating nerve. This conclusion, however, opposes the findings of Westgaard (380) who showed that direct stimulation of denervated rat soleus muscle can restore the passive membrane resistance to normal over a period of 14 days.

The idea of a trophic substance maintaining chloride permeability is attractive but remains unproven.

4. Primary membrane defect. In the absence of any

other convincing theory the possibility of a primary membrane defect must remain open. The only evidence for this is the observation, reported by Peter and Campion (309), that patients with myotonia congenita have difficulty concentrating their urine, suggesting a generalized membrane problem that may be apparent in tissues where chloride permeability is important.

TREATMENT OF MYOTONIA CONGENITA. The treatment of myotonia congenita is generally with substances that reduce muscle excitability by blocking the g_{Na^+}. Quinine was the first substance used; others that have been tried are phenytoin and procainamide. Procainamide has been a common treatment (239), but phenytoin is now generally preferred (184). None of the current treatments increase the muscle g_{Cl^-}. The weakness that is a feature of the severe recessive form of myotonia appears to be improved by drugs relieving the myotonia (318).

PARAMYOTONIA CONGENITA. Paramyotonia congenita is an autosomal dominant condition and has symptoms that are very similar to those of myotonia congenita. The myotonic symptoms are often only seen in the cold, and the patients have an additional problem of transitory weakness. In one woman (a dancer) whom we studied, the weakness was most noticeable in the morning and was accentuated if she had been dancing the previous evening. The weakness wore off during the day. Myotonia, particularly of eye muscle, was worse in the cold. Unlike myotonia congenita it is reported that the myotonic discharges in this condition become worse with repeated contractions.

There have been no studies of muscle membrane properties, but it seems likely that the condition is a variant of hyperkalemic periodic paralysis. If this is so then the primary membrane defect is probably not an altered g_{Cl^-}, as in myotonia congenita, but a change in properties of the Na^+ or K^+ conductances.

Periodic Paralysis

The familial periodic paralyses (FPP), as their name implies, are characterized by periodic attacks of weakness. There are two main types; their final muscle symptoms are similar, but they appear to have quite separate causes.

HYPOKALEMIC PERIODIC PARALYSIS. Hypokalemic periodic paralysis is an autosomal dominant condition, which is sometimes associated with thyrotoxicosis. Attacks of weakness first occur during the second decade of life, often during the night, and are precipitated by carbohydrate meals especially after exercise. The attacks may last up to 24 h and in severe cases most of the skeletal muscles of the body may be involved in a flaccid paralysis, which may go as far as impairing coughing and speech. Insulin will provoke an attack of paralysis, and attacks, regardless of the provocation, can be aborted by giving 10–15 g of oral potassium chloride or potassium citrate. Mild exercise of the affected muscles may also help reduce attacks.

Characteristically the weakness is accompanied or preceded by a fall in serum K^+ (to as low as 1.5 mM). The degree of weakness, however, is not directly related to the serum K^+ because this may return to normal before the muscle strength is restored. The serum K^+ is not lost to the body during an attack, but rather moves into the muscle tissue. Between attacks the muscle K^+ content is low and the intracellular Na^+ higher than normal. Vacuolation of the muscle fibers is a prominent feature seen both on light and electron microscopic examination. The vacuoles may be swollen T system or sarcoplasmic reticulum and may be empty or contain periodic acid–Schiff-positive material (5, 8, 89, 164, 253, 305, 342).

Muscle strength between attacks is fairly normal, but with time and repeated episodes of paralysis the vacuoles in the muscle tend to persist with loss of myofibrillar material and consequent weakness.

During an attack the muscle becomes inexcitable to either indirect or direct stimulation (187) although the contractile system is intact because skinned fibers can be made to contract with added Ca^{2+} (141). Although Shy et al. (342) found no change in the membrane potential during an attack, it is now generally accepted that the paralysis is accompanied by a large depolarization. Evidence for this comes from recordings both in vivo (319) and in vitro (195). Riecker and Bolte (319) also showed that relief of paralysis by oral KCl was accompanied by repolarization of the muscle fibers.

Hofmann and Smith (195) undertook an extensive investigation of the membrane properties of isolated intercostal muscle preparations from three patients. They found that low external K^+ by itself, and insulin in the presence of normal medium K^+, produced a large depolarization with the muscle becoming inexcitable. Normal human muscle fibers showed only small changes in membrane potential and remained excitable in these circumstances. In K^+-free medium, the addition of insulin caused FPP muscle fibers to repolarize, whereas normal fibers showed an additional small depolarization. Treatments that reduced Na^+ conductance, such as adding procaine or replacing external Na^+ with choline, caused the FPP fibers to repolarize when in a low-K^+ medium. Repolarization, however, did not always restore excitability.

ANIMAL MODEL. Much of the more recent speculation about the cause of hypokalemic periodic paralysis has been stimulated by work on muscle from rats maintained on a low-K diet. The symptoms show many similarities to those of the human condition. The skeletal muscle has a low K^+ content and higher than normal Na^+ (74), and the fibers show prominent vacuolation (222). Offerijus et al. (298) first used K^+-deficient rats in an investigation of the mechanisms by which insulin sometimes causes weakness in diabetics. They found that strips of rat diaphragm from deficient animals remained excitable when placed in K^+-free medium but the addition of insulin resulted in loss of excitability. This was reversed by the addition of K^+ to the medium. Strips of normal rat diaphragm continued to contract normally in normal or K^+-free medium both with and without insulin. Otsuka and Ohtsuki (299) showed that these changes were associated with depolarization and repolarization of the muscle membranes. They also showed that the muscles could be repolarized by replacing the external Na^+ with choline.

In the animal model muscle paralysis occurs because the surface membranes are depolarized to a point where there is inactivation of the Na^+-conductance channels and the muscle becomes refractory. Two mechanisms have been suggested to account for the depolarization. Otsuka and Ohtsuki (299) proposed that depolarization was the result of an increased g_{Na^+}, based on their finding that reducing the g_{Na^+} repolarized the membrane. Kao and Gordon (221, 222) have argued against this view, suggesting that the primary defect is a decrease in K^+ permeability that leads to depolarization and the increased g_{Na^+} is secondary to this. They were able to show an effect of insulin on g_K, decreasing the permeability by 39%, while excluding any major change in g_{Na} (221).

The membrane potential is determined by the relative permeabilities of the membrane for Na^+ and K^+, and because resting muscle g_K is very much greater than g_{Na}, the normal resting membrane potential is close to the equilibrium potential for K^+. If g_K is reduced, however, then the membrane potential will be influenced more by the Na^+ gradient across the membrane.

There are a number of ways in which g_K may be decreased:

1. Reduced extracellular K^+. Above about 25 mM the membrane potential is close to that expected from the ratio of intracellular to extracellular K. In the physiological range, however, the measured potential is about 10 mV less than expected (1, 73), and below the physiological range of external K^+ concentrations the deviation becomes even more marked. Horowicz et al. (196) have shown that K^+ fluxes both in and out of the muscle are much reduced at low external K^+ concentrations and have provided a theoretical framework for their findings.
2. Internal Na^+. Muscles from FPP patients and from K^+-deficient animals have a raised intracellular Na^+ content. Bezanilla and Armstrong (21), from experiments with squid axon, suggested that the inner openings of the K^+-conductance channels are accessible to a number of ions including Na^+ that cannot pass through to the exterior and consequently tend to block the g_{K^+}. A raised intracellular Na^+ could act in this way in affected muscle.
3. Direct effect of insulin. Insulin causes a depolarization of muscle from K-deficient rats that does not depend on the presence of glucose in the external medium, and the action of insulin is not inhibited by ouabain (221). Because insulin does not appear to work by stimulating either glucose or cation transport, some direct action on the K^+-conductance channels seems to be indicated.

In the isolated animal muscle preparation the sequence of events leading to paralysis appears fairly clear. In low-K^+ medium, g_K is already low, partly because of the low external K^+ concentration and also because of a raised intracellular Na^+. Addition of insulin may therefore make things worse by stimulating K^+ uptake, further reducing the external K^+ concentration [although in the case of the experiments of Kao and Gordon (221), where the external K^+ was 0.5 mM, it is unlikely that uptake would have significantly reduced the extracellular pool]. In addition the insulin may act directly to reduce the K^+ permeability.

Because normal muscle in low-K^+ medium does not respond to insulin, the inexcitability of the affected muscle must be more than just a normal physiological response to rather abnormal circumstances. The essential difference could be the raised intracellular Na^+, which may maintain g_K permanently near some critical value so that a normal response to insulin is sufficient to depolarize the muscle membrane. Another explanation is that there may be an abnormal response to insulin. Because insulin receptors are known to be very plastic, a change in either their number or affinity as the result of a K^+-deficient diet could result in abnormal insulin sensitivity.

Mechanisms similar to those described for the animal model could account for the symptoms of patients with hypokalemic periodic paralysis. The induction of paralysis by carbohydrate meals or insulin and the beneficial effects of oral KCl (which may help to raise muscle g_K) are all compatible with the hypothesis based on the animal model. Despite this the animal model may not be identical to the human condition. Although Hofmann and Smith (195) demonstrated insulin sensitivity of the diseased muscle with isolated human intercostal preparations, their findings differ in two important respects from the findings with animal muscles: *1)* affected animal muscles are only sensitive to insulin when in low-K^+ medium, whereas the human preparations depolarized when insulin was added to normal medium containing 5 mM K^+; *2)* in K^+-free medium the affected human muscle repolarized when insulin was added. For the animal muscle that had been depolarized with insulin, increasing the K^+ led to repolarization, whereas for the human muscle decreasing the external K^+ led to repolarization. The reported behavior of the isolated human muscle preparation is thus somewhat at odds with the known protective effects of oral K^+ in patients.

ETIOLOGY OF THE HUMAN CONDITION. By analogy with the animal model the patients could be effectively

K^+ deficient as the result of faulty electrolyte handling. This is supported by the fact that paralysis may occur with severe hypokalemia due to conditions such as diuretic or carbenoxolone overdosage. There could also be a primary defect in the nature or number of insulin receptors or in their interaction with the K^+-conductance channels.

TREATMENT OF HYPOKALEMIC PERIODIC PARALYSIS. Potassium supplementation, restriction of Na^+ intake, and avoidance of insulin, carbohydrates, and heavy exercise all help the patient with hypokalemic periodic paralysis to avoid attacks of paralysis. Mild acidosis appears to be useful (165), and it has been suggested that the raised $[H^+]$ may help by blocking Na^+ channels. Acetazolamide, which is a carbonic anhydrase inhibitor and K^+ diuretic, has proved valuable in the treatment of this condition.

HYPERKALEMIC PERIODIC PARALYSIS. One of the drawbacks of treating patients with periodic paralysis with potassium salts was that in a number of cases the potassium actually made the condition worse. This led to the description of hyperkalemic periodic paralysis as a condition quite separate from the hypokalemic variety.

Attacks of weakness generally begin in the first decade of life; these are provoked by potassium and can be relieved by glucose and insulin. In these respects the condition is the reverse of hypokalemic periodic paralysis. During attacks serum K^+ usually rises (although the extent is variable), with the K^+ moving out of the muscle and possibly other tissues as well. Although the factors that provoke attacks are opposite to those of hypokalemic periodic paralysis, there are similar chronic changes in the muscle. Muscle Na^+ increases and K^+ decreases during attacks and there is evidence that the abnormality of ionic content persists between attacks. Vacuolation of the muscle fibers, very similar to that in hypokalemic periodic paralysis, is seen in the affected muscles (31, 32, 68, 153, 154, 242, 253, 259, 305).

Ever since the condition was first described it was known to be closely linked to paramyotonia. Layzer et al. (236) suggested that myotonia is the primary expression of the muscular abnormality and weakness a secondary feature. Other investigators, however, have not found myotonia to be such a common feature (31), and it appears that symptoms may vary from myotonia alone to paralysis with all possible combinations of the two.

Microelectrode studies have shown a lowered resting potential between attacks with a further large depolarization occurring during an attack (32, 78, 262). Although the raised serum K^+ and the decreased intracellular K^+ reduce the resting membrane potential, it is unlikely that this is the complete explanation of the depolarization because the change in cation gradient is not sufficient to account for the degree of depolarization (78). The weakness often occurs before the serum K^+ begins to rise (44). Hyperkalemia may therefore be a consequence rather than a cause of muscle depolarization.

The cause of the depolarization remains unknown. Because the precipitating factors are quite different from those in hypokalemic paralysis, it is unlikely to be caused by a decrease in g_{K^+}. Creutzfeldt et al. (78) have suggested an increase in g_{Na^+}, and in the absence of experimental evidence this seems a likely hypothesis. Because the attacks are periodic, there must be not only an increased resting conductance but also a mechanism inducing change. Raised external K^+ is the only stimulus that has been identified; a possible sequence of events leading to paralysis would be a small rise in serum K^+ as the result of diurnal variation, ingestion of K^+ or of muscle activity that may trigger a further increase in membrane sodium conductance, depolarization of the muscle membrane, and movement of K^+ out of the muscles. As membrane depolarization develops and the potential approaches the electrical threshold, the membrane becomes hyperexcitable and shows myotonic behavior. With further depolarization the muscle becomes inexcitable and paralysis ensues. There is some evidence that as an attack develops, the muscle goes through a myotonic phase (52), although it has not been confirmed whether patients suffering predominantly from myotonic symptoms should have a lesser degree of depolarization than those suffering from the paralytic symptoms.

TREATMENT OF HYPERKALEMIC PERIODIC PARALYSIS. Management and treatment of acute attacks of hyperkalemic periodic paralysis are the exact opposite of those for hypokalemic paralysis. High carbohydrate intake, glucose, and insulin all help to minimize attacks, probably by encouraging K^+ uptake by the muscles. Acetazolamide is very effective in the long-term management of hyperkalemic periodic paralysis (260) just as it is in the management of the hypokalemic variety. It may act similarly by preventing K^+ flux across the muscle membrane; alternatively, it could promote K^+ excretion and thus reduce serum K^+ levels (171). Griggs (171) reports that acetazolamide in paramyotonia has a beneficial effect on the myotonic symptoms but causes profound weakness, indicating that hyperkalemic periodic paralysis and paramyotonia may not, after all, be the same condition. The β-adrenergic stimulant, salbutamol, is reported to be an effective treatment for hyperkalemic periodic paralysis (375).

Malignant Hyperpyrexia

Malignant hyperpyrexia is a rare condition but one that presents considerable problems for anesthetists; apparently healthy individuals undergoing routine surgery can develop an alarming and often fatal hyperpyrexia, which was first described in Australia in the 1960s [see Denborough and Lovell (92)]. Typically after anesthesia is induced, muscle stiffness is noted in the patient, accompanied by a rapid rise in body temperature, increase in plasma potassium and lactate, and subsequent cardiac failure. Myoglobinuria and renal damage are additional problems. Unless the signs are recognized early during anesthesia and treatment begun promptly, the prognosis is poor, death resulting in about 50% of cases. It is now clearly established that the precipitating factors are the use of halothane as an anesthetic agent and/or the use of suxamethonium as a muscle relaxant.

The condition is inherited as an autosomal dominant although the incidence is twice as high in males as in females; this may reflect the high incidence of traumatic accidents requiring surgery in young males (135). The incidence of this disease has been variously reported as 1:20,000 (41) or 1:200,000 persons subjected to anesthesia (135). The latter authors suggest that the discrepancy in incidence may be due to differing anesthetic techniques in Canada and the United Kingdom.

Although apparently healthy and athletic by nature, susceptible individuals have muscles that, when examined on biopsy, frequently have a number of abnormal features, most noticeably internal nuclei, small angular fibers, target fibers, and "moth-eaten" fibers. With electron-microscope examination, areas of sarcomere disruption and Z-band streaming can be seen (185, 205).

The diagnosis of susceptible individuals can be made with reasonable confidence by use of an in vitro muscle preparation, which, when compared with normal human muscle, shows a greater propensity to contracture in the presence of caffeine (136, 284, 285, 295). An alternative diagnostic technique may be to measure the proportion of the active form of phosphorylase in muscle. Willner et al. (388) have shown this to be considerably raised in muscle from susceptible subjects.

Hyperpyrexic attacks are not an inevitable consequence of halothane anesthesia; many susceptible subjects are anesthetized with apparently no ill effects. Halsall et al. (183) estimated that the probability of pyrexia developing in susceptible subjects was 44%. This type of observation has led to the suggestion that there may be unidentified stress factors, which render the subjects more susceptible to the ill effects of halothane (389). It has also created some debate as to whether the abnormality in this condition resides primarily in the muscle or is a reflection of abnormal somatic or sympathetic nervous activity.

A condition similar to human hyperpyrexia has been described in Pietrain and Landrace pigs. These animals are particularly sensitive to stress and develop muscle rigidity, acidosis, and hyperkalemia and die of heart failure in stressful conditions. This condition is of considerable economic importance because the meat from such animals tends to go into rapid contracture post mortem, extruding water and leaving a pale and unattractive product. Like humans, susceptible pigs are sensitive to halothane and depolarizing muscle relaxants (for review see ref. 386). In pigs, however, stress plays a much greater part in precipitating attacks; although stress may sensitize susceptible human subjects, it is not the primary precipitating factor. Nonetheless the muscle abnormalities of pigs and humans appear to be very similar (294).

Isolated muscle from susceptible pigs is abnormally sensitive to halothane and to caffeine, generating contractures at lower than normal concentrations of these substances. In the whole animal there is some dispute as to the role that α- and β-agonists play in precipitating pyrexic attacks (173, 180). With the perfused hindquarters of a pig that is free from nervous or hormonal influences, Gronert et al. (173) have shown that the muscles of affected animals give an abnormal response to halothane but not to α- or β-agonists. They also found that the affected muscles were abnormally sensitive to temperatures above 41°C, showing a rapid rise in oxygen consumption and lactate production. It is suggested that the observed beneficial effects of α-antagonists in the whole animal (247, 248) may be explained by the better control of pyrexia brought about by vasodilation.

The major defect of muscle in malignant hyperpyrexia appears to be in the control of intracellular calcium and the mechanisms involved in the control of excitation-contraction coupling (40). Other reported changes in mitochondria and sarcoplasmic reticulum are probably of a secondary nature.

The only effective treatment for the muscle abnormality is the use of dantrolene, a peripheral muscle relaxant, which is thought to act by interfering with the mechanisms responsible for calcium release (137, 294). When used in vitro on isolated preparations, dantrolene has been shown to be effective in preventing halothane-induced contractures in affected human and pig muscles (14, 135).

The management of susceptible patients requires careful monitoring of body temperature and the avoidance of known precipitating agents and stress. If a hyperpyrexic attack develops, intravenous dantrolene should be administered, and strenuous efforts made to limit the rise in body temperature, plasma lactate, and potassium concentrations.

Muscle Pain, Cramps, and Contractures

It is common knowledge that discomfort can arise from muscle as a result of excessive or unaccustomed physical activity. Although the cause of such pain is still far from understood, it may be related to injury in the muscle (13). Ischemic muscle pain has been extensively studied ever since the classic work of Lewis and Pickering on intermittent claudication (238). Ischemia is a potent cause of pain, and its effects may potentiate pain produced by other factors. There is, however, no simple relationship between the perception of pain and the accumulation of a metabolic product, e.g., lactic acid. Another possibility is that muscle contractions result in the release of some pain-producing substance that excites the Aδ and C nociceptive nerve fibers (267). Various suggestions have been made as to the nature of the nociceptive substance; these include peptides such as bradykinin, prostaglandins, histamine, ATP, phosphate, and an increase in hydrogen ion concentration resulting from anaerobic glycolysis. Oxygen lack does not appear to be the most important factor because prolonged ischemia before exercise does not bring on pain any sooner than it does during activity (238). This type of study, however, may not be sufficiently discriminating in view of the fact that resting muscle metabolism is very low. Needle biopsy studies of ischemic muscle at rest show only very slow changes in muscle metabolite levels (186).

Cramp is an involuntary contraction of the muscle that may involve individual fibers, motor units, or groups of motor units. The mechanism underlying such activity may be a disturbance at any level from the central nervous system via the peripheral motor nerve to the muscle cell itself. This type of contraction is commonly associated with electrical activity of the muscle membranes, in contrast to the electrically silent contractures seen in patients with metabolic disorders such as myophosphorylase deficiency. The mechanisms responsible for cramps and contractures have been well reviewed by Layzer and Rowland (237), as have the mechanisms and clinical conditions associated with muscle pain (279).

DRUG-INDUCED MYOPATHIES

Apart from the effect of steroids and hormones on muscle, there are a number of myopathies that are thought to result from drug administration [Table 3; (233)]. The drugs may be divided into those that produce destructive lesions in the muscle, by an unknown mechanism, and those that act by affecting the normal mechanisms of muscle contraction. An example of the latter category are drugs resulting in hypokalemia, which leads to altered function and structure (see HYPOKALEMIC PERIODIC PARALYSIS, p. 655).

The principal characteristics of drug-induced myopathies are pain and weakness, which may be analyzed on the basis of the mechanisms described previously. Less severe than in myopathy are the conditions of fasciculation and slight cramplike discomfort, which may be produced by drugs such as clofibrate, isoetharine, salbutamol, and some cytotoxic agents. As yet little is known of the changes in these less severe, though still painful, myopathies, because it is unusual to carry out muscle biopsies to investigate muscle pathology or chemistry in such cases. In practice most drug-induced changes cease to exist when the offending substance is withdrawn. Therefore the approach has been simply to deal with the problem pragmatically rather than to investigate underlying mechanisms.

There is no simple relationship between the severity of the myopathy and the presence of pain. Some of the more striking conditions associated with muscle wasting, e.g., steroid myopathy, are entirely painless.

MECHANISMS UNDERLYING MUSCLE DISEASE

This section is a brief introduction to a very large literature. Fortunately there are several recent and comprehensive reviews of experimental myopathies and studies relevant to human disease (251, 291, 324).

Vascular and Humoral Influences

Vascular changes have been considered important in muscular dystrophy because there are abnormalities in the microcirculation that could reduce oxygenation of the muscle cells (91, 143). None of these changes is thought to be of primary importance. All may play secondary roles as factors aggravating the initial damage.

Influence of Nerve on Muscle

The importance of an intact and active nerve supply is beyond doubt. Denervation leads to a number of functional changes in the muscle, including fiber atrophy and a change in membrane chemosensitivity, changes that are reversed by reinnervation. Consequently the idea arose that nerve exerts a trophic influence on muscle (177, 361). This subject has been reviewed by Vrbová (370) and, with particular reference to the muscular dystrophies, by McComas (261).

In all studies concerning the influence of nerve on muscle the question arises as to whether the maintenance of a particular function is the result of a trophic influence from the nerve or a direct consequence of the muscle contractile activity. It was first suggested that the localization of acetylcholine sensitivity as the result of innervation was due either to a trophic substance other than acetylcholine released from the motor end plate (271) or to acetylcholine itself (357). Vrbová (370) commented that it is unlikely that a substance coming from a motor end plate, which suppresses acetylcholine sensitivity, would exert its influence on parts of the fiber several centimeters away and yet not affect the high sensitivity of the muscle fiber at the motor end plate. Most likely muscle activity itself is the cause of the reduced extrajunctional activity. Evidence favoring this view was provided by experiments in which denervated muscle was directly stimulated (108, 213, 250, 380).

Another major influence of nerve on muscle is determining the contractile speed and metabolic characteristics of the individual muscle fibers. Buller et al.

TABLE 3. *Features of Major Drug-Induced Muscular Syndromes*

Disorder	Drugs Implicated	Clinical Features
Acute/subacute painful proximal myopathy	Clofibrate, ε-aminocaproic acid, emetine, heroin, alcohol	Muscle pain, tenderness, proximal or generalized weakness; reflexes usually preserved
	Vincristine	Proximal pain, atrophy, weakness, absent reflexes
	Drugs causing hypokalemia, diuretics, purgatives, licorice, carbenoxolone, amphotericin B	Weakness may be periodic; reflexes may be depressed or absent
	Clofibrate, isoetharine, denazol, cimetidine, metolazone, bumetanide, lithium, cytotoxics	Myalgia, cramps, myokymia, weakness
Acute rhabdomyolysis	Heroin, amphetamine, phencyclidine, alcohol	Severe muscle pain, tenderness, swelling, flaccid quadriparesis, areflexia, gross myoglobinuria, renal failure
Subacute/chronic painless proximal myopathy	Corticosteroids	Predominantly proximal weakness and atrophy
	Chloroquine, alcohol, heroin, perhexiline	Reflexes may be lost through associated neuropathy
	Drugs causing hypokalemia (see above)	Weakness may be periodic; reflexes may be depressed or absent
Myasthenic syndromes	Aminoglycosides, polymyxins, tetracyclines succinylcholine, D-penicillamine, propranolol, practolol (? other β-blockers), phenytoin, chlorpromazine, procainamide, trimethadione	Postoperative apnea; oculobulbar and limb paralysis; typical myasthenia gravis
Polymyositis/dermatomyositis	D-Penicillamine	Proximal muscle pain, weakness, skin changes
Myotonic syndrome	20,25-Diazacholesterol, suxamethonium, propranolol (? other β-blockers)	Myotonia
Malignant hyperpyrexia	Suxamethonium, halothane, diethyl ether, cyclopropane, chloroform, methoxyflurane, ketamine, enflurane, psychotropics	Rigidity, hyperpyrexia, acidosis, hyperkalemia, disseminated intravascular coagulation, renal failure

[Adapted from Lane and Mastaglia (233).]

(54) in their classic cross-innervation experiments first demonstrated that these factors were under nervous control. Subsequent work shows that in this type of experiment there are changes in contractile proteins (55, 379) and regulatory proteins (9).

Buller et al. (54) originally suggested that the influence of nerve on muscle might be mediated by a trophic substance. Subsequent work has shown, however, that as with denervation changes, patterns of contractile activity themselves exert powerful controlling influences. Slow-twitch motor units are active for long periods of time, firing at relatively low frequencies, whereas fast-twitch motor units are active only intermittently, firing at high frequencies. Experiments in which fast-twitch leg muscles of rabbits were stimulated by implanting electrodes around the motor nerves showed that prolonged periods of 10-Hz stimulation had a dramatic effect on the muscles (331). Changes in speed are accompanied by corresponding changes in the contractile proteins (349), the sarcoplasmic reticulum (313), and enzymes of glycolysis and the citric acid cycle (370).

The influence of nerve on muscle in humans can be demonstrated in those neuropathies where, as the result of reinnervation by collateral sprouting of motor axons, large areas of the muscle are composed entirely of one fiber type. The situation is analogous to the artificial cross-innervation experiments because the reinnervated fibers assume characteristics dictated by the new motoneuron. Changes in myotonic muscle have been attributed to defective trophic influence in maintaining chloride conductance (see ETIOLOGY OF MYOTONIA, p. 654), but at present the main source of speculation regarding the influence of nerve on muscle centers on the pathogenesis of the muscular dystrophies. There are some electrophysiological abnormalities in the dystrophies: slowing of conduction, evidence of denervation (fibrillation potentials), reinnervation (enlarged motor unit potentials), and reduced motor unit counts in the affected muscles (15, 261). In light of these findings McComas et al. (264) proposed the "sick neurone" theory, which stated in essence that dystrophic changes in muscle were due to the lack of some trophic factor normally produced by the motoneuron. McComas and co-workers (263) have recently examined the evidence both for and against this theory and conceded that it is unlikely to be a generalized mechanism in the dystrophies. An objection to the neurogenic theory is that there is little histochemical evidence of neurogenic change in the muscle. Although the neurogenic theory does not provide a complete explanation for dystrophic changes, some neural influence cannot be ruled out in every case and may well play a role in myotonic dystrophy. Interestingly, the Kugelberg-Welander form of spinal muscular atrophy (neurogenic in origin) results in clinical features that are very similar to those seen in limb-girdle dystrophy. Differential diagnosis is made more difficult by the fact that features of an inflammatory myopathy may be seen in scapuloperoneal atrophy with cardiopathy (208).

A possible explanation for the electrophysiological changes seen in the dystrophies may be that they are a consequence of some influence of the muscle on the nerve. There is evidence that muscle does exert some trophic influence on nerve tissue. Denervated fibers cause branching of nearby motor axons, and there can be centripetal transport of proteins from the muscle to the motoneuron cell body (158, 229, 378). Part of the problem with dystrophic muscle might be, therefore, an inadequate trophic influence of the muscle on the nerve, which is required to maintain normal innervation and function.

Disorders of the Cell Membrane

Muscle enzymes such as CK leak out of dystrophic muscle, which clearly indicates that the dystrophic muscle membrane is abnormal. There is currently much debate as to whether membrane abnormality is the primary defect that leads ultimately to the destruction of the fiber, or whether it is secondary to other changes taking place (for reviews see refs. 251, 324, 337).

The membrane hypothesis is based on the supposition that a genetic fault affects an enzyme or structural protein that is either functionally abnormal or decreased in amount, giving rise to an abnormal sarcolemmal membrane (324). The theory is rooted in the observation first made in the 1950s that certain enzymes, for example, aldolase (109, 110) and CK (120), are considerably raised in the serum of dystrophic children. Because these are relatively large molecules, this implies a markedly altered permeability of the muscle membrane.

Direct evidence of altered membrane structure is not easy to obtain because little is known about plasma membranes from normal human muscle. In making membrane preparations from dystrophic muscle it is very difficult to exclude membranes from fat cells, which often form a large proportion of the apparent muscle mass. It is also difficult to separate surface membranes from those of the T tubules. Despite these difficulties there have been reports of structural abnormalities in the sarcoplasmic membranes of dystrophic muscle; freeze-fracture techniques (336, 338) allow one to visualize the fine details of membrane ultrastructure. In normal muscle, orthogonal arrays of particles and caveolae are seen on the protoplasmic face of the fractured membrane, whereas in material from dystrophic muscle far fewer of these arrays are seen. The significance of these findings is not known but it has been suggested that they may indicate a stage preceding the production of a focal defect at the cell surface. Such defects have been demonstrated on the surface of nonnecrotic fibers (62, 276) and electron-cytochemical studies have shown peroxidase entering the muscle fiber through these holes (276). Partly as a consequence of the difficulties in obtaining muscle membranes a great deal of work has been done with erythrocyte membranes. Finding abnormalities in a tissue other than muscle has strengthened the view that the primary cause of dystrophy may lie in a generalized membrane defect. Abnormally shaped erythrocytes have been observed in patients with myotonic dystrophy and also in Duchenne carriers (272). There is also an increased tendency for the red cells in Duchenne sufferers and carriers to form echinocytes (168). Physical examination of erythrocyte cell membrane fluidity has demonstrated small differences; these have been reviewed and commented on by Plishker and Appel (311) and Barachi (19).

Bodensteiner and Engel (25) suggest that the damage seen in dystrophic muscle is due to the accumulation of intracellular calcium that can occur as a result of abnormal membrane permeability.

Muscle Protease Activity

Interest in the role of extraneous calcium in the pathogenesis of the muscular dystrophies was first stimulated by the description of calcium-activated neutral protease in muscle (58, 86, 87, 314). This enzyme has the interesting property of specifically degrading the Z-line material (changes in Z-line structure such as streaming are notable features of dystrophic muscle when examined under the electron microscope). The protease requires high concentrations of calcium for activation (10^{-4} M), so it is unlikely that it is involved in the normal processes of protein turnover. In Duchenne muscle, where there may be leaky surface membranes that cause calcium influx from the extracellular fluid, it is possible that this enzyme becomes activated (223). Measuring calcium-activated and neutral protease activity is difficult, and reported results are confusing. Kar and Pearson (224) reported elevated levels in dystrophic muscle, whereas Ebashi and Sugita (119) could find only minimally raised levels in Duchenne muscle but approximately a fourfold increase in a single case of the milder Becker-type dystrophy.

In light of the current interest in the role of proteases in the dystrophic process, attempts have been made to modify these changes with specific protease inhibitors. In murine dystrophy, treatment with leupeptin was found to decrease muscle protein degradation. The extent of this inhibition was similar to that seen in control and denervated rat muscle (240). Pepstatin has also been used for this purpose (71, 353). Attempts to modify the disease process by inhibiting protein degradation, although interesting, may be counterproductive because the normal processes of regeneration most certainly require a parallel increase in degradation as muscle structure is remodelled (see *Factors Affecting Protein Turnover in Muscle*, p. 644). Proteolytic mechanisms in muscle and their possible involvement in disease have been reviewed by Kar and Pearson (225) and Libby and Goldberg (241).

Inflammatory Disorders of Muscle

A considerable literature now exists on the probable role of autoimmunity in the etiology of both polymyositis and dermatomyositis (304, 322). Most investigators think a cell-mediated defect is likely to be of primary importance. Experimental models of myositis have been established in rats (303) and guinea pigs (84) and used to study possible lymphocyte dysfunction. Good evidence for this is now available (219, 220) showing lymphocytes from rats with experimental polymyositis to be cytotoxic to normal rat muscle in culture. Cytotoxicity of human lymphocytes from patients with polymyositis has been demonstrated against human fetal muscle preparations. Johnson et al. (209) produced a lymphotoxin active against human fetal muscle monolayers by incubating lymphocytes with autologous muscle from patients with polymyositis. Experimental allergic myositis (reviewed by Sloper in ref. 347), however, differs in several respects from human polymyositis and dermatomyositis.

Overuse and Disuse as Causes of Muscle Damage

The effect of exercise, alteration of muscle length, nutrition, and general metabolism all seem to be factors that might be influencing the eventual time course of protein turnover and cell integrity in muscular dystrophy. In dystrophic muscle there is a considerable amount of regeneration taking place (17) and evidence of enhanced protein synthesis (278).

In the search for the underlying cause of dystrophic changes, possible abnormalities in membrane function and protein synthesis must be considered in relation to the contractile activity of muscle. It is important to discover whether exercise is harmful or beneficial to the integrity of dystrophic cells. Studies in animals suggest that dystrophic muscle may be stronger if subjected to activity (199), but in a study of children with Duchenne dystrophy there was no evidence to suggest that strength-training exercise could alter the progress of the dystrophic changes (90).

PROSPECTS FOR TREATMENT OF MUSCLE DISEASE

The forms of treatment available for specific diseases have been discussed in the relevant sections, and agents used in the treatment of the dystrophies have been reviewed by Heckmatt and Dubowitz [Table 4; (191)]. So far no treatment has proved satisfactory on a carefully controlled clinical trial. Although not curable, muscular dystrophy is treatable; the main emphasis is directed toward weight control, maintenance of good posture, and the avoidance of contractures (343).

The history of attempted drug treatment for Duchenne dystrophy has been one of enthusiastic uncontrolled trials whose results, after carefully controlled clinical trials, have proved to be untenable. A particular difficulty is the variable time course of the pathological process, and it is evident that any controlled trial needs to be fairly long (at least 2 yr) before a clear answer can be expected. An alternative to randomized clinical trials would be to make measurements monitoring the effects of drugs with the patient as his own control. This would have considerable advantages but depends on having a wide range of techniques available for following the course of the disease and for relating any changes observed to the normal growth patterns of a healthy child.

TABLE 4. *Theoretical Basis of Drug Trials in Muscular Dystrophy*

Epinephrine	Muscular dystrophy thought due to a defect in sympathetic innervation of muscle sarcoplasm.
Amino acids	Muscular dystrophy thought due to protein malabsorption or a failure of muscle protein synthesis.
Glycine	Glycine administration increased creatinuria in normal subjects and therefore thought to encourage creatine synthesis in muscle.
Vitamin E	Muscle weakness in offspring of female rats partially deprived of vitamin E, due to necrosis and cellulitis of voluntary muscle.
Vitamin B_6	Degeneration of muscle fibers among the many lesions produced by depriving rats of vitamin B_6
Butyl-Sympathol	Dystrophic process thought secondary to abnormalities in regulation of muscle microcirculation leading to ischemia.
Anabolic steroids	17-Ethyl-19-nortestosterone adminstration increases urinary excretion of creatine in normal subjects, a possible result of increased synthesis in muscle. Same steroid prolongs survival of dystrophic mice.
Corticosteroids	Corticosteroids of value in inflammatory myopathy.
Nucleotides (ATP)	Nucleotides may be depleted in myopathy. Decreased concentration and increased turnover of nucleotides found in dystrophic mouse muscle.
Allopurinol	Muscle concentrations of ATP reduced in Duchenne dystrophy. Allopurinol may shift purine from uric acid pathway (catabolism) to pathway of purine manufacture, thus increasing concentrations of muscle nucleotides.
Penicillamine	Penicillamine may protect enzymes of glycolytic and anabolic pathways and also prevent collagen cross linkage and deposition in muscle.
Superoxide dismutase	Prevents free radical damage to muscle cell membranes.

[Adapted from Dubowitz and Heckmatt (113).]

At present many drugs are known to damage muscle (233), but only a few appear to affect its function in a positive manner; those that do, e.g., catecholamines (30), appear to have different effects on skeletal muscle according to whether the muscle is slow or fast twitch, fresh or fatigued. Perhaps a search could be made for agents that influence skeletal muscle in one or more of the following ways: by influencing membrane function, by altering contractile properties, by influencing energy exchanges, or by influencing protein synthesis.

A systematic search along these lines may reveal some agents that, either by correcting the underlying defect or by alleviating clinical symptoms, may prove therapeutically useful.

We are most grateful to Dr. J. M. Round for her help in preparing the chapter.

For the last 11 years our work on muscle has been continuously supported by the Wellcome Trust and the Muscular Dystrophy Group of Great Britain. Support for individual projects has also been provided by the Medical Research Council of Great Britain and the Muscular Dystrophy Association of America.

REFERENCES

1. Adrian, R. H. The effect of internal and external potassium concentration on the membrane potential of frog muscle. *J. Physiol. London* 133: 631–658, 1956.
2. Adrian, R. H., and S. H. Bryant. On the repetitive discharge in myotonic muscle fibres. *J. Physiol. London* 240: 505–515, 1974.
3. Adrian, R. H., and M. W. Marshall. Action potentials reconstructed in normal and myotonic muscle fibres. *J. Physiol. London* 258: 125–143, 1976.
4. Adrian, R. H., and L. D. Peachey. Reconstruction of the action potential of frog sartorius muscle. *J. Physiol. London* 235: 103–131, 1973.
5. Aitken, R. S., E. N. Allott, L. I. M. Castelden, and M. Walker. Observations on a case of familial periodic paralysis. *Clin. Sci.* 3: 47–57, 1937.
6. Albuquerque, E. X., J. E. Rash, R. F. Mayer, and R. Sutterfield. An electrophysiological and morphological study of the neuromuscular junction in patients with myasthenia gravis. *Exp. Neurol.* 51: 536–563, 1976.
7. Albuquerque, E. X., and S. Thesleff. A comparative study of membrane properties of innervated and chronically denervated fast and slow skeletal muscles of the rat. *Acta Physiol. Scand.* 73: 471–480, 1968.
8. Allott, E. N., and B. McArdle. Further observations on familial periodic paralysis. *Clin. Sci.* 3: 229–239, 1938.
9. Amphlett, G. W., S. V. Perry, H. Syska, M. D. Brown, and G. Vrbová. Cross innervation and the regulatory protein system of rabbit soleus muscle. *Nature London* 257: 602–604, 1975.
10. Andersen, D. M. Familial cirrhosis of the liver with storage of abnormal glycogen. *Lab. Invest.* 5: 11–20, 1956.
11. Angelini, C., and A. G. Engel. Subcellular distribution of acid and neutral α-glucosidase in normal, acid maltase deficient and myophosphorylase deficient human skeletal muscle. *Arch. Biochem.* 156: 350–355, 1973.
12. Angelini, C., S. Lucke, and F. Cantarutti. Carnitine deficiency of skeletal muscle: report of a treated case. *Neurology* 26: 633–637, 1976.
13. Asmussen, E. Observations on experimental muscular soreness. *Acta Rheumatol. Scand.* 2: 109–116, 1956.
14. Austin, K. L., and M. A. Denborough. Drug treatment of malignant hyperpyrexia. *Anaesth. Intensive Care* 5: 207–213, 1977.
15. Ballantyne, J. P., and S. Hansen. Neurogenic influence in muscular dystrophies. In: *Pathogenesis of Human Muscular Dystrophies*, edited by L. P. Rowland. Amsterdam: Excerpta Med., 1978, p. 187–199.
16. Ballard, F. J., F. M. Tomas, and L. M. Stern. Increased turnover of muscle contractile proteins in Duchenne muscular dystrophy as assessed by 3-methylhistidine and creatinine excretion. *Clin. Sci.* 56: 347–352, 1979.
17. Baloh, R., P. A. Cancilla, K. Kalyanaraman, T. Munsat, C. M. Pearson, and R. Rich. Regeneration of human muscle. A morphologic and histochemical study of normal and dystrophic muscle after injury. *Lab. Invest.* 26: 319–328, 1972.
18. Bank, W. J., S. DiMauro, and L. P. Rowland. Renal failure in McArdle's disease. *N. Engl. J. Med.* 287: 1102, 1972.
19. Barchi, R. L. Molecular structure and biophysical aspects of the sarcolemma. In: *Current Topics in Nerve and Muscle Research*, edited by A. J. Aguayo and G. Karpati. Amsterdam: Excerpta Med., 1979, p. 3–15. (Int. Congr. Ser. 455.)
20. Bergström, J. Muscle electrolytes in man: determined by neutron activation analysis on needle biopsy specimens: a study in normal subjects, kidney patients and patients with chronic diarrhoea. *Scand. J. Clin. Lab. Invest. Suppl.* 68: 1–110, 1962.
21. Bezanilla, F., and C. M. Armstrong. Negative conductance caused by entry of sodium and cesium ions into potassium channels of squid axon. *J. Gen. Physiol.* 60: 588–608, 1972.
22. Bigland-Ritchie, B., D. A. Jones, G. P. Hosking, and R. H. T. Edwards. Central and peripheral fatigue in sustained maximum voluntary contractions of human quadriceps muscle. *Clin. Sci. Mol. Med.* 54: 609–614, 1978.
23. Bigland-Ritchie, B., D. A. Jones, and J. J. Woods. Excitation frequency and muscle fatigue: electrical responses during human voluntary and stimulated contractions. *Exp. Neurol.* 64: 414–427, 1979.
24. Blass, J. P. Pyruvate dehydrogenase deficiencies. In: *Inherited Disorders of Carbohydrate Metabolism*, edited by D. Burman, J. B. Halton, and C. A. Pennock. Lancaster, UK: MTP, 1980, p. 239–268.
25. Bodensteiner, J. B., and A. G. Engel. Intracellular calcium accumulation in Duchenne dystrophy and other myopathies: a study of 567,000 muscle fibers in 114 biopsies. *Neurology* 28: 439–446, 1978.
26. Bohmer, T., H. Bergrem, and K. Eiklid. Carnitine deficiency induced during intermittent haemodialysis for renal failure. *Lancet* 1: 126–128, 1978.
27. Border, J. R., U. P. Burns, C. Rumph, and W. G. Schenk. Carnitine levels in severe infection and starvation; a possible key to the prolonged catabolic state. *Surgery* 68: 175–179, 1970.
28. Borenstein, S., and J. E. Desmedt. Local cooling in myasthenia: improvement of neuromuscular failure. *Arch. Neurol. Chicago* 32: 152–157, 1975.
29. Bouwsma, G., and G. K. Van Wijngaarden. Spinal muscular atrophy and hypertrophy of the calves. *J. Neurol. Sci.* 44: 275–279, 1980.
30. Bowman, W. C., and M. W. Nott. Action of sympathomimetic amines and their antagonists on skeletal muscle. *Pharm. Rev.* 21: 27–72, 1969.
31. Bradley, W. G. Adynamia episodica hereditaria. Clinical, pathological and electrophysiological studies in an affected family. *Brain* 92: 345–378, 1969.
32. Bradley, W. G. Ultrastructural changes in adynamia episodica hereditaria and normokalaemic familial periodic paralysis. *Brain* 92: 379–390, 1969.
33. Bradley, W. G. The neuropathies. In: *Disorders of Voluntary Muscle*, edited by J. N. Walton. Edinburgh: Churchill Livingstone, 1974, p. 804–851.
34. Bradley, W. G., P. Hudgson, D. Gardner-Medwin, and J. N. Walton. Myopathy associated with abnormal lipid metabolism in skeletal muscle. *Lancet* 1: 495–498, 1969.
35. Bradley, W. G., M. Jenkinson, D. C. Park, P. Hudgson, D. Gardner-Medwin, R. J. T. Pennington, and J. N. Walton. A myopathy associated with lipid storage. *J. Neurol. Sci.* 16: 137–154, 1972.
36. Bradley, W. G., and P. K. Thomas. The pathology of peripheral nerve disease. In: *Disorders of Voluntary Muscle*, edited by J. N. Walton. Edinburgh: Churchill Livingstone, 1974, p. 234–275.
37. Brandt, N. J., F. Buchthal, F. Ebbesen, Z. Kamieniecka, and C. Krarup. Post-tetanic mechanical tension and evoked action potentials in McArdle's disease. *J. Neurol. Neurosurg. Psychiatry* 40: 920–925, 1977.
38. Bremer, J. Carnitine and its role in fatty acid metabolism. *Trends Biochem. Sci.* 2: 207–209, 1977.
39. Bressler, R., and B. Wittles. The effect of diphtheria toxin on carnitine metabolism in the heart. *Biochim. Biophys. Acta* 104: 39–45, 1965.
40. Britt, B. A. Etiology and pathophysiology of malignant hyperthermia. *Federation Proc.* 38: 44–48, 1979.
41. Britt, B. A., and W. Kalow. Malignant hyperthermia: etiology unknown. *Can. Anaesth. Soc. J.* 17: 316–330, 1970.
42. Brooke, M. H. *A Clinician's View of Neuromuscular Diseases.* Baltimore, MD: Williams & Wilkins, 1977.

43. BROOKE, M. H., J. E. CARROLL, J. E. DAVIES, AND J. M. HAGBERG. The prolonged exercise test. *Neurology* 29: 636–643, 1979.
44. BROOKS, J. E. Hyperkalemic periodic paralysis. Intracellular electromyographic studies. *Arch. Neurol. Chicago* 20: 13–18, 1969.
45. BROWN, G. L., AND A. M. HARVEY. Congenital myotonia in the goat. *Brain* 62: 341–363, 1939.
46. BRYANT, S. H. Muscle membrane of normal and myotonic goats in normal and low external chloride (Abstract). *Federation Proc.* 21: 312, 1962.
47. BRYANT, S. H. Cable properties of external intercostal muscle fibres from myotonic and nonmyotonic goats. *J. Physiol. London* 204: 539–550, 1969.
48. BRYANT, S. H. The electrophysiology of myotonia; with a review of congenital myotonia of goats. In: *New Developments in Electromyography and Clinical Neurophysiology. New Concepts of the Motor Unit Neuromuscular Disorders, Electromyographic Kinesiology*, edited by J. E. Desmedt. Basel: Karger, 1973, vol. 1, p. 420–450.
49. BRYANT, S. H. Myotonia in the goat. *Ann. NY Acad. Sci.* 317: 314–325, 1979.
50. BRYANT, S. H., AND D. CAMERINO. Chloride conductance of denervated gastrocnemius fibers from normal goats. *J. Neurobiol.* 7: 229–240, 1976.
51. BRYANT, S. H., AND A. MORALES-AGUILERA. Chloride conductance in normal and myotonic muscle fibers and the action of monocarboxylic aromatic acids. *J. Physiol. London* 219: 367–383, 1971.
52. BUCHTHAL, F., L. ENGBAECK, AND I. GAMSTORP. Some aspects of the pathophysiology of adynamia episodica hereditaria. *Dan. Med. Bull.* 5: 167–169, 1958.
53. BULCKE, J. A., J. DEMEIRSMAN, AND J. L. TERMOTE. The influence of skeletal muscle atrophy on needle electromyography. As demonstrated by computed tomography. *Electromyogr. Clin. Neurophysiol.* 19: 269–279, 1979.
54. BULLER, A. J., J. C. ECCLES, AND R. M. ECCLES. Interactions between motoneurones and muscles in respect of the characteristic speeds of their responses. *J. Physiol. London* 150: 417–439, 1960.
55. BULLER, A. J., W. F. H. M. MOMMAERTS, AND K. SERAYDARIAN. Enzymic properties of myosin in fast and slow twitch muscles of the cat following cross-innervation. *J. Physiol. London* 205: 581–597, 1969.
56. BURACK, R., R. H. T. EDWARDS, M. GREEN, AND N. L. JONES. The response to exercise before and after treatment of myxedema with thyroxine. *J. Pharmacol. Exp. Ther.* 176: 212–219, 1971.
57. BURKE, D., N. F. SKUSE, AND A. K. LETHLEAN. Isometric contraction of the abductor digiti minimi muscle in man. *J. Neurol. Neurosurg. Psychiatry* 37: 825–834, 1974.
58. BUSCH, W. A., M. H. STROMER, D. E. GOLL, AND A. SUZUKI. Ca^{2+}-specific removal of Z lines from rabbit skeletal muscle. *J. Cell Biol.* 52: 367–381, 1972.
59. CAMERINO, D., AND S. H. BRYANT. Effects of denervation and colchicine treatment on the chloride conductance of rat skeletal muscle fibers. *J. Neurobiol.* 7: 221–228, 1976.
60. CAMPBELL, E. J. M., R. H. T. EDWARDS, D. K. HILL, D. A. JONES, AND M. K. SYKES. Perception of effort during partial curarisation. *J. Physiol. London* 263: 186P–187P, 1976.
61. CAMPBELL, H., AND E. BRAMWELL. Myasthenia gravis. *Brain* 23: 277–336, 1900.
62. CARPENTER, S., AND G. KARPATI. Duchenne muscular dystrophy: plasma membrane loss initiates muscle cell necrosis unless it is repaired. *Brain* 102: 147–161, 1979.
63. CARRIER, H. N., AND G. BERTHILLIER. Carnitine levels in normal children and adults and in patients with diseased muscles. *Muscle Nerve* 3: 326–334, 1980.
64. CARROLL, J. E., M. H. BROOKE, D. C. DEVIVO, K. K. KAISER, AND J. M. HAGBERG. Biochemical and physiologic consequences of carnitine palmityltransferase deficiency. *Muscle Nerve* 1: 103–110, 1978.
65. CARROLL, J. E., M. H. BROOKE, D. C. DEVIVO, J. B. SHUMATE, R. KRATZ, S. P. RINGEL, AND J. M. HAGBERG. Carnitine 'deficiency': lack of response to carnitine therapy. *Neurology* 30: 618–626, 1980.
66. CARROLL, J. E., D. C. DEVIVO, M. H. BROOKE, G. J. PLANER, AND J. H. HAGBERG. Fasting as a provocative test in neuromuscular diseases. *Metabolism* 28: 683–687, 1979.
67. CARROLL, J. E., J. M. HAGBERG, M. H. BROOKE, AND J. B. SHUMATE. Bicycle ergometry and gas exchange measurements in neuromuscular diseases. *Arch. Neurol. Chicago* 36: 457–461, 1979.
68. CARSON, M. J., AND C. M. PEARSON. Familial hyperkalemic periodic paralysis with myotonic features. *J. Pediatr.* 64: 853–865, 1964.
69. CHALOVICH, J. M., C. T. BURT, M. J. DANON, T. GLONEK, AND M. BÁRÁNY. Phosphodiesters in muscular dystrophies. *Ann. NY Acad. Sci.* 317: 649–669, 1979.
70. CHARVIÈRE, M., AND G. B. DUCHENNE. Emporte pièce histologique. *Bull. Acad. Natl. Med. Paris* 30: 1050–1051, 1865.
71. CHELMICKA-SCHORR, E. E., B. G. W. ARNASON, K. E. ASTROM, AND Z. DARZYNKIEWICO. Treatment of mouse muscular dystrophy with the protease inhibitor pepstatin. *J. Neuropathol. Exp. Neurol.* 37: 263–269, 1978.
72. CHUI, L. A., T. L. MUNSAT, AND J. R. CRAIG. Effect of ethanol on lactic acid production by excised normal muscle. *Muscle Nerve* 1: 57–61, 1978.
73. CONWAY, E. J. Nature and significance of concentration relations of potassium and sodium ions in skeletal muscle. *Physiol. Rev.* 37: 84–132, 1957.
74. CONWAY, E. J., AND D. HINGERTY. Relations between potassium and sodium levels in mammalian muscle and blood plasma. *Biochem. J.* 42: 372–376, 1948.
75. COSTILL, D. L., W. J. FINK, AND M. L. POLLOCK. Muscle fiber composition and enzyme activities of elite distance runners. *Med. Sci. Sports* 8: 96–100, 1976.
76. COX, R. A., AND C. L. HOPPEL. Biosynthesis of carnitine and 4-N-trimethylaminobutyrate from lysine. *Biochem. J.* 136: 1075–1082, 1973.
77. CRESSHULL, I., M. J. DAWSON, R. H. T. EDWARDS, D. G. GADIAN, G. K. GORDON, D. SHAW, AND D. R. WILKIE. Human muscle analysed by 31P nuclear magnetic resonance in intact subjects. *J. Physiol. London:* 317: 18P, 1981.
78. CREUTZFELDT, O. B., B. C. ABBOT, W. M. FOWLER, AND E. M. PEARSON. Muscle membrane potentials in episodic adynamia. *Electroencephalogr. Clin. Neurophysiol.* 15: 508–519, 1963.
79. CULL-CANDY, S. G., R. MILEDI, AND A. TRAUTMANN. Endplate currents and acetylcholine noise at normal and myasthenic human end-plates. *J. Physiol. London* 287: 247–265, 1979.
80. CULLEN, M. J., AND J. J. FULTHORPE. Stages in fibre breakdown in Duchenne muscular dystrophy. An electron-microscopic study. *J. Neurol. Sci.* 24: 179–200, 1975.
81. DAHLBACK, D., D. ELMQVIST, T. R. JOHNS, S. RUDNER, AND S. THESLEFF. An electrophysiologic study of the neuromuscular junction in myasthenia gravis. *J. Physiol. London* 156: 336–343, 1961.
82. DASTUR, D. K., B. M. GAGRAT, N. H. WADIA, M. M. DESAI, AND E. P. BHARUCHA. Nature of muscular change in osteomalacia: light- and electron-microscope observations. *J. Pathol.* 117: 211–228, 1975.
83. DAU, P. C. Plasmapheresis therapy in myasthenia gravis. *Muscle Nerve* 3: 468–482, 1980.
84. DAWKINS, R. L. Experimental myositis associated with hypersensitivity to muscle. *J. Pathol. Bacteriol.* 90: 619–625, 1965.
85. DAWSON, M. J., D. G. GADIAN, AND D. R. WILKIE. Mechanical relaxation rate and metabolism studied in fatiguing muscle by NMR. *J. Physiol. London* 299: 465–484, 1980.
86. DAYTON, W. R., D. E. GOLL, M. G. ZEECE, R. M. ROBSON, AND W. J. REVILLE. A Ca^{2+}-activated protease possibly involved in myofibrillar protein turnover. Purification from porcine muscle. *Biochemistry* 15: 2150–2158, 1976.
87. DAYTON, W. R., W. J. REVILLE, D. E. GOLL, AND M. H. STROMER. A Ca^{2+}-activated protease possibly involved in myo-

fibrillar protein turnover. Partial characterization of the purified enzyme. *Biochemistry* 15: 2159–2167, 1976.

88. DECOURSEY, T. E., S. G. YOUNKIN, AND S. H. BRYANT. Neural control of chloride conductance in rat extensor digitorum longus muscle. *Exp. Neurol.* 61: 705–709, 1978.
89. DEGRAEFF, J., AND L. D. F. LAMEIJER. Periodic paralysis. *Am. J. Med.* 39: 70–80, 1965.
90. DELATEUR, B. J., AND R. M. GIACONI. Effect on maximal strength of submaximal exercise in Duchenne muscular dystrophy. *Am. J. Phys. Med.* 58: 26–36, 1979.
91. DEMOS, J. Measure des temps de circulation chez 79 myopathies étude statistique des résultats; rôle du degré de l'atteinte musculaire clinique du mode evolutif de la maladie du sexe du malade des saisons. *Rev. Fr. Étud. Clin. Biol.* 6: 876–887, 1961.
92. DENBOROUGH, M. A., AND R. R. H. LOVELL. Anaesthetic deaths in a family. *Lancet* 2: 45, 1960.
93. DENNY-BROWN, D., AND S. NEVIN. The phenomenon of myotonia. *Brain* 64: 1–18, 1941.
94. DESMEDT, J. E. The neuromuscular disorder in myasthenia gravis. 1. Electrical and mechanical response to nerve stimulation in hand muscles. In: *New Developments in Electromyography and Clinical Neurophysiology. New Concepts of the Motor Unit, Neuromuscular Disorders, Electromyographic Kinesiology*, edited by J. E. Desmedt. Basel: Karger, 1973, vol. 1, p. 241–304.
95. DESMEDT, J. E. The neuromuscular disorder in myasthenia gravis. 2. Presynaptic cholinergic metabolism, myasthenia-like syndromes and a hypothesis. In: *New Developments in Electromyography and Clinical Neurophysiology. New Concepts of the Motor Unit, Neuromuscular Disorders, Electromyographic Kinesiology*, edited by J. E. Desmedt. Basel: Karger, 1973, vol. 1, p. 305–342.
96. DESMEDT, J. E., AND S. BORENSTEIN. Diagnosis of myasthenia gravis by nerve stimulation. *Ann. NY Acad. Sci.* 274: 174–188, 1976.

96a. DESMEDT, J. E., B. EMERYK, P. RENOIRTE, AND K. HAINANT. Disorder of muscle contraction processes in sex-linked (Duchenne) muscular dystrophy, with correlative electromyographic study of myopathic involvement in small hand muscles. *Am. J. Med.* 45: 853–872, 1968.

97. DIDONATO, S., F. CORNELIO, L. PACINI, D. PELUCHETTI, M. RIMOLDI, AND S. SPREAFICO. Muscle carnitine palmityltransferase deficiency: a case with enzyme deficiency in cultured fibroblasts. *Ann. Neurol.* 4: 465–467, 1978.
98. DIMAURO, S. Metabolic myopathies. In: *Handbook of Clinical Neurology. Diseases of the Muscle*, edited by P. J. Vinken and G. W. Bruyn. Amsterdam: Elsevier, 1979, vol. 41, p. 175–234.
99. DIMAURO, S., S. ARNOLD, A. MIRANADA, AND L. P. ROWLAND. McArdle disease: the mystery of reappearing phosphorylase activity in muscle culture—a fetal isoenzyme. *Ann. Neurol.* 3: 60–66, 1978.
100. DIMAURO, S., AND P. M. M. DIMAURO. Muscle carnitine palmityltransferase deficiency and myoglobinuria. *Science* 182: 929–931, 1973.
101. DIMAURO, S., AND A. B. EASTWOOD. Disorders of glycogen and lipid metabolism. *Adv. Neurol.* 17: 123–142, 1977.
102. DIMAURO, S., L. Z. STERN, M. MEHLER, R. B. NAGLE, AND C. PAYNE. Adult-onset acid maltase deficiency: a postmortem study. *Muscle Nerve* 1: 27–36, 1978.
103. DIMAURO, S., C. TREVISAN, AND A. HAYS. Disorders of lipid metabolism in muscle. *Muscle Nerve* 3: 369–388, 1980.
104. DONALDSON, S. K. B., L. HERMANSEN, AND L. BOLLES. Differential, direct effects of H^+ on Ca^{2+}-activated force of skinned fibres from the soleus, cardiac and adductor magnus muscles of rabbits. *Pfluegers Arch.* 376: 55–65, 1978.
105. DONS, B., K. BOLLERUP, F. BOND-PETERSEN, AND S. HANCKE. The effect of weight-lifting exercise related to muscle fibre composition and muscle cross-sectional area in humans. *Eur. J. Appl. Physiol. Occup. Physiol.* 40: 95–106, 1979.
106. DRACHMAN, D. B., C. W. ANGUS, R. N. ADAMS, AND I. KAO. Effect of myasthenic patients' immunoglobulin on acetylcholine receptor turnover: selectivity of degradation process. *Proc. Natl. Acad. Sci. USA* 75: 3422–3426, 1978.
107. DRACHMAN, D. B., C. W. ANGUS, R. N. ADAMS, J. D. MICHELSON, AND G. J. HOFFMAN. Myasthenia antibodies cross-link acetylcholine receptors to accelerate degradation. *N. Engl. J. Med.* 298: 1116–1122, 1978.
108. DRACHMAN, D. B., AND F. WITZKE. Trophic regulation of acetylcholine sensitivity of muscle: effect of electrical stimulation. *Science* 176: 514–516, 1972.
109. DREYFUS, J. C., AND G. SCHAPIRA. Biochemistry of progressive muscular dystrophy. In: *Biochemistry of Hereditary Myopathies*. Springfield, IL: Thomas, 1962.
110. DREYFUS, J. C., G. SCHAPIRA, AND F. SCHAPIRA. Biochemical study of muscle in progressive muscular dystrophy. *J. Clin. Invest.* 33: 794–797, 1954.
111. DUBOWITZ, V. *Muscle Disorders in Childhood.* Philadelphia, PA: Saunders, 1978.
112. DUBOWITZ, V., AND M. H. BROOKE. *Muscle Biopsy: A Modern Approach.* Philadelphia, PA: Saunders, 1973. (Major Problems in Neurology, Ser. 2.)
113. DUBOWITZ, V., AND J. HECKMATT. Management of muscular dystrophy. *Br. Med. Bull.* 36: 139–144, 1980.
114. DUBOWITZ, V., AND A. G. E. PEARCE. Enzymic activity of normal and diseased human muscle: a histochemical study. *J. Pathol. Bacteriol.* 81: 365–378, 1961.
115. DUCHENNE, G. B. *De électrisation localisée et son application à la pathologie et à la thérapeutique* (2nd ed.). Paris: Baillière, 1861.
116. DUCHENNE, G. B. *Physiologie des mouvements demontrée à l'aide de l'expérimentation électrique et de l'observation clinique et applicable a l'étude des paralysies et deformation* (1867), transl. by E. B. Kaplan. Philadelphia, PA: Saunders, 1959.
117. DUCHENNE, G. B. Recherche sur la paralysie musculaire pseudohypertrophique ou paralysie myo-sclérosique. *Arch. Gen. Med.* 2: 200–209, 1868.
118. DYKEN, M. L., D. M. SMITH, AND R. L. PEAKE. An electromyographic diagnostic screening test in McArdle's disease and a case report. *Neurology* 17: 45–50, 1967.
119. EBASHI, S., AND H. SUGITA. The role of calcium in physiological and pathological processes of skeletal muscle. In: *Current Topics in Nerve and Muscle Research*, edited by A. J. Aguayo and G. Karpati. Amsterdam: Excerpta Med., 1979, p. 73–84. (Int. Congr. Ser. 455.)
120. EBASHI, S., Y. TOYOKURAY, H. MOMOI, AND H. SUGITA. High creatine phosphokinase activity of sera of progressive muscular dystrophy patients. *J. Biochem. Tokyo* 46: 103–104, 1959.
121. EDSTRÖM, L. Selective atrophy of red muscle fibers in the quadriceps in long-standing knee-joint dysfunction. Injuries to the anterior cruciate ligament. *J. Neurol. Sci.* 11: 551–558, 1970.
122. EDSTRÖM, L., AND B. EKBLOM. Difference in sizes of red and white muscle fibers in vastus lateralis of muscular quadriceps femoris of normal individuals and athletes: relation to physical performance. *Scand. J. Clin. Lab. Invest.* 3: 155–160, 1974.
123. EDSTRÖM, L., AND R. NORDEMAR. Differential changes in type I and type II muscle fibers in rheumatoid arthritis. A biopsy study. *Scand. J. Rheumatol.* 3: 155–160, 1974.
124. EDWARDS, R. H. T. Studies of muscular performance in normal and dystrophic subjects. *Br. Med. Bull.* 36: 159–164, 1980.
125. EDWARDS, R. H. T., R. C. HARRIS, AND D. A. JONES. The biochemistry of muscle biopsy in man: clinical application. In: *Recent Advances in Clinical Biochemistry, No. 2*, edited by K. G. M. M. Alberti and C. Price. Edinburgh: Churchill Livingstone, 1981, vol. 2, p. 242–269.
126. EDWARDS, R. H. T., D. K. HILL, AND D. A. JONES. Effect of fatigue on the time course of relaxation from isometric contractions of skeletal muscle in man. *J. Physiol. London* 227: 26P–27P, 1972.
127. EDWARDS, R. H. T., D. K. HILL, AND D. A. JONES. Metabolic changes associated with slow relaxation in fatigued mouse muscle. *J. Physiol. London* 251: 287–301, 1975.
128. EDWARDS, R. H. T., D. K. HILL, D. A. JONES, AND P. A. MERTON. Fatigue of long duration in human skeletal muscle after exercise. *J. Physiol. London* 272: 769–778, 1977.

129. Edwards, R. H. T., C. M. Maunder, P. D. Lewis, and A. G. E. Pearse. Percutaneous needle biopsy in the diagnosis of muscle diseases. *Lancet* 2: 1070–1071, 1973.

130. Edwards, R. H. T., C. M. Wiles, K. Gohil, S. Krywawych, and D. A. Jones. Energy metabolism in human myopathy. In: *Disorders of the Motor Unit*, edited by D. Schottland. Boston, MA: Wiley, 1981, p. 715–728.

131. Edwards, R. H. T., C. M. Wiles, J. M. Round, M. J. Jackson, and A. Young. Muscle breakdown and repair in polymyositis: a case study. *Muscle Nerve* 2: 223–228, 1979.

131a. Edwards, R. H. T., D. R. Wilkie, M. J. Dawson, R. E. Gordon, and D. Shaw. Clinical use of nuclear magnetic resonance in the investigation of myopathy. *Lancet* 2: 725–731, 1982.

132. Edwards, R. H. T., A. Young, G. P. Hosking, and D. A. Jones. Human skeletal muscle function: description of tests and normal values. *Clin. Sci. Mol. Med.* 52: 283–290, 1977.

133. Edwards, R. H. T., A. Young, and C. M. Wiles. Needle biopsy of skeletal muscle in the diagnosis of myopathy and the clinical study of muscle function and repair. *N. Engl. J. Med.* 302: 261–271, 1980.

134. Ekstedt, J. Human single fiber action potentials. *Acta Physiol. Scand. Suppl.* 226: 1–96, 1964.

135. Ellis, F. R., and P. J. Halsall. Malignant hyperpyrexia. *Br. J. Hosp. Med.* 24: 318–327, 1980.

136. Ellis, F. R., D. G. F. Harriman, S. Currie, and S. Cain. Screening for malignant hyperthermia in susceptible patients. In: *International Symposium on Malignant Hyperthermia, 2nd: Proceedings*, edited by J. A. Aldrete and B. A. Britt. New York: Grune & Stratton, 1978, p. 273–285.

137. Ellis, K. O., and S. H. Bryant. Excitation-contraction uncoupling in skeletal muscle by dantrolene sodium. *Naunyn-Schmiedeberg's Arch. Pharmacol.* 274: 107–109, 1972.

138. Elmqvist, D. Neuromuscular transmission defects. In: *New Developments in Electromyography and Clinical Neurophysiology. New Concepts of the Motor Unit, Neuromuscular Disorders, Electromyographic Kinesiology*, edited by J. E. Desmedt. Basel: Karger, 1973, vol. 1, p. 229–240.

139. Elmqvist, D., W. W. Hofman, J. Kugelberg, and D. M. J. Quastel. An electrophysiological investigation of neuromuscular transmission in myasthenia gravis. *J. Physiol. London* 174: 414–434, 1964.

140. Engel, A. G., and C. Angelini. Carnitine deficiency of human skeletal muscle with associated lipid storage myopathy: a new syndrome. *Science* 179: 899–902, 1973.

141. Engel, A. G., and E. H. Lambert. Calcium activation of electrically inexcitable muscle fibers in primary hypokalemic periodic paralysis. *Neurology* 19: 851–858, 1969.

141a. Engel, A. G., E. H. Lambert, and F. M. Howard. Immune complexes IgG and C_3 at the motor end-plate in Myasthenia Gravis. *Mayo Clin. Proc.* 52: 267–280, 1977.

141b. Engel, A. G., J. M. Lindstrom, E. H. Lambert, and V. A. Lennon. Ultrastructural localization of the acetylcholine receptor in myasthenia gravis and in its experimental autoimmune model. *Neurology* 27: 307–315, 1977.

142. Engel, A. G., and R. G. Siekert. Lipid storage myopathy responsive to prednisone. *Arch. Neurol. Chicago* 27: 174–181, 1972.

143. Engel, W. K. Investigative approach to the muscular dystrophies. In: *Treatment of Neuromuscular Disease*, edited by R. C. Griggs and R. T. Moxley III. New York: Raven, 1977, p. 197–226. (Advances in Neurology Ser. 17.)

144. Engel, W. K., and M. H. Brooke. Histochemistry of the myotonic disorders. In: *Progressive Muskeldystrophie Mytonie Myasthenie*, edited by E. Kuhn. Stuttgart: Springer-Verlag, 1966, p. 203–209.

145. Engel, W. K., N. A. Vick, C. J. Glueck, and R. I. Levy. A skeletal muscle disorder associated with intermittent symptoms and a possible defect of lipid metabolism. *N. Engl. J. Med.* 282: 697–704, 1970.

146. Fambrough, D. M., D. B. Drachman, and S. Satyamurti. Neuromuscular junction in myasthenia gravis: decreased acetylcholine receptors. *Science* 182: 293–295, 1973.

147. Feng, T. P. Heat-tension ratio in prolonged tetanic contractions. *Proc. R. Soc. Med.* 108: 522–537, 1931.

148. Fetell, M. R., P. E. Duffy, and L. P. Rowland. Infiltrating lipoma: a cause of monomelic hypertrophy. *Muscle Nerve* 1: 75–80, 1978.

149. Fick, A. *Mechanische arbeit und Wärmeentwicklelung bei der Muskelhätigkeit.* Leipzig, East Germany: Brockhaus, 1882.

150. Flacke, W. Studies on veratrum alkaloids. XXXIII. The action of some esters of germine with acetic acid on the sartorius muscle of the frog. *J. Pharmacol. Exp. Ther.* 137: 62–69, 1962.

151. Floyd, W. F., P. Kent, and F. Page. An electromyographic study of myotonia. *Electroencephalogr. Clin. Neurophysiol.* 7: 621–630, 1955.

152. Gage, P. W., and R. S. Eisenberg. Action potentials, afterpotentials, and excitation-contraction coupling in frog sartorius fibers without transverse tubules. *J. Gen. Physiol.* 53: 298–310, 1969.

153. Gamstorp, I. Adynamia episodica hereditaria. *Acta Paediatr. Uppsala Suppl.* 108: 1–120, 1956.

154. Gamstorp, I. A study of transient muscle weakness. *Acta Neurol. Scand.* 38: 3–19, 1962.

155. Gandevia, S. C., and D. I. McCloskey. Changes in motor commands, as shown by changes in perceived heaviness, during partial curarisation and peripheral anaesthesia in man. *J. Physiol. London* 272: 673–689, 1977.

156. Gandevia, S. C., D. I. McCloskey, and E. K. Potter. Alterations in perceived heaviness during digital anaesthesia. *J. Physiol. London* 306: 365–375, 1980.

157. Gardner-Medwin, D. Clinical features and classification of the muscular dystrophies. *Br. Med. Bull.* 36: 109–115, 1980.

158. Glatt, H. R., and C. G. Honegger. Retrograde episodal transport for cartography of neurones. *Experientia* 29: 1515–1517, 1973.

159. Gohil, K., D. A. Jones, and R. H. T. Edwards. Analysis of muscle mitochondrial function with techniques applicable to needle biopsy samples. *Clin. Physiol.* 1: 195–207.

160. Goldberg, A. L., G. N. DeMartino, and P. Libby. The influence of thyroid hormones and proteinease inhibitors on protein degradation in skeletal muscle. In: *Current Topics in Nerve and Muscle Research*, edited by A. J. Aguayo and G. Karpati. Amsterdam: Excerpta Med., 1979, p. 53–60. (Int. Congr. Ser. 455.)

161. Gollnick, P. D., R. B. Armstrong, C. W. Saubert IV, K. Piehl, and B. Saltin. Enzyme activity and fiber composition in skeletal muscle of untrained and trained men. *J. Appl. Physiol.* 33: 312–319, 1972.

162. Goodgold, J., and A. Eberstein. An electromyographic study of induced myotonia in rats. *Exp. Neurol.* 21: 159–166, 1968.

163. Goodgold, J., and A. Eberstein. *Electrodiagnosis of Neuromuscular Diseases.* Baltimore, MD: Williams & Wilkins, 1972.

164. Gordon, A. M., J. R. Green, and D. Lagunoff. Studies on a patient with hypokalemic familial periodic paralysis. *Am. J. Med.* 48: 185–195, 1970.

165. Gordon, A. M., and L. I. Kao. Disorders of muscle membranes. The periodic paralyses. In: *Physiology of Membrane Disorders*, edited by T. E. Andreoli, J. F. Hoffman, and D. D. Fanestil. New York: Plenum, 1978, p. 817–829.

166. Gowers, W. R. Pseudohypertrophic muscular paralysis. *Lancet* 2: 113–116, 1879.

167. Grampp, W., J. B. Harris, and S. Thesleff. Inhibition of denervation changes in skeletal muscle by blockers of protein synthesis. *J. Physiol. London* 221: 743–754, 1972.

168. Grassi, E., B. Lucci, C. Marchini, S. Ottonello, M. Parma, R. Reggiani, G. L. Rossi, and J. Tagliavini. Deformed erythrocytes in muscular dystrophies. *Neurology* 28: 842–844, 1978.

169. Graystone, J. E. Creatinine excretion during growth. In: *Human Growth: Body Composition, Cell Growth Energy, and Intelligence*, edited by D. B. Cheek. Philadelphia, PA: Lea & Febiger, 1968, p. 182–197.

170. Griggs, R. C. Hypertrophy and cardiomyopathy in the neuro-

muscular diseases. *Circ. Res.* 35, Suppl. 2: 145–151, 1974.

171. GRIGGS R. C. The myotonic disorders and the periodic paralyses. In: *Treatment of Neuromuscular Diseases*, edited by R. C. Griggs and R. T. Moxley III. New York: Raven, 1977, p. 143–159. (Advances in Neurology Ser. 17.)
172. GRIMBY, G., C. BROBERG, I. KROTKIEWSKA, AND M. KROTKIEWSKA. Muscle fibre composition in patients with traumatic cord lesion. *Scand. J. Rehabil. Med.* 8: 37–42, 1976.
173. GRONERT, G. A., J. H. MILDE, AND S. R. TAYLOR. Porcine muscle responses to carbachol, α- and β-adrenoceptor agonists, halothane or hyperthermia. *J. Physiol. London* 307: 319–333, 1980.
174. GROSS, D., A. GRASSINO, W. R. D. ROSS, AND P. T. MACKLEM. Electromyogram pattern of diaphragmatic fatigue. *J. Appl. Physiol: Respirat. Environ. Exercise Physiol.*: 46: 1–7, 1979.
175. GROSS, M. Proximal spinal muscular atrophy. *J. Neurol. Neurosurg. Psychiatry* 29: 29–34, 1966.
176. GRUENER, R., L. Z. STERN, C. PAYNE, AND L. HANNAPEL. Hyperthyroid myopathy. Intracellular electrophysiological measurements in biopsied human intercostal muscle. *J. Neurol. Sci.* 24: 339–349, 1975.
177. GUTMANN, E. (editor). *The Denervated Muscle* (translation). New York: Consultants Bureau, 1962, p. 13–56.
178. HÄGGMARK, T., AND E. ERIKSSON. Cylinder or mobile cast brace after knee ligament surgery. A clinical analysis and morphologic and enzymatic studies of changes in the quadriceps muscle. *Am. J. Sports Med.* 7: 48–56, 1979.
179. HÄGGMARK, T., AND E. ERIKSSON. Hypotrophy of the soleus muscle in man after Achilles tendon rupture. Discussion of findings obtained by computed tomography and morphologic studies. *Am. J. Sports Med.* 7: 121–126, 1979.
180. HALL, G. M., J. N. LUCKE, AND D. LISTER. Porcine malignant hyperthermia. V. Fatal hyperthermia in the Pietrain pig, associated with the infusion of α-adrenergic agonists. *Br. J. Anaesth.* 49: 855–863, 1977.
181. HALL, K., AND R. LUFT. Growth hormone and somatomedin. In: *Advances in Metabolic Disorders*, edited by R. Levine and R. Luft. New York: Academic, 1974, vol. 7, p. 1–36.
182. HALLIDAY, D., AND R. O. MCKERAN. Measurement of muscle protein synthetic rate from serial muscle biopsies and total body protein turnover in man by continuous intravenous infusion of L-[α-^{15}N]lysine. *Clin. Sci. Mol. Med.* 49: 581–590, 1975.
183. HALSALL, P. J., AND F. R. ELLIS. A screening test for the malignant hyperpyrexia phenotype using suxamethonium-induced contracture of muscle treated with caffeine and its inhibition by dantrolene. *Br. J. Anaesth.* 51: 753–756, 1979.
184. HARPER, P. S. *Myotonic Dystrophy*. Philadelphia, PA: Saunders, 1979. (Major Problems in Neurology, Ser. 9.)
185. HARRIMAN, D. G. F., F. R. ELLIS, A. J. FRANKS, AND D. W. SUMNER. Malignant hyperthermic myopathy in man: an investigation of 75 families. In: *International Symposium on Malignant Hyperthermia, 2nd: Proceedings*, edited by J. A. Aldrete and B. A. Britt. New York: Grune & Stratton, 1978, p. 67–87.
186. HARRIS, R. C., R. H. T. EDWARDS, E. HULTMAN, AND L. O. NORDESJÖ. The time course of phosphorylcreatine resynthesis during recovery of the quadriceps muscle in man. *Pfluegers Arch.* 367: 137–142, 1976.
187. HARTING, H. Über einen fall von intermittierender Paralysis Spinalis. *Zentralbl. Med. Wiss.* 13: 428–429, 1875.
188. HAY, A. M., AND J. C. WATERLOW. The effect of alloxan diabetes on muscle and liver protein synthesis in the rat, measured by constant infusion of L-[^{14}C]lysine. *J. Physiol. London* 191: 111P–112P, 1967.
189. HAYWARD, M. Automatic analysis of the electromyogram in healthy subjects of different ages. *J. Neurol. Sci.* 33: 397–413, 1977.
190. HAYWARD, M., AND R. G. WILLISON. Automatic analysis of the electromyogram in patients with chronic partial denervation. *J. Neurol. Sci.* 33: 415–423, 1977.
191. HECKMATT, J. Z., V. DUBOWITZ, AND S. LEEMAN. Detection of pathological change in dystrophic muscle with B-scan ultrasound imaging. *Lancet* 1: 1389–1390, 1980.
192. HENRIKSSON, J., AND J. S. REITMAN. Time course of changes in human skeletal muscle succinate dehydrogenase and cytochrome oxidase activities and maximal oxygen uptake with physical activity and inactivity. *Acta Physiol. Scand.* 99: 91–97, 1977.
193. HILL, D. K., M. J. MCDONNELL, AND P. A. MERTON. Direct stimulation of the adductor pollicis in man. *J. Physiol. London* 300: 2P–3P, 1980.
194. HJALMARSON, A. C., D. E. RANNELS, R. KAO, AND H. E. MORGAN. Effects of hypophysectomy, growth hormone, and thyroxine on protein turnover in heart. *J. Biol. Chem.* 250: 4556–4561, 1975.
195. HOFMANN, W. W., AND R. A. SMITH. Hypokalemic periodic paralysis: studies in vitro. *Brain* 93: 445–474, 1970.
196. HOROWICZ, P., P. W. GAGE, AND R. S. EISENBERG. The role of the electrochemical gradient in determining potassium fluxes in frog striated muscle. *J. Gen. Physiol. Suppl.* 51: 193S–203S, 1968.
197. HOSKING, G. P., U. S. BHAT, V. DUBOWITZ, AND R. H. T. EDWARDS. Measurements of muscle strength and performance in children with normal and diseased muscle. *Arch. Dis. Child.* 51: 957–963, 1976.
198. HOSKING, G. P., N. P. C. CAVANAGH, D. P. L. SMYTH, AND J. WILSON. Oral treatment of carnitine myopathy [letter]. *Lancet* 1: 853, 1977.
199. HUDECKI, M. S., C. POLLINA, A. K. BHARGAVA, J. E. FITZPATRICK, C. A. PRIVITERA, AND D. SCHMIDT. Effect of exercise on chickens with hereditary muscular dystrophy. *Exp. Neurol.* 61: 65–73, 1978.
200. HULTMAN, E. Studies of muscle metabolism of glycogen and active phosphate in man with special reference to exercise and diet. *Scand. J. Clin. Lab. Invest. Suppl.* 94: 1–63, 1967.
201. HURWITZ, L. J., D. MCCORMICK, AND I. V. ALLEN. Reduced muscle and α-glucosidase (acid maltase) activity in hypothyroid myopathy. *Lancet* 1: 67–69, 1970.
202. IKAI, M., AND T. FUKUNAGA. Calculation of muscle strength per unit cross-sectional area of human muscle by means of ultrasonic measurement. *Int. Z. Angew. Physiol.* 26: 26–32, 1968.
203. IKAI, M., AND T. FUKUNAGA. A study on training effect on strength per unit cross-sectional area of muscle by means of ultrasonic measurement. *Int. Z. Angew. Physiol.* 28: 173–180, 1970.
204. IONASESCU, V., H. ZELLWEGER, AND T. W. CONWAY. A new approach for carrier detection in Duchenne muscular dystrophy. Protein synthesis of muscle polyribosomes in vitro. *Neurology* 21: 703–709, 1971.
205. ISAACS, H. Myopathy and malignant hyperthermia. In: *International Symposium on Malignant Hyperthermia, 2nd: Proceedings*, edited by J. A. Aldrete and B. A. Britt. New York: Grune & Stratton, 1978, p. 89–102.
206. ITO, Y., R. MILEDI, A. VINCENT, AND J. NEWSOM-DAVIS. Acetylcholine receptors and end-plate electrophysiology in myasthenia gravis. *Brain* 101: 345–368, 1978.
207. JACOB, A., E. R. CLACK, AND A. E. H. EMERY. Genetic study of sample of 70 patients with myasthenia gravis. *J. Med. Genet.* 5: 257–261, 1968.
208. JENNEKENS, F. G. I., H. F. M. BUSCH, N. M. VAN HEMEL, AND R. A. HODGLAND. Inflammatory myopathy in scapulo-ilio-peroneal atrophy with cardiopathy. A study of two families. *Brain* 98: 709–722, 1975.
209. JOHNSON, R. L., C. W. FINK, AND M. ZIFF. Lymphotoxin formation by lymphocytes and muscle in polymyositis. *J. Clin. Invest.* 51: 2435–2449, 1972.
210. JONES, D. A., B. BIGLAND-RITCHIE, AND R. H. T. EDWARDS. Excitation frequency and muscle fatigue: mechanical responses during voluntary and stimulated contractions. *Exp. Neurol.* 64: 401–413, 1979.
211. JONES, N. L., E. J. M. CAMPBELL, R. H. T. EDWARDS, AND D. G. ROBERTSON. *Clinical Exercise Testing: A Guide to the Use of Exercise Physiology in Clinical Investigation*. Philadelphia, PA: Saunders, 1975.

212. JONES, P. R. M., AND J. PEARSON. Anthropometric determination of leg fat and muscle plus bone volumes in young male and female adults. *J. Physiol. London* 204: 63P–66P, 1969.
213. JONES, R., AND G. VRBOVÁ. Can denervation hypersensitivity be prevented? *J. Physiol. London* 217: 67P–68P, 1971.
214. JULIEN, J., C. VITAL, J. M. VALLAT, M. VALLAT, AND M. LE BLANC. Oculopharyngeal muscular dystrophy. A case with abnormal mitochondria and "fingerprint" inclusions. *J. Neurol. Sci.* 21: 165–169, 1974.
215. KADEFORS, R., E. KAISER, AND I. PETERSEN. Dynamic spectrum analysis of myo-potentials and with special reference to muscle fatigue. *Electromyography* 8: 39–74, 1968.
216. KAGEN, L. J. Myoglobinemia in inflammatory myopathies. *J. Am. Med. Assoc.* 237: 1448–1452, 1977.
217. KAGEN, L. J., S. MOUSSAVI, S. L. MILLER, AND P. TSAIRIS. Serum myoglobin in muscular dystrophy. *Muscle Nerve* 3: 221–226, 1980.
218. KAISER, E., AND I. PETERSÉN. Muscle action potentials studied by frequency analysis and duration of measurement. *Acta Neurol. Scand.* 41: 213–235, 1965.
219. KAKULAS, B. A. Destruction of differentiated muscle cultures by sensitised lymphoid cells. *J. Pathol. Bacteriol.* 91: 495–503, 1966.
220. KAKULAS, B. A. In vitro destruction of skeletal muscle by sensitised cells. *Nature London* 210: 1115–1118, 1966.
221. KAO, I., AND A. M. GORDON. Mechanism of insulin-induced paralysis of muscles from potassium-depleted rats. *Science* 188: 740–741, 1975.
222. KAO, I., AND A. M. GORDON. Alteration of skeletal muscle cellular structures by potassium depletion. *Neurology* 27: 855–860, 1977.
223. KAR, N. C., AND C. M. PEARSON. A calcium-activated neutral protease in normal and dystrophic human muscle. *Clin. Chim. Acta* 73: 293–297, 1976.
224. KAR, N. C., AND C. M. PEARSON. Muscular dystrophy and activation of proteases. *Muscle Nerve* 1: 308–313, 1978.
225. KAR, N. C., AND C. M. PEARSON. Proteolytic mechanisms in muscular dystrophies and other neuromuscular diseases. In: *Degradative Processes in Heart and Skeletal Muscle*, edited by K. Wildenthal. Amsterdam: Elsevier, 1980, p. 257–269.
226. KARPATI, G., S. CARPENTER, A. G. ENGEL, G. WATTERS, J. ALLEN, S. ROTHMAN, G. KLASSEN, AND O. A. MAMER. The syndrome of systemic carnitine deficiency. Clinical, morphologic, biochemical, and pathophysiologic features. *Neurology* 25: 16–24, 1975.
227. KENNELLY, A. E. An approximate law of fatigue in the speeds of racing animals. *Proc. Am. Acad. Arts Sci.* 42: 275–331, 1906.
228. KREITZER, S. M., M. EHRENPREIS, E. MIGUEL, AND J. PETRASEK. Acute myoglobinuric renal failure in polymyositis. *NY State J. Med.* 2: 295–297, 1978.
229. KRISTENSSON, K., AND Y. OLSSON. Retrograde axonal transport of protein. *Brain Res.* 29: 363–365, 1971.
230. LANAVI, A. La contracción miotónica en el hombre despríes de curarización. *Medicina Buenos Aires* 7: 21–26, 1947.
231. LAND, J. M., AND J. B. CLARK. Mitochondrial myopathies. *Biochem. Soc. Trans.* 7: 231–245, 1979.
232. LANDOUZY, L., AND J. DÉJÈRINE. De la myopathie atrophique progressive (myopathie héréditaire), débutant, dans l'enfance par la face, sans altération du système nerveux. *C. R. Acad. Sci.* 98: 53–55, 1884.
233. LANE, J. M., AND F. L. MASTAGLIA. Drug-induced myopathies in man. *Lancet* 2: 562–565, 1978.
234. LAYZER, R. B. Glycolysis and glycogen. In: *Pathogenesis of Human Muscular Dystrophies*, edited by L. P. Rowland. Amsterdam: Excerpta Med., 1977, p. 395–403. (Int. Congr. Ser. 404.)
235. LAYZER, R. B., R. J. HAVEL, AND M. B. MCILROY. Partial deficiency of carnitine palmityltransferase: physiologic and biochemical consequences. *Neurology* 30: 627–633, 1980.
236. LAYZER, R. B., R. E. LOVELACE, AND L. P. ROWLAND. Hyperkalemic periodic paralysis. *Arch. Neurol. Chicago* 16: 455–472, 1967.
237. LAYZER, R. B., AND L. P. ROWLAND. Cramps. *N. Engl. J. Med.* 285: 31–40, 1971.
238. LEWIS, P. O., G. W. PICKERING, AND P. ROTHSCHILD. Observations on muscular pain in intermittent claudication. *Heart* 15: 359–383, 1931.
239. LEYBURN, P., AND J. N. WALTON. The treatment of myotonia: a controlled trial. *Brain* 82: 81–91, 1959.
240. LIBBY, P., AND A. L. GOLDBERG. Leupeptin, a protease inhibitor, decreases protein degradation in normal and diseased muscles. *Science* 199: 534–536, 1978.
241. LIBBY, P., AND A. L. GOLDBERG. The control and mechanism of breakdown in striated muscle: studies with selective inhibitors. In: *Degradative Processes in Heart and Skeletal Muscle*, edited by K. Wildenthal. Amsterdam: Elsevier, 1980, p. 201–222.
242. LILJESTRAND, A. Fall av adynamia episodica hereditaria. *Opusc. Med.* 7: 183–193, 1957.
243. LINDSTROM, J. M., M. E. SEYBOLD, V. A. LENNON, S. WHITTINGHAM, AND D. D. DUANE. Antibody to acetylcholine receptor in myasthenia gravis. Prevalence, clinical correlates, and diagnostic value. *Neurology* 26: 1054–1059, 1976.
244. LIPICKY. R. J. Studies in human myotonic dystrophy. In: *Pathogenesis of Human Muscular Dystrophies*, edited by L. P. Rowland. Amsterdam: Excerpta Med., 1977, p. 729–738. (Int. Congr. Ser. 404.)
245. LIPICKY, R. J., AND S. H. BRYANT. Sodium, potassium, and chloride fluxes in intercostal muscle from normal goats and goats with hereditary myotonia. *J. Gen. Physiol.* 50: 89–111, 1966.
246. LIPICKY, R. J., S. H. BRYANT, AND J. H. SALMON. Cable parameters, sodium, potassium, chloride, and water content, and potassium efflux in isolated external intercostal muscle of normal volunteers and patients with myotonia congenita. *J. Clin. Invest.* 50: 2091–2103, 1971.
247. LISTER, D., G. M. HALL, AND J. N. LUCKE. Porcine malignant hyperthermia. III. Adrenergic blockade. *Br. J. Anaesth.* 48: 831–838, 1976.
248. LISTER, D., R. A. SAIR, J. A. WILL, G. R. SCHMIDT. R. G. CASSENS, W. G. HOEKSTRA, AND E. J. BRISKEY. Metabolism of striated muscle of stress-susceptible pigs breathing oxygen or nitrogen. *Am. J. Physiol.* 218: 102–107, 1970.
249. LIVERSEDGE, L. A., AND M. J. CAMPBELL. The central neuronal muscular atrophies and other dysfunctions of the anterior horn cells. In: *Disorders of Voluntary Muscle* (3rd ed.), edited by J. N. Walton. Edinburgh: Churchill Livingstone, 1974, p. 775–803.
250. LOMO, T., AND J. ROSENTHAL. Control of ACh sensitivity by muscle activity in the rat. *J. Physiol. London* 221: 493–513, 1972.
251. LUCY, J. A. Is there a membrane deficit in muscle and other cells? *Br. Med. Bull.* 36: 187–192, 1980.
252. LUFT, R., D. EKKOS, G. PALMRIERI, L. ERNSTER, AND B. AFZELIUS. A case of severe hypermetabolism of nonthyroid origin with a defect in maintenance of mitochondrial respiratory control. A correlated clinical biochemical and morphological study. *J. Clin. Invest.* 41: 1776–1804, 1962.
253. MACDONALD, R. D., N. B. REWCASTLE, AND J. G. HUMPHREY. The myopathy of hyperkalemic periodic paralysis. An electron microscopic study. *Arch. Neurol. Chicago* 19: 274–283, 1968.
254. MACDONALD, R. D., N. B. REWCASTLE, AND J. G. HUMPHREY. Myopathy of hypokalemic periodic paralysis. An electron microscopic study. *Arch. Neurol. Chicago* 20: 565–585, 1969.
255. MAHLER, R. F. Disorders of glycogen metabolism. In: *Clinics in Endocrinology and Metabolism*, edited by K. G. M. M. Alberti. London: Saunders, 1976, vol. 5, p. 579–598.
256. MANCHESTER, K. L. The hormonal control of protein metabolism. In: *Protein Metabolism and Nutrition*, edited by D. J. A. Cole, K. M. Borrman, P. J. Buttery, D. Lewis, R. J. Neale, and H. Swan. London: Butterworths, 1976, p. 35–47.
257. MARUYAMA, K., M. L. SUNDE, AND R. W. SWICK. Growth and muscle protein turnover in the chick. *Biochem. J.* 176: 573–582, 1978.
258. MAYER, M., E. SHAFRIR, N. KAISER, R. J. MILHOLLAND, AND

F. ROSEN. Interaction of glucocorticoid hormones with rat skeletal muscle: catabolic effects and hormone binding. *Metabolism* 25: 157–167, 1976.

259. MCARDLE, B. Myopathy due to a defect in muscle glycogen breakdown. *Clin. Sci.* 10: 13–25, 1951.

260. MCARDLE, B. Adynamic episodica hereditaria and its treatment. *Brain* 85: 121–148, 1962.

261. MCCOMAS, A. J. *Neuromuscular Function and Disorders.* London: Butterworths, 1977.

262. MCCOMAS, A. J., K. MROZEK, AND W. G. BRADLEY. The nature of the electrophysiological disorder in adynamia episodica. *J. Neurol. Neurosurg. Psychiatry* 31: 448–452, 1968.

263. MCCOMAS, A. J., R. E. P. SICA, AND M. E. BRANDSTATER. Further motor unit studies in Duchenne muscular dystrophy. *J. Neurol. Neurosurg. Psychiatry* 40: 1147–1151, 1977.

264. MCCOMAS, A. J., R. E. P. SICA, AND S. CURRIE. Muscular dystrophy: evidence for a neural factor. *Nature London* 226: 1263–1264, 1970.

265. MCKERAN, R. O., D. HALLIDAY, AND P. PURKISS. Increased myofibrillar protein catabolism in Duchenne muscular dystrophy measured by 3-methylhistidine excretion in the urine. *J. Neurol. Neurosurg. Psychiatry* 40: 979–981, 1977.

266. MCKERAN, R. O., G. SLAVIN, T. M. ANDREWS, P. WARD, AND N. G. P. MAIR. Muscle fibre type changes in hypothyroid myopathy. *J. Clin. Pathol.* 28: 659–663, 1975.

267. MENSE, S. S. Muscle nociceptors. *J. Physiol. Paris* 73: 233–240, 1977.

268. MERTON, P. A. Voluntary strength and fatigue. *J. Physiol. London* 123: 553–564, 1954.

269. MERYON, E. On granular and fatty degeneration of the voluntary muscle. *Med. Chir. Trans. Edinburgh* 35: 73–84, 1852.

270. MERYON, E. *Practical and Pathological Researches on the Various Forms of Paralysis.* London: Churchill, 1864, p. 200–215.

271. MILEDI, R. Properties of regenerating neuromuscular synapse in the frog. *J. Physiol. London* 154: 190–205, 1960.

272. MILLER, S. E., A. D. ROSES, AND S. H. APPEL. Scanning electron microscopy studies in muscular dystrophy. *Arch. Neurol. Chicago* 33: 172–174, 1976.

273. MILLWARD, D. J. Protein turnover in skeletal and cardiac muscle during normal growth and hypertrophy. In: *Degradative Processes in Heart and Skeletal Muscle*, edited by K. Wildenthal. Amsterdam: Elsevier, 1980, p. 161–199.

274. MILLWARD, D. J., P. C. BATES, J. G. BROWN, S. R. ROSOCHACKI, AND M. J. RENNIE. Protein degradation and the regulation of protein balance in nature. In: *Protein Degradation in Health and Disease.* Amsterdam: Excerpta Med., 1980, p. 307–309. (Ciba Found. Symp. 75.)

275. MILLWARD, D. J., P. C. BATES, G. K. GRIMBLE, J. G. BROWN, M. NATHAN, AND M. J. RENNIE. Quantitative importance of non-skeletal muscle sources of N^2-methylhistidine in urine. *Biochem. J.* 90: 225–228, 1980.

276. MOKRI, B., AND A. G. ENGEL. Duchenne dystrophy: electron microscopic findings pointing to a basic or early abnormality in the plasma membrane of the muscle fiber. *Neurology* 25: 1111–1120, 1975.

277. MOMMAERTS, W. F. H. M., B. ILLINGWORTH, C. M. PEARSON, R. J. GUILLORG, AND K. SERAYDARIAN. A functional disorder of muscle associated with the absence of phosphorylase. *Proc. Natl. Acad. Sci. USA* 45: 791–797, 1959.

278. MONCKTON, G., AND H. MARUSYK. The incorporation of ^{3}H[G]-L-leucine into single muscle fibres in Duchenne dystrophy and Charcot-Marie-Tooth disease. *Can. J. Neurol. Sci.* 6: 53–57, 1979.

279. MORGAN-HUGHES, J. A. Painful disorders of muscle. *Br. J. Hosp. Med.* 22: 362–365, 1979.

280. MORGAN-HUGHES, J. A., P. DARVENIZA, S. N. KAHN, D. N. LANDON, R. M. SHERRATT, J. M. LAND, AND J. B. CLARK. A mitochondrial myopathy characterized by a deficiency in reducible cytochrome b. *Brain* 100: 617–640, 1977.

281. MORGAN-HUGHES, J. A., AND W. G. P. MAIR. Atypical muscle mitochondria in oculoskeletal myopathy. *Brain* 96: 215–224, 1973.

282. MOSER, H. VON, U. WEISMANN, R. RICHTERICH, AND E. ROSSI. Progressive muskeldystropie Haufigkeit, Klinik und Genetik der Duchenne-Form. *Schweiz. Med. Wochenschr.* 94: 1610–1621, 1966.

283. MOSSO, A. *Fatigue*, translated by M. Drummond and W. G. Drummond. London: Allen & Unwin, 1915, p. 78–80.

284. MOULDS, R. F. W., AND M. A. DENBOROUGH. A study of the action of caffeine, halothane, potassium chloride and procaine on normal human skeletal muscle. *Clin. Exp. Pharmacol. Physiol.* 1: 197–209, 1974.

285. MOULDS, R. F. W., AND M. A. DENBOROUGH. Identification of susceptibility to malignant hyperpyrexia. *Br. Med. J.* 2: 245–247, 1974.

286. MOULDS, R. F. W., A. YOUNG, D. A. JONES, AND R. H. T. EDWARDS. A study of the contractility, biochemistry and morphology of an isolated preparation of human skeletal muscle. *Clin. Sci. Mol. Med.* 52: 291–297, 1977.

287. MOXHAM, J., A. J. R. MORRIS, S. SPIRO, R. H. T. EDWARDS, AND M. GREEN. The contractile properties and fatigue of the diaphragm in man. *Clin. Sci.* 58: 6P, 1979.

288. MOXHAM, J., C. M. WILES, D. NEWHAM, AND R. H. T. EDWARDS. Sternomastoid muscle function and fatigue in man. *Clin. Sci.* 59: 463–468, 1980.

289. MOXLEY, R. T., III. Metabolic studies in muscular dystrophy, a role for insulin. In: *Treatment of Neuromuscular Diseases*, edited by R. C. Griggs and R. T. Moxley III. New York: Raven, 1977, p. 161–173. (Advances in Neurology Ser. 17.)

290. MUNCK, A. Glucocorticoid inhibition of glucose uptake by peripheral tissues: old and new evidence, molecular mechanisms, and physiological significance. *Perspect. Biol. Med.* 14: 265–269, 1971.

291. MUNSAT, T. L. Pharmacologic therapy of dystrophy in man and animals. *Ann. NY Acad. Sci.* 317: 400–408, 1979.

292. NAESS, K., AND A. STORM-MATHISON. Fatigue of sustained tetanic contractions. *Acta Physiol. Scand.* 34: 351–366, 1956.

293. NEEDHAM, D. M. *Machina Carnis: the Biochemistry of Muscular Contraction in Its Historical Development.* Cambridge, UK: Cambridge Univ. Press, 1972.

294. NELSON, T. E. Excitation contraction coupling, a common etiological pathway for malignant hyperthermia susceptible muscle. In: *International Symposium on Malignant Hyperthermia, 2nd: Proceedings*, edited by J. A. Aldrete and B. A. Britt. New York: Grune & Stratton, 1978, p. 23–36.

295. NELSON, T. E., E. W. JONES, J. H. VENABLE, AND D. D. KERR. Malignant hyperthermia of Poland China swine: studies of a myogenic etiology. *Anesthesiology* 36: 52–56, 1972.

296. NEWSOM-DAVIS, J., A. J. PINCHING, A. VINCENT, AND S. G. WILSON. Function of circulating antibody to acetylcholine receptor in myasthenia gravis: investigation by plasma exchange. *Neurology* 28: 266–272, 1978.

297. O'DOHERTY, D. S., D. SCHELLINGER, AND V. RAPTOPOULOS. Computed tomographic patterns of pseudohypertrophic muscular dystrophy: preliminary results. *J. Comput. Assist. Tomography* 1: 482–486, 1977.

298. OFFERIJUS, F. G. J., D. WESTERINK, AND A. F. WILLEBRANDS. The relationship of potassium deficiency to muscular paralysis of insulin. *J. Physiol. London* 141: 377–384, 1958.

299. OTSUKA, M., AND I. OHTSUKI. Mechanism of muscular paralysis by insulin with special reference to periodic paralysis. *Am. J. Physiol.* 219: 1178–1182, 1970.

300. PATHEN, B. M., J. M. SHABOT, J. ALPERIN, AND R. F. DODSON. Hepatitis associated with lipid storage myopathy. *Ann. Intern. Med.* 87: 417–421, 1977.

301. PATRICK, J., AND J. LINDSTROM. Autoimmune response to acetylcholine receptor. *Science* 180: 871–872, 1973.

302. PATTERSON, S., AND L. KLENERMAN. The effect of pneumatic tourniquets on the ultrastructure of skeletal muscle. *J. Bone Jt. Surg.* 61B: 178–183, 1979.

303. PEARSON, C. M. Development of arthritis, periarthritis and periostitis in rats given adjuvants. *Proc. Soc. Exp. Biol. Med.* 91: 95–101, 1956.

304. PEARSON, C. M. Mechanisms involved in polymyositis and dermatomyositis. In: *Infection and Immunology in the Rheumatic Diseases*, edited by D. C. Dumonde. Oxford, UK: Blackwell Scientific, 1976, p. 489–493.
305. PEARSON, C. M., AND K. KALYANARAMAN. The periodic paralyses. In: *The Metabolic Basis of Inherited Disease* (3rd ed.), edited by J. B. Stanbury, J. B. Wyngaarden, and D. S. Fredrickson. New York: McGraw-Hill, 1972, p. 1181–1203.
306. PENNINGTON, R. J. T. Clinical biochemistry of muscular dystrophy. *Br. Med. Bull.* 36: 123–126, 1980.
307. PERKOFF, G. T., P. HARDY, AND E. VELEZ-GARCIA. Reversible acute muscular syndrome in chronic alcoholism. *N. Engl. J. Med.* 274: 1277–1285, 1966.
308. PERNOW, B. B., R. J. HAVEL, AND D. B. JENNINGS. The second wind phenomenon in McArdle's syndrome. *Acta Med. Scand. Suppl.* 472: 294–307, 1967.
309. PETER, J. B., AND D. S. CAMPION. Animal models of myotonia. In: *Pathogenesis of Human Muscular Dystrophies*, edited by L. P. Rowland. Amsterdam: Excerpta Med., 1977, p. 739–746. (Int. Congr. Ser. 404.)
310. PFAU, A. Interpretation of whole body potassium measurement. In: *Human Body Composition*, edited by J. Brozek. Oxford, UK: Pergamon, 1965, p. 57–60.
311. PLISHKER, G. A., AND S. H. APPEL. An overview of erythrocyte abnormalities in muscle diseases. In: *Current Topics in Nerve and Muscle Research*, edited by A. J. Aguayo and G. Karpati. Amsterdam: Excerpta Med., 1979, p. 39–50. (Int. Congr. Ser. 455.)
312. PORTE, D., JR., D. W. CRAWFORD, D. B. JENNINGS, C. ABER, AND B. MCILROY. Cardiovascular and metabolic responses to exercise in a patient with McArdle's syndrome. *N. Engl. J. Med.* 275: 406–412, 1966.
313. RAMIREZ, B. U., AND D. PETTE. Effects of long-term electrical stimulation on sarcoplasmic reticulum of fast rabbit muscle. *FEBS Lett.* 49: 188–190, 1974.
314. REDDY, M. K., J. D. ETLINGER, M. RABINOWITZ, D. A. FISCHMAN, AND R. ZAK. Removal of Z-lines and alpha-actin from isolated myofibrils by a calcium-activated neutral protease. *J. Biol. Chem.* 250: 4278–4284, 1975.
315. REEDS, P. J., A. A. JACKSON, D. PICOU, AND N. POULTER. Muscle mass and composition in malnourished infants and children and changes seen after recovery. *Pediatr. Res.* 12: 613–618, 1978.
316. REID, C. The mechanism of voluntary muscle fatigue. *Q. J. Exp. Physiol.* 19: 17–28, 1928.
316a. RENNIE, M. J., R. H. T. EDWARDS, AND D. J. MILLWARD. Increased protein degradation in muscle disease: cause or effect. *Muscle Nerve* 5: 85–86, 1982.
316b. RENNIE, M. J., R. H. T. EDWARDS, D. J. MILLWARD, S. C. WOLMAN, D. HOLLIDAY, AND D. E. MATTHEWS. Effects of Duchenne muscular dystrophy on muscle protein synthesis. *Nature London* 296: 165–167, 1982.
317. RENNIE, M. J., S. ROSOCHACKI, M. NATHAN, P. C. BATES, R. H. T. EDWARDS, AND D. J. MILLWARD. Intracellular, plasma and urine 3-methylhistidine as an index of muscle wasting and repair. In: *Amino Acid Analysis in Clinical Chemistry and Medical Research*, edited by J. M. Rattenbury. Chichester, UK: Horwood, 1980, p. 210–224.
318. RICKER, K., A. HAAS, G. HERTEL, AND H. G. MERTENS. Transient muscular weakness in severe recessive myotonia congenita. Improvement of isometric muscle force by drugs relieving myotonic stiffness. *J. Neurol.* 218: 253–262, 1978.
319. RIECKER, G., AND H. D. BOLTE. Membran potentiale einzlaner Skeletmuskelzellen bei hypokaliamischer periodischer Muskel paralyse. *Klin. Wochenschr.* 44: 804–807, 1966.
320. RIGGS, J. E., R. C. GRIGGS, AND R. T. MOXLEY III. Acetazolamide-induced weakness in paramyotonia congenita. *Ann. Intern. Med.* 86: 169–173, 1977.
321. ROELOFS, R. I., W. K. ENGEL, AND P. B. CHAUVIN. Histochemical phosphorylase activity in regenerating muscle fibers from myophosphorylase-deficient patients. *Science* 177: 795–797, 1972.
322. ROSE, A. L., AND J. N. WALTON. Polymyositis: a survey of 89 cases with particular reference to treatment and prognosis. *Brain* 89: 747–768, 1966.
323. ROTTHAUWE, H. W., W. MORTIER, AND H. BEYER. Neuer Typ einer recessiv X-chromosomal vererbten Muskeldystrophie: Scapulo-humero-distale Muskeldystrophie mit frühzeitigen Kontrakturen und Herzrhythmusstörungen. *Humangenetik* 16: 181–200, 1972.
324. ROWLAND, L. P. Biochemistry of muscle membranes in Duchenne muscular dystrophy. *Muscle Nerve* 3: 3–20, 1980.
325. ROWLAND, L. P., S. ARAKI, AND P. CARMEL. Contracture in McArdle's disease. Stability of adenosine triphosphate during contracture in phosphorylase-deficient human muscle. *Arch. Neurol. Chicago* 13: 541–544, 1965.
326. ROWLAND, L. P., C. CLARK, AND M. OLARTE. Therapy for dermatomyositis and polymyositis. In: *Treatment of Neuromuscular Diseases*, edited by R. C. Griggs and R. T. Moxley III. New York: Raven, 1977, p. 63–97. (Advances in Neurology Ser. 17.)
327. RÜDEL, R. The mechanism of pharmacologically induced myotonia. In: *Membranes and Disease*, edited by L. Bolis, J. F. Hoffman, and A. Leaf. New York: Raven, 1976, p. 207–213.
328. RÜDEL, R., AND J. SENGES. Mammalian skeletal muscle: reduced chloride conductance in drug-induced myotonia and induction of myotonia by low-chloride solution. *Naunyn-Schmiedeberg's Arch. Pharmacol.* 274: 337–347, 1972.
329. RUDMAN, D., C. W. SEWELL, AND J. D. ANSLEY. Deficiency of carnitine in cachectic serotic patients. *J. Clin. Invest.* 60: 716–723, 1967.
330. SAHGAL, V., V. SUBRAMANI, R. HUGHES, A. SHAH, AND H. SINGH. On the pathogenesis of mitochondrial myopathies. An experimental study. *Acta Neuropathol.* 46: 177–183, 1979.
331. SALMONS, S., AND G. VRBOVÁ. The influence of activity on some contractile characteristics of mammalian fast and slow muscles. *J. Physiol. London* 201: 535–549, 1969.
332. SALTIN, B., K. NAZAR, D. L. COSTILL, E. STEIN, E. JANSSON, B. ESSÉN, AND P. D. GOLLNICK. The nature of the training response; peripheral and central adaptations of one-legged exercise. *Acta Physiol. Scand.* 96: 289–305, 1976.
333. SARGEANT, A. J., C. T. M. DAVIES, R. H. T. EDWARDS, C. MAUNDER, AND A. YOUNG. Functional and structural changes after disease of human muscle. *Clin. Sci. Mol. Med.* 52: 337–342, 1977.
334. SATYAMURTI, S., D. B. DRACHMAN, AND F. SLONE. Blockade of acetylcholine receptors: a model of myasthenia gravis. *Science* 187: 955–957, 1975.
335. SCHMID, R., AND R. E. MAHLER. Chronic progressive myopathy with myoglobinuria, demonstration of a glycogenolytic defect in the muscle. *J. Clin. Invest.* 38: 2044–2058, 1959.
336. SCHOTLAND, D. L., E. BONILLA, AND M. VAN METER. Duchenne dystrophy: alteration in muscle plasma membrane structure. *Science* 196: 1005–1007, 1977.
337. SCHOTLAND, D. L., E. BONILLA, AND Y. WAKAYAMA. Pathogenesis of muscle cell damage in the dystrophies, morphologic aspects including freeze fracture studies. In: *Current Topics in Nerve and Muscle Research*, edited by A. J. Aguayo and G. Karpati. Amsterdam: Excerpta Med., 1979, p. 29–38. (Int. Congr. Ser. 455.)
338. SCHOTLAND, D. L., E. BONILLA, AND Y. WAKAYAMA. Application of the freeze fracture technique to the study of human neuromuscular disease. *Muscle Nerve* 3: 21–27, 1980.
339. SCHOTLAND, D. L., S. DIMAURO, E. BONILLA, A. SCARPA, AND C. P. LEE. Neuromuscular disorder associated with a defect in mitochondrial energy supply. *Arch. Neurol. Chicago* 33: 475–479, 1976.
340. SCHWARZ, H. A., G. SLAVIN, AND B. ANSELL. Histological and morphometric studies in polymyositis and dermatomyositis. *Ann. Rheum. Dis.* 39: 186, 1980.
341. SERRATRICE, G., H. ROUZ, R. AQUARON, AND A. M. RECORDIER. Serum and muscle activities (glycolytic and transferase) in human cortisone myopathies. In: *Muscle Diseases*, edited by J. N. Walton, N. Canal, and G. Scarlato. Amsterdam:

Excerpta Med., 1970, p. 489-496.

342. SHY, G. M., T. WANKO, P. T. ROWLEY, AND A. G. ENGEL. Studies in familial periodic paralysis. *Exp. Neurol.* 3: 53-121, 1961.

343. SIEGEL, I. M. The management of muscular dystrophy: a clinical review. *Muscle Nerve* 1: 453-460, 1978.

344. SIMPSON, J. A. Myasthenia gravis: a personal view of pathogenesis and mechanism, part 1. *Muscle Nerve* 1: 45-56, 1978.

345. SIMPSON, J. A. Myasthenia gravis: a personal view of pathogenesis and mechanism, part 2. *Muscle Nerve* 1: 151-156, 1978.

346. SĬRCA, A., AND M. SUSEC-MICHIELI. Selective type II fibre muscular atrophy in patients with osteoarthritis of the hip. *J. Neurol. Sci.* 44: 149-159, 1980.

347. SLOPER, J. C., T. A. PARTRIDGE, P. D. SMITH, AND D. MANGHANI. The pathogenesis of experimental allergic myositis. In: *Infection and Immunology in the Rheumatic Diseases*, edited by D. C. Dumonde. Oxford, UK: Blackwell Scientific, 1979, p. 495-501.

348. SMITH, J. B., AND A. PATEL. The Wohlfart-Kugelberg-Welander disease; review of the literature and report of a case. *Neurology* 15: 469-473, 1965.

349. SRÉTER, F. A., J. GERGELY, S. SALMONS, AND F. ROMANUL. Synthesis by fast muscle of myosin light chains characteristic of slow muscle in response to long-term stimulation. *Nature London New Biol.* 241: 17-19, 1973.

350. STÅLBERG, E., J. EKSTEDT, AND A. BROMAN. Neuromuscular transmission in myasthenia gravis studied with single-fibre electromyography. *J. Neurol. Neurosurg. Psychiatry* 37: 540-547, 1974.

351. STÅLBERG, E., J. V. TRONTELJ, AND M. JANKO. Single fibre EMG findings in muscular dystrophy (Abstract). In: *Symposium on Structure and Function of Normal and Diseased Muscle and Peripheral Nerve.* Kazimierz, Poland: 1972.

352. STEPHENS, J. A., AND A. TAYLOR. Fatigue of maintained voluntary muscle contraction in man. *J. Physiol. London* 220: 1-18, 1972.

353. STRACHER, A., E. B. MCGOWAN, AND S. A. SHAFIO. Muscular dystrophy: inhibition of degeneration in vivo with protease inhibitors. *Science* 200: 50-51, 1978.

354. SWASH, M., M. S. SCHWARTZ, AND M. K. SARGEANT. Pathogenesis of longitudinal splitting of muscle fibers in neurogenic disorders and in polymyositis. *Neuropathol. Appl. Neurobiol.* 4: 99-115, 1978.

355. TARUI, S., G. OKUNO, Y. IKURA, Y. TANAKA, T. TANAKA, M. SUDA, AND M. NISHIKAWA. Phosphofructokinase deficiency in skeletal muscle. A new type of glycogenosis. *Biochem. Biophys. Res. Commun.* 19: 517-523, 1965.

356. TEVAARWERK, G. J. M., K. P. STRICKLAND, C. H. LIN, AND A. J. HUDSON. Studies on insulin resistance and insulin receptor binding in myotonia dystrophica. *J. Clin. Endocrinol. Metab.* 49: 216-222, 1979.

357. THESLEFF, S. Supersensitivity of skeletal muscle produced by Botulinum toxin. *J. Physiol. London* 151: 598-607, 1960.

358. THOMAS, P. K., D. B. CALNE, AND C. F. ELLIOTT. X-linked scapuloperoneal syndrome. *J. Neurol. Neurosurg. Psychiatry* 35: 208-215, 1972.

359. THORSTENSSON, A., G. GRIMBY, AND J. KARLSSON. Force-velocity relation and fiber composition in human knee extensor muscles. *J. Appl. Physiol.* 40: 12-16, 1976.

360. TORNVALL, G. Assessment of physical capabilities with special reference to the evaluation of maximum voluntary isometric strength and maximal working capacity. *Acta Physiol. Scand. Suppl.* 201: 1-102, 1963.

361. TOWER, S. Trophic control of non-nervous tissues by the nervous system: a study of muscle and bone innervated from an isolated and quiescent region of spinal cord. *J. Comp. Neurol.* 67: 241-267, 1937.

362. TOYKA, K. V., D. B. DRACHMAN, D. E. GRIFFIN, A. PESTRONK, J. A. WINKELSTEIN, K. H. FISCHBECK, AND I. KAO. Myasthenia gravis. Study of humoral immune mechanisms by passive transfer to mice. *N. Engl. J. Med.* 296: 125-131, 1977.

363. TOYKA, K. V., D. B. DRACHMAN, A. PESTRONK, AND I. KAO. Myasthenia gravis: passive transfer from man to mouse. *Science* 190: 397-399, 1975.

364. TRENKLE, A. Hormonal and nutritional interrelationships and their effects on skeletal muscle. *J. Anim. Sci.* 38: 1142-1152, 1974.

365. TSUKAGOSHI, H., T. NAKANISHI, K. KONDO, AND T. TSUBAKI. Hereditary proximal neurogenic muscular atrophy in adult. *Arch. Neurol. Chicago* 12: 597-603, 1965.

366. ULBRICHT, W. The effect of veratridine on excitable membranes of nerve and muscle. *Ergeb. Physiol. Biol. Chem. Exp. Pharmakol.* 61: 18-71, 1969.

367. UTHNE, K., C. R. REAGAN, L. P. GIMPEL, AND J. L. KOSTYO. Effects of human somatomedin preparations on membrane transport and protein synthesis in the isolated rat diaphragm. *J. Clin. Endocrinol. Metab.* 39: 548-554, 1974.

368. VICTOR, M., R. HAYES, AND R. D. ADAMS. Oculopharyngeal muscular dystrophy. *N. Engl. J. Med.* 267: 1267-1272, 1962.

369. VIETS, H. R. A historical review of myasthenia gravis from 1672-1900. *J. Am. Med. Assoc.* 153: 1273-1280, 1953.

370. VRBOVÁ, G. The influence of the motor nerve on the characteristic properties of skeletal muscle. In: *The Biochemistry of Myasthenia Gravis and Muscular Dystrophy*, edited by G. G. Lunt and R. M. Marchbanks. New York: Academic, 1978, p. 3-21.

371. WALKER, M. B. Treatment of myasthenia gravis with physostigmine. *Lancet* 1: 1200-1201, 1934.

372. WALKER, M. B. A case showing the effect of prostigmin on myasthenia gravis. *Proc. R. Soc. Med.* 28: 759-761, 1935.

373. WALLER, A. D. The sense of effort: an objective study. *Brain* 14: 179-249, 1891.

374. WALTON, J. N., AND F. J. NATRASS. On the classification, natural history and treatment of the myopathies. *Brain* 77: 169-231, 1954.

375. WANG, P., T. CLAUSEN, AND H. ORSKOV. Salbutamol inhalations suppress attacks of hyperkalemia in familial periodic paralysis. *Monogr. Hum. Genet.* 10: 62-65, 1978.

376. WARTHIN, A. S. The myocardial lesions of diphtheria. *J. Infect. Dis.* 35: 32-66, 1924.

377. WATERLOW, J. C., P. J. GARLICK, AND D. J. MILLWARD. *Protein Turnover in Mammalian Tissues and in the Whole Body.* Amsterdam: Elsevier, 1978.

378. WATSON, W. E. Centripetal passage of labelled molecules along mammalian motor axons. *J. Physiol. London* 196: 122P-123P, 1968.

379. WEEDS, A. G., D. R. TRENTHAM, C. J. C. KEAN, AND A. J. BULLER. Myosin from cross-reinnervated cat muscles. *Nature London* 247: 135-139, 1974.

380. WESTGAARD, R. H. Influence of activity on the passive electrical properties of denervated soleus muscle fibres in the rat. *J. Physiol. London* 251: 683-697, 1975.

381. WILES, C. M. The Determinants of the Relaxation Rate of Human Muscle in Vivo. London: Univ. of London, 1980. Dissertation.

382. WILES, C. M., AND R. H. T. EDWARDS. Weakness in myotonic syndromes. *Lancet* 2: 598-601, 1977.

383. WILES, C. M., D. A. JONES, AND R. H. T. EDWARDS. Fatigue in human metabolic myopathy. In: *Human Muscle Fatigue: Physiological Mechanisms*, edited by R. Ponter and J. Whelan. London: Putman Med., 1981, p. 264-282. (Ciba Found. Symp.)

384. WILES, C. M., A. YOUNG, D. A. JONES, AND R. H. T. EDWARDS. Muscle relaxation rate, fibre-type composition and energy turnover in hyper- and hypothyroid patients. *Clin. Sci.* 57: 375-384, 1979.

385. WILLEMS, J. C., L. A. H. MANNEIS, J. M. F. TRIJBELS, J. H. VERRKAPS, A. E. R. H. MEYER, D. VAN DAM, AND V. VAN HAESLIT. Leigh's encephalomyopathy in a patient with cytochrome c oxidase deficiency in muscle tissue. *Pediatrics* 60: 850-857, 1977.

386. WILLIAMS, C. H., M. D. SHANKLIN, H. B. HEDRICK, M. MUHRER, D. STUBBS, G. F. KRAUSE, C. G. PAYNE, J. D. BENEDICT, D. P. HUTCHESON, AND J. F. LASLEY. The fulmi-

nant hyperthermia-stress syndrome: genetic aspects, hemodynamic and metabolic measurements in susceptible and normal pigs. In: *International Symposium on Malignant Hyperthermia, 2nd: Proceedings*, edited by J. A. Aldrete and B. A. Britt. New York: Grune & Stratton, 1978, p. 113–140.

387. WILLNER, J. H., S. GINSBURG, AND S. DIMAURO. Active transport of carnitine into skeletal muscle. *Neurology* 28: 721–724, 1978.

388. WILLNER, J. H., D. S. WOOD, C. CERRI, AND B. BRITT. Increased myophosphorylase in malignant hyperthermia. *N. Engl. J. Med.* 303: 138–140, 1980.

388a. WINER, N., D. M. KLACHKO, R. D. BAER, P. L. LANGLEY, AND T. W. BARNES. Myotonic response induced by inhibitors of cholesterol biosynthesis. *Science* 153: 312–313, 1966.

389. WINGARD, D. W. Malignant hyperthermia: a human stress syndrome (Letter)? *Lancet* 2: 1450–1451, 1974.

390. WOOD, D. S. Human skeletal muscle: analysis of Ca^{2+} regulation in skinned fibers using caffeine. *Exp. Neurol.* 58: 218–230, 1978.

391. WOOD, D. S., M. M. SORENSON, A. B. EASTWOOD, W. E. CHARASH, AND J. P. REUBEN. Duchenne dystrophy: abnormal generation of tension and Ca^{2+} regulation in single skinned fibers. *Neurology* 28: 447–457, 1978.

392. YOUNG, A., D. P. BRENTON, AND R. H. T. EDWARDS. Analysis of muscle weakness in osteomalacia. *Clin. Sci. Mol. Med.* 54: 31P, 1978.

393. YOUNG, A., I. HUGHES, P. RUSSELL, AND M. J. PARKER. Measurement of quadriceps muscle wasting. *Ann. Rheum. Dis.* 38: 571, 1979.

394. YOUNG, V. R., AND H. N. MUNRO. Muscle protein turnover in human beings in health and disease. In: *Degradative Processes in Heart and Skeletal Muscle*, edited by K. Wildenthal. Amsterdam: Elsevier, 1980, p. 271–291.

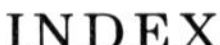

INDEX

Index